Optical Fiber
Communications

for BTech, MSc (Electronics), BSc (Electronics) Hons/Pass, GATE, NET/SLET, UGC–CSIR

Optical Fiber Communications

for BTech, MSc (Electronics), BSc (Electronics) Hons/Pass, GATE, NET/SLET, UGC–CSIR

SL Kakani

MSc (Physics), PhD

Former Executive Director
Institute of Technology and Management
(Affiliated to Rajasthan Technical University, Kota)
Bhilwara 311001, Rajasthan, India
E-mail: slkakani28@gmail.com

Shubhra Kakani

MSc (Physics), PhD

MLV Government College
Bhilwara 311001, Rajasthan, India

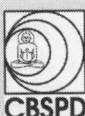

CBSPD

CBS Publishers & Distributors Pvt Ltd

New Delhi • Bengaluru • Chennai • Kochi • Kolkata • Lucknow • Mumbai
Hyderabad • Jharkhand • Nagpur • Patna • Pune • Uttarakhand

Optical Fiber Communications

ISBN: 978-93-88178-86-0

First Edition: 2019

Reprint: 2023

Published by **Satish Kumar Jain** and produced by **Varun Jain** for

CBS Publishers & Distributors Pvt Ltd

4819/XI Prahlad Street, 24 Ansari Road, Daryaganj, New Delhi 110 002, India.
Ph: 011-23289259, 23266861

Website: www.cbspd.com
e-mail: delhi@cbspd.com

Corporate Office: 204 FIE, Industrial Area, Patparganj, Delhi 110 092
Ph: 011-4934 4934   Fax: 011-4934 4935

e-mail: publishing@cbspd.com; publicity@cbspd.com

Branches

- **Bengaluru:** Seema House 2975, 17th Cross, KR Road, Banasankari 2nd Stage, Bengaluru 560 070, Karnataka, India
  Ph: +91-80-26771678/79   Fax: +91-80-26771680   e-mail: bangalore@cbspd.com
- **Chennai:** 7, Subbaraya Street, Shenoy Nagar, Chennai 600 030, Tamil Nadu, India
  Ph: +91-44-26680620, 26681266   Fax: +91-44-42032115   e-mail: chennai@cbspd.com
- **Kochi:** 42/1325, 1326, Power House Road, Opp KSEB, Power House, Ernakulum Kochi 682 018, Kerala, India
  Ph: +91-484-4059061-65,67   Fax: +91-484-4059065   e-mail: kochi@cbspd.com
- **Kolkata:** 147, Hind Ceramics Compound, 1st Floor, Nilgunj Road, Belghoria, Kolkata-700056, West Bengal, India
  Ph: +033-25633055, 033-25633056   e-mail: kolkata@cbspd.com
- **Lucknow:** Basement, Khushnuma Complex, 7 Meerabai Marg (Behind Jawahar Bhawan),Lucknow-226001, UP, India
  Ph: +0522-4000032   e-mail: tiwari.lucknow@cbspd.com
- **Mumbai:** PWD Shed, Gala no 25/26, Ramchandra Bhatt Marg, Next to JJ Hospital Gate no. 2, Opp. Union Bank of India,
  Noorbaug, Mumbai-400009, Maharashtra, India
  Ph: 022-66661880/89   e-mail: mumbai@cbspd.com

Representatives

- Hyderabad   0-9885175004
- Patna   0-9334159340
- Jharkhand   0-9811541605
- Pune   0-9923910676
- Nagpur   0-9421945513
- Uttarakhand   0-9716462459

Printed at:

Rashtriya Printers, Dilshad Garden, Delhi, India

Preface

The field of optical fiber communications has advanced significantly over the last three decades. In the early days, most of the usable bandwidth was significantly underutilized as the transmission capacity was quite low and hence, there was no need to apply techniques developed in nonoptical communication systems to improve the spectral efficiency. However, with the recent revival of coherent detection, high spectral efficiency can be realized using advanced modulation formats.

The book is aimed at BTech and MSc (Electronics), BSc (Electronics) Hons/Pass and three year diploma students. Written in a simple language, gives adequate information and instructions to enable students to achieve maximum comprehension. The book covers the basic theoretical principles, essential mathematics, applications of the optical fiber communications, is suitable for students, professionals and teachers. This book is a self-sufficient text in itself and students will be able to master the subject with a little help from other supplementary books on similar topics. The book also covers courses under optoelectronics, photonics.

The book is structured into 13 chapters and appendices. Chapter 1 to chapter 12 cover introduction, electromagnetic optics, optical fibers, fiber optic materials, cables and connectors, fiber optic waveguides and mode analysis, transmission characteristics of optical fibers, optical sources 1: laser, optical sources 2: light emitting diode (LED), optical receivers, optical and photonic components—optical amplifiers, advanced optical communication systems and optical networks—wavelength division multiplexing (WDM) technology, fiber optic communications. Chapter 13 describes fiber optic measurement and testing in detail. The topics are all drawn from many works previously published and given in the suggested reading.

The *salient features* of the book are:

- Extensive coverage of topics related to optical fiber communication.
- Each chapter is followed by a good number of worked out problems, summary, review questions, problems, short-answer questions and multiple choice questions with answers.

We hope that this student-friendly text will definitely cater to the needs of students, teachers and engineers working in this field.

We are extremely thankful and grateful to Mr SK Jain, Managing Director, CBS Publishers and Distributors, New Delhi, for his continued support. We are thankful to Mr YN Arjuna, Sr. Vice President Publishing, Editorial and Publicity and his team comprising Ms Ritu Chawla, Ms Sanjubala, Mr Kuldeep, Ms Baljeet Kaur and Mr Manish Raj for bringing out the book in the present form.

Inspite of our best efforts, some mistakes and misconceptions might have crept into the text, for which we beg to be pardoned.

We welcome suggestions and corrections from the readers.

SL Kakani
Shubhra Kakani

Contents

Preface   v

1. **Introduction**   1

  1.1 Historical Perspectives 1
  1.2 General Optical Fiber Communication System 3
  1.3 Digital Modulation for Advanced Optical Transmission System 7
  1.4 Demodulation Techniques 9
  1.5 Advantages of Optical Fiber Communication 10

2. **Electromagnetic Optics**   23

  2.1 Introduction 23
  2.2 Nature of Light 23
  2.3 Fundamental Laws of Optics 24
  2.4 Polarization of Light 27
  2.5 Polarization of Sensitive Materials 28
  2.6 Electromagnetic Waves 30
    2.6.1 Maxwell's Equations and Boundary Conditions 31
    2.6.2 Maxwell's Equations in a Source-Free Region 33
    2.6.3 Boundary Conditions 34
  2.7 Wave Equation 35
  2.8 Time Harmonic Fields 37
  2.9 Polarized Waves 38
    2.9.1 Linearly Polarized Waves 38
    2.9.2 Circularly and Elliptically Polarized Waves 39
    2.9.3 Fresnel Coefficients and Phases 40
    2.9.4 TE Polarization 40
    2.9.5 TM Polarization 41
    2.9.6 Polarization by Reflection from Dielectric Surfaces 42
    2.9.7 Expression for Brewster's Angle 43
  2.10 Antireflection Coating 43
  2.11 Bragg Mirrors 44
  2.12 Poynting Theorem 44

3. **Optical Fibers**   62

  3.1 Introduction 62
  3.2 Optical Fiber 64
  3.3 Optical Fiber as Waveguide: Principle of Propagation 65
  3.4 Principle of Optical Fiber: Total Internal Reflection 66
    3.4.1 Meridional and Skew Rays 70
    3.4.2 Acceptance Angle for Skew Rays 72

3.5 Modes of Propagation: V-Parameter 73
3.6 Index Profile or Refractive Index Profile 76
3.7 Types of Optical Fibers 77
3.8 Ray propagation in Graded-Index Fibers 86
3.9 Effect of Material Dispersion 88
3.10 The Combined Effect of Multipath and Material Dispersion 90
3.11 Calculation of RMS Pulse Width 91
3.12 Advantages of Optical Fiber 91
3.13 Signal Degradation 92
3.14 Fiber Losses 92
    3.14.1 Attenuation 93
    3.14.2 Dispersion Shifted Fiber 94
3.15 Optical Fiber Cables 95
    3.15.1 Fiber Strength and Durability 95
    3.15.2 Fiber-Optic Connectors 96
3.16 Fiber Fabrication 96
    3.16.1 Liquid Phase Melting Techniques 97
    3.16.2 Vapour Phase Deposition Technique 98
    3.16.3 Modern Fiber Optic Processes 99
    3.16.4 Advanced Fiber Optic Cables 99
    3.16.5 Fiber Optic Cables vs Copper Cables 100
3.17 Polarization 101
3.18 Optical Fiber Amplification 103
3.19 Optical Nonlinearities in Fibers 104
3.20 Solitons in Optical Fiber 106
3.21 Applications of Fiber Optic Cables 107
    3.21.1 Applications of Advanced Fiber Cables 108

4. **Fiber Optic Materials, Cables and Connectors—Power Launching and Fiber Coupling**   130

  4.1 Introduction 130
  4.2 Fiber Materials 130
    4.2.1 Glass Fibers 131
    4.2.2 Fluoride Fibers 133
    4.2.3 Active Glass Fibers 134
    4.2.4 Chalcogenide Glass Fibers 135
    4.2.5 Plastic Optical Fiber (POF) 135
    4.2.6 Plastic Clad Silica (PCS) Fibers 136
  4.3 Fiber Fabrication Methods 137

4.4 Mechanical Properties of Optical Fibers *142*

4.5 Optical Fiber Cables *143*

4.6 Fiber-Optic Connections and Related Losses *146*

4.7 Connectors and Splices *149*

4.8 Applications of Connectors and Splices *150*

4.9 Requirements of Connectors and Splices *150*

4.10 Fiber Connectors *151*

4.11 Mechanical Considerations *152*
    4.11.1 Durability *152*
    4.11.2 Environmental Consideration *153*
    4.11.3 Compatibility *153*

4.12 Fiber-Optic Connector Types *153*

4.13 Adapters for Different Fiber-Optic Connector Types *154*

4.14 Fiber-Optic Connector Structures *154*

4.15 Fiber-Optic Connector Assembly Techniques *154*
    4.15.1 Common Fiber Connector Assembly *155*
    4.15.2 Hot-Melt Connector *155*
    4.15.3 Epoxyless Connector *155*
    4.15.4 Butt-Jointed Connectors *155*
    4.15.5 Expanded-Beam Connectors *156*
    4.15.6 Multifiber Connectors *156*
    4.15.7 Automated Polishing *156*
    4.15.8 Fluid Jet Polishing *157*
    4.15.9 Fiber-Optic Connector Cleaning *157*
    4.15.10 Connector Testing *157*

4.16 Fiber splicing *158*
    4.16.1 Fusion Splices *159*
    4.16.2 Mechanical Splices/V-Groove *159*
    4.16.3 Multiple Splices *161*

4.17 Connectors verses Splices *162*

4.18 Characterization of Optical Fibers *162*
    4.18.1 Measurement of Optical Attenuation *162*
    4.18.2 Measurement of Dispersion *165*
    4.18.3 Measurement of Numerical Aperture (NA) *165*
    4.18.4 Measurement of Refractive Index (RI) Profile *166*
    4.18.5 Field Measurements: Optical Time Domain Reflectometry (OTDR) *167*

4.19 Applications of the Fiber Optic Cables *168*

5. Optical Fiber Waveguides and Mode Analysis　　183

5.1 Introduction *183*

5.2 Concept of Electromagnetic Waves *183*

5.3 Solution in an Inhomogeneous Medium *185*

5.4 Planar Optical Waveguide *188*

5.5 Modes in Cylindrical Optical Fibers *191*
    5.5.1 Bound or Guided Modes *191*
    5.5.2 Cladding Modes *192*
    5.5.3 Leaky Modes *192*
    5.5.4 Formulation of Waveguide Equations *192*

5.6 The Modes of a Symmetric Step Index Fiber *195*

5.7 Power Distribution and Confinement Factor *199*

5.8 Cylindrical Waveguides *202*
    5.8.1 Modal Analysis of an Ideal Step-Index Optical Fiber *202*
    5.8.2 Fraction Modal Power Distribution *209*
    5.8.3 Graded Index (GI) Fibers *211*
    5.8.4 Limitations of Multimode Fibers *213*

5.9 Photonic Crystal Fibers *213*
    5.9.1 Index-Guided Microstructures *214*
    5.9.2 Photonic Band Gap Fibers *215*

6. Transmission Characteristics of Optical Fibers　　237

6.1 Introduction *237*

6.2 Attenuation *238*

6.3 Absorption Loss *239*
    6.3.1 Intrinsic Absorption *239*
    6.3.2 Extrinsic Absorption *242*
    6.3.3 Defect Loss *243*
    6.3.4 Scattering Loss *243*

6.4 Mid-Infrared and Far-Infrared Transmission *250*

6.5 Dispersion *253*
    6.5.1 Interamodal Dispersion or Chromatic Dispersion or Group Velocity Dispersion (GVD) *256*

6.6 Signal Distortion in Optical Fibers *256*
    6.6.1 Group Velocity Dispersion *258*

6.7 Waveguide Dispersion in a Single Mode Fiber *264*
    6.7.1 Profile Dispersion *264*
    6.7.2 Polarization Mode Dispersion (PMD) *266*

6.8 Intermodal Dispersion *268*
    6.8.1 Pulse Broadening in a Multimode Step-Index Fiber *269*
    6.8.2 RMS Pulse Broadening *271*
    6.8.3 Intermodal Dispersion in a Multimode Graded Index Fiber *272*
    6.8.4 Mode Coupling *277*

6.9 Dispersion Optimization of Single Mode Fibers *278*

   6.9.1 Dispersion-Shifted Fibers (DSFs) *278*

   6.9.2 Dispersion-Flattened Fibers (DFFs) *279*

   6.9.3 Polarization Maintaining Fibers *282*

6.10 Nonlinear Effects *283*

6.11 Soliton Propagation *284*

7. Optical Sources 1—The LASER   311

7.1 Introduction *311*

7.2 Semiconductors *313*

   7.2.1 Energy Band Diagram *313*

   7.2.2 The *pn* Junction *320*

   7.2.3 Spontaneous and Stimulated Emission at the *pn* Junction *321*

   7.2.4 Direct and Indirect Band Gap Semiconductors *321*

   7.2.5 Compound Semiconductors *325*

7.3 Spontaneous and Stimulated Emission *327*

7.4 Relation between Einstein's Coefficients *328*

7.5 Laser Components *329*

7.6 Population Inversion *331*

7.7 Optical Feedback *332*

7.8 Conditions for Laser Oscillations *333*

7.9 Laser Rate Equations *337*

7.10 Characteristics of Laser Radiation *340*

7.11 Types of Lasers *341*

7.12 Laser Oscillations and Resonant Modes *342*

7.13 Semiconductor Lasers *343*

   7.13.1 Semiconductor Laser Diode or Semiconductor Injection Laser *343*

   7.13.2 Population Inversion and Optical Feedback in a Laser Diode *344*

   7.13.3 Distributed–Feedback Lasers *345*

   7.13.4 Heterojunction Lasers *347*

   7.13.5 Radiative and Nonradiative Recombination *350*

   7.13.6 Laser Rate Equations *351*

   7.13.7 Steady-State Solutions of Rate Equations *352*

   7.13.8 Lasing Conditions and Resonant Frequencies *355*

7.14 Laser Diode Structures and Radiation Patterns *357*

7.15 Quantum-Well Lasers *361*

7.16 Quantum-Dot Lasers *362*

7.17 Vertical Cavity Surface Emitting Lasers (VCSELs) *364*

7.18 Distributed-Feedback Lasers: FP Laser, DBR Laser, and DFB Laser *366*

7.19 Electron Transitions in Semiconductors *367*

7.20 Homogeneous *pn* Junction *368*

   7.20.1 Heterostructures *368*

   7.20.2 Optical Gains *369*

   7.20.3 Determination of Optical Gain *371*

7.21 Rate Equations *372*

   7.21.1 Carriers *373*

   7.21.2 Photons *374*

   7.21.3 Rate Equation Parameters *374*

   7.21.4 Derivation of Rate Equation for Electric Field *375*

7.22 Analysis Based on Rate Equations *377*

   7.22.1 Steady-State Analysis *377*

   7.22.2 Small-Signal Analysis with the Linear Gain Model *378*

   7.22.3 Small-Signal Analysis with Gain Saturation *379*

   7.22.4 Large-Signal Analysis for QW Lasers *382*

   7.22.5 Frequency Chirping *382*

   7.22.6 Equivalent Circuit Model for a Bulk Laser *383*

   Appendix 7.1: Semiconductor Heterojunctions *423*

   Appendix 7.2: Parameters of Selected Semiconductors and Semiconductor Compounds *426*

8. Optical Sources 2— The Light Emitting Diode (LED)   427

8.1 Introduction *427*

8.2 Photoelectric Effect *428*

   8.2.1 Photoemissive Effect *428*

   8.2.2 Photoconductive Effect *429*

   8.2.3 Photovoltaic Effect *430*

8.3 Photodetectors *431*

   8.3.1 Photoconductor *432*

   8.3.2 Quantum Efficiency (η) *433*

   8.3.3 Bandwidth *434*

   8.3.4 Noise Equivalent Power (NEP) *435*

8.4 Light Emitting Diodes (LEDs) *437*

   8.4.1 LED Construction and Working *438*

   8.4.2 Internal and External Quantum Efficiency of an LED *440*

   8.4.3 LED Structures: Homojunction and Heterojunction *441*

   8.4.4 Characteristics of LED *447*

8.5 Advanced LED Structures *454*

   8.5.1 LED Indicator Circuits *457*

   8.5.2 Multicolour LEDs *457*

   8.5.3 LED Testing *458*

   8.5.4 Quantum Efficiency and LED Power *458*

   8.5.5 Modulation of an LED *461*

9. Optical Receivers   488

9.1 Introduction *488*

9.2 Principle of Optoelectronic Detection *490*

9.3 Optical Receiver *491*
  9.3.1 Sensitivity *491*
  9.3.2 Dynamic Range *491*
  9.3.3 Bit-Rate Transparency *491*
  9.3.4 Bit-Pattern Independency *491*
  9.3.5 Optical Receiver Configuration *491*
9.4 Photodetectors *505*
9.5 Principles of Photodetection *505*
9.6 Properties of Semiconductor Photodetectors *507*
  9.6.1 Quantum Efficiency (η) *507*
  9.6.2 Responsivity (R) *507*
  9.6.3 Long-Wavelength Cut-off *509*
  9.6.4 Response Time *509*
  9.6.5 Sensitivity *510*
9.7 Performance Parameters of Photodetectors *510*
  9.7.1 Dark Current or Leakage Current *510*
  9.7.2 Quantum Efficiency *511*
  9.7.3 Responsivity (R) *511*
  9.7.4 Speed of Response *511*
9.8 Types of Optical Detectors *511*
  9.8.1 Phototransistors *511*
  9.8.2 Photovoltaics *512*
  9.8.3 Metal-Semiconductor-Metal (MSM) Detectors *513*
  9.8.4 *pn* Photodiode *515*
  9.8.5 *p-i-n* (PIN) Photodiodes *516*
  9.8.6 Avalanche Photodiodes *520*
9.9 Photodetector Noise *521*
  9.9.1 Shot Noise *523*
  9.9.2 Thermal Noise *523*
  9.9.3 Quantum Noise *525*
  9.9.4 Quantum Limit *525*
9.10 Receiver Analysis *526*
9.11 BER of an Ideal Optical Receiver *527*

10. **Optical and Photonic Components— Optical Amplifiers**   **546**

10.1 Introduction *546*
10.2 Semiconductor Optical Amplifiers *547*
  10.2.1 General Properties of Optical Amplifiers *549*
  10.2.2 Gain Spectrum and Bandwidth *549*
  10.2.3 Gain Saturation *551*
  10.2.4 Amplifier Noise *552*
  10.2.5 Gain Formula for SOA with Facet Reflectivities *554*
  10.2.6 The Effect of Facet Reflectivities *555*
  10.2.7 SOA Rate Equations for Pulse Propagation *556*
  10.2.8 Pulse Amplification *558*
  10.2.9 Design of SOA *559*
  10.2.10 Some Amplifications of SOA *560*

10.3 Rare Earth Doped Fiber Amplifiers *566*
  10.3.1 Erbium-Doped Fiber Optical Amplifiers *566*
  10.3.2 Steady-State Analysis *569*
  10.3.3 Effective Two-Level Approach *569*
  10.3.4 Gain Characteristics of Erbium-Doped Fiber Amplifiers *571*
  10.3.5 Typical EDFA Characteristics *571*
  10.3.6 Alternative Model of EDFA *572*
  10.3.7 Other Rare Earth Doped Fiber Optical Amplifiers *574*
10.4 Raman Fiber Optical Amplifiers or Fiber Raman Amplifiers (FRA) *574*
10.5 Planer Waveguide Optical Amplifiers *578*
10.6 Linear Optical Amplifiers *578*
10.7 Basic Applications of Optical Amplifiers *578*
  Appendix: Optical Switches *595*
  A10.1 Introduciton *595*
  A10.2 Opto-Mechanical Switches *595*
  A10.3 Electro-Optic Switches *603*
  A10.4 Thermo-Optic Switches *606*
  A10.5 Acousto-Optic Switches *610*
  A10.6 Micro-Electromechanical System (MEMS) *611*
  A10.7 3D MEMS Based Optical Switches *613*
  A10.8 Micro-Optic Mechanical System (MOMS) *614*

11. **Advanced Optical Communication Systems and Optical Networks— Wavelength Division Multiplexing (WDM) Technology**   **615**

11.1 Introduction *615*
11.2 Time Division Multiplexing *619*
11.3 Frequency Division Multiplexing (FDM) *619*
11.4 Dense Wavelength Division Multiplexing (DWDM) *619*
11.5 Coarse Wavelength Division Multiplexing (CWDM) *620*
11.6 Passive Components *620*
  11.6.1 Couplers *620*
11.7 Multiplexers and Demultiplexers *628*
  11.7.1 Multiplexing and Demultiplexing Using a Prism *630*
  11.7.2 Multiplexing and Demultiplexing Using a Diffraction Grating *631*
  11.7.3 Optical Add/Drop Multiplexers/ Demultiplexers *631*
  11.7.4 Arrayed Waveguide Gratings (AWGs) *632*
  11.7.5 Fiber Bragg Grating (FBG) *633*
  11.7.6 Thin Film Filters or Multilayer Interference Filters *634*

11.7.7 Periodic Filters, Frequency Slicers, Interleavers Multiplexing 634

11.7.8 Mach–Zehnder Interferometer 635

11.8 Active Components 636

11.9 Topologies and Architectures 640

11.9.1 Point-to-Point WDM Links 640

11.9.2 Wavelength-Routed Networks 640

11.9.3 WDM Star, Ring, and Meshes 641

11.9.4 Network Reconfigurability 644

12. **Fiber Optic Communications** 664

12.1 Introduction 664

12.2 Essential Components of Fiber Communication System 665

12.3 Basic Communication System 677

12.4 Types of Topologies 677

12.5 Types of Networks 678

12.6 Submarine Cables 682

12.7 Open system Interconnection (OSI) 683

12.8 System Architectures 685

12.8.1 Point-to-Point Links 685

12.8.2 Distributed Networks 685

12.9 Line Coding in Optical Links 688

12.10 Error Control or Correction 689

12.11 Performance of Passive Linear Optical Networks 690

12.11.1 Power Budget Calculation 691

12.11.2 Nearest-Distance Power Budget 691

12.11.3 Largest-Distance Power Budget 691

12.12 Performance of Star Optical Networks 692

12.13 SONET and SDH 693

12.13.1 Purposes and Features of SONET/SDH 694

12.14 Multiplexing Terminology and Signaling Hierarchy 695

12.14.1 Existing Multiplexing Terminology and Digital Signalling Hierarchy 695

12.14.2 SONET Multiplexing Terminology and Optical Signaling Hierarchy 695

12.14.3 SDH Multiplexing Terminology and Optical Signalling Hierarchy 696

12.15 SONET and SDH Transmission Rates 696

12.16 SONET Systems 698

12.17 Metro and Long-Haul Optical Networks 699

12.18 Network Configuration 700

12.18.1 Automatic Protection Switching (APS) 700

12.18.2 SONET/SDH Ring Configurations 700

12.19 Nonlinear Effects 704

12.19.1 Stimulated Raman Scattering 705

12.19.2 Stimulated Brilliaun Scattering (SBS) 706

12.19.3 Four-Wave Mixing 707

12.19.4 Self- and Cross-Phase Modulation 707

12.20 Dispersion 708

12.20.1 Information Capacity Determination 708

12.20.2 Group Delay 708

12.20.3 Modal Dispersion 712

12.20.4 Signal Distortion in Single Mode Fibers 712

12.20.5 Higher Order Dispersion 713

12.20.6 Dispersion Induced Limitations 713

12.20.7 Basic Propagation Equation 713

12.20.8 Chirped Gaussian Pulses 713

12.20.9 Limitations of Bit Rate 713

12.20.10 Dispersion Management 713

12.21 Solitons 715

12.21.1 Nonlinear Effects, i.e. Nonlinear Optical Susceptibility 715

12.21.2 Main Nonlinear Effects 716

12.21.3 Stimulated Raman Scattering 716

12.21.4 Derivation of the Nonlinear Schödinger Equation 716

13. **Fiber Optic Measurement and Testing** 745

13.1 Introduction 745

13.2 Measurement Standards 745

13.3 Testing Photonic Components 746

13.4 Optical Power Measurements (Intensity) 748

13.4.1 Optical Power Measurement Units 748

13.4.2 Optical Power Loss Measurements 748

13.4.3 Crosstalk 749

13.4.4 Polarization Dependent Loss (PDL) 750

13.4.5 Return Loss (RL) or Backreflection 751

13.4.6 Temperature Dependent Loss 751

13.4.7 Wavelength Dependent Loss 752

13.4.8 Chromatic Dispersion 752

13.4.9 Optical Frequency Measurements 754

13.5 Testing Optical Fiber Switches 754

13.5.1 Mechanical Tests 754

13.5.2 Environmental Tests 755

13.5.3 Repeatability Test 755

13.5.4 Speed Test 756

13.6 Light Wavelength Measurements *757*

13.7 Device Power Handling Tests *757*

13.8 Troubleshooting *757*

13.9 Sources of Error During Fiber Optic
Measurements *758*
   13.9.1 Resolution *758*
   13.9.2 Accuracy *758*
   13.9.3 Stability (Drift) *758*
   13.9.4 Linearity *759*
   13.9.5 Repeatability Error *759*
   13.9.6 Reproducibility *759*

13.10 Optical System Test Equipment/
Instruments *760*
   13.10.1 Optical Power Meter *760*
   13.10.2 Fiber Optical Power
        Attenuators *761*
   13.10.3 Test-Support Lasers: Tunable Laser
        Sources *762*
   13.10.4 Optical Spectrum Analyzer
        (OSA) *762*
   13.10.5 Optical Time Domain
        Reflectometer (OTDR) *764*

13.11 Characterization Techniques of
Optical Fiber *765*
   13.11.1 Attenuation and Its
        Measurement *766*
   13.11.2 Dispersion Measurement *767*
   13.11.3 Measurements with Optical Time
        Domain Reflectometer
        (OTDR) *771*

13.12 Eye Diagram Tests *772*

Suggested Reading 775

Appendices 777

Appendix A: List of Abbreviations 777

Appendix B: Physical Constants 779

Appendix C: Standard International (SI)
Units 779

Appendix D: Bessel Functions 780

Appendix E: Some Useful Mathematical
Relations 782

Index 785

Introduction

1.1 HISTORICAL PERSPECTIVES

Optical fiber communications has advanced at a tremendous pace since its inception in 1966. Its technological development has progressed through three principal phases. The *multimode fiber era* at the initial stage when silica fiber was first fabricated and manufactured in the early 1970s. Then at the end of the 1970s, *single-mode fibers* were manufactured, and the laser sources at a wavelength of 1300 nm were also available for research laboratories. At this wavelength, the fiber dispersion is almost zero, and the transmission system is limited by the attenuation of the lightwaves. Figure 1.1 shows the increase of the transmission capacity and distance as optical communications progressed during 1975–2010. A significant increase in the capacity–distance product after 1990 is due to the invention of *in-line optical amplifiers using erbium-doped silica-based fibers*. Prior to this, a certain improvement in the transmission capacity due to a change from the use of multimode to single-mode fibers allowed the distance between repeaters to increase to about 40 km.

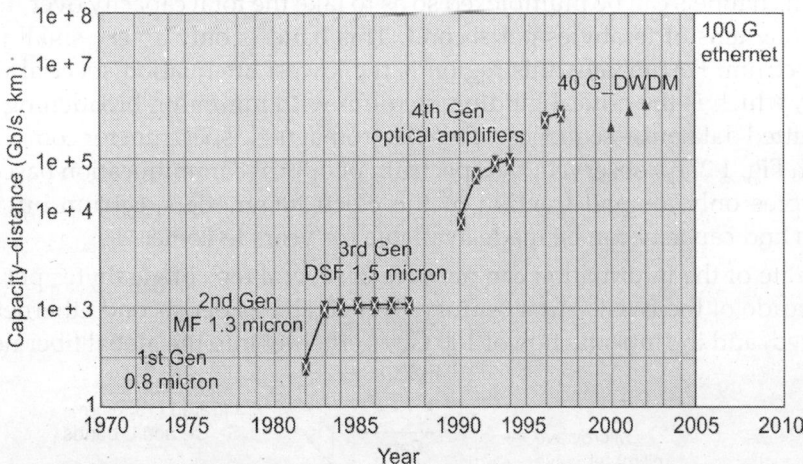

Fig. 1.1: Demonstrates the progress of optical communications (1975–2010) with transmission capacity–distance product increase with year

Since then single-mode optical fibers with low loss at 1550 nm were used with sources in this region. The loss is nearly half of that at 1300 nm, so the repeater distance, in practice, was limited to 40 km. This scenario did not improve until the late 1980s, when optical amplifiers were invented, in particular, the Er-doped fiber amplifier that offers significant optical gain in the 15,530–1,565 nm range. Amplification for the L-band would also be available using different doped agents in the silica fiber. However, Raman amplification can also be available, and the gain is distributed along the length of the propagation of the optical signals. These optical amplifiers have since then revolutionized the design and the implementation of optical transmission systems and networks in which the attenuation factor was no longer a major obstacle.

The advancement of single-mode optical fibers of transmission and dispersion compensating types and single frequency source as well as wideband and low-noise optical receivers have permitted the transmission of high-quality signals over an extremely long haul (in the order of more than a few thousands) at bit rates reaching 40–100 Gb/s. Dispersion management techniques can be exploited to further extend the transmission distance.

Since the linewidth of laser sources can now be narrowed so as to be considered as single-frequency sources, the modulation by direct modulating the electron density in the lasing cavity is seldom employed for a bit rate equal to or greater than 10 Gb/s. External modulation via the use of electro-optic effects and the interference of the continuously turned-on lightwaves is the technique that is commonly used currently. Thus, modulation formats have been used to achieve effective bandwidth in the optical passband and to combat effects of nonlinearity and dispersion. Thus, in this book we concentrate on models for external modulation of the continuous wave operation of the lasers and on advanced methods of detection and transmission of information over optically amplified multi-span single-mode optical fiber systems.

Optical communication systems employ lightwaves to transmit information from one place to another separated by a few kilometers to thousands of kilometers for delivery to homes and from central exchanges between major cities. Furthermore, the reach can now be extended to transoceanic distances covering several thousands of kilometers. The lightwave frequency is in the range of nearly 200 THz for 1550 nm wavelength and several wavelength channels can be multiplexed so as to take the total capacity over this spectral band to a few tens of terabytes per second. This band is only a very small part of the optical spectrum. Fortunately, this region is the lowest attenuation spectral window of silica fiber, which is the critical guiding medium with minimum broadening effects on the transmitted data pulse sequences. This electromagnetic spectrum for communications is shown in Fig. 1.2. As observed, the spectrum of optical communication based on silica fiber occupies only a small fraction of the electromagnetic spectrum but extensive bandwidth and capacity can be made available for years to come.

The bit rate of the information can now reach several tens of gigabytes per second in the first decade of the twenty-first century. Ten gigabytes per second ethernet has been standardized, and the introduction of 100 Gb/s ethernet into the global fiber networks is

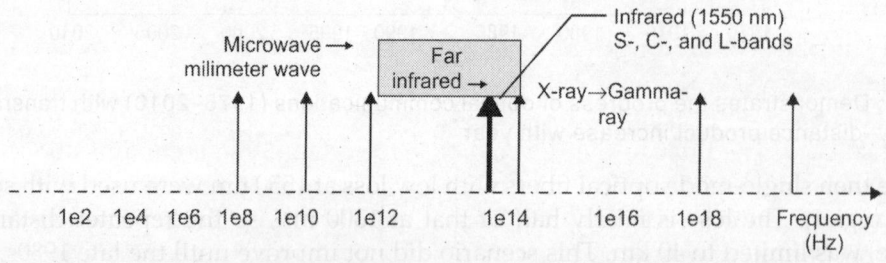

Fig. 1.2(a): Electromagnetic spectrum of waves for communications and lightwave region for silica-based fiber optical communications

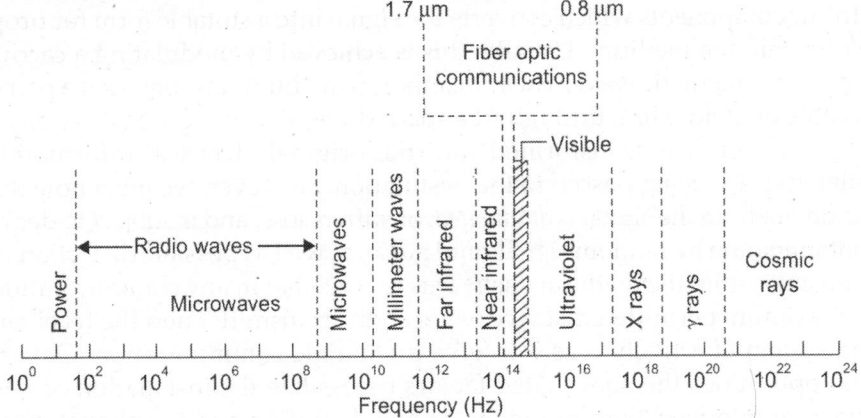

Fig. 1.2(b): Electromagnetic spectrum

inevitable. Similarly, for transmission rates under synchronous digital hierarchy (SDH), OC-192 and OC-768 for 10 and 40 Gb/s have been demonstrated over the last decade. Recently, the possibility of 1 Tb/s per wavelength channel has also been proposed but is yet to be demonstrated. The modulated lightwaves are guided through single-mode optical fibers and compensated over several spans that are made up by cascading dispersive and compensating fibers as well as optical amplifiers through which direct amplification of photons is achieved.

An important development, however, concerns the discovery of photonic band gaps which can be created in structures which propagates light, such as crystals or optical fibers. As the ultimate optical dispersion compensation devices, photonic bandgap fibers (holey fibers) are an interesting class in themselves. These are fibers with a hollow structure, with holes engineered to achieve a particular functionality. Instead of being drawn from a solid perform, holey fibers are drawn from a group of capillary tubes fused together. This way, dispersion, disperson slope, and the nonlinear coefficients could in principle, be all precisely designed and controlled upto a very small or very large values, well outside the range of those of the solid fiber.

Although several technologies have emerged that meet some or all of the above requirements, no technology is a clear winner. The trend is towards tunable devices, or even actively self-tunable devices, or even actively self-tunable compensators, and such devices will allow system designers to cope with the shrinking system margins and with the emerging rapidly reconfigurable optical networks.

1.2 GENERAL OPTICAL FIBER COMMUNICATION SYSTEM

An optical fiber communication system is similar in basic concept to any type of communication system. Figure 1.3 (a) shows a block schematic of a general communication system, the function of which is to convey the signal from the information source over the transmission medium to the destination. This is why, the communication system consists of a transmitter or modulator linked to the information source, the transmission medium, and a receiver or demodulator at the destination point. In *electrical communication system*, the information source provides an electrical signal, usually derived from a message signal which is not electrical (e.g. sound) to a transmitter comprising electrical and electronic components which converts the signal into a suitable form for propagation over the transmission medium. Usually, this is achieved by modulating a carrier, which may be an electromagnetic wave. The transmission medium can consist of a pair of wires, a coaxial cable or a radio link through free space down which the signal is transmitted to the receiver, where it is transformed into the original electrical information signal (demodulated) prior being passed to the destination. However, we must note that in any transmission medium the signal is *attenuated*, or suffers loss, and is subject to degradations due to contamination by random signals and noise, as well as possible distortions imposed by mechanisms within the medium itself. This reveals that in any communication system there is a maximum permitted distance between the transmitter and the receiver beyond which the system effectively ceases to give intelligible communication. Obviously, for long-haul applications the above cited factors necessitate the installation of *repeaters* or *line amplifiers* at intervals, both to remove signal distortion and to enhance signal level, prior transmission is continued down the link.

In optical fiber communication system [Fig. 1.3(b)], the information source provides an electrical signal usually derived form a message signal which is not generally an electrical signal (e.g. picture, sound). The electrical signal from the information source is fed to a transmitter comprising an electrical stage which drives an optical source to give modulation of the lightwave carrier. We may note that in IM/DD system, the modulating signal is used to modulate the intensity of the light source only. We may note that unlike conventional electrical modulation scheme where the amplitude, frequency or phase of the carrier is altered in accordance with the modulating signal, the frequency or the phase of the optical signal from the optical source remain unaltered. Obviously, the function of the optical source in a way is to provide electrical (E)-to-optical (O) [(E/O)] conversion. The optical source which provides the electrical–optical conversion may be either a *semiconductor laser* or *light-emitting diode* (LED) or *injection laser diode* (ILD). These optical sources are *lightweight*, *compact*, and most importantly, quite compatible in size with the optical fiber which is used as *waveguide* for subsequent transmission of the signal. Further, both LED and ILD optical sources consume low electrical power and at the same time

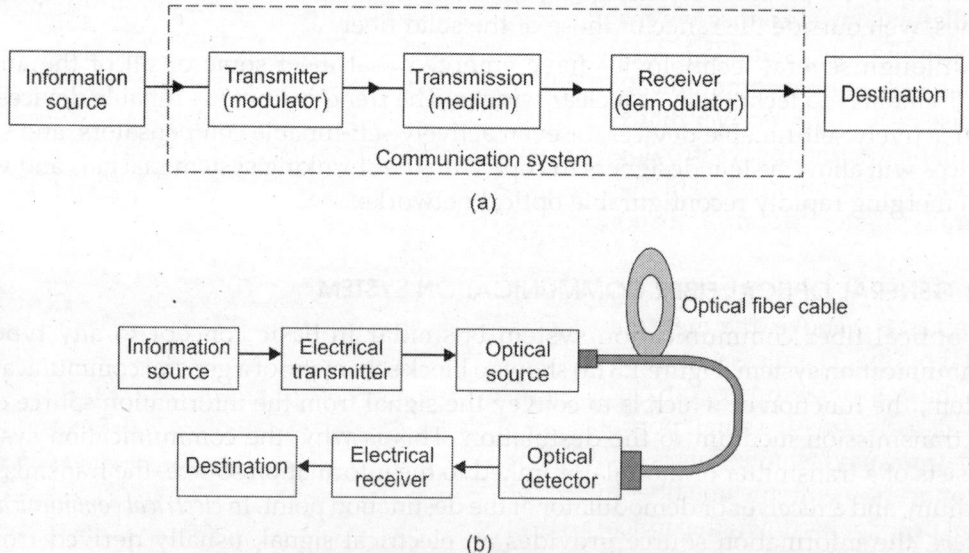

Fig. 1.3: Block diagram of the general communication system

can generate light-wave at different wavelength regions of the optical spectrum where the optical fibers made of silica offer less attenuation. The modulated lightwave output from the optical source is coupled to the transmission medium consisting of optical fiber cable and the receiver consists of an optical detector which drives a further electrical stage and hence provides demodulation of the optical carrier. Usually, the fiber cable contains a group of optical fibers which are generally long thin strands (~ 100 μm diameter) of ultrapure glass that provides low-loss at the transmitting wavelength.

An optical fiber consists of two coaxial solid cylinders made of slightly different refractive index. The inner solid cylinder called the *core* has higher refractive index as compared to the outer cylinder called as *cladding*. The optical signal propagates through the optical fiber by *total internal reflection*. As the optical signal propagates down the length of the optical fiber, signal gets attenuated due to absorption, scattering, etc. within the fiber and at the same time signal gets distorted and broadened because of various dispersion mechanism. The weak distorted optical signal is received by the receiver at the destination. As stated above, the key component of the receiver is an *optical detector* which converts the weak and distorted information bearing signal to an electrical signal that is a replica of the modulated signal. Photodiodes (*p-n*, *p-i-n*, or avalanche) and, in some instances, phototransistors and photoconductors are utilized for the detection of the optical signal and the optical-electrical conversion. This reveals that there is a requirement for electrical interfacing at either end of the optical link and at present signal processing is usually performed electrically. However, significant developments have taken place in devices for optical signal processing which have started to alter this situation. The signal is processed by an electrical receiver and the output is finally sent to the destination.

The optical carrier may be modulated using either an *analog* or *digital* information signal. Figure 1.4 shows the block diagram of an practical optical communication system. Like electrical communication, the optical carrier may be modulated using either an *analog* or *digital* information signal. In the system shown in Fig. 1.3(b) analog modulation involves the variation of the light emitted from the optical source in a continuous manner. A practical digital optical communication link appears like shown in Fig. 1.4. With digital modulation, however, discrete changes in the light intensity are obtained (i.e. on-off pulses representing bits 1s and 0s). Although often simpler to implement, analog modulation with an optical fiber communication system is less efficient, requiring a far higher signal-to-noise ratio at the receiver than digital modulation. Also, the *linearity* needed for analog modulation is not always provided by semiconductor optical sources, especially at high modulation frequencies. This is why, analog optical fiber communication links are generally limited to shorter distances and lower bandwidth operation with digital links.

The basic components of a practical communication link are *optical transmitter, optical repeater, optical receiver, optical fiber waveguide, connector, splice, splitter, optical amplifier,* etc. As stated above, the message signal may in a continuous analog or in the form of digital pulses. The message signal is used to modulate the intensity of the optical source with the help of modulator (an electrical drive circuit). Usually the manufacturers provide optical sources with a small portion of an optical fiber (about 1-2 m length) attached to it in an optimum fashion. This is called *fiber digital flylead* and this can be easily plugged in for connection with the line fiber by making use of a demountable connector. The optical signal propagates down the optical fiber towards the receiver end. The signal propagates along the optical fiber gets attenuated due to absorption of optical signal by fiber material and also signal gets distorted due to dispersion phenomenon. The weak and distorted

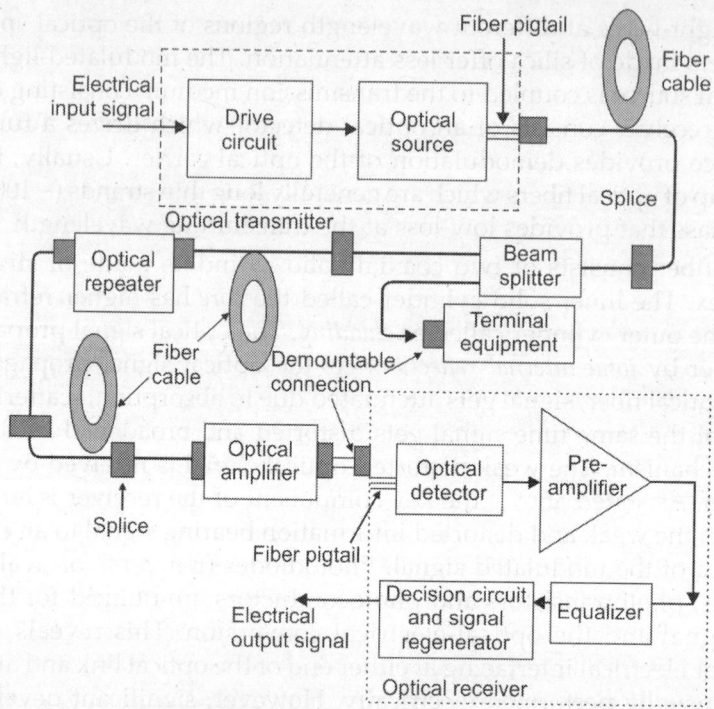

Fig. 1.4: Practical block diagram of an optical communication system

optical signal is subsequently allowed to travel along the optical fiber and prior to this, the signal gets distorted beyond recognition, the signal is reconstructed and boosted to travel further over the transmission link with the help of regenerative repeaters. In Fig. 1.4, only one repeater unit is shown. We may note that the actual number of repeaters needed along a transmission line depends on the transmission characteristics of optical fiber channel and the total distance to the covered.

At the end of the link, the received optical signal which is attenuated and distorted during transmission down the optical fiber is reconverted from optical to electrical signal for further electrical processing and extraction of the original electrical message signal. At the receiving end, the key element is an optical detector (*p-i-n* or avalanche photodiode) which converts the intensity variation in the recovered optical signal into a corresponding electrical signal. We must remember that the size of the optical detector have to be compatible to optical fiber size. Figure 1.5 shows a block schematic of a typical digital optical fiber link.

Initially, the input digital signal from information source is suitably encoded for optical transmission. The laser drive circuit directly modulates the intensity of the semiconductor laser with the encoded digital signal. Hence a digital optical signal is launched into the optical fiber cable. The avalanche photodiode (APD) detector is followed by a front-end amplifier and equalizer or filter to provide gain as well as linear signal processing and noise band-width reduction.

The important requirements of photodector characteristics include linearity, high-speed of response, high responsivity and low-noise behaviour. We may note that in a practical optical communication system, there are also additional components used such as optical connectors, splices, couplers and optical amplifiers. The connectors and splices are used

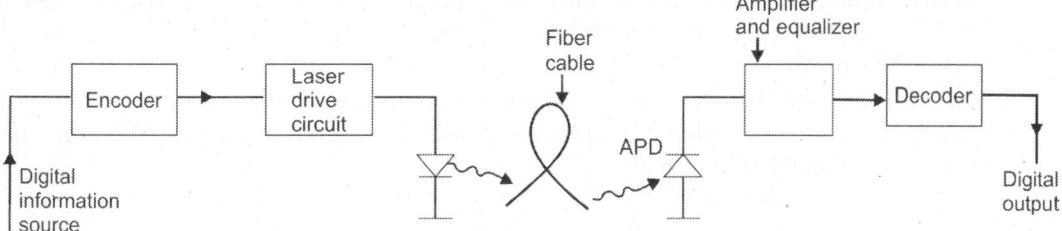

Fig. 1.5: A digital optical fiber link using a semiconductor laser source and an avalanche photodiode detector

for joining two optical fibers. The connectors are generally demountable whereas the splices provide permanent joints. The couplers are in-line bus that are basically used at terminal points to remove a portion of the optical signal from the trunk line at intermediate points or inject additional optical signals into the trunk. Interestingly optical amplifiers provide on-line amplification to the propagating optical signal. We may note that such amplifiers are useful for compensating the attenuation caused by the optical fiber during propagation of the signal. To provide amplification of the signal in the optical domain both semiconductor laser amplifier as well as erbium doped fiber amplifier are used. We may note that a practical optical communication system is actually much more complex than that is apprently shown by simple block diagrams (Figs 1.4 and 1.5).

1.3 DIGITAL MODULATION FOR ADVANCED OPTICAL TRANSMISSION SYSTEM

Depending on the modulation of the carrier by amplitude, frequency or phase, the following four digital modulation formats form the basis of modulation formats in advanced optical fiber communication systems.

The optical signal field has the ideal form during the duration of 1 bit period given as

$$E_s(t) = E_p(t)\, a(t)\, \cos\,[\omega(t)\, t + \theta(t)] \quad [0 \le t \le T] \tag{1.1}$$

where

$E_s(t)$: optical signal field

$E_p(t)$: polarized field coefficient as a function of time

$a(t)$: amplitude variation

$\omega(t)$: optical frequency change with respect to time

$\theta(t)$: phase variation with respect to time

- For amplitude shift keying (ASK), the amplitude $a(t)$ takes the value $a(t) > 0$ for a "ONE" symbol and the value of 0 for a "ZERO" symbol. Other values such as the angular frequency and the phase parameter remain unchanged over a 1 bit period.
- For phase shift keying (PSK), the phase angle $\theta(t)$ takes a value of π radian for a "ONE" symbol and 0 rad for the symbol "ZERO" so that the distance between these symbols on the phase plane is at maximum and hence minimum interference or error can be obtained. These values are changed accordingly if the number of phase states is increased as shown in Fig. 1.6. The values of $a(t)$, $\omega(t)$, and $E_p(t)$ remain unchanged.
- For frequency shift keying (FSK), the value of $\omega(t)$ takes the value ω_1 for the "ONE" symbol and ω_2 for the "ZERO" symbol. The values of $a(t)$, $\theta(t)$, and $E_p(t)$ remain unchanged. Indeed FSK is a form of phase modulation, provided that the phase is continuous. Sometimes, continuous phase modulation is also used as the term for FSK.

In the case where the frequency spacing between ω_1 and ω_2 equals a quarter of the bit rate, the FSK is called minimum shift keying (MSK).

- For polarization shift keying (PolSK), we have $E_p(t)$ taking one direction for the "ONE" symbol and the other for the "ZERO" symbol. Sometimes, continuous polarization of lightwave is used to multiplex two optically modulated signal sequences to double the transmission capacity (Figs 1.6 and 1.7).

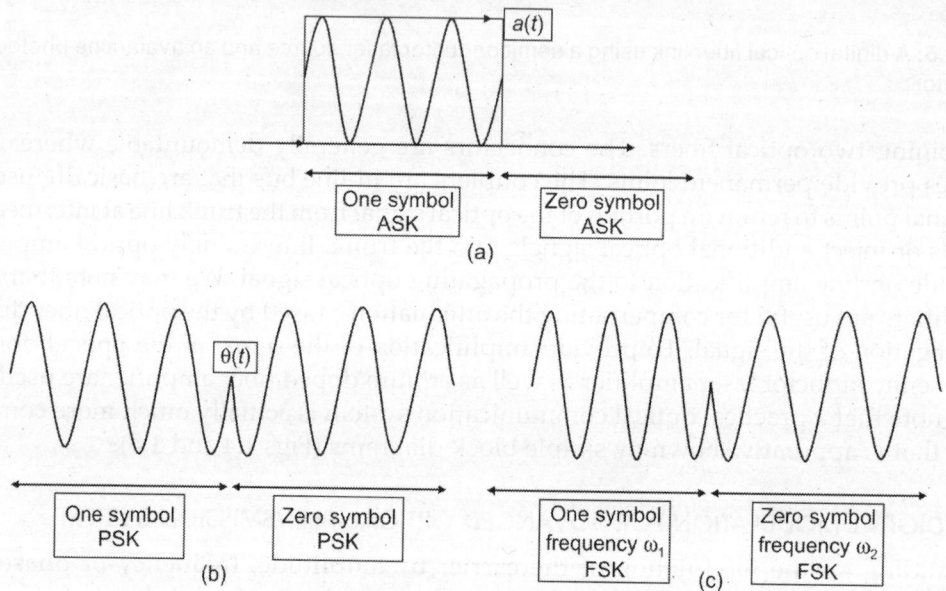

Fig. 1.6: Illustration of ASK, PSK and FSK with the symbols and the variation of the optical carrier (a) amplitude (b) phase and (c) frequency

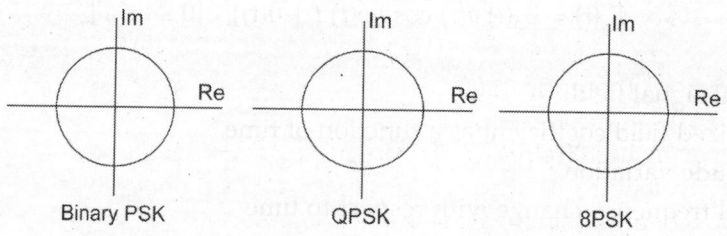

Fig. 1.7: Phase of the carrier under modulation with π phase shift of the binary phase shift keying (BPSK) at the edge of the pulse period

Besides the above mentioned formats, the pulse shaping also plays an important role in these advanced systems. They include non-return-to-zero (NRZ), return-to-zero (RZ), and duobinary (DuoB). RZ and NRZ are binary-level formats taking two levels "0 and 1" while DuoB is a tri-level shaping taking the values of "−1 0 1." The −1 in optical waves can be taken care of by an amplitude of "1" and a phase of π phase shift with respect to the "+1" which means a differential phase is used to distinguish between the +1 and −1 states.

The modulated lightwaves at the output of the optical transmitter are then fed into the transmission fibers and fiber spans, as shown in Fig. 1.8.

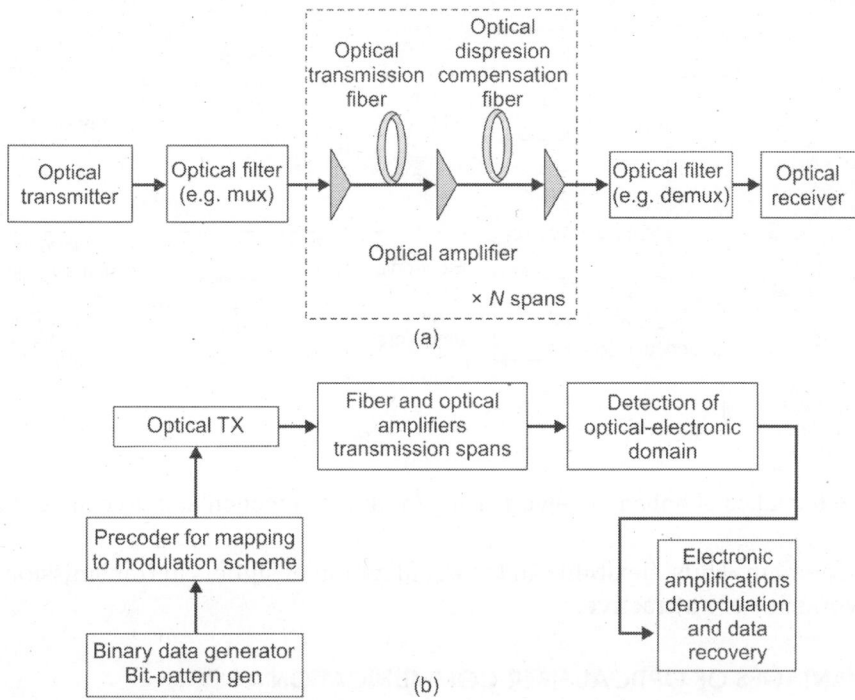

Fig. 1.8: (a) Generalized diagram of optical transmission systems and (b) details of the optical transmission system

1.4 DEMODULATION TECHNIQUES

The output transmitted signals, which are normally distorted, are then detected by a digital optical receiver. The main function of this optical receiver is to recognize whether the current received and thence the "bit symbol" voltage at the output of the amplifiers following the detector is a ONE or a ZERO. The modulation of the amplitude, the phase, or the frequency of the optical carrier requires an optical demodulation, that is, the demodulation of the optical carrier is implemented in the optical domain. This is necessary due to the extremely high frequency of the optical carrier (in the order of nearly 200 THz for 1550 nm wavelength) it is impossible to demodulate in the electronic domain by direct detection using a single photodetector. Indeed it is quite straightforward to demodulate in the optical domain using optical interferometers to compare the phases of the carriers in two consecutive bits.

However, the phase and the frequency of the lightwave signals can be recovered via an intermediate step by mixing the optical signals with a local oscillator, a narrow linewidth laser, to beat it to the baseband or an intermediate frequency region. This is coherent detection technique. Figure 1.9 shows the schematic of optical receivers using direct detection and coherent detection.

The main difference between these detection systems and those presented in several textbooks is the electronic signal processing subsystem following the detection circuitry. In the first decade of the twenty-first century, we have witnessed tremendous progress in the speed of *electronic ultra-large-scale integrated circuits*, with the number of samples per second reaching a few tens of giga-samples. This has permitted considerations for applications of digital signal processing of distorted received optical signals in the

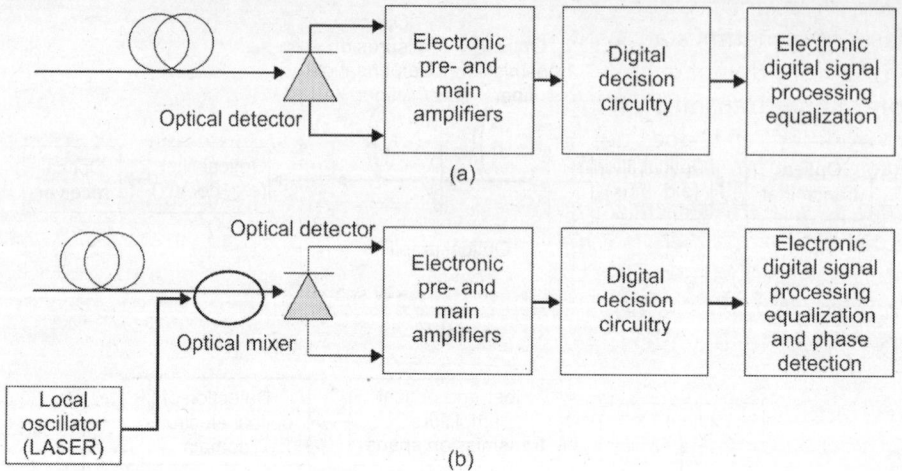

(a)

(b)

Fig. 1.9: Schematics of optical receivers using (a) direct detection and (b) coherent detection

electronic domain. Thus, flexibility in the equalization of signals in transmission systems and networks is very attractive.

1.5 ADVANTAGES OF OPTICAL FIBER COMMUNICATION

An optical communication system using an optical carrier wave guided along a glass fiber has a number of extremely attractive features over the conventional electrical communication system that uses copper cable as waveguide. Some of the features of optical fiber communication were apparent when the technique was originally conceived. Furthermore, the advances in the related technology till date have surpassed even the most optimistic predictions, creating additional advantages. Some of the most distinct advantages of optical fiber communication are following:

i. *Small size and light weight*: Optical fibers have small diameters which are often no greater than the diameter of human hair (~ 100 mm). Hence, the optical fibers coated with protecting layers are far smaller and much lighter than corresponding copper cables. The small size and light weight of optical fibers make them especially attractive for an expansion of signal transmission within mobiles such as aircraft, satellites and even ships. They have proved a tremendous boon towards the alleviation of duct congestion in cities.

ii. *Enormous potential bandwidth*: The frequency of the optical carrier in the range 10^{13} to 10^{16} Hz (generally in the near infrared around 10^{14} Hz or 10^{5} GHz) yields a far greater potential transmission bandwidth as compared to conventional metallic cable systems (i.e. coaxial cable bandwidth typically around 20 MHz over distances upto 10 km) or even millimeter wave radio systems (i.e. systems currently operating with modulation bandwidths of 700 MHz over a few hundreds of meters). Obviously, the information carrying capacity of an optical fiber is far superior to the best available copper cable systems. We may note that the full potential bandwidth of optical fibers (~ 50 THz) is yet not being utilized due to technological constraints. However, with the advent of *wavelength division multiplexing* (WDH), particularly with dense packing of optical wavelengths (of, essentially, fine frequency spacing), it would be possible to enhance the bandwidth utilization significantly in near future.

iii. *Electrical isolation*: Optical fibers which are fabricated from dielectric material, e.g. glass, or sometimes a plastic polymer, are electrical insulators. As a result, these waveguides do not exhibit earth loop and interface problems. This property makes optical fiber transmission ideally suited for communication in electrical hazardous environment as it does not create spark. This feature of optical fibers also enables easy interfacing of equipment.

iv. *Immunity to interference and crosstalk*: Optical fibers are made from dielectric materials form a *dielectric waveguide* and are therefore free from electromagnetic interference (EMI), *radio-frequency interference* (RFI), or *switching transients* giving *electromagnetic pulses* (EMPs). Further, unlike metallic cables, optical fiber cables are free from inductive pick-up from other electrical signal carrying wires or lightning, i.e. the function of fiber optic communicated system remains unaffected even in electrically noisy environment. The optical fiber cable is also not susceptible to lightning strikes it used overhead rather than underground. Moreover, the optical interference between individual fibers in an optical fiber cable is also absent and as a result cross-talk effect is negligible which is quite common in conventional electrical communication that uses metallic cables.

v. *Signal security*: The light from optical fiber cable does not radiate significantly and, as a result, there is practically no leakage of optical power from the fiber. Clearly, optical fibers provide a high degree of signal security. Emanations, if any, get absorbed in opaque jackets surrounding the fibers. Unlike the situation with copper cables, a transmitted optical signal cannot be obtained from a optical fiber in a noninvasive manner (i.e. without drawing optical power from the fiber). Therefore, in theory, any attempt to acquire a message signal transmitted optically may be detected. This feature is obviously very attractive for military, banking and general secure data transmission (i.e. computer network) applications.

vi. *Low transmission loss*: Optical fiber cables exhibit very low attenuation or transmission loss as compared to conventional copper cables. The development of the optical fiber fabrication over the past 28 years has resulted in the production of very high quality optical fibers which provide extremely low loss (as low as 0.15 dB/km) and this feature has become a major advantage of optical fiber communication. The low loss optical fibers have considerably enhanced the repeater spacing and significantly reduced the system cost. This property of fiber has provided a totally compelling case for the adoption of optical fiber communications in the majority of long-haul telecommunication applications, replacing not only copper cables, but also satellite communications, as a consequence of very noticeable delay incurred for voice transmission when using this latter approach.

vii. *Ruggedness and flexibility*: With proper protecting layers and cabling structures, optical fibers may be manufactured with very high tensile strengths, i.e. fiber cables remain flexible yet rugged enough to bear stresses during instalation. Optical fibers may also be bent to quite small radii or twisted without damage. As compared to metallic cables, optical fiber cable is quite superior in respect to transportation, storage, handling and installation, while exhibiting atleast comparable strength and durability. The optical fiber cables can be used for under-sea installation and other abusive environment without causing any damage.

viii. *System reliability and easy maintaince*: These feathers primarily stem from the availability of extremely low-loss and low dispersion single mode optical fiber cables which has improved the reliability of long-haul optical links with lesser number of repeaters or line amplifiers as compared to the conventional metal cable systems. Furthermore, the average life time of the state-of-the-art optical fiber system is about 20 to 30 years, i.e. the reliability of the optical components is no longer a problem. Both these factors also tend to reduce maintaince time and cost, i.e. optical communication subsystems require minimum maintenance in the long run.

ix. *Potential low cost*: The cost of overall system of optical communication link for long-haul application is considerably less than its electrical counterpart using copper conductors as cables. Extremely low loss and large bandwidth of the optical fiber communication system are primarily responsible for the development of low-cost system using lightwave technology. No doubt, the high quality light sources, e.g. ILD and optical fiber connectors, couplers are still very expensive. However, the glass which generally provides the optical fiber transmission medium is made from sand is abundantly available in nature. This significantly reduces the cost of this waveguide used in optical fiber communication system in comparison with copper cables.

The above mentioned advantages of optical fiber communication have made this technology almost indispensible for long-haul optical links, but it is not always the case in short-haul applications where the additional cost incurred, due to the electrical-optical conversion (and vice versa) may be a deciding factor. Nevertheless, there are also other possible cost advantages in relation to shipping, handling, installation and maintenance, etc.

The reducing cost of optical fiber communications have made this technology almost indispensible for long-haul links and not only preferred over conventional electrical communication with electrical line transmission systems, but also for microwave and millimeter radio transmission systems. Initially, optical fiber communication link were used only in intercity and intercontinental trunk lines but with increasing demand of larger bandwidth and advent of *integrated service digital network* (ISDN) involving transmission of voice, video, facsimile, computer data, etc. optical fibers have finally made its place into subscribers loop.

SUMMARY

1. Optical fiber communications technology has developed rapidly since the early 1970s and has, in combination with the advancement of digital processing technology, revolutionized global communications.

2. Fiber optic cables transmit data through very small cores at the speed of light. Significantly different from copper cables, fiber optic cables offer high bandwidths and low losses, which allow high data transmission rates over long distances. Light propagates throughout the fiber cables according to the principle of total internal reflection.

3. Optical communication is an interdisplinary field that combines photonic/opto-electric devices and communication systems.

4. There are three common types of fiber optic cables: *single-mode, multimode,* and *graded index*. Each has its advantages and disadvantages. There are also several different designs of fiber optic cables, each made for different applications. In addition, new fiber optic cables with different core and cladding designs have been emerging; these are faster and can carry more modes.

5. Although fiber optic cables are used mostly in communication systems, they also have established medical, military, scanning, imaging, and sensing applications. They are also used in optical fiber devices and fiber optic lighting.

6. There are specific situations in which fiber has advantages over copper cable. First the fiber cable is immune to electrical interference and tapping. It also carries high data capacity over long distances and is small and lightweight. When it comes to testing, fiber may still require some fairly sophisticated equipment but the newer standards for copper cabling present the same issues.

REVIEW QUESTIONS

1. Briefly write the evolution of today's optical fiber communication and major milestones that paved the way for the incredible expansion of optical fiber communication network all over the globle.

2. Draw a block schematic of a general communication system as well as of optical fiber communication system and explain briefly the function of each part.

3. Explain analog and digital information signals. Why analog modulation with an optical fiber communication system is less efficient?

4. Draw a block schematic of a typical digital optical fiber link and explain briefly.

5. Mention advantages of optical fiber communication.

SHORT ANSWER QUESTIONS

1. Why in the early days, most of the fiber's usable bandwidth remain significantly under-utilized?

   Ans. Due to quite low transmission capacity.

2. Briefly mention the major milestones towards the evolution of optical fiber communication.

   Ans.
• 1790s	Claud Clappe	Optical telegraph
• 1841	Daniel Colladen and Jacques Babinet	Light could be guided along jets of water for fountain displays
• 1870	John Tyndall	Light-pipe phenomenon demonstration
• 1880	Alexander Graham Bell	Optical telephone system
• 1920s	John Logie Baired, UK Clarence W. Hansell, USA	Patented the idea of using arrays of hollow pipes or transparent rods to transmit images for television or facsimile systems
• 1930	H. Lamm	Demonstration of light transmission through fibers
• 1951	A.C.S. van Heel, Holland Harold H. Hopkins, and Narinder S. Kabany, UK	Light transmission through bundles of fibers
• 1955	Lawrence Curtiss	Glass-clad fibers
• 1958	Alec Reeves	Digital pulse-code modulation
• 1960	Maiman (USA)	First Laser (Ruby) operation of He-Ne Laser

• 1962	USA	Semiconductor laser
• 1967	Charles K. Kao and George A. Hockham	Cladded optical fiber for long distance transmission
• 1969	Uchida (Japan)	Graded index fiber
• 1970	Kapron and Keck (USA)	Fiber transmission loss < 20 dB/km
• 1972	Gambling et al. (UK)	GHz bandwidth over 1 km optical link.
• 1978	USA	Commercial optical fiber link
• 1980	Bell Labs (USA)	Single-mode 1.3 µm technology for the first transatlantic fiber optic-cable, TAT-8
• 1985	Bell Labs (USA)	Single-mode fiber across USA to carry long-haul telephone signal at 400 Mbps and even more
• 1987	Dave Payne	First Erbium-doped fiber amplifier operating at 1.55 µm
• 1988	Linn Mollenaur	First *soliton* transmission through 4000 km of single mode fiber
• 1990	AT and T	Laid a fiber cable that spanned the Atlantic Ocean.
• 1993	TAT-8	Transmission of first soliton signals over 180 million km
• 1996	Nakazawa Fujitsu, NTT Labs and Bell Labs	Transmission of one trillion bits per second through single through single optical fibers.

3. What are fiber optic cables?

Ans. Fiber optic cable is a filament of transparent material used to transmit light. The centre of the cable is referred to as the core. It has a higher refractive index than the cladding, which surrounds the core. The contact surface between the core and the cladding creates an interface surface that guides the light, the difference between the refractive index of the core and cladding is what causes the mirror like interface surface, which guides light along the core. Light bounces through the core from one end to the other according to the principle of total internal reflection. The cladding is then covered with a protective plastic or PVC jackets. The diameters of the core, cladding, and jacket can vary widely; e.g. a single fiber optic cable can have core, cladding, and jacket diameters of 9, 125, and 250 µm respectively.

4. How many types of fiber optic cables are there?

Ans. There are three common type of fiber optic cables: Single mode, multimode, and graded index. Each has its advantages and disadvantages. There also are several different designs of fiber optic cables, each made for different applications. In addition, new fiber optic cables with different core and cladding designs have been emerging; these are faster and can carry more modes.

5. How many main components of an optical transmitter?

Ans. There are two main components of an optical transmitter: (i) Optical source, e.g. laser, and (ii) the optical modulator.

6. What do you understand by 'bandwidth'?

Ans. To transmit more bits of information in a given time period, the transmission medium should have a high bandwidth. Typically, the bandwidth is of the order of the carrier frequency. In the case optical signals, the carrier frequency is 200 THz and the bandwidth of the fiber is several THz, whereas the bandwidth of the copper cable is typically several GHz or MHz.

7. What is attenuation?

Ans. Attenuation or loss, in an optical fiber, primarily decides the maximum transmission distance (distance between the optical transmitter and the receiver) without using any repeater, which generally restores the signal at intermediate points in a long haul communication system. The loss of silica optical fiber is around 0.2 dB/km, which is much lower than that of copper cable. Because of the lower loss, optical signals can propagate over a longer distance without requiring repeaters.

8. Why, optical fibers are not affected by radio-frequency interference (RFI) and electromagnetic interference (EMI)?

Ans. Optical fibers are insulators, as they are made up of glass or plastic, i.e. optical fibers are purely dielectric waveguides with no metal parts. This property of optical fibers is useful for many applications. Particularly, it makes the optical signal traversing through the fiber free from RFI and EMI. RFI is caused by radio or television broadcasting station, radars, and other signals originating in electronic equipment. EMI may be caused by these sources of radiation as well as from industrial machinery, or from naturally occuring phenomena such as lightning or unintensional sparking. Optical fibers do not pick up or propagate electromagnetic pulses (EMPs). Thus, fiber-optic systems may be employed for reliable monitoring and telemetry in industrial environments, where EMI or EMPs cause problems for metallic cables. In the case of copper cables, electromagnetic noise fields set up conduction currents which interfere with the signal transmission.

9. What is the role of fiber optics technology in our life?

Ans. Today, we are living in an "information society" where the efficient transfer of information is highly relevant to our well-being. Fiber-optic systems are going to form the very means of such information transfer and hence they are destined to have very important role, directly or indirectly, in the development of every sphere of life. The areas in which fiber optic technology is going to have a major impact are: voice communication, video communication, data transfer, internet, sensor systems for industrial development, etc.

10. What is photonics?

Ans. The invention of laser in 1960 has brought new ideas and new methods to many areas of science and technology. Starting from the consideration that, in a simplified view, a light beam can be seen as a stream of energy quanta, known as photons, the name "photonics" has been coined, in analogy to electronics, to indicate the generation and use of photon streams for engineering applications. The applications of photonics are everywhere around us from long-distance communications to DVD players, from industrial manufacturing to health care, from lighting to image formation and display.

11. What are photonic band gap fibers (holey fibers)?

Ans. These are fibers with a hollow structure, with holes engineered to achieve a particular functionality. Instead of being drawn from a solid perform, holey fibers are drawn from a group of capillary tubes fused together. This way, the dispersion, dispersion slope, and the nonlinear coefficients could in principle all be precisely designed and controlled, upto very small or very large values, well outside the range of those of slid fiber.

12. Explain channel capacity.

Ans. Channel capacity is an important factor in the analysis of any communication network. This is the maximum rate at which data can be sent across a channel from the message source to the user destination. A fundamental and important theorem for this is the *Shannon capacity formula*. This theorem states that if a channel has a bandwidth B (measured in Hz), then the maximum information transmission capacity C of that channel is given in bits per second by the relationship

$$C = B \log_2 \left(1 + \frac{S}{N} \right)$$

Here $\log_2$ represents the base-2 logarithm, and S and N are the average signal power and noise power, respectively. Typically these powers are measured at the receiver, since it is at this point that a signal is extracted from the channel and processed.

The parameter S/N is the *signal-to-noise ratio* (SNR), which is the ratio of power in a signal to the power contained in the noise at a particular measurement point. This ratio is often expressed in decibles:

$$SNR_{dB} = 10 \log \frac{\text{signal power}}{\text{noise power}}$$

$$= 10 \log \left(\frac{S}{N} \right)$$

The Shannon formula indicates the theoretical maximum capacity that can be achieved. In practice this capacity cannot be reached, since the formula only takes into account thermal noise and does not consider factors such as impulse noise, attenuation, attenuation distortion, or delay distortion. Further more, intuitively it might seem that the capacity can be increased merely by raising the signal strength. However, raising the signal level also increases *nonlinear effects* in the system, which leads to higher noise powers. We may also note that increasing the bandwidth B decreases the ratio S/N, since the wider the bandwidth the more noise is introduced into the system.

13. Define decibel.

Ans. The decibel which is used for comparing two power levels, may be defined for a particular optical wavelength as the ratio of the input (transmitted) optical power P_i into a fiber to the output (received) optical power P_o from the fiber as:

$$\text{Number of decibels (dB)} = 10 \log_{10} \frac{P_i}{P_o}$$

This logarithmic unit having the nature of the decibel allows a large ratio to be expressed in a fairly simple manner. Power levels differing in many orders of magnitude can be compared easily when they are in decibel form. Another attractive feature of the decibel is that to measure the changes in the strength of a signal, one merely adds or subtracts the decibel numbers between two different points.

14. The last decade of the twentieth century witnessed highly advanced and intricate communication systems. Justify this statement.

Ans. The last decade of 20th century witnessed highly and intricate communication systems, such as:

- Fax
- Optical fiber communication
- Cellular mobile communication
- Personal mobile communication
- Computer networks
- Integrated services digital network (ISDN)
- Intelligent networks (IW)
- Cordless phones
- Paging
- The Internet

15. How many types of signals are there?

Ans. There are two types of signals: analog and digital

i. *Analog signal*: An analog signal is a function of time, and has a continuous range of values. There is a definite function value of the analog signal at each point of time.

A *pure sine wave* is an example of an analog signal or analog waveform. A voice signal is a practical example of an analog signal. When a voice signal is converted to electrical form by a microphone, you get a corresponding electrical analog signal. This electrical signal can be seen on an oscilloscope. Being an analog signal, this waveform has definite values at all points of time (Fig. 1.10).

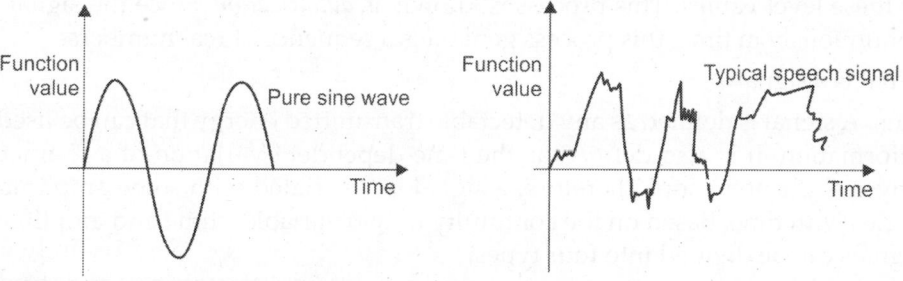

Fig. 1.10: Analog signals

ii. *Digital signal*: A digital signal does not have continuous function values on a time scale. It is discrete in nature, i.e. it has some values at discrete timings. In between two consecutive values, the signal value is either zero or different value. The sound signal produced by drum beats is an example of a digital signal. A digital signal is graphically represented in Fig. 1.11.

16. What do you understand by digitization of analog signals?

Ans. To send a signal in an analog format, the transmission

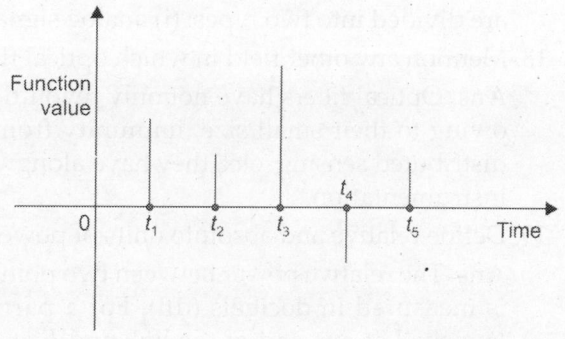

Fig. 1.11: Digital signal

channel typically cannot achieve perfect reproduction of the signal at the destination, so there always will be some degree of distortion. Furthermore, different types of analog signals may require different channel responses. This puts a strain on the design of multipurpose analog link. In addition, noises that get added to the analog signal as it passes through multiple repeaters cannot be eliminated, which further degrades the signal.

In contrast, digital signals can undergo a great amount of distortion and still allow the information to be extracted with a high degree of fidelity. To avoid the shortcomings of analog signals and to create networks that can multiplex and switch any type of information, most information is sent in a digital format. In order to achieve this network flexibility, most analog signals need to be converted to a digital format. However, there are a number of situations in which it is advantageous to send high-speed analog signals in their native form over relatively short distances, e.g. the transmission of microwave signals from a satellite dish to a processing station located less than a kilometer away.

An analog signal can be transformed into a digital signal through a process sampling and the assignment of quantized values to represent the intensity of the signal at regular intervals of time. In order to convert an analog signal to a digital form, one starts by taking instantaneous measures of the height of the signal wave at regular intervals, which is called *sampling* of the simple. The simplest, but not necessarily the best, way to convert these analog samples to a digital format is to divide the amplitude excursion of the analog signal into N equally spaced levels and assign a discrete binary word to each level. Each analog sample is then assigned one of these level values. This process is known as *quantization*. Since the signal varies continuously in time, this process generates a sequence of real numbers.

17. What is a signal?

Ans. A signal is defined as any detectable transmitted energy that can be used carry information. It is also defined as the time-dependent variation of a characteristic physical phenomenon. Therefore, a signal is associated with some amplitude that varies with time. Based on the continuity of two variables, time and amplitude, the signals can be divided into four types:

   i. Continuous time, continuous sample
   ii. Continuous time, discrete amplitude
   iii. Discrete time, continuous amplitude
   iv. Discrete time, discrete amplitude

The communication signals based on the continuous nature of time and amplitude are divided into two types: (i) analog signal (ii) digital signal.

18. Mention any other field in which optical fibers invaded significantly?

Ans. Optical fibers have not only revolutionized communication systems but also, owing to their small size, immunity from EMI and RFI, compatibility with fully distributed sensing, etc., they have alongwith lasers, invaded the field of industrial instrumentation.

19. Define relative and absolute units of power.

Ans. The relative power between two points along a fiber-optic communication link is measured in decibels (dB). For a particular wavelength λ, if P_0 is the power launched at one end of the link and P is the power received at the other end, the efficiency of the transmission of the link is P/P_o. When P and P_o are both measured in the same units, their ratio in the decibels is expressed as follows:

$$dB = 10 \log_{10} (P/P_o)$$

There is always some loss in the communication link. Hence the ratio P/P_o is always less than 1 and the logarithm of this ratio is negative.

In order to make absolute measurements, P_o is given a reference value, normally 1 mW. The value of power (say P) *relative* to P_o = (1 mW) is denoted by dB_m. Thus, we have

$$dB_m = 10 \log_{10} \frac{P\,(mW)}{P_o\,(1mW)} = 10 \log_{10} P$$

20. Explain bandwidth and channel capacity of a fiber-optic system.

Ans. The optical bandwidth of a fiber-optic system is the range of frequencies (transmitted by the system between two points (f_1 and f_2 on a frequency scale) where the output optical power drops to 50% of its maximum value (Fig. 1.12). This corresponds to a loss of –3 dB. Normally f_1 is taken to be zero.

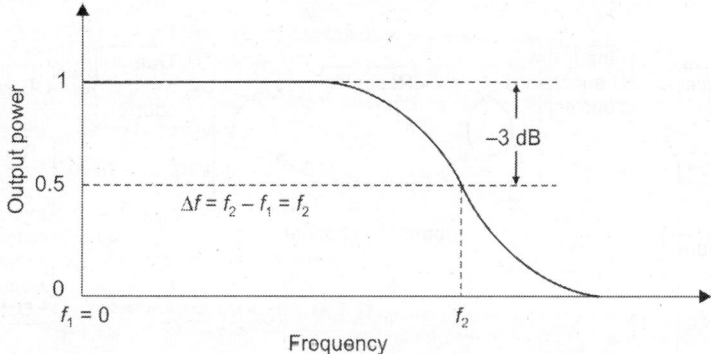

Fig. 1.12

It is important to note that in an all-electrical systems, the power is proportional to the square of the root-mean-square value of the current. Thus the 0.5 (or –3 dB) point on a power scale corresponds to 0.707 on a current scale. The electrical bandwidth for such systems (with $f_1 = 0$) is defined as the frequency for which the output current amplitude drops to 0.70 of its maximum value. In a fiber-optic system, the power supplied by the optical source is normally proportional to the current supplied to it (and not to the square of the current as in an all-electrical system). In this case, therefore, the half-power point is equivalent to half-current point. Thus the electrical bandwidth $(\Delta f)_{el}$ of a fiber-optic system is less than its optical bandwidth $(\Delta f)_{opt}$. Actually,

$$(\Delta f)_{el} = (\Delta f)_{opt} (1/2)^{1/2}$$

or $\quad\quad\quad (\Delta f)_{el} = 0.707\,(\Delta f)_{opt}$

The term 'channel capacity' is used in connection with a digital system or a link. It is the highest data rate (in bps) a system can handle. It is related to the bandwidth Δf and is limited by the S/N ratio of the received signal. Employing information theory, it can be shown that the channel capacity or the maximum bit rate B of a communication channel which is able to carry analog signals covering a bandwidth

Δf (in Hz) is given by Shannon's formula.

The term 'channel capacity' is used in connection with a digital

$$B \text{ (bps)} = \Delta f \log_2 [1 + (S/N)^2]$$

where S is the average signal power and N is the average noise power. If $S/N \gg 1$,

$$B \approx 2\Delta f \log_2 (S/N) \approx 6.64 \, \Delta f \log_{10} (S/N)$$

We may note that when analog signals are transmitted digitally, the bit rate will depend on the sampling rate of the analog signal and the coding scheme. The Nyquist criterion suggests that an analog signal can be transmitted accurately if it is sampled at a rate of atleast twice the highest frequency contained in the signal, i.e., if the sampling frequency $f_1 \gg 2f_2$. Clearly, a voice channel of 4 kHz bandwidth would require $f_s = 8$ kHz. However, a standard coding procedure requires 8 bits to describe the amplitude of each sample, so that the amplitude data rate required to transmit a single voice message would be 8×8000 bps $= 64$ kbps.

21. Draw a block diagram of generalized configuration of a fiber-optic communication system.

Ans. Figure 1.13 shows a generalized configuration of a fiber-optic communication system.

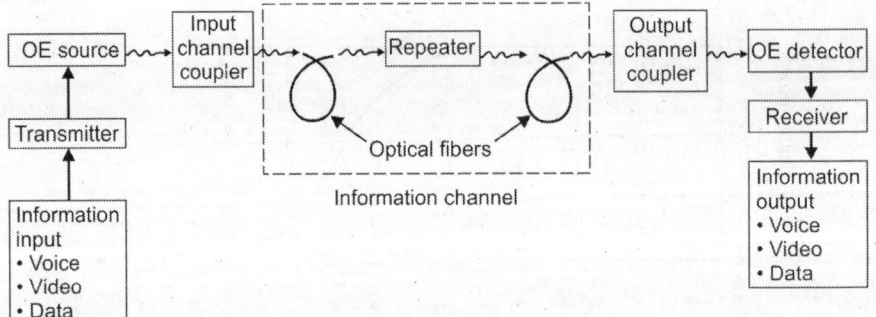

Fig. 1.13: Generalized configuration of a fiber optic communication system (OE → optoelectronic)

22. Explain, how an analog signal is converted to a digital signal.

Ans. The two basic processes of converting an analog signal to a digital signal are sampling and quantization.

An analog-to-digital converter consists of:

- The sampler
- The quantizer
- The coder

Figure 1.14 shows functional block diagram of an analog-to-digital converter.

The analog signal is passed to the first block, the sampler, which samples the continuous analog signals at discrete times making the signal discrete in time. At this point, the signal is a discrete time signal only, since its amplitude is still continuous and can take any value within the limit of the analog waveform. This discrete time continuous amplitude signal is passed to the next block known as the quantizer, which quantizes the amplitude. The quantization of amplitude is done at different levels of amplitude. The individual discrete time waveform samples are assigned the amplitudes based on the level of amplitude that is nearest to their current amplitude. Suppose the number of different levels of amplitude is fixed

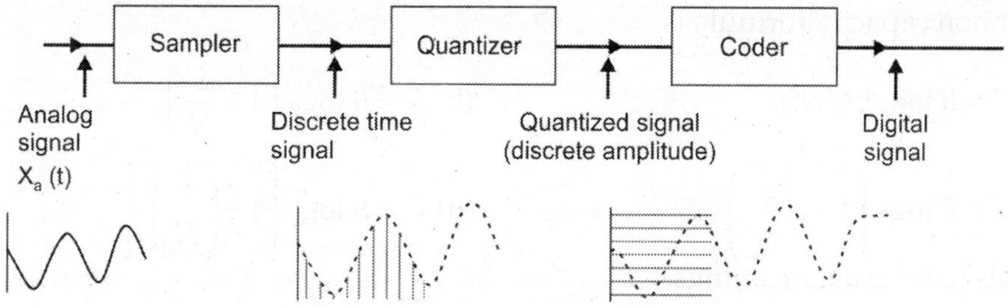

Fig. 1.14: Analog-to-digital converter

at 8, then the total range of the possible amplitude is divided into eight values and each sample is assigned one of these amplitudes close to it. The resulting discrete time discrete amplitude signal is passed to the third and final block, the coder. The coder effectively converts this discrete time discrete amplitude signal into an information sequence containing only binary digits. Therefore, the analog-to-digital converter (ADC or A/D) takes an analog waveform and outputs a sequence of binary digits, which is understood by the digital circuitry following the analog-to-digital converter. The ADC is usually placed before the source encoder and after the information source if the source is analog in nature.

MULTIPLE CHOICE QUESTIONS

1. A digital transmission system consists of
   (a) the transmitter only
   (b) the channel only
   (c) the receiver only
   (d) all the above
2. The time period of following analog sinusoid signal $x(t) = 10 \sin (10\pi t + 10°)$ is
   (a) 0.1 s
   (b) 0.2 s
   (c) 0.4 s
   (d) 0.8 s

   [**Hint.** Standard equation is $x(t) = A \cos (2\pi f + \theta)$. Comparing it with the given equation, we have

   $$2\pi f = 10 \pi$$
   $$\therefore \qquad f = 5 \text{ Hz}$$

   $\therefore \qquad$ Time period $T = \dfrac{1}{f} = \dfrac{1}{5} = 0.2 \text{ s}$]

3. An analog to digital converter consists of
   (a) the sampler only
   (b) the quantizer only
   (c) the coder only
   (d) all the above
4. The process of converting a continuous time signal into a discrete time signal by taking samples of the continuous time signal at discrete times is called
   (a) quantization
   (b) coding
   (c) sampling
   (d) none of the above
5. The process of converting a discrete time continuous amplitude signal into a digital signal is called
   (a) sampling
   (b) coding
   (c) quantization
   (d) none of the above

6. Shannon capacity formula is

(a) $C = B \log_2 (S/N^2)$

(b) $C = B \log_2 \left(1 + \dfrac{S}{N}\right)$

(c) $C = B \log_2 \left(1 + \sqrt{\dfrac{S}{N}}\right)$

(d) $C = B \log_2 \left[1 + \left(\dfrac{S}{N}\right)^2\right]$

Symbols have usual meanings.

ANSWERS

1. (d)   2. (b)   3. (d)   4. (c)   5. (c)   6. (b)

2

Electromagnetic Optics

2.1 INTRODUCTION

The study of optical communication requires a background in electromagnetics. Therefore, this chapter is devoted to a review of electromagnetics and optics.

2.2 NATURE OF LIGHT

The term *light* is born to indicate electromagnetic radiation having wavelength within the interval 0.4–0.75 μm, which is the interval spanned by the radiation emitted by the sun. As a result of biological adaption, this is also the wavelength range to which the retina of our eyes is sensitive. In contemporary scientific terminology, the term *light* is also applied to infrared and ultraviolet radiation.

Historically, the nature of light has been subjected to a considerable debate. Some scientists like Huygens and Young, posited the *"wave-like"* nature of light, while others, like Newton, had a *"corpuscular"* point of view. The highly successful description of light provided by Maxwell's equations seemed to end the debate, by providing a strong validation of wave-like interpretation. However, the controversy reopened in the last part of 19th century, because the wave-like interpretation was inconsistent with experimental observations of certain phenomena such as the *photoelectric effect* and the *spectral radiance of blackbody emission*. Planck and Einstein clearly demonstrated that electromagnetic energy is emitted and absorbed in discrete units, or fundamental quanta of energy, called *photons*.

Quantum theory provides a unified view that combines both the *wave-like* and the *corpuscular* aspects of light. Mathematically, the energy E, of a photon is related to the frequency, v, of the emitted light as

$$E = hv = \frac{hc}{\lambda} \tag{2.1}$$

where h is constant of proportionality, the universal constant, called Planck's constant, has value 6.23×10^{-34} Js, c is the velocity of light in free space, and is related to the wavelength and frequency, i.e. $c = \lambda v$, where λ is the wavelength of the emitted light. Quantum theory of light formed the basis for *wave–particle duality*, i.e. everything has both a *particle nature* and a *wave nature*, and several experiments demonstrate their coexistence and manifestation in form or the other. Louis de Broglie in 1924, proposed that even electrons exhibits wave–particle duality, governed by the relation

$$\lambda = \frac{h}{mv} = \frac{h}{p} \tag{2.2}$$

where $p = mv$ is the momentum of the electron. This was later experimentally demonstrated by Davisson and Germer in 1927.

We may note that the various theories pertaining to light such as rectilinear propagation of light which is only an approximation of generalized theory of light due to Fresnel, *Fresnel's wave theory of light*. Further, Maxwell's electromagnetic theory and quantum theory of light coexist. Interestingly, the apparent contradictions are largely overcome with the application of *wave–particle duality*. However, each of theories has some limitation when it is applied to explain a particular optical phenomenon, i.e. the most appropriate theory is largely dependent on the type of the optical phenomenon under consideration. For example, in order to explain large-scale optical phenomenon, one finds that it is sufficient to consider that is emitted from the source in the form of rays which travel in a straight line. We may note that the *rectilinear propagation of light* is the basis of *geometrical optics*.

When we consider more finer optical phenomena such as *interference* and *diffraction*, we find that these phenomena can only be explained with the help of wave theory of light. In order to explain the polarization of light one has to take the help of Maxwell's electromagnetic theory of light. Further, to explain the *interaction of light with matter*, one has to apply quantum theory of light.

When light is incident on an atom, a photon can transfer its energy to an electron within this atom, thereby exciting it to a higher energy level. In this process either all or none of the photon energy is imparted to the electron. The energy *absorbed* by the electron must be exactly equal to that required to excite the electron to higher energy level E_2 from lower energy level E_1, i.e.:

$$E_2 - E_1 = h\nu \tag{2.3}$$

Conversely, an electron in an excited state can fall to a lower energy state separated from it by an energy $h\nu$ by *emitting* a photon of exactly this energy.

In view of these developments, light must be regarded as having a *dual nature*. Light exhibits the characteristics of a wave in some situations and characteristics of a particle in other situations.

Now, it is well established that *light is an energy-carrying electromagnetic wave that emanates from vibrating electrons in atoms*. When light is transmitted through matter, some of the electrons in the matter are forced into vibration. In this way, vibrations in the emitter are transmitted to vibrations in the receiver.

2.3 FUNDAMENTAL LAWS OF OPTICS

According to *wave theory of light* or principle of physical optics, a point optical source radiates electromagnetic waves in the form of a train of spherical wavefronts with the point source at the centre [Fig. 2.1(a)]. According to Huygen, a *wavefront* is the locus of all points in the wavetrain which have the same phase. In general, wavefronts are obtained by joining the maxima (crests) or minima (troughs) of the wave. Since all points in a given wavefront have the same phase, a wavefront is often referred to as a *phase front*. Further, the wavefronts are separated by one wavelength (λ). Thus, a wavefront or phasefront is defined as the locus of all points in the wave train which have the same phase.

When the wavelength of light is much smaller than the object (or opening) which it encounters, the wavefront appears as straight lines to this object or opening. In this case, the light wave can be represented as a *plane wave*, and its direction of travel can be shown by a *light ray* which is drawn perpendicular to the phase front [Fig. 2.1(b)]. The light rays concept allows large-scale optical effects, e.g. reflection and refraction to be analyzed by

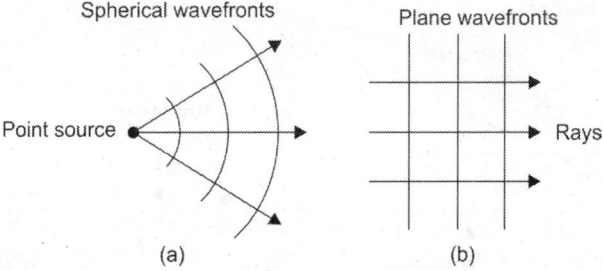

Fig. 2.1: Representations of spherical and plane wavefronts and their associated rays

the simple geometrical process of *ray tracing*. The concept of light ray is very useful because these rays show the direction of energy flow in the light beam.

These light rays obey following rules:

i. In a medium, light rays travel with velocity v given by:

$$v = \frac{\text{velocity of light in free space}}{\text{velocity of light in medium}} = \frac{c}{n} \tag{2.4}$$

where $c = 3 \times 10^8$ ms^{-1} is the velocity of light in vacuum and n is known as refractive index of the medium. Table 2.1 shows some typical values of refractive indices. As v is always less than c, n is always greater than 1. For air $n = n_a \approx 1$.

Table 2.1: Refractive index for some materials

Material	Refractive index (n)
Air	1.0
Water	1.33
Silica glass	1.5
GaAs	3.35
Silicon	3.5
Germanium	4.0

ii. In a uniform medium, rays travel in a straight path.

iii. The phenomenon of *refraction* of light at the interface between two transparent media of uniform indices of refraction is governed by **Snell's law**. Consider a ray of light passing from a medium of refractive index n_1 into a medium of refractive index n_2 [Fig. 2.2(a)]. Assume that $n_1 > n_2$ and that the angles of incidence and refraction with respect to the normal to the interface are ϕ_1 and ϕ_2 respectively. Then, according to Snell's law:

$$n_1 \sin \phi_1 = n_2 \sin \phi_2 \tag{2.5}$$

As $n_1 > n_2$, if we increase the angle of incidence ϕ_1, the angle of refraction ϕ_2 will go on increasing until a critical situation is reached, when for a certain value of $\phi_1 = \phi_c$, ϕ_2 becomes $\pi/2$, and the refracted ray passes along the interface. This angle $\phi_1 = \phi_c$ is the *critical angle*. The limiting value of the angle of incidence $\phi_1 (= \phi_c)$ in the denser medium for which the refracted ray grazes the interface between the two media is called the critical angle (ϕ_c). Substituting the values of $\phi_1 = \phi_c$ and $\phi_2 = \pi/2$, in Eq. (2.5), we find

$$n_1 = \sin \phi_c = n_2 \sin (\pi/2) = n_2.$$

Thus,

$$\sin \phi_c = \frac{n_2}{n_1} \tag{2.6}$$

$$\Rightarrow \qquad \phi_c = \sin^{-1} (n_2/n_1) \tag{2.6a}$$

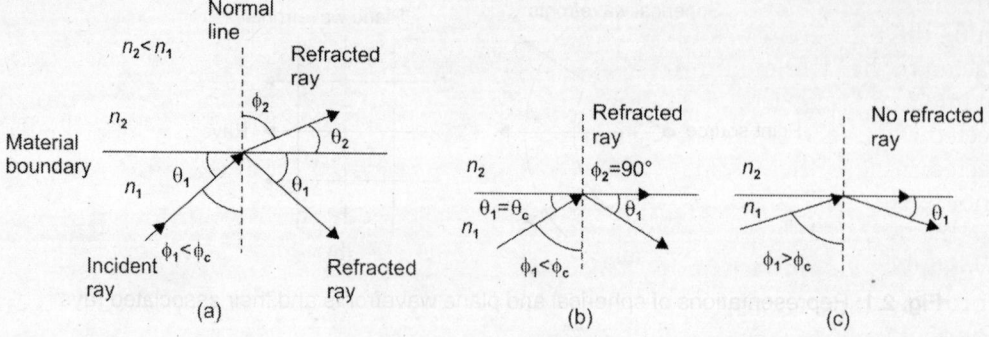

Fig. 2.2: Representation of the critical angle and total internal reflection at a glass–air interface (a) refraction of a ray of light (b) critical ray incident at $\phi_1 = \phi_c$ and refracted at $\phi_2 = \pi/2$ (c) total internal reflection ($\phi_1 > \phi_c$)

If the angle of incidence ϕ_1 is further increased beyond ϕ_c, the ray is no longer refracted but is reflected back into the same medium [Fig. 2.2(c)], this is ideally expected. In practice, however, there is always some tunneling of optical energy through this interface. The wave carrying this energy is called *evanescent wave*. One can explain this in terms of electromagnetic theory.

It is often convenient to measure the angle of incidence and reflection with respect to the interface of the two media rather than the normal drawn on the plane at the point of incidence. These angle made by the incident and the refracted rays with respect to the interface of the two media are represented by θ_1 and θ_2 respectively in Fig. 2.2(c). Now, if the angles are measured with respect to the interface plane, the critical condition of refraction would be reached when θ_1 is decreased. One can write Snell's law in terms of θ_1 and θ_2 as

$$n_1 \sin\left(\frac{\pi}{2} - \theta_1\right) = n_2 \sin\left(\frac{\pi}{2} - \theta_2\right)$$

$$\Rightarrow \qquad n_1 \cos\theta_1 = n_2 \cos\theta_2 \qquad\qquad (2.6b)$$

One can obtain the critical angle of incidence θ_c with respect to the boundary of this two media by putting $\theta_2 = 0$ in Eq. (2.6b). Thus, the measured critical angle with respect to the interface plane of the media can be expressed as

$$\theta_c = \cos^{-1}\left(\frac{n_2}{n_1}\right) \qquad\qquad (2.6c)$$

When the angle of incidence (with respect to interface) is decreased below the *critical angle θ_c*, there would be no refraction and light would be total internally reflected as illustrated with the help of ray diagram in Fig. 2.2(d).

When the angle of incidence θ_1 (measured with respect to the interface boundary plane of the two media, is equal to the critical angle θ_c, the refracted ray grazes the interface (becomes parallel to the plane of interface), i.e. θ_c is the minimum value of the angle of incidence for refraction to occur at the interface. When the angle of incidence is less

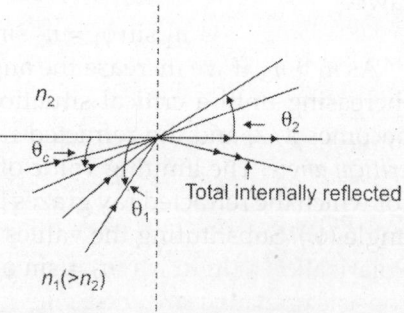

Fig. 2.2: (d) illustration of total internal reflection with the help of ray diagram

than θ_c, the total energy is reflected back into the original medium and no part of it is refracted in the rarer medium. This phenomenon is termed as *total internal reflection*. The total internally reflected ray is shown in Fig. 2.2(d) with the help of double arrow on the reflected ray. We may note that in actual practice, nearly 99.9% of the incidence light is reflected back to the original medium when total internal reflection takes place. One cannot explain the small loss at the interface with the help of ray analysis. However, wave theory can account for this small loss at the interface. One can easily extend the above simplistic approach underlying the concept of total internal reflection to understand the propagation of light through an optical fiber. However, this simplistic approach does not apply to all types of optical fibers particularly for single mode fibers or a few modes fiber. We will study this in detail in Chapter 4.

In addition, when light is totally internally reflected, a phase change δ occurs in the reflected wave. This phase change depends on the angle $\theta_1 < \dfrac{\pi}{2} - \phi_c$ according to relationships:

$$\tan\frac{\delta_N}{2} = \frac{\sqrt{n^2 \cos^2 \theta_1 - 1}}{n \sin \theta_1} \tag{2.7}$$

$$\tan\frac{\delta_P}{2} = n\frac{\sqrt{n^2 \cos^2 \theta_1 - 1}}{\sin \theta_1} \tag{2.8}$$

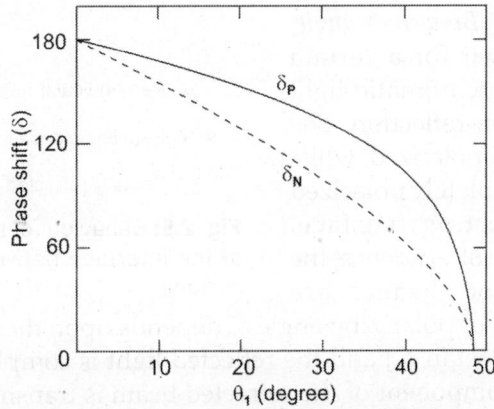

Fig. 2.3: Phase shifts occurring from the reflection of wave components normal (δ_N) and parallel (δ_P) to the plane of incidence

Here, δ_N and δ_P are the phase shifts of the electric-field wave components normal and parallel to the phase of incidence, respectively, and $n = n_1/n_2$. Figure 2.3 shows these phase shifts for a glass–air interface ($n = 1.5$ and $f_c = 42.5°$). The values range from zero immediately at the critical angle to $\dfrac{\pi}{2} - \phi_c$, when $\phi_c = 90°$.

2.4 POLARIZATION OF LIGHT

Polarization of light waves demonstrates that they are *transverse*. An ordinary light wave consists of many transverse electromagnetic waves that vibrate in a variety of directions, i.e. in more than one plane is called *unpolarized light*. One can pictorially represent any arbitrary direction of vibration as a combination of a parallel vibration and a perpendicular vibration (Fig. 2.4).

In an unpolarized light, all directions of vibration at right angles to that of propagation of light consists of two orthogonal plane polarization components, one that lies in the plane of incidence (the plane containing the incident ray and reflected ray) and the other of which lies in a plane perpedicular to the plane of incidence. These are termed the *parallel polarization* and the *perpendicular polarization* components, respectively.

Unpolarized light can be split into separate polarization component either by reflection of nonmetallic surface or by refraction when the light beam passes from one material to another. Figure 2.5 shows that when an unpolarized light beam travelling in air impinges on a nonmetallic surface such as glass, part of the beam is reflected and part is refracted into a glass. The reflected beam is partially· polarized and at a specific angle, i.e. *Brewster's angle*, [Brewster discovered that for a certain angle of incidence, monochromatic light was 100% polarized upon reflection. The refracted beam is partially polarized, while the reflected beam is completely polarized parallel to the reflecting surface. Furthermore, at this angle of incidence, the reflected and refracted beams are

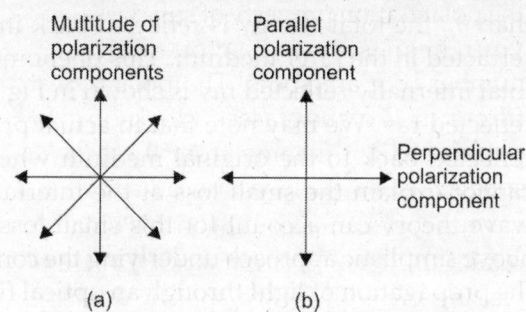

Fig. 2.4: Polarization of light represented as a combination of a parallel vibration and a perpendicular vibration

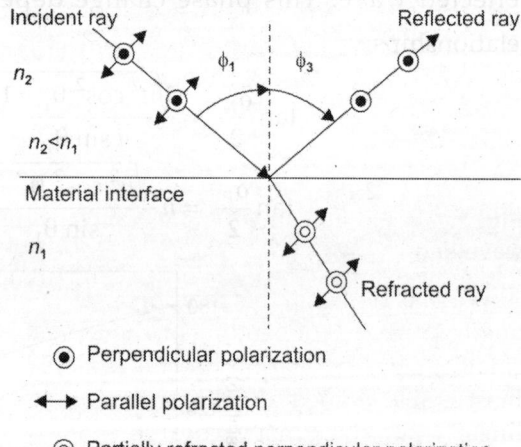

Fig. 2.5: Behaviour of an unpolarized light beam at the interface between air and nonmetallic surface

perpendicular. The value of polarizing angle ϕ_p depends upon the refractive index of the refractive medium, i.e. $n = \tan \phi_p$] and the reflected light is completely perpendicularly polarized. The parallel component of the refracted beam is transmitted entirely into the glass, whereas the perpendicular component is only partially refracted. How much of the refracted light is polarized depends on the angle at which the light approaches the surface and on the material composition.

2.5 POLARIZATION OF SENSITIVE MATERIALS

The polarization characteristics of light are important when one examining the behaviour of components such as *optical isolators* and *light filters*. We shall restrict to the study of three polarization – sensitive materials or devices that are used in such components. These devices are *polarizers*, *Faraday rotators*, and *birefringent crystals*.

(i) *Polarizer*: This is a material or device that transmits only one polarization component and blocks the other, e.g. when unpolarized light enters a polarizer that has a vertical transmission axis (Fig. 2.6), only the vertical polarization component passes through the polarizer (device). This concept is used in polarizing sunglasses to reduce the glare of partially polarized sunlight reflections from the road or water surfaces. In order to see the polarization property of sunglasses, tilt your head sideways, you will see a number of glare spots. The polarization filters in the sunglasses block out the polarized light coming from these glare spots when you held your head normally.

(ii) *A Faraday rotator*: This is a device that rotates the *state of polarization* (SOP) of light passing through it by a specific angle. A popular device rotates the SOP clockwise by 45° or λ/4 (Fig. 2.7).

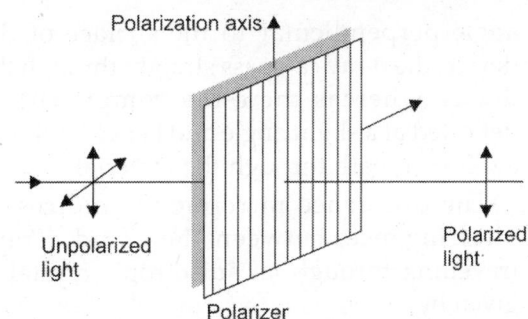

Fig. 2.6: Only the vertical polarization component passes through a vertically oriented polarizer

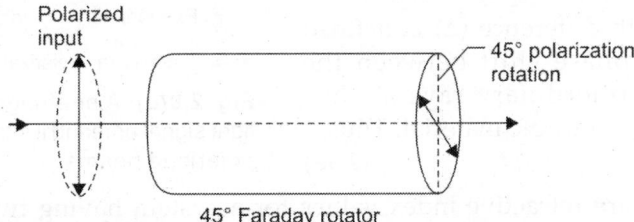

Fig. 2.7: A Faraday rotator rotates the state of polarization clockwise by 45° or a quarter of a wavelength (λ/4)

We may note that this rotation is independent of the SOP of input light, but the rotation angle is different depending on the direction in which the light passes through the Faraday rotator, e.g. the rotation process is not reciprocal. In this process, the SOP of the input light is maintained after the rotation, e.g. if the input light to a 45° Faraday rotator is linearly polarized in a vertical direction, then the rotated light existing the crystal is also linearly polarized at 45° angle. The Faraday rotator material is usually an asymmetric crystal, e.g. yttrium iron garnet (YIG) and the degree of angular rotation is proportional to the thickness of the device.

(iii) *Double-refractive crystals or Birefringent*: These crystals have a property called double refraction, or birefringent which is defined as the double refraction of light in a transparent, molecularly ordered material, which is manifested by the existence of orientation-dependent difference in refractive index.

The phenomenon of double refraction [Fig. 2.8(a)] is based on the laws of electromagnetism due to Maxwell. One of the most familiar example of double refraction occurs with calcium carbonate (calcite) crystals. Birefringent splits the light signals entering it into two orthogonally (perpendicularly) polarized beams [Fig. 2.8(b)]. One of the beams is called an *ordinary* (o) – ray, since it obeys Snell's law of refraction at the surface of crystals. The second ray is called the *extraordinary* (e) ray, since it refracts at an angle that deviates from the prediction of the standard form of Snell's law.

As shown in Fig. 2.8(b), each of the two orthogonal polarization components refracted at different angle, e.g. if the incident unpolarized light arrives at an

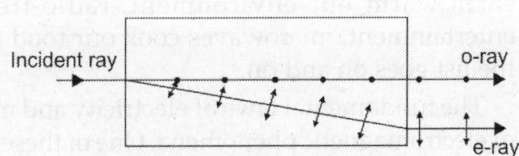

Fig. 2.8(a): Phenomenon of double refraction exhibited by a birefringent crystal. The electric-field vectors of the o-ray and e-ray are shown to vibrate perpendicular and parallel to the plane of the figure, respectively

angle perpendicular to the surface of the device, the o-ray can pass straight through the device whereas the e-ray component, is deflected at a slight angle and hence it follows a different path through the material.

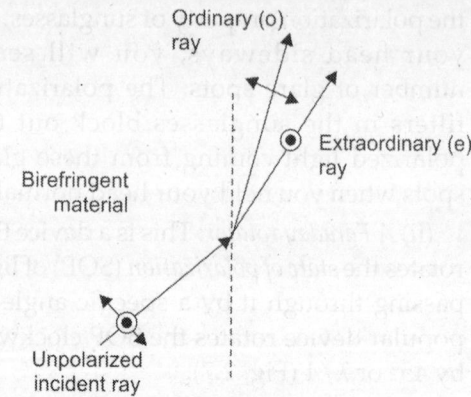

The difference in refractive indices or birefringence, between the e and o rays travelling through an anisotropic crystal is given by:

$$\text{Birefringence } (B) = [n_e - n_o] \qquad (2.9)$$

where n_e and n_o are the refractive indices experienced by the e and o rays respectively.

The optical path difference (Δ) is defined by the relative phase shift between the ordinary and extraordinary rays as they emerge from an anisotropic material. Thus,

$$\Delta = (n_1 - n_2)\, t \qquad (2.9a)$$

Fig. 2.8(b): A birefringent crystal splits the light signal entering it into two perpendicularly polarized beams

where n_1 and n_2 are refractive index values for a system having two values and t is thickness of the system.

There are some birefringent crystals that are used in optical communication components. Table 2.2 lists n_o and n_e of some of these birefringent crystals along with their applications.

Table 2.2: Common birefringent crystals and some of their applications				
Crystal name	Symbol	n_o (ordinary index)	n_e (extra-ordinary index)	Applications
Calcite	$CaCO_3$	1.658	1.486	Polarization controllers and beam splitters
Lithium niobate	$LiNbO_3$	2.286	2.200	Light signal modulators
Rutile	TiO_2	2.616	2.903	Optical isolators and circulator
Yttrium vanadate	YVO_4	1.945	2.149	Optical isolators, circulators, and beam displacers

2.6 ELECTROMAGNETIC WAVES

Although, we are not always aware of the presence of electromagnetic (em) waves, but these waves permeate our environment regularly. In the form of *visible light*, they enable us to view the world around us with our eyes. Infrared waves from the surface of the earth warm our environment, radio-frequency waves carry our favourite radio entertainment, microwaves cook our food and are used in communication systems and the list goes on and on.

The fundamental laws of electricity and magnetism—*Maxwell's equations* form the basis of electromagnetic phenomena. One of these equations predicts that a time-varying electric field produces a magnetic field just as a time-varying magnetic field produces an electric field. From this generalization, Maxwell provided the final important link between electric and magnetic fields. The most *dramatic prediction of his equations is the existence of electro-magnetic waves that propagate through empty space with the speed of light* ($c = 3 \times 10^8$ ms^{-1}). This discovery led to many practical applications, such as radio and television, and to

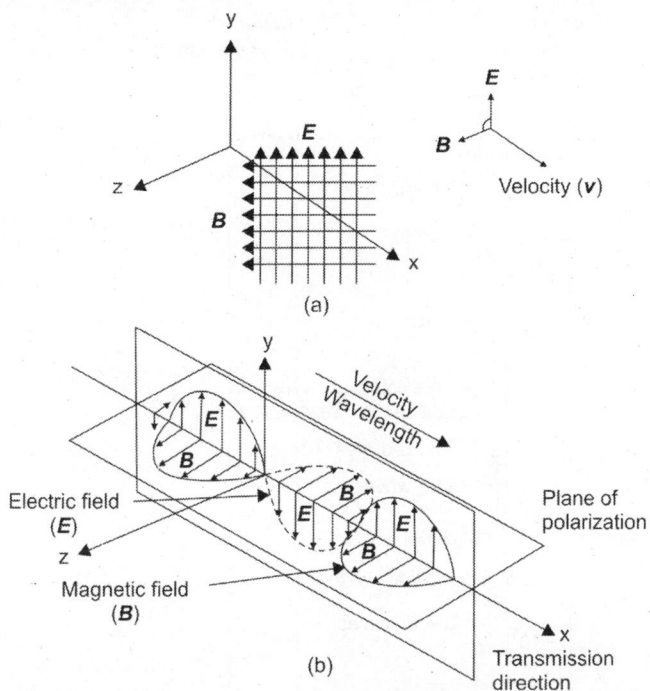

Fig. 2.9: Propagation of a plane wave, **E** and **B** vectors

the realization that light is one form of electromagnetic radiations. Figure 2.9 shows the propagation of electromagnetic wave at one instant.

We may note that:

    i. the two fields E and B are perpendicular to each other, and

    ii. both the fields E and B are perpendicular to the direction of propagation of the wave.

The second fact is a property characteristic of *transverse wave*. This means an electromagnetic wave is a transverse wave.

The following properties are associated with an electromagnetic wave travelling through *free space*:

    i. Electromagnetic waves travel with the speed of light ($c = 3 \times 10^8 \text{ ms}^{-1}$ in vacuum).

    ii. Electromagnetic waves are transverse waves.

    iii. The ratio of electric (E) to magnetic field (B) in an electromagnetic wave equals the speed of light ($E/B = c$).

    iv. Electromagnetic waves carry both energy and momentum which can be delivered to a surface. Figure 2.10 shows the electromagnetic radiation spectrum.

2.6.1 Maxwell's Equations and Boundary Conditions

The space variations of electric and magnetic field components are related to time variations of magnetic and electric field components respectively. This interdependence gives rise to the phenomenon of electromagnetic wave propagation.

Maxwell in 1873 published his original findings of the electromagnetic theory of light. This theory has led to many important discoveries, including the existence of electromagnetic waves. Based on his theory, all electric, magnetic, electromagnetic, and optical phenomena are governed by the same fundamental laws of electromagnetism. These laws are written mathematically in terms of *Maxwell equations* (in MKS units):

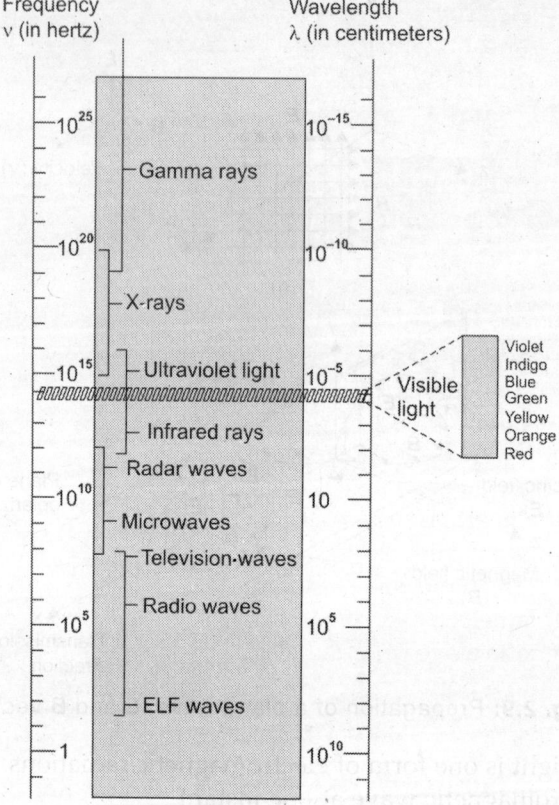

Fig. 2.10: Spectrum of electromagnetic radiation

$$\nabla \times E = -\frac{\partial B}{\partial t} \tag{2.10}$$

$$\nabla \times H = J + \frac{\partial D}{\partial t} \tag{2.11}$$

$$\nabla \cdot D = \rho \tag{2.12}$$

$$\nabla \cdot B = O \tag{2.13}$$

where

E is electric field intensity (Vm^{-1} or NC^{-1}),

B is magnetic field (T or tesla),

J is electric current density (Am^{-2}),

ρ is volume charge density (Cm^{-3}).

where $D = P + \varepsilon_0 E$.

The operator ∇ in cartesian coordinates

$$= \hat{i}\frac{\partial}{\partial x} + \hat{j}\frac{\partial}{\partial y} + \hat{k}\frac{\partial}{\partial y} \tag{2.14}$$

The above relations are supplemented with constitutive relations:

$$D = \varepsilon E \tag{2.15}$$

$$B = \mu H \tag{2.16}$$

$$J = \sigma E \tag{2.17}$$

where $\varepsilon = \varepsilon_0 \varepsilon_r$ is the dielectric permittivity (Fm^{-1}), $\mu = \mu_0 \mu_r$ is permeability (Hm^{-1}), σ is electrical conductivity and ε_r is relative dielectric constant. For optical problems, one may take $\mu_r = 1$. The permittivity of a vacuum, $\varepsilon_0 = 8.854 \times 10^{-12}\ Fm^{-1}$ and permeability of a vacuum, $\mu_0 = 4\pi \times 10^{-7}\ Hm^{-1}$.

From Eqs (2.10) and (2.11), we see that a time-changing magnetic field produces an electric field and a time-changing electric field or current density produces a magnetic field. The charge distribution ρ and current density J are the *source* for generation of electric and magnetic fields. For the given charge and current distribution, Eqs (2.10) to (2.13) may be solved to obtain the electric and magnetic field distributions. The terms on the right hand sides of Eqs (2.10) and (2.11) may be viewed as the sources for generation of field intensities appearing on the left hand sides of Eqs (2.10) and (2.11). As an example, consider the alternating current $I_0 \sin (2\pi ft)$ flowing in the transmitter antenna. From Ampere's law, we find that the current leads to a magnetic field intensity around the antenna (first term of Eq. (2.11)). From Faraday's law, it follows that the time-varying magnetic field induces an electric field intensity [Eq. (2.10)] in the vicinity of the antenna. Consider a point in the neighbourhood of the antenna (but not on the antenna). At this point $J = 0$, but the time-varying electric field intensity or displacement current density (second term on the right hand side of Eq. (2.11)) leads to a magnetic field intensity, which in turn leads to an electric field intensity (Eq. (2.10)). This process continues and generated electromagnetic wave propagates outward just like the water wave generated by throwing a stone into a pond. If the displacement current density were to be absent, there would be no coupling between electric and magnetic fields and we would not have had electromagnetic waves.

First, we recall two mathematical theorems, Gauss's theorem:

$$\oint_S F \cdot dS = \int_V \nabla . F dV \tag{2.18}$$

where S is the closed surface area defining volume V, and Stokes's theorem:

$$\oint_L F \cdot dl = \oint_S \nabla \times F \cdot dS \tag{2.19}$$

where contour L define surface area A. With the help of the above theorem, Maxwell's equations in *differential form can be transformed into an integral form*. Integral forms of Maxwell's equation are:

$$\oint_S D \cdot dS = \int_V \rho dV \tag{2.20}$$

$$\oint_S B \cdot dS = 0 \tag{2.21}$$

$$\oint_L E.dl = -\int_S \frac{\partial B}{\partial t} \cdot dS \tag{2.22}$$

$$\oint_L H \cdot dl = \oint_S \left(J + \frac{\partial D}{\partial t} \right) \cdot dS \tag{2.23}$$

Properties of the medium are mostly determined by ε, μ and σ. Further, for the dielectric medium the main role is played by ε. The medium is known as *linear*, if ε is independent of E; otherwise it is nonlinear. If it does not depend on position in space, the medium is said to be *homogeneous*; otherwise it is *inhomogeneous*. If properties are independent of direction, the medium is *isotropic*; otherwise it is *anisotropic*.

2.6.2 Maxwell's Equations in a Source-Free Region

In free space or dielectric, if there is no charge or current in the neighbourhood, we can set $\rho = 0$ and $J = 0$ in Eqs (2.10) to (2.13). We may note that the above equations describe the relations between electric field, magnetic field and the sources at a space-time point and therefore, in a region sufficiently far away from the sources, we can set $\rho = 0$ and $J = 0$ in that region. However, on the antenna, we cannot ignore the source terms ρ or J in Eqs (2.10) to (2.13). Setting $\rho = 0$ and $J = 0$ in the source-free region, Maxwell's equations takes the form

$$\nabla \times E = \frac{-\partial B}{\partial t} \qquad (2.23a)$$

$$\nabla \times H = \frac{-\partial D}{\partial t} \qquad (2.23b)$$

$$\nabla \cdot D = 0 \qquad (2.23c)$$

$$\nabla \cdot B = 0 \qquad (2.23d)$$

In the source-free region, the time-changing electric/magnetic field (which was generated from a distance source ρ or J) acts as a source for a magnetic/electric field.

2.6.3 Boundary Conditions

Boundary conditions are derived from an integral form of *Maxwell's equations*. For this purpose, we separate all vectors into two components, one parallel to the interface and other normal to the interface. The derivation of boundary conditions is facilitated by using the contour and cylindrical shapes as shown in Fig. 2.11. It will be done independently for the electric and magnetic fields.

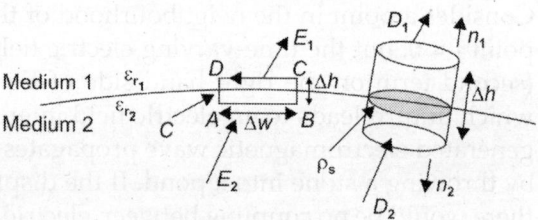

Fig. 2.11: An interface between two media. Contour and volume used to derive boundary conditions for fields between two different dielectrics are shown

(i) Electric Boundary Conditions

First, analyse transversal components. Integrate Eq. (2.22) over closed loop C (Fig. 2.11) and then set $\Delta h \to 0$:

$$\int_{ABCDA} E \cdot dl = -E_1 \cdot dl + E_2 \cdot dl$$
$$= -E_{1t}\Delta W + E_{2t}\Delta W$$
$$= 0$$

Therefore

$$E_{1t} = E_{1t} \qquad (2.24)$$

The tangenital component of the electric field is therefore continuous across the boundary between any two dielectric media. Using general relation [Eq. (2.15)], one obtains the boundary conditions for tangenital component of vector D.

$$\frac{D_{1t}}{\varepsilon_{r1}} = \frac{D_{2t}}{\varepsilon_{r2}} \qquad (2.25)$$

In order to obtain conditions for normal components, consider the cylinder shown in Fig. 2.11. Here n_1 and n_2 are normal vectors pointing outwards of the top and bottom surfaces into corresponding dielectrics. Apply Gauss's law with integration over surface S of the cylinder.

$$\int_{s} D \cdot dS = \int_{op} D_1 \cdot n_1 dS + \int_{bottom} D_2 \cdot n_2 dS = \rho_s \Delta S \qquad (2.26)$$

The contribution from the outer surface of the cylinder vanishes in the limit $\Delta h \to 0$. Use the face that $n_2 = -n_1$ and have:

$$n_1 \cdot (D_1 - D_2) = \rho_s \tag{2.27}$$

or $\qquad\qquad \varepsilon_{r1}E_{2n} - \varepsilon_{r2}E_{1n} = \rho_s \tag{2.28}$

Here, we have used general relation [Eq. (2.15)]. Normal component of vector D is not continuous across boundary (unless $\rho_s = 0$).

(ii) Magnetic Boundary Conditions

When deriving boundary conditions for magnetic field, we use approach similar as for electric fields, we use Eq. (2.21) where integration is over the cylinder.

$$\int_S B \cdot dS = 0$$

or $\qquad\qquad B_{1n} = B_{2n} \tag{2.29}$

Using general relation [Eq. (2.16)], one obtains conditions for magnetic field H:

$$\mu_{r1}H_{1n} = \mu_{r2}H_{2n} \tag{2.30}$$

The above relations tell us that normal component B is continuous across the boundary.

To obtain how transversal magnetic components behave across interface, apply Ampere's law for contour C and then let $\Delta h \to 0$, one obtains:

$$\int_S H \cdot dl = \int_A^B H_2 \cdot dl - \int_C^D H_1 \cdot dl = I$$

Here I is the net current crossing the surface of the loop. Let Δh approach zero, the surface of the loop approaches a thin line of length ΔW. Hence, the total current flowing through this thin line is $I = J_s \cdot \Delta W$, where J_s is the magnitude of the normal component of the surface current density traversing the loop. We can therefore express the above equation as:

$$H_{2t} - H_{1t} = J_s \tag{2.31}$$

Utilizing unit vector $\hat{n}_2$, the above relation can be written as:

$$n_2 \times (H_1 - H_2) = J_s \tag{2.32}$$

where n_2 is the normal vector pointing away from medium 2 (Fig. 2.11). J_s is the surface current.

In Table 2.3, we summarize boundary conditions between two dielectrics for the electric and magnetic fields. The behaviour of various field components is shown schematically in Fig. 2.12.

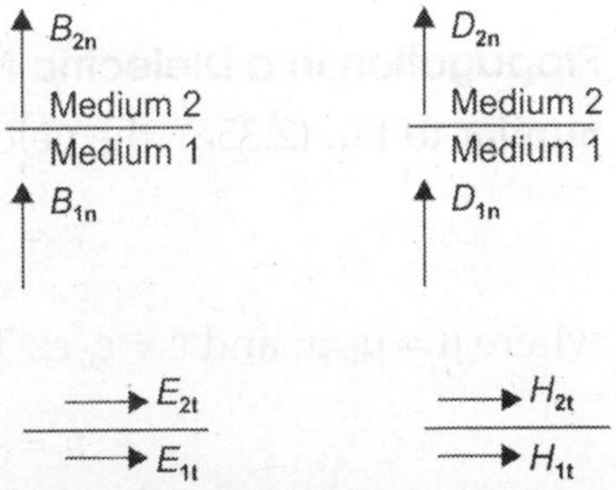

Fig. 2.12: Boundary conditions for fields

Table 2.3: Summary of boundary conditions for electric and magnetic fields

Field components	General form	Specific form
Tangential E	$n_2 \times (E_1 - E_2) = 0$	$E_{1t} = E_{2t}$
Normal D	$n_2 \cdot (D_1 - D_2) = \rho_s$	$D_{1t} = D_{2t} = \rho$
Tangential H	$n_2 \times (H_1 - H_2) = J_s$	$H_{2t} = H_{1t}$
Normal B	$n_2 \times (B_1 - B_2) = 0$	$B_{1n} = E_{2n}$

2.7 WAVE EQUATION

Here, we will derive the wave equation. The wave equation for a source-free medium where $\rho_v = 0$ and $J = 0$. The wave equation is obtained by applying curl operation to both sides of Eq. (2.10).

$$\nabla \times \nabla \times E = -\frac{\partial}{\partial t}(\nabla \times B)$$

$$= -\mu \frac{\partial}{\partial t}(\nabla \times H)$$

$$= -\mu \frac{\partial}{\partial t}\frac{\partial D}{\partial t} = -\mu\varepsilon \frac{\partial}{\partial t}\frac{\partial^2 D}{\partial t^2}$$

where we have used Maxwell Eqs (2.11) and (2.15). Next apply the following mathematical formula:

$$\nabla \times \nabla \times E = \nabla(\nabla . E) - \nabla^2 E \tag{2.33}$$

With the help of Maxwell Eq. (2.12), one finds finally:

$$\nabla^2 E = \mu\varepsilon \frac{\partial^2}{\partial t^2} E \tag{2.34}$$

which is the *desired wave equation*.

Similarly, we can get general form of wave equation of *H* as:

$$\nabla^2 E = \mu\varepsilon \frac{\partial^2 H}{\partial t^2} \tag{2.35}$$

Equation (2.34) is called the wave equation and it forms the basis for the study of electromagnetic wave propagation.

The wave described by Eq. (2.34) transports both energy and momentum.

Free Space Propagation

For free space, $\varepsilon = \varepsilon_0 = 8.854 \times 10^{-12} \, C^2/Nm^2$, $\mu = \mu_0 = 4\pi \times 10^{-7} \, N/A^2$, and

$$c = \frac{1}{\sqrt{\mu_0 \varepsilon_0}} \approx 3 \times 10^8 \, m/s \tag{2.35a}$$

where c is the velocity of light in free space. Before Maxwell's time, electromagnetics, magnetostatics, and optics were unrelated. Maxwell unified these three fields and showed that the light wave is actually an electromagnetic wave with velocity in vacuum given by Eq. (2.35a).

Propagation in a Dielectric Medium

Similar to Eq. (2.35a), the velocity of light in a medium can be written as

$$v = \frac{1}{\sqrt{\mu\varepsilon}} \tag{2.35b}$$

where $\mu = \mu_0 \mu_r$ and $\varepsilon = \varepsilon_0 \varepsilon_r$. Therefore,

$$v = \frac{1}{\sqrt{\mu_0 \varepsilon_0 \mu_r \varepsilon_r}} \tag{2.35c}$$

Using Eq. (2.35b) in Eq. (2.35c), we have

$$v = \frac{c}{\sqrt{\mu_r \varepsilon_r}} \tag{2.35d}$$

For dielectrics, $\mu_r = 1$ and the velocity of light in a dielectric medium can be written as

$$v = \frac{c}{\sqrt{\varepsilon_r}} = \frac{c}{n} \tag{2.35e}$$

where $n = \sqrt{\varepsilon_r}$ is called the refractive index of the medium. The refractive index of a medium is greater than 1 and the velocity of light in a medium is less than that in free space.

2.8 TIME HARMONIC FIELDS

In many practical situations, fields have sinusoidal time dependence and are known as *time-harmonic*. This fact is expressed as:

$$E(r, t) = \text{Re}\{E(r)\, e^{j\omega t}\} \tag{2.36}$$

where $E(r)$ is the phasor form of $E(r, t)$ and is in general complex. Re{....} indicates "taking the real part in" quantity in brackets. Finally, ω is the angular frequency in rad/s. In what follows, all fields will be represented in phasor notation.

Applying the time-harmonic assumption Eq. (2.36) to source free Maxwell's equations results in:

$$\nabla \times E = -j\omega\mu H \tag{2.37}$$
$$\nabla \times H = -j\omega\varepsilon E \tag{2.38}$$

Applying the time harmonic assumption again to wave equation [Eq. (2.34)] gives:

$$\nabla^2 E + k^2 E = 0 \tag{2.39}$$

where $k = \omega\sqrt{\mu\varepsilon}$. Explicitly, the above wave equation is:

$$\left(\frac{\partial^2}{\partial x^2} + \frac{\partial^2}{\partial y^2} + \frac{\partial^2}{\partial z^2} + k^2 \right) E_i = 0 \tag{2.40}$$

with $i = x, y, z$.

As an example, let us consider propagation of a uniform plane wave characterized by uniform electric field with nonzero component E_x. Assume also:

$$\frac{\partial^2 E_x}{\partial x^2} = 0, \frac{\partial^2 E_x}{\partial y^2} = 0 \tag{2.41}$$

The wave equation reduces to:

$$\frac{\partial^2 E_x}{\partial z^2} + k^2 E_x = 0 \tag{2.42}$$

and has the following forward propagating solution:

$$E_x(z) = E_0 e^{jkz} \tag{2.43}$$

Magnetic field is determined from the Maxwell's equation [Eq. (2.37)]:

$$\nabla \times E = \begin{vmatrix} \hat{a}_x & \hat{a}_y & \hat{a}_z \\ 0 & 0 & \dfrac{\partial}{\partial z} \\ E_x(z) & 0 & 0 \end{vmatrix} \tag{2.44}$$

$$= -j\omega\mu(\hat{a}_x H_x + \hat{a}_y H_y + \hat{a}_z H_z)$$

Here $\hat{a}_x, \hat{a}_y, \hat{a}_z$ are unit vectors along x, y, z axes, respectively. From Eq. (2.44), one finds:

$$H_x = 0 \tag{2.45}$$

$$H_y = \frac{1}{j\omega\mu} \frac{\partial E_x(z)}{\partial z}$$

$$H_z = 0$$

Using the solution for $E_x(z)$, one finally obtains the expression for magnetic field:

$$H_x = \hat{a}_y H_y(z) \qquad (2.46)$$

or

$$H_x = \frac{1}{-j\omega\mu}(-jkE_x)\hat{a}_y \qquad (2.47)$$

$$= \hat{a}_y \frac{k}{\omega\mu} E_x(z)$$

$$= \hat{a}_y \frac{1}{Z} E_x(z)$$

where the impedance Z of the medium is defined as $Z = \sqrt{\dfrac{\mu}{\varepsilon}}$. The propagating wave is shown in Fig. 2.13.

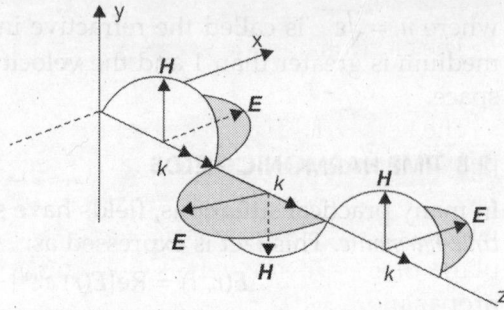

Fig. 2.13: Visualization of the electric and magnetic fields

We finish this section by providing a useful relation between electric and magnetic fields. Assuming time-harmonic and plane-wave dependence of both fields as:

$$E \sim \exp(i\omega t - i k \cdot r)$$

and using constitutive relation [Eq. (2.16)], Maxwell equation [Eq. (2.10)] takes the form

$$k \times E = \omega\mu_0 H$$

Introducing unit vector $\hat{k}$ along wave vector k and the expression for wave number:

$$k = \omega n \sqrt{\mu_0 \varepsilon_0} \text{, one finds}$$

$$n\hat{k} \times E = Z_0 H$$

where Z_0 is the *impedance* of the free-space.

2.9 POLARIZED WAVES

Let us now discuss the concept of polarization of electromagnetic waves. Polarization characterizes the curve which E vector makes (in the plane orthogonal to the direction of propagation) at a given point in space as a function of time. In the most general case, the curve produced is an ellipse and, accordingly, the wave is called elliptically polarized. Under certain conditions, the ellipse may be reduced to a circle or a segment of a straight line. In those cases it is said that the wave's polarization is circular or linear, respectively. Since the magnetic field vector is related to the electric field vector, it does not need separate discussion. First consider a single electromagnetic wave.

2.9.1 Linearly Polarized Waves

Consider an electromagnetic wave characterized by electric field vector E directed along the x-axis.

$$E = \hat{a}_x E_0 \cos(\omega t - kz + \phi) \qquad (2.48)$$

It is known as a linearly polarized plane wave with the electric field vector oscillating in the x direction. Wave propagates in the $+z$ direction. In Eq. (2.48), $\omega = 2\pi\nu$ is the angular frequency and k is the propagation constant defined as:

$$k = \frac{\omega}{v}$$

where $v = c/n$ is the velocity of the electromagnetic wave in the medium having refractive index n, ϕ is known as a phase of electromagnetic wave.

The electromagnetic wave can also be written in the complex representation as:

$$E = \hat{a}_x E_0 e^{i(\omega t - kz + \phi)} \tag{2.49}$$

The actual field as described by Eq. (2.48) is obtained from Eq. (2.49) by taking *real* part. A more general expression for the electromagnetic wave is:

$$E = \hat{e} E_0 e^{i(\omega t - \mathbf{k} \cdot \mathbf{r} + \phi)}$$

which is known as the *plane polarized wave*. Here unit vector $\hat{e}$ lies in the plane known as plane of polarization. It is perpendicular to vector $\mathbf{k}$ which describe direction of propagation:

$$\mathbf{k} . \hat{e} = 0$$

2.9.2 Circularly and Elliptically Polarized Waves

In general, when we have an arbitrary number of plane waves propagating in the same direction they add up to a complicated wave. In the simplest case, one has only two such plane waves. To be specific, consider two plane waves oscillating along orthogonal direction. They are linearly polarized having the same frequencies and propagating in the same direction:

$$E_1 = E_x \hat{a}_x = \hat{a}_x E_{0x} \cos(\omega t - kz) \tag{2.50}$$
$$E_2 = E_y \hat{a}_y = \hat{a}_y E_{0y} \cos(\omega t - kz) + \phi) \tag{2.51}$$

We want to know the type of the resulting wave and the curve traced by the tip of the total electric vector $E = E_1 + E_2$

$$E = E_1 + E_2$$
$$= E_0 \{\cos(\omega t - kz) + \cos(\omega t - kz + \phi)\}$$

First, eliminate $\cos(\omega t - kz)$ term. From Eq. (2.50), we have

$$\cos(\omega t - kz) = \frac{E_x}{E_{0x}} \tag{2.52}$$

Using trigonometric indentify

$$\cos(\alpha - \beta) = \cos\alpha \cos\beta + \sin\alpha \sin\beta$$

We can express Eq. (2.51) as follows

$$E_y = E_{0y}\{\cos(\omega t - kz)\cos\delta + [1 - \cos^2(\omega t - kz)]^{1/2}\sin\delta\}$$

Substitute Eq. (2.52) in the above and have:

$$\frac{E_y}{E_{0y}} = \frac{E_x}{E_{0x}}\cos\phi + \left(1 - \frac{E_x^2}{E_{0x}^2}\right)^{1/2}\sin\phi$$

Squaring both sides gives

$$\left(\frac{E_y}{E_{0y}} = \frac{E_x}{E_{0x}}\cos\phi\right)^2 = \left(1 - \frac{E_x^2}{E_{0x}^2}\right)^{1/2}\sin\phi$$

or $\quad \dfrac{E_y^2}{E_{0y}^2} - 2\cos\phi\,\dfrac{E_y}{E_{0y}}\dfrac{E_x}{E_{0x}} + \dfrac{E_x^2}{E_{0x}^2}\cos^2\phi + \dfrac{E_x^2}{E_{0x}^2}\sin^2\phi = \sin^2\phi$

Finally, the above equation gives:

$$\left(\frac{E_y}{E_{0y}}\right)^2 + \left(\frac{E_x}{E_{0x}}\right)^2 - 2\left(\frac{E_y}{E_{0y}}\right)\left(\frac{E_x}{E_{0x}}\right)\cos\phi = \sin^2\phi \tag{2.53}$$

This is *general equation of an ellipse*. Thus the endpoint of $E(z, t)$ will trace an ellipse at a given point in space. It is said that the wave is *elliptically polarized*.

When phase $\phi = \pi/2$ the resultant total electric field is:

$$\left(\frac{E_y}{E_{0y}}\right)^2 + \left(\frac{E_x}{E_{0x}}\right)^2 = 1$$

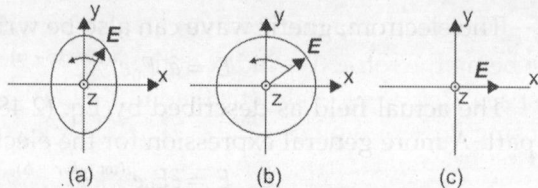

which describes *right elliptically polarized wave* since as time increases the end of electric vector E rotates clockwise on the circumference of an ellipse. Typical situa-

Fig. 2.14: Typical states of polarization: (a) elliptic (b) circular (c) linear

tions are illustrated in Fig. 2.14 where we show elliptic, circular and linear polarizations.

2.9.3 Fresnel Coefficients and Phases

In this section, we discuss electromagnetic wave undergoing reflection at the boundary between two dielectrics (Fig. 2.15). The plane of incidence is defined as the plane formed by unit vector $\hat{n}$ normal to the interface between two media and the directions of propagation of the incident and reflected waves.

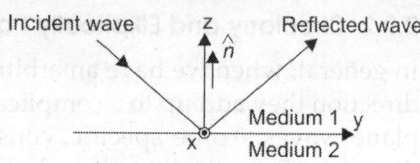

Fig. 2.15: Plane of incidence

We will derive so-called *Fresnel coefficients* which are reflection and transmission coefficients expressed in terms of the angle of incidence and material properties (ε–dielectric constants) of the two dielectrics. Further, Fresnel phases are determined from Fresnel coefficients using the following definition:

$$r = e^{-2j\phi} \tag{2.54}$$

Both reflection coefficients r and phases ϕ will be be calculated for both types of modes, TE and TM.

2.9.4 TE Polarization

Referring to Fig. 2.16 the E_{1i}, E_{1r}, E_{2t} complete values of incident, reflected and transmitted electric fields in medium 1 and 2. The incident electric field in medium 1(E_{1i}) is parallel to the interface between both media. Such orientation is known as TE polarization. It is often said that electric field vector E is normal to the plane of incidence. Such configuration is also known as *s-polarization*.

Boundary conditions require that the tangential component of the total field E and the total field H on both sides of the interface be equal. These conditions result in the following equations:

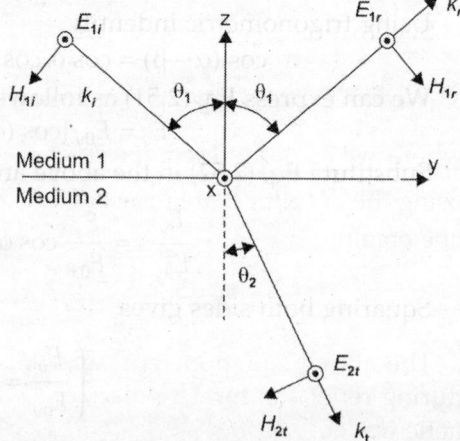

Fig. 2.16: Fresnel reflection for TE polarization. Directions of vector for TE polarized wave

$$E_{1i} + E_{1r} = E_{2t}$$

$$-H_{1i} \cos \phi_1 + H_{1r} \cos \theta_1 = -H_{2t} \cos \theta_2 \tag{2.55}$$

We also have the following relations involving impedances in both media:

$$\frac{E_{1i}}{H_{1i}} = Z_1, \frac{E_{1r}}{H_{1r}} = Z_1, \frac{E_{2t}}{H_{2t}} = Z_2 \tag{2.56}$$

For a nonmagnetic medium ($\mu_r = 1$) the impedance can be written as $Z_0 = \sqrt{Z_0/n}$, with n being the refractive index of the medium and $Z_0 = \sqrt{\mu_0/\varepsilon_0}$, is the impedance of a free space. Replacing magnetic field in the second equation of Eq. (2.55) by the electric fields using Eq. (2.56) gives:

$$E_{1i} + E_{1r} = E_{2t} \tag{2.57}$$

$$-\frac{E_{1i}}{Z_1}\cos\theta_1 + \frac{E_{1r}}{Z_1}\cos\theta_1 = -\frac{E_{2t}}{Z_2}\cos\theta_2$$

Reflection coefficient is defined as:

$$r_{TE} = \frac{E_{1r}}{E_{1i}} \tag{2.58}$$

From Eq. (2.57) by eliminating E_{2t} and using definition (2.58), one obtains:

$$r_{TE} = \frac{Z_2\cos\theta_1 - Z_1\cos\theta_2}{Z_2\cos\theta_1 + Z_1\cos\theta_2}$$

Replacing impedances Z by refractive indices n, we finally have:

$$r_{TE} = \frac{n_1\cos\theta_1 - n_2\cos\theta_2}{n_1\cos\theta_1 + n_2\cos\theta_2}$$

$$= \frac{n_1\cos\theta_1 - \sqrt{n_2^2 - n_1^2\cos\theta_2}}{n_1\cos\theta_1 + \sqrt{n_2^2 - n_1^2\cos\theta_2}} \tag{2.59}$$

using Snell's law. For angles θ_1 such that $n_2^2 - n_1^2\cos\theta_2 < 0$, the reflection becomes complex. For such cases, we write it as:

$$r_{TE} = \frac{n_1\cos\theta_1 - j\sqrt{n_1^2\cos\theta_1 - n_2^2}}{n_1\cos\theta_1 + j\sqrt{n_1^2\cos\theta_1 - n_2^2}} \equiv \frac{a - jb}{a + jb} \tag{2.59a}$$

Such complex number can be expressed as:

$$r_{TE} = \frac{e^{-j\phi_{TE}}}{e^{j\phi_{TE}}} = e^{-2j\phi_{TE}} \tag{2.59b}$$

where we have defined $a + jb = e^{-j\phi_{TE}}$. Finally using the definition of Fresnel phase, Eq. (2.54) one obtains:

$$\tan\phi_{TE} = \frac{\sqrt{n_1^2\cos\theta_1 - n_2^2}}{n_1\cos\theta_1} \tag{2.60}$$

The above equation represents phase shift during reflection for TE polarized electromagnetic wave.

2.9.5 TM Polarization

Field configuration used to analyse reflection for TM polarization (magnetic field parallel to the interface) is shown in Fig. 2.17. Here, electric field vector E is parallel to the plane of incidence. Such configuration is also known as p-polarization.

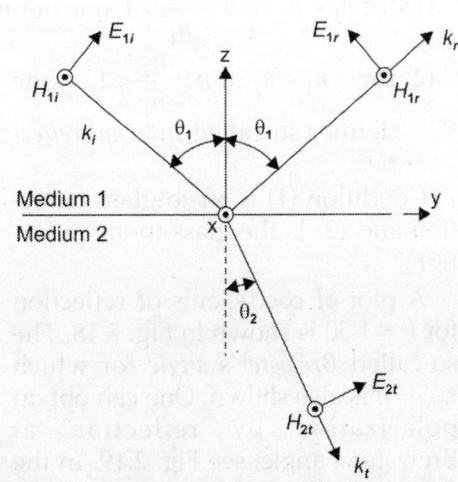

Fig. 2.17: Fresnel reflection for TM polarization. Directions of vectors for a TM polarized wave

We will drive coefficient of reflection r_{TM} for TM mode. As before E_{1i}, E_{1r}, E_{2t} are (complex) values of incident, reflected and transmitted electric fields in medium 1 and 2. Similar notation holds for magnetic vectors. Boundary conditions require that tangenital components which are continuous across interface. The relevant conditions are

$$E_{1j} \cos \theta_1 - E_{1r} \cos \theta_1 = E_{2t} \cos \theta_2 \tag{2.61}$$

Using Eq. (2.56) for impedances to eliminate magnetic field in the previous equations results in the following:

$$E_{1i} \cos \theta_1 - E_{1r} \cos \theta_1 = E_{2t} \cos \theta_2 \tag{2.62}$$

$$\frac{E_{1i}}{Z_1} + \frac{E_{1r}}{Z_1} = \frac{E_{2t}}{Z_2} \tag{2.63}$$

Reflection coefficient is defined as:

$$r_{TM} = \frac{E_{1r}}{E_{1i}} \tag{2.64}$$

From Eq. (2.62):

$$r_{TM} = \frac{Z_1 \cos \theta_1 - Z_2 \cos \theta_2}{Z_1 \cos \theta_1 + Z_2 \cos \theta_2}$$

It can be also expressed in terms of refractive index:

$$r_{TM} = \frac{n_2 \cos \theta_1 - n_1 \cos \theta_2}{n_2 \cos \theta_1 + n_1 \cos \theta_2}$$

$$= \frac{n_2 \cos \theta_1 - \sqrt{n_1^2 - n_2^2} \cos \theta_1}{n_2 \cos \theta_1 + \sqrt{n_1^2 - n_2^2} \cos \theta_1} \tag{2.65}$$

TM phase is obtained in the same way as for TE polarization. Final result is:

$$\tan \phi_{TM} = \frac{n_1^2}{n_2^2} \times \frac{\sqrt{n_1^2 \cos \theta_1 - n_2^2}}{n_1 \cos \theta_1} \tag{2.66}$$

2.9.6 Polarization by Reflection from Dielectric Surfaces

In interpreting the formulas for r_{TE} and r_{TM}, we distinguish between two situations:

(1) for $n_1 < n_2$ or $n = \frac{n_2}{n_1} > 1$, one defines so-called *external reflection*.

(2) for $n_1 < n_2$ or $n = \frac{n_2}{n_1} < 1$, one defines so-called *internal reflection*.

Condition (1) is air-to-glass reflection and (2) is the glass-to-air reflection.

A plot of coefficients of reflection for $n = 1.50$ is shown in Fig. 2.18. The so-called *Brewster's angle* for which $r_{TM} = 0$ is also shown. One can obtain polarization by reflection at Brewster's angle, see Fig. 2.19. In the figure we illustrate properties of the reflected and transmitted light incident at the surface at Brewster's angle.

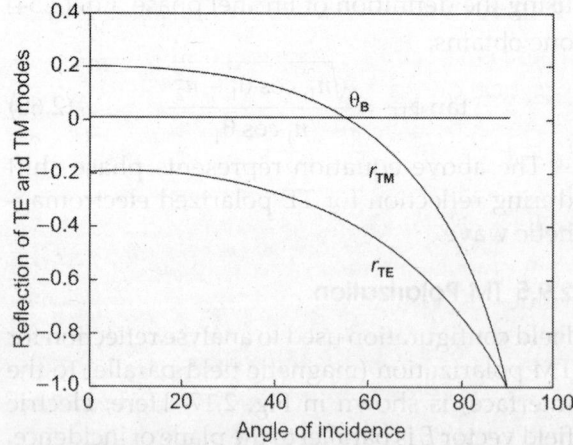

Fig. 2.18: Reflection of TE and TM modes for external reflection with $n = 1.50$ (Brewster's angle is also shown)

Unpolarized light is incident at the interface at *Brewster's angle* θ_B. Upon reflection, one obtains polarized TM light. At the same time, the refracted light is only partially polarized since r_{TE} is nonzero.

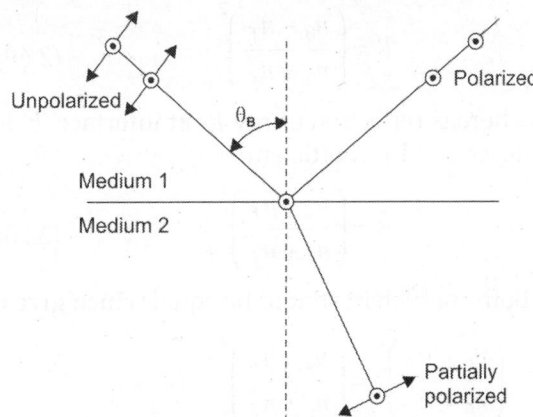

Fig. 2.19: Polarization at Brewster's angle

At *Brewster's angle* θ_B of incidence, coefficient of reflection r_{TM} (also known as r_{11} since E is parallel to the plane of incidence) is zero, i.e. $r_{11} = 0$. The above happens when the sum of the angles of incidence and refraction is equal to $\pi/2$, i.e.:

$$\theta_1 + \theta_2 = \frac{\pi}{2}$$

No such angle exists for the s polarization (TE). Thus if an unpolarized light is incident at Brewster's angle, the reflected light will be linearly polarized, in fact s-polarized.

2.9.7 Expression for Brewster's Angle

Expression for r_{TM} is:

$$r_{TM} = \frac{n_2 \cos \theta_1 - \frac{n_1}{n_2} \sqrt{n_2^2 - n_1^2 \sin^2 \theta_1}}{n_2 \cos \theta_1 + \frac{n_1}{n_2} \sqrt{n_2^2 - n_1^2 \sin^2 \theta_1}} \qquad (2.67)$$

Vanishing for r_{TM} corresponds to $\theta_1 = \theta_B$. We have

$$n_2 \cos \theta_B - \frac{n_1}{n_2} \sqrt{n_2^2 - n_1^2 \sin^2 \theta_B} = 0$$

from which we find an expression for Brewster's angle

$$\tan \theta_B = \frac{n_2}{n_1} \qquad (2.68)$$

2.10 ANTIREFLECTION COATING

There is a need to reduce (or completely eliminate) the effect of reflections. Therefore, the practical question is how to eliminate reflections at the interface between two dielectrics.

As seen before, light passing through a boundary between two dielectrics is lost due to reflection. The effect depends on the difference of the values of refractive indices between neighbouring layers. One can observe that for an equal refractive indices there will be no reflection but also no refraction, which is not a very interesting possibility.

A practical method of reducing reflections is to use several layers with properly selected values of refractive indices. For a single layer, interference of two reflected waves can lead to elimination of reflection, but only at a particular wavelength.

Let us analyse this situation in more detail. Consider reflections of two waves R_1 and R_2 (Fig. 2.20). One of the conditions for destructive interference is that the amplitudes of both reflected waves should be equal. The reflection of ray R_1 at interface 'a' is described by reflection coefficient.

$$R = \left(\frac{n_0 - n_f}{n_0 + n_f} \right)^2 \qquad (2.69)$$

whereas reflection of ray R_2 at interface 'b' is described by coefficient:

$$R = \left(\frac{n_s - n_f}{n_s + n_f} \right)^2 \qquad (2.70)$$

Both coefficient should be equal which gives:

$$\left(\frac{n_0 - n_f}{n_0 + n_f} \right)^2 = \left(\frac{n_s - n_f}{n_s + n_f} \right)^2$$

Assuming that the upper medium is air, i.e. $n_0 = 1$, from the above one finds expression for the value of refractive index for a layer as:

$$n_f = \sqrt{n_s} \qquad (2.71)$$

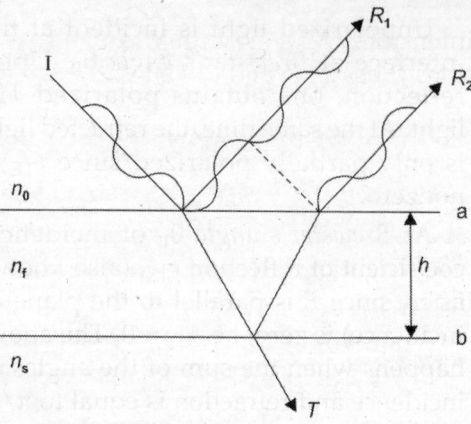

Fig. 2.20: Illustration of reflection from single dielectric film layer (case of destructive interference is shown)

Therefore, at a particular wavelength there will be no reflection once the refractive index of coating layer is given by Eq. (2.67). If there is a need to design structures producing no reflection over some frequency band, one must design multilayer structure consisting of layers with different refractive indices. In order to design such structures a more realistic description is necessary.

2.11 BRAGG MIRRORS

The *Bragg mirror*, also known as the *Bragg reflector*, consists of identical layers of dielectrics with high and low values of refractive indices as shown in Fig. 2.21. The main interest in fabricating such structures is that they have extremely high reflectivities at optical and infrared frequencies. They are important elements of VCSELs

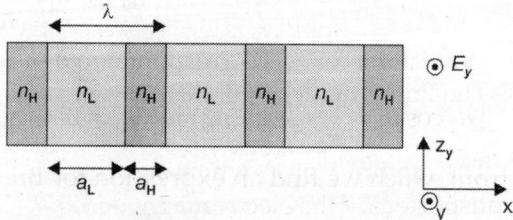

Fig. 2.21: Schematic of a seven-layer dielectric (Bragg) mirror; shown are N = 3 periods

where high reflectivity and bandwidth are required. A typical structure forming Bragg mirror consists of N layers of dielectrics with refractive indices n_L (low refractive index) and n_H (high refractive index). The ratio of those values, the so-called *contrast ratio*, plays an important role.

The structure is known as a quarter-wave dielectric stack, which means that the optical thicknesses are quarter-wavelength long; that is $n_H . a_H = n_L . a_L = \lambda_0 / 4$ at some wavelength λ_0. The structure consists of an odd number of layers with the high index layer being the first and the last layers.

Spectrum of reflectivity of a Bragg mirror is shown in Fig. 2.22 for $N = 10$ periods of Bragg reflector.

2.12 POYNTING THEOREM

Electromagnetic waves carry with them electromagnetic power. We will now derive a relation between the rate of such energy transfer and the electric and magnetic field intensities. We start with Maxwell's equations [Eqs (2.11) and (2.12)].

$$\nabla \times E = -\frac{\partial B}{\partial t} \qquad (2.72)$$

$$\nabla \times H = \frac{\partial D}{\partial t} + J \qquad (2.73)$$

Using the following mathematical indentify:

$$\nabla \cdot (E \times H) = H \cdot (\nabla \times E) - E (\nabla \times H) \qquad (2.74)$$

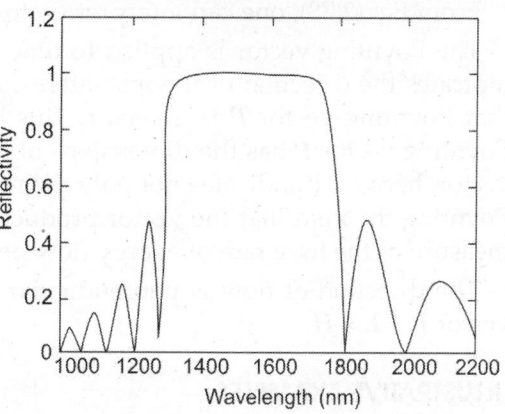

Fig. 2.22: Spectrum of reflectivity of Bragg mirror for $N = 10$ periods of Bragg reflector

Substituting Maxwell's equations into Eq. (2.74) and using constitutive relations, one obtains:

$$\nabla \cdot (E \times H) = -H \cdot \mu \frac{\partial H}{\partial t} - E \cdot J - E \cdot \mu \frac{\partial E}{\partial t}$$

$$= -\mu \frac{1}{2} \frac{\partial H \cdot H}{\partial t} - \sigma E^2 - \varepsilon \frac{1}{2} \frac{\partial E \cdot E}{\partial t}$$

$$= -\frac{\partial}{\partial t} \left(\frac{1}{2} \varepsilon E^2 + \frac{1}{2} \mu H^2 \right) - \sigma E^2 \qquad (2.75)$$

Integrate Eq. (2.75) over volume V and apply Gauss's theorem, one finds:

$$\int_V \nabla \cdot (E \cdot H) dV = -\frac{\partial}{\partial t} \int_V \left(\frac{1}{2} \varepsilon E^2 + \frac{1}{2} \mu H^2 \right) - dV - \int_V \sigma E^2 dV \qquad (2.76)$$

The Poynting vector P is defined as:

$$P = E \times H \qquad (2.77)$$

The modulus of P, which has dimension Wm^{-2}, represents the power per unit area transported by the electromagnetic wave. Further, the time average of the modulus of P, which is the intensity of the wave is given by

$$I = c \frac{\varepsilon_0}{2} E_0^2 \qquad (2.77a)$$

The electric field can be described by using complex exponentials of the type

$$E = E_0 \exp \left[-i \left(\omega t - k \cdot r + \phi \right) \right] \qquad (2.77b)$$

We see that in complex notation, the average power density is proportional to the absolute square of the field amplitude.

Equation (2.76) can be written as:

$$\oint_S P \cdot dS = \frac{\partial}{\partial t} \int_V (w_e + w_m) dV + \int_V p_\sigma dV \qquad (2.78)$$

where

$w_e = \frac{1}{2} \varepsilon E^2$ is electric energy density

$w_m = \frac{1}{2} \mu H^2$ is magnetic energy density

$p_\sigma = \sigma E^2$ is Ohmic power density

From Eq. (2.78), one can interpret vector P as representing the power flow unit area.

The Poynting vector is applied to time constant fields. The direction of the vector P indicates the direction of the instantaneous power flow at the point. Many of us think that Poynting vector P is a vector. This homogeneous is accidental, but correct. The Poynting vector P has the dimensions of *power per unit area* and its unit is Wm^{-2}. It is a vector, because it indicates not only the magnitude of energy but also its direction. It is Poynting theorem that the vector product or cross product $P = E \times H$ at any point is a measure of the time rate of energy flow per unit area of that point.

The direction of flow is perpendicular to E and H and is the direction of Poynting vector $P = E \times H$.

ILLUSTRATIVE EXAMPLES

Example 1

(a) Consider normal incidence of light on an air-silica interface. Compute the fraction of reflected and transmitted power. Also, express the transmitted loss in decibels. Assume refractive index of silica to be 1.45. (b) Repeat the calculation for Si which has $n = 3.50$. (c) Consider coupling of GaAs optical source with a refractive index of 3.6 to a silica fibre which has refractive index of 1.48. Assume close physical contact of the fibre end and the source.

Solution

(a) The corresponding coefficient known as reflectance

$$R = |r|^2 = \left(\frac{n_1 - n_2}{n_1 + n_2} \right)^2 \tag{i}$$

Substituting values for air and silica, one obtains:

$$R = \left(\frac{1.45 - 1.00}{1.45 + 1.00} \right)^2 = 0.033 \tag{ii}$$

so about 3% of the light is reflected. The remainder, 97% is transmitted.

The transmission loss in dB is:

$$\log_{10} 0.97 = 0.13 \text{ [dB]}$$

This result shows that there is about 0.2 dB loss when light enters glass from air.

(b) For Si, using the same procedure we obtain:

$$R = \left(\frac{1.00 - 3.50}{1.00 + 3.50} \right)^2 = 0.309$$

This means that about 31% of light is reflected.

(c) The Fresnel reflection at the interface is:

$$R = \left(\frac{3.60 - 1.48}{3.60 + 1.48} \right)^2 = 1.704$$

Therefore, about 17.4% of the created optical power is emitted back into the source. The power coupled into optical fibre is:

$$P_{\text{coupled}} = (1 - R) \, P_{\text{emitted}}$$

The power loss, α in decibels is:

$$\alpha = -10 \log_{10} = \frac{P_{coupled}}{P_{emitted}}$$

$$= -10 \log_{10} (1 - R)$$

$$= -10 \log_{10} (1 - 0.174) - 10 \log_{10} (0.826)$$

$$= 0.83 \text{ dB}$$

Example 2

A lossless dielectric medium has $\sigma = 0$, $\mu_r = 1$ and $\varepsilon_r = 4$. An electromagnetic wave has magnetic field components expressed as:

$$H = -0.1 \cos(\omega t - z)\,\hat{i} + 0.5 \sin(\omega t - z)\,\hat{j} \text{ A/m}$$

Determine:

(a) the phase constant β,

(b) the angular velocity,

(c) the wave impedance, and

(d) the components of the electric field intensity of the wave.

Solution

Here:

$$\sigma = 0, \qquad \mu_r = 1$$

$$\varepsilon_r = 4, \qquad \alpha = 0 \quad \text{for lossless dielectric}$$

(a) Looking at the equations of H, we can find β directly. $\beta = 1$ rad/m [as

$$H = H_m \cos(\omega t - \beta_z) \text{ type}].$$

(b) $\beta = \omega\sqrt{\mu\varepsilon} = \omega\sqrt{\mu_0\varepsilon_0}\,\sqrt{\varepsilon_r\mu_r} = \dfrac{\omega}{c}\sqrt{4} = \dfrac{2\omega}{c}$

$$\therefore \omega = \frac{\beta c}{2} = \frac{1 \times 3 \times 10^8}{2} = 1.5 \times 10^8 \text{ rad/s}$$

(c) Wave impedance:

$$\eta = \sqrt{\frac{\mu}{\varepsilon}} = \sqrt{\frac{\mu_0}{\varepsilon_0}}\,\sqrt{\frac{\mu_r}{\varepsilon_r}} = 377 \times \sqrt{\frac{1}{4}} = \frac{377}{2}\ 60\pi\Omega$$

(d) $H = -0.1\cos(\omega t - z)\,\hat{j} \text{ Am}^{-1}$

The wave is travelling in z-direction and has components of H in $\hat{i}$ and $\hat{j}$-direction, H_x and H_y, respectively, varying with respect to z. For finding E, we use Maxwell's equation for a lossless medium.

$$\nabla \times H = \varepsilon\frac{\partial E}{\partial t}$$

$$\nabla \times H = \begin{vmatrix} \hat{i} & \hat{j} & \hat{k} \\ \dfrac{\partial}{\partial x} & \dfrac{\partial}{\partial y} & \dfrac{\partial}{\partial z} \\ H_x & H_y & H_z \end{vmatrix} = -\frac{\partial H_y}{\partial z}\hat{i} + \frac{\partial H_y}{\partial z}\hat{j}$$

$$E = \frac{1}{\varepsilon}\int(\nabla \times H)\,dt = \frac{0.5}{\varepsilon\omega}\sin(\omega t - z)\,\hat{i} + \frac{0.1}{\varepsilon\omega}\cos(\omega t - z)\hat{j}$$

or

$$E = 94.12\sin(\omega t - z)\,\hat{i} + 18.83\cos(\omega t - z)\,\hat{j} \text{ V/m}$$

Example 3

The electric field intensity of a uniform plane wave in air is 7500 Vm^{-1} in the $\hat{j}$ direction.

The wave is propagating in the $\hat{i}$ direction at a frequency of 2×10^9 rad/s. Determine: (a) the wavelength of the wave (b) the frequency (c) the time period, and (d) the amplitude of **H**. (Take $v = 3 \times 10^8$ ms^{-1}).

Solution

Here: $E_y = 7500 \cos (2 \times 10^9\ t - \beta x)$ in air

$\varepsilon_0 = 8.854 \times 10^{-12}$ F/m, $\mu_0 = 4\pi \times 10^{-7}$ Hm^{-1}

(a) $\lambda = \dfrac{v}{\nu} = \dfrac{3 \times 10^8}{(2 \times 10^9 / 2\pi)} = 0.943$ m

(b) $\nu = \dfrac{\omega}{2\pi} = \dfrac{2 \times 10^9}{2\pi} = 318.3$ MHz

(c) $T = \dfrac{1}{\nu} = \dfrac{10^{-6}}{318.3} = 3.142$ ns

(d) $\dfrac{E}{H} = \eta = \sqrt{\dfrac{\mu_0}{\varepsilon_0}} \cong 377\Omega$

E_y and H_z components shall exist.

$|H| = \dfrac{7500}{377} = 19.9$ A/m

This gives $H_z = 19.9 \cos (2 \times 10^9 t - \beta x)$.

Example 4

The electromagnetic wave intensity received on the surface of the earth from the sun is found to be 1.33 kW/m^2. Find the amplitude of electric field vector associated with sunlight as received on earth surface. Assume sun's light to be monochromatic ($\lambda = 6000$Å).

Solution

The energy transported by an electromagnetic wave per unit area per second during propagation is represented by Poynting vector **P** as:

$$P = E \times H$$

The energy flux per unit area per second is:

$$|P| = |E \times H| = EH \sin 90° = EH$$

The energy flux per unit area per second at the earth surface:

$$|P| = 1.33 \text{ kW/m}^2$$
$$= 1.33 \times 10^3 \text{ Jm}^{-2}\text{ s}^{-1}$$

or $\qquad EH = 1330 \text{ Jm}^{-2}\text{ s}^{-1}$ (i)

We know that:

$$\eta = \frac{E}{H} = \frac{\mu_0}{\varepsilon_0} = \sqrt{\frac{4\pi \times 10^{-7} \text{ Wb/A·m}}{8.854 \times 10^{-12} \text{ C}^2/\text{Nm}^2}}$$

or $\qquad \dfrac{E}{H} = 376.72\Omega \cong 377\Omega$ (ii)

Multiplying Eqs (i) and (ii), one obtains:

$$EH \times \frac{E}{H} = 1330 \times 37$$

or

$$E^2 = 501410 \text{ or } E = 708.1 \text{ VM}^{-1}$$

Substituting this value in Eq. (i), one obtains:

$$H = \frac{1330}{708.1} = 1.878 \text{ Am}^{-1}$$

∴ The amplitude of electric and magnetic fields of radiation are:

$$E_0 = E\sqrt{2} = 708.1\sqrt{2} = 1001.4 \approx 1001 \text{ Vm}^{-1}$$

and

$$H_0 = H\sqrt{2} = 1.878\sqrt{2} = 2.65 \text{ Vm}^{-1}$$

Example 5

For a lossy dielectric material having $\mu_r = 1$, $\varepsilon_r = 48$, $\sigma = 20$ S/m, calculate the attenuation constant, phase constant and intrinsic impedance at a frequency of 16 GHz.

Solution

We have:

$$\frac{\sigma}{\omega\varepsilon} = \frac{20 \times 10^{12}}{2\pi \times 16 \times 10^9 \times 48 \times 8.856} = 0.47$$

$$\begin{aligned}
\gamma &= i\omega\sqrt{\mu\varepsilon}\sqrt{1 - i\frac{\sigma}{\omega\varepsilon}} \\
&= i(2\pi)16 \times 10^9 \sqrt{4\pi \times 10^{-7} \times 48 \times 8.854 \times 10^{-12}} \times \sqrt{1 - i(0.47)} \\
&= i2323.25\sqrt{1.0966} \angle -24.23° \\
&= 2432.88 \angle 77.89° = 510.4 + i2378.7 \text{ m}^{-1}
\end{aligned}$$

$$\alpha = 510.4 \text{ Np/m}$$
$$\beta = 2378.7 \text{ rad/m}$$

The intrinsic impedance:

$$\eta = \sqrt{\frac{i\omega\mu}{\sigma + i\omega\varepsilon}} = \sqrt{\frac{\mu}{\varepsilon\left(1 + \frac{\sigma}{i\omega\varepsilon}\right)}}$$

$$= \sqrt{\frac{4\pi \times 10^{-7}}{48 \times 8.854 \times 10^{-12}}} \times \sqrt{\frac{1}{1 - j(0.47)}}$$

$$= \frac{54.377}{\sqrt{1.0966} \angle -24.23°}$$

$$= 51.93 \angle 12.12° \Omega$$

The electric field (E_y) leads the magnetic field (H_z) by 12.12° at every point.

Example 6

Find the skin depth δ of an electromagnetic wave in copper at $\nu = 60$ Hz. For copper $\sigma = 5.8 \times 10^7$ mho/m, and $\mu_r = 1$.

Solution

For copper at $\nu = 60$ Hz:

$$\frac{\sigma}{\omega\varepsilon} = \frac{5.8 \times 10^7}{2\pi \times 60 \times 8.854 \times 10^{-12}}$$

$$= 1.74 \times 10^{14} \gg 1$$

Therefore, at $\eta = 60$ Hz, copper is a very good conductor. The depth of penetration

$$\delta = \frac{1}{\beta} = \sqrt{\frac{2}{\omega\mu\sigma}}$$

$$= \sqrt{\frac{2}{2\pi \times 60 \times 4\pi \times 10^{-7} \times 5.8 \times 10^7}}$$

$$= 8.53 \times 10^{-3} \text{ m.}$$

Example 7

Estimate the values of the phase-shift encountered by the normal and parallel components of the reflected waves in total internal reflection when the angle of incidence (with respect to the interface) is 20°. Assume that the light travels from glass ($n_1 = 1.458$) to water ($n_2 = 1.33$). Estimate the value of the angle of incidence for which the phase-shift encountered by each component is zero. **[PTU, RTU]**

Solution

The value of phase shift for the normal component can be estimated as

$$\delta_\perp = 2\tan^{-1}\left(\frac{\sqrt{\dfrac{(1.458)^2}{(1.33)^2}\cos^2 20° - 1}}{\dfrac{1.458}{1.33}\sin 20°}\right) = 66°.81$$

and that for the parallel component can be estimated as

$$\delta_\| = 2\tan^{-1}\left(\frac{\sqrt{\dfrac{(1.458)^2}{(1.33)^2}\cos^2 20° - 1}}{\dfrac{1.33}{1.458}\sin 20°}\right) = 76°.80$$

The phase-shift undergone by each component is zero, when

$$\theta_1 = \theta_c = \cos^{-1}\left(\frac{1.33}{1.458}\right) = 24°.19$$

Example 8

The critical angle for the glass-air interface is 0.7297 rad. Show that the refractive index of glass is 1.5. **[B Tech]**

Solution

We have

$$\sin\phi_c = \frac{n_2}{n_1}$$

Here $n_2 = 1$. Now, refractive index of glass n_1 is

$$n_1 = \frac{1}{\sin\phi_c} = \frac{1}{\sin 0.7297} = 1.5$$

Example 9

The output of laser operating at 190 THz is incident on a dielectric medium of refractive index 1.45. Calculate (a) the speed of light, (b) the wavelength in the medium, and (c) the wave number in the medium.

Solution

(a) The speed of light in the medium

$$v = \frac{c}{n} = \frac{3 \times 10^8 \text{ m/s}}{1.45} = 2.069 \times 10^8 \text{ m/s}$$

(b) Speed = frequency × wavelength

$$v = f\lambda$$

Here $f = 190$ THz, $v = 2.069 \times 108$ m/s

$$\therefore \qquad \lambda = \frac{2.069 \times 10^8}{190 \times 10^{12}} \text{ m} = 1.0889 \text{ μm}$$

(c) The wave number in the medium is

$$k = \frac{2\pi}{\lambda} = \frac{2\pi}{1.088 \times 10^{-6}} = 5.77 \times 10^6 \text{ m}^{-1}$$

Example 10

An optical signal of bandwidth 100 GHz is transmitted over a dispersive medium with β_2 (group velocity dispersion parameter) = 10 ps^2/km. The delay between minimum and maximum frequency components is found to be 3.14 ps. Find the length of the medium.

Solution

$$\Delta\omega = 2\pi\,100 \text{ Grad/s}, \Delta T = 3.14 \text{ ps}, \beta_2 = 10 \text{ ps}^2/\text{km}$$

Now, $$\Delta T = L\,|\beta_2|\,\Delta\omega$$

or $$L = \Delta T / |\beta_2|\,\Delta\omega$$

$$= \frac{3.14 \text{ ps}}{10\,\dfrac{\text{ps}^2}{\text{km}} \times 2\pi \times 100} = 500 \text{ m}$$

SUMMARY

- **Light:** The form of electromagnetic radiation to which the human eye is sensitive and on which our visual awareness of the universe and its contents relies (colour).

  Light may be regarded as a form of *electromagnetic radiation* consisting of interdependent mutually perpendicular transverse oscillations of an electric and magnetic field. It forms a narrow section of the electromagnetic spectrum, the wavelength range (for normal vision) being approximately 390 nm (violet) to 740 nm (red). According to *quantum theory*, light is absorbed in packets of light quanta or photons (energy = $h\nu$).

  The existence of two theories, i.e. wave theory and quantum theory to account for light is referred to as the *wave particle duality*. The wave theory and quantum theory of light are regarded as complementary; phenomena involving the propagation of light can be interpreted adequately on the wave basis, but when interactions of light (e.g. photoelectric effect, etc.) are under consideration, the quantum theory has to be employed.

  During the course of evolution of wave mechanics it has become evident that *electrons* and other *elementary particles* have dual wave and quantum properties.

- The observed behaviour of light as it travels from one place to another, and its interaction with matter had led to the development of a lot of technological tools, e.g. microscope, telescope, high speed cameras, etc. All these instruments use the intricate behaviour of light as it travels from one place to another, and as it interacts with material objects.

- *Electromagnetic (em) spectrum*: An orderly arrangement of radiation according to wavelength (λ), frequency (ν), or energy is known as spectrum. The em spectrum is such a spectrum. In it, the components of radiation are arranged in order of frequency and wavelength.

  All the radiations constituting the e.m. spectrum travel at the same speed in vacuum ($c = 3 \times 10^8$ ms^{-1}).

- According to *Maxwell's* electromagnetic theory, the changing fields produced by the oscillating charges result in electromagnetic disturbances that travel through space as waves. The waves sent out by oscillating charges are viewed as fluctuating electric and magnetic fields, and hence, they are called em waves. These waves travel with the speed of light ($c = 3 \times 10^8$ ms^{-1}) in vacuum.

- EM waves are transverse waves.

  $\dfrac{E}{B} = c$ (velocity of light in vacuum).

- EM waves carry both energy and momentum, which can be delivered to the surface.

- *Maxwell's equations*: A series of classical equations that govern the behaviour of em waves in all practical situations. They connect vector quantities applying to any point in a varying electric or magnetic field. The equations are:

$$\nabla . D = \rho \tag{1}$$

$$\nabla . B = 0 \tag{2}$$

$$\nabla \times E = -\frac{\partial B}{\partial t} \tag{3}$$

$$\nabla \times H = J + \frac{\partial B}{\partial t} \tag{4}$$

where $D = \epsilon E$
$B = \mu H$
$J = \sigma E$

From the above equations, Maxwell demonstrated that each field vector E or B obeys a wave equation, he showed that when a varying electric field exists, it is accompanied by a varying magnetic field induced at right angle, and *vice versa*, and the two form an electromagnetic field that could propagate as a transverse wave. He showed that in vacuum, the speed of the wave, $c = 1/\sqrt{\epsilon_0 \mu_0}$, where ϵ_0 and μ_0 are the permittivity and permeability of vacuum respectively.

Maxwell's equation [Eq. (1)] represents Coulomb's law; Eq. (2) represents the absence of *magnetic monopoles*; Eq. (3) represents Faraday's laws of electromagnetic induction and Eq. (4) represents a generalization of Ampere's law.

- Integral forms of Maxwell's equations:

$$\oint_S D.dS = \int_V \rho dV$$

$$\oint_S B.dS = 0$$

$$\oint_L E.dl = -\int_S \frac{\partial B}{\partial t}$$

$$\oint_L H.dl = -\int_S \left(J + \frac{\partial D}{\partial t} \right) d.S$$

- Solving Maxwell's equation, one obtains wave equations of E and H as:

$$\nabla^2 E = \mu\varepsilon \frac{\partial^2 E}{dt^2}$$

$$\nabla^2 H = \mu\varepsilon \frac{\partial^2 H}{dt^2}$$

In general case, em wave propagation involves electric and magnetic fields having more than one components, each dependent on all three coordinates.

- The ratio of E and H in a wave is denoted by η, and is called *intrinsic impedance*.

$$\eta = \frac{E}{H} = \sqrt{\frac{\mu}{\varepsilon}}$$

For free space:

$$\eta = \sqrt{\frac{\mu_0}{\varepsilon_0}} \cong 377 \text{ or } 120\pi$$

- *Maxwell's equations when the material is lossy*, i.e. it will have finite conductivity σ:

$$\nabla \cdot D = 0$$
$$\nabla \cdot E = 0$$
$$\nabla \times E = -i\omega\mu H$$
$$\nabla \times H = (\sigma + i\omega\varepsilon)E$$
and $\nabla \times (\nabla \times E) = \nabla \cdot (\nabla \cdot E) - D^2 E$

On solving, one gets intrinsic impedance:

$$\eta = \frac{E_y}{H_z} = \frac{i\omega\mu}{\gamma}$$

where $\gamma = i\omega\sqrt{\mu\varepsilon} \sqrt{1 - \frac{i\sigma}{\omega c}}$

$$\therefore \qquad \eta = \sqrt{1 - \frac{i\omega\mu}{(\sigma + i\omega\varepsilon)}}$$

Obviously, η is a complex quantity.

In the loss dielectrics, the electric field leads the magnetic field in time phase.

- In electromagnetics, materials are roughly divided into two classes: (i) *conductors*, and (ii) *dielectrics* or *insulators*. We may note that the dividing line between two classes of materials in not sharp and some media are considered as conductors in one part of radio frequency range, and as dielectric (with loss) in another part of the range.

- *Skin death*: In a medium of high conductivity, the wave is attenuated as its progress due to those losses which occur in the medium. In a good conductor, the rate of attenuation is very great and the wave may penetrate only a very short distance before being reduced to a negligible small percentage of its original strength. The *depth of penetration* or *skin depth* (δ) is defined as the depth in which the wave has been attenuated to $1/e$ or approximately 37% of its original value.

$$\delta = \frac{1}{\omega\sqrt{\frac{\mu\varepsilon}{2}\left[1 + \frac{\sigma^2}{\omega^2\varepsilon^2} - 1\right]}}$$

For good conductor

$\dfrac{\sigma}{\omega\varepsilon} \gg 1$, so

$$\delta = \sqrt{\dfrac{2}{\omega\mu\sigma}} = \sqrt{\dfrac{1}{\pi\nu\mu\sigma}}$$

For copper $\sigma = 5.8 \times 10^7\,\mathrm{Sm^{-1}}$, $\mu = \mu_0$ at $f = 1$ MHz:

$$\therefore \delta = \dfrac{1}{\sqrt{\pi \times 10^6 \times 4\pi \times 10^{-7} \times 5.8 \times 10^7}} = 0.0661\,\mathrm{mm}$$

Value at 50 Hz

$$\delta = \dfrac{1}{\pi \times 50 \times 4\pi \times 10^{-7} \times 5.8 \times 10^7} = 9.35\,\mathrm{mm}$$

At *microwave* frequency 10,000 MHz, $\delta = 6.61 \times 10^{-4}$ mm, which is about 1/8th of the wavelength of visible light.

- *Poynting vector*: The vector P giving the direction and magnitude of energy flow in an electromagnetic field

  $P = E \times H$,

  where E and H are mutually orthogonal vectors of the electric and magnetic fields, respectively. If energy dissipation takes place during the propagation, this vector becomes complex with a real part equal to the average energy flow.

REVIEW QUESTIONS

1. What is the nature of light? Explain briefly.
2. What do you understand by dual nature of light? Explain with examples.
3. Write Maxwell's equations in differential and integral forms. Derive the wave equation from these equations for free space and charge free region.
4. Show that for uniform plane waves in a perfect dielectric medium, E and H are normal to each other and also show that the ratio of their magnitude is constant of the medium. Write the name of the constant and explain its significance.
5. Define skin depth (δ). Show that in case of a semifinite solid conductor δ is given by:

   $$\delta = \sqrt{\dfrac{2}{\omega\mu\sigma}}$$

   Symbols have their usual meanings.
6. State Poynting theorem and show that Poynting vector:

   $P = E \times H$
7. Using Maxwell's equations, show that in free space, the electro-magnetic wave propages with the speed of light, i.e.:

   $$v = \dfrac{1}{\sqrt{\mu_0\varepsilon_0}} = 3 \times 10^8\,\mathrm{ms^{-1}} = c$$
8. Enumerate Maxwell's equations and show that they predict existence of electromagnetic waves.
9. What are polarization sensitive materials?

   Give examples of few common birefrigent crystals with their applications.

PROBLEMS

1. If the earth receives 2 cal min^{-1} cm^{-2} solar energy, calculate the amplitudes of the electric and magnetic fields of radiation?

   [**Ans.** $E_0 = E/\sqrt{2} = 1024.3 \text{ Vm}^{-1}$,

   $\quad H_0 = H/\sqrt{2} = 2.717 \text{ Am}^{-1}$]

2. Show that a linearly polarized plane wave can be decomposed into a right hand and a left-hand circularly polarized waves of equal amplitudes.

3. Assume that for some materials refractive index at a particular wavelength is negative. Discuss the consequences of such an assumption. Consider modification of Snell's law.

4. A uniform plane wave in a medium having $\sigma = 10^{-3}$ Sm^{-1}, $\varepsilon_r = 80\ \varepsilon_0$ and $\mu_r = \mu_0$ is having a frequency 10 kHz. Calculate the various parameters of the wave.

   [**Ans.** $\alpha = 2\pi \times 10^{-3} \text{ Np m}^{-1}$

   $\quad \beta = 2\pi \times 10^{-3} \text{ rad m}^{-1}, \eta = 2\pi\,(1+j)\Omega$

   $\quad \lambda = 1000 \text{ m}, v = 10^7 \text{ ms}^{-1}$

5. The relative permeability of distilled water is 81. Show that the refractive index and the velocity of light in it are $n = 9.0$ and $v = 3.33 \times 10^7 \text{ ms}^{-1}$ respectively.

6. Calculate the skin depth (δ) for an e.m. wave of frequency 1 MHz travelling through copper. Given $\alpha = 5.8 \times 10^7$ Sm^{-1} and $n = 4\pi \times 10^{-7}$.

   [**Ans.** $\delta = 66\ \mu m$]

7. A plane em wave is travelling in the positive z direction in an unbounded lossless dielectric medium with relative permeability $\mu_r = 1$ and relative permittivity $\varepsilon_r = 3$ has an electric field intensity $E = 6 \text{ Vm}^{-1}$. Calculate.

   (i) the speed of em waves in the given medium, and

   (ii) the impedance of the medium.

   [**Ans.** (i) $v = 1.732 \times 10^8 \text{ ms}^{-1}$

   $\quad$ (ii) $\eta = 2.17 \times 10^2\ \Omega$]

SHORT ANSWER QUESTIONS

1. What is the basis of Maxwell's electromagnetic theory?

   Ans. The theory developed by Maxwell is based on the following statements:

   (i) Electric fields originate on positive charges and terminate on negative charges. The electric field due to point charges can be determined at a location by applying Coulomb's force law to positive test charge placed at that location.

   (ii) Magnetic field line always form closed loops, i.e. they do not begin or end anywhere.

   (iii) A varying magnetic field induces an emf and hence, an electric field. This is Faraday's law.

   (iv) Magnetic fields are generated by moving charges (or currents), as summarized in Ampere's law.

2. What is quantum nature of light?

   Ans. Light energy is always emitted or absorbed in discrete units called *quanta* or *photons*. Energy of photon depend only on frequency v of a photon and is given by:

   $$E = h\nu$$

3. Write basic optical laws.

Ans. (i) *Refractive index (n)*: The ratio of the speed of light in a vacuum to that in matter is the index of refraction of material and is given by:

$$n = c/v$$

(ii) *Snell's law*: The relationship at the interface is known as Snell's law and is given by:

$$n_1 \sin \phi_1 = n_2 \sin \phi_2$$

where n_1 and n_2 are refractive indices of medium 1 and medium 2 respectively. ϕ_1 is the angle of incidence between the incident ray and the normal to the surface in medium 1 and angle ϕ_2 is angle of refraction between the normal and refracted ray in medium 2.

4. Write the important properties of em waves propagating through free space.

Ans. (i) EM waves travel with speed of light in vacuum
$(c = 3 \times 10^8 \text{ ms}^{-1})$

(ii) EM waves are transverse in nature

(iii) $E/B = c$ (velocity of light)

(iv) EM waves carry both energy and momentum.

5. What is intrinsic impedance? What is its value for free space?

Ans. $\eta = \dfrac{E}{H} = \sqrt{\dfrac{\mu}{\varepsilon}}$

For free space $\eta = \sqrt{\dfrac{\mu_0}{\varepsilon_0}} \cong 377$ or 120π

6. In electromagnetics, how materials are divided?

Ans. (i) Conductors (ii) Dielectrics or insulators.

The dividing line between two classes is not sharp and some media are considered as conductors in one part of radio frequency range, and as dielectric (with loss) in another part of the range.

7. What is Poynting vector?

Ans. $P = E \times H$

P is interpreted as an instantaneous power density that is measured in Wm^{-2}, P can be used to determine total power crossing the surface in an outward sense.

The Poynting vector is applied to time constant fields.

8. Draw a figure of plane polarized em wave and mention its important features.

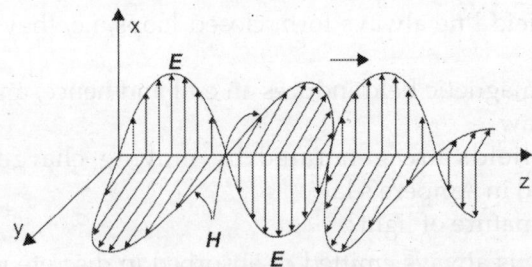

Fig. 2.23: An instantaneous snapshot of a plane-polarized transverse wave showing the electric and magnetic field vectors **E** and **H**, with the wave moving to the right

Ans. Figure 2.23 shows plane-polarized electromagnetic wave. We observe that:

(i) Vibrations of its electric field vector E are parallel to each other for all points in the wave.

(ii) At all these points (i) the vibrating E vector and the direction of propagation form a plane called the *plane of vibration* or the *plane of polarization*. All such planes are parallel in a plane-polarized wave.

(iii) In this case, the resultant electric-field vector may be resolved in two components which have a random phase difference. If the wave is propagating along the z-axis and the two components are along the x and y axes and have the same amplitudes with a phase difference of $\pi/2$, the wave is said to be circularly polarized. However, if the amplitudes of the two components are not same, but their phase difference is still $\pi/2$, the resultant wave is said to be elliptically polarized.

9. How velocity of propagation of light is affected in anisotropic materials, e.g. KDP, etc.?

Ans. In optically anisotropic materials, the velocity of propagation of light depends on the direction as well as the state of polarization. Thus, there are two principal refractive indices: One corresponding to the ordinary (o) ray (which follows Snell's law) and other corresponding to the extraordinary (e) ray (which does not follow Snell's law).

10. What are uniaxial crystals? Give two examples.

Ans. Crystals, which have two principal refractive indices and one optic axis (the direction along which the velocity of both the rays is same) are termed *uniaxial crystals*. Example are calcite and quartz.

11. What is Pockel's electro-optic effect?

Ans. When an electric field is applied across a birefringent crystal, e.g. KDP, this may change its refractive indices. When this change is linearly proportional to the electric field, the effect is called the *Pockel's electro-optic effect*. This can be used for phase modulation.

12. What happens when a voltage V is applied along the optic axis of KDP crystal?

Ans. KDP is a birefringent crystal. When a voltage V is applied along the optic axis of this crystal, the incident plane-polarized light splits into two components and the net phase shift between them is given by:

$$\phi = \frac{2\pi}{\lambda} r_{63} n_0^3 V$$

MULTIPLE CHOICE QUESTIONS

1. The mass of photon of wavelength λ is given by:

(a) $hc\lambda$ (b) $h/\lambda c$

(c) $\dfrac{hc}{\lambda}$ (d) $\dfrac{h\lambda}{c}$

[**Hint.** We have $hc = mc^2$ or $\dfrac{hc}{\lambda} = mc^2$ ($\because c = \nu\lambda$). Hence $m = h/\lambda c$)

2. A photon has energy $E = h\nu$ and momentum $p = \dfrac{h}{\lambda}$. The speed of light in terms of E and p is:

(a) Ep

(b) $\sqrt{EP}$

(c) p/E

(d) E/p

[**Hint.** $\dfrac{E}{p} = \dfrac{h\nu}{h/\lambda} = \nu\lambda = c$]

3. The momentum of a photon of wavelength λ is:

(a) $\dfrac{h}{c\lambda}$

(b) $\dfrac{hc}{\lambda}$

(c) $h\lambda$

(d) h/λ

[**Hint.** $E = h\nu = mc^2$ $\therefore m = \dfrac{h\nu}{c^2} = \dfrac{h}{c\lambda}$

$\therefore$ Momentum of photon, $mc = h/\lambda$]

4. The momentum of a particle of mass m and charge q is equal to that of photon of wavelength λ. The speed of particle is given by:

(a) $qh\lambda$

(b) $\dfrac{mh}{\lambda}$

(c) $\dfrac{h}{m\lambda}$

(d) $\dfrac{h\lambda}{m}$

[**Hint.** We have $mv = \dfrac{h}{\lambda}$ $\therefore v = \dfrac{h}{m\lambda}$]

5. The concept that a changing electric field in a conductor produces induced magnetic field was proposed by:

(a) Faraday

(b) Biot–Savart

(c) Maxwell

(d) Oersted

6. The concept of displacement current was proposed by:

(a) Maxwell

(b) Faraday

(c) Ampere

(d) Gauss

7. Maxwell's modified Ampere's law is valid:

(a) only when electric field does not change with time

(b) only when electric field varies with time

(c) in the above situations

(d) none of the above

8. The dimensions of Planck's constant (h) are:

(a) ML^2T^{-2}

(b) $ML^{-3}T^{-5}$

(c) ML^2T^{-1}

(d) being a constant, h has no dimension

[**Hint.** Dimensions of h = dimensions of energy × dimensions of time = $ML^2T^{-2}T$ = ML^2T^{-1}]

9. Which is the incorrect statement about the electromagnetic waves:

(a) the electromagnetic field vector E and B are mutually perpendicular and they are also perpendicular to the direction of propagation of the electromagnetic wave

(b) the field vector E and H are in same phase

(c) the field vector E and H are along the same direction

(d) electromagnetic waves are transverse in nature

10. Which one is the incorrect statement about the electromagnetic waves:

(a) the energy density associated with the electromagnetic wave in free space propagates with a speed less than the speed of light

(b) in free space, the electromagnetic waves travel with the speed of light

(c) the direction of flow of electromagnetic energy along the direction of propagation of wave

(d) the electrostatic energy density is equal to magnetic energy density

11. Poynting vector P is:

(a) $E \cdot H$

(b) $E \times H$

(c) E/H

(d) $\oint (E \times H) \cdot dS$

12. Intrinsic impedance of dielectric with $\sigma = 0$ is:

(a) μ/ε

(b) $\sqrt{\dfrac{\mu}{\varepsilon}}$

(c) $\sqrt{\mu\varepsilon}$

(d) $1\sqrt{\mu\varepsilon}$

13. For good dielectrics:

(a) $\dfrac{\sigma}{\omega\varepsilon} = 0$

(b) $\dfrac{\sigma}{\omega\varepsilon} \gg 1$

(c) $\dfrac{\sigma}{\omega\varepsilon} = 1$

(d) $\dfrac{\sigma}{\omega\varepsilon} \ll 1$

14. The skin depth for a good conductor is:

(a) $\sqrt{\dfrac{2}{\omega\mu\sigma}}$

(b) $\sqrt{2\,\omega\mu\sigma}$

(c) $\sqrt{\dfrac{\omega\mu\sigma}{2}}$

(d) $\dfrac{2}{\sqrt{\omega\mu\sigma}}$

15. The intrinsic impedance of good conductor is given by:

(a) $\sqrt{\dfrac{\mu}{\varepsilon}}\left(1 + \dfrac{i\sigma}{\sqrt{2\omega\varepsilon}}\right)$

(b) $\sqrt{\dfrac{i\omega\mu}{\sigma}}$

(c) $\sqrt{\dfrac{i\omega\mu}{\sigma + i\omega\mu}}$

(d) $\sqrt{i\omega\mu\sigma\left(1 + i\dfrac{\omega\mu}{\sigma}\right)}$

16. A monochromatic electromagnetic wave means that:

(a) the field strength at a point varies with time according to sine and cosine function

(b) the wave always travels in the same direction

(c) electric field vector E lies in one direction only

(d) magnetic field vector B must be perpendicular to the direction of propagation

17. "The net power flowing out of a given volume V is equal to the time rate of decrease in energy stored within V minus the ohmic losses" is the statement of:
    (a) Gauss's theorem
    (b) Stoke's theorem
    (c) Poynting theorem
    (d) none of these

18. The depth of penetration is the depth in which the electro-magnetic wave has been attenuated to:
    (a) e of the original value
    (b) $1/e$ of the original value
    (c) 50% of the original value
    (d) 100% of the original value

19. A half-wave plate will introduce a path difference (between two emerging beams) of:
    (a) $\lambda/4$
    (b) $\lambda/2$
    (c) $3\lambda/4$
    (d) λ

20. In a longitudinal electro-optic modulator, half-wave voltage is that voltage which introduces the following phase shift between two polarization components:
    (a) $\pi/4$
    (b) $\pi/2$
    (c) π
    (d) 2π

21. In a transverse electro-optic modulator:
    (a) V_π is independent of the length l and width d of the modulator crystal
    (b) V_π is dependent on the length l but not on the width d of the crystal
    (c) V_π is dependent on the width d but not on the length l of the crystal
    (d) V_π is dependent on the ratio d/l

22. In a Raman-Nath modulator, the acousto-optic grating is:
    (a) so thin that it behaves almost like a plane transmission grating
    (b) so thick that it behaves almost like Bragg's crystal grating
    (c) analogous to a concave Rowland's grating
    (d) quite complicated

23. Consider an electromagnetic wave travelling in the z-direction. The orthogonal components of its resultant E-vector are along the x- and y-direction. Assume that the two components have same amplitudes but a phase difference of $\pi/2$. The resultant E-vector at any point in space:
    (a) is constant in amplitude but rotates with an angular frequency ω
    (b) changes in amplitude but rotates with an angular frequency ω
    (c) remains stationary
    (d) varies randomly

24. The electromagnetic wave of Question 23, is said to be:
    (a) unpolarized
    (b) plane-polarized
    (c) circularly polarized
    (d) elliptically polarized

25. In a birefringent crystal:
    (a) the o-ray follows Snell's law but the e-ray does not
    (b) the e-ray follows Snell's law but the o-ray does not
    (c) both o-ray and e-ray follow Snell's law
    (d) both the o-ray and e-ray do not follow Snell's law

26. In a doubly refracting crystal, the optic axis is the direction in which:
    (a) v_0 is greater than v_e
    (b) v_0 is equal to v_e
    (c) v_0 is less than v_e
    (d) v_0 and v_e vary randomly

27. A uniaxial crystal has:
    (a) one principal refractive index and no optic axis
    (b) one principal refractive index and one optic axis
    (c) two principal refractive indices and one optic axis
    (d) three principal refractive indices and two optic axes

28. A quarter-wave plate will introduce a phase difference (between two emerging beams) of:
    (a) $\pi/4$
    (b) $\pi/2$
    (c) π
    (d) $3\pi/2$

ANSWERS

1. (b)	2. (d)	3. (d)	4. (c)	5. (c)	6. (a)	7. (c)	8. (c)	9. (c)	10. (a)
11. (b)	12. (b)	13. (d)	14. (a)	15. (b)	16. (a)	17. (c)	18. (b)	19. (b)	20. (c)
21. (d)	22. (a)	23. (a)	24. (c)	25. (a)	26. (b)	27. (c)	28. (b)		

3

Optical Fibers

3.1 INTRODUCTION

It has been known and understood by the time of Isaac Newton that light beams could be trapped and guided in a medium of higher index of refraction material surrounded by lower index of refraction material (Fig. 3.1). Three hundred years later, we figured out how to use this observation and revolutionized the telecommunication industry.

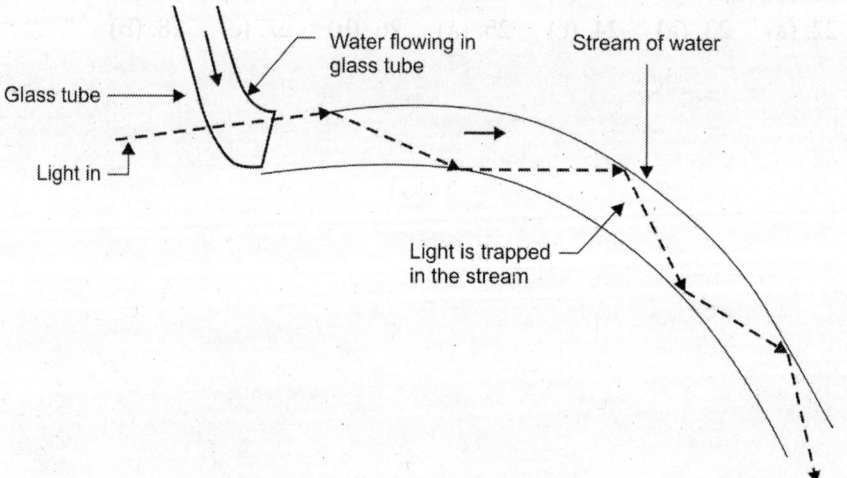

Fig. 3.1: Schematic diagram of the experimental demonstration by Newton which shows that light can be guided in a stream of water

In 1870, Tyndall, first studied transmission in a confined path. In 1930, H Lamm conducted experiments on image transmission through quartz fibres. In 1936, GC Southworth studied theoretically and experimentally, the behaviour of electromagnetic waves in cylindrical nonconductive materials; similar to today's optical fibre laser light transmission. In the early 1960s, Bell Laboratories (BS) and Standard Telephone Laboratories (UK) demonstrated optical transmission through low loss glass fibres useful for long distance communications.

In 1966, Charles Kao and Charles Hockham proposed that an *optical fibre* might be used as a means of telecommunication, provided the signal loss could be made less than 20 decibles per kilometer (dB/km). At that time optical fibres exhibited losses of the order of 1000 dB/km.

At this point, it is important to know why the need for optical fibres as a transmission medium was felt. Truly speaking, the transfer of information from one point to another, i.e. communication is achieved by superimposing (or modulating) the information onto an electromagnetic wave, which acts as a carrier for the information signal. The modulation carrier is then transmitted through the information channel (open or guided) to the receiver, where it is demodulated and the original information sent to the destination. Now, the carrier frequencies present certain limitations in handling the volume and speed of information transfer. These limitations generated the need for *increased carrier frequency*. In fibre optic systems, the carrier frequencies are selected from the optical range (particularly the infrared part of the spectrum (Fig. 3.2).

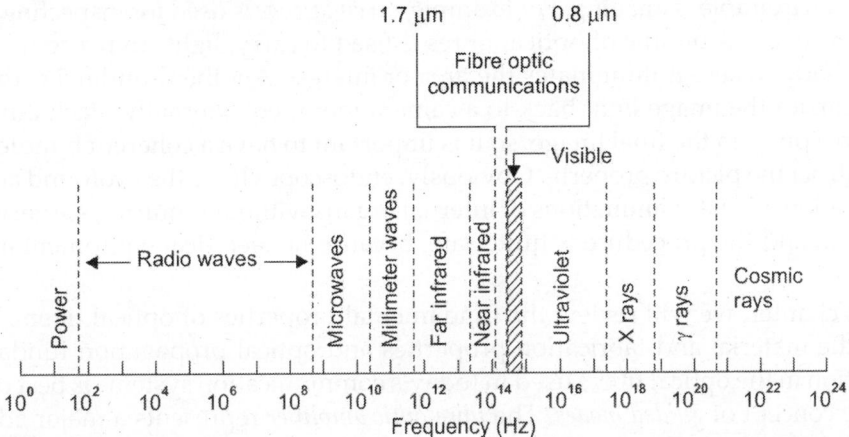

Fig. 3.2: Electromagnetic spectrum showing carrier frequencies of IR part

We can see that the typical frequencies are of the order of 10^{14} Hz, which is 10,000 times greater than that of microwaves. Obviously, optical fibres are the most suitable medium for transmitting these frequencies, and hence optical fibres present theoretically unlimited possibilities. Thus, we can say that:

(i) Optical fibres deals with study of propagation of light through transparent dielectric waveguides. The optical fibres are used for transmission of data from point to point location. Currently, the optical fibre systems are extensively used as the transmission line between terrestrial hardwired systems.

(ii) The carrier frequencies used in conventional systems had the limitations in handling the volume and rate of data transmission. The greater the carrier frequency, larger the available bandwidth and information carrying capacity.

The more general term used for an optical fibre is *light wave guide* and for fibre optics communication as *light wave communication*. However, the name *photonics* for fibre optic communications is becoming popular day to day. *Photonics* is very much helping the technology for fibre optic communication to enhance its performance and become more cost effective. Today, optical fibres are finding use in large number of areas, e.g. *sensors, display systems, copying machines, defence services* due to high privacy, etc. In telecommunications, modulating a beam of light (LED or LASER) as a source of light and using optical fibre waveguides have the inherent advantage of very large bandwidth, small dimensions, low loss bandwidth and insensitivity to electrical interference.

Optical fibres are dielectric waveguides, which are fabricated from glass or plastic. A fibre is as thin as human hair designed to guide light wave along their length. They are operated on optical frequencies. Usually an optical fibre is a cylindrical waveguide system through which the optical wave can propagate. The principle by which light wave travels through the fibre is 'total internal reflection' without loss of incident intensity.

An important structure used in optical systems is the layered structure or waveguide structure. These structures are used to confine optical waves in a well defined region and guide their propagation. One can make layered structures from non-crystalline or crystalline materials. For example, glass is used to produce optical fibres for use in optical communication, whereas semiconductor waveguides are used in semiconductor lasers.

In short, we can say that fibre optics have revolutionised the modern world. Two areas in which optical fibres are used extensively are *communications* and *imaging*. Optical fibres have made it possible to perform internal medical examinations with minimal intrusion, an example is imaging. For example, an *endoscope* is used for inspecting different parts of the body. A bundle of optical fibres is used to carry, light from a source into the patient's body, where it illuminates the area of interest. Another bundle, i.e. the output bundle, carries the image light back to a camera mounted externally. Each output fibre turns into a pixel in the final image, so it is important to have a coherent bundle in order to reconstruct the picture properly. Obviously, endoscopes have the profound advantage that they allow visual examinations of internal organs without requiring surgery, or even an incision, and the procedure is quite safe, because no electrical equipment enters the body.

In this chapter, we will review the fundamental properties of optical fibers. This will include the material and fabrication properties and optical propagation fundamentals. Propagation in the optical fibers used in today's communication systems is best described using the concept of *guided modes*. The *fibre-optic amplifier* represents a major advance in fiber-optic technology. Commercialization of this device is in the initial stages. The promise of optical communication using many wavelengths and exploiting *nonlinearities*, such as *soliton* propagation is indeed exciting.

3.2 OPTICAL FIBER

Optical fibers are the dielectric waveguides, which are fabricated from glass or plastic and are operated on optical frequencies. These are normally cylindrical in form. The optical fiber cable (Fig. 3.3) has three principal sections: (i) Core (ii) Cladding and (iii) Jacket or Sheath.

(i) **Core:** Core is the innermost region of the fiber. Core has specific property of conducting an optical beam. Core is usually made of glass ($n_1 = 1.5$) or plastic. Glass is used as core material for low and medium loss fibers, whereas plastic core is used for relatively higher loss fibers. Quartz ($n_1 = 1.46$) is also used for core material. The diameter of core varies from 8 to 200 μm. We may note that the core is the actual working structure of the optical fiber, which is covered with another layer of glass or plastic having slightly different chemical composition known as cladding.

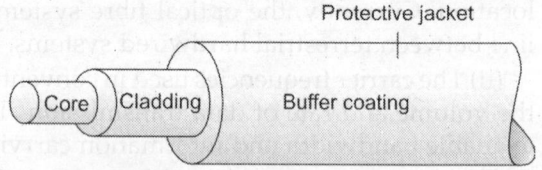

Fig. 3.3: A single fibre structure

(ii) **Cladding:** The core is surrounded by a solid dielectric cladding having refractive index n_2 which is less than n_1 of core ($n_2 < n_1$). The cladding material is either glass or plastic. Although cladding is not mandatory for light propagation along the core, however, it has the following advantages:

    (a) It reduces scattering loss arising due to dielectric discontinuities at the boundary of core surface and air ($n = 1$).

(b) It adds mechanical strength to the fiber.

(c) It protects the core from absorbing surface contaminants.

We can have three types of core and cladding: (i) Plastic core and cladding (ii) Glass (silica) core and cladding and (iii) Glass core with plastic cladding.

Although glass has low loss, plastic provides more flexibility and ruggedness to fiber, less expensive, also 60% less heavy than glass and is stress tolerant. Hence plastic fiber is preferred for small distance communication. The optical fiber may have an abrupt boundary core between cladding, i.e. they may exhibit a gradual change in material between them.

(iii) **Jacket or sheath:** The outermost section of optical fiber is made up of plastic or special kind of polymer and other material usually opaque in nature. This is known as jacket or sheath. A typical single fiber cable is shown in Fig. 3.4.

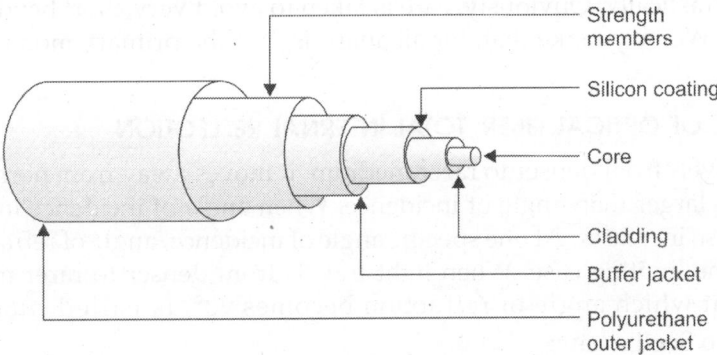

Fig. 3.4: A schematic representation of typical fiber cable

Jacket protects the core from abrasion, interaction with environment, crushing, absorption, moisture and all other adversities of the terrestrial atmosphere. Obviously, jacket enhances tensile strength of fiber.

Apart from its use as communication channel, optical fibers find wide uses in many other areas. Sensors for detecting electrical, mechanical and thermal energies are made using optical fibers. Copier machines, simple display systems, medical diagnostic, fibroscopes, etc. also utilize fiber optics.

The optical properties of cladding are different from those of the core. Jacket protects the fiber structure from moisture, abrasion, mechanical shocks and other environmental hazards.

The core forms the actual working structure of optical fiber. An incident (wave) ray of light entering the core suffers a number of total internal reflections at the core-cladding interface. Obviously the interface between core and cladding acts as a mirror at which total internal reflection of the transmitted light takes place.

3.3 OPTICAL FIBER AS WAVEGUIDE: PRINCIPLE OF PROPAGATION

A waveguide is a tubular structure through which energy of sort could be guided in the form of waves. As light waves can be guided through a fiber, it is called *light guide*. Usually, it is also called as *fiber wave guide* or *fiber light wave*.

As stated earlier, the cladding in an optical fiber always has a lower refractive index than that of core. The light signals which enters into the core can strike the interface of the core and cladding only at large angles of incidence, because of the ray geometry (Fig. 3.5). We can see that the light signal undergoes reflection after reflection within the fiber core. Since each reflection is a total internal reflection, the signal sustains its strength and also confines itself completely within the core during propagation. Clearly the optical fiber functions as a waveguide.

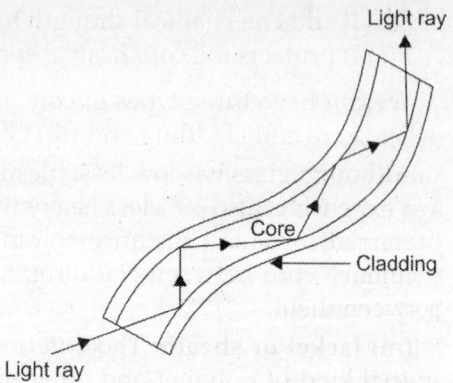

Fig. 3.5: Optical fiber as a waveguide

The propagation of light continues as long as the fiber is not bent too sharply, since for sharp bends, the light fails to undergo total internal reflection because of which the signal strength comes down drastically. Obviously, care is taken to avoid very short bends in the signal carrying fiber. We may make that, for all analysis, it is the primary mode of use.

3.4 PRINCIPLE OF OPTICAL FIBER: TOTAL INTERNAL REFLECTION

When light travels from denser to rarer medium, it moves away from normal. The angle of refraction is larger than angle of incidence. When angle of incidence increases, angle of refraction also increases. At one specific angle of incidence, angle of refraction becomes 90° and it is the limiting case. When light travels from denser to rarer medium, angle of incidence at which angle of refraction becomes 90°, is called *critical angle* (θ_c).

According to Snell's Law:

$$n_1 \cdot \sin \theta_1 = n_2 K \cdot \sin \theta_2 \quad \text{or} \quad \frac{\sin \theta_1}{\sin \theta_2} = \frac{n_2}{n_1} \tag{3.1}$$

where θ_1 is the angle of incidence in the medium of refractive index n_1 and θ_2 is the angle of refraction in the medium of refractive index n_2. In this case $n_1 > n_2$. When $\theta_1 = \theta_c$, $\theta_2 = 90°$, therefore $\sin \theta_c = n_2/n_1$.

When the angle of incidence is greater than critical angle, the angle of refraction becomes greater than 90° and it is no more refraction. The light comes back in the same (original) medium and it is called *total internal reflection*. This principle is used in optical fiber ray transmission.

As stated earlier, optical fiber consists of *core* of refractive index n_1 and cladding of refractive index n_2 ($n_1 > n_2$). At the interface of core-cladding (Fig. 3.3), there occurs total internal reflection and ray travels through core of the fiber. Figure 3.6(a) shows the geometry of launching a light ray into an optical fiber.

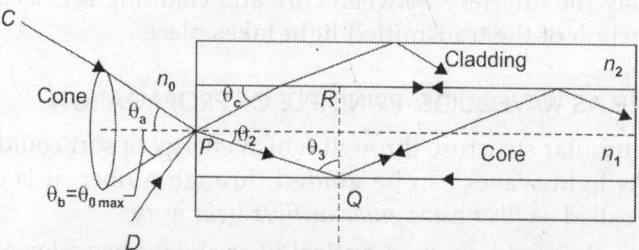

Fig. 3.6(a): Ray transmission through an optical fiber

The incident rays with angle of incidence greater than θ_c at the core cladding surface are transmitted by total internal reflection. A ray travelling parallel to axis (or making relatively small angle with axis) is called *meridional* ray. For example, CP is the meridional ray. The ray CP makes an angle of incidence θ_a at air-core interface. The rays making an angle greater than θ_a at air-core interface, make angle of incidence of core-cladding interface, less than θ_c and they are lost as they do not undergo total internal reflection. For example, ray DP. The rays entering the fiber core within the *acceptance cone* specified by conical half-angle θ_a are transmitted and others are lost. The maximum angle of incidence at air-core (or any other medium and core) interface, specified by the conical half-angle, for the light rays to be transmitted through the optical fiber is called *acceptance angle* for the fiber.

In optical fiber ray transmission, generally a term *numerical aperture* (NA) is used. This term is used in optics: where it *defines the light-gathering power of lens or express the angle of view of lens. The NA is the product of the refractive index of the surrounding medium and sine of half the angle of view of the lens.*

In optical fiber, *NA* gives the relation between the acceptance angle and refractive index of three media involved, viz. core, cladding and air (or any other medium). Suppose θ_a is the *acceptance angle*, or the acceptance cone half angle refractive index of air or any other medium present at core interface is n_0 and refractive index of core is n_1 and that of cladding is n_2 $(n_1 > n_2)$.

From Snell's law:

$$n_0 \sin \theta_1 = n_1 \sin \theta_2 \qquad (3.1a)$$

In triangle PQR, $\theta_3 = [(\pi/2) - \theta_2]$. Here $\theta_3 > \theta_c$, therefore:

$$n_0 \sin \theta_1 = n_1 \cos \theta_3$$

$$= n_1 \sqrt{1 - \sin^2 \theta_3}$$

For limiting case, $\theta_1 \rightarrow \theta_a$ and $\theta_3 \rightarrow \theta_c$

hence

$$n_0 \sin \theta_a = n_1 \sqrt{1 - \sin^2 \theta_c}$$

$$= n_1 \sqrt{1 - \left(\frac{n_2}{n_1}\right)^2}$$

$$= \sqrt{n_1^2 - n_2^2}$$

$$NA = n_0 \sin \theta_a = \sqrt{n_1^2 - n_2^2} \text{ or } \sin \theta_a = \sqrt{\frac{n_1^2 - n_2^2}{n_0}} \qquad (3.2)$$

we have:

$$\sin \theta_a = \sin (\theta_1)_{max}$$

$$= \left(\frac{n_1}{n_0}\right) \cos \phi_c$$

We know that:

$$\theta_c = \frac{n_2}{n_1}$$

If surrounding medium is air, $n_0 = 1$ and $NA = \sin \theta_a = \sqrt{n_1^2 - n_2^2}$ or $\theta_a = \sin^{-1} \sqrt{n_1^2 - n_2^2}$

Sometimes the NA is expressed in terms of relative refractive index Δ, between core and cladding. Δ is also called as index difference:

$$\Delta = \frac{n_1 - n_2}{n_1}$$

$$n_1^2 - n_2^2 = (n_1 + n_2)(n_1 - n_2)$$

$$= \left(\frac{n_1 + n_2}{2}\right)\left(\frac{n_1 - n_2}{n_1}\right)2n_1 \quad \left(\because \frac{n_1 + n_2}{2} \approx n_1\right)$$

$$= 2n_1^2 \cdot \Delta$$

Thus,
$$NA = n_1\sqrt{2\Delta} = \sqrt{n_1^2 - n_2^2} \qquad (3.3)$$

The derivation of the above relation [Eq. (3.3)] is based on the approximation, $n_1 \approx n_2$ which is valid when Δ is very small. This approximation is generally valid for all practical fibers as Δ is generally 0.01 or less.

We may note that all rays having entrance angles less than $\theta_{0\,max}$ [Fig. 3.6(b)] will be totally internally reflected at the core-cladding interface and guided along the fiber. On the other hand, the rays making an angle larger than $\theta_{0\,max}$ at the entrance would be refracted out into the cladding region and lost. Obviously, $\theta_{0\,max}$ is the maximum angle to the fiber axis at which light may enter the fiber and propagate subsequently. This is illustrated in Fig. 3.6(a). This conical half angle $\theta_b = \theta_{0\,max}$ is referred to as maximum acceptance angle or simply acceptance angle of the optical fiber. One can write the acceptance angle for a step index fiber as

$$\theta_{max} = \sin^{-1}\left(\frac{NA}{n_0}\right) = \sin^{-1}\frac{\sqrt{n_1^2 - n_2^2}}{n_0} \qquad (3.3a)$$

When light enters the fiber from air, i.e. $n_0 = 1$, Eq. (3.3a) reads as

$$(\theta_{max})_{air} = \sin^{-1}(NA) = \sin^{-1}\sqrt{n_1^2 - n_2^2} \qquad (3.3b)$$

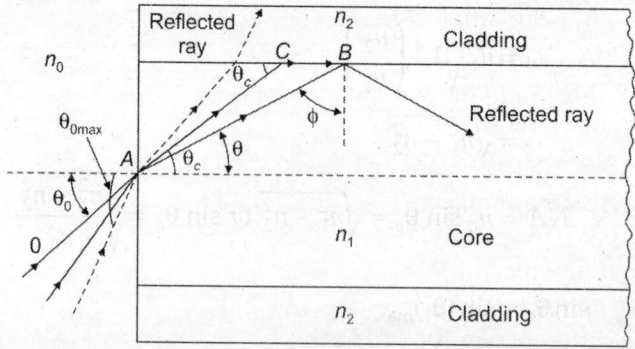

Fig. 3.6(b): Meridional ray path through a step index fiber

However, in actual practice, the light enters the fiber cone from another medium (usually termed as *index matching fluid*) having nearly the same refractive index. This reduces the Fresnel's loss at the entrance.

Since $\theta_{0\,max}$ is very small and hence one may approximate

$$\sin\theta_{0\,max} \approx \theta_{0max} = \sqrt{n_1^2 - n_2^2} \qquad (3.3c)$$

For small value of $\theta_{0\,max}$, one can approximate the maximum solid angle of the fiber as

$$\Omega = \int_0^{\theta_{0max}} \int_0^{2\pi} \sin\theta_0 d\theta_0 d\phi \approx 2\pi \int_0^{\theta_{0max}} \theta_0 d\theta_0$$

$$= \pi\theta_c^2 \max = \pi(n_1^2 - n_2^2) \tag{3.3d}$$

Clearly, NA represents a figure of merit used to find the light gathering capability of a fibre. Higher the NA, higher is θ_a and higher the amount of light coupled to the fiber. Obviously, NA is a measure of the ability of the fiber to accept light for transmission. NA is effectively depending only on the refractive indices of the core and cladding of materials and is not a function of fiber dimension.

NA is a *dimension-less quantity* lying typically between 0.14 and 0.50 depending on the index difference between the core and the cladding. The maximum value of NA for step index fiber occure for air cladding, i.e. without any solid cladding, which can be determined from Fig. 3.7.

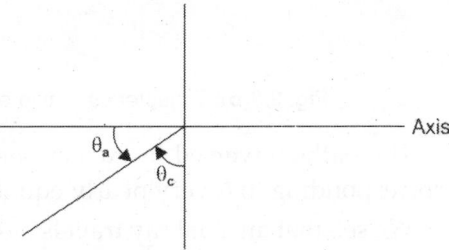

Fig. 3.7: Acceptance angle for air cladding

The plastic fibers usually have a large difference between the refractive index of the core and that of cladding. As a result, plastic fibers have a large value of NA. Further, the importance of NA is that it measures the light gathering power of the optical fiber from a source, e.g. the light coupled from an LED source to a step index fiber is proportional to the square of the NA. This clearly reveals that a larger value of NA will mean a larger light gathering power of the fiber. Apparently one may prefer to have optical fibers with large NA. However from optical fiber communication point of view, one finds that there is an adverse consequence of using fibers with a large NA. A large NA demands for a large difference between refractive indices of the core and the cladding. However, this large difference in refractive index value results in large *intermodal dispersion* which severely restricts the bandwidth of transmission.

For air cladding:

Acceptance angle, $\theta_a = 90° - \theta_c$

$$NA = \sin\theta_a = \sin(90° - \theta_c) \tag{3.4}$$

Acceptance angle θ_a for grade index fibre is given as:

$$NA = \sin\theta_c \tag{3.5}$$

Variation of NA with acceptance angle (θ_a) is shown in Fig. 3.8(a). We may note that:

(i) The larger the diameter of the core, the larger is the acceptance angle.

(ii) The larger the difference in the refractive indices of the core and cladding, the large is the acceptance angle.

(iii) If $\theta_1 > (\theta_1)_{max}$ (or $\theta_1 > \theta_0$), the ray refracts through the cladding and the corresponding optical signal is lost.

So far, we have considered only the propagation of a single ray of light. However, a pulse

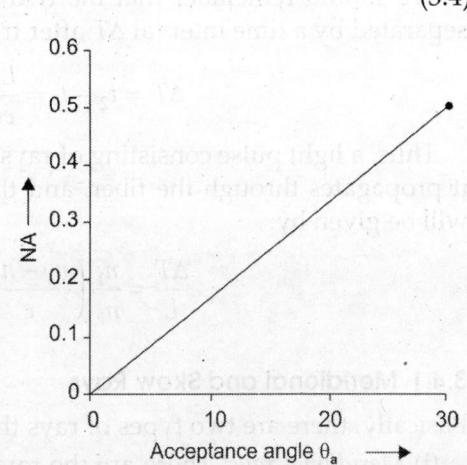

Fig. 3.8(a): Variation of NA with acceptance angle

of light consists of several rays, which may propagate at all values of α [Fig. 3.8(b)], varying from 0 to α_m.

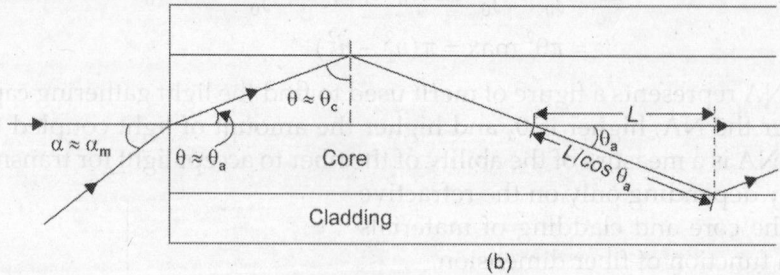

Fig. 3.8(b): Trajectories of two extreme rays inside the core of a step-index fiber

The paths traversed by two extreme rays, one corresponding to α = 0 and other ray corresponding to α very nearly equal to (but less than) α_m, are shown in Fig. 3.8(b).

We see that an axial ray travels a distance L inside the core of index n_1 with velocity v in time:

$$t_1 = \frac{L}{v} = \frac{ln_1}{c}$$

where $n_1 = c/v$, c is velocity of light.

The most oblique ray corresponding to $\alpha \approx \alpha_m$ will cover the same length of fiber (axial length L, but actual distance $L/\cos\theta_a$) in time t_2 given by:

$$t_2 = \sin^{-1}\left(\frac{NA}{\cos\gamma}\right) = \frac{\sqrt{n_1^2 - n_2^2}}{\cos\gamma}$$

$$= \frac{Ln_1}{c\left(\dfrac{n_2}{n_1}\right)} = \frac{Ln_1^2}{cn^2}$$

We should remember that the two rays are launched at the same time, but will be separated by a time interval ΔT after travelling the length L of the fiber, given by:

$$\Delta T = t_2 - t_1 = \frac{Ln_1^2}{cn_2} - \frac{Ln_1}{c} = \frac{Ln_1}{c}\left(\frac{n_1 - n_2}{n_2}\right)$$

Thus, a light pulse consisting of rays spread over α = 0 to α = α_m will be broadened as it propagates through the fiber, and the pulse broadening per unit length of traversal will be given by:

$$\frac{\Delta T}{L} = \frac{n_1}{n_2}\left(\frac{n_1 - n_2}{c}\right) \tag{3.5}$$

3.4.1 Meridional and Skew Rays

Basically, there are two types of rays that can propagate in an optical fiber:

(i) *Meridional rays*: These are the rays confined to the meridional planes of the fiber. Meridional planes are those which contain the axis of symmetry, i.e. the fiber core axis. Since a particular meridional ray lies in a single plane and hence it is easy to

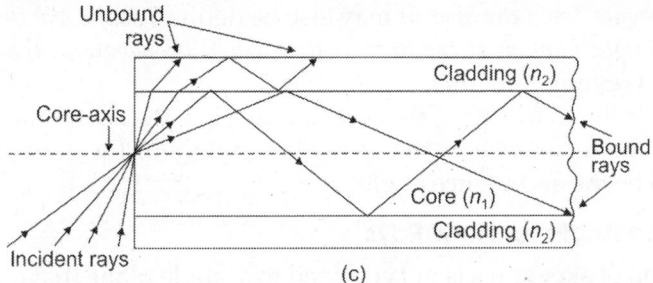

Fig. 3.8(c): Bound and unbound meridional rays in an SI optical fiber

track its path as it propagates through the fiber. Meridional rays are further divided into two categories: *bound rays* or *trapped rays* and *unbound rays*. The bound rays propagate along the fiber core following the laws of total internal reflection and unbound rays are refracted out of the core into the cladding region. Figure 3.8(c) illustrates the paths of both categories of meridional rays in a step index (SI) fiber.

(ii) *Skew rays*: These are the meridional rays that propagate through the core without passing through the fiber axis. Skews are actually larger in number as compared to meridional rays and follow a helical path along the fiber. Since these rays do not lie in the same plane and hence it is very difficult to track them. However, the skew rays constitute a large section of the total bound rays propagating through the fiber. Skew rays circulate along the core following a zig zag path and it is not easy to visualize them in two-dimensions. Figure 3.8(d) shows the helical path followed by skew rays down the fiber as well as its appearance at cross-section of the fiber. The skew rays change direction by 2γ at each reflection [Fig. 3.8(e)], where γ is the angle between the projection of ray in two dimensions and the radius of the fiber core at the point of reflection.

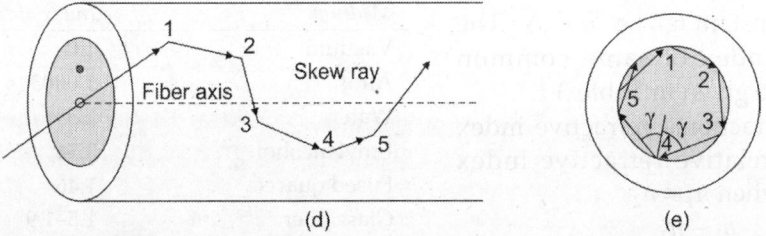

Fig. 3.8(d) and (e): The helical trajectory path followed by a skew ray (a) down the fiber (b) cross-sectional view of the fiber

Note 1: θ_a or $(\theta_1)_{max}$, i.e. acceptance angle or acceptance cone half angle [Eq. (3.2)] defines the maximum angle in which external light rays couple at air-fiber interface and travel down the fiber with a response maximum 10 dB down the peak value. Rotating the acceptance angle around the fiber axis, we get the acceptance cone of the fiber as shown in Fig. 3.9.

Note 2: *Acceptance angle is defined as the maximum angle that a ray can have relative to the axis of the fiber*

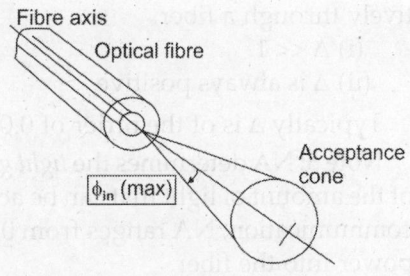

Fig. 3.9: Acceptance cone of a fiber cable

so that is may propagate down the fiber. It may also be defined as *the maximum angle from the fiber axis at which light may enter the fiber so that it will propagate in the core through total internal reflection.* We may note that:

(i) The larger is the diameter of the core, the larger is the acceptance angle.

(ii) The large the difference in the refractive indices of the core and cladding, the larger will be the acceptance angle.

3.4.2 Acceptance Angle for Skew Rays

As the propagation of skew rays is not confined to a single plane that contains the axis of symmetry of the fiber and hence it is essential to define the direction of the ray in two perpendicular planes. One can estimate the maximum acceptance angle for the skew rays in a *step-index fiber* from the following relation.

$$\sin (\theta_{0\,max})_{skew} = \frac{NA}{\cos \gamma} = \frac{\sqrt{n_1^2 - n_2^2}}{\cos \gamma}$$

or

$$(\theta_{0\,max})_{skew} = \sin^{-1}\left(\frac{NA}{\cos \gamma}\right) \qquad (3.5a)$$

where γ is the angle between the core radius and projection of the skew ray in two dimensions. The *helical path* followed by a skew ray through an optical fiber when viewed in two dimensions appears to give a change in direction by 2γ. This reveals that the skew rays are accepted by the fiber at large acceptance angle than the meridian rays depending on the value of $\cos \gamma (\leq 1)$. We may also note that a particular skew ray is characterized by the angle γ which may vary between $0°$ for meridian rays and $30°$ for skew rays entering at the core-cladding rays and giving a maximum acceptance angle of $\pi/2$. We may also note that for meridian rays, $\cos \gamma = 1$ and the acceptance angle of skew rays reduces to that for meridian rays.

Note 3: The refractive index (n) of a dielectic material depends on its dielectric constant (ε), i.e. $n = \sqrt{\varepsilon}$. The refractive index of same common materials are given in Table 3.1.

Note 4: Fractional refractive index change or relative refractive index difference when $n_1 \neq n_2$:

$$\Delta = \frac{n_1 - n_2}{n_1}$$

For the internal reflection $n_1 > n_2$. Obviously, to guide light ray effectively through a fiber:

(i) $\Delta << 1$.

(ii) Δ is always positive

Typically Δ is of the order of 0.01.

Table 3.1: Typical indices of refraction (at 589 nm)

Medium	Index of refraction (n)
Vacuum	1.0
Air	1.0003 (= 1.0)
Water	1.33
Ethyl alcohol	1.36
Fused quarts	1.46
Glass fiber	1.5–1.9
Diamond	2.0–2.42
Silicon	3.4
Gallium arsenide	3.6

Note 5: NA determines the *light gathering ability* of the fiber. This means NA is a measure of the amount of light that can be accepted by the fiber. When fibers used in short distance communication, NA ranges from 0.1 to 0.3. When NA is too small, it is difficult to launch power into the fiber.

Larger the value of NA means more is the amount of light accepted from the fiber.

NA is not a function of fiber dimensions and NA effectively depends only on refractive indices of core and cladding.

Note 6: Decibels (dB): The relative power level between two points along a fiber-optic communication link is measured in decibels (dB). For a particular wavelength λ, if P_0 is the power launched at one end of the link and P is the power received at the other end, then the efficiency (η) of transmission of the link is:

$$\eta = P/P_0$$

When the measure P and P_0 both in the same units, then P/P_0 ratio is expressed in decibels as:

$$dB = 10 \log_{10} (P/P_0)$$

We may note that there is always some loss in the communication link. This means that P/P_0 is always less than 1 and $\log_{10} (P/P_0)$ is always negative.

In order to make absolute measurements, P_0 is assigned a reference value, normally 1 mW. The value of power (say, P) relative to P_0 (= 1 mW) is denoted by dB_m. Obviously:

$$dB_m = 10 \log_{10} \frac{P\,(mW)}{P_0\,(1mW)} = 10 \log_{10} P \tag{3.6}$$

Note 7: To prevent energy losses via absorption and scattering, the cladding should be at least a few wavelengths thick. One can see that a typical value for n_2/n_1 is 0.09. For this value, one finds the critical angle as 0.142 radius or 8.11°. Thus, rays travelling at an angle less than 8.11° relative to the reference axis will be totally internally reflected and guided by the fiber. Higher angle rays will enter the cladding and be lost due to high levels of scattering and absorption.

We may note that dielectric cladding on glass core reduces scattering loss, protects core from absorbing external optical disturbances and provides mechanical strength to main core glass fiber. Sometimes, there is buffer coating over cladding which adds further strength to main fiber and protects it from mechanical vibrations and impact.

If ray AB is rotated around the fiber axis keeping θ_a same, it describes a conical surface as shown in Fig. 3.10. Now only those rays that are funneled into the fiber within this cone having a full angle $2\theta_a$ will only be total internally reflected and thus confined within the fiber propagation, i.e. only rays within the cone are accepted. Therefore, the cone is called acceptance cone. Light incident at an angle beyond θ_a will be refracted though the cladding and the corresponding optical energy is lost.

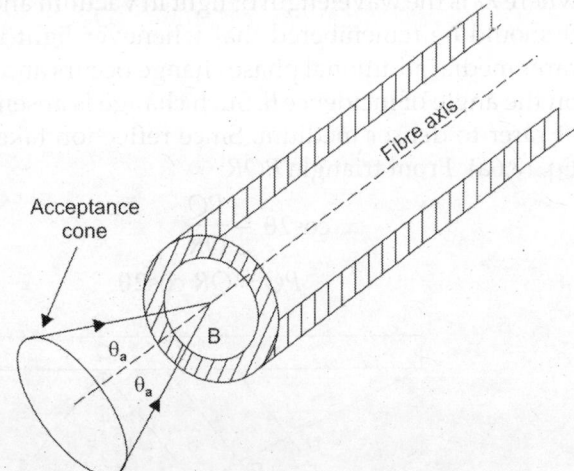

Fig. 3.10: Conical surface described by a ray due to rotation around the fiber axis

3.5 MODES OF PROPAGATION: V-PARAMETER

Light transmitted through one end of the fiber propagate down the fiber in the form of transverse magnetic (TM) and transverse electric (TE) modes. Let us first understand

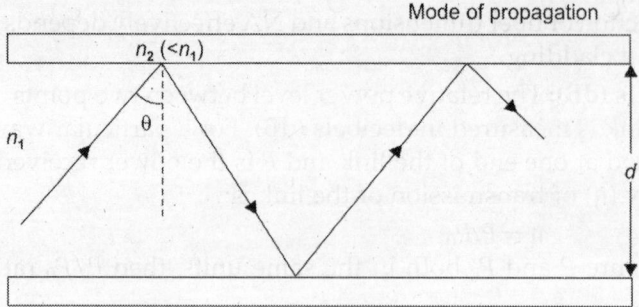

Fig. 3.11: Path of a light ray down a planar dielectric waveguide that results when the angle of incidence at the boundary is $\theta_1 > \theta_c$

how the modes are formed. A ray of transmitted light propagates down the fiber as shown in Fig. 3.11.

Due to the total internal reflection provided the angle of incidence at the core–cladding interface is greater than the critical angle ($\theta > \theta_c$). A ray indicated in reality represents infinite number of such parallel rays, all are very close to each other since the beam transmitted has some cross-section.

If a line is drawn normally as shown in Fig. 3.12(a), it represents plane wavefront and all points along the same wavefront must be in phase with each other. The PQ after reflection at Q travels to R and then travels parallel to PQ from R, i.e. $UTPR$ represents a plane wavefront and, hence, the points P and R must be in phase with each other. If they are out of phase with each other, destructive interference takes place and propagation is not possible. Now, moving from P to R along the ray the phase change is given by:

$$(PQ + QR)\frac{2\pi n_1}{\lambda_0} - 2\psi \tag{3.6a}$$

where λ_0 is the wavelength of light in vacuum and ψ is the phase change due to reflection. It should be remembered that whenever light is reflected at the interface of denser to rarer media, additional phase change occurs and the magnitude of the change ψ depends on the angle of incidence θ. Such change is absent if reflection takes place at the interface of rarer to denser medium. Since reflection takes place both at Q and R, 2ψ appears in Eq. (3.6a). From triangle PQR:

$$\cos 2\theta = \frac{PQ}{QR}$$

$$PQ = QR \cos 2\theta$$

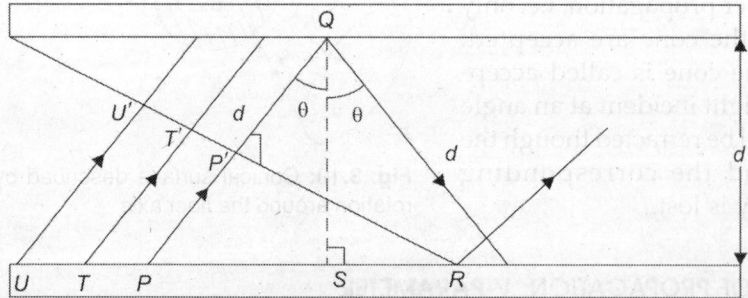

Fig. 3.12(a): Ray paths having the same internal angle θ within a planar waveguide. A wavefront is shown connecting the points UTPR must, therefore, have the same phase

or $\qquad PQ + QR = QR(1 + \cos^2\theta)$

$\therefore \qquad\qquad\qquad\quad = 2QR\cos^2\theta$

From triangle QSR: $\cos\theta = \dfrac{QS}{QR}$

$$QS = PQ\cos\theta = d\cos\theta$$

$\therefore \qquad PQ + QR = 2d\cos\theta$

Hence, Eq. (3.6a) can be written as:

$$\text{Phase change} = \frac{4\pi n_1 d\cos\theta}{\lambda_0} - 2\psi = 2\pi m$$

or $$\frac{2\pi n_1 d\cos\theta}{\lambda_0} - \psi = 4\pi m \qquad (3.6b)$$

where m is an integer.

For each value of m, there will be a corresponding value of θ, i.e. θ_a. Rearranging Eq. (3.6b), we have:

$$\cos\theta_a = \frac{(m\pi + \psi)\lambda_0}{2\pi d\, n_1} \qquad (3.7)$$

We may note that it is not possible to obtain an explicit expression for θ in terms of m (m can have only few specific integer values, since θ_a can take values in the range θ_c to $\pi/2$.)

Now, rearranging Eq. (3.6b), one obtains:

$$m = \frac{2d\, n_1 \cos\theta_a}{\lambda_0} - \frac{\psi}{\pi} \qquad (3.8)$$

Further, we know that $\sin\theta_c = n_2/n_1$. Since $\theta_a \geq \theta_c$ to maintain total internal reflection (TIR) condition:

$$\sin\theta_a \geq \frac{n_2}{n_1}$$

and $$\cos\theta_a = \sqrt{(1 - \sin^2\theta_a)}$$

$$\leq \sqrt{\left(1 - \frac{n_2^2}{n_1^2}\right)}$$

$$\leq \sqrt{\frac{n_1^2 - n_2^2}{n_1}}$$

Now, one can write Eq. (3.8) as:

$$m \leq \frac{2dn_1}{\lambda_0}\frac{\sqrt{n_1^2 - n_2^2}}{n_1} - \frac{\psi}{\pi} \qquad (3.9)$$

or $$m \leq \frac{2V}{\pi} - \frac{\theta}{\pi} \qquad (3.10)$$

where $$V = \frac{\pi d}{\lambda_0}\sqrt{n_1^2 - n_2^2}$$

or $$V = \frac{\pi d}{\lambda_0} NA \qquad (3.11)$$

where V is called as the *normalized frequency* or *cutoff parameter* or *V parameter*.

V parameter depends on:
  (i) Characteristics of optical fiber, and
  (ii) The wavelength of light propagating.

We see that each value of m is associated with a distinct wave pattern or mode within the waveguide. When $m > \left(\dfrac{2V}{\pi} - \dfrac{\psi}{\pi} \right)$, the condition for TIR will not be satisfied, the mode is said to be beyond "cutoff".

From Eq. (3.11), one finds that if $2V < \psi$, no mode can be propagated. However, for any value of V, one finds that it is always possible to find an angle θ such that the corresponding value of ψ is less than $2V$, consequently, at least one mode can always be propagated. In general, one finds that the light launched at the fiber and within, the acceptance cone meets the core cladding interface at an angle θ varying between θ_c and $\pi/2$. Of all the three rays only those which satisfy Eq. (3.10) alone propagate forming modes as shown in Fig. 3.12(a).

We can write Eq. (3.11) as:

$$C = \frac{2\pi r}{\lambda_0} \sqrt{n_1^2 - n_2^2} \quad (\because d = 2r) \tag{3.12}$$

where r is the radius of the core.

Eq. (3.12) can also be expressed in terms of fractional index change (Δ) as:

$$V = n_1 \sqrt{2\Delta}\, kr \tag{3.13}$$

where $k = 2\pi/\lambda_0$ is the radial wave vector.

The total number of modes can be obtained as:

$$N = \int V dV = \frac{V^2}{2}$$

$$= \frac{1}{2} \left(NA \times \frac{2\pi r}{\lambda_0} \right)^2 \tag{3.14}$$

We may note that V parameter actually determines the number of modes supported by optical fiber.

We may also note that *mode* refers to the number of paths for the light rays in the fibre cable. In single mode follows single path through core. In multimode, the light takes many paths through the core [Fig. 3.12(b)].

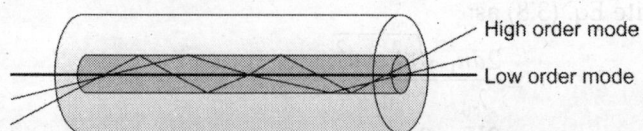

Fig. 3.12(b): Modes in optical fibers

3.6 INDEX PROFILE OR REFRACTIVE INDEX PROFILE

An *index profile* for an optical fiber is a plot of refractive index (n) drawn on horizontal axis versus the distance from the core axis drawn on the vertical axis as shown in Fig. 3.13.

The index profile of multimode fiber can be either a step index type of graded index type. The index profile of a single mode fibre is usually a step index type.

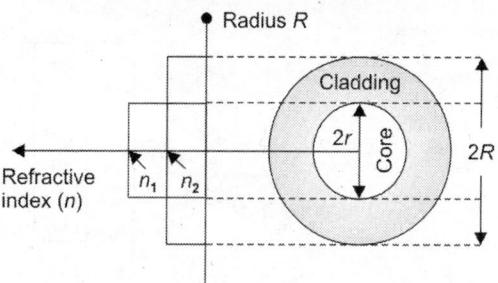

Fig. 3.13: Index profile for an optical fiber

3.7 TYPES OF OPTICAL FIBERS

There are *two basic ways of classifying* fiber optic cables. The first way is how the refractive index varies across the cross-section of the cable. The second way by its mode. The mode refers to the various paths that rays can take in passing through the fiber.

There are two basic ways of defining the index of refraction variation across a cable, i.e. their step index and graded index. Step index refers to the fact that there is a sharply defined step in the index of refraction (n) where the fiber core and the cladding interface. It means that the core has one constant refractive index n_1 while the cladding has another constant refractive index n_2. In other type of cable that has a graded index, the refractive index of core is not constant. Instead, the refractive index varies smoothly and continuously over the diameter of the core. As we get closer to the centre of the core, the refractive index gradually increases, reaching a maximum at the centre of the core and declining as the other outer edge of the core is reached. The refractive index of the cladding is constant.

Each type of optical fiber cable is classified by one of these methods of *rating*, i.e. the *index* or *mode*. In practice, there are three commonly used types of fiber optic cable:

(a) Single mode step index fiber (SMF)
(b) Multimode step index fiber (MMF)
(c) Multimode graded index fiber (GRIN)

(a) Single Mode Step Index Fiber (SMF)

A single mode fiber has a *core material of uniform refractive index* value. Similarly, cladding also has a material of uniform index but of lesser value. This result in a sudden increase in the value of refractive index profile takes the shape of a step. The diameter value of core is about 2 μm to 15 μm and external diameter of cladding is 60 μm to 70 μm.

Because of its narrow core, it can guide just a *single mode* as shown in Fig. 3.14. This is why, it is called *single mode fiber*.

The refractive index profile for SMF makes a step change at the core-cladding interface. One may define the refractive index as:

$$n(r) = n_1 \text{ for } r < a \text{ (core)}$$
$$n_2 \text{ for } r \geq \text{ (cladding)}$$

where r is the distance from the center of core along the radius, a is the core radius and n_1 core refractive index and n_2 the cladding refractive index.

Single mode fibres are the most extensively used ones and they constitute 80% of all the fibers that are manufactured world today. They need lasers as the source of light. Though less expensive, it is very difficult to splice them. They find particular application in submarine cable system.

(b) Multimode Step Index Fiber (MMF)

The geometry of a multimode step index fiber is shown in Fig. 3.15. Its construction is similar to that of the single mode step index fiber, but differs in its core that has a much

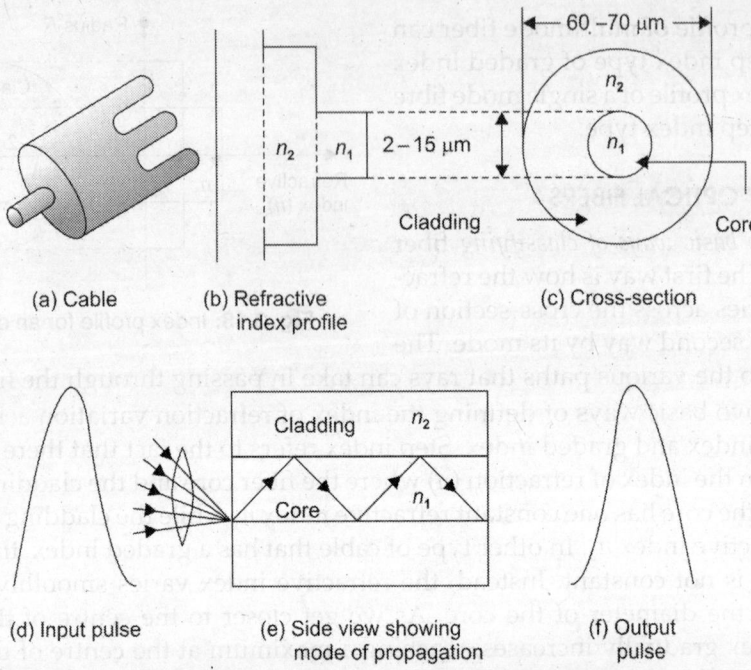

(a) Cable   (b) Refractive index profile   (c) Cross-section

(d) Input pulse   (e) Side view showing mode of propagation   (f) Output pulse

Fig. 3.14: Single mode step-index fiber

larger diameter, by virtue of which it will be able to support propagation of large number of modes as shown in Fig. 3.15. Its refractive index profile is also similar to that of a single mode fiber, but with a larger plane region for the core.

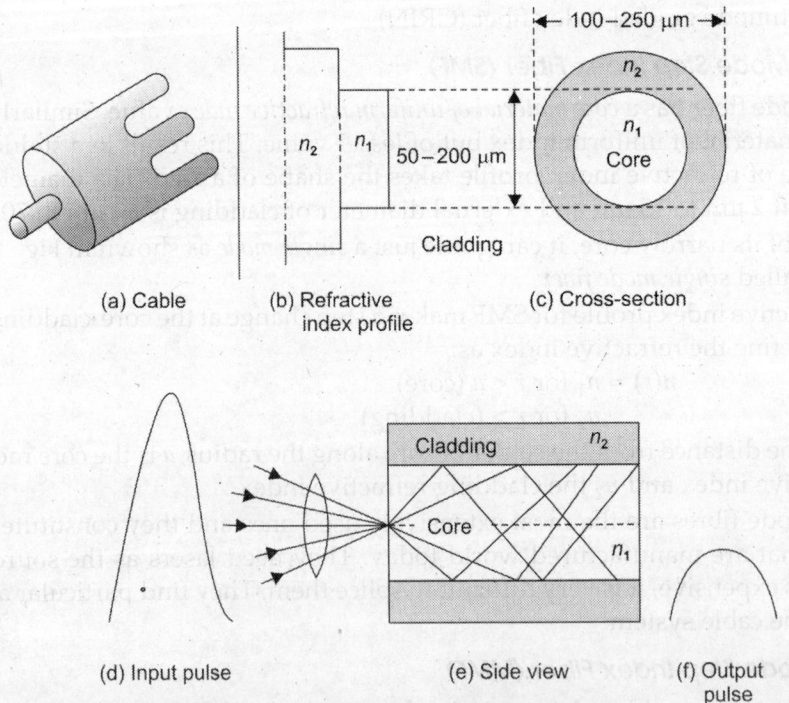

(a) Cable   (b) Refractive index profile   (c) Cross-section

(d) Input pulse   (e) Side view   (f) Output pulse

Fig. 3.15: Multimode step index fiber

The multimode step index fiber can accept either a laser or a light emitting diode (LED) as source of light. It is least expensive of all. Its typical application is in the *data links*, which has lower bandwidth requirements.

Multimode step index fibers allow the propagation of a finite number of guided modes along the channel. The number of guided modes is dependent upon the physical parameter (i.e. relative refractive index difference, core radius) of the fiber and the wavelengths of the transmitted light which are included in the normalized frequency v for the fiber. There is a cutoff value of normalized frequency v_c for guided modes below which they cannot exist. However, mode propagation does not entirely cease below cutoff. Modes may propagate as unguided or leaky modes which can travel considerable distances along the fiber. Nevertheless, it is the guided modes which are of paramount importance in optical fiber communication as these are confined to the fiber over its full length. The total number of guided modes or mode volume M_s for a step index fiber is related to the V value for the fiber by the expression

$$M_s = \frac{V^2}{2}$$ (3.15)

which allows an estimate of the number of guided modes propagating in a particular multimode step index fiber.

The total number of modes M entering the fiber depends on wavelength (λ), radius of fiber (r) and refractive indices (n_1, n_2) and is given by the relation:

$$M = \frac{2\pi^2 r^2}{\lambda^2}(n_1^2 - n_2^2) = \frac{1}{2}\left[\frac{\pi d}{\lambda} NA\right]^2$$ (3.15a)

where d is the core diameter ($d = 2r$ or $2a$). An important parameter connected with cut off conditions for fiber modes is normalized frequency V (or V-number or V-parameter) given by the relation

$$V^2 = 2M$$ (3.15b)

A model is referred to as being cutoff when it is no longer bound to the core of the fiber. V-number is a dimensionless number that determines how many modes a fiber can support. The percentage of power flow in cladding depends on M and hence V as given by the relation:

$$\frac{P_{clad}}{P} = \frac{4}{3}M^{1/2}$$ (3.15c)

Therefore, the optical power is launched into a large number of guided modes, each having different spatial field distribution, propagation constants etc. In an ideal multimode step index fiber with properties (i.e. relative index difference, core diameter) which are independent of distance, there is no mode coupling, and the optical power launched into a particular mode remains in that mode and travels independently of the power launched into the other guided modes. Also, the majority of these guided modes operates far from the cutoff and is well confined to the fiber core. Thus most of the optical power is carried in the core region and not in the cladding. The properties of the cladding (e.g. thickness) do not, therefore, signiticantly affect the propagation of these modes.

Note 1: Single mode supports only one mode (fundamental mode) of propagation for waveguiding, whereas multimode fibers may contain a few modes to hundreds of modes for propagation along the fiber.

Note 2: The core diameter of single mode fiber is extremely small (8–12 μm) as compared to that of multimode fiber which varies between 50–200 μm for Si fiber and 50–100 μm for GI fiber. Because of larger dimension, it is easier to launch power from an optical source to a multimode fiber. Single mode fibers require highly directive source for launching of power, e.g. source like injection laser diode (ILD), whereas a diffuse source like a light emitting diode (LED) can be used to launch optical power to a multimode fiber.

Note 3: A major disadvantage associated with a multimode fiber arises from *intermodal dispersion* (sometimes referred to simply as modal or mode dispersion). This causes the pulse to spread out in time, i.e. the width of the received pulse becomes larger than the time allocated to the pulse at the time of transmission. The spreading of pulse causes interference with adjacent bits causing *intersymbol interference* (ISI). ISI causes by intermodal dispersion highly restricts the rate at which we can transmit optical pulse through a multimode fiber. To minimize intermodal dispersion, multimode fiber is generally made to have a graded-index profile. However, in a single mode fiber only one mode is present and, as a result, it is free from intermodal dispersion. This is why a single mode fiber with a much larger bandwidth is attractive for use in long-haul optical communication. Further, single mode fibers are sometimes deliberately designed to have graded-index profiles, not to combat intermodal dispersion but to have additional flexibility in the design in terms of a larger allowable diameter at a given wavelength of operation.

(c) Multimode Graded Index Fiber (GRIN)

Multimode graded index fiber is also denoted as GRIN. The geometry of the GRIN multimode fiber is same as that of the MMF. Its core material has a special feature that its refractive index value decreases in the radially outward direction from the axis, and becomes equal to that of the cladding at the interface. But the refractive index of the cladding remains uniform. Its refractive index profile is shown in Fig. 3.16. Either a laser or light emitting diode (LED) can be the source for the GRIN multimode fiber. It is the

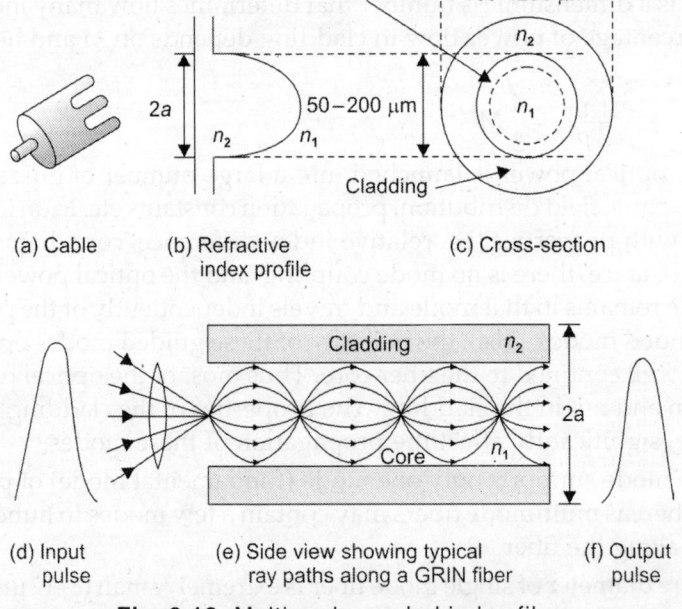

(a) Cable

(b) Refractive index profile

(c) Cross-section

(d) Input pulse

(e) Side view showing typical ray paths along a GRIN fiber

(f) Output pulse

Fig. 3.16: Multimode graded index fibre

most expensive of all. Its splicing could be done with some difficulty. Its typical application is the *telephone trunk* between central offices.

In the graded index fiber, the acceptance angle and the numerical aperture decrease with radial distance from the axis. The numerical aperture of the graded index multimode fiber is given by:

$$NA = n_1 \sqrt{2\Delta \left[1 - \left(\frac{r}{a}\right)^2\right]} \tag{3.15d}$$

where a is the total radius of the core and r is the varying radius of the core.

The index variation in these fibers may be represented as:

$$n(r) = n_1 \left[1 - 2\Delta (r/a)^\alpha\right]^{1/2} \qquad r < a \text{ (core)}$$

$$= n_1 \left[(1 - 2\Delta)^{1/2}\right] = n_2 \qquad r \geq a \text{ (cladding)}$$

where Δ is relative refractive index difference and α is the profile parameter which gives the characteristic refractive index profile of the fiber core (Fig. 3.17).

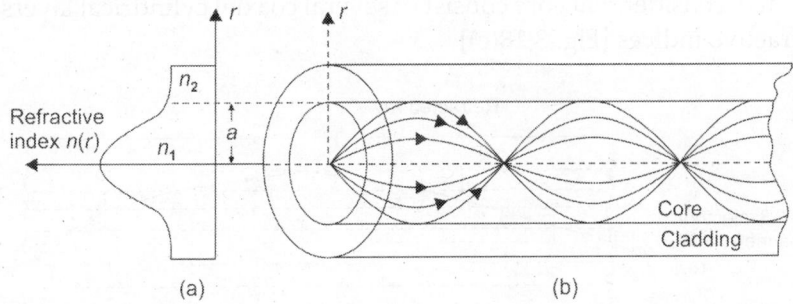

(a) (b)

Fig. 3.17: The refractive index profile and ray transmission in a multimode graded index fiber

When $\alpha = \infty$ the fiber represents a step index profile, a parabolic profile when $\alpha = 2$ and a triangular profile when $\alpha = 1$.

Fibers with $\alpha = 2$ produce propagation having a near parabolic profile (Fig. 3.18a).

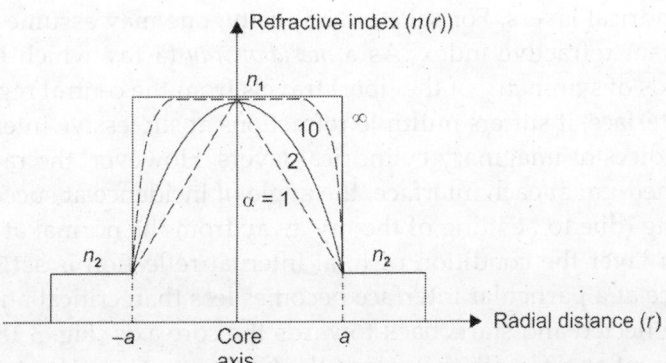

Fig. 3.18(a): Fiber refractive index profile for different values of α

The path of light rays through multimode step-index fiber, single mode step index fiber and multimode graded index fiber are shown in Fig. 3.18(b). With the help of Fig. 3.18(b), one can easily visualize the transmission of light through a multimode step index fiber by considering multiple total internal reflection episodes at different points along the core-cladding interface for all rays those make angles less than the critical angle (θ_c) with the interface. As the ray picture presented in Fig. 3.18(b) does not hold for a small geometry fiber, e.g. single mode fiber, the propagation through a single fiber is indicated in Fig. 3.18(b)(ii) by using an axial beam. Moreover, in a graded index fiber the refractive index decreases progressively along the radius of the fiber as one moves from the centre of core towards core-cladding interface. As a result, an incident ray making a certain angle with the core axis gets bent continuously as it moves towards the cladding. This is why the rays propagating through GI fibers are, therefore, indicated with the help of curved

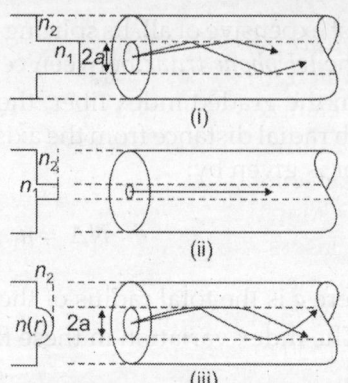

Fig. 3.18(b): The path of light rays through (i) multimode step-index fiber (ii) single mode step-index fiber and (iii) multimode graded-index fiber

ray paths [Fig. 3.18(b)(iii)]. In order to appreciate the propagation of light rays through a GI fiber, one may consider that core consist of several coaxial cylindrical layers of slightly different refractive indices [Fig. 3.18(c)].

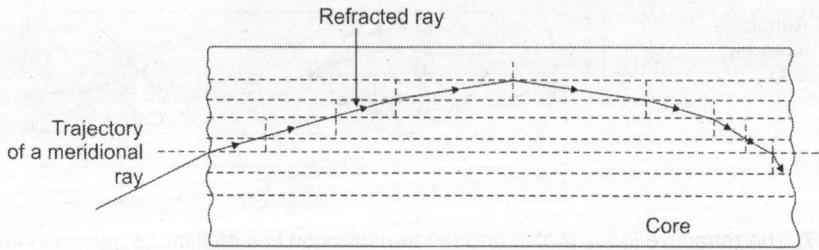

Fig. 3.18(c): The trajectory of a meridional ray through the core of a graded-index fiber approximated by several coaxial solid cylinders of different refractive indices

The refractive index of the central cylinder is the highest and it decreases progressively in the outer cylindrical layers. For sake of simplicity, one may assume each cylindrical layer have constant refractive index. As a *meridian ray* (a ray which lies in the plane containing the axis of symmetry of the fiber) travels from the central region towards the core-cladding interface, it suffers multiple refractions at successive interfaces of high to low refractive indices of imaginary cylindrical layers. However, the ray travels from a denser to rarer medium at each interface, the angle of incidence at successive interfaces goes on increasing (due to bending of the ray away from the normal at each refraction) until at a certain layer the condition of total internal reflection is satisfied. When the angle of incidence at a particular interface becomes less than critical angle, the ray gets total internally reflected and starts back towards the core axis (Fig. 3.18c). The incident ray making different angles with the axis of the GI fiber is thus reflected from different radial distance from the axis (refer to Fig. 3.17)

Multimode and Single Mode Fibers

These two types of fibers are in common use. Both these fibers are 125 microns in outside diameter.

Multimode fiber optic cable has a large diameter core that is much larger than the wavelength of light transmitted, and therefore has multiple pathways of light. Several wavelengths of light are used in the fiber core.

Multimode fiber has light travelling in the core in many rays, called modes. It has a bigger core, almost always 62.5 microns, but sometimes 50 microns and is used with LED source at wavelengths of 850 and 1300 mm for slower local area networks (LANs) and lasers at 850 and 1310 mm for network running at gigabits per second or more.

Singlemode fiber has a much smaller core, only about 9 microns, so that the light travels in only one ray. It is used for telephone and CATV with laser sources at 1300 nm and 1550 nm.

Plastic optical fiber (POF) is large core (about 1 mm) fiber that can only be used for short, low speed networks. Step index multimode was the first fiber design but is too slow for most uses, due to the dispersion caused by the different path lengths of the various modes. Step index fiber is rare. Only POF uses a step index design today.

Graded index multimode fiber uses variations in the composition of the glass in the core to compensate for the different path lengths of the modes. It offers hundreds of times more bandwidth than step index fiber, i.e. up to about 2 gigahertz over 1 km.

Singlemode fiber shrinks the core down so small that the light can only travel in one ray. This increases the bandwidth to almost infinitely. But it is particularly limited to about 100,000 gigahertz.

The size of an optic fiber matters. Fiber comes in two types, single-mode and multimode. Except for fibers used in specialty applications, singlemode fiber can be considered as one size and type. When dealing with long haul telecom or submarine cases, especially single mode fibers are used.

Multimode fibers originally came in several sizes, optimized for various networks and sources, but the data industry standardized on 62.5 core fibers. 62.5/125 fiber has a 62.5 micron core and a 125 micron cladding. Multimode fiber optic cable can be used for most general fiber applications. Multimode cable comes with two different core sizes: 50 micron or 62.5 micron. Although 50-micron fiber features a smaller core, which is the light-carrying portion of the fiber, both 62.5- and 50-micron cable feature the same glass cladding diameter of 125 microns. Both can be used in the same types of networks, although 50-micron cable is used more often for premise applications such as backbone, horizontal, and intrabuilding connections. Both types can use either LED or laser light sources.

The main difference between 50 micron and 62.5 micron cable is in bandwidth. 50 micron cable features three times the bandwidth of standard 62.5 micron cable, particularly at 850 nm. The 850 nm wavelength is becoming more important as lasers are being used more frequently as a light source.

Other differences are distance and speed. 50 micron cable provides longer link lengths and higher speeds in the 850 nm wavelength.

Fiber type	Bandwidth (minimum)	at 850 nm	at 1310 nm
50/125 μm	50 MHz/km	500 m	500 m
62.5/125 μm	160 MHz/km	220 m	500 m

Singlemode fiber optic cable has a small core and only one pathway of light. With only a single wavelength of light passing through its core, singlemode realigns the light toward the centre of the core instead of simply bouncing it off the edge of the core as with multimode. Singlemode is typically used in long-haul network connections spread out over extended areas, longer than a few miles. For example, they can be used for connections between switching offices. Singlemode cable features a 9-micron glass core.

Duplex cable consists of two fibers, usually in a zipcord (side-by-side) style. Use duplex multimode or singlemode fiber optic cable for applications that require simultaneous, bi-directional data transfer. Workstations, fiber switches and servers, fiber modems, and similar hardware require duplex cable. Duplex fiber is available in singlemode and multimode.

Simplex fiber optic cable consists of a single fiber, and is used in applications that only require one-way data transfer. For instance, an interstate trucking scale that sends the weight of the truck to a monitoring station or an oil line monitor that sends data about oil flow to a central location. Simplex fiber is available in singlemode and multi-mode.

Although it may seem from what we have discussed about total internal reflection that any ray of light can travel down the fiber, in fact, because of the wave nature of light, only certain ray directions can actually travel down the fiber. These are called the *fiber mode*. In a multimode fiber many different modes are supported by the fiber.

Because its core is so narrow that singlemode fiber can support only one mode. This is called the *lowest order mode*. Singlemode fiber has some advantages over multimode fiber.

Graded index fiber has a different core structure from single mode and multimode fiber. Whereas in a step-index fiber fiber the refractive index of the core is constant throughout the core, in a graded index fiber the value of the refractive index changes from the centre of the core onwards. It has a quadratic profile. This means that the *refractive index of the core is proportional to the square of the distance from the centre of the fiber*.

The two main types of fiber in use today are *step-index multimode* and *step-index singlemode* fiber. The step-index part of the name can be understood from Fig. 3.19 which shows the cross-section of the fiber. Step-index refers to the abrupt change in refractive index between the core and cladding materials in contrast to graded-index fibers where refractive index changes gradually over the diameter of the fiber (Fig. 3.20).

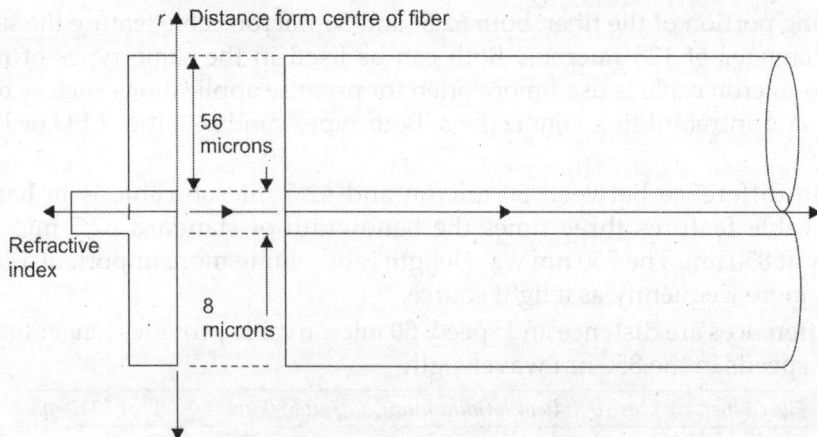

Fig. 3.19: Single mode optical fiber

Multimode fibers have cores of around 50 μm and outside diameters of about 125 μm. Singlemode fiber has a core reduced to below 10 μm to allow only one mode of propagation to be supported.

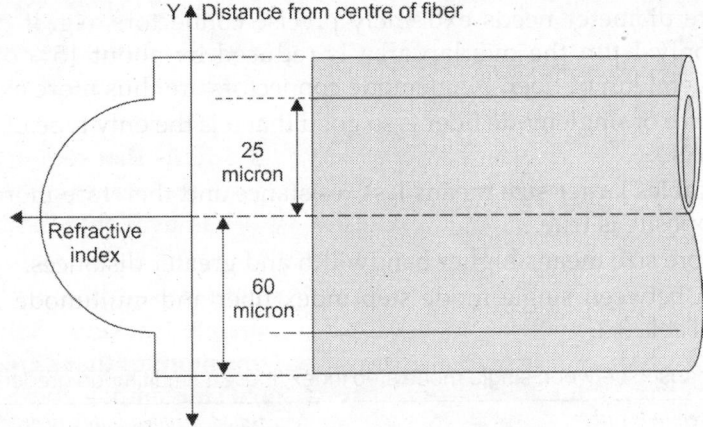

Fig. 3.20: Graded index optical fiber

Multimode fiber can capture light from the light source and pass light to the receiver with high efficiency, so can be used with low-cost light emitting diodes (LEDs). High precision connectors are not required because the large core diameter allows wide-tolerance on mechanics. Multimode modal dispersion severely limits the usable bandwidth. Multimode fibers suffer from higher losses than singlemode fibers.

Multimode fiber has found some application in *cost-sensitive areas* such as LAN but even here, it is too costly compared to copper solutions and local-loop applications. But its poor bandwidth and high-loss characteristics means that its application in high-data rate links has been very limited.

Singlemode fiber exhibits lower attenuation. Attenuation of single-mode fiber is specified at 0.37 dB/km at 1310 nm, in effect allowing a non-repeated run to be increased by a factor of two over multimode fiber. The use of singlemode fiber completely eliminates modal-dispersion which is the key cause of bandwidth limitation in multimode optical fiber, but this does not mean that it has infinite bandwidth. The dispersion left is called chromatic dispersion (so called as it is wavelength dependent). Chromatic dispersion is caused by the core material itself and is actually negative at short wavelength and moves positive at longer wavelengths. This creates a *'magic' wavelength* at which dispersion is actually zero.

This is, interestingly enough, at about 1310 nm which explains the wide use of this particular wavelength. If 1310 nm is used on a singlemode fiber, it is easy to achieve a bandwidth of several Gbit/s with losses of around 37 dB/km. Thus, in a singlemode fiber, attenuation is the limiting factor for long-distance transmission.

The sizes of these two main types of fibers are shown in Fig. 3.21.

The characteristics of singlemode fiber: Bandwidth can be in the order of many Gbit/s with very low attenuation. This allows long-distance unrepeated transmission up to around 50 km.

The small diameter (10 μm) of the core necessitates the use of expensive laser diodes to enable efficient light coupling and pass sufficient light into the fiber.

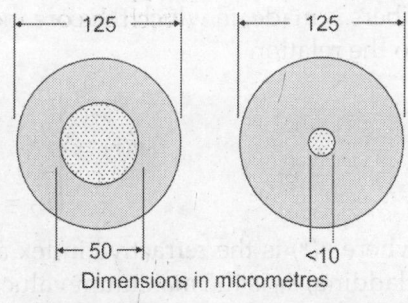

Fig. 3.21: Sizes of the two main types of fiber

The small core diameter needs extremely precise connectors, e.g. if two fibers are misaligned by only 1 μm the overlap area is reduced by about 15% or attenuation equivalent to several km of fiber. Singlemode connectors are thus more expensive.

The performance of singlemode fiber is so good that it is the only type of fiber used for long distance links.

With copper cables larger size means less resistance and therefore more current, but with fiber the opposite is true.

So a smaller core size means higher bandwidth and greater distances.

A comparison between single mode step index fiber and multimode graded index fiber is given in Table 3.2.

Table 3.2: Comparison between single mode step index fiber and multimode graded index fiber

S. No.	*Single mode step index fiber*	*Multimode graded index fiber*
1.	In single mode fibre, the diameter of core is very small. Only one mode is allowed to propagate through it. Core diameter ~ 2–15 μm, cladding diameter ~ 60–70 cm	In multimode fiber, the diameter of core is comparatively large so that more mode can propagate through it. Core diameter ~50–200 μm clading diameter ~100–250 μm
2.	Difference in refractive indices of core and cladding is usually very small	Difference in refractive indices of core and cladding is larger
3.	A very narrow source of light, i.e. either laser or LED can only be used to launch light in the fiber	Light source should not necessarily be very narrow
4.	Numerical aperture NA of single mode fiber is usually small	Numerical aperture of multimode fiber is large
5.	Refractive index of core is constant and changes abruptly at core-cladding interface	Refractive index of core decreases parabolically from the centre of core-cladding interface
6.	Single mode fiber are expensive but more efficient	Multimode fibers are comparatively cheap, but have low information carrying capability

3.8 RAY PROPAGATION IN GRADED-INDEX FIBERS

In a step-index fiber, the refractive index of the core is constant, n_1, and that of the cladding is also constant, n_2; n_1 being greater than n_2. The refractive index n is a step function of the radial distance. A pulse of light launched in such a fiber will get broadened as it propagates through it due to multipath time dispersion. Therefore, such fibers cannot be used for long-haul applications. In order to overcome this difficulty, another class of fibers is made, in which the core index is not constant but varies with radius r according to the relation

$$n(r) = \begin{cases} n_1 = n_0 \left[1 - 2\Delta \left(\dfrac{r}{a} \right)^{\alpha} \right]^{1/2} & \text{for } r \leq a \\ n_2 = n_0 \left[1 - 2\Delta \right]^{1/2} = n_c & \text{for } b \geq r \geq a \end{cases} \tag{3.16}$$

where $n(r)$ is the refractive index at radius r, a is the core radius, b is the radius of the cladding, n_0 is the maximum value of the refractive index along the axis of the core, Δ is the relative refractive index difference, and α is called the *profile parameter*. Such a fiber is called a *graded-index* (GI) fiber. For $\alpha = 1$, the index profile is triangular; for $\alpha = 2$, the profile is parabolic; and for $\alpha = \infty$, the profile is that of a Si fiber (Fig. 3.22).

For a parabolic profile, which reduces the modal dispersion considerably, the expression for NA can be obtained as follows:

$$NA = (n_1^2 - n_2^2)^{1/2}$$

$$= \left[n_0^2 \left\{ 1 - 2\Delta 1 - 2\Delta \left(\frac{r}{a} \right)^2 \right\} - n_0^2 (1 - 2\Delta) \right]^{1/2}$$

$$= n_0 \left[2\Delta \left(1 - \frac{r^2}{a^2} \right) \right]^{1/2} \qquad (3.17)$$

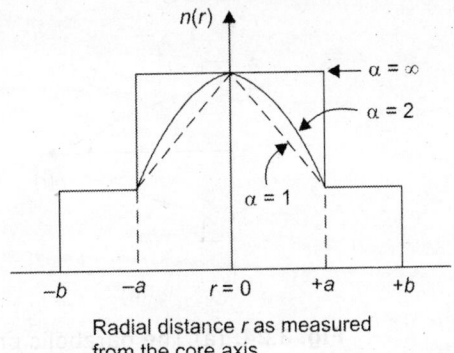

Radial distance r as measured from the core axis

Fig. 3.22: Variation of n(r) with r for different refractive index profiles

Therefore axial $NA = n_0 \sqrt{2\Delta}$. This means that the NA decreases with increasing r and becomes zero at $r = a$.

In order to apreciate ray propagation through a GI fiber, let us first visualize the core of this fiber as having been made up of several coaxial cylindrical layers (Fig. 3.23).

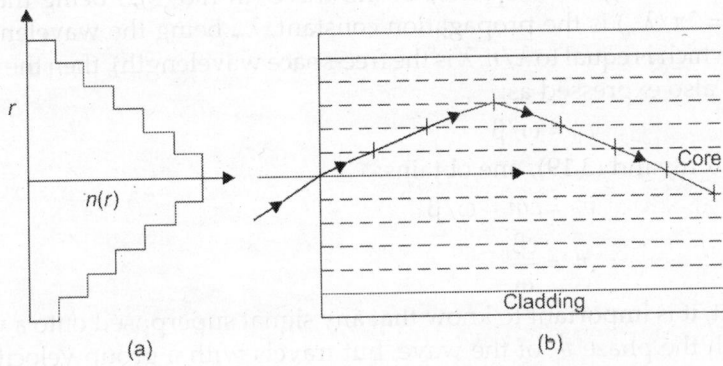

Fig. 3.23: (a) Variation of n with r (b) ray traversal through different layers of the core

The refractive index of the central cylinder is the highest, and it goes on decreasing in the successive cylindrical layers. Thus, the meridional ray shown takes on a curved path, as it suffers multiple refractions at the successive interfaces of high to low refractive indices. The angle of incidence for this ray goes on increasing until the condition for total internal reflection is met; the ray then travels back towards the core axis. On the other hand, the axial ray travels uninterrupted.

In this configuration, the multipath time dispersion will be less than that in Si fibers. This is because the rays near the core axis have to travel shorter paths compared to those near the core-cladding interface. However, the velocity of the rays near the axis will be less than that of the meridional rays because the former have to travel through a region of high refractive index ($v = c/n$). Thus, both the rays will reach the other end of the fiber almost simultaneously, thereby reducing the multipath dispersion. If the refractive index profile is such that the time taken for the axial and the most oblique ray is same, the multipath dispersion will be zero. In practice, a parabolic profile ($\alpha = 2$), (Fig. 3.24) reduces this type of dispersion considerably.

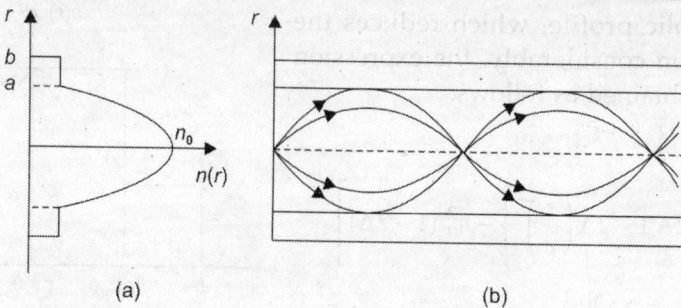

Fig. 3.24: (a) The parabolic profile of a GI fiber (b) ray path in such a fiber

3.9 EFFECT OF MATERIAL DISPERSION

The refractive index n of any transparent medium is given by $n = c/v$, where c is the velocity of light in vacuum and v is its velocity in the medium. In terms of wave theory, v is called the *phase velocity* v_p of the wave in the medium. Thus, we have:

$$v = v_p = c/n \tag{3.18}$$

If $\omega(= 2\pi f)$ is the angular frequency of the wave (in rad/s), f being the frequency in hertz, and β ($= 2\pi/\lambda_m$) is the propagation constant, λ_m being the wavelength of light in the medium (which is equal to λ/n; λ is the free-space wavelength), then the phase velocity of the wave is also expressed as:

$$v_p = \omega/\beta \tag{3.19}$$

Using Eqs (3.18) and (3.19), one obtains:

$$v_p = c/n = \omega/\beta$$

or

$$n = \frac{c\beta}{\omega} \tag{3.20}$$

At this point, it is important to know that any signal superposed onto a wave does not propagate with the phase v_p of the wave, but travels with a group velocity v_g given by the following expression:

$$v_g = \frac{d\omega}{d\beta} = \frac{1}{d\beta/d\omega} \tag{3.21}$$

In a nondispersive medium, v_p and v_g are same, as v_p is independent of the frequency ω; but in a dispersive medium, where v_p is a function of ω:

$$v_g = \frac{1}{d\beta/d\omega} = \frac{v_p}{1 - (\omega/v_p)(dv_p/d\omega)} \tag{3.22}$$

Thus a signal, which is normally a light pulse, will travel through a dispersive medium (e.g., the core of the optical fiber) with speed v_g. Therefore, for such a pulse, we may define a group index n_g such that:

$$n_g = c/v_g \tag{3.23}$$

Let us substitute for v_g from Eq. (3.21) in Eq. (3.23) to get:

$$n_g = c\frac{d\beta}{d\omega} = c\frac{d}{d\omega}\left(\frac{\omega n}{c}\right) = \frac{d}{d\omega}(n\omega)$$

$$= n + \omega\frac{dn}{d\omega} \tag{3.24}$$

This is an *important expression, relating the group index* n_x *with the ordinary refractive index or the phase index n.*

Since
$$\frac{dn}{d\omega} = \frac{dn}{d\lambda} = \frac{d\lambda}{d\omega}$$

and
$$\omega = \frac{2\pi c}{\lambda}$$

$$\frac{d\omega}{d\lambda} = -\frac{2\pi c}{\lambda^2}$$

We have from Eq. (3.24):

$$n_g = n + \frac{2\pi c}{\lambda}\frac{dn}{d\lambda}\left(-\frac{\lambda^2}{2\pi c}\right) = n - \lambda\frac{dn}{d\lambda} \tag{3.25}$$

Thus
$$v_g = \frac{c}{n_g} = \frac{c}{(n - \lambda\, dn/d\lambda)} \tag{3.26}$$

Obviously, a light pulse, therefore, will travel through the core of an optical fiber of length L in time t given by:

$$t = \frac{L}{v_g} = \left[n - \lambda\frac{dn}{d\lambda}\right]\frac{L}{c} \tag{3.27}$$

If the spectrum of the light source has a spread of wavelength $\Delta\lambda$ about λ and if the medium of the core is dispersive, the pulse will spread out as it propagates and will arrive at the other end of length L, over a spread of time Δt. If $\Delta\lambda$ is much smaller than the central wavelength λ, we can write:

$$\Delta t = \frac{dt}{d\lambda}\Delta\lambda = \frac{L}{c}\left[\frac{dn}{d\lambda} - \frac{dn}{d\lambda} - \lambda\frac{d^2n}{d\lambda^2}\right]\Delta\lambda$$

$$= -\frac{L}{c}\lambda\frac{d^2n}{d\lambda^2}\Delta\lambda \tag{3.28}$$

If $\Delta\lambda$ is the full width at half maximum (FWHM) of the peak spectral power of the optical source at λ, then its relative spectral width γ is given by:

$$\gamma = \left|\frac{\Delta\lambda}{\lambda}\right| \tag{3.29}$$

If an impulse of negligible width is launched into the fiber, then Δt will be the half power width τ of the output (or the broadened pulse). Thus, the pulse broadening due to material dispersion may be given by:

$$\tau = \frac{L}{c}\gamma\left|\lambda^2\frac{d^2n}{d\lambda^2}\right|$$

or
$$\frac{\tau}{L} = \frac{\gamma}{c}\left|\lambda^2\frac{d^2n}{d\lambda^2}\right| \tag{3.30}$$

The material dispersion of optical fibers is quoted in terms of the material dispersion parameter D_m given by:

$$D_m = \frac{1}{L}\frac{\tau}{\Delta\lambda} = \frac{\lambda}{c}\left|\frac{d^2n}{d\lambda^2}\right| \tag{3.31}$$

D_m has the units of ps nm^{-1} km^{-1}. Variation of D_m with wavelength (λ) for pure silica is shown in Fig. 3.25. We may note that majority of fibers are manufactured using silica as the host material.

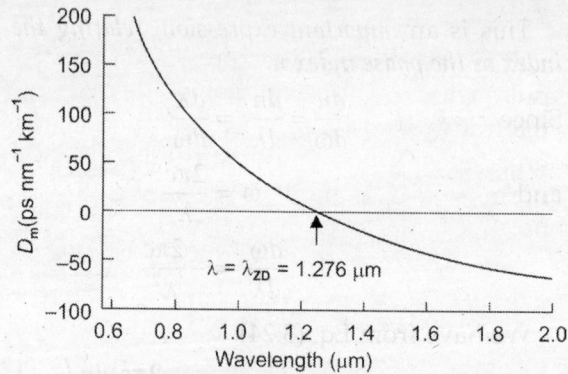

Fig. 3.25: Material dispersion parameter D_m as a function of λ for pure silica

We may note that D_m changes sign at $\lambda = \lambda_{ZD} = 1.276$ µm (for pure silica). This point has been frequently referred to as the *wavelengh of zero material dispersion*. This wavelength can be changed slightly by adding other dopants to silica. Clearly, the use of an optical source with a narrow spectral width (e.g. injection laser) around λ_{ZD} would substantially reduce the pulse broadening due to material dispersion.

3.10 THE COMBINED EFFECT OF MULTIPATH AND MATERIAL DISPERSION

In a fiber-optic communication system, the optical power generated by the optical source, e.g. LED, is proportional to the input current to the transmitter. The optical power received by the detector is proportional to the power launched into and propagated by the optical fiber. This, in turn, gives rise to a proportional current at the receiver end, thus giving an overal linearity to the system.

We have alreay seen that multipath and material dispersion lead to the broadening of the pulse launched into a fiber. Thus, the received pulse represents the impulse response of the fiber. If we assume that the FWHM of the transmitted pulse is τ_0, and the impulse responses due to multipath and material dispersion lead to approximately Gaussian pulses of FWHM τ_1 and τ_2, respectively, as shown in Fig. 3.26, and that the two mechanisms are almost independent of each other, then the received pulse width at half maximum power, τ, will be given by:

$$\tau = \left[\tau_0^2 + \tau_1^2 + \tau_2^2 \right]^{1/2} \tag{3.32}$$

$$\frac{\tau}{L} = \left(\frac{\tau_0}{L} \right)^2 + \left(\frac{\tau_1}{L} \right)^2 + \left(\frac{\tau_2}{L} \right)^{1/2} \tag{3.33}$$

where L is the total length of the fiber.

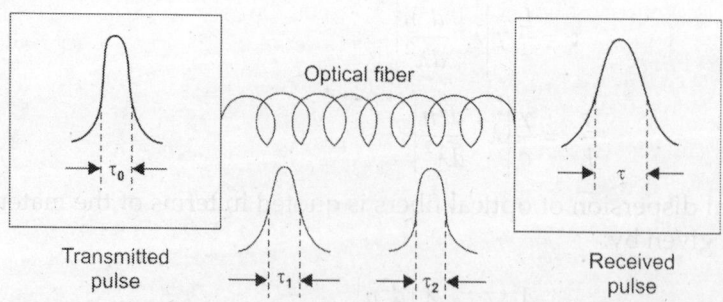

Fig. 3.26: The combined effect of multipath and material dispersion

It is also possible to express the same result in terms of the root mean square (rms) pulse widths. The calculation of the rms pulse width is given in the next section. Thus, if the transmitted pulse is Gaussian in shape and has an rms width σ_0 and this pulse is broadened by both multipath and material dispersion leading to nearly Gaussian pulses of rms width σ_1 and σ_2, respectively, then the rms width σ of the received pulse is given by:

$$\frac{\sigma}{L} = \left[\left(\frac{\sigma_0}{L}\right)^2 + \left(\frac{\sigma_1}{L}\right)^2 + \left(\frac{\sigma_2}{L}\right)^2\right]^{1/2} \qquad (3.34)$$

3.11 CALCULATION OF RMS PULSE WIDTH

The rms width σ of a pulse is defined as follows. If $p(t)$ is the power distribution in the pulse as a function of time t and the total energy in the pulse is:

$$\varepsilon = \int_{-\infty}^{\infty} p(t)\, dt \qquad (3.35)$$

then its rms width σ is given by:

$$\sigma^2 = \frac{1}{\varepsilon} \int_{-\infty}^{\infty} t^2\, p(t)\, dt - \left[\frac{1}{\varepsilon} \int_{-\infty}^{\infty} tp(t)\, dt\right]^2 \qquad (3.36)$$

3.12 ADVANTAGES OF OPTICAL FIBER

The transmission and reception of large amount of data/information at the fastest rate is a fundamental requirement of communication technology. This data may be in any form, viz. text, sound, pictures etc.

The information-carrying capacity is directly related to the bandwidth (or frequency extent) of the modulated carrier, which is generally limited to a fixed fraction of the carrier frequency. Theoretically, greater the carrier frequency, larger is the available transmission bandwidth and thus the information-carrying capacity of the system. Therefore, radio frequency communication was developed at VHF and UHF. The communication at optical frequency, 10^{14} Hz, offers an increase in the bandwidth by a factor of 10^4, over high frequency microwave transmission of 10^{10} Hz.

The invention of laser in 1960 provided a powerful coherent light source together with the possibility of modulation at high frequency. The semiconductor lasers (1962) and low loss optical fibre waveguides boosted the development of optical fiber communication in 1960s and 1970s.

The theoretical transmission loss of a silica fiber at a wavelength of 1.55 μm is 0.13 dB/km. It is limited by Rayleigh scattering and vibrational absorption of Si–O bonds. The best transmission reported for infrared fibers is 0.73 dB/km using a fluoride glass. Two major factors are associated with this; one, if the losses are less, efficiency increases and two, the spacing of repeaters also increases, which reduces cost and complexity of system. For conventional metal cables, losses are around 5 dB/km.*

The diameter of optical fiber is very small, of the order of μm. Even including protective coating, size is small compared to conventional metal cables. Due to small size and low weight, they are used in aircrafts, ships, satellites, automobiles etc. for internal communications.

The fibers are made of glass or plastic polymers, therefore, they are electrical insulators. There are no problems of short circuit, sparks, earth loop and interface, electromagnetic interferences, switching transients resulting from electromagnetic pulses, radio frequency

---

* Signal attenuation in number of decibels per unit length $\alpha_{dB} = 10 \log_{10}(P_i/P_o)/L$, where P_i is the input transmitted optical power, P_o is the output optical power and L is the fiber length

interference, susceptibility to lightning stroke, cross talk, etc. The signal transmission of optical fiber is safe because it does not radiate much and it is almost impossible to tap the signal in non-invasive manner (non-invasive means without drawing optical power from the fiber). Tapping can be immediately detected. Therefore, this type of communication is very useful in military or bank or defence or high security related communications.

The technological progress made it possible to manufacture fiber with high tensile strengths. They can be twisted or bent into small radii without damage. Hence, these cables are superior to copper cables in terms of size, weight, storage, handling, transportation and installation. The cost of manufacturing glass fiber cables is also low compared to metal cables. Due to low loss, line amplifiers or repeaters are widely separated. It reduces the cost of equipments, installation, maintenance etc. The overall cost and benefits of optical fiber communications are better than metal cable or radio wave communications.

There are some problems also. For example, fragility of bare and small size create problems in splicing (means forming permanent joints), connectors, losses in couplers, complex testing procedure, stress corrosion etc. But engineering and technological advancements are expected to overcome these problems.

3.13 SIGNAL DEGRADATION

When a light signal modulated by analogue or digital information propagates through a fiber, it is degraded at other end in the sense that power loss and shape distortions takes place in the signal. Loss or signal attenuation weakens the strength of light signal after travelling a certain distance. A repeater is required at a distance where the signal is not severely attenuated. Similarly, due to distortion, optical signal pulses (in digital communication) are broadened as they travel along the fiber. The excessive broadening may cause overlapping with neighbouring pulses, thereby, creating error ('1' may be replaced by '0' or *vice versa*) in the receiver output. Obviously, signal degradation is mainly due to two reasons: (i) attenuation (loss) and (ii) distortion (broadening of pulses).

Fiber loss and distortion depends on the material used and structural defects during fiber manufacturing. Materials used in making the fiber are glasses and plastics. The most common optically transparent glasses from which fiber is made is silica which has refractive index $n_1 = 1.458$ at 850 nm. The cladding material (having slightly lower index (n_2) is made by adding 'dopants' such as B_2O_3, GeO_2 or P_2O_5 in silica.

3.14 FIBER LOSSES

The basic mechanisms responsible for fiber losses are:

(i) *Absorption:* Absorption depends on fiber material and wavelength. Glass introduces less absorption loss as compared to plastic. Absorption of energy may be caused by atomic defects, impurity atom or basic constituent atoms of fiber material. This loss includes ultraviolet absorption, infrared absorption and ion-resonance absorption. Absorption loss due to impurities is the major source of loss in optical fiber. There are two important types of impurities: (i) the transition metal ions and hydroxyl (OH) ions. The transient metal impurities, i.e. Cu, Fe, Co, V, Cr, Ni and Mn absorb strongly in the region of interest. This means that the fiber be free from these impurities in the electronic absorption. The trapped OH^- ions in the fiber material absorb at 0.95 μm and 1.39 μm. These regions corresponds to region of interest and hence the presence of OH^- ion should be minimized and as far as possible should be kept below 0.01 part per million (ppm). There are certain wavelength ranges at which attenuation is minimum. Such a range of wavelength is called as optical window or transmission window. These windows are quite suitable for transmission of information.

(ii) *Scattering losses:* Light scattering (Rayleigh scattering) is caused by structural imperfection in the guided mode besides the fiber material. The order of losses introduced per kilometer due to scattering is 2.5 dB at 8.20 nm, 0.24 dB at 1300 nm, and 0.012 dB at 1550 nm. This reveals that loss

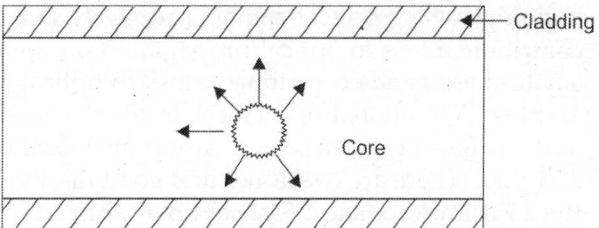

Fig. 3.27: Scattering losses

reduces with increasing wavelength. This loss arises due to microscope irregularities in material density, structural inhomogeneities or defects during manufacture process. Light is refracted by imperfection and some of it is spread out to escape through the cladding (Fig. 3.27). For Rayleigh scattering proportional to λ^{-4}, this sets a lower limit on wavelength that can be transmitted through a glass fiber to about 0.8 μm. Below this wavelength, scattering loss is quite high.

(iii) *Radiative losses:* These originate from peturbations in fiber, geometry, e.g. bends (microscopic or macroscopic) of finite radius. Bends can arise when cable turns a corner or when fiber is incorporated in cable.

(iv) *Coupling losses (splicing losses):* These losses occurs at junctions connecting source to fiber, fiber to fiber and fiber to photodetector. Losses at the junction of two fiber sections are caused mainly due to misalignment. There are four types of misalignment, namely lateral misalignment, gap displacement, angular misalignment and imperfect finish of surface.

(v) *Loss due to geometrical effects:* During manufacture and/or installation, bending (microscopic or macroscopic) causes loss of power (Fig. 3.28(a)). Due to small cracks in glass, microbending is caused. When the cracks extend to a large distance along the length of the optical fiber, microbending occurs. However, coupling can occur due to microbending but microbending obstructs more propagation.

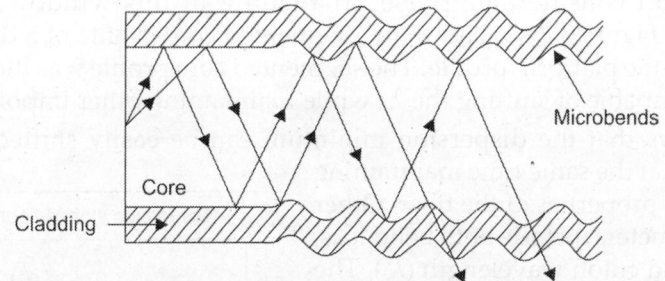

Fig. 3.28(a): Losses due to tight bending of fiber

3.14.1 Attenuation

In addition to the requirement of minimum pulse broadening during pulse propagation, minimum loss in optical power is also required. The optical fiber fabrication process minimize the introduction of common transition-metal impurities, such as iron, copper, cobalt, etc., into the glass. The important source of attenuation in fiber can be classified as due to molecular vibrational resonance, vibrational resonances of the OH ion, and Rayleigh scattering. The molecular vibrational resonance in optical fiber glasses occurs in the infrared region beyond 5 μms, but these bands have tails that extend into the region at which optical signals propagate (0.8–1.6 µms). Although small, these bands contribute a loss to optical propagation on the order of 0.5 dB/km and less. Although small, these bands contribute a loss to optical propagation on the order of 0.5 dB/km and less. Vibrational resonances in fibers can also result from the inclusion of the OH ions in the silica matrix. An important vibrational resonance of the OH ion occurs at 2.71 µms. There are overtones and combination bands at 0.95, 1.25, and 1.38 µms due to the 2.71-µm resonance. Optical fiber fabrication processes limit the amount of OH ions through proper doping procedures, and it is possible to fabricate fibers with OH ion inclusions on the order of parts per billion. The window of transmission of 0.8, 1.3 and 1.55 µm are chosen so that losses due to OH ion vibrational resonances are limited.

Rayleigh scattering of light is strongly wavelength-dependent and varies inversely with the fourth power of the wavelength. This source of optical loss results from concentration fluctuations at high temperatures that are frozen in place as the glass cools through the transformation region. One can calculate an effective loss coefficient due to Rayleigh scattering by the expression.

$$\alpha_R = \frac{8\mu^3}{3\lambda^4}(n^2 - 1)\,kTB \tag{3.37}$$

Here, B represents the isothermal compressibility of the glass, T is the effective temperture and k is Boltzman's constant. At 1550 nm, losses resulting from Rayleigh scattering are on the order of 0.13 dB/km. This window is minimum with respect to optical attenuation as it is optimized with respect to the losses resulting from Rayleigh scattering (which increase with lower wavelength). Losses in this window are as low as 0.2 dB/km, whereas in the 1310 nm window, they are on the order of 0.35 dB/km.

3.13.2 Dispersion Shifted Fiber

The attenuation of silica-based fibers is a minimum near 1.55 µms. For this reason, there is considerable interest in transmitting information at this wavelength. Also, with the recent availability of erbium-doped fiber amplifiers at 1.55 µms, this window of operation is most advantageous for long distance communication. Step-index, single-mode fibers, however, exhibit considerable pulse broadening in this window, approximately 18 ps/(nm·km). Figure 3.28(b) shows the segmented core profile of a dispersion-shifted fiber and that of the platform profile. The segmented core profile was the first dispersion-shifted profile capable of shifting the λ_0 while maintaining other important parameters.

Studies shows that the dispersion minimum can be easily shifted to the 1.55 µm window., while at the same time maintaining other important properties of the fiber. Other important parameters include both bend loss, spot size (r_0), and cutoff wavelength (λ_c). The cutoff wavelength refers to the wavelength below which multimode propagation exists. These dispersion-shifted profiles are now finding application in *transoceanic communication* and the *trunk lines*. The use of dispersion-shifted fibers with erbium-doped amplifiers requires a minimum dispersion, on the order of 0.2 ps (nm·km) because optical nonlinearities distort the signal at the zero dispersion wavelength λ_0 thus, of particular concern is the four-wave mixing.

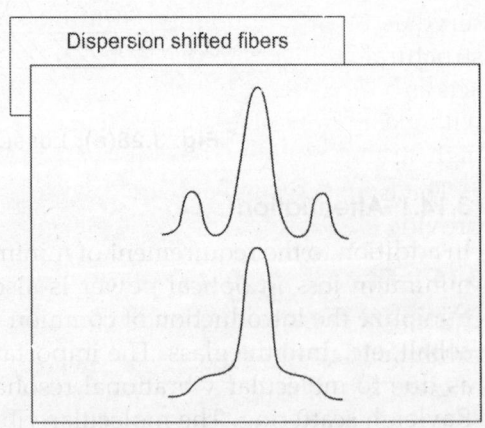

Dispersion shifted fibers

Fig. 3.28(b): Dispersion shifted profiles

Some standard optical fibers are listed in Table 3.3.

Table 3.3: Standard optical fibers

Optical fiber (type)	Cladding diameter (μm)	Core cladding (μm)	D	Applications
Single mode (8/125)	125	8	0.1% to 0.2%	(i) Long distance (ii) High data rate
Multimode (50/125)	125	50	1% to 2%	(i) Short distance (ii) Low data rate
Multimode (62.5/125)	125	62.5	1% to 2%	LAN
Multimode (100/140)	140	100	1% to 2%	LAN

3.15 OPTICAL FIBER CABLES

Where optical fibers are to be installed in a working environment and their *mechanical properties* are of prime importance. Bare glass fibers are brittle and have small sectional areas which make them susceptible to damages when employing normal transmission line handling procedures. It is, therefore, necessary to cover the fibers to improve their tensile strength and to protect them against external influences. This is done by surrounding the fiber with protective layers referred to as coating and cabling. A plastic coating with high elastic modulus is applied directly to the fiber cladding. This coated fiber is incorporated to an optical cable to increase its resistance to mechanical strain, stress and environmental conditions.

The optical cable gives:
  (i) *Fiber protection*: The optical cable protects the fiber against damage and breakage during installation and also throughout the life of the fiber.
 (ii) *Stability of the fiber* must have good stable transmission characteristic such that attenuation due to cabling is minimized.
(iii) *Cable strength*: The mechanical properties such as tension, torsion, and compression, etc. of optical cables must be similar to electrical transmission cables.
(iv) *Identification and joining of the fibers within the cable*: If the fibers are arranged in a suitable geometry, it may be possible to use multiple jointing techniques rather than jointing each fiber individually.

One or more structural members are usually included in the optical fiber cable to serve as a core foundation around which the buffered fibers may be wrapped. The structural members may also be strength member. In certain cases, a central steel wire acts as both a structural and a strength member. Structural members may be non-metallic with plastic, fiberglass. Strength members are preferred to have a high Young's modulus, high strain capability, flexibility and low weight per unit length.

The cable is usually covered with an outer plastic sheath to reduce abrasion and to provide extra protection against external mechanical effects such as crushing.

3.15.1 Fiber Strength and Durability

Optical fibers are fabricated from silica or a compound of glasses that are brittle and exhibit perfect elasticity until their breaking point is reached. The bulk material strength of glass is high and is given by the following expression:

$$S_t = \left(\frac{\gamma_p E}{4la} \right)^{1/2} \tag{3.38}$$

where S_t is the cohesive strength, γ_p is the surface energy of the material, E the Young's modulus and l_a is the atomic spacing or bond distance.

3.15.2 Fiber-Optic Connectors

The interconnection of optical components is a vital part of an optical system, having a major effect on performance. *Interconnection* between two fiber-optic cables is achieved either by *connectors* or *splices* which link the ends of the fiber cables optically and mechanically.

Connector are devices used to connect a fiber-optic cable to an optical fiber device, such as a detector, optical amplifier, optical light power meter, or link to another fiber cable. They are designed to be easily and reliably connected and disconnected. The connector create an intimate contact between the mated halves to minimise the power loss across the junction. They are appropriate for *in-door* applications.

Splices are used to permanently connect one fiber-optic cable to another. Splices are suitable for outdoor and indoor applications. Some types of splices are used to temporarily connect for *quick testing* purposes.

The key to a fiber-optic interconnection is precise alignment of the mated fiber cable cores so that the couples from one fiber, across the junction, into the other fiber. This precise alignment creates a challenge for designers. There are many applications for fiber connectors and splices in fiber systems, such as:

 (i) Connecting between a pair of fiber cables, using connectors or a splice, is an essential part of any fiber system.
 (ii) Interfacing devices to local area network.
(iii) Connecting and disconnecting fiber cables to patch panels where signals can be checked and routed in a fiber system.
(iv) Connecting and splicing may be required on short fiber cables for wiring, testing devices, and at other intermediate points between transmitters and receivers.
 (v) Dividing a fiber system into subsystems which simplifies the selection, installation, and maintenance of fiber systems.
(vi) Temporarily connecting remote mobile systems and recording equipment in many fiber systems.

3.16 FIBER FABRICATION

From the consideration of *optical wave guiding*, it is clear that a variation of refractive index inside the optical fiber (i.e. between the core and the cladding) is a fundamental necessity in the fabrication of fibers for light transmission. Hence, at least two different materials which are transparent to light over the current operating wavelength range (0.8 to 1.6 µm) are required. In practice, these materials must exhibit relatively low optical attenuation and they must, therefore, havge low intrinsic absorption and scattering losses. A number of organic and inorganic substances meet these conditions in the visible and near infrared regions of the spectrum. In order to avoid scattering losses in excess of the fundamental intrinsic losses, scattering centers such as bubbles, strains and grain boundaries must be eradicated. This limits the choice of suitable materials for the fabrication of optical fibers to either glasses or certain plastics.

In case of graded index fibers, it is essential that the refractive index of the material may be varied by suitable doping with another compatible material. Hence, these two materials should have mutual solubility over a relatively wide range of concentrations that can be only achieved in glasses and glass-like materials. Glass exhibit the best material characteristics for use in low loss optical fibers. Plastic fibers find some use in short-haul, low band width applications.

Generally, there are two methods of preparing optical glasses:
(1) Liquid phase melting techniques
(2) Vapour phase deposition methods

3.16.1 Liquid Phase Melting Techniques

In the liquid phase melting technique, the glass is processed in the molten state producing a multicomponent glass structure.

The first stage is the preparation of material powders usually in oxides or carbonates of the required constituents. These include oxides such as SiO_2, B_2O_2, Al_2O_3, and carbonates such as Na_2CO_3, $CaCO_3$ and $BaCO_3$ which will decompose into oxides during the glass melting. Very high purity is essential which is attained by fine filtration and co-precipitation, followed by solvent extraction before recrystalization and final drying in a vacuum to remove any residual OH ions.

These high purity powdered glass materials are melted to form a homogeneous, bubble free multicomponent glass.

The refractive index may be varied by either a change in the composition of the various constituents or by ion exchange when materials are in the molten phase. Communication may arise during melting from several sources, e.g. furnace environment and the crucible.

A technique for avoiding this contamination involves melting the glass directly into a radio frequency (~5 MHz) induction furnace while cooling the silica by gas or water flow.

The glass is homogenized and dried by bubbling pure gases through the melt, while protecting against any airborne dust particles, the melt is then cooled and formed into long rods of multicomponent rods.

To produce fine optical fiber waveguides, a preform is made using the rod in tube process. A rod of core glass is inserted into a tube of cladding glass and the preform is drawn in a vertical muffle furnace (Fig. 3.29). This technique is useful for the production of step index fibers with large core and cladding diameters.

Another technique suitable for the production of large core diameter step index fibers is called the *stratified melt process*. This process involves pouring a layer of cladding glass over the core glass in a platinum crucible. A bait glass rod is dipped slowly into the molten combination and slowly withdrawn giving a composite core-clad preform which may then be drawn into a fiber.

The double crucible method is used in the drawing of optical fibers.

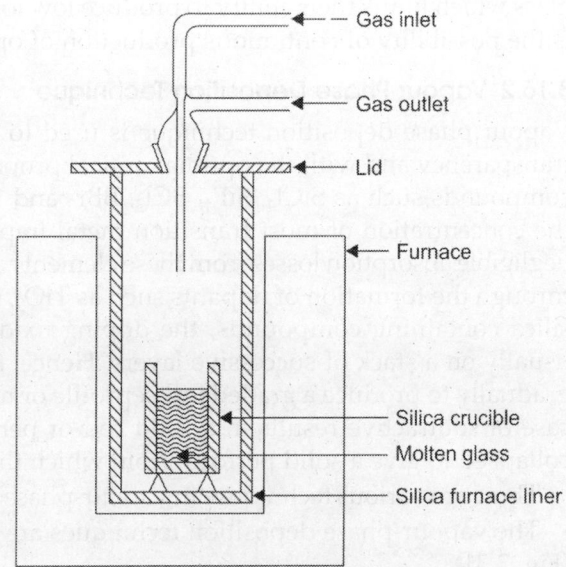

Fig. 3.29: Schematic of glass making furnace for the production of high purity glasses

The core and cladding glass in the form of separate rods is fed into two concentric platinum crucible m which is located in a muffle furnace capable of heating the crucible content to a temperature of between 800° and 1200°C. The crucibles have nozzles in their bases from which the clad fiber is drawn directly from the melt. Index grading may be achieved through the diffusion of mobile ions across the core cladding interface within the molten glass. It is possible to produce fibers with a reasonable refractive index profile using this process, hence graded index fibers produced by this technique are subsequently less dispersive than step index but do not have the bandwidth-length products of optimum profile fibers.

Using very high purity melting techniques and the *double crucible drawing method* (Fig. 3.30), step index and graded index fibers with attenuation as low as 3.4 dβ·km^{-1} and 1.1 dβ·km^{-1} respectively have been produced. Liquid-phase tech-

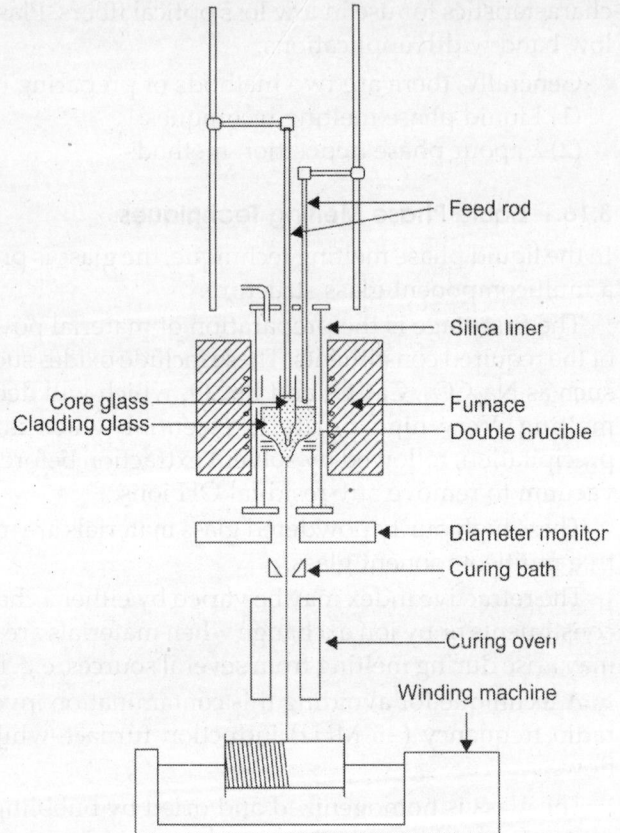

Fig. 3.30: Schematic of double crucible method for fiber drawing

niques have the inherent disadvantage of obtaining and maintaining extremely pure glass which limits their ability to produce low loss fibers, the advantage of this technique is the possibility of continuous production of optical fibers.

3.16.2 Vapour Phase Deposition Technique

Vapour phase deposition technique is used to produce silica rich gases of the highest transparency and with the optimal optical properties. The starting materials are volatile compounds such as $SiCl_4$, SiF_4, BCl_3, BBr_3 and $POCl_3$ which may be distilled to reduce the concentration of most transition metal impurities to below one part in 10^9, giving negligible absorption losses from these elements. Refractive index modification is achieved through the formation of dopants such as TiO_2, GeO_2, P_2O_5 and F. Gases mixtures of the silica containing compounds, the doping oxidation reaction where the deposition is usually on a stack of successive layers. Hence, the dopant concentration may be varied gradually to produce a graded index profile or maintained to give a step index profile. In case of subtractive results in a solid rod or perform whereas the hollow tube must be collapsed to give a solid perform from which the fiber may be drawn.

There are various techniques in vapour-phase deposition which produce low loss fiber.

The vapour-phase deposition techniques are broadly categorized into two categories (Fig. 3.31):

(1) Flame hydrolysis
(2) Chemical vapour deposition

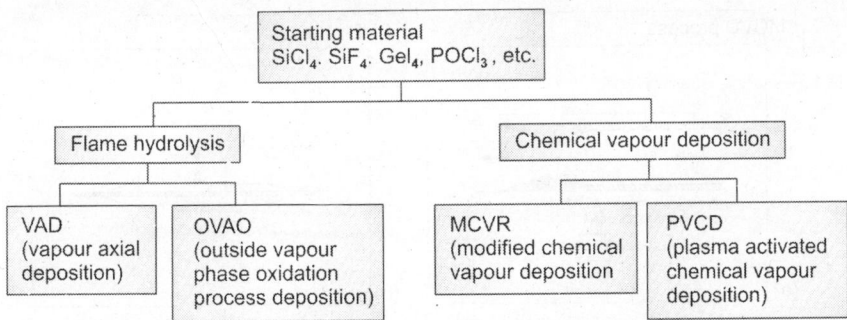

Fig. 3.31: Flame hydrolysis and chemical vapour deposition techniques

These techniques have all demonstrated relatively similar performance for the fabrication of both multimode and single mode fiber of stand step and graded index designs.

3.16.3 Modern Fiber Optic Processes

Modern fiber optic processes enable the fabrication of low-cost fibers of excellent quality. In all glass-forming processes, silica tetrachloride and the dopants, such as germanium tetrachloride, are delivered to the reaction region as vapors, where silica and germania are formed. The byproduct is chlorine gas, Cl_2. In addition to glass blank fabrication, high-speed draw (greater than one meter per second) are used to draw and coat the fiber with an organic material that protects the fiber from handling and from the environment.

There are basically three methods used to form the glass blank. The modified chemical vapor deposition process (MCVD), the outside vapor deposition process (OVD), and the vapor-axial deposition process (VAD). In the MCVD process, successive layers of SiO_2 and dopants, which include germania, phosphorous, and fluorine, are deposited on the inside of a fused silica tube by mixing the chloride vapors and oxygen at a temperature on the order of 1800°C. The temperature is maintained using a burner which traverses the outside of the tube. After the dopants are deposited, the temperature of the tube is raised, via the burner, to collapse the tube. In the OVD process, the core and cladding layers are deposited on a rotating mandrel by the flame hydrolysis process. Upon completing the deposition process, the mandrel is removed from the preform, and the preform is sintered in a furnace to form the fiber blank. The VAD process is also a flame hydrolysis process, but, in this technique, the soot is deposited axially. Figure 3.32 is a schematic of the three blank fabrication processes.

In the drawing process, the blank is fed from above into the drawing portion of the furnace while being drawn from the bottom using tractors. The fiber is then wound onto a drum while being monitored for tensile strength. The temperature during draw is on the order of 2000°C. After exciting the furnace, the fiber is coated with a UV-curable coating before winding on the drum.

3.16.4 Advanced Fiber Optic Cables

The scaling down of fiber light sources brings the benefits of fiber technology to wide range of applications. These developments have led to a surge of interest in advanced fiber cables for both military and industrial applications. Advanced fiber cables are also used for transmitting high volumes of data in communication systems over long distances for getting *very clear images*, and in building many sophisticated instruments for a variety

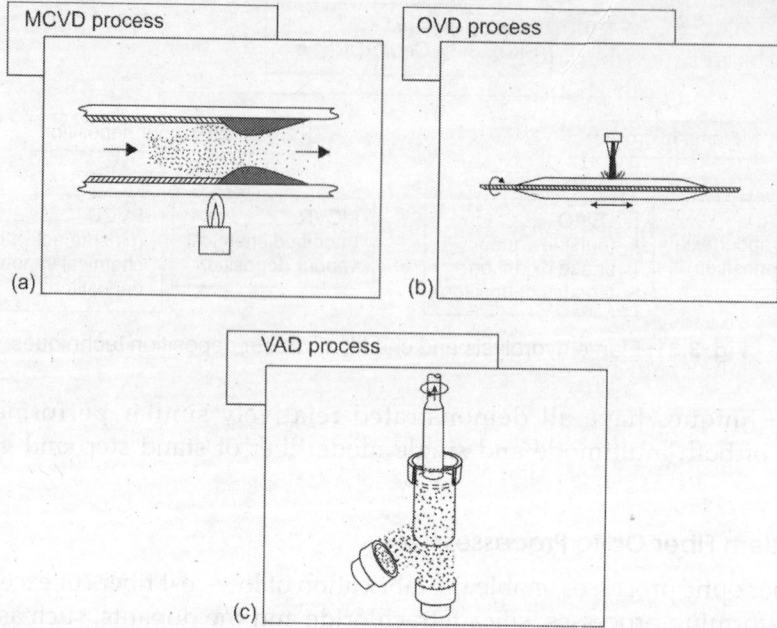

Fig. 3.32: Schematic of three blank fabrication processes: (a) MCVD; (b) OVD; (c) VAD

of applications. By creating new core designs, adding dopants to the fiber core and cladding, and developing advanced fiber optic cable technology. For example, the core of the *holey fiber* consists of many air holes acts as a single fiber. This fiber enables a high data transmission rate and capacity, and consequently, reduces the cost of network. The holey fibers have tubes or spaces in the core along the fiber's length. Some types of these advanced fiber optic cables are listed below:

   (i) Dual-core fiber for high power laser
  (ii) Fiber-Bragg gratings
 (iii) Chirped fiber Bragg gratings
 (iv) Blazed fiber Bragg gratings
  (v) Nonzero-dispersion fiber-optic cables
 (vi) Photonic crystal fiber cables
(vii) Polymer-Holey-fiber cables
(viii) Liquid crystal photonic bandgap fiber cables
 (ix) Lenses and trapped fiber cables
  (x) Bend-insensitive fiber cables
 (xi) Nanoribbon fiber optic cables

3.16.5 Fiber Optic Cables vs Copper Cables

There is still a place for fiber optic and copper cables in communication systems, but the shrinking price gap, coupled with increasing bandwidth demands, make fiber cables worth using in more situations than ever before. The customers of small and large communication providers are dispersed all over the world, and they need to send and receive lots of data. Customers require large amounts of bandwidth, and fiber cables are the only medium that can support this. Some of those customer's bandwidth requirements have been growing exponentially since the beginning of the twenty-first century. In reality, all fiber networks have a lot of room for future growth. The ultimate choice is whether to use fiber optic cables. As mentioned above, the fiber optic technology is moving forward to create high-capacity fibers with low production and installation costs and increasing bandwidths. The overall cost difference between optical fiber and twisted-pair copper cabling has been reduced. Now the choice between optical fiber and twisted-pair copper cabling has shifted in favour of the fiber cable.

Desktop computers require very high bandwidths. One way to meet this need is to wire them with fiber optic cables. However, copper cable has continued to prove more capable than expected; every time that new, higher-speed network standards appear to be forcing a move to fiber cable, someone has found a way to pump more data through the old copper cables.

Still, fiber cables can be made even more economically attractive by rethinking the way the network is physically laid out. Because fiber cable can be run for longer distance than copper, the network could be laid out without the wiring closets full of additional gear that are common in copper-based networks. Instead, fiber might run directly from the desktop back to the server or to the backbone connecting floors of a building, and the savings on the intermediate gear might more than cancel out the higher cost of installing the fiber cable. Running fiber cable to small enclosures close to users, and then covering the last short distances with copper, provides an economical alternative that minimizes the length of the twisted-pair cable used.

The increasing use of wireless networking also opens up a variation on the fiber cable network layout. Fiber can be run to a wireless access point that can then be used to serve a group. Thus, the copper cable can be eliminated altogether without actually taking fiber cable to every machine.

Many companies are removing existing copper cables and replacing them with fiber cables. When facilities are built or refurnished, fiber cables are installed. The choice between copper and fiber cables depends on several factors, including the applications being run on the network, the company's future plans, and the demands of costumers.

In particular, there are some specific situations in which fiber has advantages over copper cable. First, fiber cable is immune to electrical interference and tapping. It also carries high data capacity over long distances and is small and lightweight. When it comes to testing, fiber may still require some fairly sophisticated equipments—but the newer standards for copper cabling present the same issues.

In the end, the choice between fiber and copper cables comes down to the company's networking requirements, the needs of individual users, and the budget. Table 3.4 presents a side-by-side comparison of the important differences between fiber and copper cables.

3.17 POLARIZATION

Single-mode fibers capable of maintaining an input linear polarization are known as *polarization-preserving fibers*. These fibers employ either an elliptical core or stress rods placed 180° from each other and outside the core. The elliptical core and/or stress rods introduce a birefringence that removes the degeneracy of the orthogonally polarized mode. The *birefringence* is defined as the difference between the effective indices of the two orthogonal modes and is on the order of 10^{-4}. Figure 3.33 shows the index profile for stress rod and elliptical core polarization-maintaining fibers. Polarization-preserving fibers are not used at present in telecommunication system but rather find application in the area of fiber-optic sensors. As an example, fiber-optic gyroscopes use polarization-

Table 3.4: Fiber optic cables vs copper cables

S.No.	Fiber optic cables	Copper cables
1.	Fiber-based systems are more expensive to buy and install	Copper-based systems are less expensive to buy and install
2.	Fiber is clearly the superior technologically. Installing fiber ensures performance, as even higher speed networks will emerge in the future	Installing copper cable ensures performance for low-speed networks
3.	Carry high data capacity over long distances	Carry low data capacity over short distances
4.	Wide bandwidth	Limited bandwidth
5.	Low loss per cable length	Conventional loss per cable length
6.	Immune to electrical interference and tapping	Not immune to electrical interference and tapping
7.	Small size and lightweight	Large size and heavyweight
8.	New technology reduces installation time	Conventional technology keeps the same installation time
9.	High safety	Low safety
10.	Fast-developing technology	Steady-state developing technology

preserving fiber to prevent coupling from one polarization to the other in the gyroscope coil. Such coupling leads to inaccurate sensing and is eliminated by using only one polarization. An important parameter for these fibers is the *beat length*, defined as the wavelength divided by the birefringence (δn). This parameter describes the beating which results from the fact that the propagation speed along the fast axis is considerably larger than that along the slow axis. Highly polarized fiber exhibits beat lengths on the order of less than a centimeter. Standard fibers have

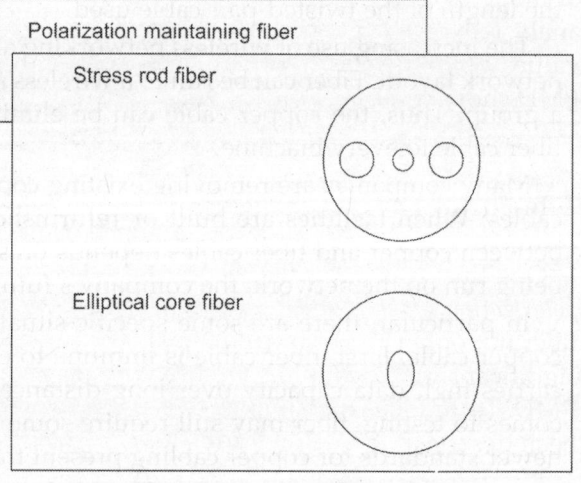

Fig. 3.33: Polarization maintaining fibers, index profiles

very small birefringence and exhibit beat lengths greater than ten meters.

The slight differences in propagation speeds for the two polarization modes in standard single-mode fiber lead to PMD. Polarization-mode dispersion for standard fiber is, typically, significantly less than $1\,\text{ps}/\sqrt{(\text{km})}$. The inverse square root length dependence results from the fact that the polarization randomly couples as the light propagates through the fiber. Transoceanic systems using optical amplifiers eliminate the need for expensive electronic regenerators. Without signal regeneration, polarization-mode dispersion can become significant over hundreds of kilometers. Also, CATV analog transmission systems can be sensitive to PMD when component polarization-dependent loss and significant laser chirping occur. In this situation, composite second-order distortion (CSO) can significantly degrade the signal.

As mentioned, small-core eccentricities, on the order of a few percent, can be the source of PMD. Significant literature exists on the effect of core ellipticity on polarization dispersion for step index fibers. However, these perturbation models predict that the polarization dispersion increases linearly with length. The square root length dependence that is experimentally observed results from random coupling of the polarization modes. In step index fibers, polarization dispersion results from both form *birefringence* and *stress birefringence*, both of which depend on core ellipticity and are approximated in the low ellipticity limit as:

$$e = \frac{A - B}{A + B} \tag{3.39}$$

and

$$E = 1 - \frac{B^2}{A^2}, \tag{3.40}$$

where A and B are the major and minor diameters. The stress birefringence depends on the expansion differences of the core and cladding, $\Delta\alpha$, which, in turn, depend on the dopant concentrations. The stress birefringence also depends on the fictive temperature T which is used to approximate a point below which the glass structure cannot change on the same time scale as the cooling rate, a stress optic coefficient C_s, and Poisson's ratio σ.

The measured value of PMD can be sensitive to fiber deployment. This is because the amount of mode coupling varies with deployment and with the environment. The effect of mode coupling on PMD is modeled using the statistics of random occurrences. This analysis explains the square root length dependence of PMD and the distribution of PMD values with changes in the environment and the fact that repeated measurements of PMD show that the observed values obey a Maxwellian process:

$$P(\Delta\tau) = \frac{2\tau}{\sqrt{2\pi}\, q^3}\, e^{-(\Delta\tau^2 / 2q^2)} \tag{3.41}$$

In Eq. (3.41), q^2 is the variance. Another aspect of the random coupling of the polarization modes is a significant wavelength dependence of PMD.

One final and important aspect of polarization modes in fibers is the *evolution of the polarization states as light propagates through a fiber*. Light linearly polarized as it enters the fiber not only evolves into circularly or elliptically polarized light, as it propagates, but significant mode coupling occurs. This complicates the analysis and measurement of PMD. Techniques to minimize the effects of mode coupling on the stability of PMD have been described in 1994 by Judy.

3.18 OPTICAL FIBER AMPLIFICATION

An important aspect of optical fiber research is rare-earth doping for amplification and lasing. Amplification in optical fiber has not only renewed interest in the materials and propagative aspects of fiber research, but it has also significantly affected the systems aspects of optical communication. Doping of fibers for optical amplification has been under study since the 1960s, when neodymium was used as a dopant. Interest in rare-earth doping was renewed in the 1980s when research scientists showed amplification in the 1.55 μm region, which coincidentally is the low-loss transmission window. The fact that erbium-doping enables amplification in the transmission window of lowest loss has attracted much interest in this aspect of optical fiber research.

In the erbium-doped fiber amplifier (in its simplest form), Fig. 3.34, an erbium-doped fiber with lengths on the order of meters and dopant levels on the order of 2 ppm, is spliced to a wavelength-dependent, fiber-optic coupler. The coupler enables one to continuously pump the erbium-doped fiber with light emitted from a high-power semiconductor laser diode at 980 or 1480 nm. Filters and optical isolators are often included

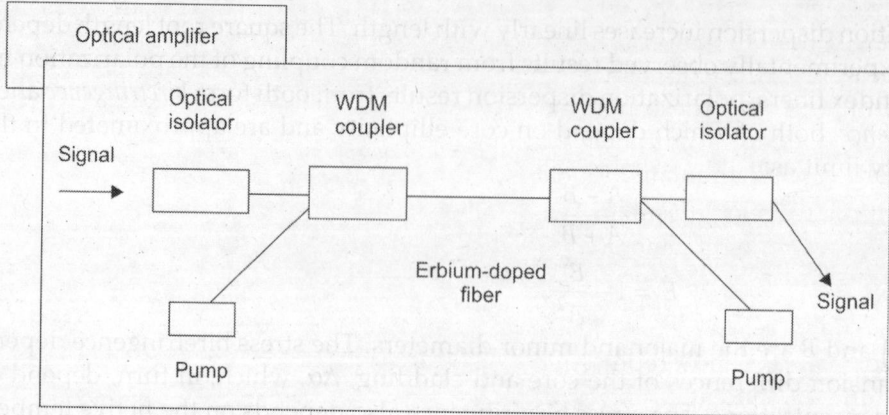

Fig. 3.34: Schematic (simple) of the optical amplifier

to minimize spontaneous emission noise and reflections. The pump light is used to excite ions from the ground state to an excited state. Signal light entering the fiber initiates stimulated emission and is coherently amplified. Years of research at many laboratories has led to the development of *erbium amplifiers*. Such technical issues as wavelength dependence of gain, gain saturation, polarization dependence and spontaneous emission, among others, have been carefully studied. Spontaneous emission occurs when ions in the excited state spontaneously relax to the ground state contributing to noise. This phenomenon in itself significantly affects the signal-to-noise ratio of an amplifier-based communication system. Another important parameter of the optical amplifier is the concentration of erbium ions. An optimum concentration of erbium ions avoids clustering which alters the excited states and results in elevating one ion to a higher state and emission to the ground of neighbouring ions.

Research in the area of rare-earth doped optical fibers is far from complete. Issues, such as multiple wavelength amplification, need to be further addressed. Research into the possibilities of using erbium-doped fibers in a lasing configuration is useful for picosecond pulse sources. Another aspect of rare-earth doping is the interest in amplification at 1.3 µm. Amplification in the low-loss transmission windows requires dopants other than erbium (praseodymium, co-doped with neodymium, for example), and also requires th use of a fluoride glass host. In a silica glass, the phonon vibrational spectrum affects the amplification process. In a fluoride-based glass, however, the phonon edge is shifted to higher frequencies, thereby, enabling reasonable amplification in the 1.3 µm window. Other issues remain, however, including the amount of gain and the wavelength dependence of the gain.

Fluoride fibers are melted at temperatures far below that of silica and, therefore, cannot be fused to silica fibers. The index is not well matched to silica and, therefore, leads to strong back reflections. More importantly, the fabrication technology of fluoride-based fibers is less advanced than that of silica. Nonetheless, interest in amplification at 1.3 µm remains because there is a huge installed base of optical fiber that is optimized for minimum pulse distortion at 1.3 µm rather than 1.55 µms.

3.19 OPTICAL NONLINEARITIES IN FIBERS

Nonlinear effects in silica fibers have been considered unimportant. However, the use of optical amplifiers and the promise of dense wavelength-division multiplexing imposes a number of limitations on the ultimate bandwidth of optical communication. Optical nonlinearities will be discussed in detail in other chapters, but it is important to mention the limitation that these nonlinearities impose on communication bit rates. These nonlinearities are stimulated Brillouin scattering, four-wave mixing, cross-phase modulation, and stimulated Raman scattering.

Multiple wavelength mixing was first observed in optical fibers by Hill in 1978. The output power of light generated at a fourth wavelength can be written as:

$$P_R(L) = \frac{1024\pi^6}{n^4 \lambda^2 c^2}(D_x)^2 \frac{P_i(0)P_j(0)P_k(0)}{A_{eff}^2} e^{-\alpha L} \frac{(1-e^{-\alpha L})^2}{\alpha^2} \eta \tag{3.42}$$

In Eq. (3.42), i, j and k represent the three input wavelengths at $Z = 0$, P_F is the power at wavelength F and at $Z = L$. A_{eff} is the effective area of the guide, α is the loss, and D_x is a degeneracy factor. The efficiency factor is given by:

$$\eta = \frac{\alpha^2}{\alpha^2(\Delta\beta)^2} 1 + \frac{4e^{-\alpha L}\sin^2(\Delta\beta L/2)}{(1-e^{-\alpha L})^2} \tag{3.43}$$

where

$$\Delta\beta = \beta(f_i) + \beta(f_j) + \beta(f_k) - \beta(f_F). \tag{3.44}$$

In Eq. (3.44), $\Delta\beta$ is the difference in propagation constants, which depends on the dispersion of the fiber. Numerical and systems studies have shown the importance of using a finite amount of dispersion to avoid generating new wavelengths while depleting the signal wavelength. Finite dispersion is also important at single channel operation very long lengths because multiple wavelength mixing occurs through the wavelengths generated with amplifiers by amplified spontaneous emission. A major impact of four-wave mixing is that it forces designers to operate their signal wavelength away from a dispersion zero. Over long distances, this require chromatic or dispersion compensation.

Brillouin scattering is the interaction of light with acoustical vibrations in fiber. The signal or carrier wave is shifted to longer wavelengths (Stoke's shift) with the simultaneous emission of an acoustical phonon. The amount of power generated can be characterized with an exponential gain coefficient, g_B:

$$g_B = 4 \times 10^{-9} \text{ cm/W}. \tag{3.45}$$

The gain coefficient enables one to calculate the amount of stimulated *Brillouin scattering* with length as a function of incident light power. The wavelengths generated are separated from the carrier by less than one thousandth of a nanometer. This slight shift in wavelength would not be expected to cause problems, except for the fact that the generated light is scattered backwards, depleting the carrier signal and, at times, affecting the transmission laser. It is estimated that Brillouin scattering becomes an issue when the power in an optical fiber is on the order of a milliwatt.

Raman scattering results from an interaction of the incident light with molecular vibrations in the fiber. As with Brillouin scattering, Raman scattering can be characterized with a gain coefficient:

$$g_B = 7 \times 10^{-12} \text{ cm/W}. \tag{3.46}$$

Comparison of Eqs (3.45) and (3.46) shows that the threshold for Raman scattering occurs at power levels three orders of magnitude higher than that for *Brillouin scattering*. Raman scattering can be a problem, however, because the wavelength or bandwidth of interaction is greater than a hundred nanometers. Raman scattering can cause serious cross-talk for multiple channel systems of significant power and will ultimately limit the information transmission capacity of optical fiber systems. It is estimated that

Raman scattering becomes an issue when the total power in an optical fiber is on the order of 1 W.

Self- and cross-phase modulation refers to the fact that the index of glass is intensity-dependent:

$$n = n_0 + n_2 I \tag{3.47}$$

where n_0 represents the linear index and the second term includes the intensity-dependent refractive index n_2 and the optical intensity I.

In silica, n_2 is on the order of $3 \times 10^{-16} \, \text{cm}^2/\text{W}$ and $6 \times 10^{-16} \, \text{cm}^2/\text{W}$ for self- and cross-phase modulation, respectively. Both cross- and self-modulation affect the phase and, hence, the arrival time of a pulse. Changes in power and the modulation of power with other carriers limit the amount of power in fibers. It is estimated that self- and phase-modulation becomes an issue when the power in a fiber is on the order of 10 mW.

3.20 SOLITONS IN OPTICAL FIBER

Now, we will briefly introduce the concept of *soliton pulses in optical fiber*. This is a fascinating and current research topic, and it is expected that the use of soliton pulses in optical fibers will enable transmission over transoceanic distance at the highest of possible bit rates.

Soliton propagation in fiber is a nonlinear phenomenon, and such pulses are sensitive to the amount of optical power. Attenuation severely limits the distances over which a soliton pulse can travel without significant distortion. The development of the *erbium-doped optical amplifier* has spurred research activity toward commercializing transoceanic soliton systems. The coincidence of minimum fiber attenuation in the 1550 nm telecommunication window and the strong gain in this same window with the erbium amplifier is, indeed, encouraging. In fact, by amplifying the signal every 30 kms, soliton pulses can travel thousands of kilometers without distortion. One can also use multiple wavelengths *wavelength division multiplexing* (WDM) without the imposition of a number of the nonlinearities. For these reasons, it is expected that, ultimately, soliton trans-mission will be the technique of choice for *transoceanic communication*. However, more research is required before the potential of soliton communication can be fully realized.

Solitons occur in nature in many different ways, optical pulses being one of them. Scott Russel is credited with first observing and recording solitary waves in a barge canal in Great Britain in 1938. He followed the "large solitary elevation" on horseback and noted that it did not change in form or speed for miles. He derived equations describing the velocity of the waves and reported on his work at the Liverpool meeting of the British Association for the Advancement of Science. In 1967, a group of mathematical physicists from Princeton University solved the so-called Kortewegde Vries equations describing the nonlinear hydrodynamic wave. The Russian pair, Zahkharov and Shabat in 1971 considered the nonlinear propagation of optical waves in a two-dimensional medium. They showed that the nonlinear Schroedinger equation could be solved using the inverse scattering theorem and pointed out the relationship between spatial dispersion and optical intensity.

Hasegawa and Tappert in 1973 showed, theoretically, that temporal solitons should exist in fiber and pointed out the possibility of using them for optical communication. Mollenauer and collaborators in 1980 observed solitons experimentally in fiber. They built a "color center" laser that enabled them to generate and launch narrow temporal pulses of power levels significant enough to develop into soliton pulses. This experimental observation can be considered to mark the beginning of a new technology aimed at enabling dispersionless transmission over transoceanic distances. There are, however, many obstacles yet to be overcome before this technology can be fully utilized.

Nonlinear pulse propagation in fiber is described with the so-called nonlinear Schroedinger equation:

$$-i\frac{\partial u}{\partial z} = \frac{\lambda^2 D}{4\pi c}\frac{\partial^2 u}{\partial t^2} + \frac{2\pi n_2}{\lambda A_{\text{eff}}}|u|^2 u. \tag{3.48}$$

Here, D is the dispersion and u is the pulse amplitude which varies both spatially and temporally. The soliton pulse has both a temporal and spectral width, both of which are described with hyperbolic secant functions:

$$u(t) = (\sec h t)\, e^{iz/2} \tag{3.49}$$

and

$$\bar{u}(w) = \frac{1}{2}\sec h\left[(w - w_0)\frac{\pi t_c}{2}\right]. \tag{3.50}$$

In Eq. (3.48), t_c is the temporal width and w_0 the center frequency. An important parameter is the power P_c at which the nonlinearity and dispersion balance:

$$P_c = \frac{\lambda A_{\text{eff}}}{2\pi n_2 Z_c} \tag{3.51}$$

$$Z_c = \frac{2\pi c}{\lambda^2 D}t_c^2. \tag{3.52}$$

The parameter Z_c characterizes the distance at which the pulse begins to spread. Another important parameter is the soliton period, characterized by Z_c times $p/2$.

The possibility of switching light at ultrafast speeds using solitons is also a topic for current research. Soliton pulses have properties that make them attractive in this regard.

3.21 APPLICATIONS OF FIBER OPTIC CABLES

Since the discovery of the laser, fiber optic cables and optical fiber devices have seen increased applications in every sector of industry. Light is a very important element in our lives, controlling and operating many types of devices, instruments, and systems. Fiber optics has emerged as a practical technology that is easy to work with. Fiber optic cables with other optic components are used in building optical fiber devices and systems. One of the large-scale applications of fiber optics is its use in communication systems. The small sizes and wide bandwidths, as well as their capacity to carry large amounts of information, make optical fibers very attractive for use in these systems. Later chapters in this book will explain in more detail communication systems that use optical fiber technology. Video, including broadcast television, is one of the main telecommunication applications. Other applications include cable television, is one of the main telecommunication applications. Other applications include cable television, high-speed internet, wireless transition, remote monitoring, and surveillance. Fiber optic video transmission is successfully used around the world in surveillance and remote monitoring systems with many applications. Fiber optics applications in the military include communications, command-and-control links on ships and aircrafts, data links for satellite earth stations, and transmission lines for tactical command-post communications.

Fiber cables can be used throughout the communication network, including in the final link into the subscriber's home to wall outlets. This field has continued to develop since the discovery of optical amplifiers, dense wavelength division multiplexes (DWDM), fiber Bragg grating, and photonics crystal fibers.

One particular advantage of fiber optic cables is that they are immune to electromagnetic interference (EMI) from electricity. Therefore, optic cables can be placed near high-voltage power cables without any effect on data transmission. Similarly, the cables also can be laid along railway lines without suffering from EMI.

Optical fibers are applied in building *night-vision viewing devices, scanning and sensing instruments*, and *vibration sensors*, which are extensively used in military, medical, and other applications. Imaging techniques have been rapidly developed for a variety of medical applications, such as viewing inside human tissues and scanning microscopic particles.

Fibers are also used in monitoring and sensing technology. They are used as sensors to monitor the vibration in the structures of bridges and high buildings. They are also used as gas and DNA sensors.

The use of fiber optic cables in lighting systems can reduce energy consumption. Fiber optic lighting systems are developing quickly, with wide applications. Fiber optic lighting systems can be applied to the interior and exterior of commercial, retail, and residential buildings. New applications are being explored in landscaping, waterscaping, medical lighting instruments, and theme environments.

Fiber optic cables can also be coated for special handling requirements and resistance to temperature, chemicals, or radiation. Radiation-resistant fiber is suitable for use in environments where electronics-based optical solutions are not viable, such as monitoring nuclear waste disposal in storage facilities. To make the fibers heat resistant, a chemical-reistant polyimide coating that can withstand temperatures of up to 300°C is applied. This is especially useful for manufacturers designing medical equipment for applications in which autoclave sterilization is necessary.

3.21.1 Applications of Advanced Fiber Cables

Fiber-optic cables are used in many applications. One of many applications for different fiber cable types is fiber-optic sensing. Fiber-optic sensing can be classed as intrinsic and extrinsic. In intrinsic sensors, the fiber simply conducts light from a sensing head to a detector; the interaction between light and the environment takes place outside the fiber cable. In intrinsic sensors, the interaction between the environment, the fiber, and the light itself generates information about a specific measurement. The key advantage of intrinsic fiber-optic sensors is the fundamental ability of a fiber to guide light around bends and over long distances. This enables the fiber to be confined within small physical volumes and magnifies the effects of very fine environment changes to a level that can be measured accurately and quantified.

Fiber Bragg gratings are commonly employed as passive temperature and pressure sensors. The ability to adjust these optical devices introduces a new dimension for the design of very fast, precise, and multifunctional fiber sensors without compromising their intrinsic advantages. As explained in the previous section, an FBG consists of a short length of fiber-optic having a periodic modulation of refractive index along it length. This periodic structure causes the FBG to act as a narrowline filter with a peak reflectivity at a specific wavelength, called Bragg wavelength (λ_B), which is determined by the period length of the FBG and the refractive index of the fiber. If the refractive index of the FBG is changed by a temperature shift, or the period is altered in some way (e.g. by compression or expansion), a shift in the peak reflected wavelength results. Detecting this shift is the basis of fiber sensing.

Fiber Bragg gratings are also used in many other applications, such as tunable FBGs. Tuning can be accomplished by several mechanisms, such as electric heating, the piezoelectric effect, mechanical stretching and bending, and acoustic modulation. These sensors are available in the market in different types, sizes, and wavelength ranges.

Photonics bandgap and photonics crystal fibers are both members of the family of MOFs, called *holey fibers*. Both types can be used in gap sensors. The sensors are made of a holey fiber for the 1550 nm spectral range. One end of the fiber is spliced to conventional single mode fiber from an optical source, such as a laser or an LED, and placed on the outer end in a V-groove in a vacuum chamber, as shown in Fig. 3.35. A multi-mode fiber leading to a detector is installed 50 μm away from the end in the V-groove. The separation allows gas to flow into or out of the hollow core of the bandgap fiber, while still allowing for efficient optical coupling between the fibers. A 1-meter length of the fiber is filled with acetylene (C_2H_2) to a pressure of 10 m bar and illuminated with a tunable laser source. The expected spectral changes of acetylene are observed and displayed on a monitor.

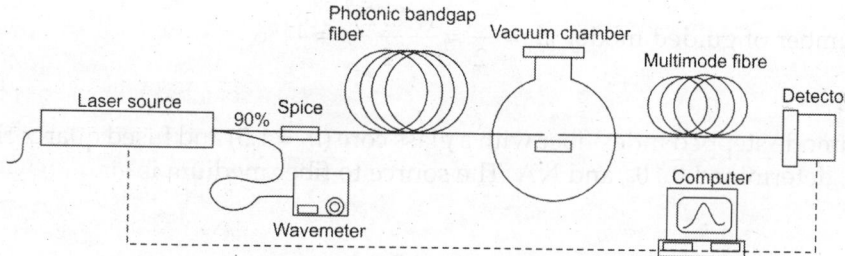

Fig. 3.35: Band gap fiber used in gas sensor

Beyond pressure and temperature sensor technology, advanced fiber sensors types include chemical, strain, biomedical, electrical and magnetic, rotation, vibration, and displacement as major applications. One more application of the advanced fiber sensor technology is in the area of DNA analysis. Fiber-optic biosensors have the ability to detect the presence of short DNA sequences called *oligonucleotides*. This ability gives the diagnostic some excellent tools for early and accurate diagnosis. These fibers are efficiently constructed as waveguides with novel properties for communications and sensing applications.

Example 1

For a 3 μm diameter optical fiber with core and cladding indexes of refraction of 1.545 and 1.510 respectively, determine the cutoff wavelength.

Solution

$$\lambda_c = \frac{2\pi a n_1 \sqrt{2\Delta}}{2.405}$$

where, λ_c – cutoff wavelength (μm),

$\quad n_1$ – core index of refraction (unit less)

$\quad n_2$ – cladding index of refraction (unit less)

$\quad a$ – core radius (μm)

$$\Delta = \frac{n_1 - n_2}{n_1}$$

$$\Delta = \frac{1.545 - 1.510}{1.545} = 0.023, \quad a = \frac{3}{2} = 1.5 \ \mu m$$

$$\lambda_c = \frac{(2\pi)(1.5)(1.545)\sqrt{2(0.023)}}{2.405} = 1.29 \ \mu m$$

Example 2

For a multimode index fiber $n_1 = 1.53$, $n_2 = 1.50$ and $\lambda = 1 \ \mu m$. If core radius is 50 μm, calculate the normalized frequency of the fiber (v) and the number of guided mode.

Solution

Normalized frequency,

$$v = \frac{2\pi a (NA)}{\lambda}$$

$$= \frac{2 \times 3.14 \times 50 \times 10^{-6} \times \sqrt{(1.53)^2 - (1.50)^2}}{1 \times 10^{-6}} = 94.72$$

Total number of guided mode, $m_s = \dfrac{v^2}{2} = \dfrac{(94.72)^2}{2} = 4486$

Example 3

For a multimode stepped index fiber with a glass core ($n_1 = 1.5$) and fused quartz cladding ($n_2 = 1.46$), determined θ_c, θ_m and NA. The source to fiber medium is air.

Solution

Critical angle, $\qquad \theta_c = \sin^{-1} \dfrac{n_2}{n_1} = \sin^{-1} \dfrac{1.46}{1.5} = 76.7°$

$$\theta_m = \sin^{-1} \frac{\sqrt{n_1^2 - n_2^2}}{n_0}$$

$$\theta_{m(max)} = \sin^{-1} \sqrt{n_1^2 - n_2^2} = \sin^{-1} \sqrt{(1.5)^2 - (1.46)^2} = 20.2°$$

$$NA = \sin \theta_m = \sin 20.2 = 0.344$$

The maximum diameter a single-mode optical fiber can have is proportional to the wavelength of light ray entering the cable and numerical aperture of the fiber. Mathematically, the maximum radius of core of a single-mode fiber is:

$$r_{max} = \frac{0.383 \ \text{Å}}{NA} = \frac{0.383 \ \text{Å}}{0.344} = 1.113 \text{Å}$$

where $r_{max} \rightarrow$ maximum core radius, NA $\rightarrow$ numerical aperture (unitless), $\lambda \rightarrow$ light ray wavelength.

Example 4

The numerical aperture of an optical fiber is 0.5 and core refractive index 1.54. Determine (i) Refractive index (RI) of cladding (ii) change in core cladding refractive index per unit RI of the core.

Solution

(i) $NA = \sin \theta_m = \sqrt{n_1^2 - n_2^2}$

$\therefore (0.5)^2 = (1.54)^2 - n_2^2$ or $n_2 = 1.456$

(ii) RI of the core = $\dfrac{n_1 - n_2}{n_1} = \dfrac{1.54 - 1.456}{1.54} = 0.0542$

Example 5

Determine the numerical aperture of a step index fiber when core refractive index $n_1 = 1.5$ and cladding refractive index $n_2 = 1.48$. Find the maximum angle for entrance of light if the fiber is placed in air.

Solution

(i) $NA = \sqrt{(n_1^2 - n_2^2)} = \sqrt{(1.5)^2 - (1.48)^2} = \sqrt{(2.98 \times 0.02)} = 0.24413$

(ii) The maximum entrance angle i_0 can be found from:

$$i_0 = \sin^{-1}\left(\frac{NA}{n}\right) = \sin^{-1}\frac{0.24413}{1} = 14.13°$$

Example 6

An optical fiber has NA of 0.20 and cladding refractive index of 1.59. Determine acceptance angle for the fiber in water with refractive index 1.33.

Solution

$$NA = \frac{\sqrt{(n_1^2 - n_2^2)}}{n_0}$$

When the fiber is in air, $n_0 = 1$, then:

$$NA = \sqrt{(n_1^2 - n_2^2)} = 0.20$$

$$n_0 = \sqrt{(NA)^2 + n_2^2} = \sqrt{(0.20)^2 + (1.59)^2} = 1.6025$$

When the fiber is in water, $n_0 = 1.33$.

Now, $$NA = \frac{\sqrt{(n_1^2 - n_2^2)}}{n_0} = \frac{\sqrt{(1.6025)^2 - (1.59)^2}}{1.33} = 0.15$$

∴ $$i_0 = \sin^{-1}(NA) = \sin^{-1}(0.15) = 8.6°.$$

Example 7

Calculate the refractive indices of core and cladding material of a fiber from the following data: NA = 0.22 and $\Delta = 0.012$.

Solution

$$NA = n_1\sqrt{2\Delta}$$

∴ $$n_1 = \frac{NA}{\sqrt{2\Delta}} = \frac{0.22}{\sqrt{2 \times 0.012}} = 1.42$$

∵ $$\Delta = \frac{n_1 - n_2}{n_1}$$

∴ $$0.012 = \frac{1.42 - n_2}{1.42} \text{ or } n_2 = 1.40$$

Example 8

Calculate numerical aperture, acceptance angle and critical angle of an optical fiber, having refractive index of core 1.52 and refractive index of cladding 1.46.

Solution

We have,
$$\Delta = \frac{n_1 - n_2}{n_1} = \frac{1.52 - 1.46}{1.52} = 0.0395$$

Now,
$$NA = n_1\sqrt{(2\Delta)} = 1.52 \times \sqrt{(2 \times 0.0395)} = 1.52 \times 0.281 = 0.427$$

Acceptance angle, $i_0 = \sin^{-1}(NA) = \sin^{-1}(0.427)$

Critical angle, $\theta_c = \sin^{-1}(n_2/n_1) = \sin^{-1}(1.46/1.52) = \sin^{-1}(0.96)$

Example 9

A step index in air has NA of 0.16, core refractive index of 1.45 and core diameter of 60 cm. Determine the normalized frequency for the fiber when light at a wavelength of 0.9 μm is transmitted.

Solution

$$V = \frac{\pi d}{\lambda}\sqrt{(n_1^2 - n_2^2)} = \frac{\pi d}{\lambda}(NA)$$

Substituting the given values, one obtains:

$$V = \frac{3.14 \times 0.60 \text{ m}}{9 \times 10^{-7} \text{ m}} \times 0.16 = 335103 = 3.35 \times 10^5$$

Example 10

Calculate the numerical aperture, acceptance angle and critical angle of an optical fiber, having refractive index of the core is 1.5 and refractive index of the cladding is 1.45.

Solution

Numerical aperture $NA = n_1\sqrt{2\Delta}$

where
$$\Delta = \frac{n_1 - n_2}{n_1} = \frac{1.5 - 1.45}{15} = 0.0333$$

∴ $NA = n_1\sqrt{2\Delta} = 1.5\sqrt{2 \times 0.0333} = 0.387$

Maximum acceptance angle:
$$\sin\alpha_m = 0.387$$
$$\alpha_m = \sin^{-1}(0.387) = 22.8°$$

Let θ_c be the critical angle:
$$\alpha_m = \sin^{-1}(0.387) = 22.8°$$

Example 11

A glass fiber is made with core material whose refractive index is 1.5 and the cladding is doped to give a fractional index difference of 0.0005. Calculate the refractive index of the cladding, the numerical aperture and critical internal angle.

Solution

The fractional difference of refractive index:

$$\Delta = \frac{n_1 - n_2}{n_1}$$

$$0.0005 = \frac{1.5 - n_2}{1.5}$$

$$n_2 = 1.49925$$

Numerical aperture $NA = n_1\sqrt{2\Delta} = 1.5\sqrt{2 \times 0.0005} = 0.0474$

Let θ_c be the critical angle:

$$\therefore \qquad \sin \theta_c = \frac{n_1}{n_2} = \frac{1.49925}{1.5} - 0.9995$$

$$\theta_c = \sin^{-1}(0.9995) = 88.2°$$

Thus, numerical aperture (NA) is 0.0474 and critical angle (θ_c) is 88.2°.

Example 12

The angle of incidence for a ray in a step-index fiber for which $n_1 = 1.5$ is 11°.
Compute the refractive index of the cladding material.

Solution

$$i + \theta_c = 90°$$

$$\theta_c = 90 - 11 = 79°$$

Now: $\qquad 79° = \sin^{-1}\left[\dfrac{n_2}{n_1}\right]$

or $\qquad \left(\dfrac{n_2}{n_1}\right) = \sin 79° = 0.982$

$$n_2 = n_1 \times 0.982 = 1.5 \times 0.982 = 1.472$$

Thus, the refractive index of cladding (n_2) is 1.472.

Example 13

A fiber has diameter of 5 μm and its core refractive index is 1.45 and cladding refractive index is 1.447. If $\lambda = 1$ μm, how many modes can be propagated inside the fiber?

Solution

The number of modes in Si fiber is given by:

$$N = 4.9\left(\frac{d \times NA}{\lambda}\right)^2 = 4.9\left[\frac{5 \times 10^{-6} \times 0.092}{1 \times 10^{-6}}\right] = 1.04$$

where $\qquad NA = \sqrt{n_1^2 - n_2^2} = \sqrt{1.45^2 - 1.447^2} = \sqrt{0.0085} = 0.092$

Therefore, there is a single mode propagation through this fiber.

Example 14

Calculate the V number and number of modes propagating through the fiber of diameter 100 μm having core and cladding refractive indices of 1.53 and 1.50 respectively? The propagating wave has a wavelength of 1 μm.

Solution

The $\qquad V$ number $= \dfrac{2\pi a}{\lambda}(NA)$

$$NA = \sqrt{(n_1^2 - n_2^2)} = \sqrt{(1.53)^2 - 1.50^2} = 0.301$$

$\therefore \qquad V$ number $= \dfrac{2\pi \times 50 \times 10^{-6}(0.301)}{1 \times 10^{-6}} = 94.6$

The maximum number of modes propagating through the step index fiber is:

$$N = \frac{V^2}{2} = \frac{(94.6)^2}{2} = 4474$$

V number is 94.6; number of modes propagating through the step index fiber is 4474.

Example 15

Calculate the fractional index change for a given optical fiber if the refractive indices of the core and the cladding are 1.563 and 1.498 respectively.

Solution

Fractional index change:

$$\Delta n = \frac{n_1 - n_2}{n_1} = \frac{1.563 - 1.498}{1.563} = 0.0416$$

Fractional index change is 0.0416.

Problem 16

A step-index has a diameter for 200 mm and numerical aperture 0.3. Calculate the number of propagating modes at wavelength of 0.85 mm.

Solution

The number of modes:

$$N = \frac{V^2}{2} = \frac{1}{2}\left[\frac{2\pi a}{\lambda}(NA)\right]^2$$

$$= \frac{1}{4}\frac{4\pi^2 a^2}{\lambda^2}(NA)^2 = \frac{2\pi^2 a^2}{\lambda^2}(NA)^2$$

$$= \frac{2 \times (3.14)^2 \times (100 \times 10^{-6})^2 \times (0.3)^2}{(0.85 \times 10^{-6})^2}$$

$$= 24{,}560$$

Taking into account the two possible polarization, the number of modes = 2 × 24,560 = 49,120.

Example 17

Calculate the total number of guided modes propagating in the multimode step index fiber having core diameter of 50 µm and numerical aperture of 0.2 and operating at wavelength of 1 µm and also calculate the number of modes of graded index fiber having the same parameter.

Solution

Let N be the number of modes in a step index:

$$N_{SI} = 4.9\left[\frac{d \times NA}{\lambda}\right]^2$$

where d = core dia = 50 × 10⁻⁶ meter

λ = wavelength = 1 × 10⁻⁶ meter

$$\therefore \qquad N_{SI} = 4.9\left[\frac{50 \times 10^{-6} \times 0.2}{1 \times 10^{-6}}\right]^2 = 4.9[10]^2 = 490$$

Thus, the number of modes propagated in a step index is 490. Number of modes propagated in a graded index fiber is 245.

Example 18

If the core and cladding, refractive indices for a step index fiber are 1.47 and 1.46 respectively, what will be the broadening of a pulse after a distance of 5 km?

Solution

Given: $L = 5 \times 10^3$ m, $n_1 = 1.47$, $n_2 = 1.46$, $c = 3 \times 10^8$ m/s

We know that the pulse broadening is given by:

$$\Delta t = \frac{n_1 L}{c n_2}(n_1 - n_2) = \frac{1.47 \times 5 \times 10^3}{3 \times 10^8 \times 1.46}(1.47 - 1.46)$$

$$= \frac{7.35 \times 10^3 \times 0.01}{4.38 \times 10^8} \simeq 0.17 \text{ ms}$$

Example 19

Calculate the index difference between the core and the cladding of a fiber with an NA of 0.1.

Solution

We will solve this in two ways. First we will make as estimate:

$$\sin(\theta_a) = \sqrt{n_1^2 - n_2^2} = NA = 0.1$$

$$n_1^2 - n_2^2 = 0.01$$

$$(n_1 - n_2)(n_1 + n_2) = 0.01$$

$$\Delta(n_1 + n_2) = 0.01$$

$$\Delta = \frac{0.01}{n_1 + n_2} \cong \frac{0.01}{2.90} = 0.003448$$

In this case, we assume that $n_1 \cong n_2 = 1.45$.

In the second case, we will evaluate the approximation made above, taking the index of the cladding to be 1.45:

$$\Delta(n_1 + n_2) = 0.01$$

$$\Delta(n_1 - 2n_2 + 2n_2 + n_2) = \Delta^2 + 2\Delta n_2 = 0.01$$

$$\Delta = \frac{-2n_2 \pm \sqrt{4n_2^2 + 0.04}}{2} = -1.45 + 1.453445 = 0.003444$$

The index difference is less, much less the 1%. The accuracy of the approximation is better than three significant figures.

Example 20

It is given that for a GaAs LED, the relative spectral width γ at $\lambda = 0.85$ μm is 0.035. This source is coupled to a pure silica fiber (with $|\lambda^2(d^2n/d\lambda^2)| = 0.021$ for $\lambda = 0.85$ mm) Calculate the pulse broadening per kilometer due to material dispersion.

Solution

The pulse broadening per unit length due to material dispersion is given by:

$$\frac{\tau}{L} = \frac{\gamma}{c}\left|\lambda^2 \frac{d^2n}{d\lambda^2}\right| = \frac{0.035}{3 \times 10^8 \text{ ms}^{-1}} \times 0.021 = 2.45 \times 10^{-12} \text{ s m}^{-1} \quad \text{or} \quad \frac{\tau}{L} = 2.45 \text{ ns} \cdot \text{km}^{-1}$$

Example 21

Calculate the total pulse broadening due to material dispersion for a graded index fiber of total length 80 km when a LED emitting at (a) $\lambda = 850$ nm and (b) $\lambda = 1300$ nm is coupled to the fiber. In both the cases, assume that $\Delta\lambda = 30$ nm. The material dispersion parameters of the fiber for the two wavelengths are 105.5 ps nm^{-1}·km^{-1} and 2.8 ps nm^{-1}, respectively.

Solution

(a) We have: $\tau = D_m L \Delta\lambda = 105.5 \times 80 \times 30 = 253{,}200$ ps $= 253.2$ ns
(b) $\tau = 2.8 \times 80 \times 30 = 6720$ ps $= 6.72$ ns

This example shows that proper selection of wavelength can reduce pulse broadening considerably.

Example 22

The core diameter of multimode step index fiber is 46 μm and numerical aperture is 0.3. Determine number of guided modes at operating wavelength of 0.8 μm.

Solution

$$f = \frac{2\pi}{\lambda} a \, (NA) = \frac{2\pi}{0.8 \times 10^{-6}} \times 23 \times 10^{-6} \times 0.3 \approx 54.16$$

$$N_g = \frac{f^2}{2} \approx 1466$$

Example 23

The mean optical power launched into an optical fiber 150 μW. The mean optical power at the fiber output is 10 μW. The length of the fiber is 5 km. Calculate the signal attenuation per kilometer for the fiber.

Solution

$$\alpha_{dB} = 10 \log_{10} \frac{P_i}{P_o} = 10 \log_{10} \frac{150 \times 10^{-6}}{10 \times 10^{-6}} = 11.76 \text{ dB}$$

$$\alpha_{dB} \div L = \frac{11.76}{5} = 2.352 \text{ dB/km}$$

Example 24

For a step index fiber, the normalized frequency (V parameter) is 26.6 at a wavelength of 1300 nm. Determine the numerical aperture (NA), if the core radius is 25 μm.

Solution

Given: $V = 26.6$, $\lambda = 1300$ nm $= 1.3$ mm, $r = 25$ μm.

The normalized frequency for a step index fiber is given by:

$$V = \frac{2\pi r}{\lambda} (NA)$$

$$NA = \frac{V\lambda}{2\pi r} = \frac{26.6 \times 1.3}{2 \times 3.14 \times 25} = \frac{24.58}{157} = 0.22$$

Example 25

An optical fiber has an attenuation 3.5 dB/km. If 0.5 mW of optical power is mainly launched into the fiber, what is the power level in μW after 4 km?

Solution

Given: $\alpha = 3.5$ dB/km, $P_i = 0.5$ mW, $L = 4$ km.

We know that the attenuation of an optical fiber is given by:

$$\alpha = \frac{10}{L} \log \frac{P_i}{P_o}$$

$$3.5 = \frac{10}{4} \log \left(\frac{0.5}{P_o} \right)$$

or

$$\frac{3.5 \times 4}{10} = \log \frac{0.5}{P_o}$$

or

$$1.4 = \log \frac{0.5}{P_o}$$

or

$$10^{1.4} = \frac{0.5}{P_o}$$

$$P_o = \log \frac{0.5}{10^{1.4}} = \frac{0.5}{25.11} = 19.9 \text{ mW}$$

Example 26

If the core and cladding, refractive indices for a step index fiber is 1.47 and 1.46 respectively, what will be the broadening of a pulse after a distance of 5 km?

Solution

Given: $L = 5 \times 10^3$, $n_1 = 1.47$, $n_2 = 1.46$, $c = 3 \times 10^8$ m/s

We know that the pulse broadening is given by:

$$\Delta t = \frac{n_1 L}{c n_2} (n_1 - n_2) = \frac{1.47 \times 5 \times 10^3}{3 \times 10^8 \times 1.46} (1.47 - 1.46)$$

$$= \frac{7.35 \times 10^3 \times 0.01}{4.38 \times 10^8}$$

$$= 0.17 \text{ μs}$$

Example 27

The relative refractive index difference of a silica fiber is 1%. Calculate the solid acceptance angle of the fiber in air assuming the core refractive index to be 1.458.   **[DTU]**

Solution

The NA of the fiber is given by the relation

$$NA = n_1 \sqrt{2\Delta} = 1.458\sqrt{0.02} = 0.21$$

The solid acceptance angle of the fiber can be obtained from

$$\Omega_{max} = \pi(NA)^2 = 3.14 \times (0.21)^2 = 0.15 \ sr \text{ (steradian)}$$

Example 28

A step-index silica fiber with a core radius much longer than the operating wavelength of light has a core refractive index of 1.50 and a cladding refractive index of 1.48. Estimate the value of (i) numerical aperture of the fiber, (ii) maximum acceptance angle in air, and (iii) maximum acceptance angle in water having a refractive index of 1.33.   **[RTU]**

Solution

The large dimension of the core in comparison with the operating wavelength allows one to apply the ray analysis approach for computation of numerical aperture and acceptance angle.

(i) The numerical aperture of the fiber is given by the relation

$$\text{NA} = \sqrt{n_1^2 - n_2^2} = \sqrt{(1.50)^2 - (1.48)^2} = 0.24$$

(ii) The acceptance angle of the fiber in air is

$$(\theta_{0\,max})_{air} = \sin^{-1}(\text{NA}) = \sin^{-1}(0.24) = 14°13'$$

(iii) The acceptance angle of the fiber in water is

$$(\theta_{0\,max})_{air} = \sin^{-1}\left(\frac{\text{NA}}{n_0}\right) = \sin^{-1}\left(\frac{0.24}{1.33}\right) = 10°39'$$

Example 29

A GI fiber with a parabolic profile has a refractive index of 1.458 at the centre of the core. Estimate the value of the numerical aperture of the fiber at a point exactly midway between the axis of the core and the core cladding interface assuming $\Delta = 0.01$.　　**[KTU]**

Solution

The axial numerical aperture of the GI fiber is

$$\text{NA}(0) = n_1\sqrt{2\Delta} = 1.458\sqrt{2 \times 0.01} = 0.206$$

For a GI fiber with parabolic-index profile, $\alpha = 2$. Therefore, the local NA at $r = a/2$ is obtained as

$$\text{NA}(r = a/2) = NA(0)\sqrt{1 - \left(\frac{r}{a}\right)^2} = 0.206\sqrt{1 - \left(\frac{1}{2}\right)^2} = 0.178$$

Example 30

The cutoff wavelength for a step index fiber is 1.1 μm. The core index $n_1 = 1.45$ and $\Delta = 0.005$. Find the core radius. Is this fiber single-moded at 1.55 μm?　　**[KTU]**

Solution

We have

$$n_2 = n_1(1 - \Delta) = 1.14(1 - 0.005) = 1.4428$$

Core radius

$$a = \frac{2.4048\lambda_c}{2\pi(n_1^2 - n_2^2)^{1/2}} = \frac{2.4048 \times 1.1\,\mu m}{2\pi[(1.45)^2 - (1.4428)^2]^{1/2}} = 2.907\,\mu m$$

Since the operating wavelength $\lambda = 1.55\,\mu m > \lambda_c$, it is single moded at this wavelength.

SUMMARY

- The refractive index (n) of a transparent medium is the ratio of the speed of light in vacuum (c) to the speed of light in the medium (v), thus $n = c/v$.
- The phenomenon of refraction of light is governed by *Snell's law*: $n_1 \sin\theta_1 = n_2\sin\theta_2$.
- An optical fiber is a thin dielectric waveguide made up of a solid cylindrical core of glass (silica) or plastic of refractive index (RI), n_1, surrounded by a coaxial cylindrical cladding of RI, n_2. When n_1 and n_2, both are constant, the fiber is said to be a step-index fiber.
- Within an optical fiber, light is guided by *total internal reflection* (TIR). For light guidance, two conditions have to be satisfied: (i) n_1 must be greater than n_2 ($n_1 > n_2$),

and (ii) at the core–cladding interface, the light ray must strike at an angle greater than the critical angle θ_c, where $\theta_c = \sin^{-1}(n_2/n_1)$.

This requires that the ray of light must enter the core of the fiber at an angle less than the acceptance angle θ_a: $n_a \sin \theta_a = n_1 \sin \theta_c$.

- The light gathering capacity of a fiber is expressed in terms of the *numerical aperture* (NA), which is expressed as: $NA = n_a \sin \theta_a = \sqrt{(n_1^2 - n_2^2)} = n_1 2\Delta$.
- When a pulse of light propagates through the fiber, it gets broadened. *Pulse broadening* is caused due to following two mechanisms:

  (i) *Multipath time dispersion*, given by $\dfrac{\Delta T}{L} = \dfrac{n_1}{n_2}\left(\dfrac{n_1 - n_2}{c}\right)$. To some extent, one can reduce this type of dispersion by *index grading*, i.e. by varying the RI of the core in a specific manner. It is reported that the *parabolic profile* gives best results.

  (ii) *Material dispersion*, caused by change in the RI of the fiber material with wavelength. This is given by $\dfrac{\tau}{T} = \dfrac{r}{c}\left|\lambda^2 \dfrac{d^2 n}{d\lambda^2}\right|$.

- Fiber optics is a technology related to the transportation of optical energy (light energy) in guiding media, specifically glass fiber.
- In case of optical fibers, there must be very little absorption of light as it travels through a long distance inside the fiber. One can achieve this by purification and special preparation of the material used.
- Fibers that are used in optical communication are wave guides made of transparent dielectrics. Its function is to guide visible and infrared light over long distances.
- Optical fibers are classified into two categories based on: (i) number of modes, and (ii) refractive index.
- On the basis of number of modes of propagation, optical fibers are classified into two types: (i) single mode fiber (SMF) and (ii) multi-mode fiber (MMF).
- On the basis of refractive index, fibers can be classified into two types: (i) step-index optical fiber, and (ii) graded-index optical fiber.
- The condition for propagation of light within the optical fiber is $\sin i < NA$.
- *V*-number is an important parameter for optical fiber and is generally called normalized frequency of the fiber $V = \dfrac{2\pi a}{\lambda}(NA) = \dfrac{2\pi a}{\lambda} n_1 \sqrt{2\Delta}$, where $\Delta = \dfrac{n_1 - n_2}{n_1}$ is fractional refractive index change.

  The wavelength corresponding to the value of $V = 2.405$ is known as cutoff wavelength.
- Losses occurring in optical fibers may be mainly due to the following mechanisms: (i) absorption, (ii) scattering, and (iii) fiber bends.
- The index of refraction in graded index fibers varies gradually from the axis of fiber.
- Mode of fiber refers to the number of paths the light ray can travel down the optical fiber.
- The single mode propagation of LP_{01} mode in step index optical fiber is possible over the region $0 < V < 2.405$.
- *Step index fibers* are those fibers where the refractive index (RI) of the core is constant throughout and steps down to the refractive index of the cladding. The light in these fibers travels down the fibers by bouncing off the core-cladding interface.

- *Graded index fibers* have a core with a RI which varies quadratically according to the distance out from the center of the fiber, decreasing as you move further out. Ligfht travelling in these fibers actually follows a curved path due to the continuously varying RI. In these fibers, ray of light follows sinusoidal paths.

REVIEW QUESTIONS

1. Define an optical fiber system. What is numerical aperture of an optical fiber? What is its significance?
2. Obtain the expression for NA in terms of RI of the core and cladding of an optical fiber.
3. Outline the primary building blocks of a fiber optic system.
4. Draw a block diagram for optical communication through fiber optic cables. Mention the advantages of optical communication.
5. Explain the working of monomode and multimode optical fibers. For long distance communication which optical fiber is preferred and why?
6. Contrast glass and plastic fiber cables.
7. Explain the principle and working of fiber optic sensors.
8. Write short notes on:
     (i) Fiber optic cable
     (ii) Step index fiber
     (iii) Graded index fiber
     (iv) Fiber optic communication system
9. What are the functions of the core and cladding in an optical fiber? Why should their refractive indices be different? Can it be possible for the light to be guided without cladding?
10. Explain total internal reflection? Why it is necessary to meet the condition of total internal reflection at the core-cladding interface.
11. Define NA of a fiber. On what factors it depend?
12. What is acceptance angle? What is the condition for propagation of light through an optical fiber?
13. Explain how right propagates through a graded index fiber.
14. Differentiate between single mode and multimode fibers.
15. Differentiate between step index fiber and graded index fiber.
16. Explain multipath time dispersion and material dispersion. How can these be minimized?
17. Distinguish between step index multimode fiber and graded index multimode fiber.

PROBLEMS

1. A multimode step index fiber has $n_1 = 1.53$, $n_2 = 1.50$ and $\lambda = 1$ μm. In order to make this fiber single mode, what will be core radius?

[**Hint:** $a \leq \dfrac{2.405\lambda}{2\pi(NA)}$, $NA = \sqrt{(1.53)^2 - (1.50)^2}$

$a \leq \dfrac{2.405 \times 1 \times 10^{-6}}{2 \times 3.14 \times \sqrt{(1.53)^2 - (1.50)^2}}$, or $a \leq 1.27$ μm]

2. Numerical aperture of an optical fiber is 0.5 and core refractive index is 1.48. Show that cladding refractive index is 1.393 and acceptance angle is 30°.

[Hint: NA = $\sqrt{n_1^2 - n_2^2}$ = 0.5, RI of core = n_1 = 1.48; that is n_2 = 1.393; RI of cladding = n_2 = 1.393; Acceptance angle θ = $\sin^{-1}$ (NA) = 30°]

3. A step index fiber in air has NA of 0.16, core refractive index of 1.45 and core diameter of 60 cm. Show that the normalized frequency for the fiber when light at a wavelength of 0.9 mm transmitted is 3.35×10^5.

$$\left[\textbf{Hint}: v = \frac{\pi d}{\lambda_0} \sqrt{n_1^2 - n_2^2} = \frac{3.143 \times 0.6 \text{ m}}{9 \times 10^{-7} \text{ m}} \times 0.16 = 3.35 \times 10^5 \right]$$

4. An optical fiber has NA of 0.20 and cladding refractive index of 1.59. Show that the acceptance angle for the fiber in water which has a refractive index of 1.33 is 8.6°.

[Hind: NA = $\dfrac{\sqrt{(n_1^2 - n_2^2)}}{n_0}$

When the fiber is in air, n_0 = 1 and NA = $\sqrt{(n_1^2 - n_2^2)}$ = 0.20

∴ $n_1 = \sqrt{(NA)^2 + n_2^2} = \sqrt{(0.20)^2 + (1.59)^2}$ = 1.6026

When the fiber is in water, n_0 = 1.33

NA = $\dfrac{\sqrt{(n_1^2 - n_2^2)}}{n_0} = \dfrac{\sqrt{(1.6025)^2 - (1.59)^2}}{1.33}$ = 0.15

θ_0 (max) = $\sin^{-1}$ (NA) = $\sin^{-1}$ (0.15) = 8.6°]

5. Show that the core radius necessary for single mode operation at 850 nm Si fiber with n_1 = 1.480 and n_2 = 1.47 is 1.89 μm. Also show that NA and maximum acceptance angle of this fiber are 0.1717 and 9° 53′ 12″ respectively.

[Hint:

(i) $\quad v = \dfrac{\pi d}{\lambda_0} \sqrt{n_1^2 - n_2^2}$

$\quad 2.405 = \dfrac{\pi d}{450 \times 10^{-9} \text{ m}} \times 0.1717$

or $\quad d$ =3.79 mm, ∴ r = 1.89 mm

(ii) NA = $\sqrt{n_1^2 - n_2^2} = \sqrt{(1.48)^2 - (1.47)^2}$ = 0.1717

(iii) $\sin \theta_0$ (max) = NA

∴ θ_0 (max) = $\sin^{-1}$ (NA) = $(n_1^2 - n_2^2)^{1/2}$

$\quad = \sin^{-1}$ (0.1717) = 9°53′12″]

6. A fiber cable has index of refraction core 1.52 and cladding 1.31. Show that numerical aperture is 0.77.

7. For a multimode step index fiber with glass core (n_1 = 1.5), acceptance angle is required to be 20.2°. Find numerical aperture and refractive index of cladding (n_2).

[Hint: NA = sin (θ_{in}), Here θ_{in} = 20.2°, hence NA = sin 20.2° = 0.344, NA = $\sqrt{n_1^2 - n_2^2}$

Hence, 0.344 = $\sqrt{1.5^2 - n_2^2} = \sqrt{2.25 - n^2}$. By solving, we get n_2 = 1.45]

8. A light ray travels from a medium of refractive index n_1 = 1.5 to another with refractive index n_2 = 1.46. Calculate the critical angle of incidence measured from normal at the boundary. What will be this angle if the second medium is air?

[**Hint:** For $n_1 = 1.5$ and $n_2 = 1.46$:

Critical angle, $\theta_c = \text{arc sin}\left(\dfrac{n_2}{n_1}\right) = \text{arc sin}\left(\dfrac{1.46}{1.5}\right) = \text{arc sin }(0.9733) = 76.7°$

When second medium is air:

$n_2 = 1.0003$, $\theta_c = \text{arc sin}\left(\dfrac{1.0003}{1.5}\right) = 41.8$]

9. A step index fiber has an acceptance angle (θ_a) of 20° in air and relative refractive index difference of 3%. Calculate the NA and the critical angle at the core-cladding interface. [**Ans.** 0.34, 76°]

10. The speed of light in vacuum and in the core of a Si fiber is 3×10^8 ms^{-1} and 2×10^8 ms^{-1} respectively. When the fiber is placed in air, the critical angle (θ_c) at the core-cladding interface is 75°. Calculate the (i) NA of the fiber, and (ii) multipath time dispersion per unit length. [**Ans.** (i) 0.388, (ii) 1.7×10^{-10} sm^{-1}]

11. A Si fiber has NA = 0.17 and a cladding refractive index of 1.46. Determine the (a) the acceptance angle of the fiber when it is placed in water (the refractive index of water = 1.33), and (b) the critical angle (θ_c) at the core-cladding interface. [**Ans.** (a) 7.34°, (b) 83.35°]

12. A step index fiber in air has a numerical aperture of 0.22. Calculate the acceptance angle in air for skew rays that change direction by 110° at each reflection.
[**Hint:** The skew rays under consideration change direction by 110° at each reflection. Therefore
$$2\gamma = 110°$$
i.e. $\gamma = 55°$

We have $(\theta_{0\,max})_{skew} = \sin^{-1}\left(\dfrac{NA}{\cos \gamma}\right) = \sin^{-1}\left(\dfrac{0.22}{\cos 55°}\right)$

$= 22°·55$]

13. A step index fiber in air accepts skew rays at a maximum axial angle of 45°. If the skew rays change direction by 90° at each reflection within the fiber core, estimate the acceptance angle for the meridional rays for the fiber in air.
[**Hint:** In the case, we have
$$2\gamma = 90°$$
i.e. $\gamma = 45°$

Now $\sin 45° = \dfrac{NA}{\cos 45°}$

i.e. NA $= \sin 45° \cos 45° = \dfrac{1}{\sqrt{2}}\dfrac{1}{\sqrt{2}} = 0.5$

The maximum acceptance angle if the fiber in air ($n_0 = 1$) for the meridional rays is
$$\theta_{max} = \sin^{-1}(0.5) = 30°]$$

14. A step index fiber has core and cladding reactive indices of 1.45 and 1.43 respectively. Calculate the maximum acceptance angle of the fiber in air meridional rays. Compare this value with that for skew rays that change direction with in the core by 100° at each reflection.

[**Hint:** $q_{max} = \sin^{-1}(0.24) = 13°·88$

As the skew rays change direction by 100° at each reflection, we have

$$2\gamma = 100°$$

i.e. $$\gamma = 50°$$

We have $$(\theta_{max})_{skew} = \sin^{-1}\left(\frac{NA}{\cos\gamma}\right) = \sin^{-1}\left(\frac{0.24}{\cos 50°}\right) = 21°\cdot92$$

Thus the acceptance angle for the skew rays is nearly 8° greater than that for meridional rays.]

15. The power transmitted in a fiber-optic system is 0.012 W. (a) Convert this into dBm units (b) The received power is –5 dBm. Convert this into mW units.
    [**Hint:**

    (a) $$P_{tr}\,(dBm) = 10\log_{10}\left[\frac{12\,mW}{1mW}\right] = 10.79\,dBm$$

    (b) Power received $= P_{rec}\,(dBm) = -5\,dBm$
    $$\therefore \qquad P_{rec}\,(mW) = 10^{-5/10}\,mW = 0.3162\,mW]$$

SHORT ANSWER QUESTIONS

1. To prevent energy losses via absorption and scattering, what should be the order of cladding in an optical fiber?
   Ans. At least a few wavelengths thick.

2. How numerical aperture (NA) of an optical fiber is defined?
   Ans. NA $= \sqrt{n_1^2 - n_2^2}$, where n_1 is refractive index of the core of a fiber and n_2 is that of cladding ($n_1 > n_2$): One can define the numerical aperture of a fiber as the physical area that light must enter in order to propagate through the fiber. The numerical aperture for light sources can be calculated in terms of angle involved with the output.

3. How will you define acceptance angle (θ_a) for an optical fiber?
   Ans. $\theta_a = \sin^{-1}\sqrt{n_1^2 - n_2^2}$.

4. What is major economic benefit offered by fiber optics in information technology?
   Ans. Very high information transmission rate at low cost per circuit-km.

5. What type of reflection is expected from an optical fiber?
   Ans. Total internal reflection.

6. How is an optical fiber fabricated?
   Ans. In the fabrication of optical fibers one can use either different glasses with different refractive indices for core and cladding or use fused silica (quartz, glass) whose refractive index is modified by doping. The type of glass used will also vary with application, but purity (lack of foreign materials as well as imperfections such as cracks or bubbles) must also be kept very high.

7. What is kevlar?
   Ans. It is a yarn type material having high tensile strength. It is used in fiber construction to provide additional strength to the cable.

8. Explain the relationship between information capacity and bandwidth.
   Ans. The information carrying capacity of a communication system is directly proportional to its bandwidth, i.e. higher the bandwidth, the greater its information carrying capacity.

9. Explain the purpose of cladding in optical fiber.

Ans. Due to its lower refractive index than core, cladding helps in retaining light with the core. Moreover, it provides mechanical strength, reduces scattering loss and also protects the core from absorbing surface contaminates with which is could come in contact.

10. Mention the advantages of optical fiber communication over metallic cable communication.

Ans. (i) Extremely wide bandwidth
    (ii) Light in weight and small in size
    (iii) Immune to electrostatic interference
    (iv) More secured, greater safety and no crosstalk.

11. Can light propagate through an optical fiber cable with the angle of incidence at entrance end greater than acceptance angle?

Ans. No. Only when light enters at an angle less than the acceptance angle, light can propagate through the cable by undergoing total internal reflection.

12. What is an optical fiber sensor?

Ans. It is a transducer which can convert various input variables (physical quantities) into an electrical signal in measurable form.

13. What are the advantages of optical sensors in sensing applications?

Ans. (i) They are electrically passive
    (ii) They have good geometrical flexibility
    (iii) They are light in weight and small in size
    (iv) Chemical and environmental ruggedness is high

14. What are the characteristics of wave that may get modulated in fiber optic sensors?

Ans. Amplitude or intensity, phase, polarisation, frequency and direction of propagation may get modulated.

15. Which type of optical fiber (single mode or multimode) tends to have lower loss and produces less signal distortion?

Ans. Single mode fiber.

16. Which properties of optical fibre reduce connection loss in short distance systems?

Ans. (i) Higher fiber numerical aperture, and (ii) Large fiber core.

17. Which basic optical material property is considered relevant for optical fiber light communication?

Ans. Index of refraction.

18. Out of core or cladding, which optical fiber has a higher index of refraction?

Ans. Core.

19. Multimode step index fibers have a core and cladding of constant refractive index n_1 and n_2 respectively. Out of these, which refractive index core or cladding is lower?

Ans. Cladding.

20. What is the benefit of having large core diameters and large NA for multimode step index fibres?

Ans. This makes it easier to couple light from an LED into the optical fiber.

21. Meridional rays are classified as either bound or unbound rays. While propagating through the fiber, the bound rays follow what property of light?

Ans. Total internal reflection.

22. What are the advantages of optical fiber over copper wire conductors?

Ans. Optical fiber transmission has following advantages over convention copper wire system:

   (i) More data can be sent over the long distances through optical fiber due to its lower transmission losses

  (ii) The light weight and the small thin hair-szied dimension of the optical fibers are quite advantageous, e.g. in aircraft

 (iii) Dielectric nature of optical fiber provides optical immunity to the electro-magnetic interferences

 (iv) The principal material for the optical fiber, i.e. silica, whose source is sand, is abundantly available

23. What are the advantages of optical fibers?

Ans. See text.

24. What are fiber lasers?

Ans. Fiber lasers also called as fiber sources are light sources made from fiber. They are built around fiber cores, which are doped with materials that can be stimulated to emit light.

25. What are the advantages of fiber optic systems?

Ans. Fiber optic systems offer several advantages. Few of them are as follows:

   (i) Optical fibers are light in weight and occupy less space than coaxial (bundles of twisted pair) cables.

  (ii) Optical fibers are composed of dielectric materials, and therefore, these are totally immune to extraneous interfering electromagnetic signals.

 (iii) There is virtually no signal leakage from optical fibers and hence cross-talk is not possible.

 (iv) Attenuation of signals in optical fibers is much smaller than in coaxial cables or twisted pair.

  (v) Optical fibers are immune to electromagnetic interference and do not pick up line currents. Obviously, these can be safely used in high voltage environments, e.g. power station, and can be laid alongside metallic power cables.

 (vi) The basic raw material used in the fabrication of low loss fibers is silica, which is abundantly available in nature (although in impure form), whereas copper constitutes the basic raw material in coaxial cables.

 (vii) Optical fibers can withstand environmental hazards in a better manner and also have longer life compared to copper cables.

(viii) Optical fibers are non-conductive and non-inductive. This reveals that there is no interference with other communi-cation systems.

 (ix) The speed of transmission through optical fibers is very high because the signals are carried by light.

  (x) The channel capacity of optical fibers is very large as compared to the audio band (5 to 10 Hz); the frequency of carrier light wave is very high ($\sim 10^{14}$ Hz). Obviously, one can accommodate a large number of speed signal channels in fibers whose bandwidth is larger than that of a wire transmission line.

26. What are the disadvantages of optical fiber systems?

Ans. The major disadvantages of optical fiber systems are as follows:

    (i) Optical fiber systems are virtually of less use unless they are connected to standard electronic facilities which often require expensive interfaces.

    (ii) Optical fibers have significantly lower tensile strength than coaxial cables. This can be improved by coating the fiber with standard Kevlar and a protective jacket of PVC.

    (iii) Occasionally, it is necessary to provide electrical power to remote interface or regenerating equipment. Thus, additional metallic cables have to be included in the cable assembly.

    (iv) Optical fibers require special tools to splice and repair cables and special test equipments to make routine measurements. Repairing fiber cables is also difficult and expensive and working on optical fiber cables also requires special skills and training.

27. Show that NA of a graded-index (GI) fibers is given by $NA(r) = NA(0)\sqrt{1 - (r/a)^\alpha}$, where $N(0) = n_1\sqrt{2\Delta}$ is the numerical aperture at the centre of the core. How NA of GI fibers varies with radial distance from the centre of the core?

Ans. The refractive index of a GI fiber is a function of radial distance r from the centre of the core and is constant in cladding. Therefore, we expect that the *NA* of GI fiber will also be a function of radial distance. NA of GI fiber can be defined in an analogous way to NA to Si fiber is

$$NA(r) = \sqrt{n^2(r) - n_2^2} \qquad\qquad (i)$$

Using the relation for the variation of refractive index along the radial distance of a graded index fiber

$$n(r) = \begin{cases} n_1\left[1 - 2\Delta\left(\dfrac{r}{a}\right)^\alpha\right]^{1/2} & (r < a) \\[2mm] n_1(1 - 2\Delta)^{1/2} \approx n_1(1 - \Delta) = n_2 & (r \geq a) \end{cases}$$

where r is the distance measured from the centre of the core along the radius and a is the core radius, we obtain

$$NA(r) = \sqrt{n_1^2\left[1 - 2\Delta\left(\frac{r}{a}\right)^\alpha\right] - n_2^2}$$

$$= \sqrt{n_1^2 - n_2^2}\left[1 - \frac{2n_1^2\Delta}{n_1^2 - n_2^2}\left(\frac{r}{a}\right)^\alpha\right]^{1/2}$$

$$= NA(0)\sqrt{1 - \left(\frac{r}{a}\right)^\alpha} \qquad\qquad (ii)$$

where NA (0) is the numerical aperture at the centre of the core, also called the axial NA of the GI fiber, given by

$$NA(0) = \sqrt{n^2(0) - n_2^2} = \sqrt{n_1^2 - n_2^2} \approx n_1\sqrt{2\Delta} \qquad\qquad (ii)$$

The NA of a GI fiber has a maximum value NA (0) at the centre of the core and radius to zero at the core-cladding interface ($r = a$). Figure 3.36 shows the variation of NA of GI fiber with radial distance. We may note that the local NA of GI fiber at a particular point depends on the value of α which defines the shape of the index profile. We have $\alpha = \infty$ for an SI fiber and NA is constant and equal to NA (0) of a corresponding GI fiber and drops abruptly to zero at the core-cladding interface as shown in Fig. 3.36.

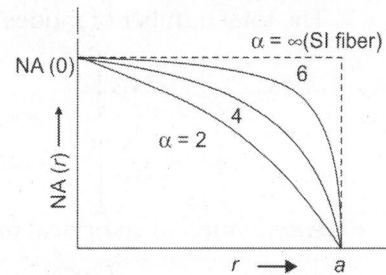

Fig. 3.36: Variation of numerical aperture (NA) of a GI fiber with radial distance from the centre of the core

MULTIPLE CHOICE QUESTIONS

1. In fiber-optic communication, the propagation of light through the fiber is based on the principle of:
   (a) diffraction of light
   (b) interference of light
   (c) total internal reflection
   (d) polarization of light

2. The refractive index in a graded index fiber:
   (a) increases throughout the core
   (b) remains constant throughout the core
   (c) decreases parabolically throughout the core
   (d) None of the above

3. The acceptance angle or acceptance cone half angle for the optical fiber is:
   (a) $\theta_m = \sin^{-1}(n_1 - n_2)$
   (b) $\theta_m = \sin^{-1}\sqrt{n_1^2 - n_2^2}$
   (c) $\theta_m = \sqrt{n_1^2 - n_2^2}$
   (d) $\theta_m = n_1^2 / n_2^2$

4. Numerical aperture of step index optical fiber is:
   (a) $NA = n_1\sqrt{2\Delta}$
   (b) $NA = n_1^2\sqrt{2\Delta}$
   (c) $NA = n_1^2 - n_2^2$
   (d) $NA = n_1 2\Delta$

5. The jacket of an optical fiber enables:
   (a) to prevent from moisture trapping
   (b) to prevent from mechanical abrasions
   (c) to prevent from interaction with internal atmosphere
   (d) All of the above

6. When V parameter is less than 2.405, then optical fiber will support:
   (a) three modes
   (b) two modes
   (c) one mode
   (d) none of the above

7. The optical fibers are made of:
   (a) dielectrical material
   (b) metallic material
   (c) magnetic material
   (d) plastic doped with metallic impurities

8. Pulse broadening can be minimised by making use of:
   (a) multimode graded index fiber
   (b) single mode index fiber
   (c) multimode step index fiber
   (d) none of the above

9. The total number of modes in a multimode fiber is given by:

(a) $M = \dfrac{1}{2}\left[\dfrac{\pi d}{\lambda} NA\right]^2$

(b) $M = \left[\dfrac{2\pi d}{\lambda} NA\right]$

(c) $M = \dfrac{1}{2}\left[\dfrac{\pi d}{\lambda} NA\right]^{1/2}$

(d) $M = \dfrac{1}{2}\left[\dfrac{\pi d}{\lambda} NA\right]^3$

10. Attenuation in an optical fiber is measured by:

(a) $loss = 10 \log_{10}\left(\dfrac{P_i}{P_o^2}\right)$

(b) $loss = -10 \log_{10}\left(\dfrac{P_o}{P_i}\right)$

(c) $loss = 10 \log_{10}\left(\dfrac{P_i^2}{P_o}\right)$

(d) $loss = -10 \log_{10}\left(\dfrac{P_i}{P_o}\right)$

11. Information signals are transmitted from optical fiber in the form of:
    (a) analogue signals
    (b) digital signals
    (c) binary and hexadecimal bits
    (d) None of the above

12. Dispersion in optical fibers is due to:
    (a) chromatic dispersion
    (b) material dispersion
    (c) intermodal dispersion
    (d) All of the above

13. The propagation of light along the wavelength is decided by the:
    (a) interference
    (b) dispersion
    (c) modes of the waveguides
    (d) None of the above

14. In multimode propagation the light propagates the fiber in:
    (a) straight line
    (b) zig zag fashion
    (c) circular path
    (d) elliptical path

15. In order that mode remain guided, the propagation factor β must safisfy:

(a) $n_2 < \beta < n_1$

(b) $n_2 \dfrac{2\pi}{\lambda} < \beta < n_1 \dfrac{2\pi}{\lambda}$

(c) $n_2 < \beta = n_1$

(d) $n_2 = \beta < n_1$

16. A ray of light is passing from a silica glass of refractive index 1.48 to another silica glass of refractive index 1.46. What is the range of angles (measured with respect to the normal to the interface) for which this ray will undergo total internal reflection?

[B Tech]

(a) 0°–80°
(b) 81°–90°
(c) 90°–180°
(d) 180°–360°

17. Light is guided within the core of a step-index fiber by:
    (a) refraction at the core-air-interface
    (b) total internal reflection at the core-cladding interface
    (c) total internal reflection at the outer surface of the cladding
    (d) change in the speed of light within the core

18. A step-index fiber has a core with a refractive index of 1.50 and a cladding with a refractive index of 1.46. Its numerical aperture is: [B.Tech.]
    (a) 0.156
    (b) 0.244
    (c) 0.344
    (d) 0.486

19. The optical fiber of Question 18 is placed in water (refractive index 1.33). The acceptance angle of the fiber will be approximately:

    (a) 10°   (b) 15°

    (c) 20°   (d) 25°

20. The axial refractive index of the core, n_0 of a graded-index fiber is 1.50 and the maximum relative refractive index difference Δ is 1%. What is the refractive index of the cladding? **[B Tech]**

    (a) 1.485   (b) 1.50

    (c) It will depend on the profile parameter

    (d) It will depend on the radius of the core

21. An impulse is launched into one end of a 30 km optical fiber with a rated total dispersion of 20 ns/km. What will be the width of the pulse at the other end? **[B Tech]**

    (a) 20 ns   (b) 100 ns

    (c) 300 ns   (d) 600 ns

22. For a typical LED, the relative spectral width γ is 0.030. This source is coupled to a pure silica fiber with $|\lambda^2(d^2n/d\lambda^2)| = 0.020$ at the operating wavelength. What is the pulse broadening per km due to material dispersion? **[B Tech]**

    (a) 2 ps·km^{-1} (b) 2 ns·km^{-1}

    (c) 2 ms·km^{-1} (d) 0.2 ms·km^{-1}

23. A pulse of 100 ns half-width is transmitted through an optical fiber of length 20 km. The fiber has a rated multipath time dispersion of 10 ns·km^{-1} and a material dispersion of 2 ns·km^{-1}. What will be the half-width of the received pulse? **[B Tech]**

    (a) 100 ns   (b) 227 ns

    (c) 240 ns   (d) 340 ns

24. A LED is emitting a mean wavelength of $\lambda = 0.90$ μm and its spectral half-width $\Delta\lambda = 18$ nm. What will be the half-width of the received pulse? **[B Tech]**

    (a) 0.02   (b) 0.05

    (c) 0.90   (d) 18

25. A laser diode has a relative spectral width of 2×10^{-3} and is emitting a mean wavelength of 1 μm. What is its spectral half-width? **[B Tech]**

    (a) 1 μm   (b) 0.2 μm

    (c) 20 nm   (d) 2 nm

ANSWERS

1. (c)	2. (c)	3. (b)	4. (b)	5. (d)	6. (c)	7. (a)	8. (a)	9. (a)	10. (b)
11. (b)	12. (d)	13. (c)	14. (b)	15. (b)	16. (b)	17. (b)	18. (c)	19. (b)	20. (a)
21. (d)	22. (b)	23. (b)	24. (a)	25. (d)					

CHAPTER

4

Fiber Optic Materials, Cables and Connectors—Power Launching and Fiber Coupling

4.1 INTRODUCTION

The production, application and installation of optical fibers within a line transmission system are of paramount importance if optical fiber communication systems are to be considered as viable replacements for conventional metallic line communication systems. It is, therefore, essential that:

(i) Optical fibers may be produced with good stable transmission characteristics in long lengths at a minimum cost with maximum reproducibility.

(ii) A range of optical fiber types with regard to size, refractive indices and index profiles, operating wavelengths, materials etc. be available in order to fulfill many different system applications.

(iii) The fibers may be converted into practical cables which can be handled in a similar manner to conventional electrical transmission cables without problems associated with the degradation of their characteristics or damage.

(iv) The fibers and fiber cables may be terminated and connected together (jointed) with excessive practical difficulties and in ways which limit the effect of this process on the fiber transmission characteristics to keep them within acceptable operating levels. It is important that these joining techniques may be applied with ease in the field locations where cable connection take place.

(v) The fiber optic cables are to be used under a variety of situations such as underground, outdoor poles or submerged under water. The structure of cable depends on the situation where it is to be used, but the basic cable design principles remains same.

(vi) Mechanical property of cable is one of the important factor for using any specific cable. Maximum allowable axial load on cable decides the length of the cable can be reliably installed.

(vii) Also the fiber cables must be able to absorb energy from impact loads. The outer sheath must be designed to protect glass fibers from impact loads and from corrosive environmental elements.

4.2 FIBER MATERIALS

Light guidance through a step index optical fiber requires the refractive indices of the core and cladding to be different. Hence, two compatible materials that are transparent in the operating wavelength range are required. For graded-index fibers, in order to produce a particular index profile, a variation of the refractive index within the core is also required. This is possible only by varying the dopant concentration. Here again two compatible materials, which are mutually soluble and have similar transmission characteristics, will be required. Further, these materials should be such that long, thin, flexible fibers can be drawn. We summarize these requirements of fiber optic material as follows:

   (i) The material must be transparent for efficient transmission of light.

   (ii) It must be possible to draw long thin fibers from the material.

 (iii) Fiber material must be compatible with the cladding material.

Glass and plastics fulfills the above mentioned requirements of fiber materials.

Most fiber consists of silica (SiO_2) or silicate. Various types of high loss and low loss glass fibers are available to suit the requirements. Plastic fibers are not popular because of high attenuation but they have better mechanical strength.

Silica glass is especially attractive because of its following properties:

   (i) In the near infrared (NIR) wavelength region ranging from 0.85 µm to 1.65 mm, silica (SiO_2) has good optical transparency. Further, high quality silica glass exhibits lowest attenuation of 0.2 dB/km around 1.5 µm wavelength.

  (ii) At reasonably high temperatures, long strands of fibers can be drawn from molten silica.

 (iii) Silica based optical fibers can be *spliced* and cleaved without much of practical difficulties.

 (iv) A silica optical fiber has an extremely high mechanical strength against pulling and even bending, provided that silica fiber is not too thick and also its surfaces are well prepared. We can further improve the mechanical strength of a fiber with a suitable polymer jacket. Further, simple cleaving (breaking) of silica fiber ends can provide nicely flat surfaces with sufficient optical quality.

  (v) Silica fibers can be used even in abusive environment because they are chemically very stable and does not react with most of the chemicals.

 (vi) To increase or decrease the refractive index precisely, silica glass can be doped with various materials. This property of silica glass enables one to achieve compatible materials with a slight difference in the values of refractive indices for creating core and cladding regions.

 (vii) Low *Kerr nonlinearity* of silica make them suitable for optical communication since non-linear effects are often detrimental for such applications.

     There are number of polymers, generally referred to as *plastics* also exhibit many of the above properties. These polymers are also used in making plastic optical fiber (POF). However, plastic fibers have substantially higher attenuation as compared to silica fibers and hence they have limited application. Application of POF is generally restricted to short-distance optical communication system designed for low-bit rate purpose. Further, silica fibers exhibit larger dispersion due to its large NA.

4.2.1 Glass Fibers

Glass is a noncrystalline solid (NCS) or amorphous solid made by fusing mixtures of metal oxides having refractive index of 1.458 at 850 nm. Glass in general is a hard substance, usually brittle and transparent, mainly composed of silicates and alkali fused at high temperature. Usually glass is obtained by fusing mixtures of elements, metal oxides, halides, sulfides, tellurides or selenides. Most of the available glasses are prepared by melting and quanching. Alternatively glass can also be obtained by decomposition from a vapour or a liquid solution.

We may note that technically, glass formation is a property of any material but in practice limited to a small number of substances. The major glass forming substances are listed in Table 4.1.

For changing the refractive index different oxides such as B_2O_3, GeO_2 and P_2O_5 are added as dopants (Table 4.2). Figure 4.1(a) shows variation of refractive index with doping concentration.

Figure 4.1(a) shows that addition of dopants GeO_2 and P_2O_5 increases refractive index, while dopants fluorine (F) and B_2O_3 decreases refractive index. One important criteria is that the refractive index of core is greater than that of the cladding, hence some important compositions are used as in Table 4.2.

Table 4.1: Major glass forming substances

Constituents	Particulars
Elements	S, Se, P, etc.
Oxides	SiO_2 : GeO_2, P_2O_5, B_2O_3, PbO_3, etc.
Halides	BeF_2, AlF_3, NaF, $ZnCl_2$, etc.
Sulfides	As_2S_3, CS_2, Sb_2S_3, etc.
Selenides	SnSe, PbSe, As_2Se_3, etc.
Tellurides	SnTe, PbTe, Sb_2Te_3, As_2Te_3, etc.
Nitrides	KNO_3, $Ca(NO_3)_2$, etc.
Sulphates	$KHSO_4$
Carbonates	K_2CO_3, $MgCO_3$, etc.
Polymers	Polystyrene, polycarbonate, nylon, etc.

Table 4.2: Silica based fibers with composition

Core	Cladding
SiO_2	SiO_2 : B_2O_3
SiO_2	SiO_2 : F
SiO_2 : GeO_2	SiO_2 : GeO_2 : B_2O_3
SiO_2 : B_2O_3 : P_2O_5	SiO_2 : B_2O_3
SiO_2 : B_2O_3 : P_2O_5	SiO_2 : B_2O_3

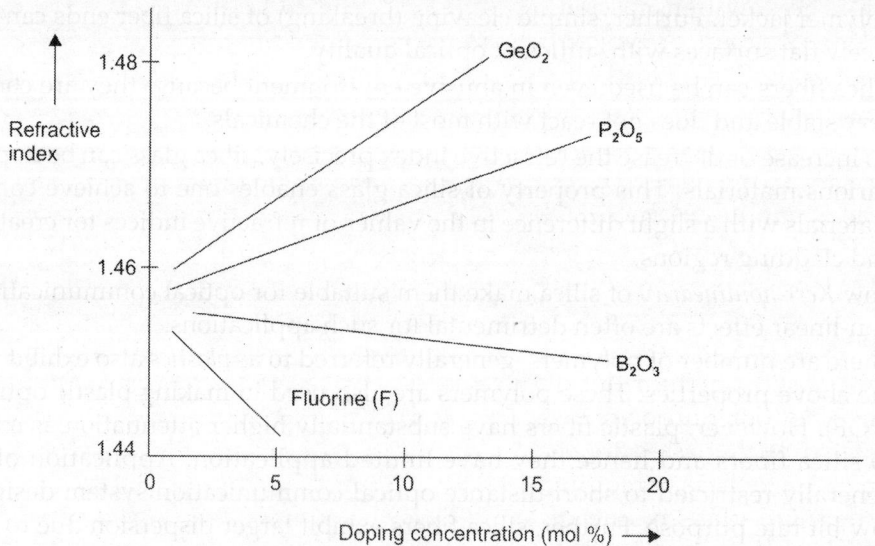

Fig. 4.1(a): Variation of refractive index of silica glass with doping concentration

Structure of glass is not well defined like crystalline materials but instead glass has a randomly oriented molecular network. This is why, it has a fixed melting point. Glass is generally hard at room temperature and it continues to stay in that state when heated to several hundred degrees of celsius depending on its constituents. Beyond 1000°C, silica glass generally softens and further rise in temperature around 1400–1600°C, glass enters into a viscous state. This extended range of temperature is usually referred to as melting temperature of glass rather than melting point. One can reduce the melting temperature of silica glass by adding sodalime. For making optical fiber, the most widely used glass is generally oxide glass and particularly silica (SiO_2) having refractive index of 1.458 at a wave length of 850 nm.

One of the major advantages of glass is that one can change its properties by changing the composition of glass. In case of glass fiber, the core and cladding can be created by controlling the dopant property to maintain a small difference in fractive index between the two. The refractive index of the core in an optical fiber is higher than the cladding refractive index and one can design silica based fibers by suitably controlling the dopant. Table 4.2 shows a few possible options where in $SiO_2 : GeO_2$ indicates GeO_2 doped silica glass, and so on.

The principal raw materials for silica is sand and glass. The fiber composed of pure silica is called as *silica glass*. The desirable properties of silica glass are:
- Resistance to deformation even at high temperature.
- Resistance to breakage from thermal shocks (low thermal expansion).
- Good chemical durability.
- Better transparency.

Other types of glass fibers are:
(i) Halide glass fibers.
(ii) Active glass fibers.
(iii) Chalcogenide glass fibers.
(iv) Plastic optical fibers.

A relatively newer class of fibers is being developed using fluoride glasses, which have extremely low transmission losses at mid-infrared wavelengths (0.2–8 µm), with least loss at ~2.55 µm. A typical core glass consists of ZBLAN glass (named after its constituents ZrF_4, BaF_2, LaF_3, AlF_3, and NaF) and ZHBLAN cladding glass (H standing for HaF_4).

Another class of fibers, called *active fibers*, incorporates some rare-earth elements into the matrix of passive glass. These dopant ions absorb light from the optical source, get excited, and emit fluorescence. Erbium and neodymium have been widely used. Thus, it is possible to fabricate fiber amplifiers, using selective doping. Now, we study these fibers in detail.

4.2.2 Fluoride Fibers

These are based on fluoride glasses, e.g. fluoroaluminate or fluorozirconate glasses. The cations of such glasses are usually from heavy metals such as zirconium or lead. Fluorozirconate glass is one of a typical member of the halide glass family having ZrF_4 as the major component or principal consti-tuents. In order to provide moderate resistance to crystallization, other constituents

Table 4.3: Various constituents of ZBLAN glass with molecular percentage

Constituent	Molecular percentage
ZrF_4	54
BaF_2	20
LaF_3	4.5
AlF_3	3.5
NaF	18

are added. As stated earlier ZBLAN glass (ZrB_4–BaF_2–LaF_3–AlF_3–NaF) is most extensively investigated halide glass. Table 4.3 shows the detailed composition of ZBLAN glass.

ZBLAN glass is used for making the core of the optical fiber and to create the cladding of a lower refractive index ZBLAN is usually doped with HaF_4·HaF_4 replaces partially ZrF_4 in ZBLAN and results in a suitable reduction of refractive index. Clearly, a halide fiber thus constitute ZBLAN core with ZBLAN:HaF_4 cladding. It is reported that heavy metal fluoride constituents lead to low phonon energies and as a result fluoride fibers exhibit a optical transparency, i.e. extremely low optical absorption in mid-infrared (MIR) wavelengths region (2–8 μm) unlike common silica fiber which absorb light significantly beyond 2 μm wavelength. To make low-loss fluoride glass, a combination of fluorozirconate (ZrF_4) and fluorohafnate (HfF_4) has been extensively used. Table 4.4 lists a host of fluoride fibers using various constituent components.

Table 4.4: Composition of fluoride glass-based optical fiber

Glass	Composition (mol %)							
	ZrF_4	BaF_2	GdF_3	LaF_3	YF_3	AlF_3	LiF	NaF
ZBG	63	33	4	–	–	–	–	–
ZBGA	60	32	4	–	–	4	–	–
ZBLAL	52	20	–	5	–	3	20	–
ZBLYAL	49	22	–	3	3	3	20	–
ZBLYAN	47.5	23.5	–	2.5	2	4.5	–	20

A major problem faced with pure halide fiber is that fluoride glass has a tendency to form microcrystallites which increases scattering of light resulting in increase in attenuation. However, other possible applications of fluoride fibers have also been explored subsequently. The mid-infrared (MIR) transparency of fluoride glasses have been exploited to develop mid-infrared spectroscopy, fiber optic sensors, MIR imaging, etc. Fluoride fibers have also been used to transport light over a short distance from Er:YAG laser operating at 2.9 μm wavelength in a several medical appliances.

Hallide glass is also found to be quite useful for realization of various kinds of fiber lasers and fiber amplifiers in view of suppressed multi-phonon transitions in fluoride glasses. It is reported that heavy metal hallide glasses in the family of $ZrF_4 - BaF_2 - LaF_3 - NaF - AlF_3$ system offer extremely low loss in the longer wavelength and are quite suitable for operation in mid-infrared region. Further, ZBLNA system is reasonably stable to be drawn into fibers continuously without devitrification. The value of the transmission loss reported for the fluoride fiber are 0.001 dB/km at 3.2 μm and 0.005 dB/km at 3.5 μm.

4.2.3. Active Glass Fibers

Optical fibers used as channel in guided optical communication is usually viewed as a passive component in the sense that the output power available at the receiver end is always less than the power launched at the input end (transmitter) of the fiber. However, by incorporating rare-earth elements into a normally passive fiber, one may induce new optical and magnetic properties in the fiber. One can subsequently exploit these properties to obtain amplification, phase retardation and other non-linear behaviour of light propagating through such fibers. Usually, this kind of fibers are called as *active fibers*. A variety of glasses can be suitably doped to act as active fibers for making fiber lasers as well as fiber amplifiers.

Fiber lasers and fiber amplifiers are nearly based on active glass fibers which are doped with trace-amount (0.005–0.05 mole%) of laser-active rare earth elements, e.g. erbium, neodymium, ytterbium, etc. (in the fiber core). These rare-earth dopant ions create metastable states in the energy gap of the principal glass material so as to create a situation for *stimulated emission*. Further, the active fibers in fiber laser or amplifier act as *gain media* to provide high gain efficiency, resulting from strong optical confinement in the waveguide structure. Table 4.5 shows some commonly used rare-earth elements and host glasses with emission wavelength from corresponding active fibers.

Table 4.5: Laser active rare-earth dopants and host glass alongwith desired wavelength of emission

Rare-earth ions	Host glass	Laser wavelength
Neodymium (Nd^{3+})	Silica glass and phosphate glass	1.03–1.1 µm, 0.9–0.95 µm, 1.32–1.35 µm
Erbium (Er^{3+})	Silica glass, fluoride glass and phosphate glass	1.5–1.6 µm, 2.7 µm, 0.55 µm
Ytterbium (Yb^{3+})	Silica glass	1.0–1.1 µm
Thulium (Tm^{3+})	Silica glass, fluoride glass	1.7–2.1 µm, 1.45–1.53 µm, 0.48 µm, 0.8 µm
Neodymium (Nd^{3+})	Chalcogenide glass	1.08 µm
Praseodymium (Pr^{3+})	Chalcogenide glass	1.3, 1.6, 2.9, 3.4, 4.5, 4.8, 4.9, and 7.2 µm
Holmium (Ho^{3+})	YAG, YLF, silica	2.1 µm, 2.8–2.9 µm

However, for rare-earth doped active fibers, the material composition of core is normally modified by putting additional dopants. To facilitate the lasing action, in place of using pure silica, some form of aluminosilicate, germanosilicate, or phosphosilicate glass is used. Halide fibers are also used extensively for making fiber lasers and fiber amplifiers. Generally, ytterbium and neodymium-doped gain media are generally used for making lasers while erbium-doped fibers are widely used for making erbium-doped fiber amplifiers (EDFA).

4.2.4 Chalcogenide Glass Fibers

Chalcogenide glass contain atleast one of the Chalcogens elements, e.g. S, Se or Te. These glasses exhibit high optical nonlinearity and, as a result, have found wider applications in nonlinear optics ranging from amplifiers to all optical switches. Usually, Chalcogenide glass containing one of the Chalcogens, i.e., S or Se or Te are generally co-doped with a number of other elements such as P, I, Cl, Br, Cd, Si, etc., for tailoring the refractive index and other optical properties and improving thermal and mechanical stability. The most widely investigated material from the Chalcogenide glass family is As_2S_3. It is reported that Chalcogenide glass based single mode fiber with $As_{40}S_{58}Se_2$ (core) and As_2S_3 (cladding) exhibit a loss as low as a 1 dB/km. However, delicate nature, complicated fabrication methodology and usually excessive cost of Chalcogenide glasses have restricted their widespread application as well as commercialization. However, the Chalcogenide glass fibers are reported to be an excellent host for rare-earth ions, not only for the near infrared region (1.3–1.55 µm) telecommunication systems, but also for applications at the longer wavelengths. In past few years, special Chalcogenide glasses have been prepared for doping with rare-earth elements for laser emission in the mid-infrared wavelength region and beyond (2–12 µm).

4.2.5 Plastic Optical Fiber (POF)

These are manufactured from a variety of polymers usually referred to as plastic materials such as polystyrene, polycarbonates, and polymethylmethacrylate (PMMA). These materials exhibit transmission windows usually in the visible wavelength region (500–800 nm). However, the attenuation of optical signal in plastic optical fibers at these wavelengths is very high typically in the range from 150 dB/km for PMMA to 1,000 dB/km for polystrene. The attenuation in these fibers is much higher than that of high quality single mode glass fibers, which have a loss only in the tune of 0.2 dB/km. Moreover, dispersion in these fibers is also very high in view of larger NA as compared to glass fibers arising out of large differences between the refractive indices of core and cladding. However, the large dispersion in POF severely restricts the transmission speed of data through POFs. The POFs are limited to short-distance applications at low data rate. Nevertheless, POFs have several advantages that make them suitable for applications in areas such as industrial controls, sensors for detecting high-energy particles, automobiles, general illumination purpose including short-haul data links. A special type of POF have been made from an amorphous fluorinated polymer called CYTOP which exhibit even lower attenuation (~ 50 dB/km).

These fibers offer several advantages over glass fibers. A large value of NA enables light to be easily coupled even from inexpensive diffused optical sources, e.g. light emitting diodes (LEDs). Low cost of these fibers and other associated optical components makes POF-based communication system cheaper compared to glass fibers-based optical fiber communication systems. These fibers also have other advantages, e.g. lighter weight, operation in the visible region, greater flexibility, and resiliency to bending, shock and vibration, ease in handling and connecting (POF diameters are 1 mm compared with 8–100 mm for glass), require simple and inexpensive test equipment, splices and connectors. However, lack of industrial standards and high loss make these fibers less attractive for sophisticated applications. The attenuation in POF is caused by the molecular vibrational absorption of the groups C-H, N-H and O-H and further by the absorption due to electronic transitions between energy levels within molecular bonds. Additional factors include scattering arising from composition, orientation, and density fluctuations.

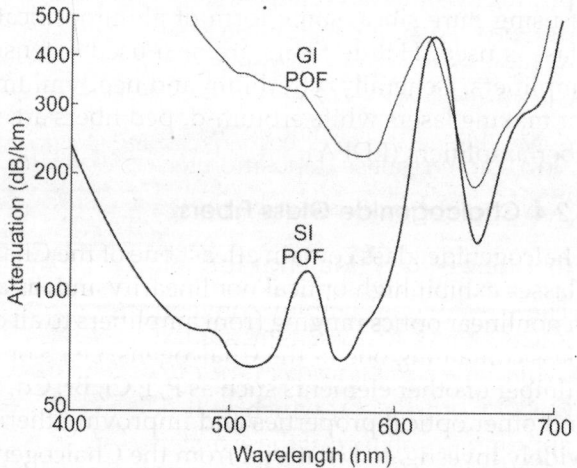

Fig. 4.1(b): Attenuation profiles of a standard Si-POF and a GI-POF

Figure 4.1(b) shows the attenuation profiles of step-index (SI) and graded-index of POFs. These fibers exhibit attenuation windows usually in the visible region. Figure 4.1(c) shows the attenuation characteristics of a typical POF fiber. However, the POF fiber exhibits a low value of attenuation in the near infrared (IR) region.

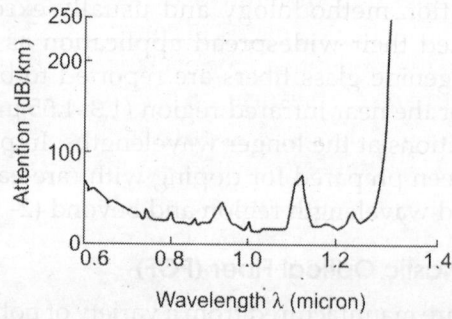

Fig. 4.1(c): Variation of attenuation of POF fiber with wavelength (λ)

4.2.6 Plastic Clad Silica (PCS) Fibers

Plastic clad fibers are multimode and have either a step index or a graded index profile. Basically, PCS is a compromise between high performance silica fiber and less efficient plastic fibers. PCS consists of a core made of silica glass and cladding made of compatible polymer of lower refractive index. Commercial PCS fibers consist of a pure silica core, a soft silicon cladding and a protective jacket. The PCS fibers exhibit lower radiation-induced losses than silica-clad-silica fibers and, therefore, have an improved performance in certain environments. We may note

Table 4.6: Specifications of a typical commercial PCS fiber

Parameter	Values
Core diameter	200 mm to 1500 mm
Number Aperture	0.40
Core to clad ratio	1.1, 1.2, 1.4
Cladding material	Silicone
Jacket material	Nylon, Tefzel

that PCS fibers are an economical alternative to all-silica fibers. The advantages of PCS fibers include their high light collection efficiency, insensitivity to bending excellent transmission. Table 4.6 shows the parameters of a typical commercial PCS fibers.

4.3 FIBER FABRICATION METHODS

Fabrication of all glass-fibers is a two-stage process in which initially the pure glass is produced and converted in a form (rod or preform) suitable for making the fiber. A drawing or pulling technique is then employed to acquire the end product. The methods of preparing extremely pure optical glasses may be placed into following two major categories:

(i) Liquid-phase (melting) techniques, and

(ii) Vapour-phase deposition techniques.

Now, we briefly describe these techniques.

(i) Liquid-Phase (Melting) Techniques

These techniques employ conventional glass refining techniques for ultra pure material powders which are usually oxides or carbonates of required constituents. These include oxides such as SiO_2, GeO_2, B_2O_2 and Al_2O_3, and carbonates such as Na_2CO_3, K_2CO_3, $CaCO_3$, and $BaCO_3$ which will decompose into oxides during the glass melting. An appropriate mixture of these materials is then melted at temperatures varying from 900°C to 1300°C in silica or platinum crucibles. After the melt has been processed suitably, it is cooled and drawn into rods or tubes (or about 1 m in length) of multi-component glass. The rod of core glass is then inserted into a tube of cladding glass to make a perform.

Figure 4.2 shows the apparatus used for drawing fiber from this preform. Here, the preform is precision-fed into a cylindrical furnace capable of maintaining high temperature, normally called a drawing furnace. During its passage through the hot zone, its end is softened to the extent that a vary thin fiber can be drawn from it. The outer diameter of the fiber is monitored through a feedback mechanism, which controls the feed rate of the preform

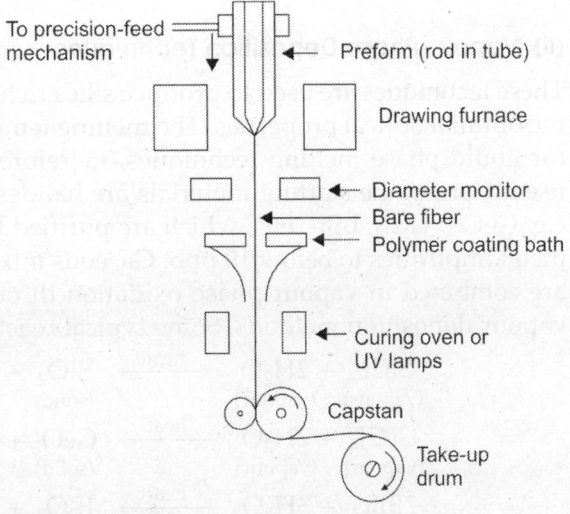

Fig. 4.2: Schematic of a fiber-drawing apparatus

and also the winding rate of the fiber. The bare fiber is then given a primary protective coating of polymer by passing it through the coating bath. This coating is cured either by UV lamps or thermally. The furnished fiber is then wound on a take-up drum.

A fiber about 20–30 km long can be drawn from a preform of about 1 m in 2–3 h. Higher pulling rates are limited by the pulling process as well as the subsequent primary coating operation. This method of preparing fibers tends to be a bach process and hence continuous production is not possible.

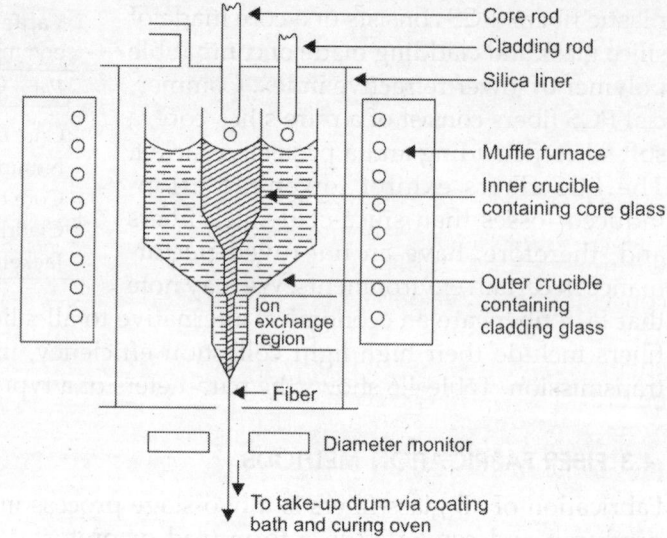

Fig. 4.3: Double crucible apparatus for continuous production of fibers

Continuous manufacture is possible using another technique, which is called the *double crucible method*. Figure 4.3 shows the double crucible apparatus.

Double crucible consists of two concentric platinum crucibles mounted inside a vertical cylindrical muffle furnace whose temperature may be varied from 800°C to 1200°C. The starting material—core and cladding glasses, either directly in the powdered form or in the form of preformed rods—is fed into the two crucibles separately. Both the crucibles have nozzles at their bases from which a clad fiber may be drawn from the melt in a manner similar to that shown in the Fig. 4.2. Index grading may be achieved by diffusion of dopant ions across the core-cladding interface, within the melt. Relatively inexpensive fibers of large core diameters and, therefore, large numerical apertures may be produced continuously by this method. An attenuation level of the order of 3 dB/km for sodium borosilicate glass fiber, which is prepared using this technique, has been reported in the literature.

(ii) Vapour-Phase Deposition Techniques

These techniques are used to produce silica rich glasses of highest transparency and with the optimal optical properties. The melting temperature of silica-rich glasses are too high for liquid-phase melting techniques, therefore, vapour-phase deposition methods are used. Herein, the starting materials are halides of silica (e.g. $SiCl_4$) and of the dopants, e.g. $GeCl_4$, $TiCl_4$, BBr_3, etc., which are purified to reduce the concentration of transition-metal impurities to below 10 ppb. Gaseous mixtures of halides of silica and the dopants are combined in vapour-phase oxidation through either flame hydrolysis or chemical vapour deposition methods. Some typical reactions are as follows:

$$SiCl_4 + 2H_2O \xrightarrow{\text{heat}} SiO_2 + 4HCl \tag{4.1}$$
$$\text{(vapour)} \quad \text{(vapour)} \qquad \text{(solid)} \quad \text{(gas)}$$

$$GeCl_4 + 2H_2O \xrightarrow{\text{heat}} GeO_2 + 4HCl \tag{4.2}$$
$$\text{(vapour)} \quad \text{(vapour)} \qquad \text{(solid)} \quad \text{(gas)}$$

$$2BBr_3 + 3H_2O \xrightarrow{\text{heat}} B_2O_3 + 4HBr \tag{4.3}$$
$$\text{(vapour)} \quad \text{(vapour)} \qquad \text{(solid)} \quad \text{(gas)}$$

$$\underset{\text{(vapour)}}{SiCl_4} + \underset{\text{(gas)}}{O_2} \xrightarrow{\text{heat}} \underset{\text{(solid)}}{SiO_2} + \underset{\text{(gas)}}{2Cl_2} \tag{4.4}$$

$$\underset{\text{(vapour)}}{GeCl_4} + \underset{\text{(gas)}}{O_2} \xrightarrow{\text{heat}} \underset{\text{(solid)}}{GeO_2} + \underset{\text{(gas)}}{2Cl_2} \tag{4.5}$$

$$\underset{\text{(vapour)}}{TiCl_4} + \underset{\text{(gas)}}{O_2} \xrightarrow{\text{heat}} \underset{\text{(solid)}}{TiO_2} + \underset{\text{(gas)}}{2Cl_2} \tag{4.6}$$

The oxides resulting from these reactions are normally deposited onto a substrate or within a hollow tube, which is built up as a stack of successive layers. Thus, the concentration of the dopant may be varied gradually to produce the desired index profile. This process results in either a solid rod or a hollow tube of glass, which should be collapsed to produce a solid perform. Using the apparatus shown in Fig. 4.2, fibers may be drawn from this perform.

Based on above principle, various techniques have been developed. We will discuss a few of them here.

(a) Outside-Vapour-Phase Oxidation (OVPO) Process

This process which uses flame hydrolysis stems from work on 'soot' processes originally developed by Hyde in 1942. Figure 4.4 shows the flame hydrolysis to deposit the required glass composition onto a rotating mandrel (an aluminium rod). The mixtures of vapours of the starting materials, e.g. $SiCl_4$, $GeCl_4$, BBr_3, etc. is blown through the oxygen-hydrogen flame. The soot produced by the oxidation of halide vapours is deposited on a cool mandrel. The flame is moved back and forth over the length of the mandrel so that a sufficient number of layers is deposited on it. The concentration of the dopant

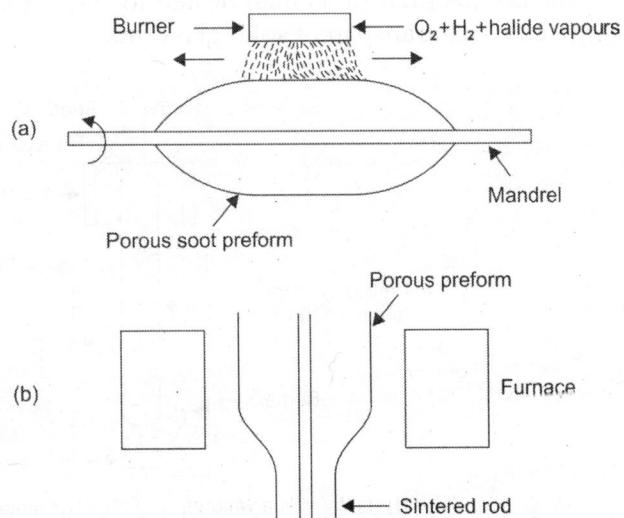

Fig. 4.4: Schematic of glass deposition by the OVPO method: (a) soot deposition (b) preform sintering

halides is either varied gradually, if index grading is required, or maintained constant, if step index is required.

After the deposition of the core and cladding layers is complete, the mandrel is removed. The hollow and porous preform left behind is then sintered in a furnace to form a solid transparent glass rod. This is then drawn into a fiber by the apparatus discussed earlier. With a single preform, 30–40 km of fiber can be easily prepared. Nevertheless, a number of proprietary approaches to scaling up the process have provided preforms capable of producing 250 km of fiber. The index profile can be controlled well using this method, as the flow rate of vapours can be adjusted after the deposition of each layer. An attenuation of less than 1 dB/km at an operating wavelength of 1.3 μm has been reported, but the fibers exhibit an axial dip in the refractive index.

The index profile can be controlled well using this method, as the flow rate of vapours can be adjusted after the deposition of each layer. An attenuation of less than 1 dB/km at an operating wavelength of 1.3 µm has been reported, but the fibers exhibit an axial dip in the refractive index.

The purity of the glass fiber depends on the purity of the feeding materials and also upon the amount of OH impurity from the exposure of the silica to the water vapour in the flame following the reactions described earlier.

(b) Vapour Axial Deposition (VAD) Process

This process was developed by Zaw in 1977. The VAD technique uses an end-on deposition onto a rotating fused silica target. In this process, core and cladding glasses are simultaneously deposited onto the end of a speed rod, which is rotated to maintain azimuthal homogeneity and also pulled up, as illustrated in Fig. 4.5. The porous preform so deposited, while the seed rod is being pulled up, is heated to about 1100°C in an electric furnace in an atmosphere of O_2 and thionyl chloride. Any water vapour in the preform is removed through the following reaction:

$$SOCl_2 + H_2O \rightarrow SO_2 + 2HCl \tag{4.7}$$

The porous preform is then heated to about 1500°C in a carbon furnace, where it is sintered into a transparent solid glass rod.

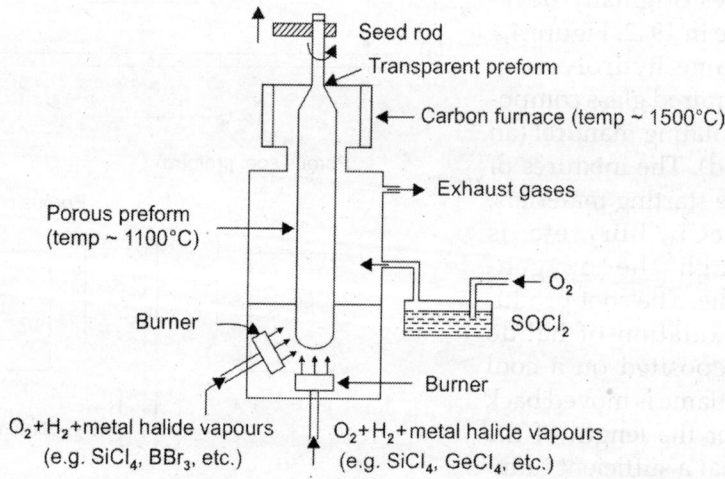

Fig. 4.5: Schematic of the apparatus for the VAD technique

A good control over the index profile may be achieved with germanium-doped cores. Graded-index with an attenuation level less than 0.5 dB/km at 1.3 µm has been produced by this method. In principle, this process may be adopted to draw fiber continuously, although at present, it tends to be operated as a batch process partly because the resultant performs can yield more than 100 km of fiber.

Modified chemical vapour deposition (MCVD method): Chemical vapour deposition processes are generally used at very low deposition rates in the semiconductor industry to produce protective SiO_2 films on silicon semiconductor devices. Basically MCVD is a vapour-phase oxidation process taking place inside a hollow silica tube as shown in Fig. 4.6. The tube has a length of about 1 m and a diameter of about 15 mm. It is horizontally mounted and rotated on a glass-working lathe, with an arrangement (normally an oxygen-hydrogen flame) for heating the outer surface of the tube to about 1500°C. The reactants in the form of halide vapours and oxygen are passed at a controlled rate through the tube. The halides are oxidized in the hot zone of the tube and the generated soot (glass particles) is deposited on the inner wall. The hot zone (i.e. the flame) is moved back and forth allowing the layer-by-layer deposition of the soot. Index grading may be achieved by varying the concentration of the dopants layer by layer. The tube can form a cladding material or serve as a support structure only for the porous preform. After the deposition is complete, the tube or the porous preform is sintered at a higher temperature (1700–1900°C) to form a transparent glass rod. Fiber is then drawn from this rod in the usual manner.

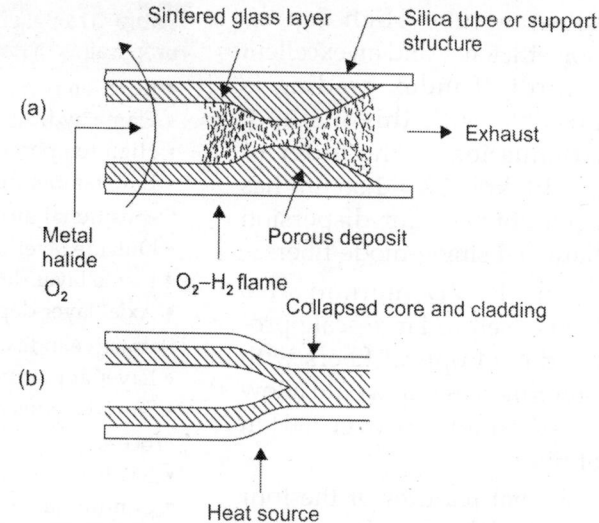

Fig. 4.6: Schematic diagram: (a) apparatus for the MCVD process (b) preform sintering

Presently, this is a widely used method for fabricating fibers, as it permits the deposition to occur in a clean environment, with reduced OH impurity. This method is suitable for preparing a variety of glass compositions for multimode or single-mode step-index (SI) or graded-index fibers. Typically, attenuation of the order of 0.2 dB/km at a wavelength of 1.55 μm has been reported for single-mode germania-doped silica fibers prepared by this method. Further, this technique is also suitable for preparing polarization-maintaining single-mode fibers.

Although, MCVD is not a continuous process, but this technique has proved suitable for the widespread mass production of high-performance of optical fibers. Further, it can be scaled up to produce preforms which provide 100 km to 200 km of fiber.

(c) Plasma-Activated Chemical Vapour Deposition (PCVD) Method

A variation on the MCVD technique is the use of various types of plasma to supply energy for the vapour-phase oxidation of halides. This method involves plasma-induced chemical vapour deposition inside a silica. The deposition rates of the MCVD process may be increased if microwave-frequency plasma is created in the reaction zone. This process is illustrated in Fig. 4.7. Herein, a microwave cavity (operating at 2.45 GHz) surrounds the substrate tube.

The halide vapours of the silica-based compound or the

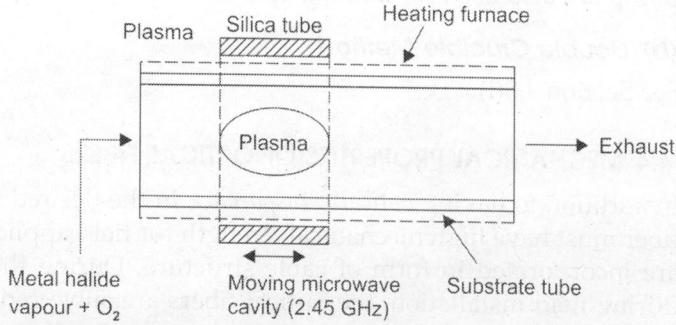

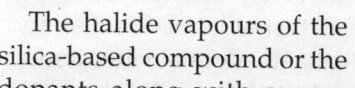

Fig. 4.7: Schematic of the apparatus used for the PCVD process

dopants along with oxygen are introduced into the tube where they react in the microwave-excited plasma zone. The tube temperature is maintained at about 1900°C using a stationary furnace. The reaction zone is moved back and forth along the tube enabling circularly symmetrical deposition of glass layers onto the inner wall of the substrate tube. High deposition efficiency and an excellent control of index grading is possible with this method. Attenuation of the order of 0.3 dB/km at $\lambda = 1.55$ μm has been obtained for dispersion flattened single-mode fibers.

The PCVD method also lends itself to large-scale production of optical fibers with preform sizes that would allow the preparation of over 200 km of fiber.

Salient features of the four vapour-phase deposition (VPD) techniques discussed above are summarized in Table 4.7.

Table 4.7: Salient features of VPD techniques used in the preparation of low-loss optical fibers

• Reaction type	OVPO, VAD
• Flame hydrolysis	MCVD
• High-temperature oxidation	PCVD
• Low-temperature oxidation	
Depositional direction	
• Outside layer deposition	OVPO
• Inside layer deposition	MCVD, PCVD
• Axial layer deposition	VAD
Refractive index profile formation	
• Layer approximation	OVPO, MCVD, PCVD
• Simultaneous formation	VAD
Process	
• Batch	OVPO, MCVD, PCVD
• Continuous	VAD

(iii) Fiber Fabrication Method Without Involving Performs

There are atleast two common methods of fiber fabrication which do not require formation of fiber performs:

(a) Rod in Tube Method

In this method of fiber fabrication, a solid rod of a glass (say, $SiO_2 : GeO_2$) having higher refractive index is inserted into a glass tube (say, SiO_2) with a lower refractive index. When the outer tube is heated to a high temperature both the rod and tube get well connected with each other. The combination of rod and tube is then heated strongly so that it melt and the bottom of the tube collapses due to surface tension. Long fibers can be drawn from the molten material. The material of the rod constitutes the core whereas the material of the cladding comes from the tube. However, utmost care is required to avoid trapping of air bubbles during fiber drawing. Casting methods where the molten core glass is poured into the cladding tube, or sucked into the tube using a vacuum pump are also used for making optical fibers without using a perform.

(b) Double Crucible Method

See Section 4.3(i).

4.4 MECHANICAL PROPERTIES OF OPTICAL FIBERS

In addition to having *optical transparency* in the desired wavelength regions, the optical fiber must have high mechanical strength for field applications. Generally, optical fibers are incorporated in form of cable structure. During the process of cabling as well as during field installation, the optical fibers are subjected to a variety of stresses. This is why, fibers have to be designed in such a way that they can withstand erratic stress and strain during cabling, installation and servicing. We may note that inadequate mechanical strength may lead to rupture of fibers leading to failure of fiber. Generally, the fibers encounter loads which can be either impulsive or slowing varying in nature. Slowly varying loads, generally, arise out of the variation of temperature or during initially settling following installation of cables. Generally, the mechanical behaviour of optical fibers are determined by two characteristic parameters: (i) strength and (ii) static fatigue. Generally, glass is viewed as a fragile material and also it is less strong as compared to conducting metal wires. Usually, the intrinsic strength of a material is determined by the strength of the cohesive bonds between the constituent atoms. This is why, the strength of the glass varies with the composition. It is reported that for short-length fiber the tensile strength of 14 GPa is achievable. This value is close to 20 GPa tensile strength exhibited by steel wires. It is also reported that good quality magnesium alumino silicate glasses used for reinforcement in composite structural applications exhibit Young's modulus (Y) ~ 90 GPa, shear modulus ~ 30 GPa and Poisson's ratio (σ) ~ 0.2 at room temperature. However, one of the problems with glass fiber is that it cannot be elongated like metal wires beyond elastic limit. This is mainly unlike glass, metal can elongate plastically beyond elastic limit whereas glass has a tendency to break or develop cracks beyond elastic limit.

Generally, the mechanical strength of optical fibers is often tested by static fatigue. In this testing, a constant load higher than the threshold load is applied to the optical fiber and the rupture is observed after sometime. We may note that the fracture depends on a number of factors for a given load, e.g. quality of coating, temperature and contaminants present. Water is one of the major contaminants that severely affects the mechanical properties of the optical fiber. The OH^- bond weakens the silica bond and caused the optical fiber to rupture much below the threshold load. The initial flaws or microcracks already present in the optical fiber also cause the facture of the fibers. When the fiber is subjected to loads the microcracks already present in the fiber start propagating causing larger size cracks that finally lead to rupture of the optical fiber. The failure of fiber cable may also occur with aging without any applied load when the cables are used in abusive environment for which fibers are not actually designed. One can describe the quality of the optical fiber by fatigue susceptibility (n) given by

$$\log (\sigma_f) = \frac{\log \delta}{(1+n)} + c \qquad (4.7a)$$

where σ_f denotes the facture stress, δ is stress rate and c is constant.

In order to provide additional mechanical strength and also protection from abusive environment, generally, buffered optical fibers are sealed in the form of cable. We may note that the type of cabling largely depends on the nature of field applications.

4.5 OPTICAL FIBER CABLES

Fiber optic cables transmit data through very small cores at the speed of light. Significantly different from copper cables, fiber optic cables offer *high band width* and *low losses* which allow high data-transmission rates over long distances. Light propages throughout the fiber cables according to the principle of total internal reflection (TIR).

There are three common types of fiber optic cables: single mode, multimode, and graded index. Each has its advantages and disadvantages. There are also several different designs of fiber optic cables, each made for different applications. In addition, new fiber optic cables with different core and cladding designs have been emerging; these are faster and can carry more modes. While fiber optic cables are used mostly in communication systems, they also have established medical, military, scanning, imaging and sensing applications. They are also used in optical fiber devices and fiber opting lighting.

The scaling down of light sources brings the benefits of fiber technology to a wide range of applications. These developments have led to a surge of interest in advanced fiber cables for both industrial and military applications. Advanced fiber cables are also used for transmitting high volumes of data in communication systems over long distances for getting clear images, and in building many sophisticated instruments for a variety of applications. By creating new core designs, adding dopants to the fiber core and cladding, and developing manufacturing processes, engineers achieve advanced fiber-optic cable technology, e.g. the core of *holey fibers* consists of many air holes; each hole acts as a single fiber. This fiber enables a high data transmission rate and capacity, and consequently, reduces the cost of the network.

Optical glass fibers are brittle and have very small cross-sectional areas (typical outer diameters range from 100 to 250 μm). They are quite susceptible to damage during normal handling and use. Thus, it is necessary to improve their tensile strength and protect them from external influences. Therefore, it is necessary to encase them in cables.

The exact design of the optical-fiber cable may vary depending on the application; i.e., it will depend on whether the cable is required to be used in underground ducts, buried directly, hung from the poles, or submerged underwater, etc. Thus, one can develop a general criterion to be applied to all the designs of cables to be formulated. A cable design should be such that it (i) protect the optical fiber from damage and breakage, (ii) does not degrade the transmission characteristics of the optical fiber, (iii) prevents the fiber from being subjected to excessive strain and limits the bending radius, (iv) provides a strength member which can improve its mechanical strength, and (v) provides for (in the case of multifiber cables) the identification and jointing of optical fibers within the cable.

In the light of above factors, the primary coated fibers are given a secondary or buffer coating for protection against external influences. It is also possible to place the fibers in an oversized extruded tube normally called a *loose buffer jacket*. This structure isolates the fiber mechanically from external forces as well as microbending losses. The empty space in the loose tube may be filled with soft, self-healing material that remains stable over a wide range of temperatures. The buffered fibers are then either stranded helically around a central strength member of placed in the slots of a structural member. The structural member may also serve as a strength member if made of load-bearing material.

The common desirable features of strength and structural members are *high Young's modulus, high tolerance to strain, flexibility,* and *low weight per unit length*. An additional requirement of the strength member is that it should have *high tensile strength*. In order to provide cushion to the entire assembly consisting of buffered fiber, and structural and strength members, a coating of extruded plastic is applied or a tape is helically wound. A further thick outer sheath of plastic is necessary to provide the cable with extra protection against mechanical forces such as crushing. Some designs include copper wires in the cable. These wires are used to feed electrical power to the remote online repeaters and also to serve as voice channels during installation and repair. Some designs of cable are shown in Figs 4.8–4.11.

Some important points about the fiber optic cables are as follows:

(i) The fiber optic cables are to be used under variety of situations such as underground, outdoor poles or submerged under water. The structure of cable depends on the situation where it is to be used, but the basic cable design principles remains same.

(ii) *Mechanical property* of the cable is one of the important factor for using any specific cable. Maximum permissible axial load on cable decides the length of the cable that can be reliably installed.

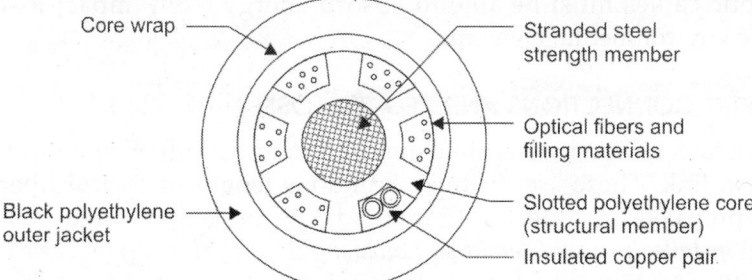

Fig. 4.8: Schematic of a slotted core cable. Here, a slotted polyethylene core is extruded over the stranded steel strength member. The buffered fibers are placed in the slots. The design is quite easy to fabricate and may be adopted for a variety of applications

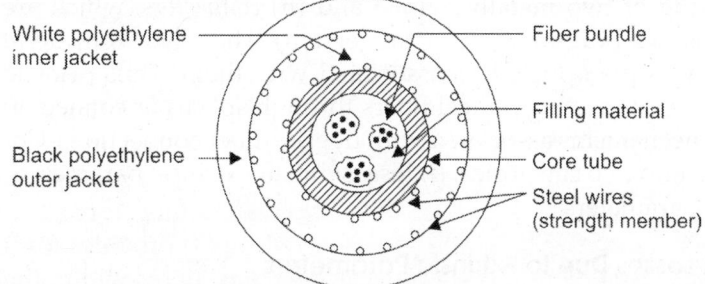

Fig. 4.9: Schematic of a loose bundle cable. Here, a tube is extruded over the fiber bundles, each bundle containing several fibers. The steel wires surrounding this tube serve as strength members. This permits a large number of fibers to be accommodated in a compact design

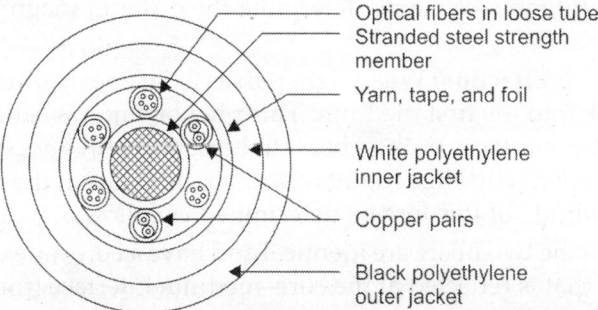

Fig. 4.10: Schematic of a multifiber cable. Here, buffered fibers are placed in loose tubes. Out of the six tubes shown, four contain optical fibers and two contain insulated copper pairs. A central steel strength member has been provided. This cable is suitable for underground ducts

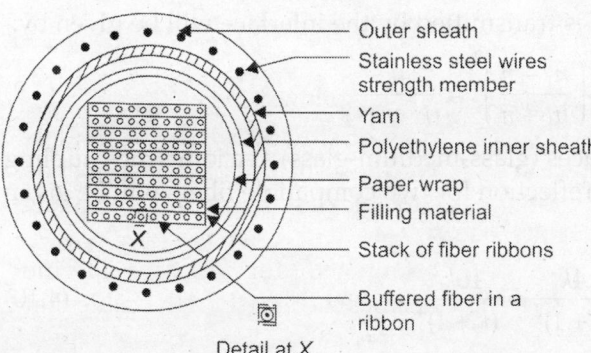

Detail at X

Fig. 4.11: Schematic of a multifiber ribbon cable. This design allows a large number of fibers to be placed in a single cable. The cable design by AJ and T can accommodate 144 fibers in the form of a stack of 12 ribbons, each ribbon containing 12 optical fibers. Ribbon cables are being developed, which can accommodate several hundred fibers

(iii) Fiber optic cables must be able to absorb energy from impact loads and from corrosive environmental elements.

4.6 FIBER-OPTIC CONNECTIONS AND RELATED LOSSES

There are three factors which determine the continuous length of an optical fiber along a communication link. These are: (i) the continuous length of optical fiber that can be produced by prevalent manufacturing methods (ii) the length of the cable that can be produced and *installed as a continuous section along the link* and (iii) *the cable length between the repeaters.* This uninterrupted length of optical fiber along a link, therefore, is not more than 10 km. Obviously, for establishing long-haul transmission links, optical fibers are required to be connected. The fiber-to-fiber connection may be achieved in two ways: (i) *splices,* which are permanent joints between two fibers (splicing is analogous to the electrical soldering of two metallic wires) and (ii) *connectors,* which are demountable joints (analogous to a plug-in-socket arrangement). The major consideration in making these connections is the optical loss associated with them. Thus prior to discussion of technique used for connecting optical fibers through splices or connectors, let us briefly review the loss mechanisms associated with fiber-to-fiber connections. Connection losses may be grouped into two categories: (i) losses due to extrinsic parameters, and (ii) losses due to intrinsic parameters.

(i) Connection Losses Due to Extrinsic Parameters

There are some factors extrinsic to the fibers that contribute to coupling losses. The important ones among these are: (i) Fresnel reflection (e.g. at glass-air-glass interfaces), (ii) longitudinal, lateral, and angular misalignment of fibers, and (iii) lack of parallelism and flatness in the end faces. We now determine the order of magnitude of joint losses due to these parameters.

Loss due to Fresnel reflection: When light passes from one medium to another, a part of it is reflected back into the first medium. This phenomenon is called *Fresnel reflection.* Therefore, even if the end faces of the fibers (to be connected) are perfectly flat and the axes of the fibers are perfectly aligned; there will be some loss at the joint due to Fresnel reflection. The magnitude of this loss be determined as follows:

Let us assume that the two fibers are identical and have a core index n, then the fraction of optical power, R, that is reflected at the core–medium interface (for normal incidence) is given by:

$$R = \left(\frac{n_1 - n}{n_1 + n}\right)^2 \tag{4.8}$$

Therefore, the fraction of power that is transmitted by the interface will be given by:

$$T = 1 - R = 1 - \left(\frac{n_1 - n}{n_1 + n}\right)^2 = \frac{4k}{(k+1)^2} \tag{4.9}$$

where $k = n_1/n$. As there are two interfaces (glass-medium-glass) at a joint, the coupling efficiency η_F in the presence of Fresnel reflection for two compatible fibers will be given by:

$$\eta_F = \frac{4k}{(k+1)^2} \frac{4k}{(k+1)^2} = \frac{16k^2}{(k+1)^4} \tag{4.10}$$

However, if the cores of the two fibers have the same size (i.e. same core diameter) but different refractive indices, say, n_1 and n_1' then the coupling efficiency η_F' in this case will be given by:

$$\eta_F' = \frac{4k}{(k+1)^2} \frac{4k'}{(k'+1)^2} \tag{4.11}$$

where $k = n_1/n$ and $k' = n_1'/n$.

Thus the loss, in decibels (dB), at a joint due to Fresnel reflection will be given by:

$$L_F = -10 \log_{10}(\eta_F) \tag{4.12}$$

or

$$L_F' = -10 \log_{10}(\eta_F') \tag{4.12a}$$

Typically, if $n_1 = 1.5$ and $n = 1$ (for air), $L_F = 0.36$ dB. Normally, in order to minimize such losses, index-matching fluid is used in the gap between fiber ends.

Fiber-to-fiber misalignment losses: In an optical fiber connection, the alignment of the two fibers to be connected is very important. The three types of misalignment that may occur are shown in Fig. 4.12. It is possible that there is (i) separation between the fiber ends along the common axis (end separation or longitudinal misalignment) (ii) a lateral offset between the axes of the two fibers (lateral misalignment), and (iii) an angle between the axes of the two fibers (angular misalignment). In each of these cases, the loss at a joint is determined by

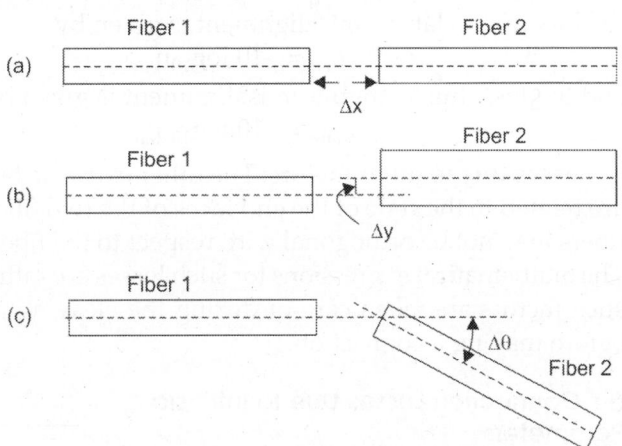

Fig. 4.12: Schematic of (a) longitudinal (b) lateral (c) angular misalignment of fiber 2 with respect to fiber 1

the optical coupling efficiency between the two fibers. It has been shown that for the three types of misalignment shown in parts (a), (b), and (c) of Fig. 4.12, the coupling efficiencies for two compatible multimode step-index fibers are given by Eqs (4.13), (4.14), and (4.15), respectively. The coupling efficiency η_{long} for a longitudinal misalignment Δx between the two fibers is given by:

$$\eta_{\text{long}} = \left[1 - \frac{\Delta x \text{NA}}{4an}\right] \tag{4.13}$$

where a is the core radius and NA is the numerical aperture of both fibers. The coupling efficiency η_{lat} for a lateral offset Δy between the axes of the two fibers is expressed as:

$$\eta_{\text{lat}} \approx \frac{2}{\pi}\left[\cos^{-1}\left(\frac{\Delta y}{2a}\right) - \left(\frac{\Delta y}{2a}\right)\left\{1 - \left(\frac{\Delta y}{2a}\right)^2\right\}^{1/2}\right] \tag{4.14}$$

Here $\cos^{-1}(\Delta y/2a)$ is expressed in radians. Finally, the coupling efficiency η_{ang} for an angular misalignment $\Delta\theta$ between the axes of the two fibers is given by:

$$\eta_{\text{ang}} \approx \left[1 - \frac{n\Delta\theta}{\pi\text{NA}}\right] \tag{4.15}$$

The main assumptions in deriving these formulae are as follows: (i) All the modes are uniformly excited. (ii) In Eq. (4.13), the optical wave propagating through the fiber is assumed to be expressed by a meridional ray and the gap (Δx) between the two fibers is assumed to be less than $a/\tan\phi_0$, where $\phi_0 = NA/n$. (iii) In Eq. (4.14), it has been assumed that the overlapped area between both the cores gives the coupling efficiency η_{lat} approximately, and the change in the optical ray angular component is small. This relation is valid for $0 \leq \Delta y \leq 2a$. (iv) In Eq. 4.15, the propagation angle (in radians) in the second fiber is restricted to $\Psi \leq (2\Delta)^{1/2}$, where Δ is the relative refractive index difference of the fiber.

The loss, in decibel, due to the three types of misalignment described above may be determined using the following relations. The loss due to longitudinal misalignment is given by:

$$L_{long} = -10 \log_{10}\eta_{long} \tag{4.16}$$

the loss due to lateral misalignment is given by:

$$L_{lat} = -10 \log_{10}\eta_{lat} \tag{4.17}$$

and the loss due to angular misalignment is given by:

$$L_{ang} = -10 \log_{10}\eta_{ang} \tag{4.18}$$

Losses due to other factors: The other extrinsic factors that may cause losses at a joint are related to the state of the end faces of the two fibers. For example, the end faces of the fibers may not be orthogonal with respect to the fiber axes. Further, they may not be flat. The mathematical expressions for such losses are rather difficult to arrive at. Nevertheless, such factors are taken care of during the cleaving and polishing of the fiber end faces before making a connection.

(ii) Connection Losses Due to Intrinsic Parameters

When the fibers to be connected are not compatible, i.e. they have different geometrical and/or optical parameters, then power may be lost at the joint. In this context, the following are quite important:
  (i) the core diameter,
  (ii) the numerical aperture or the relative refractive index difference, and
  (iii) the refractive index profile.

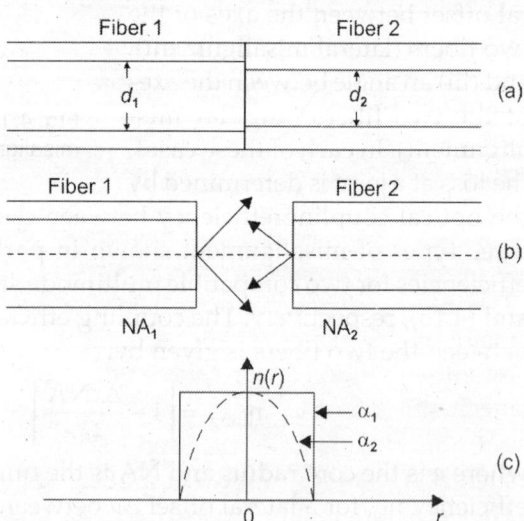

Fig. 4.13: Schematic of mismatch of intrinsic parameters: (a) core diameter (b) numerical aperture (NA) (c) refractive index profile

The mismatch of these parameters is illustrated in Fig. 4.13. In a multimode step-index or graded-index fiber, if we assume that all the modes are uniformly excited and that all the parameters of the two fibers are same except their diameters, then the coupling efficiency η_{cd} may be estimated by the ratio of the core areas. Thus, one finds:

$$\eta_{cd} = \begin{cases} \dfrac{\pi d_2^2/4}{\pi d_1^2/4} = \left(\dfrac{d_2}{d_1}\right)^2 & \text{for } d_2 < d_1 \\ 1 \text{ for } d_2 \geq d_1 \end{cases} \tag{4.19a and b}$$

where d_1 and d_2 are the core diameters of the transmitting and receiving fibers, respectively. The corresponding loss (in dB) is obtained as:

$$L_{cd} = -10 \log_{10}\eta_{cd} \qquad (4.20)$$

Diameter discrepancies of the order of 5% can result in a loss of the order of 0.42 dB. If there is a mismatch in the numerical aperture of the two fibers, the light cone transmitted by one fiber either overfills or underfills the receiving fiber. If we assume that NA_1 and NA_2 are respectively, the numerical apertures of the transmitting and receiving fibers and all their other parameters are same, then the coupling efficiency [Fig. 4.13(b)] is given by:

$$\eta_{NA} = \begin{cases} \left(\dfrac{NA_2}{NA_1}\right)^2 & \text{for } NA_1 > NA_2 \\ 1 \text{ for } NA_2 \le d_1 \end{cases} \qquad (4.21\text{a and b})$$

The corresponding loss (in dB) is given by:

$$L_{NA} = -10 \log_{10}\eta_{NA} \qquad (4.22)$$

Further, the coupling efficiency due to a mismatch of the refractive index profiles [Fig. 4.13(c)] is given by:

$$\eta_\alpha = \begin{cases} \left(\dfrac{1 + 2/\alpha_1}{1 + 2/\alpha_2}\right)^2 & \text{for } \alpha_1 > \alpha_2 \\ 1 \text{ for } \alpha_1 \le \alpha_2 \end{cases} \qquad (4.23\text{a and b})$$

and the corresponding loss is given by:

$$L_\alpha = -10 \log_{10}\eta_\alpha \qquad (4.24)$$

where α_1 and α_2 are the profile parameters for the transmitting and receiving fibers, respectively. Thus, if the transmitting fiber has a step-index profile ($\alpha = \infty$) and the receiving fiber has a parabolic profile, and if both fibers have the same core diameter and axial NA, then, for an index-matched joint ($k = 1$), there is a loss of 3 dB. However, if the direction of light propagation is reversed, there will be no loss at this joint.

4.7 CONNECTORS AND SPLICES

The interconnection of optical components is a vital part of an optical system, having a major effect on performance. Interconnection between two fiber-optic cables is achieved by either *connectors* or *splices* which link the ends of the fiber cables optically and mechanically.

Connectors are devices used to connect a fiber-optic cable to an optical fiber device, such as a detector, optical amplifier, optical light meter, or link to another fiber cable. They are designed to be easily and reliably connected and disconnected. The connectors create an intimate contact between the mated halves to minimize the power loss across the junction. They are appropriate for indoor applications. Splices are used to permanently connect one fiber-optic cable to another. Splices are suitable for outdoor and indoor applications. Some types of splices are used to temporarily connect for quick testing purposes.

The key to a fiber-optic interconnection is precise alignment of the mated fiber cable cores so that the light couples from one fiber, across the junction, into the other fiber. This precise alignment creates a challenge for designers.

There is a difference between a connection of two fiber cables and a coupling of a light source into a fiber cable. This chapter presents the operating principles of the connectors and splices, and describes their types, properties, and operations.

4.8 APPLICATIONS OF CONNECTORS AND SPLICES

Connectors and splices make optical and mechanical connections between two fiber cables. It is easy to connect and disconnect a cable with a connector from another cable or a device. There are many applications for fiber connectors and splices in fiber systems, such as:

- Connecting between a pair of fiber cables, using connectors or a splice is an essential part of any fiber system.
- Interfacing devices to local area networks.
- Connecting and disconnecting fiber cables to patch panels where signals can be checked and routed in a fiber system.
- Connecting and splicing may be required on short fiber cables for wiring, testing devices, connecting instruments and devices, and at other intermediate points between transmitters and receivers.
- Dividing a fiber system into subsystems, which simplifies the selection, installation, testing, and maintenance of fiber systems.
- Temporarily connecting remote mobile systems and recording equipment in many fiber systems.

4.9 REQUIREMENTS OF CONNECTORS AND SPLICES

It is very difficult to design a connector or a splice that meets all the requirements. A low-loss connector may be more expensive than a high-loss connector, or it may require relatively expensive application tooling. The lowest losses are desirable, but the other factors clearly influence the selection of the connector or splice as well.

The most desirable features for fiber connectors or splices required by customers and industry are as follows:

(i) *Low loss* (insertion and return): The connector or splice causes low loss of optical power across the junction between a pair of fiber cables.

(ii) *Easy installation and use*: The connector or splice should be easily and rapidly installed without the need for special tools or extensive training.

(iii) *Repeatability*: There should be no variation in power loss. Loss should be consistent whenever a connector is connected, disconnected and reconnected again, as many times as required.

(iv) *Economical*: The connector, splice, and special application tooling should be inexpensive.

(v) *Compatibility with the environment*: The connector or splice should be waterproof and not affected by temperature variations.

(vi) *Mechanical properties*: The connector or splice should have high mechanical strength and durability to withstand the application and tension forces.

(vii) *Long life*: The connector or splice should be built with a material that has a long life in various applications.

4.10 FIBER CONNECTORS

Fiber connectors are designed to be easily connected and disconnected. Fiber-optic cable can be easily connected to a transmitter, receiver, power, meters, or another fiber cable. The key optical parameter for a fiber-optic connector is its attenuation. Signal attenuation in connectors is the sum of losses caused by several factors. The major factors are as follows:

   (i) Overlap of fiber cable cores (also called lateral displacement)
  (ii) Alignment of fiber axes
 (iii) Fiber cable numerical aperture
  (iv) Reflection at the fiber cable junction/interface
   (v) Connector end polishing
  (vi) Fiber cable spacing
 (vii) Connector end face profiles
(viii) Insertion loss

When the diameter of the transmitting fiber cable is greater than that of the receiving fiber cable, as shown in Fig. 4.14, the diameter–mismatch loss (loss_{dia}) is given by:

$$\text{Loss}_{\text{dia}} \, 10 \log_{10} \frac{(\text{dia}_t^2 - \text{dia}_r^2)}{\text{dia}_t^2} \tag{4.25}$$

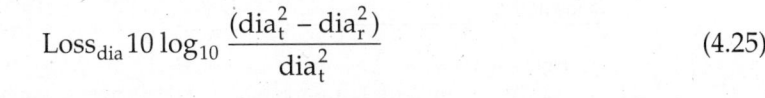

Fig. 4.14: Overlap of fiber cable cores

When the numerical aperture NA of the transmitting fiber cable is greater than that of the receiving fiber cable, as shown in Fig. 4.15, the NA–mismatch loss (loss_{NA}) is given by:

$$\text{Loss}_{\text{NA}} \, 10 \log_{10} \left(\frac{\text{NA}_r}{\text{NA}_t} \right)^2 \tag{4.26}$$

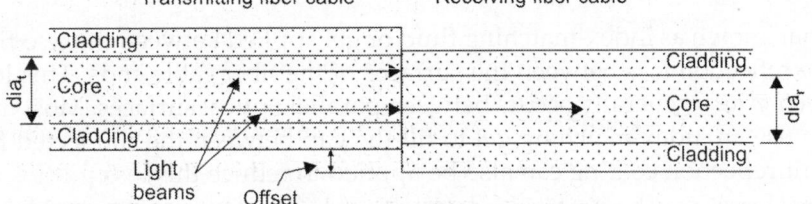

Fig. 4.15: Numerical aperture (NA)–mismatch loss

The formula for the loss due to end separation (loss$_{seperation}$) between two fiber-optic cables (at separation distance) is rather involved. Assume that the transmitting and receiving fibers are identical. Figure 4.16 illustrates the separation (some times called air gap) between a pair of fiber cables. The formula for end separation loss (loss$_{separation}$) is given by:

$$\text{Loss}_{\text{Separation}} = 10 \log_{10} \left(\frac{\dfrac{d}{2}}{\dfrac{d}{2} + S \tan (\arcsin) \left(\dfrac{\text{NA}}{n_0} \right)} \right) \tag{4.27}$$

where, d is core diameter, S is the fiber spacing, NA is the numerical aperture, n_0 is the refractive index of the material between the two fiber cables.

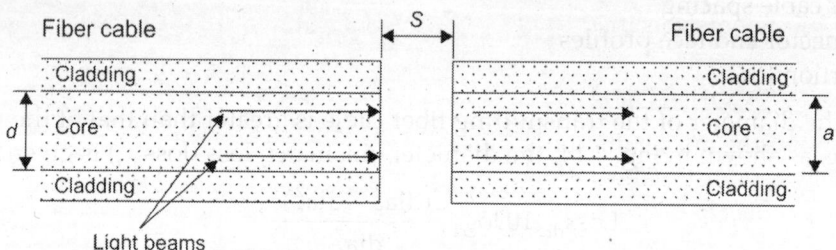

Fig. 4.16: End separation loss

A material known as index-matching fluid or gel applied between the two fiber cables reduces the reflection loss between the surfaces of the fiber cable ends. This loss, called *Fresnel reflection loss*, generally occurs between parallel optical surfaces. Most mechanical splices also use an index-matching gel to fill the gap between the connected fiber cable ends. An antireflection coating can also be applied to reduce this loss.

Additional losses may be experienced when two different types of fiber cable connectors are connected using an adapter.

Insertion loss is a measure of the performance of a connector or splice. Insertion loss is calculated by:

$$\text{loss (dB)} = 10 \log_{10} \left(\frac{P_2}{P_1} \right) \tag{4.28}$$

where P_1 is the initial power measured and P_2 is the power measured after the connector has been mated.

4.11 MECHANICAL CONSIDERATIONS

The optical characteristics of the fiber connectors are significant. However, the mechanical characteristics are also important, and in some cases critical. Virtually all fiber connectors are designed to remain in place under working conditions. Connectors must withstand physical stresses, such as forces encountered during mating and unmating, and sudden stress induced by bending and tension. Connectors must also prevent contamination caused by dirt and moisture in the fiber cable ends.

4.11.1 Durability

Durability is a concern with any type of connector. Repeated mating and unmating of the fiber connectors can cause wear in the mechanical components. Allowing dirt into the optics and straining the fiber cable will damage the exposed fiber cable ends.

4.11.2 Environmental Consideration

Fiber connectors designed for indoor applications must be protected from environmental extremes to avoid excessive connector loss and poor system performance. Special *hermetically-sealed* connectors are required for outdoor use.

4.11.3 Compatibility

Compatibility refers to the need for the connector to be compatible with other connectors or with specifications. Specifications describe the type of connector to be used in specific applications. Compatibility exists on several levels the most basic level being physical compatibility. The connector must meet certain dimensional requirements to allow it to mate with other connectors of the same style. The second level of compatibility involves connector performance, such as insertion loss, durability, operating temperature range, and other requirements specified by the customers.

4.12 FIBER-OPTIC CONNECTOR TYPES

Figure 4.17 shows the most common types of fiber-optic connectors. Fiber connectors are unique in that they must make both optical and mechanical connections. They must also allow the fiber cables to be precisely aligned to ensure that a connection is robust. Fiber connectors use various methods to achieve solid connections. Some of the types of fiber-optic connectors currently in use are listed below.

- Subscriber Connectors (SC)
- SC/APC Connectors
- FC/PC Connectors
- FC/APC Connectors
- LC Connectors
- MU Connectors
- Straight-tip Connectors (ST)
- 5685C Connectors (duplex SC)
- FDDI Connectors (MIC)
- Biconic Connectors

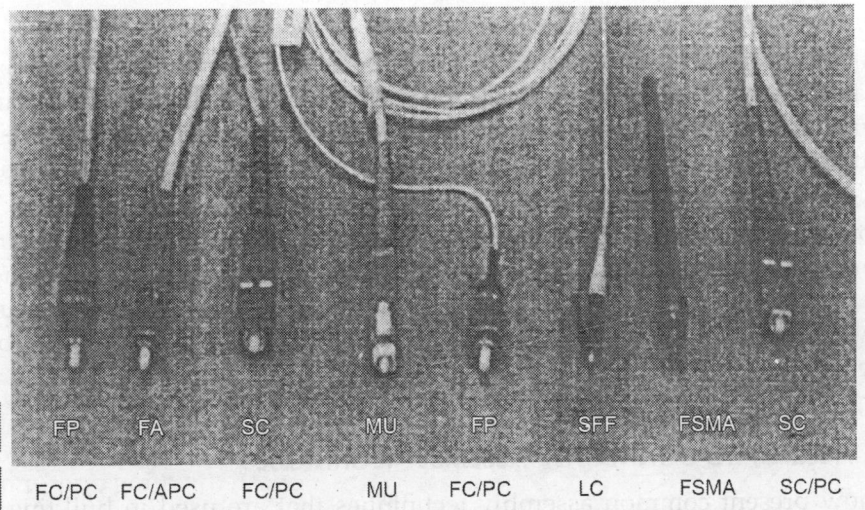

Type	FP	FA	SC	MU	FP	SFF	FSMA	SC
Name	FC/PC	FC/APC	FC/PC	MU	FC/PC	LC	FSMA	SC/PC

Fig. 4.17: Fiber-optic connector types

- SMA Connectors
- Enterprise System Connection (ESCON)
- Duplex Connectors (ST)
- Polarizing Connectors
- MT Multifiber Connectors
- MT-RJ Connectors
- D4-style Connectors
- Biconic Connectors
- MFS/MPO Connectors
- Plastic-Fiber Connectors
- E-2000 Diamond
- Fiber-Optic Connectors Self-Latch in Push/Pull System
- Special Connectors

4.13 ADAPTERS FOR DIFFERENT FIBER-OPTIC CONNECTOR TYPES

An *adapter* is a passive device used to join two different types of connectors together. The type of adapter is identified by a nomenclature, such as SC, FC, ST, or 568SC. Hybrid adapters join dissimilar connectors together, such as SC to FA. Figure 4.18 shows examples of some adapters.

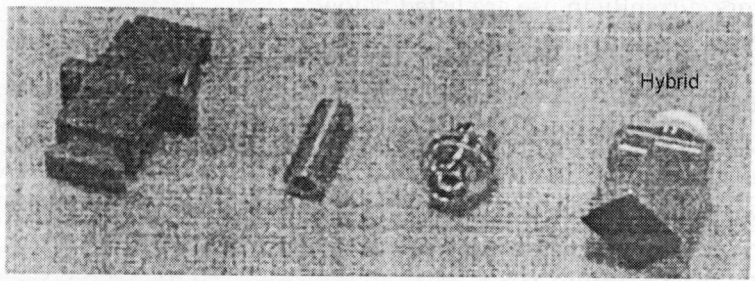

Fig. 4.18: Fiber-optic adapter types

4.14 FIBER-OPTIC CONNECTOR STRUCTURES

Most fiber-optic connectors are built from a ferrule, a connector body, an epoxy material, and a strain relief boot. Most connectors use a ferrule to hold the fiber and provide alignment. The most popular ferrule size is a 2.5 mm diameter, which is standard. Manufacturers offer a few types of ferrules made from different materials, such as ceramic, plastic, and stainless steel.

Connectors may be attached to a device-outlet box or adapter—by direct connection, by coupling a threaded nut, or by twisting a spring-loaded bayonet socket. The connector body is made from steel, ceramic, or plastic. Epoxy is usually applied to secure the fiber cable end in the connector body. A strain relief boot made from plastic or rubber is used at the junction between the connector body and the fiber cable.

4.15 FIBER-OPTIC CONNECTOR ASSEMBLY TECHNIQUES

We now present common assembly techniques that are used in building fiber-optic connectors.

4.15.1 Common Fiber Connector Assembly

The most common fiber connector assembly techniques use a fiber cable and a suitable connector. The fiber cable is most often epoxied into the connector. Epoxy provides good tensile strength to the connector to prevent the fiber cable from moving within the connector body, maintaining a good alignment. After the epoxy cures, the ferrule end is polished to a smooth finish by one of the many available procedures. Then the connector undergoes many inspections and test procedures to issue a data sheet for the customer.

4.15.2 Hot-Melt Connector

The hot-melt connectors use preloaded epoxy so that external mixing is not required. The prepared end of the fiber-optic cable is inserted into the connector ferrule. The cable (with the connector inserted) is loaded onto the connector holder and placed in an oven for a few minutes, which softens the epoxy around the fiber cable and cures the epoxy at the same time. The curing time is dependent on the type of epoxy. The end of the connector is then polished to a smooth finish. The polishing can be done by hand or by an industrial polishing machine. When such connectors are assembled in the field, a portable hand polisher is used.

4.15.3 Epoxyless Connector

Epoxyless connectors, also called crimp connectors, have been widely used for quick cable connections in telecommunication systems. When the connector is crimped, an insert compresses around the fiber cable. A front clamp on the bare fiber cable and a rear compression clamp add a higher clamping force on the fiber able buffer coating to provide the necessary tensile strength. Special gripping tools are used in the assembly of the epoxyless connectors. The end of the fiber connector is polished to a smooth finish using a portable hand polisher before the connector is assembled in the field. The main advantage of an epoxyless connector is the speed of assembly. Some customers will tolerate a slightly higher loss to achieve a fast, easy termination. The epoxyless approach is a technology that is not limited to one connector type.

4.15.4 Butt-Jointed Connectors

Butt-jointed connectors are based on the principle of aligning the two fiber ends and keeping them in close proximity (i.e. butted to each other). For this purpose, the plug-in-socket configuration shown in Fig. 4.19 is normally employed.

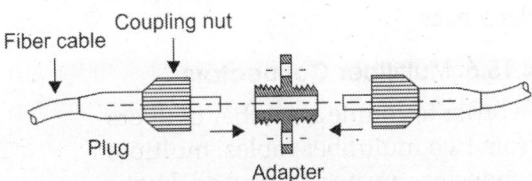

Fig. 4.19: A plug-adapter-plug configuration

The mechanical connection between the plug and the adapter on both the ends is made with the help of either threaded nuts or bayonet locks. Some connectors employ standard BNC or SMA configurations. The design of connectors differs mainly in the technique of aligning fiber ends. The simplest connector design is shown in Fig. 4.20.

It consists of metal plug (normally called ferrules), which are precision-drilled along the central axis. The prepared fiber ends (to be connected) are placed in these holes. They are then permanently bonded to the ferrules by an epoxy resin. A spring retains the ferrule in its position. The two opposite ferrules are aligned by a coaxial cylindrical alignment sleeve.

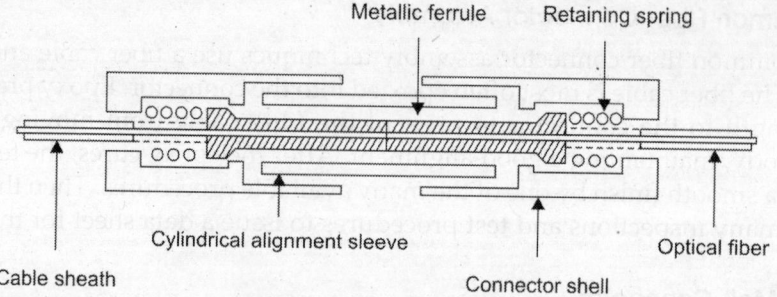

Fig. 4.20: The basic ferrule connector

Another plug-adapter-plug design is shown in Fig. 4.21. Instead of metal ferrules, it employs ceramic capillary ferrules. Ceramic has better thermal, mechanical, and chemical resistance than metal or plastic.

4.15.5 Expanded-Beam Connectors

An alternative design of connectors is based on expanded-beam coupling, illustrated in Fig. 4.22.

This technique uses two microlenses for collimating and refocusing light from one fiber end to another. As the beam diameter is expanded, the requirement of lateral alignment of the two plugs in an adapter becomes less critical as compared to butt-jointed connectors. Fresnel reflection losses may increase in this case but are normally reduced with the help of antireflection coating on the lenses.

4.15.6 Multifiber Connectors

In order to couple a number of fibers from two multifiber cables, multiple connectors are normally used. High-precision grooved silicon chips are employed to position fiber arrays. One chip can accommodate 12 fibers, and it is possible to stack many such chips. This structure is secured with the aid of spring clips and metal-backed chips as shown in Fig. 4.23.

4.15.7 Automated Polishing

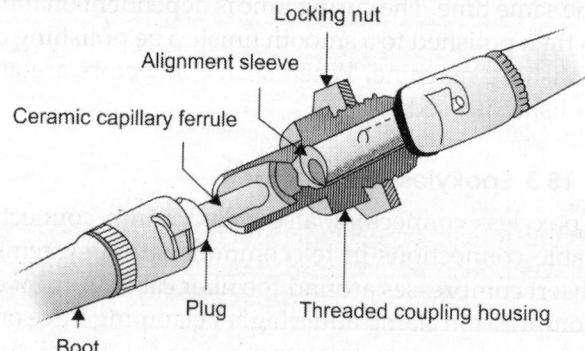

Fig. 4.21: Typical connector design employing ceramic ferrules

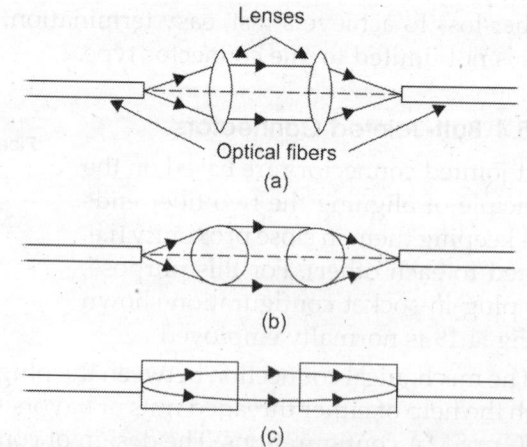

Fig. 4.22: Expanded-beam coupling using (a) a convex microlens (b) a spherical microlens (c) GRIN rod lenses

All fiber-optic connector-polishing machines are designed for accuracy, easy setup, and production efficiency. The polishing pressure, speed, and duration can be adjusted to

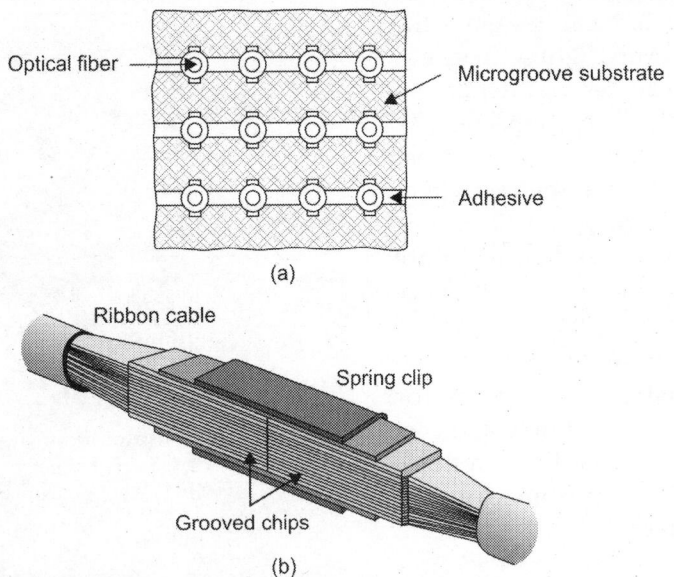

Fig. 4.23: Multiple connector (a) cross-section of a grooved chip connector (b) grooved chip assembly

meet exact requirements. These machines precisely polish the ends of fiber-optic connectors in a repeatable and reliable manner. Polishing machines are available for dry or wet polishing process.

4.15.8 Fluid Jet Polishing

Fluid jet polishing (FJP) is another technique for shaping and polishing small surface areas of complicated optics made of brittle materials. This technique uses a fluid jet system to guide pre-mixed slurry, at low pressure, onto the optical surface being machined. The surface is altered by the erosive effect of the abrasive particles in the stream.

4.15.9 Fiber-Optic Connector Cleaning

Contamination of connector ends can occur from something as simple as dust particles or fingerprints that can reduce light propagation through the fiber cable. This will degrade device performance, causing data error and loss. To avoid this, it is common practice to clean fiber connectors prior to assembly and testing.

There are three major components of the fiber-optic connector system that users must consider when cleaning, mating, and testing fiber-optic connectors: the adapter split sleeve, the outer diameter of the ferrule, and the tip of the ferrule. There are many techniques for cleaning connectors, either wet or dry, by hand with recommended cleaning chemicals, or with automated machines. Follow the cleaning procedure for each fiber connector type. Do not use the same procedure for other types of connectors. Cleaning standards for fiber-optic connectors promise savings in time and cost.

4.15.10 Connector Testing

There are many testing instruments available for testing connectors. Testing instruments range from a simple view scope to a sophisticated system. The condition of the end of the ferrule after the polishing process is usually inspected using simple instruments, as shown in Fig. 4.24. This procedure is adequate for inspecting a connector build and polished in the field.

Handheld devices can measure the losses, optical powers, light sources, etc. The basic test measures the attenuation of the fiber cable with connectors by comparing the power through the fiber cable to that of a known reference fiber cable. The power through the fiber cable under test is measured in absolute units. The power through the reference fiber cable is also measured. Figure 4.25 illustrates a connector test set-up.

Using sophisticated systems for testing connectors saved time and cost in industrial production. These systems are very accurate. Each connector type refers to a standard test.

4.16 FIBER SPLICING

The splicing process joins fibre-optic cable permanently. In general, a splice has a lower loss than a connector. Splices are typically used to join lengths of cable for outside applications. Splices may be incorporated into lengths of fiber-optic cable or housed in

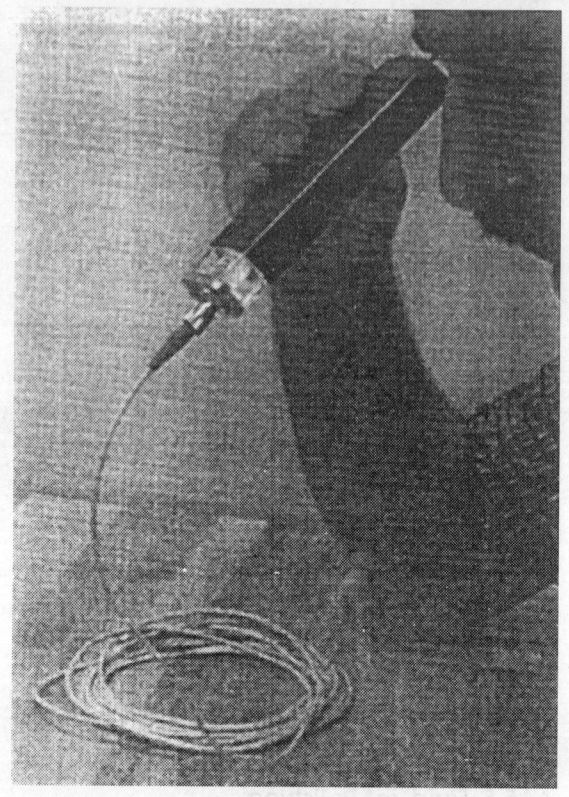

Fig. 4.24: Connector end inspection

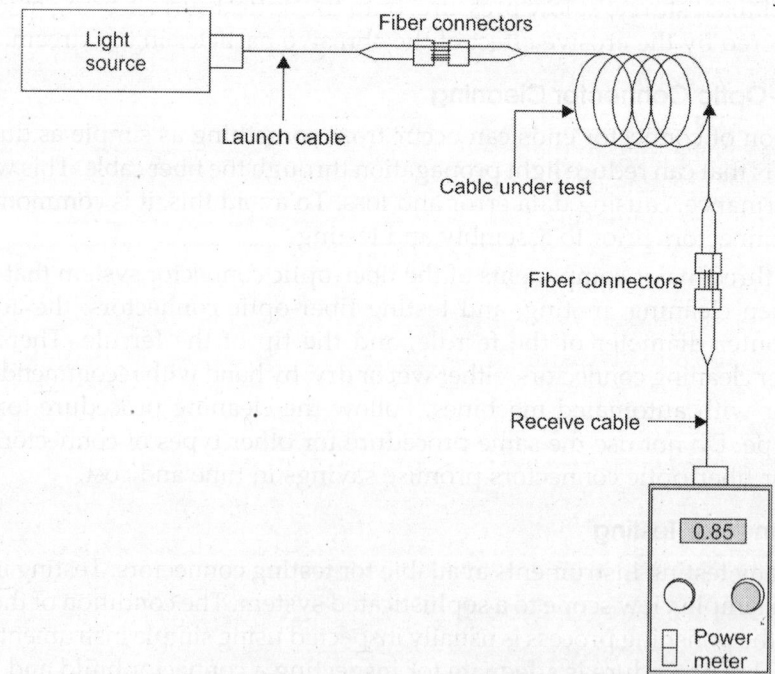

Fig. 4.25: Connector testing set-up

indoor/outdoor splice boxes, whereas connectors are typically found in patch panels or attached to equipment at fiber cable interfaces. Splicing is required (i) when the length of the system span is more than the manufactured cable length, and (ii) when the cable is broken and needs to be repaired. The primary objective of splicing is to establish transmission continuity in the fiber-optic link. This can be done in two ways, namely, through (i) *fusion splices*, or (ii) *mechanical splices*.

In order to achieve a low-loss splice, it is essential for the fiber ends (to be joined) to be smooth, flat, and perpendicular to the core axes. This is normally achieved using a cleaving tool (a blade of hard metal or diamond). The technique is called '*scribe and break*' or '*score and break*'. It involves scoring the fiber under tension with a cleaving tool, as shown in Fig. 4.26. This generates a crack in the fiber surface that propagates in the transverse direction and a flat end is produced.

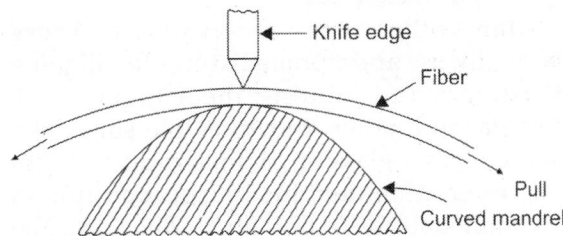

Fig. 4.26: 'Score and break' technique of cleaving optical fibers

4.16.1 Fusion splices

Fusion splice may be made by thermally bonding together prepared fiber ends as shown in Fig. 4.27.

Herein, the prepared fiber ends are placed in a precision alignment jig. The alignment is done with the help of an inspection microscope (not shown). After the initial setting, a short arc discharge is applied to 'fire polish' the fiber ends. This removes any defects due to imperfect cleaving. In the final step, the two ends are pressed together and fused with a stronger arc, thus producing a fusion splice. A possible drawback of such a splicing mechanism is that the heat produced by the welding arc may weaken the fiber in the vicinity of the splice.

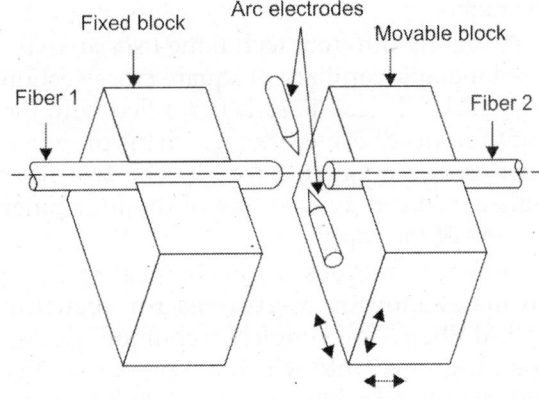

Fig. 4.27: Schematic of fusion splicing apparatus

Summarising, we have:
(i) Fusion splicing involves butting two cleaned fiber end faces and heating them until they melt together or fuse.
(ii) Fusion splicing is normally done with a fusion splice that controls the alignment of the two fibers to keep losses as low as 0.05 dB.
(iii) Fiber ends are first prealigned and butted together under a microscope with micromainpulators. The butted joint is heated with electric arc or laser pulse or melt the fiber ends so can be bonded together.

4.16.2 Mechanical Splices/V-Groove

Mechanical splices join two fiber cable ends together, both optically and mechanically by clamping them within a common structure. In general, mechanical splicing requires less expensive equipment; however, higher consumable costs are experienced.

A few important types of mechanical splices are listed below:
- Table-type splices
- Fiber lock splices
- Fastomeric splices
- Rotary or polished-ferrule splices
- Elastomeric splices
- Inner lock splices
- Key lock splices
- Twist lock splices
- Capillary splices
- V-groove splices
- Finger splices

Many other types are available. These normally use appropriate fixtures for aligning the fibers and holding them together. A popular technique, known as the snug tube splice, uses a glass or ceramic capillary with an inner diameter just large enough to accommodate the optical fibers (Fig. 4.28). The

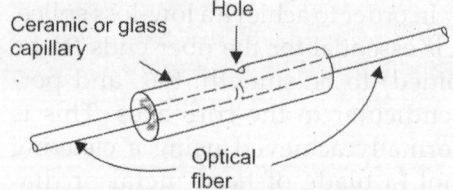

Fig. 4.28: Capillary splicing technique

prepared fiber ends are gently inserted into the capillary and a transparent adhesive (e.g. epoxy resin) is injected through a transverse hole. The adhesive ensures both mechanical bonding and index-matching. A stable low-loss splice may be obtained in this way but it poses stringent limits on the capillary diameters.

A slightly different technique uses an oversized metallic capillary of square cross-section (Fig. 4.29). The capillary is first filled with the transparent adhesive, after which the prepared fiber ends are inserted into it. The two fiber ends are forced against one of the four inner corners of the capillary.

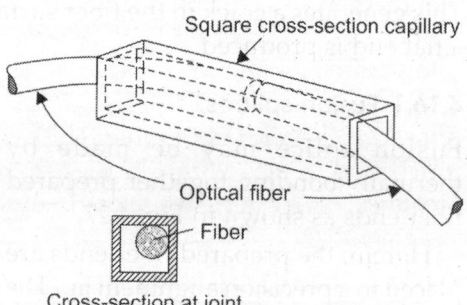

Fig. 4.29: Loose tube splicing technique

Other techniques of mechanical splicing normally employ V-grooves for securing optical fibers. The simplest technique uses an open V-groove, into which the prepared fiber ends are placed as shown in Fig. 4.30. The splice is accomplished with the aid of epoxy resin.

It is also possible to obtain a suitable groove by placing two precision pins (of appropriate diameter) close to each other. The fibers may then be placed in the cusp as shown in Fig. 4.31. A transparent adhesive ensures bonding as well as index-matching, and a flat spring on the top applies pressure ensuring that fibers remain in their positions. Such a groove is called a *spring groove*.

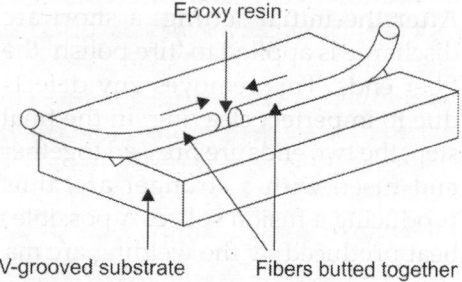

Fig. 4.30: V-groove splicing technique

There is yet another technique that utilizes the V-groove principle to realize what is known as an elastomeric splice (Fig. 4.32). In this method, the prepared fiber ends are sandwiched between two elastomeric internal parts, one of which contains a V-groove. An outer sleeve holds these two parts compressed so

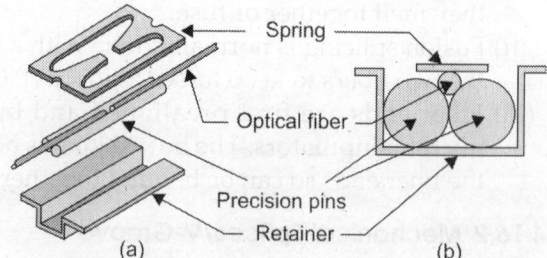

Fig. 4.31: Spring-groove splicing technique (a) exploded view illustrating the spring, fibers on pins, and retainer (b) cross-sectional view

that the fibers are held tightly in alignment. Index-matching gel is employed to improve its performance. Originally, the technique was developed for coupling multimode fibers, but it can also be used for single-mode fibers as well as fibers with different core diameters.

Splicing with most of these techniques, if properly carried out, results in splice loss of about 0.1 dB for multimode fibers. Some of these can also be used for splicing single-mode fibers.

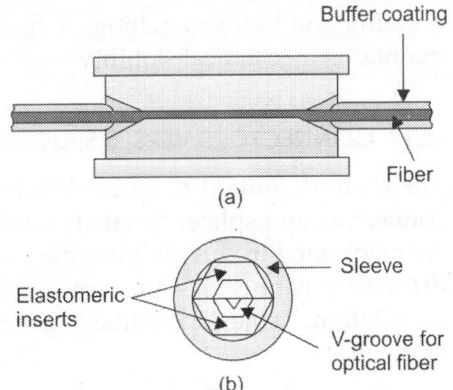

Fig. 4.32: An elastomeric splice (a) longitudinal section (b) cross-section

Key-Lock Mechanical Fiber-Optic Splices

Key-lock mechanical fiber optic splices are commonly used to quickly mate and unmate fiber optic cables. It is made for a U-shaped metal part covered by a transparent plastic body with two holes on each end. The prepared ends of the fiber cables are made longer than half of the length of the metal part. The fiber cable is inserted in the center hole. When the key is inserted in the second hole towards the edge of the splice and turned by 90°, the metal part opens and one fiber cable end can be easily inserted. This operation can be repeated on the other side to insert the second fiber cable. This type of splice provides a quick and easy way of joining two fiber cables with low signal loss. It may be used to temporarily or permanently connect fiber cables, wavelength division multiplexing components, and other fiber-optic elements.

Table-Type Mechanical Fiber-Optic Splices

A custom-made mechanical splice, used for quick mating and unmating of connections. This splice works like any other mechanical splice. The fiber cable ends are prepared and inserted into the mid-point of the block assembly. Screws are tightened to align the fiber cables on both sides. L-clamps and K-clamps (Fig. 4.33a) are placed in position to secure the fiber cables on both sides. Most fiber-

![Table-type mechanical fiber-optic splice with L-clamp, K-clamp, Screws, and Fiber cable labels]

Fig. 4.33(a): Table-type mechanical fiber-optic splice

optic companies use this kind of mechanical splice for quickly mating and unmating during manu-facturing and testing processes. The splice loss associated with these instruments is acceptable by industry standards.

4.16.3 Multiple Splices

For ribbon cables containing linear arrays of fibers, the following technique has been used. In this method (Fig. 4.33b), the fiber ends are individually prepared, and then placed in a grooved substrate. Adhesive is then used for

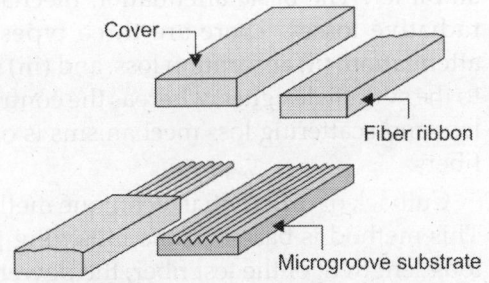

Fig. 4.33(b): Multiple splicing technique

bonding and index-matching. A cover plate retains the fibers in their position and also maintains mechanical stability.

4.17 CONNECTORS VERSES SPLICES

There are definite differences between connectors and splices. Most companies make connectors and splices to satisfy customer requirements for smaller size and lower loss. As mentioned in this chapter, fiber-optic technology is moving forward to create high-durability connectors and splices with small sizes and low cost in production and installation. Table 4.8 compares general important factors between the fiber connectors and splices.

Table 4.8: Connectors vs splices

Connectors	Splices
Provide temporary connections	Provide permanent connections
Higher loss	Lowest loss
Larger sizes	Smaller sizes
Immune, or not immune, to environmental effects (depends on the connector type)	Immune to environmental effects
It takes a long time to build a connector	It takes a very short time to build a splice
Diverse applications	Connection between a pair of fiber cables
Many types	Few types
New technology reduces installation time	Conventional technology keeps the same installation time
Building reasonable mechanical stability at the connection points	Building better mechanical stability at the connection points

4.18 CHARACTERIZATION OF OPTICAL FIBERS

There are various parameters of the optical fibers, which have to study for the evaluation of the performance of an optical fiber, e.g. optical attenuation, dispersion, numerical aperture, and refractive index profile. There are a number of methods for measuring each of these parameters. We will discuss only a few of them.

4.18.1 Measurement of Optical Attenuation

Attenuation of a light signal as it propagates along a fiber is an important consideration in the design of an optical communication system, since it plays a major role in determining the maximum transmission distance between transmitter and a receiver or an in-line amplifier. The basic attenuation mechanisms in a fiber are absorption, scattering and radiative losses. There are three types of techniques developed to measure (i) total attenuation, (ii) absorption loss, and (iii) scattering loss. The total attenuation is of interest to the system designer, whereas the contribution to this total attenuation by the absorption loss and scattering loss mechanisms is of interest in the development of low-loss optical fibers.

Cutback or differential technique method is used for measuring total fiber attenuation. This method is based on the following principle. Power P_0 is launched at one end of a long length L_1 of the test fiber; the power P_1 is received at the other end and is measured. Then, the fiber is cut back to a smaller length L_2 and the power P_2 received at the other end is measured again. Assuming wavelength λ remains same, the optical attenuation per unit length α (dB/km) may be expressed by the following relation:

$$\alpha = \frac{10}{L_1 - L_2} \log_{10}\left(\frac{P_2}{P_1}\right) \tag{4.29}$$

We now discuss the criterion for designing the equipment for studying this parameter by the cutback method.

First, a polychromatic continuous source of radiation (containing sufficient power at all the wavelengths of interest) is required. As the attenuation is to be studied for all wavelengths, a wavelength-isolation device (e.g. a monochromator) is required to follow the source. Then suitable optics has to be designed for launching the optical power at one end of the test fiber. At the other end of it, again suitable optics is required so that most of the power transmitted by the fiber is received by the detector. The detector signal should be processed and then output read on a meter or recorded on a chart recorder. Accordingly, the modules may be arranged as shown in Fig. 4.34.

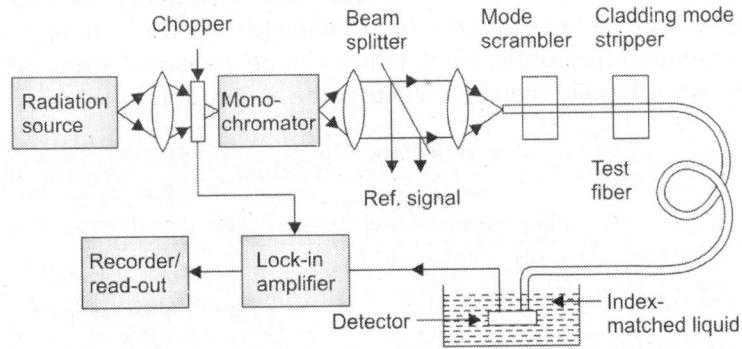

Fig. 4.34: Experimental arrangement for the measurement of total attenuation

One can understand the importance of each of these modules by investigating the dependence of the signal S developed by the detector on the pertinent variables:

$$S = P(\lambda)\, M(\theta, \lambda)\, (n_a \sin \alpha_m)\, T(\alpha_{ab}, \alpha_{sc}, L)\, D(\lambda) \tag{4.30}$$

where $P(\lambda)$ is the power furnished by the source at a specific wavelength λ; $M(\theta, \lambda)$ is a function governing the solid angle θ seen by the monochromator and its transmittance with wavelength λ; $n_a \sin \alpha_m$ gives the numerical aperture of the fiber, n_a is the refractive index of the medium surrounding the launching end of the fiber; $T(\alpha_{ab}, \alpha_{sc}, L)$ is a function determining the transmittance of the fiber. This is dependent on the absorption loss per unit length α_{ab}, the scattering loss per unit length λ_{sc}, the total length L of the fiber, and $D(\lambda)$ is the responsivity of the detector as a function of wavelength λ.

Clearly, the source should have high radiance and be continuous. A black body radiator, e.g. a tungsten halogen lamp or a high-pressure discharge lamp, e.g. a xenon arc lamp may be used. A monochromator should collect as much as possible. The components in the monochromator should have high transmittance in the regions of investigation. If a grating is used as a monochromator, overlapping orders may cause problems and hence, an order sorting filter may also be required at the exit slit of the monochromator. In order to improve the S/N ratio, the signal from the source is generally chopped at a low frequency and at the receiver end a lock-in amplifier is used to perform phase-sensitive detection.

A beam splitter is placed as shown in Fig. 4.34 for obtaining a reference signal as well as for viewing the optics. If viewing the optics is not required, a rotating sector mirror may be used in place of a beam splitter and the chopper in between the source and the monochromator may be omitted. This will provide a greater energy throughput to the optical fiber as well as a reference signal for comparison. A mode scrambler has been used to obtain equilibrium mode distribution. The fiber is also put through a cladding mode stripper, which is a device for removing the light launched into the fiber cladding. At the receiver end, the optical power is detected using either a *p-i-n* or an avalanche photodiode. The other end of the fiber terminates in an index-matched liquid so that most of the light is received by the detector.

The limitation of the cutback method is that it is destructive in nature and hence, can be used only in the laboratory. It cannot be used in field measurements.

The question arises, how does one isolate the contribution to total attenuation by the major loss mechanisms (e.g. absorption and scattering)?

In order to determine the loss due to absorption, a *calorimetric method* may be used. In this method, two similar fibers are taken and light is launched through one of them (Fig. 4.35). Absorption of light (of specific wavelength) by the bulk material of the test fiber raises the temperature of the fiber, which can be measured using a thermocouple. The rise in temperature may then be related to the absorption loss.

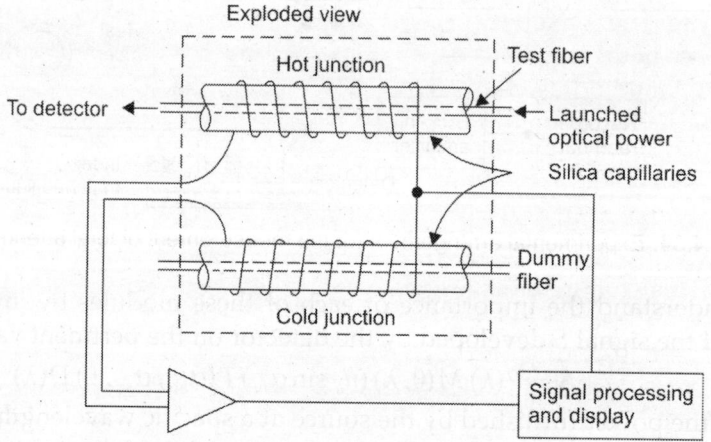

Fig. 4.35: Schematic of measurement of the temperature of an optical fiber using a thermocouple

The power loss due to scattering alone may be measured with the help of cell (Fig. 4.36). Light from a powerful source is launched into the optical fiber through

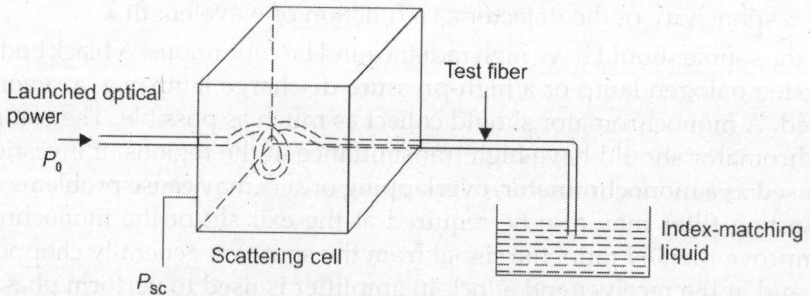

Fig. 4.36: Schematic of experimental set-up for measurement of scattering loss

appropriate launch optics. A certain length (say, L) of the fiber is enclosed inside the scattering cell. All the six inner surfaces of the cell are fitted with six photovoltaic detectors. These detectors measure the optical power (P_{sc}) scattered by the enclosed length L of the fiber. The scattering loss α_{sc} (dB/km) may be expressed as:

$$\alpha_{sc} = \frac{10}{L\,(\text{km})} \log_{10} \left(\frac{P_0}{P_0 - P_{sc}} \right) \text{dB/km} \tag{4.31}$$

where P_0 is the power launched.

4.18.2 Measurement of Dispersion

Distortion of optical signals propagating down an optical fiber is caused due to two mechanisms and this causes to limit the information-carrying capacity of the fiber. These are *intermodal* and *intramodal* dispersions.

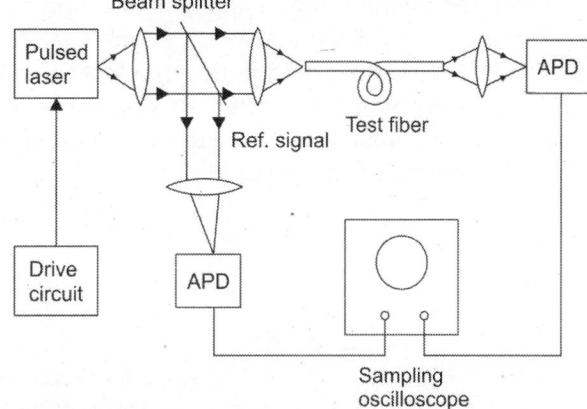

Fig. 4.37: Schematic of experimental set-up for the measurement of intermodal dispersion

One can study the dispersion effects by measuring the impulse response of the fiber in the time domain or by measuring the baseband frequency response in the frequency domain. A general method used for measuring the pulse distortion in optical fibers in the time domain is shown in Fig. 4.37. Short-duration pulses (of the order of a few hundred picoseconds) are launched at the one end of the optical fiber from a pulsed laser. As the pulses propagate through the fiber, they get broadened due to the various dispersion mechanisms. At the other end, these pulses are received by a high-speed photodetector [e.g. an avalanche photodiode (ADP)], and the detector signal is displayed on the cathode ray oscilloscope (CRO). A reference signal is utilized for triggering the CRO and also for measuring the input pulse. If τ_i and τ_o are the half-widths of the input and output pulses respectively and if the shape of the pulses is assumed to be Gaussian, then the impulse response of the fiber is given by:

$$\tau = \frac{(\tau_o^2 - \tau_i^2)^{1/2}}{L} \text{ (say, ns/km)} \tag{4.32}$$

where L is the length of the optical fiber.

In order to evaluate the the bandwidth of the fiber, measurements in the frequency domain are required. In this case, the apparatus is almost the same (Fig. 4.37), except that a sampling oscilloscope is replaced by a spectrum analyser. The latter takes the Fourier transform of the output pulse in the time domain and displays its constituent frequency components. For the measurement of the intramodal or chromatic dispersion, a polychromatic source is required in place of a laser.

4.18.3 Measurement of Numerical Aperture (NA)

NA is directly related to the light-gathering capacity of the fiber and is an important characterizing parameter. NA decides the number of modes propagating through the multimode fiber. For a step index fiber, NA is given by:

$$\text{NA} = n_a \sin \alpha_m = (n_1^2 - n_2^2)^{1/2} \tag{4.33}$$

where α_m is the angle of acceptance, n_a is the refractive index of the medium in which the fiber is placed, and n_1 and n_2 are the refractive indices of the core and cladding, respectively. For a graded-index fiber, NA is not constant but varies with the distance r from the core axis. The local NA at a radial distance r is given by:

$$NA(r) = n_a \sin\alpha_m(r) = [n_1^2(r) - n_2^2]^{1/2} \tag{4.34}$$

From Eqs (4.33) and (4.34), it becomes clear that the NA can be calculated if the refractive index profile of the fiber is known. However, this method is seldom used.

A general method, shown in Fig. 4.38 involves the measurement of the far-field pattern of the fiber. Light from a powerful source such as a laser is launched at one end of the fiber. The other end is held in the chuck of the fiber holder on a rotating stage. As the tip of the fiber is rotated, the intensity of light reaching the detector falls off on either side and an approximate Gaussian curve results. The angle at which the intensity falls to 5% of its maximum gives the value of α_m.

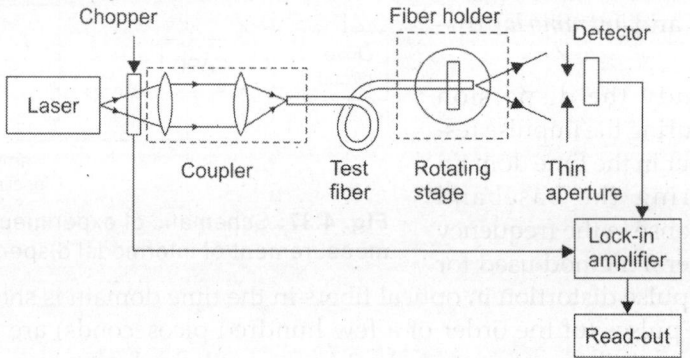

Fig. 4.38: Schematic of experimental set-up for evaluating the NA of an optical fiber

Alternatively, the light from the laser source may be made to fall a different angles on one end of the fiber and the output at the other end may be measured with the help of a detector. Again, an approximately Gaussian curve results when the output power is plotted as a function of the angle of rotation. The angle for which the power falls to 5% of its maximum gives us the value of α_m.

4.18.4 Measurement of Refractive Index (RI) Profile

RI profile of an optical fiber plays a significant role in its characterization. One can determine the NA of the fiber and the number of guided modes propagating within the fiber with the knowledge of RI profile. RI profile of the fiber also enable one to predict the response of the impulse and hence the information-carrying capacity of the optical fiber.

There are several methods to measure the RI profile. We discuss the *end-reflection method*. The method is based on the principle that when a focused beam of light is incident normally on the flat end face of a fiber, a part of the light is reflected back. The fraction R of the light reflected at the fiber-medium interface is given by the Fresnel reflection coefficient given by:

$$R = P_r / P_i = \left(\frac{n_1 - n}{n_1 + n}\right)^2 \tag{4.35}$$

where P_r and P_i are the reflected and incident powers respectively, n_1 is the RI at the striking point of the fiber, and n is the RI of the medium surrounding the fiber. For a small variation in the value of n_1, we have:

$$\Delta R = 4n \left\{ \frac{n_1 - n}{(n_1 + n)^3} \right\} \Delta n_1 \tag{4.36}$$

Clearly, the variation in the reflected light intensity can be used to calculate the RI.

The experimental set-up is shown in Fig. 4.39. A highly focused laser beam is used to measure the RI profile. The beam is first modulated by the chopper and purified by passing through a polarizer and quarter-wave plate combination. This combination also decouples the incident light from the reflected light. This light is then focused on the polished flat end of the test fiber. The other end of the fiber is dipped into an index-matching liquid so that light is not reflected back from this end. The light reflected from the flat end of the fiber is directed onto the detector via the beam splitter. The modulated output of the detector is amplified and recorded on the recorder.

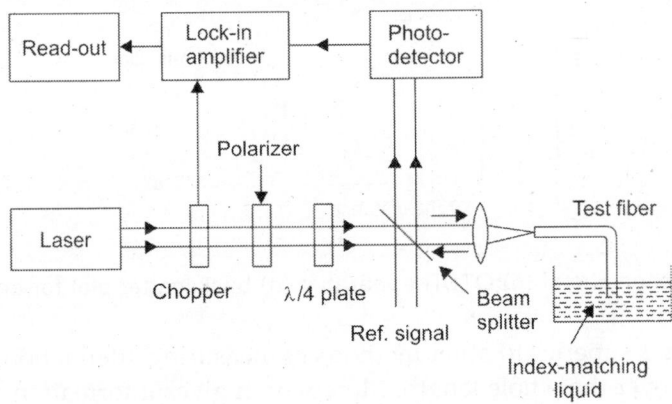

Fig. 4.39: Schematic of experimental set-up for studying the RI profile of an optical fiber

4.18.5 Field Measurements: Optical Time Domain Reflectometry (OTDR)

The method discussed above are primarily suited to the laboratory environment. However, there is a technique that can measure attenuation, connector and splicing losses, and at the same time, can also locate faults in optical fiber links in the field required. A method that finds wide applications in this field is called OTDR or the backscatter technique.

Figure 4.40 shows a schematic diagram of the OTDR apparatus. A powerful beam of light is launched through a bidirectional coupler into one end of the fiber and the backscattered light is detected with the help of an APD receiver. The received signal is integrated and amplified, and the averaged signals for successive points within the fiber are presented on the recorder or the cathode ray tube (CRT). The information displayed on the chart of the recorder or the screen of the CRT is the signal strength along the y-axis and time along the x-axis. The time is usually multiplied by the velocity of propagation to give an indication of the distance. The display expected for an ideal optical fiber of finite length is shown in Fig. 4.40(b). Any deviation from this is due to some kind of fault.

OTDR provides information about the location dependence of the attenuation. The slope of the plot shown in Fig. 4.40(b) simply provides the attenuation per unit length for

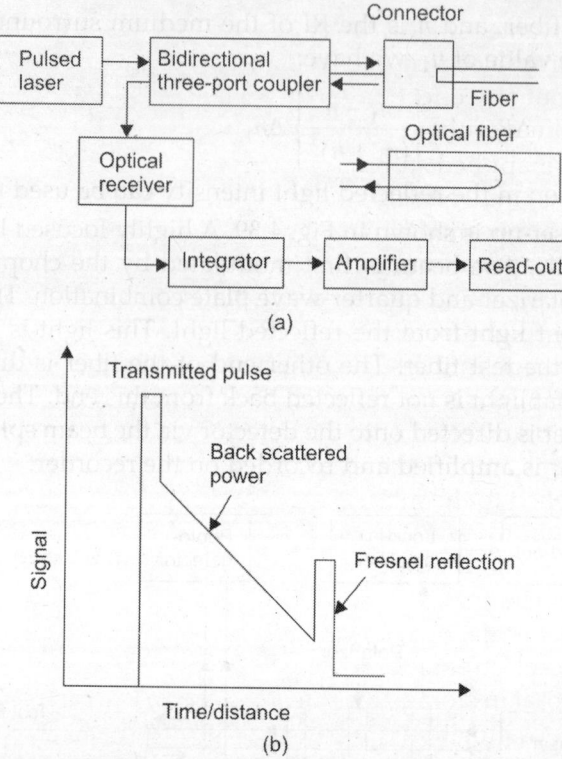

Fig. 4.40: Schematic of (a) OTDR apparatus (b) backscatter plot for an ideal fiber

the fiber. Thus, it is superior to other methods of measuring attenuation, which provide the average loss over the whole length. Moreover, it gives information about the splice or connector losses and the location of any faults on the link. Finally, the overall link length can be calculated from the time difference between the Fresnel reflections from the two ends of the fiber. Clearly, it requires access to only one end of the fiber for performing measurements.

4.19 APPLICATIONS OF THE FIBER OPTIC CABLES

Fiber optic cables with other components are used in building optical fiber devices and systems. One of large-scale applications is its use in communication systems. Video, including broadcast television, is one of the main telecommunication applications. Other applications include cable television, high-speed internet, wireless transition, remote monitoring, and surveillance. Fiber optic video transmission is successfully used around the world in surveillance and remote monitoring systems with many applications. Fiber optics applications in the military include communications, command-and-control links on ships and aircrafts, data link for satellite earth stations, and transmission lines for tactical command post communications.

Fiber cables can be used throughout the communication network, including in the final link into the subscriber's home to wall outlets. This field has continued to develop since the discovery of optical amplifiers, dense wavelength division multiplexers (DWDM), fiber Bragg grating, and photonics crystal fibers.

One particular advantage of fiber optic cables is that they are immune to electromagnetic interference (EMI) from electricity. Therefore, optic cables can be placed near high-voltage power cables without any effect on data transmission. Similarly, the cables also can be laid along railway lines without suffering from EMI.

Optical fibers are applied in building night-vision viewing devices, scanning and sensing instruments, and vibration sensors, which are extensively used in military, medical, and other applications. Imaging techniques have been rapidly developed for a variety of medical applications, such as viewing inside human tissues and scanning microscopic particles.

Fibers are also used in monitoring and sensing technology. They are used as sensors to monitor the vibration in the structures of bridges and high buildings. They are also used as gas and DNA sensors.

The use of fiber optic cables in lighting systems can reduce energy consumption. Fiber optic lighting systems are developing quickly, with wide applications. Fiber optic light systems can be applied to the interior and exterior of commercial, retail, and residential buildings. New applications are being explored in landscaping, waterscraping, medical lighting instruments, and theme environments.

Fiber optic cables can also be coated for special handling requirements and resistance to temperature, chemicals, or radiation. Radiation-resistant fiber is suitable for use in environments where electronics-based optical solutions are not viable, such as monitoring nuclear waste disposal in storage facilities. To make the fibers heat resistant, a chemical-resistant polyimide-coating that can withstand temperatures upto 300°C is applied. This is especially useful for manufacturers designing medical equipment for applications in which autoclave sterilization is necessary.

One of many applications of different fiber cable types is fiber-optic *sensing*. Fiber optic sensing can be classed as intrinsic and extrinsic. In intrinsic sensors, the fiber simply conducts light from a sensing head to a detector, the interaction between light and the environment take place outside the fiber cable. In intrinsic sensors, the interaction between the environment, the fiber, and the light itself generates information about a specific measurement. The key advantage of intrinsic fiber-optic sensors is the fundamental ability of the fiber to guide light around bends and over long distances. This enables the fiber to be confined within small physical volumes and magnifies the effects of very fine environment changes to a level that can be measured accurately.

Fiber Bragg gratings (FBGs) are employed as passive temperature and pressure sensors. The ability to adjust these optical devices introduces a new dimension for the design of very fast, precise and multifunctional fiber sensors without compromising their intrinsic advantages. Fiber Bragg gratings are also used in many other applications. Tuning can be accomplished by several mechanisms, such as electric heating, the piezoelectric effect, mechanical stretching and bending, and acoustic modulation. These sensors are available in the market in different types, sizes and wavelength ranges.

Photonic bandgap and photonic crystal fibers are both members of the family of grape fruit microstructure fibers. Both types can be used in gas sensors.

Beyond pressure and temperature sensor technology, advanced fiber sensors types include chemical strain, biomedical, electrical and magnetic, rotation, vibration, and displacement as major applications. One more application of the advanced fiber sensor technology is in the area of DNA analysis. This ability gives the diagnostic some excellent fibers are efficiently constructed as waveguides with novel properties for communications and sensor applications.

Example 1

The Si–O bond has a theoretical cohesive strength of 2.6×10^6 psi which corresponds to a bond distance of 0.16 nm. A silica optical fiber has an elliptical crack of depth 10 nm at a point along its length. Calculate (a) the fracture stress in psi for the fiber if it is dependent upon this crack, and (b) the percentage strain in the break. Given Young's modules for silica $= 9 \times 10^{10}$ N·m^{-2} and 1 psi $= 6894.76$ N·m^{-2}.

Solution

The theoretical cohesive strength for the Si–O bond is given by:

$$S_t = \left(\frac{\gamma_p E}{4 l_a}\right)^{1/2} \text{ or } \gamma_p = \frac{4 l_a S_t^2}{E}$$

where γ_p is surface energy of the material, E is Young's modulus for the material and l_a is the atomic spacing or bond distance. Substituting the values, one obtains:

$$\gamma_p = \frac{4 \times 0.16 \times 10^{-9} \, (2.6 \times 10^6 \times 6894.76)^2}{9 \times 10^{10}}$$

$$= 2.29 \text{ J}$$

(a) The fracture stress for silica fiber may be obtained from:

$$S_f = \left(\frac{2 E \gamma_p}{Y^2 C}\right)^{1/2}$$

where Y is a constant dictated by the shape of the crack (e.g. $Y = \pi^{1/2}$ for an elliptical crack) and C is the depth of the crack. For an elliptical crack:

$$S_f = \frac{2 E \gamma_p}{Y^2 C}$$

$$= \left(\frac{2 \times 9 \times 10^{10} \times 2.29}{3.14 \times 10^{-8}}\right)^{1/2}$$

$$= 3.62 \times 10^9 \text{ N·m}^{-1}$$

$$= 5.25 \times 10^5 \text{ psi}$$

(b) We may note that the fracture stress is reduced from the theoretical value for flawless silica of 2.6×10^6 psi by a factor of approximately 5.

$$\text{Young's modules, } E = \frac{\text{Stress}}{\text{Strain}}$$

$$\therefore \quad \text{Strain} = \frac{\text{Stress}}{E} = \frac{3.62 \times 10^9}{9 \times 10^{10}}$$

$$= 0.04$$

Obviously, the strain at break is 4%, which corresponds to the change in length over the original length for the fiber.

Example 2

An optical fiber has a core refractive index of 1.5. Two lengths of the fiber with smooth and perpendicular (to the core axes) end faces are butted together. Assuming the fiber axes are perfectly aligned, calculate the optical loss in decibels at the joint (due to Fresnel reflection) when there is a small air gap between the fiber end faces.

Solution

The magnitude of the Fresnel reflection at the fiber-air interface is given by:

$$\gamma = \left(\frac{n_1 - n}{n_1 + n}\right)^2$$

where n_1 is the refractive index of the fiber core and n is the refractive index of the medium between the two jointed fibers (i.e. for $n = 1$).

$$\therefore \qquad \gamma = \left(\frac{1.5 - 1}{1.5 + 1}\right)^2 = \left(\frac{0.5}{2.5}\right)^2 = 0.04$$

The value of γ obtained corresponds to a reflection of 4% of the transmitted light at the single interface. One can obtain the optical loss in decibels at the single interface from:

$$
\begin{aligned}
\text{Loss}_{\text{Fres}} &= -10 \log_{10}(1 - \gamma) \\
&= -10 \log_{10}(1 - 0.04) \\
&= -10 \log_{10} 0.96 \\
&= -0.18 \text{ dB}
\end{aligned}
$$

Similarly, we obtain the loss at the second interface also 0.18 dB.

Hence, the total loss due to Fresnel reflection at the fiber joint is approximately = 0.36 dB.

Example 3

Two compatible multimode SI fibers are jointed with a small air gap. The fiber axes and end faces are perfectly aligned. Determine the refractive index of the fiber core if the joint is showing a loss of 0.47 dB. **[B Tech]**

Solution

We have:

$$L_F = 10 \log_{10}(\eta_F) = 0.47 \text{ dB}$$

This gives

$$\eta_F = 0.897 = \frac{16k^2}{(k+1)^4}$$

For air, $n = 1$,

$$\therefore \qquad k = \frac{n_1}{n} = n_1$$

Thus $n_1^2 - 2.22n_1 + 1 = 0$ or $n_1 = 1.59$ and $n_1 = -1$

Taking the positive root, $n_1 = 1.59$. The negative root gives n_1 less than 1, which is not possible.

Example 4

Two multimode step index fibers have numerical aperture of 0.2 and 0.4 respectively, and both have the same core refractive index of 1.48. Estimate the insertion loss at a joint in each fiber caused by a 5° angular misalignment of the fiber core axes.

Solution

The angular coupling efficiency is given by:

$$\eta_{\text{ang}} = \frac{16\left(\dfrac{n_1}{n}\right)^2}{\left[1 + \left(\dfrac{n_1}{n}\right)\right]^4}\left[1 - \frac{n\theta}{\pi n_1 (2\Delta)^{1/2}}\right]$$

where $NA = n_1 (2\Delta)^{1/2}$

$$\therefore \qquad \eta_{ang} \approx \frac{16 \left(\dfrac{n_1}{n} \right)^2}{\left[1 + \left(\dfrac{n_1}{n} \right) \right]^4} \left[1 - \frac{n\theta}{\pi \times 0.2} \right]$$

For $\qquad\qquad NA = 0.2$ fiber

$$\eta_{ang} \approx \frac{16 \, (1.48)^2}{[1 + 1.48]^4} \left[1 - \frac{\dfrac{5\pi}{180}}{\pi \times 0.2} \right]$$

$$= 0.797$$

The insertion loss due to misalignment may be obtained from:

$$Loss_{ang} = -10 \log_{10} \eta_{ang}$$
$$= -10 \log_{10} (0.797) = 0.90 \text{ dB}$$

For $NA = 0.4$ fiber

$$\eta_{ang} \approx 0.926 \left[1 - \frac{\dfrac{5\pi}{180}}{\pi \times 0.4} \right]$$

$$= 0.862$$

The insertion loss due to the angular misalignment:

$$Loss_{ang} = -10 \log_{10} (0.862)$$
$$= 0.93 \text{ dB}$$

Example 5

Two compatible multimode Si fibers are jointed with a lateral offset of 3 μm, an angular misalignment of the core axes of 3°, and a small air gap (but negligible end separation). If the core of each fiber has a refractive index of 1.48, a relative refractive index difference of 2%, and a diameter of 100 μm, calculate the total insertion loss at the joint, which may be assumed to complete the sum of all the misalignment losses. **[B Tech]**

Solution

Given: $\Delta x \approx 0$ (negligible), $\Delta y = 3$ μm, $\Delta \theta = 3° = 0.052$ rad, $n_1 = 1.48$, $\Delta = 2\% = 0.02$, $2a = 100$ μm, $n = 1$ (for air), and therefore, $k = n_1/n = n_1 = 1.48$.

We have $\qquad \eta_F = \dfrac{4k}{(k+1)^2} \dfrac{4k}{(k+1)^2} = \dfrac{16k^2}{(k+1)^4}$

or $\qquad\qquad \eta_F = \dfrac{16 \times (1.48)^2}{(1.48+1)^4} = 0.9264$

Using $\qquad \eta_{lat} \approx \dfrac{2}{\pi} \left[\cos^{-1} \left(\dfrac{\Delta y}{2a} \right) - \left(\dfrac{\Delta y}{2a} \right) \left\{ 1 - \left(\dfrac{\Delta y}{2a} \right)^2 \right\}^{1/2} \right]$

We obtain: $\qquad \eta_{lat} = \dfrac{2}{\pi} \left[\cos^{-1} \left(\dfrac{3}{100} \right) - \dfrac{3}{100} \left\{ 1 - \left(\dfrac{3}{100} \right)^2 \right\}^{1/2} \right] = 0.962$

and using:
$$\eta_{ang} \approx \left[1 - \frac{n\Delta\theta}{\pi NA}\right]$$

One obtains:
$$\eta_{ang} = \left[1 - \frac{1 \times 0.052}{\pi \times 0.296}\right]$$

as
$$NA = n_1\sqrt{2D} = 1.48\sqrt{2 \times 0.02} = 0.296$$

$$\eta_{ang} = 0.944$$

Therefore the total coupling efficiency η_τ will be given by:
$$\eta_T = \eta_F\eta_{lat}\eta_{ang} = 0.9264 \times 0.962 \times 0.944 = 0.8412$$

Thus the total loss:
$$L_T = -10\log_{10}\eta_T = 0.775 \text{ dB}$$

Example 6

A single mode fiber has the following parameters: (i) normalized frequency $(V) = 2.40$, (ii) core refractive index $(n_1) = 1.46$, (iii) core diameter $(2a) = 8$ μm, and (iv) numerical aperture $(NA) = 0.1$

Estimate the total insertion loss of a fiber joint with a lateral mis-alignment of 1 mm and an angular misalignment of $1°$.

Solution

Initially, we have to determine the normalized spot size in the fiber. We have:
$$\omega = a\frac{(0.65 + 1.62\,V^{-3/2} + 2.88\,V^{-6})}{2^{1/2}}$$
$$= 4\frac{[0.65 + 1.62\,(2.4)^{-1.5} + 2.88\,(2.44)^{-6}]}{\sqrt{2}}$$
$$= 3.12 \text{ μm}$$

The loss due to lateral offset can be obtained from the relation:
$$T_1 = 2.17\left(\frac{1}{3.12}\right)^2$$

or
$$T_1 = 0.22 \text{ dB}$$

The loss due to angular misalignment may be obtained from the relation:
$$T_a = 2.17\left(\frac{\theta\omega\,n_1 V}{a\,NA}\right)^2$$
$$= 2.17\left(\frac{\left(\frac{\pi}{180}\right) \times 3.13 \times 1.46 \times 24}{4 \times 0.1}\right)$$
$$= 0.49 \text{ dB}$$

∴ Total insertion loss:
$$T_T = T_1 + T_a$$
$$= 0.22 + 0.49 = 0.71 \text{ dB}$$

Example 7

A $60/120\,\mu m$ graded-index fiber with a numerical aperture of 0.25 and a profile parameter of 1.9 is jointed with a $50/120\,\mu m$ graded-index fiber with a numerical aperture of 0.20 and a profile parameter of 2.1. If the fiber axes are perfectly aligned and there is no air gap, calculate the insertion loss at the joint in the forward and backward directions.

[B Tech]

Solution

In the forward direction:

$$\eta_{cd} = \left(\frac{50}{60}\right)^2 = 0.6944$$

$$\eta_{NA} = \left(\frac{0.20}{0.25}\right)^2 = 0.64$$

and $\qquad \eta_a = 1$

$\therefore \qquad \eta_T = 0.6944 \times 0.64 \times 1 = 0.444$

and $\qquad L_T = -10\log_{10}\eta_T = 3.52\ \text{dB}$

In the backward direction, $\eta_{cd} = 1$ and $\eta_{NA} = 1$.

But $\qquad \eta_a = \left(\frac{1 + 2/2.1}{1 + 2/1.9}\right) = 0.95$

$\eta_T = 1 \times 1 \times 0.95 = 0.95$

and $\qquad L_T = -10\log_{10}(0.95) = 0.218\ \text{dB}$

Example 8

Two single mode fibers with mode field diameters of 9.2 μm and 8.4 μm are to be connected together. Assuming no extrinsic losses, determine the loss at the connection due to the mode-field diameter mismatch.

Solution

We have the expression for intrinsic loss as:

$$\text{Loss}_{int} = -10\log_{10}\left[4\left(\frac{\omega_{02}}{\omega_{01}} + \frac{\omega_{01}}{\omega_{02}}\right)^{-2}\right]$$

where ω_{01} and ω_{02} are the spot sizes of the transmitting and receiving fibers respectively. Substituting the values in the above relation, we obtain:

Here $\omega_{01} = \dfrac{9.2}{2} = 5.6\ \mu m$, $\omega_{02} = \dfrac{8.4}{2} = 4.2\ \mu m$

$$\text{Loss}_{int} = -10\log_{10}\left[4\left(\frac{4.2}{5.6} + \frac{5.6}{4.2}\right)^{-2}\right]$$

$$= -10\log_{10} 0.922$$

$$= 0.35\ \text{dB}$$

Example 9

A four-port multimode fiber FBT coupler has 60 μW optical power launched into port 1. The measured output powers at ports 2, 3 and 4 are 0.004, 26.0 and 27.5 μW respectively.

Determine the excess loss, the insertion losses between the input and output ports, the crosstalk and the split ratio for the device.

Solution

We have the expression for excess loss (four-port coupler) as:

$$\text{Excess loss (four-port coupler)} = 10\log_{10}\left(\frac{P_1}{P_3 + P_4}\right)(\text{dB})$$

$$= 10\log_{10}\frac{60}{53.5}$$

$$= 0.5 \text{ dB}$$

$$\text{The insertion loss (parts 1 to 3)} = 10\log\frac{P_1}{P_3}(\text{dB})$$

$$= 10\log\left(\frac{60}{26}\right)$$

$$= 3.63 \text{ dB}$$

$$\text{Insertion loss (parts 1 to 4)} = 10\log_{10}\left(\frac{60}{27.5}\right)$$

$$= 3.39 \text{ dB}$$

$$\text{Cross talk (four-port coupler)} = 10\log_{10}\left(\frac{P_2}{P_1}\right)\text{ dB}$$

$$= 10\log_{10}\left(\frac{0.004}{60}\right)$$

$$= -41.8 \text{ dB}$$

$$\text{Split ratio} = \left[\frac{P_3}{(P_3 + P_4)}\right] \times 100\%$$

$$= \frac{26}{53.5} \times 100$$

$$= 48.6\%$$

SUMMARY

- Fiber optic cables are significantly different from copper cables. Fiber-optic cables transmit data through very small cores over long distances at the speed of light. These cables come in a wide variety of configurations. Important considerations in any cable installation and operation are the bending radius, tensile strength, ruggedness, durability, flexibility, environmental conditions, e.g. temperature extremes and even appearance.

- From the considerations of optical waveguiding, it is clear that variation of refractive index inside the optical fiber (i.e. between the core and the cladding) is a fundamental necessity in the fabrication of fibers for light transmission. This means at least two different compatible materials which are transparent to light over the major operating wavelength range (0.8 to 1.7 μm) are required. For most applications, silica based glass is the ultimate choice for producing optical fibers.

- Most fibers consists of silica (SiO_2) or silicate. Glass is made by fusing mixtures of metal oxides having refractive index of 1.458 at 850 nm. For changing the refractive index different oxides such as B_2O_3, GeO_2 and P_2O_5 are added.

- The fabrication of all glass fibers is a two-stage process. In the first stage, pure glass is produced and transforms it into a rod or perform. The second stage employs a pulling technique to draw fibers of required diameters.

- Vapour-phase methods are employed to produce silica-rich glass fibers whereas liquid-phase methods are used for manufacturing multicomponent glass fibers.

- The cabling of fibers requires that (i) the fiber be given primary and buffer coatings to protect against external influences (ii) a strength member be provided to improve mechanical strength and (iii) a structural member be provided to place them in multifiber cables. Several designs are available, e.g. two fiber cable, multiple fiber cables, etc.

- The basic fiber building blocks are used to form large cable. These units are bound on a buffer material which acts as strength element along with insulated copper conductor. The fiber building blocks are surrounded by paper tape, PVC jacket, yarn and outer sheath.

- Optical fiber links, in common with any communication system, have a requirement for both joining and termination of the transmission medium. The number of intermediate fiber connections or joints is dependent upon the link length (between repeaters), the continuous length of fiber cable that may be produced by the preparation methods, and the length of the fiber cable that may be practically or conveniently installed as a continuous section on the link.

- Fiber-to-fiber connection may be achieved through (i) splices (permanent joints) or connectors (demountable joints). It must be ensured that there are no misalignments in this jointing process. Connection losses may occur due to extrinsic parameters, e.g. Fresnel reflection, end separation, lateral offset, or angular misalignment of the two fiber ends. Losses can also occur due to intrinsic parameters, e.g. mismatches of core diameters, RI profiles, or numerical apertures.

- In order to evaluate the performance of an optical fiber, it is essential to measure its properties. Important among these are optical attenuation, pulse dispersion, numerical aperture, RI profile, etc. In the field, however, optical time domain reflectometry (OTDR) is an essential tool.

REVIEW QUESTIONS

1. Describe in general terms liquid-phase techniques for the preparation of multicomponent glasses for optical fibers. Discuss with the help of a suitable diagram one melting method for the preparation of multicomponent glass.

2. Indicate the major advantages of vapour-phase deposition in the preparation of glasses for optical fibers. Briefly describe the various vapour-phase techniques currently in use.

3. Compare and contrast, using suitable diagrams, the outside vapour-phase oxidation (OVPO) and the modified chemical vapour deposition (MCVD) technique for the preparation of low-loss optical fibers.

4. Describe the double crucible method for producing optical fibers. Mention the limitations of this method.

5. Distinguish between outside vapour-phase oxidation (OVPO) method and inside vapour-phase oxidation (IVPO) method for manufacturing optical fibers. Compare the salient features of these two methods.

6. Discuss the design of optical fibers from prepared glasses with regard to (a) multicomponent glass fibers (b) silica rich fibers.

7. List the silica based various optical fiber types currently on the market indicating the important features. Hence, briefly describe the general areas of applications for each type.

8. Describe the effects of stress corrosion on optical fiber strength and durability.

9. Discuss optical fiber cable design with regard to:
   (a) fiber buffering
   (b) cable strength and structural members
   (c) layered cable construction
   (d) cable sheath and water barrier.

10. State the two major categories of fiber-fiber joint, indicating the difference between them.

11. Describe the three types of fiber misalignment which may contribute to insertion. loss at an optical fiber joint.

12. Briefly outline the factors which cause intrinsic losses of fiber-fiber joints.

13. Describe with aid of suitable diagrams, three common techniques used for the mechanical splicing of optical fibers.

14. Describe with aid of suitable diagrams, the following techniques of mechanical splicing of optical fibers: (a) snug tube splice, (b) spring-groove splice, and elastomeric splice.

15. Describe with the aid of suitable diagrams, the design of the follow-ing connectors: (a) ferrule connector, and (b) expanded-beam connector.

16. The fraction of reflected light (R) at an air-fiber interface is given by:

$$R = \frac{P_r}{P_i} = \left(\frac{n_1 - n}{n_1 + n}\right)^2$$

where P_r and P_i are the reflected and incident powers, n_1 is the RI at the striking point of the fiber, and n is the RI of the medium surrounding the fiber. Show that for a small variation in the value of core index n_1, the change in R is given by:

$$\Delta R = 4n\left[\frac{n_1 - n}{(n_1 + n)^2}\right]\Delta n_1$$

17. With the aid of simple sketches, outline the major categories of multiport optical fiber coupler.

PROBLEMS

1. Silica has a Young's modulus of 9×10^{10} N·m^2 and a surface energy of 2.29 J. Estimate the fracture stress in psi for a silica optical fiber with a dominant elliptical crack of depth 0.5 μm. Also, calculate the strain at the break for the fiber. Given 1 psi = 6.894.76 N·m^{-2}.   [**Ans.** 7.43×10^4 psi, 0.6%]

2. A fusion splice is made for a multimode step index fiber. The splice exhibit a loss of 0.36 dB, which seems to be mainly due to an air gap. Show that the refractive index of fiber core is 1.5

3. Another length of the optical fiber described in problem 1 is found to break at 1% strain. The failure is due to dominant elliptical crack. Estimate the depth of this crack. **[Ans. 0.2 μm]**

4. It is reported that a 20 m length of fused silica optical fiber may be extended to 24 m at liquid nitrogen temperatures (i.e. little stress corrosion) before failure occurs. Estimate the failure stress under these conditions. Young's modulus for silica = 9×10^{10} N·m^2 and 1 psi = 6894.76 N·m^{-2}. **[Ans. 2.61 × 10^6 psi]**

5. The Fresnel reflection at a butt joint with an air gap in multimode step index fiber is 0.46 dB. Determine the refractive index of the fiber core. **[Ans. 1.59]**

6. A graded index fiber with a 50 μm core diameter has a characteristic refractive index profile (α) of 2.25. The fiber is joined with index matching and the connection exhibits an optical loss of 0.62 dB. This is found to be solely due to a lateral offset of the fiber ends. Calculate the magnitude of the lateral offset assuming the uniform illumination of all guided modes in the fiber core. **[Ans. 4.0 μm]**

7. A fiber Bragg grating assisted coupler is designed to block an incoming optical signal present at the input part of the device. When the fiber core refractive index is 1.6 and the grating period is 0.42 μm, calculate the wavelength of the blocked signal. **[Ans. 1.34 μm]**

8. A single mode step index fiber of 5 μm core diameter has a normalized frequency of 1.7, a core refractive index of 1.48 and a numerical aperture of 0.14. The loss in decibels due to angular misalignment at a fusion splice with a lateral offset of 0.4 μm is twice that due to the lateral offset. Calculate the degrees of the angular misalignment. **[Ans. 0.65°]**

9. Two compatible multimode SI fibers are jointed with a lateral offset of 10% of the core radius. The refractive index of the core of each fiber is 1.50. Estimate the insertion loss at the joint when (a) there is small air gap, and (b) an index-matching fluid is inserted between the fiber ends. **[B Tech]**

[**Hint:** We have $\Delta y/a = 10\% = 0.1$ and $n_1 = 1.50$. With the air gap ($n = 1$), $k = n_1/n = 1.5$, and with index-matching fluid ($n = n_1$), $k = 1$.

(a) We have
$$\eta_F = \frac{16k^2}{(k+1)^4}$$

$$\therefore \quad \eta_F = \frac{16(1.5)^2}{(1.5+1)^4} = 0.9216$$

Also,
$$\eta_{\text{lat}} \approx \frac{2}{\pi}\left[\cos^{-1}\left(\frac{\Delta y}{2a} - \frac{\Delta y}{2a}\right)\left\{1 - \left(\frac{\Delta y}{2a}\right)^2\right\}^{1/2}\right]$$

$$\therefore \quad \eta_{\text{lat}} = \frac{2}{\pi}\left[\cos^{-1}\left(\frac{0.1}{2}\right) - \left(\frac{0.1}{2}\right)\left\{1 - \left(\frac{0.1}{2}\right)^2\right\}^{1/2}\right]$$

Thus, the total coupling efficiency, η_T is obtained as:
$$\eta_T = \eta_F\eta_{\text{lat}} = 0.9216 \times 0.936 = 0.8629.$$
Thus the total loss $L_T = -\log_{10}\eta_T = (-10\log_{10}(0.8629)) = 0.64$ dB.

(b) Here, $\eta_F = 1$ and $\eta_{lat} = 0.936$, and hence:

$$\eta_T = \eta_F\eta_{lat} = 1 \times 0.936 = 0.936$$

and the total loss:

$$L_\tau = -\log_{10}(0.936) = 0.287 \text{ dB}$$

10. A $80/125 \, \mu\text{m}$ graded-index (GI) fiber with a NA of 0.25 and α of 2.0 is jointed with a $60/125 \, \text{mm}$ GI fiber with an NA of 0.21 and α of 1.9. The fiber axes are perfectly aligned and there is no air gap. Calculate the insertion loss at a joint for the signal transmission in the forward and backward directions.

[**Hint:**

For *Fiber 1*: Core diameter: $d_1 = 80 \, \mu\text{m}$, $\text{NA}_1 = 0.25$, $a_1 = 2.0$.

For *Fiber 2*: Core diameter: $d_2 = 60 \, \mu\text{m}$, $\text{NA}_2 = 0.21$, $a_2 = 1.9$.

In the *forward direction*, i.e. when the signal is propagating from fiber 1 to fiber 2, we have

$$\eta_{cd} = \left(\frac{d_2}{d_1}\right)^2 = \left(\frac{60}{80}\right)^2 = 0.5625$$

$$\eta_{NA} = \left(\frac{\text{NA}_2}{\text{NA}_1}\right)^2 = \left(\frac{0.21}{0.25}\right)^2 = 0.7056$$

$$\eta_\alpha = \left(\frac{1+2/\alpha_1}{1+2/\alpha_2}\right) = \left(\frac{1+2.0/2.0}{1+2.0/1.9}\right) = 0.9743$$

Thus, the total coupling efficiency at the joint, $\eta_T = \eta_{cd}\eta_{NA}\eta_a$. Substituting the values of η_{cd}, η_{NA} and η_a, one obtains

$$\eta_T = 0.5625 \times 0.7056 \times 0.9743 = 0.3867$$

Therefore, the total loss at the joint will be

$$L_T = -\log_{10}\eta_T = -\log_{10}(0.3867) = 4.1259 \text{ dB}$$

In the *backward direction*, η_{cd}, η_{NA} and η_u are all unity and hence there will be no loss.]

SHORT ANSWER QUESTIONS

1. What optical fiber properties reduce connection loss in short distance systems?
   Ans. (i) Larger fiber core, and
   (ii) Higher fiber numerical
2. What trade offs are considered by designers in fiber optic systems?
   Ans. (i) Types of connections
   (ii) Optical sources, and
   (iii) detector types in military and subscriber loop applications.
3. Which fiber part, core or cladding has a higher index of refraction?
   Ans. Core.
4. In multimode step index fibers, the majority of light propagates in the fiber core, why?
   Ans. Most modes in multimode step index fibers propagates far from cutoff.
5. What is basic requirement for light guidance through an optical fiber?
   Ans. Refractive indices of the core and cladding should be different. This is why, two compatible materials that are transparent in the operating wavelength range are required.

6. Why multimode step index fibers have relatively large core diameters and large NA?

   Ans. To make it easier to couple light from a LED into the fiber.

7. For most applications, which material is the ultimate choice for producing optical fibers?

   Ans. Silica based glass.

8. How are the source to fiber coupling and micro-bending and macro-bending losses affected by core diameter and Δ?

   Ans. Coupling efficiency increases with core diameter and Δ, whereas bending losses increases with core diameter and inversely with Δ.

9. How glass fibers are fabricated?

   Ans. The fabrication of all-glass fibers is a two-stage process. In the first stage pure glass is produced and transforms it into a rod or perform. The second stage employs a pulling technique to draw fibers of required diameters.

10. Which fiber optic component (splice, connector or coupler) makes a permanent connection in a distributed system?

    Ans. Splice.

11. Which methods produce multicomponent glass fibers?

    Ans. Liquid phase methods.

12. Which methods are employed to produce silica-rich glass fibers?

    Ans. Vapour phase methods.

13. Mention the three basic errors that occur during fiber alignment.

    Ans. (i) Longitudinal misalignment

    (ii) Lateral misalignment, and

    (iii) Angular misalignment.

14. Mention the requirements of cabling of fibers.

    Ans. (i) The fiber should be given primary and buffer coating to protect against external influences

    (ii) A strength member to be provided to improve mechanical strength, and

    (iii) A structural member be provided to place them in multifiber cable

15. When the axes of two connected fibers are no longer in parallel, what this misalignment termed?

    Ans. Angular misalignment.

16. How fiber-to-fiber connections may be achieved?

    Ans. Through splices (permanent joints) or connectors (demountable joints). One will have to ensure that there are no misalignments in this joining process. One will have to take care of connection losses. Connection losses may occur due to extrinsic parameters, e.g. Fresnel's reflection, end separation, lateral offset, or angular misalignment of the two fiber ends.

    Losses can also occur due to intrinsic parameters, e.g. mismatches of core diameters, RI profiles or aperatures.

17. Which single mode or multimode fibers are more sensitive to alignment errors?

    Ans. Single mode fibers.

18. For reliable operation quality end preparation is needed. What properties must an optical fiber end face should have to ensure proper fiber connections?

    Ans. Flat, smooth and perpendicular to the fiber axis.

19. What are the important properties of an optical fiber, which are to be measured essentially for the evaluation of its performance?

    Ans. Optical attenuation, pulse dispersion, numerical aperture (NA), RI profile, etc.

20. What is a fiber optic splice?

    Ans. A fiber optic splice is a permanent fiber joint whose purpose is to establish an optical connection between two individual optical fibers.

21. Mention the techniques used for fiber splicing.

    Ans. (i) Mechanical splicing

         (ii) Fusion splicing

22. What type of faults are produced by (a) fiber breaks, (b) fiber cracks, and (c) fiber microbends?

    Ans. (a) Reflective

        (b) Nonreflective

MULTIPLE CHOICE QUESTIONS

1. Most low-loss optical fibers are made of oxide glasses, the most widely used material is:

    (a) silica (SiO_2)   (b) germanium

    (c) arsenic   (d) none of the above

2. Optical glass fibers are brittle and have very small cross-sectional area (~100 to 250 μm). They are, therefore, highly susceptible to damage during handling and use. In order to improve their tensile strength and protect them from external influences, it is necessary to:

    (a) polish them   (b) encase them in cables

    (c) wind up them   (d) none of the above

3. In a multifiber cable, the strength member: **[B Tech]**

    (a) must be placed along the central axis of the cable

    (b) must be placed in a coaxial cylindrical configuration

    (c) can be placed anywhere within the cable

    (d) is not required at all

4. An air gap is introduced while splicing two compatible fibers with core indices of 1.46. What is the loss due to Fresnel reflection at the joint?   **[B Tech]**

    (a) Zero   (b) 0.154 dB

    (c) 0.309 dB   (d) 0.36 dB

5. Two optical fibers with numerical apertures 0.17 and 0.20 are to be spliced. What will be the loss at the joint in the forward direction?   **[B Tech]**

    (a) Zero   (b) 1.41 dB

    (c) 1.82 dB   (d) 2.50 dB

6. Increase in the concentration of GeO_2 in SiO_2 will: **[B Tech]**

    (a) decrease the RI   (b) increase the RI

    (c) change RI randomly   (d) not change RI at all

7. What type of optical fibers can be drawn from a solid perform (formed by collapsing a solid rod or hollow tube deposited by the vapour-phase oxidation method)?

                                                                [B Tech]

    (a) Multimode SI fibers   (b) Multimode GI fiber

    (c) Single-mode fibers   (d) All of these

8. Increase in the concentration of B_2O_3 in SiO_2 will:
   (a) increase the RI
   (b) decrease the RI
   (c) change RI randomly
   (d) RI remains unaffected

9. For the optical fibers of Question 5, what will be the joint loss in the backward direction? **[B Tech]**
   (a) Zero
   (b) 1.41 dB
   (c) 1.82 dB
   (d) 2.50 dB

10. A 62.5/125 μm Si fiber is to be spliced to a 50/125 μm Si fiber. Both the fibers have a core index of 1.50. What will be the joint loss in the forward direction? **[B Tech]**
    (a) Zero
    (b) 0.97 dB
    (c) 1.94 dB
    (d) 2.45 dB

11. A multimode Si fiber with a core RI of 1.50 is spliced with an identical fiber. What is the NA of the fiber if the splice loss is 0.7 dB, which is mainly due to a 5° angular misalignment of the fiber core axes? **[B Tech]**
    (a) 0.17
    (b) 0.21
    (c) 0.28
    (d) 0.30

12. If two optical fibers with different diameters are to be spliced, which of the following mechanical splices will be most suitable? **[B Tech]**
    (a) Snug tube splice
    (b) Loose tube splice
    (c) Spring-groove splice
    (d) V-groove splice

13. With an OTDR, it is possible to know:
    (a) the location dependence of attenuation
    (b) the overall link length
    (c) splice and connector losses
    (d) All of the above

14. If τ_i and τ_o are the half width of the input and output pulses and if, the shape of the pulses assumed to be Gaussian, then the impulse response of the fiber in ns/km is given by: [B.Tech.]

    (a) $\tau = \dfrac{\tau_o - \tau_i}{L}$

    (b) $\tau = \dfrac{\left(\tau_o^2 - \tau_i^2\right)^{1/2}}{L}$

    (c) $\tau^2 = \sqrt{\dfrac{\left(\tau_o^2 - \tau_i^2\right)}{L}}$

    (d) $\tau^2 = \dfrac{L}{\tau_o^2 - \tau_i^2}$

15. The refractive index profile of an optical fiber helps in:
    (a) its characterization
    (b) determination of the NA
    (c) determination of guided modes propagating within the fiber
    (d) All of the above

ANSWERS

1. (a)   2. (b)   3. (c)   4. (c)   5. (a)   6. (b)   7. (d)   8. (b)   9. (b)   10. (c)
11. (c)   12. (d)   13. (d)   14. (b)   15. (d)

5

Optical Fiber Waveguides and Mode Analysis

5.1 INTRODUCTION

In Chapter 2, we have read that a uniform plane electromagnetic (em) wave propagates in an unbounded medium as a transverse electromagnetic wave (TEM) having E and H (or B) vectors both perpendicular to each other and to the direction of propagation. We have also examined the boundary effects on the propagation of an em wave. We shall now discuss the behaviour of such waves in the vicinity of the boundaries so configured as to guide that wave along a certain path. Such systems are called *waveguides*. The most efficient way of transmitting energy over short distances is by using waveguides. Waveguides were first evolved and used in practical electronics and now assumed great importance in fiber optic communication – *optoelectronics*.

In waveguide, both electric and magnetic fields are confined to space within the waveguide. The dielectric loss within the waveguide is negligibly small because the guides are normally air filled. Within a waveguide several modes of electromagnetic waves could be propagated. The mode of propagation of a waveguide is determined from solutions of Maxwell's equations.

5.2 CONCEPT OF ELECTROMAGNETIC WAVES

We will briefly summarize the results of the electromagnetic theory discussed in Chapter 2. Maxwell's set of four equations are:

$$\nabla \times E = -\frac{\partial B}{\partial t} \tag{5.1}$$

$$\nabla \times H = J + \frac{\partial D}{\partial t} \tag{5.2}$$

$$\nabla \cdot D = \rho \tag{5.3}$$

$$\nabla \cdot B = 0 \tag{5.4}$$

where, E is the electric field vector in $V{\cdot}m^{-1}$, H is the magnetic field vector in $A{\cdot}m^{-1}$, D is electric displacement vector in $C{\cdot}m^{-2}$, it is related to E by the relation $D = \varepsilon E$, where E is the dielectric permittivity of the medium. B is the magnetic induction vector in $H{\cdot}m^{-1}$, it is related to H by the relation $B = \mu H$, where μ is the magnetic permeability of the medium. ρ is the charge density of the medium in $C{\cdot}m^{-3}$. J is the current density in $A{\cdot}m^{-2}$, it is related to E by the relation $J = \sigma E$, where σ is the conductivity of the medium in $A{\cdot}V^{-1}\,m^{-1}$. ∇ is 'del' operator defined as:

$$\nabla = \hat{i}\,\frac{\partial}{\partial x} + \hat{j}\,\frac{\partial}{\partial y} + \hat{k}\,\frac{\partial}{\partial z}$$

We have $\mu = \mu_0\mu_r$, $\mu_0 = 4\pi \times 10^{-7}$ N·A^{-2} (or H·m^{-1}) is the permeability of free space, and μ_r is the relative permeability of the material and very close to unity. For most dielectrics, $\varepsilon = \varepsilon_0\varepsilon_r$, where $\varepsilon_0 = 8.854 \times 10^{-12}$ C^{2}N^{-1}·m^{-2} is the permittivity of free space, and ε_r is the relative permittivity of the material.

Inside an ideal dielectric material ρ (free charge density) = 0 and $\sigma = 0$. Therefore, *Maxwell's equations* for a dielectric medium reduces to:

$$\nabla \times E = \frac{\partial B}{\partial t} \tag{5.5}$$

$$\nabla \times H = \frac{\partial D}{\partial t} \tag{5.6}$$

$$\nabla \cdot D = 0 \tag{5.7}$$

$$\nabla \cdot B = 0 \tag{5.8}$$

Substituting for D and B and taking the curl of Eqs (5.5) and (5.6) gives:

$$\nabla \times (\nabla \times E) = -\mu\varepsilon \frac{\partial^2 E}{\partial t^2} \tag{5.9}$$

$$\nabla \times (\nabla \times H) = -\mu\varepsilon \frac{\partial^2 H}{\partial t^2} \tag{5.10}$$

In obtaining these equations we have used:

$$\nabla \cdot E = \nabla \cdot (D/\varepsilon) = 0 \tag{5.11}$$

Using the vector identity:

$$\nabla \times (\nabla \times E) = \nabla \cdot (\nabla \cdot E) - \nabla^2 E \tag{5.12}$$

We obtain the nondispersive wave equations:

$$\nabla^2 E - \mu\varepsilon \frac{\partial^2 E}{\partial t^2} = 0 \tag{5.13}$$

$$\nabla^2 H - \mu\varepsilon \frac{\partial^2 H}{\partial t^2} = 0 \tag{5.14}$$

where, ∇^2 is the Laplacian operator. Equations (5.13) and (5.14) are the standard non-dispersive wave equations. For rectangular cartesian and cylindrical polar coordinates, the above wave equations hold for each component of the field vector, each component satisfying the scalar wave equation:

$$\nabla^2 \psi - \mu\varepsilon \frac{\partial^2 \psi}{\partial t^2} = 0 \tag{5.15}$$

or

$$\nabla^2 \psi - \frac{1}{v_p^2} \frac{\partial^2 \psi}{\partial t^2} = 0 \tag{5.15a}$$

where ψ may represents a component of E or H field and v_p is the phase velocity (velocity of propagation of a point of constant phase in the wave) in the dielectric medium. It follows that:

$$v_p = \frac{1}{(\mu\varepsilon)} = \frac{1}{\sqrt{\mu\varepsilon}} = \frac{1}{\sqrt{\mu_r\mu_0\varepsilon_r\varepsilon_0}} \tag{5.16}$$

where μ_r and ε_r are the relative permeability and permittivity of free space, respectively. The velocity of light in free space:

$$c = \frac{1}{\sqrt{\mu_o \varepsilon_o}} \tag{5.17}$$

For an *isotropic medium*, the refractive index n is related to ε by relation to ε by the relation $n = \sqrt{\varepsilon / \varepsilon_0} = \sqrt{\varepsilon_r}$, with $\mu_r = 1$. Therefore, $v_p = c/n$. Eq. (5.15a) then becomes:

$$\nabla^2 \psi - \frac{n^2}{c^2} \frac{\partial^2 \psi}{\partial t^2} = 0 \tag{5.18}$$

The solution of wave equation (5.18) can be verified by substituting:

$$\psi = \psi_0 \exp\left[i\left(\omega t - \beta z\right)\right] \tag{5.19}$$

This represents a uniform plane wave propagating in Z direction with a phase velocity $v_p = \omega/\beta$, where ω is the angular frequency of the field, t is the time, β is the propagation phase constant, and $i = \sqrt{-1}$.

5.3 SOLUTION IN AN INHOMOGENEOUS MEDIUM

We now find the solution in an isotropic, linear, nonconducting, nonmagnetic, but inhomogeneous medium. The divergence of electric displacement vector D becomes:

$$\nabla \cdot D = \nabla \cdot (\varepsilon E) = \varepsilon_0 \nabla \cdot (\varepsilon_r E) = 0$$
$$= \varepsilon_0 \left[\nabla (\varepsilon_r) \cdot E + \varepsilon_r (\nabla \cdot E)\right] = 0 \tag{5.20}$$

This gives:

$$\nabla \cdot E = -\left(\frac{1}{\varepsilon_r}\right) \nabla (\varepsilon_r) E \tag{5.21}$$

From Eq. (5.9), one finds

$$\nabla \times \nabla \times E = -\mu \frac{\partial^2 D}{\partial t^2} = -\mu \varepsilon_0 \varepsilon_r \frac{\partial^2 E}{\partial t^2} \tag{5.22}$$

since $\mu = \mu_0 \mu_r = \mu_0$ ($\because \mu_r = 1$) and $D = \varepsilon_0 E = \varepsilon_0 \varepsilon_r E$

From Eqs (5.12) and (5.22), one obtains:

$$\nabla (\nabla \cdot E) - \nabla^2 E = -\mu \varepsilon_0 \varepsilon_r \frac{\partial^2 E}{\partial t^2}$$

Rearranging, one obtains:

$$\nabla^2 E - \nabla(\nabla \cdot E) - \mu_0 \varepsilon_0 \varepsilon_r \frac{\partial^2 E}{\partial t^2} = 0 \tag{5.23}$$

Substituing for $\nabla \cdot E$ from Eq. (5.21) in Eq. (5.23), one obtains:

$$\nabla^2 E - \nabla \left\{\frac{1}{\varepsilon_r} \nabla (\varepsilon_r) \cdot E\right\} - \mu \varepsilon_0 \varepsilon_r \frac{\partial^2 E}{\partial t^2} = 0 \tag{5.24}$$

Equation (5.24) shows that for an inhomogeneous medium, the equation for the Cartesion components of E, i.e. E_x, E_y, and E_z are coupled. Now, for homogeneous medium, the second term on the L.H.S. of Eq. (5.24) will become zero ($\because \nabla \cdot E = 0$ for a homogeneous medium). In this case, the Cartesian components of E will satisfy the scalar wave equation represented by Eq. (5.18).

One can obtain a similar equation to Eq. (5.24) for H also. Taking the curl of Eq. (5.6), one obtains

$$\nabla \times \nabla \times H = \nabla \times \left(\frac{\partial D}{\partial t}\right) = \frac{\partial}{\partial y}(\nabla \times D)$$

$$= \frac{\partial}{\partial t}(\nabla \times \varepsilon E) = \varepsilon_0 \frac{\partial}{\partial t}(\nabla \times \varepsilon_r E) \qquad (5.25)$$

But, we have:

$$\nabla \times \nabla \times H = \nabla(\nabla \cdot H) - \nabla^2 H$$

From Eq. (5.8), $\qquad \nabla \cdot B = \nabla \cdot (\mu_0 H) = 0$

$$\therefore \qquad \nabla \times \nabla \times H = -\nabla^2 H \qquad (5.26)$$

Equating Eqs (5.25) and (5.26), one obtains:

$$\nabla^2 H + \varepsilon_0 \frac{\partial}{\partial t}(\nabla \times \varepsilon_r E) = 0$$

or $\qquad \nabla^2 H + \varepsilon_0 \frac{\partial}{\partial t}[(\nabla \varepsilon_r) \times E + \varepsilon_r (\nabla \times E)] = 0$

or $\qquad \nabla^2 H + \varepsilon_0 (\nabla \varepsilon_r) \times \frac{\partial E}{\partial t} + \varepsilon_0 \varepsilon_r \frac{\partial}{\partial t}(\nabla \times E) = 0$

Using Eqs (5.5) and (5.6) and rearranging, one obtains:

$$\nabla^2 H + \frac{1}{\varepsilon_r}\{(\nabla \varepsilon_r) \times (\nabla \times H)\} - \mu_0 \varepsilon_0 \varepsilon_r \frac{\partial^2 H}{\partial t^2} = 0 \qquad (5.27)$$

We again see that the equations for Cartesian components of H, i.e. H_x, H_y and H_z, are coupled. To simplify Eqs (5.24) and (5.27), let us set the z-coordinates along the direction of propagation of the wave represented by Eqs (5.24) and (5.27). Let us assume that $n = \sqrt{\varepsilon_r}$ does not vary with y and z. Then, one finds:

$$\varepsilon_r = n^2 = n^2(x) \qquad (5.28)$$

This reveals that the y- and z-dependence of the fields, in general will be of the form $\exp[[-i(\gamma y + \beta z)]$. However, we put $\gamma = 0$ without any loss of generality. Now, the equations governing the modes of propagation of E_j or H_j, where $J = x, y, z$, may be written as:

$$E_j = E_j (x) e^{i(\omega t - \beta z)} \qquad (5.29)$$

and $\qquad H_j = H_j (x) e^{i(\omega t - \beta z)} \qquad (5.30)$

Here $E_j(x)$ and $H_j(x)$ represents the transverse field distributions that do not change as the field propagates through the medium.

Now, we write Eqs (5.5) and (5.6) in Cartesian coordinates. From Eq. (5.5), i.e.

$$\nabla \times E = -\frac{\partial B}{\partial t} = -\mu_0 \frac{\partial H}{\partial t}$$

one obtains:

$$\hat{i}\left(\frac{\partial E_z}{\partial y} - \frac{\partial E_y}{\partial z}\right) + \hat{j}\left(\frac{\partial E_x}{\partial z} - \frac{\partial E_z}{\partial x}\right) + \hat{k}\left(\frac{\partial E_y}{\partial x} - \frac{\partial E_x}{\partial y}\right) = -\mu_0 \frac{\partial}{\partial t}\{\hat{i} H_x + \hat{j} H_y + \hat{k} H_z\} \qquad (5.31)$$

and from Eq. (5.6), i.e.

$$\nabla \times H = -\frac{\partial D}{\partial t} = \varepsilon_0 \varepsilon_r \frac{\partial E}{\partial t} = \varepsilon_0 n^2 \frac{\partial E}{\partial t}$$

one obtains:

$$\hat{i}\left(\frac{\partial H_z}{\partial y} - \frac{\partial H_y}{\partial z}\right) + \hat{j}\left(\frac{\partial H_x}{\partial z} - \frac{\partial H_z}{\partial x}\right) + \hat{k}\left(\frac{\partial H_y}{\partial x} - \frac{\partial H_x}{\partial y}\right) = -\varepsilon_0 n^2 \frac{\partial}{\partial t}\{\hat{i}\,E_x + \hat{j}\,E_y + \hat{k}\,E_z\}] \quad (5.32)$$

The fields E and H do not vary with y, we may take the $\partial/\partial y$ terms equal to zero. Now, substituting the values of E_j and H_j from Eqs (5.29) and (5.30) into Eq. (5.31), one obtains:

$$-\hat{i}\frac{\partial}{\partial z}\{E_y\,e^{i(\omega t - \beta z)}\} + \hat{j}\frac{\partial}{\partial z}\{E_x\,e^{i(\omega t - \beta z)}\} + \hat{k}\frac{\partial}{\partial x}\{E_x\,e^{i(\omega t - \beta z)}\}$$

$$= -\hat{i}\,\mu_0\frac{\partial}{\partial t}\,H_x\,e^{i(\omega t - \beta z)} - \hat{j}\,\mu_0\frac{\partial}{\partial t}\,H_y\,e^{i(\omega t - \beta z)} - \hat{k}\,\mu_0\frac{\partial}{\partial t}\,H_z\,e^{i(\omega t - \beta z)}$$

or $\hat{i}\,(i\beta)\,E_y - \hat{j}\left[i\beta E_x + \dfrac{\partial E_z}{\partial x}\right] + \hat{k}\,\dfrac{\partial E_y}{\partial x} = -\hat{i}\,\mu_0(i\omega)\,H_x - \hat{j}\,\mu_0\,(i\omega)\,H_y - \hat{k}\,\mu_0\,(i\omega)\,H_z$

Comparing the corresponding components on both sides, one obtains the following set of equations:

$$i\beta E_y = -i\omega\mu_0 H_x \qquad\qquad\qquad (5.33)$$

or $\qquad\qquad\qquad \beta E_y = -\mu_0\omega H_x$

$$i\beta E_x + \frac{\partial E_z}{\partial x} = i\mu_0\omega H_y \qquad\qquad\qquad (5.33a)$$

$$\frac{\partial E_y}{\partial x} = -i\mu_0\omega H_z \qquad\qquad\qquad (5.33b)$$

Now substituting the values of E_j and H_j from Eqs (5.29) and (5.30) into Eq. (5.32) and setting to zero all terms containing $\partial/\partial y$, one obtains:

$$-\hat{i}\frac{\partial}{\partial z}H_y\,e^{i(\omega t - \beta z)} + \hat{j}\left[\frac{\partial}{\partial t}\{H_x\,e^{i(\omega t - \beta z)} - \frac{\partial}{\partial t}H_z\,e^{i(\omega t - \beta z)}\right] + \hat{k}\frac{\partial}{\partial t}\{H_x\,e^{i(\omega t - \beta z)}\}$$

$$= \varepsilon_0 n^2\,\hat{i}\frac{\partial}{\partial t}\{E_x e^{i(\omega t - \beta z)} + \varepsilon_0 n^2\hat{j}\frac{\partial}{\partial t}\{E_y e^{i(\omega t - \beta z)} + \varepsilon_0 n^2\,\hat{k}\frac{\partial}{\partial t}\{E_z\,e^{i(\omega t - \beta z)}\}$$

or $\hat{i}\,(i\beta)\,H_y - \hat{j}\left\{-(i\beta H_x - \dfrac{\partial H_z}{\partial x}\right\} + \hat{k}\,\dfrac{\partial H_y}{\partial x} = \hat{i}\,(i\omega\varepsilon_0 n^2)\,E_x + \hat{j}\,(i\omega\varepsilon_0 n^2)\,E_y + \hat{k}\,(i\omega\varepsilon_0 n^2)\,E_z$

Comparing the respective components, one obtains:

$$i\beta H_y = -i\omega\mu_0 n^2\,E_x \qquad\qquad\qquad (5.34)$$

or $\qquad\qquad\qquad \beta H_y = -\varepsilon_0 n^2\omega E_x$

$$-i\beta H_x - \frac{\partial H_z}{\partial x} = i\varepsilon_0 n^2\omega E_y \qquad\qquad\qquad (5.34a)$$

$$\frac{\partial H_y}{\partial x} = i\varepsilon_0 n^2\omega E_z \qquad\qquad\qquad (5.34b)$$

where $n^2 = n^2(x)$.

The above six equations, i.e. (5.33)–(5.33b), (5.34)–(5.34b) form two independent sets. Thus, Eqs (5.33), (5.33b), and (5.34a) involve E_y, H_x, and H_z. Clearly, the field components E_x, E_z, and H_y are zero. The modes described by these equations are called *transverse electric (TE) modes* as the electric field has only the transverse component E_y.

Renumbering these equations as follows, we find:

$$\beta E_y = -\mu_0 \omega H_x \qquad (5.35)$$

$$\frac{\partial E_y}{\partial x} = -i\mu_0 \omega H_z \qquad \text{TE modes} \qquad (5.36)$$

$$-i\beta H_x - \frac{\partial H_z}{\partial x} = i\varepsilon_0 \omega n^2(x) E_y \qquad (5.37)$$

The second set of equations is formed by Eqs (5.34a), (5.34b) and (5.33c), which involve only H_y, E_x, and E_z, and the field components E_y, H_x and H_z are zero. These are called *transverse magnetic (TM) modes* because the magnetic field herein has only a transverse component H_y. The second set of equations is also renumbered, we find:

$$\beta H_y = -\varepsilon_0 \omega n^2(x) E_x \qquad (5.38)$$

$$\frac{\partial H_y}{\partial x} = -i\varepsilon_0 \omega n^2(x) E_z \qquad \text{TE modes} \qquad (5.39)$$

$$i\beta H_x + \frac{\partial E_z}{\partial x} = -i\mu_0 \omega H_y \qquad (5.40)$$

5.4 PLANAR OPTICAL WAVEGUIDE

The planar optical waveguide is the simplest form of the optical waveguide and these are important components in integrated optical devices.

Figure 5.1 shows the geometrical configuration of simplest optical waveguide. We may assume that it consists of a thin dielectric slab of refractive index n_1 and sandwiched between two symmetrical dielectric slabs of refractive index n_2 and infinite thickness ($n_2 < n_1$). The waveguide is oriented such that the wave propagates along the z-direction. The y and z dimensions of the guide are assumed to extend to infinity. The thickness of the slabs is along the x-direction (Fig. 5.1). A ray of light launched into the guide slab or layer would progress by multiple reflections as shown in Fig. 5.2. One may assume that such a ray represents a *plane TEM wave* travelling at an angle θ with the z-axis. However, TEM modes are rarely found in optical waveguides. As the refractive index within the guide layer is n_1, the wavelength of light in the layer is reduced to $\lambda_m = \lambda/n_1$, where λ is the wavelength of light in vacuum and the propagation constant is increased to:

$$\beta_2 = \frac{2\pi}{\lambda_m} = \frac{2\pi n_1}{\lambda} = kn_1$$

where $k = 2\pi/\lambda$ is the vacuum propagation constant or the propagation vector.

In Fig. 5.1, we have assumed that the constructive interference of the waves form the lowest order standing wave ($m = 0$) in which the electric field is maximum at the centre. Further, the electric field is effectively confined in the central region but decays exponentially towards zero in the cladding region beyond the interfaces on both the sides. The variation of electric field in the transverse x-direction for the lowest order mode is also shown in Fig. 5.2(a). While the wave advances in the z-direction the electric field distribution does not change in the transverse direction. This stable field distribution in the transverse x-direction with periodic-dependence is called a *mode*. Figure 5.2(b) shows the variation of electric field in the z-direction. We may note that a particular mode originates from constructive interference of the plane waves corresponding to a

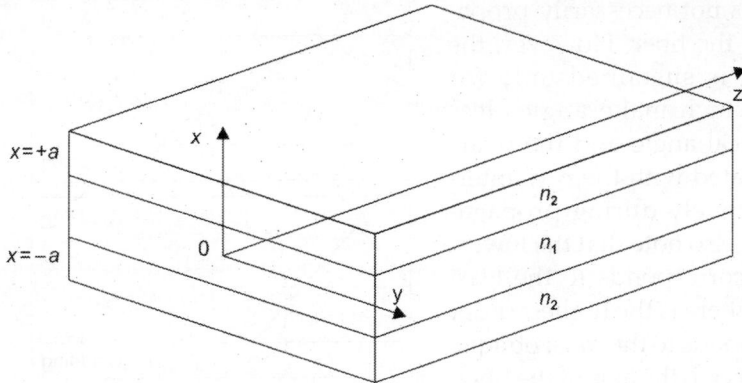

Fig. 5.1: Structure of a planar optical waveguide

ray congruence (a representative ray for this is shown in Fig. 5.2(b)) making a specific angle with the core-cladding interface or the axis of the fiber. Clearly, each representative ray propagating through the optical fiber corresponds to a mode. However, we may note that any ray making an angle less than the critical angle with the core–cladding interface does not necessarily propagate through the fiber corresponds to a mode. We may note any ray making an angle less than the critical angle with the core–cladding

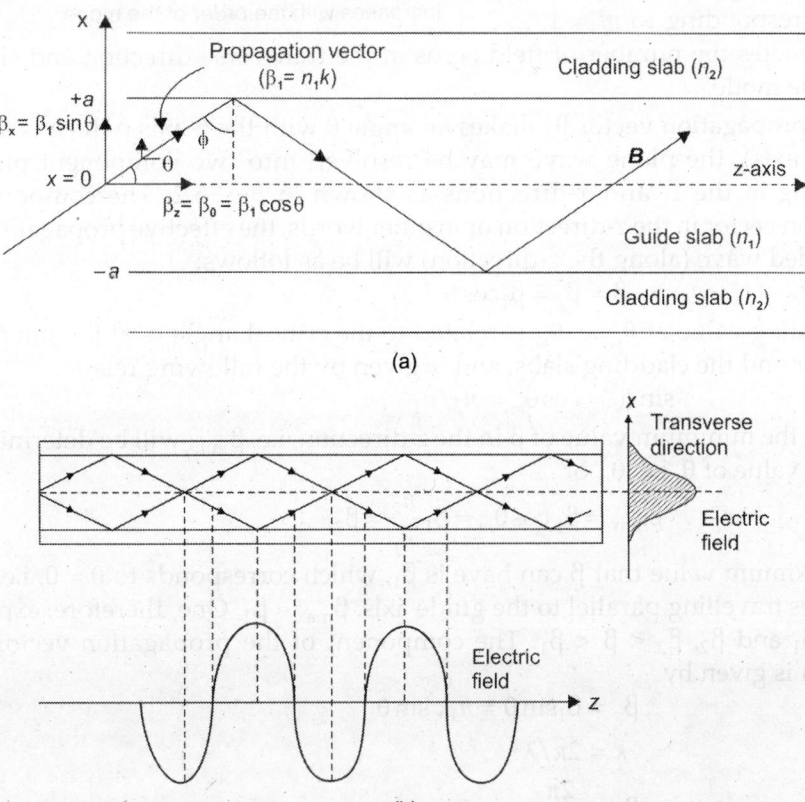

Fig. 5.2: The formation of a mode in a planar waveguide (a) plane wave propagating through the guide shown in the form of equivalent ray which correspond to the wave vector (b) formation of the lowest order mode through superposition of plane waves in the transverse direction

interface does not necessarily propagate through the fiber. However, the propagation is sustained only for those rays which make angles less than the critical angle and the plane waves associated with the rays interfere constructively during propagation. We may also note that the lowest order mode corresponds to the least oblique ray whereas the highest order mode corresponds to the most oblique ray with respect to the axis of the fiber. Clearly, the light propagating through a waveguide thus forms a discrete number of modes corresponding to discrete values ($< \theta_c$), which the equivalent rays make with the core-cladding interface. Figure 5.2(c) shows a few higher order modes with the electric field distributions in the transverse direction for different modes corresponding to $m = 1, 2, 3$.

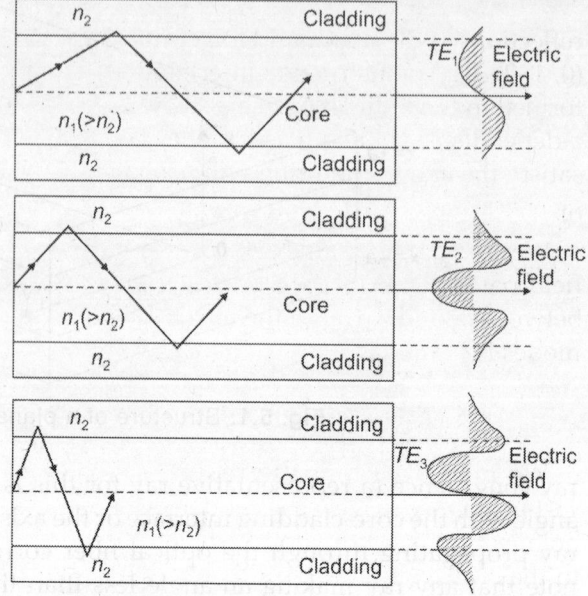

Fig. 5.2: (c) Transverse electric modes TE_m ($m = 1, 2, 3$) alongwith ray paths showing penetration in the cladding region. The penetration of the field in the cladding region increases with the order of the mode

Here m denotes the number of field zeros in the transverse direction and signifies the order of the mode.

Let the propagation vector β_1 makes an angle θ with the z-axis (which is the same as the guide axis), the plane wave may be resolved into two component plane waves propagating in the z- and x-directions as shown in Fig. 5.2. The component of the propagation vector in the z-direction or in other words, the effective propagation constant of the guided wave (along the z-direction) will be as follows:

$$\beta = \beta_2 = \beta_1 \cos\theta \tag{5.41}$$

The limiting value of θ, i.e. θ_m is related to the critical angle ϕ_c at the interface of the guide layer and the cladding slabs, and is given by the following relation:

$$\sin\phi_c = \cos\theta_m = n_2/n_1 \tag{5.42}$$

Clearly, the minimum value of β in the z-direction, i.e. β_{min}, will be determined by the maximum value of θ, i.e. θ_m or

$$\beta_{min} = \beta_1 \cos\theta_m = \beta_1 \frac{n_2}{n_1} = \beta_2 \tag{5.43}$$

The maximum value that β can have is β_1, which corresponds to $\theta = 0$, i.e. the plane TEM waves travelling parallel to the guide axis: $\beta_{max} \approx \beta_1$. One, therefore, expect β to lie between β_1 and β_2, $\beta_2 < \beta < \beta_1$. The component of the propagation vector β_1 in the x-direction is given by

$$\beta_x = \beta_1 \sin\theta = n_1 k \sin\theta$$

where

$$k = 2\pi/\lambda$$

or

$$\beta_x = \frac{2\pi}{\lambda_m} = \sin\theta \tag{5.44}$$

We see that this component of the plane wave is reflected at the interface between the guide layer and the cladding slabs. When the total phase change after two successive reflections at the upper and lower interfaces is equal to $2i\pi$ radians, where i is an integer (0, 1, 2, 3, ...), constructive interference will occur and a standing-wave pattern will be formed in the x-direction. This stable field pattern in the x-direction with only a periodic z-dependence is known as a mode. Thus, only a finite number of discrete modes which satisfy the above condition will propagate through the guide, i.e. $4a\beta_x = 2i\pi$:

or $$4a \sin \theta_i = i\lambda_m \qquad (5.45)$$

We see that each value of θ_i corresponds to a particular mode with its own characteristic field pattern and its own propagation constant β_1 in the z-direction. Obviously, β_i lies between β_1 and β_2. Since the maximum value that θ_i can take is θ_m, the number of guided modes is limited to:

$$M = i_{\max} = \frac{4a \sin \theta_m}{\lambda_m} = \frac{4an_1 \sin \theta_m}{\lambda} = \frac{4a}{\lambda} = (n_1^2 - n_2^2)^{1/2} \qquad (5.46)$$

We may note that the requirement for the ith mode to be propagated is that $i \leq (4a/\lambda)(n_1^2 - n_2^2)^{1/2}$. The mode corresponding to the highest value of i, i.e. $i_{\max}$, does not meet the condition for total internal reflection, as the value of θ_m corresponds exactly to the critical angle ϕ_c, and is refracted. Clearly, it can propagate freely in the *cladding slabs* and is said to be a *radiation mode*.

5.5 MODES IN CYLINDRICAL OPTICAL FIBERS

We may note that a longitudinal section of an optical fiber along the axis of symmetry closely resembles a planar waveguide except for the circular symmetry of the former. Further planar waveguides are also used in integrated optics as well as in optoelectronic integration for guiding light from one cycle to the other. However, in guided optical communication the channel is invariably the *cylindrical wageguide structures* based on dielectric materials called as *optical fiber*. Analysis of formation of different kinds of modes is of utmost importance to study various mechanisms of power flow, attenuation and dispersion in optical fibers, just like planar waveguides transverse electric (TE), transverse magnetic (TM) modes are created in optical fibers. In addition, hybrid modes (EH or HE) having both E_z, $H_z \neq 0$ are also created in an optical fiber. We may note that hybrid modes are a speciality of an optical fiber which is not generally found when electromagnetic wave propagates through hollow metallic waveguide. An *optical fiber* consists of a solid cylindrical core surrounded by solid coaxial cylindrical cladding and is axially symmetric. The refractive index of the core (n_1) is slightly higher than that of the cladding n_2 ($< n_1$).

5.5.1 Bound or Guided Modes

When light propagates through an optical fiber along the axis (say as z-axis), the plane-polarized electromagnetic waves get total internally reflected from the core–cladding boundary. The superposition of these plane polarized waves creates standing wave patterns in the transverse direction which remain stationary while the wave advances in the z-direction. Basically these modes are solution of Maxwell's equations under given boundary conditions. The actual number of modes created in a waveguide depends on the parameters of the waveguide and also on the wavelength of the monochromatic EM wave propating through the optical fiber. The modes, like in a planar waveguide are largely confined to the core and partly extending in the cladding. However, these modes vary harmonically in the core region and decay exponentially in the cladding region.

These modes are called as *core modes* or *bounded modes*. It is reported that lower order modes are tightly concentrated near the axis of the core while the higher order modes are tightly bounded to the axis of the core and tend to spread towards the boundary of the inner core and penetrate deeply in the cladding region.

5.5.2 Cladding Modes

When light propagates in an optical fiber it is almost inevitable that a fraction of light also enters the cladding. This is due to the fact that some light enters beyond the fiber-acceptance angle which is finally refracted out in the cladding region. Further, there exists several microbends in the fiber and other imperferction in the core-cladding interface which may cause the light to leave the core and enter the cladding. The cladding supports the formation of modes by the light entering into the cladding region being a dielectric medium. These modes which are not bound in the core region but are still solutions of the boundary-value problem are usually referred as *cladding* or *radiation* modes. As the core and cladding modes propagate through the optical fiber, the coupling of modes occur between higher order core modes and cladding modes. This is mainly because higher order core modes are less bound to the core and extend more in the cladding region. Usually, the mode coupling causes transfer of power between core and the cladding modes. The net result is a loss of power from the core mode to the cladding modes. However, in the process, higher order core modes gets eliminated and this leads to a reduction of overall *intermodal dispersion* which is a desirable effect. Further, in normal fibers the cladding is surrounded by a glossy coating of a higher refractive index. This minimises the reflection between the cladding and the coating and also minimises the guidance at the cladding-coating surface. As a result, these modes cannot propagate over a long distance, however, a few modes may manage to propagate over considerable distance. We may note that the cladding modes are also responsible for significant dispersion and hence, it is desirable to get rid of undesirable cladding modes.

5.5.3 Leaky Modes

When light enters from a source into the core of a multimode fiber there may be a few modes which generally do not strictly satisfy the conditions for being guided inside the core. Further, these modes continuously leak power from the core by quantum mechanical tunnelling process. The modes are called *leaky modes* and these modes occur when the upper and lower bounds on propagation constant β are not satisfied. However, for a mode to remain guided it is necessary that the propagation constant β satisfies the following condition

$$(n_2 k =) k_2 < \beta < k_1 (= n_1, k)$$

where n_1 and n_2 are the refractive indices of the core and the cladding and $k (= 2\pi/\lambda)$ is the free space propagation constant. This condition is called as the *cut-off condition* of the guided mode. For a particular mode, when β falls below $n_2 k$, the mode gets eliminated by leaking its power to the cladding. We may note that these leaky modes nevertheless travel there for considerable distance and also may carry significant amount of power in short length optical fibers.

5.5.4 Formulation of Waveguide Equations

Figure 5.2(d) shows the propagation of light along the axis of the optical fiber considered as z-direction. As the optical fiber is a cylindrical structure, it is most convenient to consider cylindrical coordinate system (r, ϕ, z), where z-axis is chosen along the axis of the optical fiber which is also the direction of propagation of light. In the cylindrical coordinate system the electric and magnetic field vectors of an electromagnetic wave propagating along z-direction can be expressed as

$$E\,(r, \phi, z, t) = E_0\,(r, \phi)\,\exp\,[j(\omega t - \beta z)] \tag{i}$$

$$H\,(r, \phi, z, t) = H_0\,(r, \phi)\,\exp\,[j(\omega t - \beta z)] \tag{ii}$$

where, $\qquad \boldsymbol{E} = \hat{r}E_r + \hat{\phi}E_\phi + \hat{z}E_z \tag{iii}$

$$\boldsymbol{H} = \hat{r}H_r + \hat{\phi}H_\phi + \hat{z}H_z \tag{iv}$$

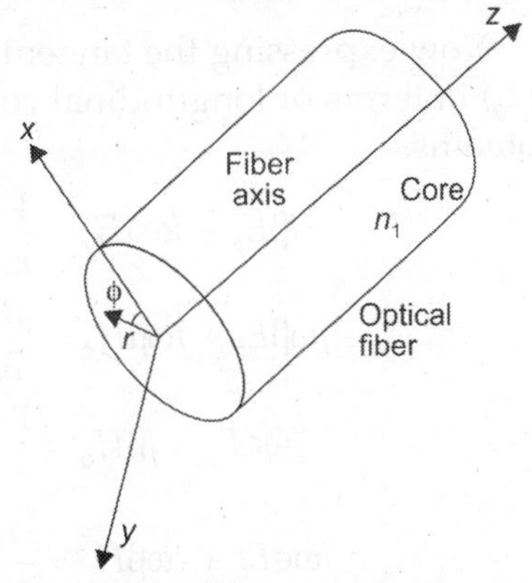

Here, $\hat{r}, \hat{\phi}, \hat{z}$ are respectively unit vectors in the radial, azimuthal, and longitudinal directions. Writing the Maxwell's curl equation: $\nabla \times \boldsymbol{E} = - \mu \dfrac{\partial \boldsymbol{H}}{\partial t}$ in cylindrical coordinates, one obtains

Fig. 5.2: (d) Optical fiber exhibits the chosen cylindrical coordinates for mode analysis. The axis of the fiber considered as z-direction

$$\begin{vmatrix} \dfrac{1}{r}\hat{r} & \hat{\phi} & \dfrac{1}{r}\hat{z} \\[2mm] \dfrac{\partial}{\partial r} & \dfrac{\partial}{\partial \phi} & \dfrac{\partial}{\partial z} \\[2mm] E_r & rE_\phi & E_z \end{vmatrix} = -j\omega\mu\,[\hat{r}H_r + \hat{\phi}H_\phi + \hat{z}H_z]$$

i.e. $\quad \dfrac{1}{r}\hat{r}\left[\dfrac{\partial E_z}{\partial \phi} + j\beta rE_\phi\right] + \hat{\phi}\left[-j\omega\beta E_r - \dfrac{\partial E_z}{\partial r}\right] + \dfrac{1}{r}\hat{z}\left[\dfrac{\partial(rE_\phi)}{\partial r} - \dfrac{\partial E_r}{\partial \phi}\right] = j\omega\mu\,[\hat{r}H_r + \hat{\phi}H_\phi + \hat{z}H_z]$

$$\tag{v}$$

Equating the components on both sides of Eq. (v), one obtains,

$$\frac{1}{r}\left[\frac{\partial E_z}{\partial \phi} + j\beta rE_\phi\right] = -j\omega\mu H_r \tag{vi}$$

$$j\omega\beta E_r + \frac{\partial E_r}{\partial r} = j\omega\mu H_\phi \tag{vii}$$

$$\frac{1}{r}\left[\frac{\partial(rE_\phi)}{\partial r} - \frac{\partial E_r}{\partial \phi}\right] = -j\omega\mu H_z \tag{viii}$$

Similarly, writing the other curl equation: $\nabla \times \boldsymbol{H} = \epsilon \dfrac{\partial \boldsymbol{E}}{\partial t}$ in cylindrical coordinates and equating the components of the radial, azimuthal, and longitudinal directions, one obtains

$$\frac{1}{r}\left[\frac{\partial H_z}{\partial \phi} + j\beta rH_\phi\right] = j\omega\epsilon E_r \tag{ix}$$

$$j\omega\beta H_r + \frac{\partial H_r}{\partial r} = -j\omega\epsilon E_\phi \tag{x}$$

$$\frac{1}{r}\left[\frac{\partial(rH_\phi)}{\partial r} - \frac{\partial H_r}{\partial \phi}\right] = j\omega\epsilon E_z \tag{xi}$$

Now expressing the tangential components of electric and magnetic fields (E_r, E_ϕ, H_r, H_ϕ) in terms of longitudinal components of electric and the magnetic field (E_z, H_z), one obtains.

$$j\beta E_\phi - j\omega\mu H_r = \frac{1}{r}\frac{\partial E_z}{\partial \phi} \tag{xii}$$

$$-j\omega\beta E_r + j\omega\mu H_\phi = \frac{\partial E_z}{\partial r} \tag{xiii}$$

$$j\omega\in E_r - j\beta H_\phi = \frac{1}{r}\frac{\partial H_z}{\partial \phi} \tag{xiv}$$

$$j\omega\in E_\phi + j\omega\beta H_r = -\frac{\partial H_z}{\partial r} \tag{xv}$$

We can obtain the radial and the azimuthal field components of the electric and magnetic fields in terms of the longitudinal components (E_z and H_z) by making use of above four equations. For example, the radial components of the electric field can be obtained by eliminating H_ϕ from Eqs (xiii) and (xiv). One can achieve this by multiplying Eq. (xiii) by β and Eq. (xiv) by $\omega\mu$ and adding the resultant equations. After algebraic manipulation, one obtains

$$E_r = -\frac{j}{\omega^2\mu\in - \beta^2}\left[\beta\frac{\partial E_z}{\partial r} + \frac{\omega\mu}{r}\frac{\partial H_z}{\partial \phi}\right] \tag{xvi}$$

Similarly, eliminating H_r from Eqs (xii) and (xv), one obtains the azimuthal component of the electric field as:

$$E_\phi = -\frac{j}{\omega^2\mu\in - \beta^2}\left[\frac{\beta}{r}\frac{\partial E_z}{\partial \phi} - \omega\mu\frac{\partial H_z}{\partial \phi}\right] \tag{xvii}$$

Now, eliminating E_ϕ from Eqs (xii) and (xv) and E_r from Eqs (xiii) and (xiv) one may express the radial and azimuthal components of the magnetic field (H_r and H_ϕ) as:

$$H_r = -\frac{j}{\omega^2\mu\in - \beta^2}\left[\beta\frac{\partial H_z}{\partial r} - \frac{\omega\in}{r}\frac{\partial E_z}{\partial \phi}\right] \tag{xviii}$$

$$H_\phi = -\frac{j}{\omega^2\mu\in - \beta^2}\left[\frac{\beta}{r}\frac{\partial H_z}{\partial \phi} + \omega\in\frac{\partial E_z}{\partial \phi}\right] \tag{xix}$$

Substituting H_r and H_ϕ from Eqs (xviii) and (xix) into Eq. (xi), one obtains,

$$\frac{\partial}{\partial r}\left[\beta\frac{\partial H_z}{\partial \phi} + \omega\in r\frac{\partial E_z}{\partial r}\right] - \frac{\partial}{\partial \phi}\left[\beta\frac{\partial H_z}{\partial r} - \frac{\omega\in}{r}\frac{\partial E_z}{\partial \phi}\right] = j\omega\in rE_z \tag{xx}$$

That is,

$$\omega\in r\frac{\partial^2 E_z}{\partial r^2} + \omega\in\frac{\partial E_z}{\partial r} + \frac{\omega\in}{r}\frac{\partial^2 E_z}{\partial \phi^2} + (\omega^2\mu\in - \beta^2)\omega\in rE_z = 0$$

The above equation can be rearranged as follows:

$$\frac{\partial^2 E_z}{\partial r^2} + \frac{1}{r}\frac{\partial E_z}{\partial r} + \frac{1}{r^2}\frac{\partial^2 E_z}{\partial \phi^2} + (\omega^2\mu\in - \beta^2)E_z = 0 \tag{xxii}$$

Similarly, substituting the values of E_r and E_ϕ from Eqs (xvi) and (xvii) into Eq. (viii), one obtains,

$$\frac{\partial^2 H_z}{\partial r^2} + \frac{1}{r}\frac{\partial H_z}{\partial r} + \frac{1}{r^2}\frac{\partial^2 H_z}{\partial \phi^2} + (\omega^2\mu\in - \beta^2)H_z = 0 \tag{xxiii}$$

From Eqs (xxii) and (xxiii), we can see that it is possible to obtain independent differential equations in terms of either E_z or H_z. This apparently suggests that E_z and H_z are uncoupled and each equation can be solved independently. However, coupling between E_z and H_z may occur as per requirement of the boundary conditions. In case the boundary conditions do not call for such coupling, Eq. (xxii) can be solved by assuming $H_z = 0$. The corresponding modes resulting from the solution of the Eq. (xxii) are called *transverse magnetic (TM) modes*. Likewise, when $E_z = 0$, Eq. (xxiii) can be solved to obtain *transverse electric modes*. However, when both E_z and H_z are non-zero, one obtains hybrid modes designated as EH or HE modes depending on whether E_z or H_z contribute respectively more towards the transverse field. Hybrid mode is a speciality of optical fibers and these modes are not found in *hollow metallic waveguides*. Clearly, analysis of propagation of light through an optical fiber is thus much more complex.

5.6 THE MODES OF A SYMMETRIC STEP INDEX FIBER

For the symmetric waveguide structure (Fig. 5.1), we have $n^2(-x) = n^2(x)$. Moreover, the structure is step index type, as the refractive index of guide layer is n_1 and the refractive index of the cladding slabs is n_2. Further, both n_1 and n_2 are constants and $n_1 > n_2$. We first take up the discussion of TE modes.

Substituting the values of H_x and H_z from Eqs (5.35) and (5.36) into Eq. (5.37), one obtains:

$$-i\beta\left(\frac{\beta}{\mu_0\omega}\right)E_y - \frac{\partial}{\partial x}\left(\frac{1}{-i\mu_0\omega}\right)\frac{\partial E_y}{\partial x} = i\varepsilon_0\omega n^2(x)E_y$$

As $E_y = E_y(x)$, the partial derivative involving E_y may as well be written as a full derivative. Thus, rearranging the above equation, one may write:

$$\frac{d^2E_y}{dx^2} - \beta^2 E_y + \mu_0\varepsilon_0\omega^2 n^2(x)E_y = 0$$

or
$$\frac{d^2E_y}{dx^2} + [k^2 n^2(x) - \beta^2]E_y = 0 \qquad (5.46a)$$

as $\qquad \mu_0\omega_0 = 1/c^2$ and $\omega/c = k$

In the waveguide of Fig. 5.1, we have:

$$n(x) = \begin{cases} n_1 \text{ for } |x| < a \\ n_2 \text{ for } |x| < a \end{cases} \qquad (5.47)$$

Moreover, E_y and H_z (and hence $\partial E_y/\partial x$) are continuous at $x = \pm a$ because E_y and H_z are tangenital components to the planes represented by $x = \pm a$, and H_z is proportional to $\partial E_y/\partial x$.

Substituting for $n(x)$ from Eq. (5.47) in Eq. (5.46), one obtains in the guide layer:

$$\frac{d^2E_y}{dx^2} + [k^2 n_1^2 - \beta^2]E_y = 0 (|x| < a) \qquad (5.48)$$

and in the cladding layer:

$$\frac{d^2E_y}{dx^2} + [k^2 n_2^2 - \beta^2]E_y = 0 (|x| < a) \qquad (5.49)$$

Les us put $\qquad\qquad u^2 = k^2 n_1^2 - \beta^2 = \beta_1^2 - \beta^2 \qquad (5.50)$

and $\qquad\qquad\qquad w^2 = \beta^2 - k^2 n_2^2 = \beta^2 - \beta_2^2 \qquad (5.51)$

Eqs (5.48) and (5.49) take the forms:

$$\frac{d^2 E_y}{dx^2} + u^2 E_y = 0 (|x| < a) \tag{5.52}$$

and

$$\frac{d^2 E_y}{dx^2} - w^2 E_y = 0 (|x| > a) \tag{5.53}$$

For the wave to be guided through the layer, both parameters u and w have to be real. Thus

$$\beta_1^2 (= k^2 n_1^2) > \beta^2 > \beta_2^2 (= k^2 n_2^2) \tag{5.54}$$

With these conditions, the solutions in the guide layer are oscillatory, while those in the cladding layers decay exponentially. This is what we exactly expected. Thus, for a guided-wave solution, the propagation constant β must lie between β_1 and β_2. The same inference is also obtained from ray analysis.

Since the refractive index $n(x)$ is symmetrically distributed about $x = 0$, the solutions are either symmetric or antisymmetric functions of x. Therefore, one must have:

$$E_y(-x) = E_y(x) \text{ symmetric modes} \tag{5.55}$$
$$E_y(-x) = E_y(x) \text{ antisymmetric modes} \tag{5.56}$$

For symmetric modes, the electric field distribution takes the form:

$$E_y(x) = \begin{cases} A \cos ux, |x| < a \\ C \exp(-w|x|), |x| > a \end{cases} \tag{5.57, 5.58}$$

where A and C are constants. The continuity of $E_y(x)$ and dE_y/dx at $x = \pm a$ gives the following equations

$$A \cos (ua) = Ce^{-wa} \tag{5.59}$$

and

$$-uA \sin(ua) = -wCe^{-wa} \tag{5.60}$$

Dividing Eq. (5.60) by Eq. (5.59), one obtains:

$$u \tan(ua) = w$$

or

$$ua \tan(ua) = wa \tag{5.61}$$

Let us now, define a new dimensionless wavelguide parameter called the *normalized frequency parameter V*. From Eqs (5.48) and (5.49), one finds:

$$u^2 + w^2 = k^2 n_1^2 - \beta^2 + \beta^2 - k^2 n_2^2 = k^2 (n_1^2 - n_2^2)$$

or

$$(ua)^2 + (wa)^2 = u^2 + w^2 = k^2 a^2 (n_1^2 - n_2^2) = \left(\frac{2\pi}{\lambda}\right)^2 a^2 (n_1^2 - n_2^2)$$

Thus, V can be defined as:

$$V = \{(ua)^2 + (wa^2)\}^{1/2} = \frac{2\pi a}{\lambda} (NA) = \frac{2\pi}{\lambda} (n_1^2 - n_2^2)^{1/2} \approx \frac{2\pi}{\lambda} n_1 \sqrt{2\Delta} \tag{5.62}$$

V-parameter is an important parameter that determines the number of modes that is supported by a particular type of fiber. From the foregoing discussion, we see that for a mode to be unbounded to the core, the parameter $U (= ua)$ must be less than the value of V.

In terms of V, Eq. (5.61) taken the form:

$$ua \tan(ua) = \{V^2 - (ua)^2\}^{1/2} \tag{5.63}$$

For antisymmetric modes, the solution take the form:

$$E_y(x) = \begin{cases} B \sin ux, |x| < a \\ \dfrac{x}{|x|} D \exp(-w|x|), |x| > a \end{cases}$$ (5.64, 5.65)

where B and D are constants. Following exactly the above procedure, one obtains:

$$-ua \cot(ua) = wa$$ (5.66)

or, in terms of the parameter V, one obtains:

$$-ua \cot(ua) = \{V^2 - (ua)^2\}^{1/2}$$ (5.67)

Equations (5.61) to (5.66) are transcendental equations and one can find their solution by plotting ua as a function of wa for $ua \tan(ua) = wa$ and $-ua \cot(ua) = wa$. Equation (5.62) is plotted as arcs of circles for constant V-values. Figure 5.3 shows the graphical solution of Eqs (5.61) and (5.62) for obtaining the propagation parameters ua and wa of TE modes for constant values of V in a planar waveguide.

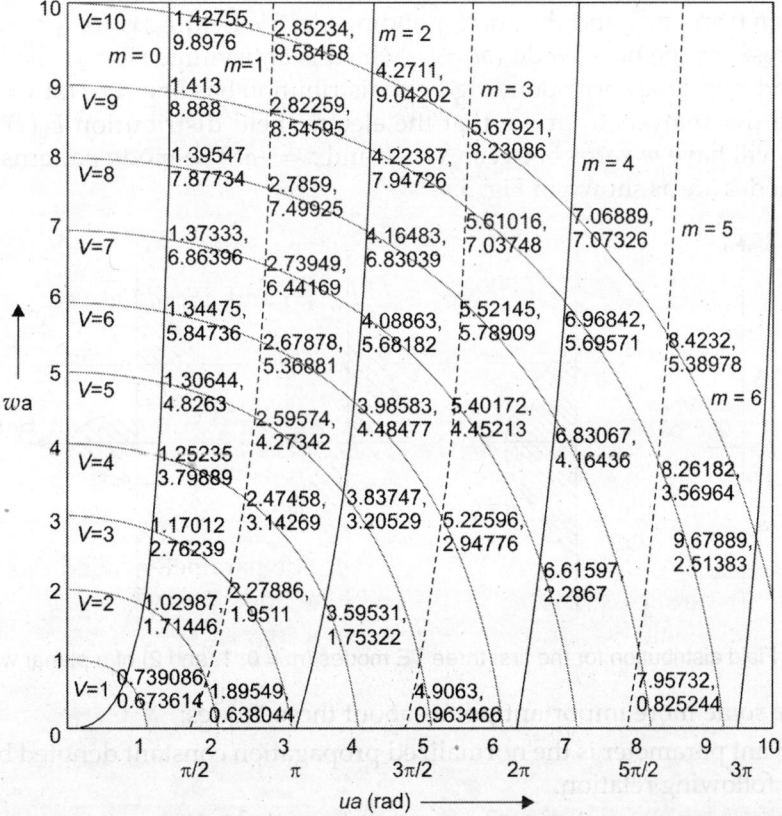

Fig. 5.3: Graphical solution of Eqs (3.61) and (3.66) for obtaining the propagation parameters ua and wa (dashed lines). $V^2 = [(ua)^2 + (wa)^2]$ = const. is plotted as arcs of circles for constant V-values (light face solid lines)

One can derive following information from Fig. 5.3:

(i) For $0 \le V \le \pi/2$ (i.e. for an arc of a circle of radius corresponding to $V < \pi/2$), there is only one intersection with the bold solid curve marked $m = 0$. This is the only solution for the guided TE mode, i.e. the waveguide supports only one discrete TE mode and this mode is symmetric in x.

(ii) For $\pi/2 \le V \le \pi$ (i.e., for an arc of circle of radius corresponding to $\pi/2 < V < \pi$), the arc intersects at two points; one on the bold solid line $m = 0$ and the other on the dashed line $m = 1$. This means that, therefore, two TE modes, one symmetric and the other antisymmetric. In general, if:

$$(2m)\frac{\pi}{2} \le V \le (2m+1)\frac{\pi}{2} \tag{5.68}$$

we will have $m + 1$ symmetric and m antisymmetric modes, and if:

$$(2m+1)\frac{\pi}{2} \le V \le (2m+2)\frac{\pi}{2} \tag{5.69}$$

we will have $m + 1$ symmetric and $m + 1$ antisymmetric modes, where $m = 0, 1, 2, ...,$ $m = 0, 2, 4, ...$ correspond to symmetric modes and $m = 1, 3, 5, ...$ correspond to antisymmetric modes. The maximum number of TE modes, M, supported by the guide would be an integer close to or greater than $2V/\pi$. This is found to be in agreement with Eq. (5.46), which was obtained on the basis of the ray model.

(iii) We may note in Fig. 5.3 that for the fundamental mode ($m = 0$), ua always lies between 0 and $\pi/2$ and the corresponding electric field $E_y(x)$ for $|x| < a$ will have no zeros. For the next mode ($m = 1$), which is antisymmetric in x, ua lies between $\pi/2$ and π and the corresponding field distribution has one zero (at $x = 0$). One can extend the analysis to prove that the electric-field distribution $E_y(x)$ for the mth mode will have m zeros between $x = -a$ and $x = +a$. The mode patterns for the first few modes are as shown in Fig. 5.4.

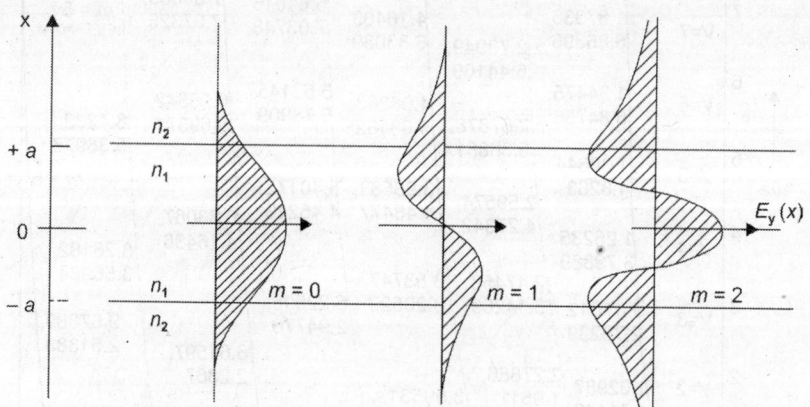

Fig. 5.4: Field distribution for the first three TE modes ($m = 0$, 1, and 2) of a planar waveguide

There are some more important points about these modes:

(i) A relevant parameter is the normalized propagation constant denoted by b, defined by the following relation:

$$b = \frac{\beta^2 - \beta_2^2}{\beta_1^2 - \beta_2^2} = 1 - \left(\frac{ua}{V}\right)^2 = \left(\frac{wa}{V}\right)^2 \tag{5.70}$$

For a given guided mode, the value of b lies between 0 and 1. The variation of b with V for first few modes is shown in Fig. 5.5. When β becomes equal to β_2, $b = 0$ and the mode is said to have reached the 'cut-off'. Clearly, at cut-off, $ua = V = V_c$ and $wa = 0$. This occurs at:

$$wa = V_c = \frac{m\pi}{2} \tag{5.71}$$

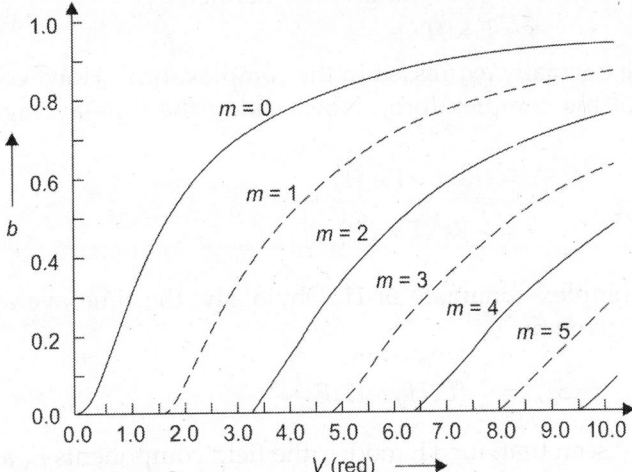

Fig. 5.5: Variation of the normalized propagation parameter b for TE modes with the V parameter for a planar waveguide

As
$$V = \frac{2\pi a}{\lambda} (n_1^2 - n_2^2)^{1/2} \qquad \text{(from Eq. 3.62)}$$

equating Eqs (5.62) and (5.71), one can obtain the thicknss of the guide layer necessary to support m modes:

$$\frac{m\pi}{2} = \frac{2\pi a}{\lambda} (n_1^2 - n_2^2)^{1/2}$$

or
$$2a = \frac{m\lambda}{2 (n_1^2 - n_2^2)^{1/2}} \qquad (5.72)$$

where $m = 0, 1, 2, ...$ We may note that fundamental mode has no cut-off frequency.

(ii) The modes for which $\beta^2 < \beta_2^2$ are called *radiation modes*. These modes are continuous. In terms of the ray model, these modes correspond to the rays for which total internal reflection does not occur, and get refracted into the cladding.

(iii) All the modes are orthogonal. If the field $E_y(x)$ corresponding to a guided mode with a propagation constant β_m is represened by $\omega_{m(x)}$ and its complex conjugate by $\omega_m(x)$, then one can show that:

$$\int_{-\infty}^{\infty} \psi_m^*(x) \, \psi_m(x) \, dx = 0 \text{ for } m \neq n$$

This is the condition of *orthogonality*.

After determining the electric-field distribution $E_y(x)$, it is possible to calculate the H_x and H_z components of the magnetic field by substituting the value of E_y in Eq. (5.35) and $\partial E_y/\partial x$ in Eq. (5.36). A similar analysis may be performed for the TM modes of a planar waveguide.

5.7 POWER DISTRIBUTION AND CONFINEMENT FACTOR

We have seen (Fig. 5.4) that the electric-field distribution of the guided modes extends beyond the boundary of the guide layer, and the extent of penetration into the cladding layer depends on the thickness and the mode number. It is important for us to know, in many situations, the fraction of guided optical power confined with the guide layer. This fraction is called the *confinement factor*.

The power flow is given by Poynting vector defined by:

$$S = E \times H$$

where E and H are normally expressed in the complex form. However, the actual fields are the real part of the complex form. Now, taking the time average of the Poynting vector, one obtains:

$$\langle S \rangle = \langle \text{Re } E \times \text{Re } H \rangle$$
$$= \frac{1}{2} \text{Re } \langle E \times H^* \rangle$$

where H^* is the complex conjugate of H. Obviously, the time average of S along the z-direction will be given by:

$$\langle S_z \rangle = \frac{1}{2} \langle E_x H_y - H_x E_y \rangle \tag{5.73}$$

We have already seen that, for TE modes, the field components E_x and E_z vanish and:

$$H_x = \frac{\beta}{\mu_0 \omega} E_y$$

Therefore

$$\langle S_z \rangle = \frac{1}{2} \frac{\beta}{\omega \mu_0} | E_y^2 | \tag{5.74}$$

For a particular mode, the power associated per unit area per unit length in the y-direction is given by:

$$P = \frac{1}{2} \frac{\beta}{\omega \mu_0} \int_{x = -\infty}^{\infty} | E_y^2 | \, dx \tag{5.75}$$

The power inside the guide layer is obtained as:

$$P_{in} = \frac{1}{2} \frac{\beta}{\omega \mu_0} \int_{-a}^{a} E_y^2 \, dx \tag{5.76}$$

and the power outside the guide layer is obtained as:

$$P_{out} = \frac{1}{2} \frac{\beta}{\omega \mu_0} \left[\int_{-\infty}^{a} E_y^2 \, dx + \int_{a}^{\infty} E_y^2 dx \right] \tag{5.77}$$

For symmetric TE modes, substituting for E_y and Eq. (5.57), one obtains:

$$P_{in} = \frac{1}{2} \frac{\beta}{\omega \mu_0} 2 \int_0^a (A \cos ux)^2 \, dx = \frac{\beta}{\omega \mu_0} A^2 \int_0^a \frac{1}{2} (1 + \cos 2ux) \, dx$$

$$P_{in} = \frac{\beta}{2 \omega \mu_0} A^2 \left[x + \frac{1}{2u} \sin 2ux \right]_0^a = \frac{\beta}{2 \omega \mu_0} A^2 \left[a + \frac{1}{2u} \sin 2ua \right] \tag{5.78}$$

Substituting the value of E_y from Eq. (5.58), one obtains:

$$P_{out} = \frac{1}{2} \frac{\beta}{\omega \mu_0} 2 \int_a^{\infty} (C e^{-wx})^2 \, dx = \frac{\beta}{\omega \mu_0} C^2 \left[-\frac{1}{2w} e^{-2wx} \right]_a^{\infty}$$

or

$$P_{out} = \frac{\beta}{\omega \mu_0} C^2 \left[\frac{1}{2w} e^{-2wx} \right] \tag{5.79}$$

From Eqs (5.78) and (5.79), one can derive the final expression for P as:

$$P = P_{in} + P_{out}$$

$$= \frac{\beta}{2\omega\mu_0} A^2 \left[a + \frac{1}{2u} \sin 2ua \right] + \frac{\beta}{\omega\mu_0} C^2 \left[\frac{1}{2w} e^{-2wa} \right]$$

$$= \frac{\beta A^2}{2\omega\mu_0} \left[a + \frac{1}{2u} \sin 2wa + \left(\frac{C}{A} \right)^2 \frac{1}{w} e^{-2wa} \right]$$

Putting the value of $C/A = e^{wa} \cos ua$ from Eq. (5.59), one obtains:

$$P = \frac{\beta A^2}{2\omega\mu_0} \left[a + \frac{1}{2u} \sin 2ua + \frac{1}{w} \cos^2 ua \right]$$

$$= \frac{\beta A^2}{4\omega\mu_0} \left[2a + \frac{2}{w} + \frac{2\sin(ua)\cos(ua)}{u} - \frac{2\sin^2 ua}{w} \right]$$

$$= \frac{\beta A^2}{4\omega\mu_0} \left[\left(2a + \frac{2}{w} \right) + \frac{2\sin(ua)\cos(ua)}{uwa} - \{wa - ua \tan ua\} \right]$$

From Eq. (5.61), the term within the braces becomes zero. This yield the following expression for P:

$$P = \frac{\beta A^2}{4\omega\mu_0} \left(a + \frac{1}{w} \right) \tag{5.80}$$

A similar expression may also be derived for power carried by antisymmetric modes.

The fraction of power confined within the guide layer, called the *confinement factor G*, is given by:

$$G = \frac{P_{in}}{P_{in} + P_{out}} \tag{5.81}$$

$$= \frac{a + \frac{1}{2} \sin 2ua}{\left[a + \frac{1}{2u} \sin 2ua \right] + \left[\frac{1}{w} e^{-2wa} \right] \left(\frac{C}{A} \right)^2} \tag{5.82}$$

Putting the value of $C/A = e^{wa} \cos ua$, from Eq. (5.59), in Eq. (5.82), one obtains:

$$G = \frac{\left[a + \frac{1}{2u} \sin 2ua \right]}{\left[a + \frac{1}{2u} \sin 2ua \right] + \left[\frac{1}{w} e^{-2wa} (e^{wa} \cos ua)^2 \right]}$$

$$= \frac{\left[a + \frac{1}{2u} \sin 2ua + \frac{1}{w} \cos^2 ua \right]}{\left[a + \frac{1}{2u} \sin 2ua \right]}$$

$$= \left[1 + \frac{\cos^2 ua}{wa \{1 + [\sin(ua)\cos(ua)/ua]} \right]^{-1} \tag{5.83}$$

A similar expression may also be derived for antisymmetric modes. Some salient features of Eq. (5.83) are as follows:

(i) As $a \to 0$, $G \to 0$; that is, for a very thin guide layer, there is no guidance of light, i.e., almost all the power is lost in the cladding.

(ii) As the G-factor depends on u and w and both these parameters in turn depend on m, G will vary with the mode number.

(iii) One can show that G increases, first rapidly and then slowly, with increase in the thickness of the guide layer for each mode.

5.8 CYLINDRICAL WAVEGUIDES

5.8.1 Modal Analysis of an Ideal Step-Index Optical Fiber

We now study the wave propagations in a cylindrical homogeneous core dielectric waveguide. This type of waveguide with a constant refractive index core is known as a *step index fiber*.

Let us consider a step-index fiber consisting of a uniform cylindrical dielectric core of radius a and refractive index n, surrounded by an infinitely thick uniform dielectric cladding of refractive index n_2. Let us find a solution of wave equation for electric and magnetic fields for the modes propagated by such a fiber.

Equations (5.24) and (5.27) shows that different components of E as well as H are coupled.

In the present case $n = \sqrt{\varepsilon_r}$ is constant $= n_1$ upto $r \leq a$ and equal to n_2 for points $r > a$ but there is a discontinuity at $r = a$. We assume that this discontinuity is small, i.e. $n_1 = n_2$. This is termed as a weakly guiding approximation. With this approximation, one may neglect the second term on the LHS of Eqs (5.24) and (5.27) and each Cartesian component of E and H satisfies the scalar wave equation; putting $\varepsilon_r = n^2$, we have

$$\nabla^2 \psi = \varepsilon_0 \mu_0 n^2 \frac{\partial^2 \psi}{dt^2} \tag{5.84}$$

where ψ represents scalar E and H field. We may note that the optical fiber boundary conditions have cylindrical symmetry and we assume that the direction of propagation of the electromagnetic waves is along the axis of the optic fiber, which is taken as z-axis. In the scalar wave approximation, the modes may be assumed to be nearly transverse and they may possess an arbitrary state of polarization. These linearly polarized modes are referred to as *LP modes*. The propagation constants of the TE and TM modes are nearly equal.

In cylindrical coordinates (r, ϕ, z), Eq. (5.84) may be expressed as

$$\nabla^2 \psi = \varepsilon_0 \mu_0 n^2 \frac{\partial^2 \psi}{\partial t^2} = \frac{\partial^2 \psi}{\partial r^2} + \frac{1}{r} \frac{\partial \psi}{\partial r} + \frac{1}{r^2} \frac{\partial^2 \psi}{\partial \phi^2} + \frac{\partial^2 \psi}{\partial z^2} - \varepsilon_0 \mu_0 n^2 \frac{\partial^2 \psi}{\partial t^2} = 0 \tag{5.85}$$

Since n may depend on the transverse coordinates (r, ϕ), though it usually depends only on r, and the wave is propagating along the z-direction, one may write the solution of Eq. (5.85) as

$$\psi(r, \phi, z, t) = \psi(r, \phi) \, e^{-i(\omega t \times \beta z)} \tag{5.86}$$

Substituting the value of ψ from Eq. (5.86) in Eq. (5.85), we obtains:

$$e^{i(\omega t - \beta z)} \frac{\partial^2 \psi}{\partial r^2} + \frac{1}{r} e^{i(\omega t - \beta z)} \frac{\partial \psi}{\partial r} + \frac{1}{r^2} e^{i(\omega t - \beta z)} \frac{\partial^2 \psi}{\partial \phi^2}$$

$$+ \psi(-\beta^2) e^{i(\omega t - \beta z)} - \varepsilon_0 \mu_0 n^2 (-\omega^2) \psi \, e^{i(\omega t - \beta z)} = 0$$

or

$$\frac{\partial^2 \psi}{\partial r^2} + \frac{1}{r} \frac{\partial \psi}{\partial r} + \frac{1}{r^2} \frac{\partial^2 \psi}{\partial \phi^2} + - [\varepsilon_0 \mu_0 \omega^2 n^2 - \beta^2] \psi = 0$$

Putting $\varepsilon_0\mu_0 = 1/c^2$ and $\omega/c = k$, the free-space wave number, in the above equation, one obtains:

$$\frac{\partial^2\psi}{\partial r^2} + \frac{1}{r}\frac{\partial\psi}{\partial r} + \frac{1}{r^2}\frac{\partial^2\psi}{\partial\phi^2} + [n^2k^2 - \beta^2]\,\psi = 0 \tag{5.87}$$

Since the fiber under consideration has cylindrical symmetry, the variables can be separated:

$$\psi(r, \phi) = R\,(r)\,\Phi(\phi) \tag{5.88}$$

where R is a function of only r and Φ is a function of only ϕ. Substituting ψ from Eq. (5.88) in Eq. (5.87), one obtains:

$$\Phi\frac{\partial^2 R}{\partial r^2} + \frac{1}{Rr}\,\Phi\frac{dR}{dr} + \frac{R}{r^2}\frac{\partial^2\Phi}{d\phi^2} + [n^2k^2 - \beta^2]\,R\Phi = 0$$

Since the derivatives involved are dependent either on r or ϕ only, the partial derivatives may be replaced by full derivatives. Further, on dividing the entire LHS by $R\Phi$, one obtains:

$$\frac{1}{R}\frac{d^2 R}{dr^2} + \frac{1}{Rr}\frac{dR}{dr} + \frac{1}{r^2}\frac{1}{\Phi}\frac{d^2\Phi}{d\phi^2} + [n^2k^2 - \beta^2] = 0$$

or

$$\frac{r^2}{R}\left(\frac{d^2 R}{dr^2} + \frac{1}{Rr}\frac{dR}{dr}\right) + r^2\,[n^2k^2 - \beta^2] = -\frac{1}{\Phi}\frac{d^2\Phi}{d\phi^2} = t^2 \quad \text{(say)} \tag{5.89}$$

where l is a constant, known as an *azimuthal eigenvalue*.

The dependence of Φ on ϕ will be of the form $e^{il\phi}$. For the function to be single-valued, i.e. $\Phi(\phi + 2\pi) = \Phi(\phi)$, the constant l is required to be an integer, i.e.:

$$l = 0, 1, 2, 3, \dots \tag{5.90}$$

Therefore the complete transverse field will be given by:

$$\psi(r, \phi, z, t) = R(r)\,e^{il\phi}\,e^{i(\omega t - \beta z)} \tag{5.91}$$

The radial part of Eq. (5.89) may be written as:

$$\frac{r^2}{R}\left(\frac{d^2 R}{dr^2} + \frac{1}{Rr}\frac{dR}{dr}\right) + r^2\,(n^2k^2 - \beta^2) = l^2$$

which after *rearrangement* gives:

$$r^2\frac{d^2 R}{dr^2} + r\frac{dR}{dr} + [r^2\,(n^2k^2 - \beta^2) = l^2]\,R = 0 \tag{5.92}$$

We know that $n = n_1$ for $r \leq a$ and $n = n_2$ for $r > a$. Thus, substituting the value of n in Eq. (5.92), we obtain for the case of a step-index fiber:

$$r^2\frac{d^2 R}{dr^2} + r\frac{dR}{dr} + [r^2\,(k^2 n_1^2 - \beta^2) - l^2]\,R = 0, r \leq a \tag{5.93}$$

and

$$r^2\frac{d^2 R}{dr^2} + r\frac{dR}{dr} + [r^2\,(k^2 n_2^2 - \beta^2) - l^2]\,R = 0, r > a \tag{5.94}$$

In order to simplify the above equations, one may put:

$$u^2 \equiv (k^2 n_1^2 - \beta^2)\,a^2 \tag{5.95}$$

and

$$w^2 \equiv (\beta^2 - k^2 n_1^2)\,a^2 \tag{5.96}$$

The normalized waveguide parameter V for the fiber can be defined by:

$$V = (u^2 + w^2)^{1/2} = ka(n_1^2 - n_2^2)^{1/2} = \frac{2\pi a}{\lambda}(n_1^2 - n_2^2)^{1/2} \tag{5.97}$$

Substituting the values of u and w in Eqs (5.93) and (5.94), one obtains:

$$r^2 \frac{d^2R}{dr^2} + r\frac{dR}{dr} + \left(\frac{u^2 r^2}{a^2} - l^2\right)R = 0, r \le a \tag{5.98}$$

and

$$r^2 \frac{d^2R}{dr^2} + r\frac{dR}{dr} + \left(\frac{w^2 r^2}{a^2} - l^2\right)R = 0, r > a \tag{5.99}$$

Equations (5.98) and (5.99) are second-order equations and hence should possess two independent solutions. The solutions corresponding to Eq. (5.98) are the *Bessel function of the first kind*. The solutions corresponding to Eq. (5.99) are the Bessel function of the second kind and the modified **Bessel function** of the *second kind*. The modified Bessel function of the first kind has a discontinuity at the origin and the Bessel function of the second kind has an asymptotic form. Hence these are discarded in the solutions for fiber modes. For the solutions to be well behaved, that is, be finite at $r = 0$ and tend to zero as $r \to \infty$, it is essential that both u and ω are real. Therefore, a valid solution of Eq. (5.98) would be given by the first kind of Bessel function of order l and that of Eq. (5.99) would be given by the second kind of modified Bessel function of order l. Thus, one finds:

$$R(r) = AJ_l\left(\frac{ur}{a}\right), r < a \tag{5.100}$$

$$R(r) = BK_l\left(\frac{wr}{a}\right), r > a \tag{5.101}$$

The Bessel function of the first kind of order l and argument x, denoted by $J_l(x)$, is defined in terms of an infinite series as follows:

$$J_l(x) = \sum_{n=0}^{\infty} \frac{(-1)^n}{n!\,\Gamma(n+l+1)}\left(\frac{x}{2}\right)^{2n+1} \tag{5.102}$$

where $x = ur/a$ and the gamma function $\Gamma(n+l+1) = (n+l)!$ (for $l = 0$)

$$J_0(x) = 1 - \frac{\left(\frac{1}{4}x^2\right)}{(1!)^2} + \frac{\left(\frac{1}{4}x^2\right)^2}{(2!)^2} + \frac{\left(\frac{1}{4}x^2\right)^3}{(3!)^2} + \dots$$

and for $l = 1$:
$$J_1(x) = \frac{1}{2}x - \frac{\left(\frac{1}{2}x\right)^3}{2!} - \frac{\left(\frac{1}{2}x\right)^5}{2!3!} - \dots$$

and so on the higher values of l.

The second kind of modified Bessel function of order l is given by:

$$K_l(\tilde{x}) = (\pi/2)\,i^{-(l+1)}\,H_l(-i\tilde{x}), \tilde{x} = \frac{wr}{a} \tag{5.103}$$

where $H_l(-i\tilde{x})$ is a Hankel function, which is a linear combination of Bessel functions of the first (J_l) and second (Y_l) kind. These functions have been chosen for $x << 1$:

$$J_1(x) = \frac{1}{l!}\left(\frac{x}{2}\right)^l, l = 0, 1, \dots \tag{5.104}$$

$$K_l(\tilde{x}) = (l-1)!\,2^{l-1}\,\tilde{x}^{-1}, l \geq 1 \tag{5.105}$$

and for $x \gg 1$:
$$J_l(\tilde{x}) = \sqrt{\frac{2}{\pi x}} \cos\left[x - \frac{\pi(2l+1)}{4}\right] \tag{5.106}$$

and
$$K_l(\tilde{x}) = \sqrt{\frac{2}{\pi x}} e^{-x}\left[1 + \frac{4l^2 - 1}{8\tilde{x}}\right] \tag{5.107}$$

Thus $J_l(x)$ is a well behaved function for $r < a$ and $K_l(\tilde{x})$ is well behaved for $r > a$.

For further analysis, some recurrence relations for these functions (with argument x) and some asymptotic forms are given as follows:

$$J_{-1} = (-1)^l J_1 \tag{5.108}$$

$$J_1' = \frac{1}{2}(J_{l-1} - J_{l+1}) = \pm J_{l\mp 1} \mp \frac{lJ_1}{x} \tag{5.109}$$

$$J_{l\mp 1} = \frac{2lJ_1}{x} - J_{l\mp 1} \tag{5.110}$$

$$J_{l\mp 2} = \frac{2(l\mp 1)J_{l\mp 1}}{x} - J_l \tag{5.111}$$

$$K_l = K_{-l} \tag{5.112}$$

$$K_l' = \frac{1}{2}(K_{l-1} - K_{l+1}) = \mp \frac{lK_l}{x} - K_{l\mp 1} \tag{5.113}$$

$$K_{l\mp 1} = \mp \frac{2lK_l}{x} + K_{l\pm 1} \tag{5.114}$$

$$K_{l\mp 2} = \mp \frac{2(l\mp 1)K_{l\mp 1}}{x} + K_l \tag{5.115}$$

Here, prime denotes the first derivative. For $\tilde{x} \ll 1$, we have:

$$\frac{K_0}{K_1} = \tilde{x}\ln\frac{2}{1.782\,\tilde{x}} \tag{5.116}$$

$$\frac{K_{l-1}}{K_l} = \frac{\tilde{x}}{2(l-1)}, l \geq 2 \tag{5.117}$$

$$\frac{K_{l+1}}{K_l} = \frac{2l}{\tilde{x}}, l \geq 1 \tag{5.118}$$

For $\tilde{x} \gg 1$, we have

$$\frac{K_{l\mp 1}}{K_l} = 1 + \frac{1 \mp 2l}{2\tilde{x}} \tag{5.119}$$

Since ψ is continuous at $r = a$, $R(r)$ must be continuous at $r = a$. Imposing this condition, one finds the values of constants A and B. Thus from Eqs (5.100) and (5.101), we have:

$$A = \frac{R(a)}{J_l(u)} \tag{5.120}$$

$$B = \frac{R(a)}{K_l(w)} \tag{5.121}$$

Substituting the values of R and Φ in Eq. (5.88), one obtains the transverse dependence of the modal fields as follows:

$$\psi(r, \phi) = A J_l \left(\frac{ur}{a} \right) \begin{bmatrix} \cos(l\phi); r < a \\ \sin(l\phi) \end{bmatrix} \tag{5.122}$$

and

$$\psi(r, \phi) = B K_l \left(\frac{wr}{a} \right) \begin{bmatrix} \cos(l\phi); r > a \\ \sin(l\phi) \end{bmatrix} \tag{5.123}$$

Now $\partial \psi / \partial r$ is also continuous at $r = a$:

$$\left. \frac{\partial \psi}{\partial r} \right|_{r=a} = A \frac{u}{a} J_l' \left(\frac{ur}{a} \right) \cos l\phi \Big|_{r=a} = A \frac{u}{a} J_l'(u) \cos l\phi$$

$$\left. \frac{\partial \psi}{\partial r} \right|_{r=a} = B \frac{w}{a} K_l' \left(\frac{wr}{a} \right) \cos l\phi \Big|_{r=a} = B \frac{w}{a} K_l'(w) \cos l\phi$$

Thus, substituting the values of A and B from Eqs (5.120) and (5.121), one obtains

$$\frac{R(a)}{J_l(u)} \frac{u}{a} J_l'(u) \cos l\phi = \frac{R(a)}{K_l(\omega)} \frac{w}{a} K_l'(w) \cos l\phi$$

or

$$\frac{u J_l'(u)}{J_l(u)} = \frac{w K_l'(w)}{K_l(w)}$$

Thus the continuity of ψ and $d\psi/dr$ at the core–cladding interface ($r = a$) leads to an eigenvalue equation of the form:

$$\frac{u J_l'(u)}{J_l(u)} = \frac{w K_l'(w)}{K_l(w)} \tag{5.124}$$

Substituting the the values of J_l' and K_l' from Eqs (5.109) and (5.110), respectively, in Eq. (5.124), one obtains:

$$\frac{u}{J_l(u)} \left[\pm J_{l \mp 1}(u) \mp \frac{l J_l(u)}{u} \right] = \frac{w}{K_l(w)} \left[\mp \frac{l K_l(w)}{w} - K_{l \mp 1}(w) \right]$$

or

$$\pm u \frac{J_{l \mp 1}(u)}{J_l(u)} \mp l = \mp l - \frac{w K_{l \mp 1}(w)}{K_l(w)}$$

One can write this equation in either of the following two forms:

$$\frac{u J_{l+1}(u)}{J_l(u)} = \frac{w K_{l+1}(w)}{K_l(w)} \tag{5.125}$$

or

$$\frac{u J_{l+1}(u)}{J_l(u)} = -w \frac{K_{l+1}(w)}{K_l(w)} \tag{5.126}$$

One can obtain, from Eqs (5.125) and (5.126), the values of u and w for various values of l and the corresponding values of the propagation constant β. For β-values lying within the range:

$$\beta_2^2 \ (= n_2^2 k^2) < \beta^2 < \beta_1^2 \ (= n_1^2 k^2) \tag{5.127}$$

the radial part of the field, $R(r)$, in the core is given by the Bessel function $J_l(x)$, $x = ur/a$, which is oscillatory in nature. Hence, there exist m allowed solutions for β for each value of l. Therefore, each allowed value of β is characterized by two integers l and m. The first integer l is associated with two circular functions $\cos l\phi$ and $\sin l\phi$ corresponding to the azimuthal part of the solution, and the second integer m is associated with the mth root of the eigenvalue equation corresponding to the radial part of the solution. These are known as guided modes.

From Eq. (5.97), we have $V^2 = u^2 + w^2$. Thus the solution of the transcendental equations (for given values of l and V) will give universal curves describing the dependence of u or w on V. The value of β can be calculated by substituting the values of u (or w) in the defining equations. Alternatively, one can define the normalized propagation constant b as follows:

$$b = \frac{\beta^2 - \beta_2^2}{\beta_1^2 - \beta_2^2} = \frac{\beta^2 - n_2^2 k^2}{n_1^2 k^2 - n_2^2 k^2} = \frac{w^2}{V^2} = 1 - \frac{u^2}{V^2} \tag{5.128}$$

Since β lies between $\beta_1 (= n_1 k)$ and $\beta_2 (= n_2 k)$ for the guided nodes, the value of b will lie between 0 (for $\beta = \beta_2$) and 1 (for $\beta = \beta_1$). The plots of b as a function of V, shown in Fig. 5.6, form universal curves.

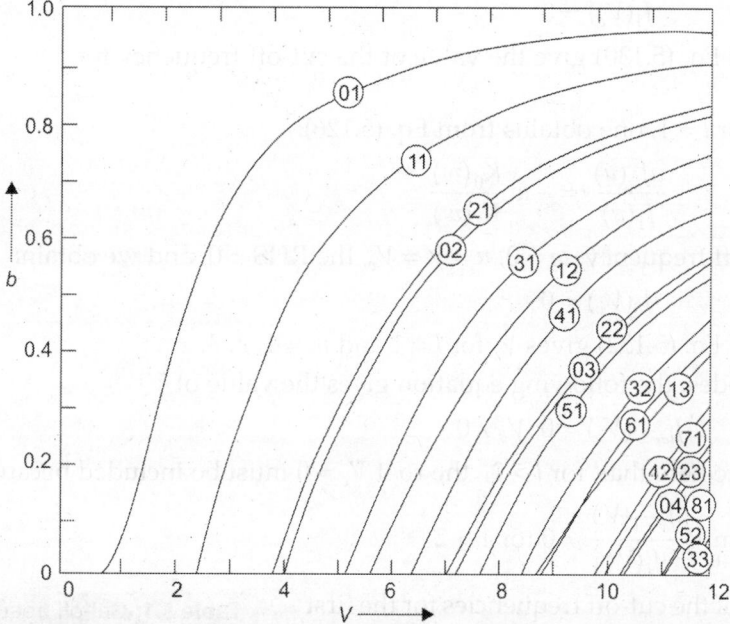

Fig. 5.6: Plots of the normalized propagation constant b as a function of the normalized frequency parameter V for a silicon (Si) fiber

A mode ceases to be guided when $\beta^2 < \beta_2^2$. Such modes are called *radiation modes*. In terms of the ray model, these modes correspond to rays that undergo refraction, rather than total internal reflection, at the core–cladding interface. When such modes are excited, they quickly leak away from the core. The condition $\beta = \beta_2$ corresponds to what is known as the *cut-off of a mode*. Thus, at $\beta = \beta_2$; $b = 0$, $w = 0$, and $u = V = V_c$, where V_c is the cut-off frequency. We may note that:

$$\lim_{w \to 0} w \frac{K_{l-1}(w)}{K_l(w)} \to 0, l = 0, 1, 2, 3, \ldots$$

Therefore, the RHS of Eq. (5.125) vanishes as $w \to 0$. Thus, Eq. (5.125) may be used for finding the cut-off frequencies of different modes.

For $l = 0$, one obtains from Eq. (5.125)

$$u \frac{J_{-1}(u)}{J_0(u)} = - w \frac{K_{-1}(w)}{K_0(w)}$$

Using Eqs (5.108) and (5.112), one obtains:

$$J_{-1}(u) = -J_1(u) \text{ and } K_{-1}(w) = -K_1(w)$$

Substituting the value of $J_{-1}(w)$ and $K_{-1}(w)$ in the above equation, one obtains:

$$\frac{uJ_1(u)}{J_0(u)} = w \frac{K_1(w)}{K_0(w)} \tag{5.129}$$

All the cuf-off frequency, $w = 0$, $u = V = V_c$, the RHS = 0, and Eq. (5.129) is transformed into:

$$\frac{V_c J_1(V_c)}{J_0(V_c)} = 0$$

or

$$J_1(V_c) = 0 \tag{5.130}$$

The roots of Eq. (5.130) give the value of the cut-off frequency for $l = 0$ and $m = 1, 2, 3, ...$

Similarly, for $l = 1$, one obtains from Eq. (5.126):

$$\frac{uJ_0(u)}{J_1(u)} = - w \frac{K_0(w)}{K_1(w)} \tag{5.131}$$

At the cut-off frequency, $w = 0$, $u = V = V_c$, the RHS = 0, and we obtain:

$$J_0(V_c) = 0 \tag{5.132}$$

The roots of Eq. (5.132) gives V_c for $l = 1$ and $m = 1, 2, 3, ...$

For $l \geq 2$ modes, the following equation gives the value of V_c.

$$J_{l-1}(V_c) = 0, V_c \neq 0$$

We may note here that, for $l > 2$, the root $V_c = 0$ must be included because:

$$\lim_{V \to 0} V \frac{J_{l-1}(V)}{J_l(V)} \neq 0 \text{ for } 1 \geq 2$$

The values of the cut-off frequencies for the first few LP modes are given in Table 5.1. Figure 5.7 shows the oscillatory nature of Bessel functions J_0 and J_1 and their roots.

Prior to proceeding further, we must remember few important points about the modes:

(i) The $l = 0$ modes have twofold degeneracy corresponding to two orthogonal linearly polarized states.

(ii) The $l \geq 1$ modes have fourfold degeneracy as each polarization state may have ϕ-dependence of the $\cos l\phi$ type or the $\sin l\phi$ type.

(iii) Total number of modes (when $V >> 1$) guided along a step-index fiber is given approximately by $M = V^2/2$. As we know from Eq. (5.97) that the V-value of the fiber is dependent on the dimensions, the numerical aperture of the fiber, and the wavelength of the light signal; the total number of guided modes in a particular fiber at a specific wavelength is fixed.

Table 5.1: Cut-off frequencies of the first few lower order LP_{lm} modes in a step index (SI) fiber

l	m			
	1	2	3	4
0	0	3.832	7.106	10.173
1	2.405	5.520	8.654	11.790
2	3.832	7.016	10.173	13.324
3	5.136	8.417	11.620	14.796

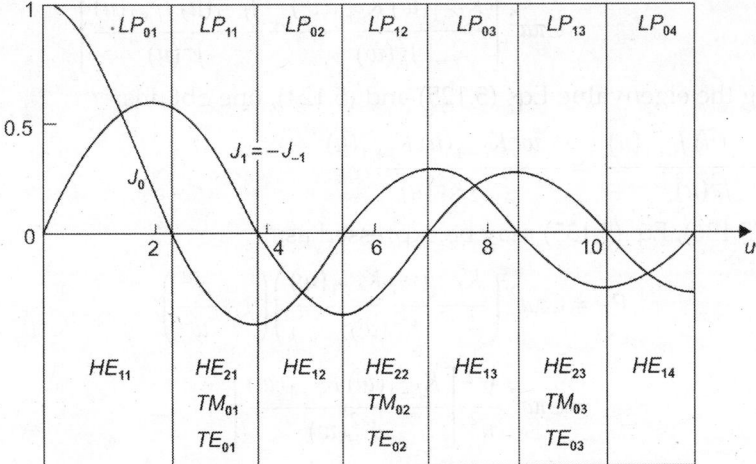

Fig. 5.7: Plot of Bessel functions J_0 and J_1, indicating the range of allowed values of u for lower order modes

5.8.2 Fraction Modal Power Distribution

Now, we calculate the fractional modal power distribution in the core and cladding of a Si fiber using a scalar approximation. In the core, power is given by:

$$P_{\text{core}} = (\text{constant}) \int_{r=0}^{a} \int_{\phi=0}^{2\pi} |\psi(r, \phi)|^2 \, r \, dr \, d\phi$$

$$= (\text{constant}) \{R(a)\}^2 \int_{r=0}^{a} \frac{J_l^2(ur/a) \, r \, dr}{J_l^2(u)} \int_{\phi=0}^{2\pi} \cos^2 l\phi d\phi$$

Here, we have substituted the value of $\psi(r, \phi)$ from Eq. (5.122) and taken the ϕ-dependence to be of the form $\cos(l\phi)$. The solution of the above integral can be shown to be:

$$P_{\text{core}} - C\pi a^2 \left[1 - \frac{J_{l-1}(u) \, J_{l+1}(u)}{J_l^2(u)}\right] \tag{5.133}$$

where C is a constant.

Similarly, one can obtain the power distribution in the cladding by solving the integral:

$$P_{\text{cladding}} = (\text{constant}) \int_{r=a}^{\infty} \int_{\phi=0}^{2\pi} |\psi(r, \phi)|^2 \, r \, dr \, d\phi$$

Substituting the value of $\psi(r, \phi)$ from Eq. (5.123) in the above relation and again taking the $\cos(l\phi)$ form, one obtains:

$$P_{\text{cladding}} = (\text{constant}) \{R(a)\}^2 \int_{r=a}^{\infty} \frac{K_l^2(wr/a)}{K_l^2(w)} \, r \, dr \int_{\phi=0}^{2\pi} \cos^2(l\phi) d\phi$$

$$= C\pi a^2 \left[\frac{K_{l-1}(w) \, K_{l+1}(w)}{K_l^2(w)} - 1\right] \tag{5.134}$$

Adding Eqs (5.133) and (5.134), one can obtain an expression for the total power P_T as follows:

$$P_T = P_{\text{core}} + P_{\text{cladding}}$$

$$= C\pi a^2 \left[1 - \frac{J_{l-1}(u) \, J_{l+1}(u)}{J_l^2(u)}\right] + C\pi a^2 \left[\frac{K_{l-1}(w) \, K_{l+1}(w)}{J_1^2(w)} - 1\right]$$

$$= C\pi a^2 \left[\frac{K_{l-1}(w)\, K_{l+1}(w)}{J_l^2(w)} - \frac{J_{l-1}(u)\, J_{l+1}(u)}{J_l^2(u)} \right] \tag{5.135}$$

Multiplying the eigenvalue Eqs (5.125) and (5.124), one obtains:

$$\frac{u^2 J_{l-1}(u)\, J_{l+1}(u)}{J_l^2(u)} = -\frac{w^2 K_{l-1}(u)\, K_{l+1}(u)}{K_l^2(u)} \tag{5.136}$$

Using Eq. (5.136), Eq. (5.135) may be expressed as:

$$P_T = C\pi a^2 \left(\frac{K_{l-1}(w)\, K_{l+1}(w)}{K_l^2(w)} \right)\left(1 + \frac{w^2}{u^2}\right)$$

$$= C\pi a^2 \frac{V^2}{u^2}\left[\frac{K_{l-1}(w)\, K_{l+1}(w)}{K_l^2(w)} \right] \tag{5.137}$$

Now, using Eq. (5.136), Eq. (5.133) may be expressed as:

$$P_{\text{core}} = C\pi a^2 \left[1 + \frac{w^2}{u^2}\, \frac{K_{l-1}(w)\, K_{l+1}(w)}{K_l^2(w)} \right] \tag{5.138}$$

Dividing Eq. (5.138) by Eq. (5.137), one obtains the fractional power propagating in the core as:

$$\frac{P_{\text{core}}}{P_T} = \frac{C\pi a^2 \left[1 + \dfrac{w^2}{u^2}\, \dfrac{K_{l-1}(w)\, K_{l+1}(w)}{K_l^2(w)} \right]}{C\pi a^2 \dfrac{V^2}{u^2}\left[\dfrac{K_{l-1}(w)\, K_{l+1}(w)}{K_l^2(w)} \right]}$$

$$= \left[\frac{u^2}{V^2}\, \frac{K_l^2(w)}{K_{l-1}(w)\, K_{l+1}(w)} + \frac{w^2}{V^2} \right] \tag{5.139}$$

The functional power propagating in the cladding is expressed as:

$$\frac{P_{\text{cladding}}}{P_T} = 1 - \frac{P_{\text{core}}}{P_T} = \frac{u^2}{V^2}\left[1 - \frac{K_l^2(w)}{K_{l-1}(w)\, K_{l+1}(w)} \right] \tag{5.140}$$

Figure 5.8 shows the plots of fractional power propagating in the core and the cladding for some lower order LP modes. It is interesting to note that for the first two lower order modes, the power flow is mostly in the cladding near cut-off. Using Eqs (5.116) to (5.118), one can show that as $V \to V_c$, $w \to 0$, and $u \to V_c$, we obtain

$$\frac{P_{\text{core}}}{P_T} \to \begin{cases} 0 & \text{for } l = 0 \text{ and } 1 \\ \dfrac{(l-1)}{l} & \text{for } l \geq 2 \end{cases} \tag{5.141}$$

However, for larger values of l, the power remains in the core even at or just beyond cut-off. Another point to be mentioned is that the power associated with a particular mode is mostly confined in the core for large values of V.

When light is launched into a fiber from an incoherent source, e.g. an LED or an incandescent lamp, it tends to excite all possible modes in the fiber with the same amount of power. One can calculate the average power by taking the sum of the power carried

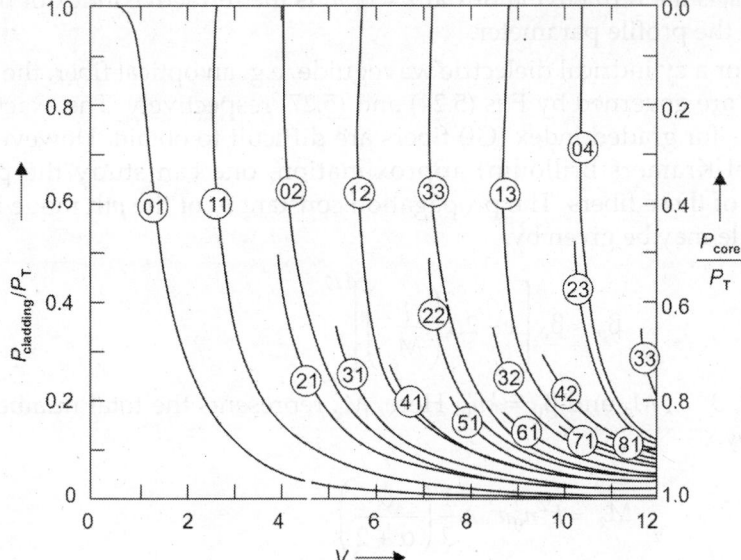

Fig. 5.8: Schematic of plots of fractional power contained in the core and cladding of a Si fiber as a function of V

by each mode and dividing it by the total number of modes. Assuming the number of modes to be very large, the average power carried by the core and cladding can be computed by integrating the power carried by the core and cladding can be computed by integrating the power carried by a single mode over all possible modes. The total average power density at the core–cladding interface under this condition is obtained as

$$\left[\frac{P_{\text{clad}}}{P_{\text{total}}}\right] = \frac{1}{2\pi a^2}$$

(3.141a)

This relation reveals that the total mean power at the core cladding interface averaged over all possible modes is independent of the total number of modes or V-number of the optical fiber. The total average cladding under this condition is obtained as

$$\left[\frac{P_{\text{clad}}}{P_{\text{total}}}\right] = \frac{4}{3}\frac{1}{\sqrt{M}}$$

(3.141b)

where M is the total number of modes. For a step index fiber the number of modes is related to the V-number as:

$$M = \frac{V^2}{2}$$

(3.141c)

Clearly, the power carried by the cladding in a multimode step index fiber decreases inversely with the V-number.

5.8.3 Graded Index (GI) Fibers

The refractive index profile for a multimode graded index (GI) fiber is given by:

$$n(r) = n_0\{1 - 2\Delta\,(r/a)^\alpha\}^{1/2},\ r \leq a$$

(5.142)

$$= n_0\{1 - 2\Delta\}^{1/2} = n_c,\ r \geq a$$

(5.143)

where

$$\Delta = (n_0^2 - n_c^2)/2n_0^2 = \frac{(n_0 - n_c)}{n_0}$$

when $\Delta << 1$, n_0 is the refractive index at $r = 0$, n_c is the refractive index of the cladding, and α is called the profile parameter.

In general, for a cylindrical dielectric waveguide, e.g. an optical fiber, the electric and magnetic field are governed by Eqs (5.24) and (5.27) respectively. The exact solution of these equations for graded index (GI) fibers are difficult to obtain. However, using the WKB (Wentzel-Kramers-Brillouin) approximation, one can study the propagation characteristics of these fibers. The propagation constant b_p of the pth mode in a GI fiber withan α-profile may be given by:

$$\beta_p \approx \beta_0 \left[1 - 2\Delta \left(\frac{p}{M_g} \right) \right]^{1/2} \tag{5.144}$$

where $p = 1, 2, 3, ..., M_g$ and $\beta_0 = kn_0$. Here, M_g represents the total number of guided modes given by:

$$M_g = k^2 n_0^2 a^2 \, \Delta \frac{1}{2} \left(\frac{\alpha}{\alpha + 2} \right) \tag{5.145}$$

Substituting the values of Δ and k, one obtains:

$$M_g = \frac{1}{2} \left(\frac{\alpha}{\alpha + 2} \right) \left[\frac{2\pi a}{\lambda} (n_0^2 - n_c^2)^{1/2} \right]^2 \tag{5.146}$$

Equation (5.146) gives the approximate modal volume or the number of modes guided by the α-profile graded-index fiber. For a step-index fiber ($\alpha = \infty$), $n = n_1$ in the core and $n = n_2$ in the cladding. Clearly, the modal volume M_s for such a fiber will be given by:

$$M_s \approx \frac{1}{2} \left[\frac{2\pi a}{\lambda} (n_1^2 - n_2^2)^{1/2} \right]^2 \tag{5.147}$$

We know that the normalized frequency parameter is given by:

$$V = \frac{2\pi a}{\lambda} (n_1^2 - n_2^2)^{1/2}$$

Therefore $\qquad M_s = \dfrac{V^2}{2} \tag{5.148}$

For a GI fiber, the numerical aperture (NA) for the guided rays varies with r as follows:

$$NA(r) = \begin{cases} \{n^2(r) - n_c^2\}^{1/2} & \text{for } r < a \\ 0 & \text{for } r \geq a \end{cases}$$

However, for small variation of $n(r)$ with r:

$$NA \approx \{n_0^2 - n_c^2\}^{1/2}$$

and $\qquad V \approx \dfrac{2\pi a}{\lambda} (n_0^2 - n_c^2)^{1/2}$

With this approximation, one finds:

$$M_g \cong \frac{\alpha}{\alpha + 2} \frac{V^2}{2} \tag{5.149}$$

We must take care when using Eqs (5.144)–(5.149) because the WKB is valid for highly multimoded fibers with V much greater than 1.

For a parabolic profile, $\alpha = 2$, and:

$$M_g \approx \frac{V^2}{4}$$

One can show that the cut-off value of the normalized frequency, V_c, to support a single mode in a graded-index fiber is given by:

$$V_c = 2.405\left(1 + \frac{2}{a}\right)^{1/2} \tag{5.150}$$

Clearly, it is possible to determine the structural and/or operational parameters of the fiber which give single-mode operation.

5.8.4 Limitations of Multimode Fibers

We have read that multimode fibers support many modes. The higher order modes (corresponding to oblique rays in terms of the ray model) travel slower and hence arrive at the other end of the fiber later than the lower order modes (corresponding to axial rays). This means that different modes travel with different group velocities. Thus, a light pulse propagating through such a fiber will get broadened. This is called *multipath dispersion* or *intermodal dispersion*. The pulse dispersion per unit length for a step-index fiber ($\alpha = \infty$) is given by:

$$\frac{\Delta T}{L} = \frac{n_1}{n_2}\left(\frac{n_1 - n_2}{c}\right) \approx \frac{n_1 \Delta}{c} \tag{5.151}$$

Similarly, one can show that the pulse dispersion per unit length for a graded index fiber with a parabolic profile ($\alpha = 2$) may be expressed as:

$$\frac{\Delta T}{L} = \frac{n_0}{2c} \Delta^2 \tag{5.152}$$

and that for a GI fiber with an optimum profile ($\alpha = 2 - 2\Delta$) may be expressed as:

$$\frac{\Delta T}{L} \approx \frac{n_0}{8c} \Delta^2 \tag{5.153}$$

Thus, pulse broadening due to intermodal dispersion, varying from about 0.05 nm/km to 80 nm/km, depending on the value of α and the core index n_0, has been observed in multimode fibers. This severely restricts the use of such fibers in long-haul communications.

Moreover, a light pulse has a number of spectral components (of different frequencies), and the group velocity of a mode varies with frequency. Therefore, different spectral components in the pulse propagate with slightly different group velocities, resulting in pulse broadening. This phenomenon is called *group velocity dispersion* (GVD) or *intramodal dispersion*.

We may note that in spite of these limitations, multimode fibers are used in local area network and short-haul communication links. However, prior to using them, the link power budget and the rise-time budget have to be analysed.

5.9 PHOTONIC CRYSTAL FIBERS

So far we have concentrated on optical fibers comprising solid silica core and cladding regions in which the light is guided by a small increase in refractive index in the core facilitated through doping the silicon with germanium. More recently, however, a new class of microstructured optical fiber containing a fine array of air holes running longitudinally down the fiber cladding has been developed. Since the microstructure within the fiber is often highly periodic due to the fabrication process, these fibers are usually referred to as *photonic crystal fibers* (PCFs), or sometimes just as holey fibers. Whereas in conventional optical fibers electromagnetic modes are guided by total internal reflection in the core region, which has a slightly raised refractive index, in PCFs two distinct guidance mechanisms arise.

Although the guided modes can be trapped in a fiber core which exhibits a higher average index than the cladding containing the air holes by an effect similar to total internal reflection, alternatively they may be trapped in a core of either higher, or indeed lower, average index by a photonic bandgap effect. In the former case the effect is often termed modified total internal reflection and the fibers are referred to as index guided, while in the latter they are called photonic bandgap fibers. Furthermore, the existence of two different guidance mechanisms makes PCFs versatile in their range of potential applications. For example, PCFs have been used to realize various optical components and devices including long period gratings, multimode interference power splitters, tunable coupled cavity fiber lasers, fiber amplifiers, multichannel add/drop filters, wavelength converters and wavelength demultiplexers. As with conventional optical fibers, however, a crucial issue with PCFs has been the reduction in overall transmission losses which were initially several hundred decibels per kilometer even with the most straightforward designs. Increased control over the homogeneity of the fiber structure together with the use of highly purified silicon as the base material has now lowered these losses to a level of a very few decibels per kilometer for most PCF types, with a loss of just 0.3dB km^{-1} at 1.55 μm for a 100 km span being recently reported.

5.9.1 Index-Guided Microstructures

Although the principles of guidance and the characteristics of index-guided PCFs are similar to those of conventional fiber, there is greater index contrast since the cladding contains air holes with a refractive index of 1 in comparison with the normal silica cladding index of 1.457 which is close to the germanium-doped core index of 1.462. A fundamental physical difference, however, between index-guided PCFs and conventional fibers arises from the manner in which the guided mode interacts withthe cladding region. Whereas in a conventional fiber this interaction is largely first order and independent of wavelength, the large index contrast combined with the small structure dimensions cause the effective cladding index to be a strong function of wavelength. For short wavelengths the effective cladding index is only slightly lower than the core index and hence they remain tightly confined to the core. At longer wavelengths, however, the mode samples more of the cladding and the effective index contrast is larger. This wavelength dependence results in a large number of unusual optical properties which can be tailored. For example, the high index contrast enables the PCF core to be reduced from around 8 μm in conventional fiber to less than 1 μm, which increases the intensity of the light in the core and enhances the nonlinear effects.

Two common index-guided PCF designs are shown diagrammatically in Fig. 5.9. In both cases a solid-core region is surrounded by a cladding region containing air holes. The cladding region in Fig. 5.9(a) comprises a hexagonal array of air holes while in Fig. 5.9(b) the cladding air holes are not uniform in size and do not extend too far from the core. It should be noted that the hole diameter d and hole to hole spacing or pitch A are critical design parameters used to specify the structure of the PCF. For example, in a silica PCF with the structure depicted in Fig. 5.9(a) when the air fill fraction is low (i.e. $d/\Lambda < 0.4$), then the fiber can be single-moded at all wavelength. This property, which cannot be attained in conventional fibers, is particularly significant for broadband applications such as *wavelength division multiplexed transmission.*

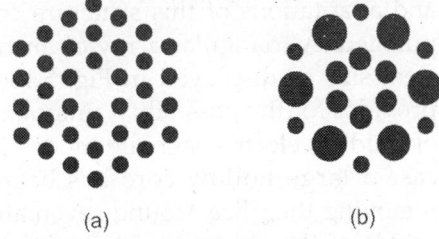

(a)　　　　　　　　(b)

Fig. 5.9: Two index-guided photonic crystal fiber structures. The dark areas are air holes while the white areas are silica

As PCFs have a wider range of optical properties in comparison with standard optical fibers, they provide for the possibility of new and technologically important fiber devices. When the hole region covers more than 20% of the fiber cross-section, for instance index-guided PCFs display an interesting range of dispersive properties which could find application as *dispersion-compensating* or *dispersion-controlling fiber components.* In such fibers it is possible to produce very high optical nonlinearity per unit length in which modest light intensities can induce substantial nonlinear effect. For example, while several kilometers of conventional fiber are normally required to achieve 2R data regeneration, it was obtained with just 3.3 m of large air-filling fraction PCF. In addition, filling the cladding holes with polymers or liquid crystals allows external fields to be used to dynamically vary the fiber properties. The temperature sensitivity of a polymer within the cladding holes may be employed to tune a Bragg grating written into the core. By contrast, index-guided PCFs with small holes and large hole spacings provide very large mode area (and hence low optical nonlinearities) and have potential applications in high-power delivery (e.g. laser welding and machining) as well as high-power fiber lasers and amplifiers. Furthermore, the large index contrast between silica and air enables production of such PCFs with large multimoded cores which also have very high numerical aperture values (greater than 0.7). Hence these fibers are useful for the collection and transmission of high optical powers in situations where signal distortion is not an issue. Finally, it is apparent that PCFs can be readily spliced to conventional fibers, thus enabling their integration with existing components and subsystems.

5.9.2 Photonic Band Gap Fibers

Photonic band gap (PBG) fibers are a class of microstructured fiber in which a periodic arrangement of air holes is required to ensure guidance. This periodic arrangement of cladding air holes provides for the formation of a photonic band gap in the transverse plane of the fiber. As a PBG fiber exhibits a two-dimensional band gap, then wavelength within this bandgap cannot propagate perpendicular to the fiber axis (i.e. in the cladding) and they can therefore be confined to propagate within a region in which the refractive index is lower than the surrounding material. Hence utilizing the photonic band gap effect light can be guided within a low-index, air-filled core region creating fiber properties quite different from those obtained without the bandgap. Although, as with index-guided PCFs, PBG fibers can also guide light in regions with higher refractive index, it is the lower index region guidance feature which is of particular interest. In addition, a further distinctive feature is that while index-guiding fibers usually have a guided mode at all wavelengths, PBG fibers only guide in certain wavelength bands, and furthermore, it is possible to have wavelengths at which higher order modes are guided while the fundamental mode is not.

Two important PBG fiber structures are displayed in Fig. 5.10. The honeycomb fiber design shown in Fig. 5.10(a) was the first PBG fiber to be experimentally realized in 1998 and adaptations of this structure continue to be pursued. A triangular array of air holes of sufficient size as displayed in Fig. 5.10(b), however, provides for the possibility, unique to PBG fibers, of guiding electromagnetic modes in air. In this case a large hollow core has been defined by removing the silica around seven air holes in the center of the structure. These fibers, which are termed *air-guiding* or *hollow-core PBG fibers*, enable more than 98% of the guided mode field energy to propagate in the air regions. Such air-guiding fibers have attracted attention because they potentially provide an environment in which

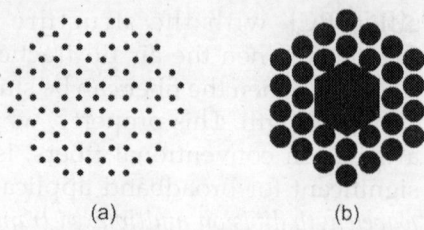

(a)   (b)

Fig. 5.10: Photonic bandgap (PBG) fiber structures in which the dark areas are air (lower refractive index) and the lighter area is the higher refractive index: (a) honeycomb PBG fiber; (b) air-guiding PBG fiber

optical propagation can take place with little attenuation as the localization of light in the air core removes the limitations caused by material absorption losses. The fabrication of hollow-core fiber with low propagation losses, however, has proved to be quite difficult, with losses of the order of 13 dB km^{-1}. Moreover, the fibers tend to be highly dispersive with narrow transmission windows and while single-mode operation is possible, it is not as straightforward to achieve in comparison with index-guiding PCFs.

More recently, the fabrication and characterization of a new type of solid silica-based photonic crystal fiber which guides light using the PBG mechanism has been reported in the literature. The fiber employed a two-dimensional periodic array of germanium-doped rods in the core region. It was therefore referred to as a nanostructure core fiber and exhibited a minimum attenuation of 2.6 dB km^{-1} at a wavelength of 1.59 μm. Furthermore, the fiber displayed greater bending sensitivity than conventional single-mode fiber as a result of the much smaller index difference between the core and the leaky modes which could provide for potential applications in the optical sensing of curvature and stress. In addition, it is indicated that the all-solid silica structure would facilitate fiber fabrication using existing technology and birefringence of the order of 10^{-4} is easily achievable with a large mode field diameter up to 10 μm, thus enabling its use within fiber lasers and gyroscope applications.

Example 1

A silica optical fiber with a core diameter large enough to be considered by ray theory analysis has a core refractive index of 1.50 and a cladding refractive index of 1.47. Calculate (a) the critical angle at the core–cladding interface (b) the NA for the fiber (c) the acceptance angle in air for the fiber

Solution

(a) $\theta_c = \sin^{-1} \dfrac{n_2}{n_1} = \sin^{-1} \dfrac{1.47}{1.50} = 78.5°$

(b) $NA = (n_1 - n_2)^{1/2} = [(1.50)^2 - (1.47)^2]^{1/2} = (2.25 - 2.16)^{1/2} = 0.30$

(c) The acceptance angle:

$\theta_a = \sin^{-1}(NA) = \sin^{-1} 0.30 = 17.4°$

Example 2

An optical fiber in air has an NA of 0.4. Compare the acceptance angle for meridional rays with that for skew rays which change by 100° at each reflection.

Solution

The acceptance angle for meridional ray is given by:

$$NA = n_0 \sin \theta_a = (n_1^2 - n_2^2)^{\frac{1}{2}}$$

With $n_0 = 1$, we have

$$\theta_a = \sin^{-1} NA = \sin^{-1} 0.4 = 23.6°$$

The skew rays change direction by 100° at each reflection, therefore $\gamma = 50°$. Hence:

$$\theta_{as} = \sin^{-1}\left(\frac{NA}{\cos \gamma}\right) = \sin^{-1}\left(\frac{0.4}{\cos 50°}\right) = 38.5°$$

In this example, the acceptance angle for the skew rays is about 15° greater than the corresponding angle for meridional rays. However, we must note that we have compared the θ_a of one particular skew ray path. When the light input to the fiber is at an angle to the fiber axis, it is possible that γ will vary from zero for meridional rays for 90° for rays which enter the fiber at the core-cladding interface giving acceptance of skew rays over a conical half angle of $\pi/2$ radians.

Example 3

A symmetric step-index (SI) planar waveguide is made of glass with $n_1 = 1.5$ and $n_2 = 1.49$. The thickness of the guide layer is 9.83 μm and the guide is excited by a source of wavelength $\lambda = 0.85$ μm. What is the range of the propagation constants? What is the maximum number of modes supported by the guide? **[B Tech]**

Solution

The phase propagation constant β lies between β_1 and β_2. Here:

$$\beta_1 = kn_1 = \frac{2\pi n_1}{\lambda} = \frac{2\pi}{(0.85 \times 10^{-6})} \times 1.50 = 11.0082 \times 10^6 \ m^{-1}$$

and

$$\beta_2 - kn_2 = \frac{2\pi n_2}{\lambda} = \frac{2\pi}{(0.85 \times 10^{-6})} \times 1.49 = 11.008 \times 10^6 \ m^{-1}$$

The maximum number of modes that the guide can support is given by Eq. (5.43), i.e.:

$$M = \frac{4a}{\lambda}(n_1^2 - n_2^2)^{\frac{1}{2}} = \frac{2 \times (9.83)}{0.85}[(1.5)^2 - (1.49)^2]^{\frac{1}{2}} \approx 4$$

Example 4

A multimode step index fiber with a core diameter of 80 μm and a relative index difference of 1.5% is operating at a wavelength of 0.85 μm. If the core refractive index is 1.48, estimate (a) the normalized frequency for the fiber (b) the number of guided modes.

Solution

(a) The normalized frequency is given by:

$$V \approx \frac{2\pi}{\lambda} an_1 (2\Delta)^{\frac{1}{2}} = \frac{2\pi \times 40 \times 10^{-6} \times 1.48}{0.85 \times 10^{-6}}(2 \times 0.015)^{\frac{1}{2}} = 75.8$$

(b) Total number of guided modes is given by:

$$M_s \approx \frac{V^2}{2} = \frac{5745.6}{2} = 2873$$

Hence this fiber has a V number of approximately 76, giving nearly 3000 guided modes.

Example 5

What should be the maximum thickness of the guide slab of a symmetrical SI planar waveguide so that it supports only the fundamental TE mode? Take $n_1 = 3.6$, $n_2 = 3.56$, and $\lambda = 0.85$ µm. **[B Tech]**

Solution

For the waveguide to support only the fundamental mode, V should be less than $\pi/2$, i.e.:

$$\frac{2\pi a}{\lambda}(n_1^2 - n_2^2)^{\frac{1}{2}} < \pi/2$$

or

$$2a < \frac{\lambda}{(n_1^2 - n_2^2)^{\frac{1}{2}}} < \frac{0.85 \text{ µm}}{2\{(3.6)^2 - (3.56)^2\}^{\frac{1}{2}}} < 0.793 \text{ µm}$$

Clearly, the thickness of the guide slab should not be more than 0.793 µm.

Example 6

The cutoff wavelength of a step index fiber is quoted as $\lambda_c = 1.20$ µm. If the fiber is operated at wavelength $\lambda = 1.55$ µm, what is V?

Solution

$$V = 2.405 \frac{\lambda_c}{\lambda} = 2.405\left(\frac{1.20}{1.55}\right) = 1.86$$

Example 7

Calculate the G-factor for the fundamental TE mode supported by the waveguide having $n_1 = 3.6$, $n_2 = 3.56$ and $\lambda = 0.85$ µm. Given $2a = 0.793$ µm. **[B Tech]**

Solution

For thickness $2a = 0.793$ µm, $V = \pi/2$. The point of intersection of an arc of $V = \pi/2$ with the curve $ua \tan ua = wa$ for $m = 0$, yield $ua = 0.934$ and $wa = 1.262$.

Using Eq. (5.83), the confinement factor G may be calculated as follows:

$$G = \left[1 + \frac{\cos^2(0.934)}{1.262\{1 + (\sin 0.934)(\cos 0.934)/0.934\}}\right]^{-1} = 0.8436$$

This means that only 84.36% of the total power carried by fundamental mode is confined within the guide layer; the remaining 15.64% extends into the cladding slabs.

Example 8

Graded index fiber with a parabolic refractive index profile core has a refractive index at the core axis of 1.5 and a relative index difference of 1%. Estimate the maximum possible core diameter which allows single mode operation at a wavelength of 1.3 µm.

Solution

The maximum value of normalized frequency for single mode operation is given by:

$$V = 2.405\left(1 + \frac{2}{\alpha}\right)^{\frac{1}{2}}$$

Here $\alpha = 2$:

∴

$$V = 2.405\left(1 + \frac{2}{2}\right)^{\frac{1}{2}} = 2.405\sqrt{2} = 2.4\sqrt{2}$$

The maximum core radius may be obtained from:

$$V = \frac{2\pi}{\lambda} a n_1 (2\Delta)^{\frac{1}{2}}$$

or
$$a = \frac{V\lambda}{2\pi n_1 (2\Delta)^{\frac{1}{2}}} = \frac{2.4\sqrt{2} \times 1.3 \times 10^{-6}}{2\pi \times 1.5 \times (0.02)^{\frac{1}{2}}} = 3.3 \ \mu m$$

Hence the maximum core diameter which allows single mode operation is approximately 6.6 μm.

Example 9

A multimode step-index fiber has a relative refractive index difference of 2% and a core refractive index of 1.5. The number of modes propagating at a wavelength of 1.3 μm is 1000. Calculate the diameter of the fiber core. **[B Tech]**

Solution

$$M_s = \frac{V^2}{2} = \frac{1}{2}\left[\frac{2\pi a}{\lambda} n_1 \sqrt{2\Delta}\right]^2 = \frac{1}{2}\frac{4\pi^2 a^2 n_1^2 2\Delta}{\lambda^2}$$

$$\therefore \qquad 2a = \frac{\lambda}{\pi n_1}\left(\frac{M_s}{\Delta}\right)^{\frac{1}{2}} = \frac{1.3}{\pi \times 1.5}\sqrt{\frac{1000}{0.02}} = 62 \ \mu m$$

Example 10

Determine the cutoff wavelength (λ_c) for a step index fiber to exhibit single mode operation when the core refractive index and radius are 1.46 and 4.5 μm, respectivity, with the relative index difference being 0.25%.

Solution

The cutoff wavelength is given by

$$\lambda_c = \frac{2\pi a n_1}{V_c}(2\Delta)^{\frac{1}{2}} = \frac{2\pi a n_1}{2.405}(2\Delta)^{\frac{1}{2}}$$

Substituting the values in the above relation, one obtains:

$$\lambda_c = \frac{2\pi \times 4.5 \times 1.46 \times (0.005)^{\frac{1}{2}}}{2.405} \ \mu m = 1.214 \ \mu m = 1214 \ nm$$

Hence the fiber is a single-mode d to a wavelength of 1214 nm.

Example 11

A step-index fiber has a numerical aperture of 0.17 and a core diameter of 100 μm. Determine the normalized frequency parameter of the fiber when light of wavelength 0.85 μm is transmitted through it. Also estimate the number of guided modes propagating in the fiber. **[B Tech]**

Solution

We have:
$$V = \frac{2\pi a}{\lambda}(n_1^2 - n_2^2)^{1/2} = \frac{2\pi a(NA)}{\lambda} = \frac{\lambda(100 \ \mu m)(0.17)}{(0.85 \ \mu m)} = 62.83$$

Therefore
$$M_s = \frac{V^2}{2} = 1974$$

Example 12

A graded index fiber with a parabolic profile supports the propagation of 700 guided modes. The fiber has a relative refractive index difference of 2%, a core refractive index of 1.45 and a core diameter of 75 µm. Calculate the wavelength of light propagating in the fiber. Further, estimate the maximum diameter of the fiber core which can give single-mode operation at the same length. **[B Tech]**

Solution

We have $M_g \cong \left(\dfrac{\alpha}{\alpha+2}\right)\dfrac{V^2}{2}$ for the mode volume to evaluate V. With $\alpha = 2$ for the parabolic profile, we have:

$$V = \sqrt{4M_g} = \sqrt{4 \times 700} = 52.91$$

and

$$\lambda = \frac{2\pi a}{V} n_1 \sqrt{2\Delta} = \frac{\pi \times (75 \ \pi m)}{52.91} \times 1.45 \times (2 \times 0.02)^{1/2} = 1.3 \ \mu m$$

The cutoff value of the normalized frequency V_c for single-mode operation in a graded-index fiber is given by the relation:

$$V_c = 2.405\left(1 + \frac{2}{\alpha}\right)^{1/2}.$$

Thus, with $\alpha = 2$: $\qquad V_c = 2.405\sqrt{2}$

The maximum core diameter may be obtained as follows:

$$2a = \frac{V_c \lambda}{\pi n_1 \sqrt{(2\Delta)}} = \frac{2.405\sqrt{2} \times (1.3 \ \mu m)}{\pi \times 1.45 \times \sqrt{(2 \times 0.02)}} = 4.85 \ \mu m$$

Example 13

Given that a useful approximation for the eigenvalue of the single-mode step index fiber cladding W is given by:
$$W(V) \approx 1.1428 \ V - 0.9960$$
Deduce an approximation for the normalized propagation constant $b(v)$. **[B Tech]**

Solution

The normalized propagation constant is given by:
$$b(V) = 1 - \frac{(V^2 - W^2)}{V^2} = \frac{W^2}{V^2}$$

Now, substituting the approximation given above, one obtains:
$$b(V) \approx \left(\frac{(1.1428V - 0.9960)}{V^2}\right)^2 = \left(1.1428 - \frac{0.9960}{V}\right)^2$$

The relative error on this approximation for $b(V)$ is less than 0.2% for $1.5 \leq V \leq 2.5$ and less than 2% for $1 \leq V \leq 3$.

Example 14

A parabolic profile graded index single-mode fiber designed for operation at a wavelength of 1.30 µm has a cutoff wavelength of 1.08 µm. From experimental measurement it is established that the first minimum in the diffraction pattern occurs at an angle of 12°. Determine the spot size at the operating wavelength (based on the ESI technique).

[B Tech]

Solution

The effective core radius is given by:

$$a_{eff} = 3.832/(k \sin \theta_{min})$$

where $\quad k = 2\pi/\lambda.$

Substituting the given values, we obtain:

$$a_{eff} = \frac{3.832 \, \lambda}{2\pi \sin \theta_{min}} = \frac{3.3832 \times 1.30 \times 10^{-6}}{2\pi \sin 12°} = 3.81 \, \mu m$$

The effective normalized frequency is given by:

$$V_{eff} = 2.405 \left(\frac{V}{V_c} \right) = 2.405 \left(\frac{\lambda_c}{\lambda} \right) = 2.405 \left(\frac{1.08}{1.30} \right) = 2.00$$

∴ The spot size can be obtained from:

$$\omega_0 = a_{eff} \left[0.6043 + 1.755 \, V_{eff}^{-1/2} + 2.78 \, V_{eff}^{-6} \right]$$

$$= 3.81 \times 10^{-6} \, [0.6043 + 1.755 \, (2.00)^{-1/2} + 2.78 \, (2.00)^{-6}] = 4.83 \, \mu m$$

Example 15

Find the core radius necessary for single mode operation at 1300 nm of a step index fiber with core and cladding refractive indices equal to 1.450 and 1.447 respectively.   [PTU]

Solution

For single mode operation, we have

$$V = V_c = \frac{2\pi a}{\lambda} (n_1^2 - n_2^2)^{1/2} = 2.405$$

or

$$a - \frac{2.405 \times 1300 \times 10^{-9}}{6.28 \times \sqrt{(1.450)^2 - (1.447)^2}} \, m - 5.24 \, \mu m$$

Example 16

Calculate the number of modes in a step-index multimode fiber at 1550 nm if the core radius of the fiber is 25 μm and the refractive index of the core is 1.46 and the relative refractive index difference is 0.2%   [UTU]

Solution

The total number of modes in the fiber can be obtained from the following relation

$$M = \frac{2\pi^2 a^2}{\lambda^2} (n_1^2 - n_2^2) = \frac{2\pi^2 a^2}{\lambda^2} (2n_1^2 \Delta)$$

or

$$M = \frac{2(3.14)^2 \, (25 \times 10^{-6})^2}{(1550 \times 10^{-9})^2} [2.(1.46)^2 \times 0.002] \approx 48$$

SUMMARY

- Maxwell's electromagnetic (em) theory is based on a set of four equations. One can derive a wave equation describing the propagation of em waves in any medium.

- In a isotropic and homogeneous dielectric medium, the wave equation is represented by $\nabla^2 \psi - \dfrac{n^2}{c^2} \dfrac{\partial^2 \psi}{\partial t^2} = 0$, where ψ represents the scalar field component of **E** and **H**. The solution of this equation is of the form: $\psi = \psi_0 \exp \{i\,(\omega t - \beta z)\}$, where the symbols have their usual meanings.

- A waveguide is used to guide electromagnetic waves through it. In waveguide, both electric and magnetic fields are confined to space within the waveguide. The dielectric loss within the waveguide is negligibly small because the guides are normally air filled. Within a waveguide several *modes* could be propagated. The mode of propagation of em waves of a waveguide is determined from solution to Maxwell's equations. If the frequency of a particular signal is above the cutoff frequency of the particular mode, then that particular signal will be passed through it or else it gets attenuated.

- A *planar guide* is the simplest form of optical waveguide. One may assume it consists of a slab of dielectric with refractive index n_1, sandwiched between two regions of lower refractive index n_2.

- A *mode* is a stable (electric or magnetic) field pattern in the transverse direction (e.g. the x-direction) with only a periodic z-dependence. In an isotropic and inhomogeneous dielectric medium, the modes of wave propagation can be described by the following sets of equations:

$$\left.\begin{aligned} \beta E_y &= -\mu_0 \omega H_x \\[4pt] \frac{\partial E_y}{\partial x} &= -i\,\mu_0 \omega H_z \\[4pt] -i\beta H_x - \frac{\partial H_z}{\partial x} &= i\varepsilon_0 \omega n^2(x)\, E_y \end{aligned}\right\} \text{TE modes}$$

$$\left.\begin{aligned} \beta H_y &= -\varepsilon_0 \omega n^2(x) E_x \\[4pt] \frac{\partial H_y}{\partial x} &= i\,\varepsilon_0 \omega n^2(x) E_z \\[4pt] -i\beta E_x + \frac{\partial E_z}{\partial x} &= i\mu_0 \omega H_y \end{aligned}\right\} \text{TE modes}$$

- The maximum number of TE modes, M, supported by a symmetrical step-index planar waveguide is an integer close to or greater than $2V/\pi$, where V is normalized frequency given by:

$$V = \frac{2\pi}{\lambda}\, a \sqrt{n_1^2 - n_2^2}$$

- The normalized propagation constant b for a fiber is given by:

$$b = \frac{\beta^2 - \beta_2^2}{\beta_1^2 - \beta_2^2} = 1 - \left(\frac{ua}{V}\right)^2 = \left(\frac{wa}{V}\right)^2$$

- For a guided mode b must lie between 0 and 1, and also β^2 must lie between $\beta_1^2 - \beta_2^2$.

- The cutoff of a mode occurs at $b = 0$, $ua = V_c = m\pi/2$ and $wa = 0$. However, the fundamental mode has no cutoff frequency.

- The thickness of a guide layer that can support m modes is given by:

$$2a = \frac{m\lambda}{2\,(n_1^2 - n_2^2)^{1/2}}$$

- The thickness of a guide layer required to support only the fundamental mode is given by:

$$2a \leq \frac{\lambda}{2\,(n_1^2 - n_2^2)^{1/2}}$$

- The fraction of guided optical power that is confined within a guide layer is called the *confinement factor*. The confinement factor depends on the thickness of the guide layer and the mode number.

- The optical fiber with a core of constant refractive index n_1 and a cladding of a slightly lower refractive index n_2 is known as *step index* fiber. This is because the refractive index profile for this type of fiber makes a step change at the core cladding index. The refractive index profile may be defined as:

$$n(r) = \begin{cases} n_1 & r \leq a \text{ (core)} \\ n_2 & r \geq a \text{ (cladding)} \end{cases}$$

in both cases.

- The wave equation, togther with the boundary conditions for cylindrical waveguides, describes the propagation of electromagnetic waves in *step-index* and *graded-index* optical fibers. Solving these equations for an ideal step-index fiber, under the weakly guiding approximation, gives a set of solutions:

$$\psi(r, \phi, z, t) = R(r)\,e^{il\phi}\,e^{i(\omega t - \beta z)}$$

where

$$R(r) = \begin{cases} A J_1\left(\dfrac{ur}{a}\right) & r < a \\ B K_1\left(\dfrac{wr}{a}\right) & r > a \end{cases}$$

The Bessel function $J_l(ur/a)$ are oscillatory in nature, and hence there exist m allowed solutions (corresponding to m roots of J_l) for each value of l. Thus, the propagation phase constant β is characterized by two integers l and m.

- The number of modes for smaller V and the propagation parameters for different modes can be found from the universal b versus V curves. However, for $V \gg 1$, the modal volumes for graded-index and step-index fibers may be calculated using the following approximate relations:

$$M_g = \frac{1}{2}\left(\frac{\alpha}{\alpha+2}\right)\left[\frac{2\pi a}{\lambda}\,(n_0^2 - n_c^2)^{1/2}\right]^2$$

$$\approx \left(\frac{\alpha}{\alpha+2}\right)\frac{V^2}{2} \tag{1}$$

and

$$M_s = \frac{1}{2}\left[\frac{2\pi a}{\lambda}\,(n_1^2 - n_2^2)^{1/2}\right]^2 \approx \frac{V^2}{2} \tag{2}$$

M_s allows an estimate of the number of guided modes propagating in a particular multimode step index fiber.

- The optical power is launched into a large number of guided modes, each having different spatial field distributions, propagation constants, etc. In an ideal multimode step index fiber with properties (i.e. relative index difference, core diameter) which are independent of distance, there is no mode coupling and the optical power launched into a particular mode remains in that mode and travels independently of the power launched into the other guided modes.

- *Graded-index fibers* do not have a constant refractive index in the core but a decreasing core index $n(r)$ with radial distance from a maximum value of n_1 at the axis to a constant value n_2 beyond the core radius a in the cladding. This index variation may be represented as:

$$n(r) = \begin{cases} n_1 \left(1 - 2\Delta \left(r/a\right)^\alpha\right)^{1/2} & r < a \, (\text{core}) \\ n_1 \left(1 - 2\Delta\right)^{1/2} & r \geq a \, (\text{cladding}) \end{cases}$$

where Δ is the relative refractive index difference and α is the profile parameter which gives the characteristic refractive index profile of the fiber core.

- For a parabolic refractive index profile fiber ($\alpha = 2$), total number of guided modes or volume $M_g \approx V^2/4$, which is half the number supported by a step index fiber ($\alpha = \infty$) with the same V value.

- The cutoff value of the normalized frequency V_c to support a single mode in a graded-index fiber is given by:

$$V_c = 2.405 \left(1 + \frac{2}{\alpha}\right)^{1/2}$$

Therefore, as in the step index case, it is possible to determine the fiber parameters which give single mode operation.

- For a step index fiber $V_c = 2.405$, the cutoff wavelength is given by:

$$\lambda_c = \frac{V\lambda}{2.405}$$

- Intermodal dispersion in multimode fibers restricts their use in long-haul communications.

REVIEW QUESTIONS

1. Explain the concept of electromagnetic modes in relation to a planar optical waveguide. Discuss the modification that may be made to electromagnetic mode theory in a planar waveguide in order to describe optical propagation in a cylindrical fiber.

2. Explain a plane TEM wave. How the wavelength of this wave change with the medium while propagating?

3. Write Maxwell's equations for the metallic and dielectric media and explain their significance.

4. Explain phase velocity and group velocity. Write expressions for these and explain the difference between them.

5. What is difference between propagation constant k, β and b? Find the interrelationship between them.

6. What do you understand by modes? Distinguish between symmetric and antisymmetric modes of a planar SI waveguide.

7. Derive the expression for the confinement factor,

$$G = \left[1 + \frac{\sin^2(ua)}{wa \left\langle 1 - \frac{\sin(ua)\cos(ua)}{ua} \right\rangle} \right]$$

for the antisymmetric TE modes of a symmetrical SI planar wavelength.

8. Mention the boundary conditions and assumptions made while solving the wave equation for an ideal step-index fiber. Also explain, how these conditions and assumptions are satisfied in a real optical fiber?

9. Define the normalized frequency for an optical fiber and explain its use in determination of the number of guided modes propagating within a step index fiber.

10. Explain, what is meant by graded index fiber, giving the expression for the possible refractive index profile?

11. What is difference between multimode step-index and graded index fibers and also between multimode and single mode fibers?

12. Explain the difference between the propagation phase constant β and the normalized propagation parameter b? Find the relation between two.

13. Derive the necessary expressions for the pulse broadening per unit length due to intermodal dispersion for a GI fiber with parabolic profile ($\alpha = 2$) and GI fiber with an optimum profile.

14. The transverse dependence of the modals:

$$\psi_z(r, \phi) = A J_l \left(\frac{ur}{a} \right) \begin{bmatrix} \cos(l\phi) : r < a \\ \sin(l\phi) \end{bmatrix}$$

and

$$\psi_z(r, \phi) = B K_l \left(\frac{wr}{a} \right) \begin{bmatrix} \cos(l\phi) : r > a \\ \sin(l\phi) \end{bmatrix}$$

give the axial components of E or H, i.e. E_z or H_z. Using the following relations, find the transverse components E_r, E_ϕ, H_r, and H_ϕ:

$$E_r = -\frac{i}{k_r^2} \left(\beta \frac{\partial E_z}{\partial r} + \omega\mu \frac{1}{r} \frac{\partial H_z}{\partial \phi} \right)$$

$$E_\phi = -\frac{i}{k_r^2} \left(\frac{\beta}{r} \frac{\partial E_z}{\partial \phi} - \omega\mu \frac{\partial H_z}{\partial r} \right)$$

$$H_r = -\frac{i}{k_r^2} \left(\beta \frac{\partial H_z}{\partial r} - \omega\varepsilon \frac{1}{r} \frac{\partial E_z}{\partial \phi} \right)$$

$$H_\phi = -\frac{i}{k_r^2} \left(\frac{\beta}{r} \frac{\partial H_z}{\partial \phi} + \omega\varepsilon \frac{\partial E_z}{\partial r} \right)$$

where K_r is the radial components of the propagation vector K in the waveguide and has an amplitude given by:

$$K_r = \sqrt{\omega^2 \varepsilon\mu - \beta^2}$$

15. Define the terms cutoff wavelength and dominant mode as applied to waveguides.

16. If the local numerical aperature (NA) of a graded-index fiber at a radial distance r is given by:

$$NA(r) = \left\{ n^2(r) - (n_c^2) \right\}^{1/2} \quad for\ r < a$$

then show that the *rms* value of the NA of the fiber for an α-profile (taken over the core area is given by the following relation:

$$(NA)_{rms} = \left[\left(\frac{\alpha}{\alpha + 2} \right) (n_0^2 - n_c^2) \right]^{1/2}$$

17. Explain the photonic crystal fiber (PCF) and also explain the guidance mechanisms for electromagnetic modes in such optical fibers.

18. Compare and contrast the performance attributors, potential drawbacks and possible applications of index-guided PCFs and photonic bandgap fibers.

PROBLEMS

1. A step index fiber has a solid acceptance angle in air of 0.115 radians and a relative refractive index difference of 0.9%. Calculate the speed of light in the fiber core.
   [**Ans.** $2.11 \times 10^8\ ms^{-1}$]

2. A step index fiber in air has a $NA = 0.16$, a core refractive index of 1.45 and a core diameter of 60 µm. Find the normalized frequency for the fiber when light as a wavelength of 0.9 µm is transmitted. Also estimate the number of guided modes propagating in the fiber. [**Ans.** 33.5, 561]

3. Perform a detailed analysis of the TM modes (which are characterized by the field components E_x, E_z, and H_y) of a symmetrical SI planar waveguide. [**B Tech**]
   [**Hint:** *Step (a)*: Substituting for E_x and E_z from Eqs (5.1) and (5.2) respectively, in Eq. (5.3), we obtain:

$$\beta \mu_y = -\varepsilon_0\, \omega n^2(x)\, E_x \tag{1}$$

$$\frac{\partial H_y}{\partial x} = i\varepsilon_0 \omega n^2(x)\, E_z \tag{2}$$

$$i\beta E_x + \frac{\partial E_z}{\partial x} = i\mu_0 \omega H_y \tag{3}$$

$$\frac{d^2 H_y}{dx^2} - \left[\frac{1}{n^2(x)} \frac{dn^2(x)}{dx} \right] \frac{dH_y}{dx} + [k^2 n^2(x) - \beta^2] H_y = 0$$

Step (b): Substitute for $n(x)$ in this equation in the region $|x| < a$ and $|x| > a$, to get two differential equations for the two regions.

Step (c): Apply the boundary conditions. Here H_y and E_z are tangenital components to the planes $x = \pm a$. Thus H_y and $[1/n^2(x)]\,(dH_y/dx)$ must be continuous at $x \pm a$.

Step (d): Write the solutions for symmetric and antisymmetric modes and arrive at the following transcendental equations:

$$ua \tan ua = \left(\frac{n_1}{n_2} \right)^2 wa \quad \text{for symmetric modes}$$

$$-ua \cot ua = \left(\frac{n_1}{n_2} \right)^2 wa \quad \text{for antisymmetric modes}$$

where the symbols have their usual meaning.

Step (e): Now, solve these equations graphically and discuss the results.]

4. A multimode graded index fiber has an acceptance angle in air of 8°. Estimate the relative refractive index difference between the core axis and the cladding when the refractive index at the core axis is 1.52. **[Ans. 0.42%]**

5. Calculate the maximum thickness of the guide slab of a symmetrical planar waveguide so that it supports the first 10 modes. Take $n_1 = 3.6$, $n_2 = 3.598$, and $\lambda = 0.90$ μm. Calculate also the maximum and minimum values of the propagation constant β. **[B Tech]**

[**Ans.** $2a = 11.875$ μm, $\beta_1 = 2.513 \times 10^5$ m^{-1}, $\beta_2 = 2.499 \times 10^5$ m^{-1}]

6. Calculate the G-factors for the modes supported by a planar waveguide whose layer has a thickness 6.523 μm, $n_1 = 1.50$, and $n_2 = 1.48$. The guide is excited by a light of wavelength $\lambda = 1.0$ mm. **[B Tech]**

[**Ans.** $G_0 = 0.98828$, $G_1 = 0.94889$, $G_2 = 0.85992$, $G_3 = 0.50960$]

7. A planar waveguide is formed from a 14 μm thick film of dielectric material of refractive index 1.46 sandwiched between two infinite dielectric slabs of refractive index 1.455. (a) Calculate the number of TE modes of propagation that the guide supports at a wavelength of 1.3 μm. (b) Estimate the propagation parameters u_m and w_m for different values of m and hence estimate b_m and β_m for each. **[B Tech]**

[**Ans.** (a) Three modes corresponding to $m = 0, 1$ and 2.

(b) Since $V = 4$, the abscissae of the intersecting points of the ua versus wa curves (see Fig. 5.3) for $m = 0, 1$ and 2 with the quadrant of a circle of radius $V = 4$ give the values of $u_m a$, and the corresponding ordinates give the values of $w_m a$. Similarly, from Fig. 5.5, one can get the values of b_m corresponding to $V = 4$. β_m can be obtained from:

$$\beta_m = \{\beta_2^2 + b_m (\beta_1^2 - \beta_2^2)\}^{1/2}, \text{ where } \beta_1 = 2\pi n_1/\lambda \text{ and } \beta_2 = 2\pi n_2 / \lambda.]$$

8. A multimode Si fiber has a core diameter of 50 μm, a core index of 1.46, and a relative refractive index difference of 1%. It is operating at a wavelength of 1.3 μm. Calculate (i) the refractive index of the cladding, (ii) the normalized frequency parameter V, and (iii) the total number of modes guided by the fiber. **[B Tech]**

[**Ans.** (i) 1.445, (ii) 25, (iii) 312]

9. The cutoff wavelength of a step index fiber is quoted as $\lambda_c = 1.20$ μm. If the fiber is operated at wavelength $\lambda = 1.55$ μm, what is normalized frequency or V number? **[B Tech]**

[**Hint:** $V = 2.405 \dfrac{\lambda_c}{\lambda} = 2.405 \dfrac{1.20}{1.55} = 1.86$]

11. A graded-index single-mode fiber has a core axis refractive index of 1.5, a triangular index profile ($\alpha = 1$) in the core, and a relative index difference of 1.3%. Calculate the core diameter of the fiber if it has to transmit (i) $\lambda = 1.3$ μm and (ii) l = 1.55 μm.

[**Ans.** (i) 7.1 μm, (ii) 8.5 μm]

12. It is reported that the effective number of modes guided by a curved multimode GI fiber of radiu a is given by:

$$(M_g)_{eff} = (M_g)\left[1 - \frac{(\alpha + 2)}{2\alpha\Delta}\left\{\frac{2a}{R} + \left(\frac{3}{2n_c kR}\right)^{2/3}\right\}\right]$$

where α is the profile parameter, Δ is the relative refractive index difference, n_c is the refractive index of the cladding, $k = 2\pi/\lambda$, and M_g is the total number of guided modes in a single fiber are given by:

$$M_g \cong \frac{\alpha}{\alpha+2} \frac{V^2}{2}$$

Calculate the radius of curvature R such that the effective number of guided model reduces to half its maximum value. Take $\alpha = 2$, $n_c = 1.48$, $\Delta = 0.01$, $a = 50$ μm, and $\lambda = 0.85$ μm. **[M Tech]**

[Ans. R ≈ 1.66 cm]

13. The refractive indices of the core and cladding of a SI fiber are 1.48 and 1.465, respectively. Light of wavelength 0.85 μm is guided through it. Calculate the minimum and maximum values of the propagation phase constant β. **[B.Tech.]**

[Ans. 10.82×10^6 m^{-1}, 10.93×10^6 m^{-1}]

14. The velocity of light in the core of a step index fiber is 2.01×10^8 ms^{-1}, and the critical angle at the core–cladding interface is 80°. Find the NA and the acceptance angle for the fiber in air. Assume that it has a core diameter suitable for consideration by ray analysis. Take $c = 3 \times 10^8$ ms^{-1} in vacuum. **[Ans. 0.263, 15.2°]**

15. A graded-index fiber with a triangular profile supports the propagation of 500 modes. The core axis refractive index is 1.46 and the core diameter is 75 μm. If the wavelength of light propagating through the fiber is 1.3 μm, calculate (a) the relative refractive index difference Δ of the fiber and (b) the maximum diameter of the fiber core which would give single-mode operation at the same wavelength. **[B Tech]**

[Ans. (a) 0.021, (b) 5.76 μm]

16. A graded-index fiber has a core diameter of 40 μm, $\alpha = 2$, $n_0 = 1.460$, and $n_c = 1.445$. If it is excited by a source of $\lambda = 1.3$ μm, calculate (a) (NA)$_{rms}$; (b) β_0, Δ, and V; and (c) the total number of propagating modes.

[Ans. (a) 0.1476, (b) 7056 mm^{-1}, 0.0102, 25.23, (c) 159]

17. A multimode step index fiber has a relative refractive index difference of 1% and a core refractive index of 1.5. The number of modes propagating at a wavelength of 1.3 μm is 1100. Find the diameter of the fiber core. **[B Tech]**

[Ans. 92 μm]

18. The relative refractive index difference between the core axis and the cladding of a graded index fiber is 7% when the refractive index at the core axis is 1.45. Calculate NA of the fiber when:

(a) the index profile is not taken into account; and

(b) the index profile is taken to be triangular.

Comment on the results. **[MSc (Ele)]**

[Ans. (a) 0.172, (b) 0.171]

19. The V-number of a step-index fiber operating at 1330 nm is 50. Estimate the number of modes that propagate through the fiber.

[Hint: The number of modes in the step-index fiber can be obtained as

$$M \approx \frac{V^2}{2} = \frac{(50)^2}{2} = 1250]$$

20. A step-index optical fiber with a core radius of 4.6 mm has a core refractive index of $n_1 = 1.465$ and index deviation of $\Delta = 0.2\%$. Estimate the cut-off wavelength for the fiber to exhibit single mode operation.

[**Hint:** The product of normalized frequency of V-number of the fiber and the wavelength of operation i.e., $V\lambda$ can be obtained from the relation

$$V\lambda = 2\pi a \left(n_1^2 - n_2^2\right)^{\frac{1}{2}} \approx 2\pi a n_1 \sqrt{2\Delta}$$

$$= 2 \times 3.14 \times 4.6 \times 10^{-6} \times 1.465 \times \sqrt{2 \times 0.002} = 2.677 \times 10^{-6}$$

The cut-off wavelength can be estimated from the relation on

$$\lambda_c = \frac{V\lambda}{2.405}$$

$$\lambda_c = \frac{2.677 \times 10^{-6}}{2.405} = 1113 \text{ nm }]$$

21. Calculate the number of modes in a graded-index fiber with a parabolic index profile operating at 1330 nm. The axial refractive index of the fiber is $n_1 = 1.49$ and that the core-cladding interface is $n_2 = 1,.47$. The core radius of the fiber is 25 mm. How many modes will be supported by a corresponding SI fiber at this wavelength?

[PTU, RTU]

[**Hint:** The value of the index deviation, D of the fiber can be estimated as

$$\Delta = \frac{n_1 - n_2}{n_1} = \frac{1.49 - 1.47}{1.49} = 0.013$$

Therefore, the number of modes supported by the parabolic index GI fiber can be estimated as

$$(M_{GI})_{\text{parabolic}} = (25 \times 10^{-6})^2 \left(\frac{2 \times 3.14}{1330 \times 10^{-9}}\right)(1.49)^2 (0.013)\left(\frac{2}{4}\right) \approx 201$$

The number of modes supported by a corresponding step-index fiber would be

$$M_{SI} \approx 2 \times 201 = 402.]$$

SHORT ANSWER QUESTIONS

1. Write the Maxwell's relations for a medium with zero conductivity.

Ans. $\nabla \times E = -\dfrac{\partial B}{\partial t}$

$\nabla \times H = -\dfrac{\partial D}{\partial t}$

$\nabla \cdot D = 0$ (no free charges)

$\nabla \cdot B = 0$ (no free poles)

2. What is a planar guide?

Ans. A planar guide is the simplest form of optical waveguide. One may assume it consists of a slab of dielectric with refractive index n_1 sandwitched between two regions of lower refractive index n_2.

3. Write the wave equation in an isotropic and homogeneous dielectric medium.

Ans. $\nabla^2 \psi - \dfrac{n^2}{c^2}\dfrac{\partial^2 \psi}{\partial t^2} = 0$

where ψ represents the scalar field components of **E** and **H**. The solution of above equation is of the form:

$$\psi = \psi_0 \exp[i\,(\omega t - \beta z)]$$

where the symbols have usual meaning.

4. What are phase and group velocities?

Ans. Within all electromagnetic waves, whether plane or otherwise, there are points of constant phase. For plane waves these constant phase points form a surface which is referred to as a wavefront. As a monochromatic light wave propagates along a waveguide in the z-direction these points of constant phase travel at a phase velocity V_p given by:

$$V_p = \omega/\beta$$

where ω is the angular frequency of the wave. However, it is impossible in practice to produce perfectly monochromatic light waves, and light energy is generally composed of a sum of plane wave components of different frequencies. Often the situation exists where a group of waves with closely similar frequencies propagate so that their resultant forms a *packet of waves*. This wave packet does not travel at the phase velocity of the individual waves but is observed to move at a group velocity of V_g given by:

$$V_g = \frac{\delta\omega}{\delta\beta}$$

The group velocity is of greatest importance in the study of transmission characteristics of optical fibers as it relates the propogation characteristics of observable wave groups or packets of light.

If propagation in an infinite medium of refractive index n_1 is considered, then the propagation constant may be written as:

$$\beta = n_1 \frac{2\pi}{\lambda} = n_1 \frac{\omega}{c}$$

Now,

$$V_p = \frac{c}{n_1}$$

Further, in the limit $\delta\omega/\delta\beta$ becomes, the group velocity:

$$V_g = \frac{d\lambda}{d\beta} \cdot \frac{d\omega}{d\lambda} = \frac{d}{d\lambda}\left(n_1 \frac{2\pi}{\lambda}\right)^{-1}\left(-\frac{\omega}{\lambda}\right)$$

$$= -\frac{\omega}{2\pi\lambda}\left(\frac{1}{\lambda}\frac{dn_1}{d\lambda} - \frac{n_1}{\lambda^2}\right)^{-1}$$

$$= \frac{c}{\left(n_1 - n\dfrac{dn_1}{dl}\right)} = \frac{c}{N_g}$$

where N_g is group index of the guide.

5. Explain the importance of the choice of cladding material.

Ans. (i) The cladding should be transparent to light at the wavelength over which the guide is to operate.

(ii) Ideally, the cladding should consist of a solid material in order to avoid both damage to the guide and accumulation of foreign matter on the guide walls. These effects degrade the reflection process by interaction with the evanescent field. This in part explains the poor performance (high losses) of early optical waveguides with air cladding.

(iii) The cladding thickness must be sufficient to allow the evanescent field to decay to a low value or losses from the penetrating energy may be encountered. In many cases, however, the magnitude of the field falls off rapidly with distance from the guide-cladding interface. This may occur within distances equivalent to a few wavelengths of the transmitted light. Therefore, the most widely used optical fibers consist of a core and cladding, both made of glass. The cladding refractive index is thus higher than would be the case with liquid or gaseous cladding giving a lower NA for the fiber, but it provides a far more practical solution.

6. What is *Goos-Haenchen* shift?

   Ans. The phase change incurred with the total internal reflection of light beam on a planar dielectric interface may be understood from physical observation. Careful examination shows that the reflected beam is shifted laterally from the trajectory predicted by simple ray theory analysis. This lateral displacement is known as the Goos-Haenchen shift.

7. What is physical interpretation of mode number *m*?

   Ans. The mode number *m* denotes the number of half-cycles of the electric field (for TE modes) or magnetic field (for TM modes) that occur over the transverse dimension. The lowest order mode ($m = 1$) is seen to have no cutoff – it will propagate from zero frequency on up. One will thus achieve single-mode operation (actually a single pair of TE and TM modes) if we can assure that $m = 2$ modes are below cutoff.

8. Write the equations for the modes of wave equation in an isotropic and inhomogeneous dielectric medium.

   Ans.

   $$\left.\begin{aligned} \beta E_y &= \mu_0 \omega H_x \\ \frac{\partial E_y}{\partial x} &= -i\mu_0 \omega H_z \\ -i\beta H_x - \frac{\partial H_z}{\partial x} &= i\varepsilon_0 \omega n^2(x)\, E_y \end{aligned}\right\} \text{TE modes}$$

   $$\left.\begin{aligned} \beta H_y &= -\varepsilon_0 \omega n^2(x)\, E_x \\ \frac{\partial H_y}{\partial x} &= -i\varepsilon_0 \omega n^2(x)\, E_z \\ i\beta E_x + \frac{\partial E_z}{\partial x} &= i\mu_0 \omega\, H_y \end{aligned}\right\} \text{TM modes}$$

9. What is normalized frequency?

   Ans. $V = ka\,(n_1^2 - n_2^2)^{1/2}$

   $$= \frac{2\pi}{\lambda} a\,(n_1^2 - n_2^2)^{1/2}$$

   $$= \frac{2\pi}{\lambda} a\,(NA) = \frac{2\pi}{\lambda} an_1\,(2\Delta)$$

The normalized frequency is a dimensionless parameter and hence is also sometimes simply called the *V* number or value of the fiber. It combines in a very useful manner the information about three important design variables for the fiber: namely, the core radius *a*, the relative refractive index difference Δ and the operating wavelength λ.

10. How waveguide perturbations affect the propagation characteristics of the fiber?

Ans. Waveguide perturbations such as deviations of the fiber axis from straightness, variations in the core diameter, irregularities at the core-cladding interface and refractive index variations may change the propagation characteristics of the fiber. These will have the effect of coupling energy travelling in one mode to another depending on the specific perturbation.

11. Write the advantages of multimode fibers over single mode fibers for lower band applications.

Ans. The advantages are:

(i) the use of spatially incoherent optical sources (e.g. most light emitting diodes) which cannot be efficiently coupled to single-mode fibers;

(ii) larger NAs, as well as core diameters, facilitating coupling to optical sources.

(iii) lower tolerance requirements on fiber connectors.

12. What are graded index fibers?

Ans. These do not have a constant refractive index in the core (this is why they are sometimes referred to as inhomogeneous core fibers) but a decreasing core index $n(r)$ with radial distance from a maximum value of n_1 at the axis to a constant value n_2 beyond the core radius a in the cladding. This index variation may be represented as:

$$n(r) = \begin{cases} n_1 \left[1 - 2\Delta \left(\dfrac{r}{a} \right)^{\alpha} \right]^{1/2} & r < a \text{ (core)} \\ n_1 (1 - 2\Delta)^{1/2} = n_2 & r \geq a \text{ (cladding)} \end{cases}$$

where Δ is the relative refractive index difference and α is the profile parameter which gives the characteristic refractive index profile of the fiber core.

13. What is the advantage of the propagation of a single mode within an optical fiber?

Ans. The signal dispersion caused by the delay differences between different modes in a multimode fiber may be avoided.

14. What are the reasons that single-mode fibers emerge as a viable communication medium and most widely used fiber type within telecommunications?

Ans. (i) They exhibit the greatest transmission bandwidths and the lowest losses of the fiber transmission media.

(ii) They have a superior transmission quality over other fiber types because of the absence of the modal noice.

(iii) They offer a substantial upgrade cabpability (i.e. future proofing) for future wide bandwidth services using either faster optical transmitters and receivers or advanced transmission techniques (e.g. coherent technology).

(iv) They are compatible with the developing integrated optics technology.

15. What is cutoff wavelength?

Ans. The single-mode operation only occurs above a theoretical cutoff wavelength λ_c given by:

$$\lambda_c = \frac{2\pi a n_1}{V_c} (2\Delta)^{1/2}$$

where V_c is the cutoff normalized frequency. Hence λ_c is the wavelength above which a particular fiber become single-moded. Thus, we have:

$$\frac{\lambda_c}{\lambda} = \frac{V}{V_c}$$

For step index fiber $V_c = 2.405$, the cutoff wavelength is given by:

$$\lambda_c = \frac{V\lambda}{2.405}$$

16. Write the design formula for obtaining a single mode fiber and explain its significance

Ans. $V = \dfrac{2\pi a}{\lambda}\left(n_1^2 - n_2^2\right) \le 2.405$

Under this condition, the optical fiber would behave as a single mode provided for given values of a, n_1 and n_2 the wavelength of the light can be so adjusted as to satisfy the above condition. Alternatively, for given values of n_1, n_2 and λ the radius of the core can be so adjusted as to satisfy the above condition allowing the fiber to support only one mode.

17. What is mode-field diameter (MFD)?

Ans. The effective value of core diameter is referred to as mode-field diameter of the fiber. We can see that the physical diameter of the core is always less than the MFD. The actual value of the MFD depends on the distribution of electric field for fundamental mode. In a multimode fiber the power mainly flow through the core region and very little fraction flows through the cladding region. From this point of view, we may consider MFD analogous to the core diameter of a multimode fiber in the sense that beyond MFD the power flowing in the remaining cladding region is negligibly small.

MULTIPLE CHOICE QUESTIONS

1. In a waveguide, suffix *mn* of the modes TE/TM denotes:
   (a) half wavelength of E field and full wavelength of H field
   (b) half wavelengths of E and H fields in directions other than guide axis
   (c) full wavelength of E field and half wavelength of H field
   (d) half wavelength of E and H fields

2. In a symmetrical SI planar waveguide, the refractive index of the guide layer is $n_1 = 1.5$ and $\Delta = 0.001$. If the thickness of the guide layer is 8.5 µm, for what wavelength will the guide support only a fundamental mode?   **[B Tech]**
   (a) 0.85 µm   (b) 1.14 µm
   (c) 1.36 µm   (d) 1.55 µm

3. A symmetrical SI planar waveguide is to be excited by a source of central wavelength $\lambda = 0.85$ µm. Assume that $n_1 = 1.5$ and $\Delta = 0.01$. What should be the thickness of the guide layer so that it supports one symmetric and one antisymmetric TE mode?   **[B Tech]**
   (a) 4.00 µm   (b) 6.00 µm
   (c) 10.00 µm   (d) 12.00 µm

4. For a given guided mode, the normalized propagation constant lies between:
   (a) $-\infty$ and $+\infty$ (b) 0 and ∞
   (c) 0 and 1   (d) -1 and $+1.5$

5. The range of the phase propagation constant $(\beta_2 < \beta < \beta_1)$ for a wave guided by a planar waveguide can be obtained if the following is known:
   (a) wavelength of the excitation source
   (b) refractive index of the guide layer

(c) refractive index of the cladding slabs

(d) all of the abve

6. Which of the following relation for NA is correct:
   (a) $NA = n_1 (2\Delta)$
   (b) $NA = n_1 (2\Delta)^{\frac{1}{2}}$
   (c) $NA = n_1^{\frac{1}{2}} (2\Delta)$
   (d) $NA = n_1^2 (2\Delta)^{\frac{1}{2}}$

7. Inside an ideal dielectric medium:
   (a) the free charge density ρ is zero but the conductivity σ is nonzero
   (b) ρ is nonzero and σ is zero
   (c) both ρ and σ are zero
   (d) both ρ and σ are nonzero

8. For symmetric TE modes supported by symmetrical SI planar waveguide, the stable electric-field distribution inside the guide layer takes: **[B Tech]**
   (a) a sinusoidal form
   (b) a cosinusoidal form
   (c) an exponential form
   (d) a tangential form

9. The maximum number of TE modes supported by a symmetrical SI planar waveguide is an integer greater than:
   (a) $2V/\pi$
   (b) $V/2\pi$
   (c) $2\pi V$
   (d) zero

10. The relation between the group velocity V_g and group index (N_g) of the guide is:
    (a) $V_g = \dfrac{c}{N_g}$
    (b) $V_g = \dfrac{c}{\sqrt{N_g}}$
    (c) $V_g = c N_g$
    (d) $V_g = \dfrac{c}{N_g^{3/2}}$

11. Mode volume or total number of guided modes M_s for a step index fiber is related to V value for the fiber by the approximate expression:
    (a) $M_s \simeq \dfrac{V}{2}$
    (b) $M_s \simeq \dfrac{V^3}{2}$
    (c) $M_s \simeq \dfrac{V^2}{2}$
    (d) $M_s = 2V^2$

12. For a typical symmetrical SI planar waveguide, the value of the V-parameter is 5. The guide which supports the following TE modes?
    (a) Two symmetric and three antisymmetric
    (b) Three symmetric and two antisymmetric
    (c) Two symmetric and two antisymmetric
    (d) One symmetric and one antisymmetric[B.Tech.]

13. The electric-field distribution $E_y(x)$ in a planar waveguide corresponding to the $m = 3$ TE mode will have the following number of zeros between $x = -a$ and $x = +a$. **[B Tech]**
    (a) Three
    (b) Two
    (c) One
    (d) Five

14. In a planar waveguide, for a typical mode, 70% of its total power remains in the guide layer and the remaining 30% extends into the cladding slabs. Its confinement factor for the mode is:
    (a) 0.40
    (b) 0.60
    (c) 0.70
    (d) 1.00

15. The effective refractive index (n_{eff}) or phase index or normalized phase change coefficient for single-mode fiber bear the following relation with the propagation constant of the fundamental mode (β) and vacuum propagation constant (k):

    (a) $n_{\text{eff}} = \beta k$

    (b) $n_{\text{eff}} = \dfrac{k}{\beta}$

    (c) $n_{\text{eff}} = \dfrac{\beta}{k}$

    (d) $n_{\text{eff}} = \sqrt{\dfrac{\beta}{k}}$

16. A step-index fiber has a core of refractive index 1.5 and a cladding of refractive index 1.49. The core diameter is 100 μm. How many guided modes are supported by the fiber if the wavelength of light is 0.85 μm?

    (a) 380

    (b) 870

    (c) 1160

    (d) 2040

17. A graded-index fiber has a triangular profile with $n_0 = 1.48$ and $\Delta = 0.02$. If it is excited by a source of $\lambda = 1.0$ μm, what is the range of phase propagation constants for the modes supported by the fiber? **[B Tech]**

    (a) 3.438–5.327 μm^{-1}

    (b) 5.289–7.142 μm^{-1}

    (c) 6.315–8.342 μm^{-1}

    (d) 8.620–9.299 μm^{-1}

18. If the core diameter of the fiber of Question 17 is 50 μm, what is the value of the normalized frequency parameter? **[B Tech]**

    (a) 19.61

    (b) 26.53

    (c) 31.41

    (d) 50.72

19. For any multimode optical fiber, what is the range of the normalized propagation parameter?

    (a) 0–1

    (b) 1–10

    (c) Cannot be calculated unless λ is known

    (d) Cannot be calculated unless the profile parameter is known

20. Single mode operation only occurs above a theoretical cutoff wavelength λ_c given by $\lambda_c = \dfrac{2\pi a n_1}{V_c}(2\Delta)^{1/2}$. For step index fiber V_c is equal to:

    (a) 1

    (b) 1.5

    (c) 2.405

    (d) 4

21. The relationship between the effective refractive index (n_{eff}) and the normalized propagation constant (b) (b is a dimensionless parameter varies between 0 and 1) is:

    (a) $b \approx n_{\text{eff}}$

    (b) $b \approx (n_{\text{eff}} - n_2)$

    (c) $b \approx \dfrac{n_{\text{eff}} - n_2}{n_1 - n_2}$

    (d) $b \approx \dfrac{n_{\text{eff}} + n_2}{n_1 + n_2}$

22. For the optical fiber of Question 18, what is the total number of modes supported by the fiber?

    (a) 94

    (b) 164

    (c) 208

    (d) 500

23. In a step-index fiber, what is the cut-off frequency of the LP_{11} mode?

    (a) 0.0

    (b) 2.405

    (c) 5.832

    (d) 8.520

24. A GI fiber with a parabolic profile has an axial refractive index of 1.46 and D of 0.5%. What is the pulse broadening per unit length due to intermodal dispersion? **[B Tech]**

(a) 50.4 mm/km

(b) 60.8 ns/km

(c) 60.8 ps/km

(d) Zero

25. In a multimode SI fiber, the higher order modes propagate within the fiber with:
    (a) lower group velocity than the lower order modes
    (b) higher group velocity than the lower order modes
    (c) same group velocity as that of lower order modes
    (d) random group velocity

26. An unclad fiber with a core refractive index of 1.46 and core diameter of 60 μm is placed in air. What is the normalized frequency for the fiber when light of wavelength 0.85 Δm is transmitted through it?
    (a) 70.74

    (b) 108.23

    (c) 221.65

    (d) 375.02

27. A 0.5 mm thick slab of glass ($n_1 = 1.45$) is surrounded by air ($n_2 = 1$). The slab guides infrared light at wavelength $\lambda = 1.0$ μm. TE and TM modes propagte will be:
    (a) 1100

    (b) 1550

    (c) 2102

    (d) 2505

28. The cutoff wavelength of a step index fiber is quoted as $\lambda_c = 1.20$ μm. If the fiber is operated at wavelength $\lambda = 1.55$ μm, then V is:
    (a) 1.1

    (b) 1.4

    (c) 1.86

    (d) 2.1

[**Hint:** $V = 2.405 \dfrac{\lambda_c}{\lambda} = 2.405 \left(\dfrac{1.20}{1.55} \right) = 1.86$)

29. The condition for single-mode operation in a step index fiber is:

(a) $\lambda > \lambda_c = \dfrac{2\pi a}{2.405} (n_1 - n_2)^{1/2}$

(b) $\lambda > \lambda_c = \dfrac{2\pi a}{2.405} (n_1^2 - n_2^2)^{1/3}$

(c) $\lambda > \lambda_c = \dfrac{2\pi a}{2.405} (n_1^2 - n_2^2)^{1/2}$

(d) $\lambda > \lambda_c = \dfrac{2\pi a}{2.405} (n_1 + n_2)$

ANSWERS

1. (b) 2. (b) 3. (b) 4. (c) 5. (d) 6. (b) 7. (c) 8. (b) 9. (a) 10. (a)
11. (c) 12. (c) 13. (a) 14. (c) 15. (c) 16. (d) 17. (d) 18. (c) 19. (a) 20. (c)
21. (c) 22. (b) 23. (b) 24. (c) 25. (a) 26. (c) 27. (c) 28. (c) 29. (c)

6

Transmission Characteristics of Optical Fibers

6.1 INTRODUCTION

In Chapters 3, 4 and 5, the basic structure and fundamental aspects of light waves propagating in optical fibers were treated, in particular, single mode fiber (SMF), which form the basic structure for standard communication transmission systems. This chapter deals with the transmission of optical signals transmitted through optical fibers, namely *attenuation* (or loss) and the *dispersion* effects.

Attenuation and dispersion are the two most important effects that play a major role in optical fiber transmission systems. *Attenuation limits the optical power transmitted through the fiber while dispersion restricts the bandwidth or rate at which data can be transmitted through the fiber*. For very low attenuation, dispersion limits the repeater spacing below what would be possible from the attenuation factor.

The fiber loss has been reduced from 100 dB/km (i.e. transmission possible over only a few meters) at 1300 nm in 1970 to about 0.25 and 0.15 dB/km, which are very close to the theoretically possible transparent limits and transmission over several hundreds of kilometers of fibers, at 1300 and 1550 nm wavelength regions, respectively, in 1980.

The dispersion of light causes temporal spreading of optical pulses and subsequently restricts the rate at which data in the form of optical pulses can be transmitted through the optical fiber. The dispersion and pulse broadening of optical fibers have also been reduced due to "*smart design*" of optical fiber structures. In the early 1970s, we saw a remarkable development of theories for understanding lightwave guiding in optical fibers of *multimode* types. The breakthrough in the reduction of loss in the optical fibers and the ability to manfacture optical fibers with a very small core diameter led to the design of SMF. The remarkable theoretical development of optical waveguiding in a "weakly guided" (i.e. a very small difference between the core and cladding regions) fiber structure led to a *plane-wavelike transmission* of lightwaves. SMFs provide extremely low dispersion making them very attractive for long haul optical communication. Special types of optical fibers such as *graded-index multimode fibers* can be designed in a suitable manner to enhance the bandwidth (or bit rate) as compared to conventional step-index optical fibers. Extensive research in the field has led to substantial improvements, giving wideband fiber bandwidths of many tens of gigahertz over a number of kilometers. Further, the availability of narrow-linewidth lasers allowed system engineers to design and implement several high-speed, long-distance fiber-optic communication systems.

In order to appreciate these advances and possible future developments in the field of fiber optic communication, the optical transmission characteristics of the fibers have to be considered in greater depth. In the present chapter, we discuss the mechanisms within optical fibers which give rise to major transmission characteristics namely attenuation and dispersion and perhaps less obvious effects, e.g. modal noise, polarization and nonlinear phenomena.

6.2 ATTENUATION

The attenuation or transmission loss in an optical fiber, primarily decides the maximum transmission distance, i.e. the distance between the optical transmitter and the receiver without using any repeaters, which generally restores the signal at intermediate points in a long haul communication system. Extremely low loss of optical fibers ($\sim$ 1 dB/km) made optical fiber communication more attractive as compared to conventional electrical communication systems based on metallic conductor cables which generally offer attenuation in the range of 3–5 dB/km.

Under general conditions of power attenuation inside an optical fiber, the attenuation coefficient of the optical power P, can be expressed as

$$\frac{dP}{dz} = -\alpha P \tag{6.1}$$

where α is the attenuation coefficient. This attenuation coefficient can include all effects of power loss when signals are transmitted through the optical fibers.

Considering optical signals with an average optical power, $P(o)$, entering at the input of the fiber length, L (z-direction), and the output optical power, $P(z)$, in relation to the attenuation coefficient α, we have

$$P(z) = P(o) \exp(-\alpha_n z) \tag{6.2}$$

where α_n is the attenuation coefficient of the optical fiber which is a function of wavelength, given by

$$\alpha_n = \frac{1}{z} \log\left[\frac{P(o)}{P(z)}\right] \tag{6.3}$$

The power ratio in *neper* (N) is expressed as

$$N = \frac{1}{2} \log\left[\frac{P(o)}{P(z)}\right] \tag{6.4}$$

Accordingly, one can express the product $2z\alpha_n$ can be expressed in terms of *nepers*.

It is customary to express α in dB/km using relation

$$\alpha(\text{dB/km}) = \frac{10}{L} \log_{10}\left[\frac{P(o)}{P(L)}\right]$$

$$= 4.343 \, \alpha \tag{6.5}$$

where L is the length (as stated above) along which the fiber traversed by the light. In terms of power ratio, Eq. (6.5) may be written as

$$\frac{P(o)}{P(L)} = 10^{\alpha L (dB)/10} \tag{6.6}$$

For an ideal fiber, we have $P(z) = P(o)$, because there is no attenuation. We may note that practical optical fibers are generally passive components (excepting active fibers) in the sense that optical power decreases as it propagates through the fiber, i.e. $P(z) < P(o)$. However, in order to obtain attenuation (in dB) as a positive quality, usually the ratio is expressed in terms of the input to output powers. Obviously, Eq. (6.6) is convenient to convert the attenuation or loss from dB to simple power ratio.

Generally, optical power is expressed in terms of dBm which corresponds to *decibel power* with respect to 1 mW reference power. Thus, power in dBm can be expressed as

$$\text{Power (in dBm)} = 10 \log \left(\frac{P}{1\,\text{mW}} \right) \tag{6.7}$$

When $P = 1$ mW, the power in dBm corresponds to zero, i.e.

$$1 \text{ mW} = 0 \text{ dBm} \tag{6.8}$$

Standard optical fibers with a small Δ would exhibit a loss of about 0.2 dB/km, i.e. the purity of silica is very high. Such purity of a bar of silica would allow us to see through a 1 km glass bar, without distortion, a person standing at the other end.

A number of mechanisms are responsible for the signal attenuation in optical fibers. These mechanisms are influenced by the material composition, the preparation and purification technique, and the wavelength structure. These may be categorized within several major areas which include material absorption, material scattering (linear and nonlinear scattering), curve and microbending losses, mode coupling radiation losses and losses due to leaky modes.

The principal material used for making optical fiber is glass. A good quality single mode fiber exhibits an attenuation of 0.5 dB/km at 1300 nm and an attenuation as low as 0.3 dB/km at 1550. However, all practical optical fibers generally exhibit attenuation peak corresponding to OH⁻ ion absorption around 1400 nm. Figures 6.1(a) and 6.1(b) shows a typical plot of attenuation versus wavelength for a standard glass optical fiber.

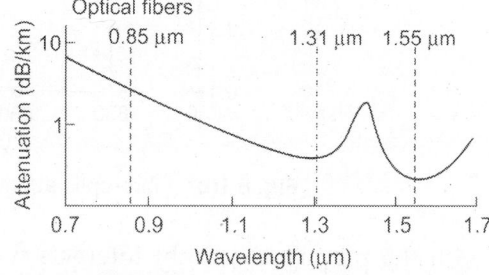

Fig. 6.1(a): Attenuation vs wavelength of a typical glass fiber exhibiting major attenuation windows and absorption peak caused by water molecules

6.3 ABSORPTION LOSS

Basically, it is a mechanism by which the light energy is lost in the propagating medium through a variety of processes. We know that light in the form of photons transfers their energy to electrons or constituent atoms of the material. Generally, the absorption of light in optical fibers is classified as *intrinsic* (caused by the interaction with one or more of the major components of the glass) or *extrinsic* (caused by impurities within glass).

6.3.1 Intrinsic Absorption

This refers to the absorption caused by basic fiber material, e.g. SiO_2, when it is in the purest form, i.e. does not contain any impurities or imperfection. We may note that this is the fundamental transmission limit of the material and no practical fiber made of this material can exhibit lower attenuation than that caused by intrinsic absorption. Basically, there are following two intrinsic absorption mechanisms:

(i) *Electron absorption*: This process involves absorption of photon that results into excitation of electron from the valence band to the conduction band of glass. The amorphous glass is an insulator having a large band gap. When a photon associated

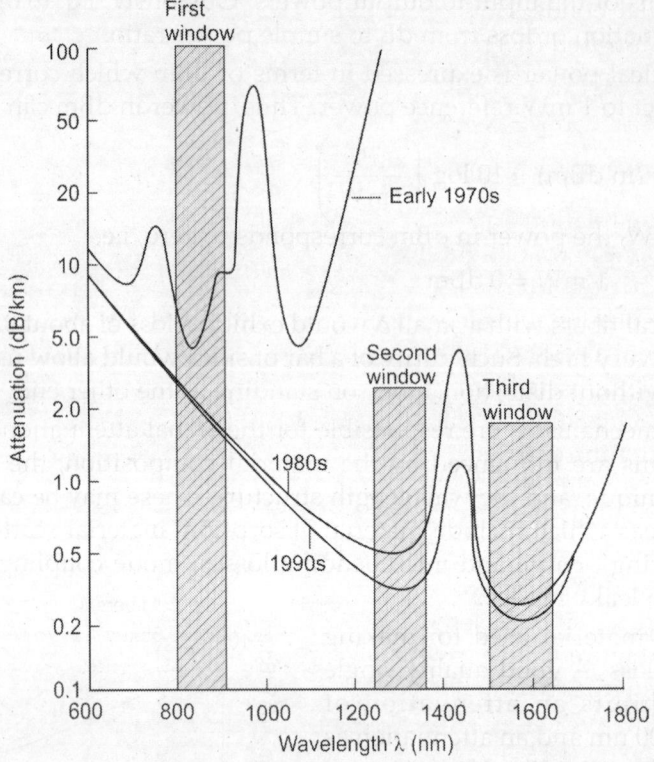

Fig. 6.1(b): Fibre-optic attenuation as a function of wavelength (λ)

with the propagating light interacts with an electron in the valence band, electronic absorption of photon takes place and transfer its energy to the electron so as to excite its energy to the electron so as to excite its higher energy state in the conduction band. Due to large bandgap, this type of absorption needs a relatively high energy photon. However, this absorption is significant in ultraviolet (UV) region (high frequency or small wavelength). The UV absorption near the absorption edge is governed by the following empirical relation

$$\alpha_{av} = C \exp (h\nu/E_0) \tag{6.9}$$

where C and E_0 are empirical constants and $h\nu$ is the energy of the photon, h is Planck's constant ($h = 6.62 \times 10^{-34}$ Js). The frequency ν of the photon is given by

$$\nu = c/\lambda \tag{6.10}$$

From Eq. (6.10), it is clear that as the wavelength of light increases, the frequency as well energy ($E = h\nu$) decreases and as a consequence absorption decreases exponentially (Fig. 6.1).

Various impurities that also lead to spurious absorption effects in the wavelength range of interest (1.2–1.6 μm) are transition metal ions and water in the form of OH ions. However, these sources of absorption have been practically reduced in recent years.

(ii) *Atomic absorption*: This is basically associated with the characteristic vibrational frequency of the chemical bond involving the constituent atoms of the material. At a particular temperature, the molecular bond vibrate with a certain characteristic frequency (ν). When light in the form of an electromagnetic wave propagates through the material, at some frequency, the former loses energy by transferring its energy to the vibrating molecular bonds. However, the loss of energy by this mechanism is generally significant in the infrared (IR) region and is manifested in the form of attenuation caused by absorption at atomic level. The IR absorption loss is governed by the relation

$$\alpha_{IR} = C \exp(-D/\lambda) \tag{6.11}$$

where C and D are empirical constants.

We can see from relation Eq. (6.11) that with increase in wavelength (λ) of light the loss due to atomic absorption increases very fast. However, the absorption wavelength depends on the constitutent bonds. The fundamental absorption wavelengths in high quality silica glass for B–O, P–O, Si–O and GeO bonds are reported in the literature to be 7.3, 8.0, 9.0 and 11.0 μm respectively. Figure 6.2 shows that the loss due to atomic absorption in the NIR region (below 1.7 μm) is very low. Basically, this is the primary reason behind the use of NIR (0.7–1.6 μm) band for silica based optical fiber communication. Figure 6.3 clearly shows that at optical wavelengths, two major absorption intrinsic mechanisms leave a low intrinsic absorption window over 0.8–1.7 μm wavelength range, which shows a possible optical attenuation against wavelength characteristic for absolute pure glass.

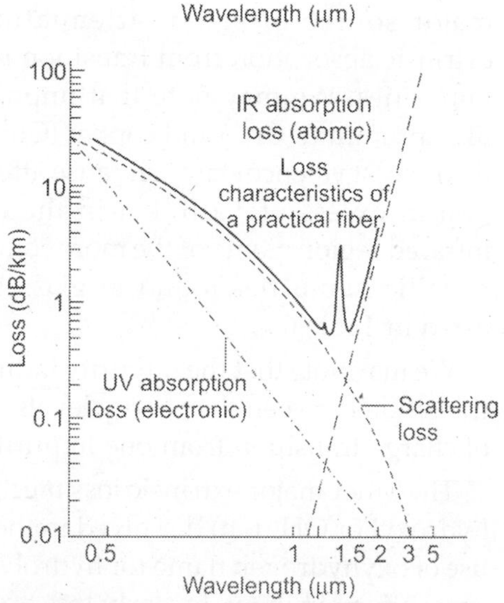

By changing the composition of glass, the absorption of optical signal by atomic and electronic absorption can be reduced significantly. Optical fibers based on heavy metal halides have been found to exhibit very low loss even far beyond the mid IR regions.

Fig. 6.2: The contribution of intrinsic absorption loss in the UV and IR region alongwith scattering loss due to Rayleigh scattering vis-a-vis measured loss in a practical optical fiber

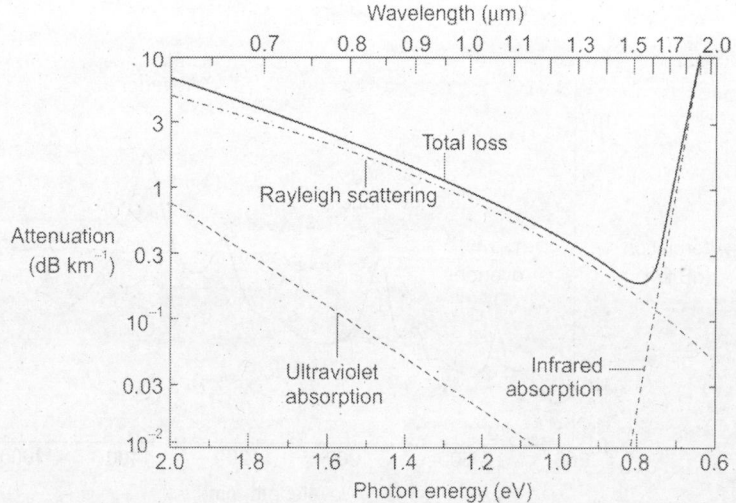

Fig. 6.3: The attenuation spectra for the intrinsic loss mechanisms in pure GeO_2–SiO_2 glass

6.3.2 Extrinsic Absorption

The impurities present in fiber material can also absorb optical signal. These impurities may come from raw material used for making optical fiber or from contamination arising out of improper processing. A major source of signal attenuation is extrinsic absorption from transition metal impurities. We may note that impurities like chromium (Cr^{3+}) and copper (Cu^{2+}), in their worst valence state can cause attenuation in excess of 1 dB/km in the near-infrared region. Some of the more common metallic impurities found in glasses are listed in Table 6.1.

Table 6.1: Absorption losses caused by some of the more common metallic ion impurities in glasses, together with the absorption peak wavelength in nm

Metal ions	Peak wavelength (nm)	Loss (dB/km) (one part in 10^9)
Cr^{3+}	625	1.6
C^{2+}	685	0.1
Cu^{2+}	850	1.1
Fe^{2+}	1100	0.68
Fe^{3+}	400	0.15
Ni^{2+}	650	0.1
Mn^{3+}	460	0.2
V^{4+}	725	2.7

We may note that the impurity induced extrinsic absorption may occur due to electronic transition between the energy levels associated with partially filled subshells or because of charge transition from one impurity ion to the other ion.

The other major extrinsic loss mechanism is caused by absorption due to water (as the hydroxyl or OH^- ion) dissolved in the glass. OH^- ion contamination may result from the use of oxyhydrogen flame for hydrolysis reactions of $SiCl_4$ and $GeCl_4$. The excess extrinsic absorption exhibited by early loss optical fibers was mainly due to the presence of large amount of OH^- ions. In order to keep the attenuation of the fiber to an acceptable limit, the number of hydroxyl have to be reduced to the order to only a few parts per billion. The OH^- ions get bonded in the glass structure and cause fundamental absorption peaks at 1380 nm, 950 nm and 720 nm (Fig. 6.4). It is possible to fabricate high quality single mode silica fiber to offer loss in the tune of 0.5 dB/km in the window near 1330 nm and about 0.2 dB/km in the window near 1550 nm which is very close to the intrinsic attenuation of 0.18/km for silica fiber by reducing the OH^- ion content to the level of 1 ppb (parts per billion).

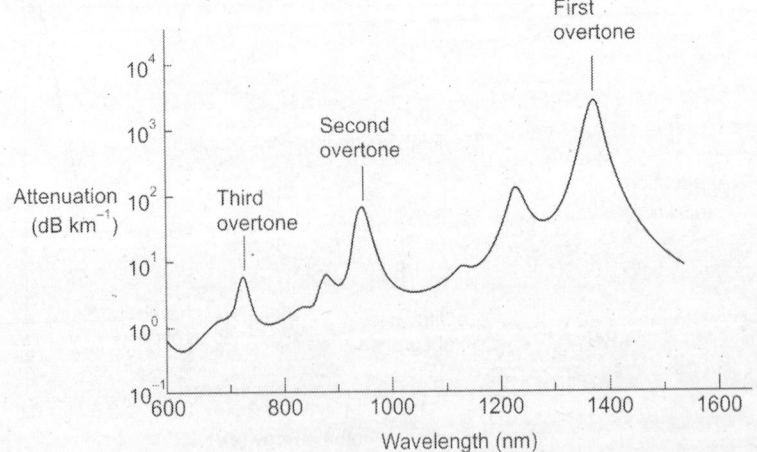

Fig. 6.4: The absorption spectrum for the hydroxyl (OH) group in silica

6.3.3 Defect Loss

A fiber may also suffer from additional loss induced by *atomic defects* arising out of imperfections in atomic structure, e.g. missing atom or a molecule, high density cluster of atoms or oxygen deficiencies, etc. However, in good quality optical fibers, the loss due to these factors is usually low. However, when the fibers are subjected to high energy ionization radiation, e.g. nuclear radiation, cosmic radiation, etc. this component of loss become quite significant. There are several practical applications where the fibers are actually subjected to this type of radiation, e.g. optical fibers sometimes used in nuclear reactors where they are exposed to numerous ionizing radiations, fibers used in satellites are also often subjected to cosmic radiation in Van Allen belt, etc. It is reported that a high radiation dose may cause a significant amount of loss by creating defect centres in the optical fiber. We express the dose of ionizing radiation received by a material in terms of the unit rad.

$$1 \text{ rad (Si)} = 100 \text{ erg g}^{-1} = 0.01 \text{ J/kg}$$

The attenuation caused by ionizing radiation increases with the increase in the total radiation dose received by the fiber and it is found that the attenuation due to this may be as high as 5 dB/km when the total radiation dose is of the order of 10^4 rad (Si).

6.3.4 Scattering Loss

This type of loss generally occur when the propagating light wave interacts with a particle in the fiber material in a manner that energy is transferred in a different direction. However, in an optical fiber, this is viewed as transfer of optical power from one mode to another. There are several cases, where the transfer of power may take place from a propagating mode to a leaky or radiation mode which do not survive over a long distance and are radiated out of the optical fiber. We may note that the scattering occurs because of microscopic variation in material density, structural non-homogeneity or compositional variation over distance of the order of wavelength of the propagating light. In general, one can classify scattering under two categories:(i) *linear scattering loss* and (ii) *non-linear scattering loss.*

(i) Linear Scattering Loss

The Optical power in linear scattering is transferred to a different mode is proportional to the power contained in the propagating mode. This process tends to result in attenuation of the transmitted light as the transfer may be to a leaky or radiation mode which does not continue to propagate within the fiber core, but is radiated from the fiber. We may note that linear scattering is characterized by the fact that there is no change in the frequency of the scattered wave because of the transfer of power from the propagating mode. Linear scattering may be categorized into two major types: *Rayleight scattering* and *Mie scattering.*

Rayleight Scattering

This type of scattering is the dominant intrinsic loss mechanism in the low-absorption window between the ultraviolet (UV) and infrared (IR) absorption tails. It is caused by inhomogeneities that occur on a small scale compared with the wavelength of the light. These microscopic variations and inhomogeneities arise from density and compositional and result in the refractive index fluctuations over distances which are much less than the value of the wavelength of light.

Rayleight scattering generally accounts for more than 95% of the attenuation in the optical fiber. When light travels in the silica core and interacts with the silica molecules, the elastic collisions lead to Rayleigh scattering. If the scattered light does not fall within the angle accepted by the optical fiber, it deviates from the propagation direction leading to loss of optical power. Further, it may so happen sometime that the scattered light is reflected back towards the source. In such cases, the scattered light may be used to detect the presence of defects in an optical fiber and is the basic principle of operation of an *optical time domain reflectometer* (OTDR). We may note that Rayleigh scattering in glass is also similar to scattering of sunlight that makes the *sky look blue*. The scattering due to density fluctuation, which is in almost all directions, produce an attenuation proportional to λ^{-4} following the Rayleigh scattering formula. For a single-component glass, the Rayleigh scattering coefficient γ_R is given by

$$\gamma_R = \frac{8\pi^3}{3\lambda^4} n^8 \cdot p^2 \cdot \beta_c \cdot k \cdot T_F \tag{6.12}$$

where λ is wavelength of the propagating light in the fiber, n is the refractive index of the medium, p is the average photoelastic coefficient, β_c is the isothermal compressibility at a fictive temperature, T_F and k are the fictive temperature and the Boltzmann constant respectively. The fictive temperature T_F is defined as the temperature at which the glass can reach a state of thermal equilibrium and is closely related the annual temperature. One can calculate the transmission loss factor (transmissivity) of the fiber L_{RS} from following the relation

$$L_{RS} = \exp(-\gamma_R L) \tag{6.13}$$

where L is the length of the fiber. We can see from relation Eq. (6.12) that the effect of Rayleigh scattering is strongly influenced by wavelength of operation and hence reduces at longer wavelength. One can calculate the corresponding attenuation in decibels *per unit length* due to scattering from the following relation

$$\alpha_{RS} = 10 \log(1/L) \tag{6.14}$$

One can also calculate the Rayleigh scattering loss (RSL) from the following relation

$$L_{RS} = (0.75 + 4.5\Delta)\lambda^{-4} \text{ dB/km} \tag{6.15}$$

where Δ is the relative index difference and λ is the wavelength in μm. Obviously, to minimise the loss, Δ should be made as low as possible.

For silica glass at $\lambda = 0.6328$ μm, L_{RS} is reported to be 3.9 dB/km. However, the loss due to Rayleigh scattering usually dominate the overall loss in an optical fiber below $\lambda = 1$ mm. Beyond 1 μm, the infrared loss dominates over loss due to Rayleigh scattering (Fig. 6.2).

Mie Scattering

This is the other form of linear scattering which is usually less common in high quality optical fibers. This type of scattering occurs due to inhomogeneities which are comparable in size to the guided wavelength. For optical fibers such inhomogeneities may arise due to imperfection caused by the manfacturing process and may also include irregularities at core-cladding interface, core-cladding refractive index difference along the fiber length, diameter fluctuations, strains and bubbles. When the scattering inhomogeneity exceed $\lambda/10$, the scattered intensity which has an angular dependence can be very large. One can control losses due to Mie scattering by controlling the irregularities.

(ii) Non-Scattering Loss

It is reported that optical fibers behave as linear waveguides in the sense that the output power increases proportionately with the increase in input optical power. However, this is always not true. There are several non-linear effects occur, which in case of scattering disproportionate attenuation, i.e. non-linear scattering become dominant at high optical power levels. The non-linear scattering results in transfer of power from one mode to at a different frequency. Further, the optical power may also be transferred from a mode in either forward or backward direction. Usually, two types of non-linear scattering, i.e. (i) *Stimulated Brillouin scattering* (SBS) and (ii) *Stimulated Raman scattering* (SRS) are observed in long single mode optical fibers at high power levels. These scattering mechanism in fact give optical gain but with a shift in frequency, thus contributing to attenuation for light transmission at specific wavelength. From this point of view, we see that non-linear scattering is undesirable so far as conventional optical communication is concerned. However, the power level required for non-linear scattering to dominate, is usually much above the level of power used in practical optical communication systems. As a result, one finds the contribution of the non-linear scattering in the total attenuation (or loss) in an optical fiber remains almost unnoticed. We may note that such non-linear scattering phenomena can also be used to provide optical amplifier which find extensive application in long distance communication systems.

Stimulated Brillouin Scattering (SBS)

SBS occurs from the scattering of the propagating light by thermal molecular vibrations of the material of the fiber. The scattered light appears as upper and lower sidebands which are separated from the incident light by the modulated frequency. In this scattering process, the incident photon produces a *phonon* (phonon is a quantum of an elastic wave in a crystal lattice. When the elastic wave has a frequency f, the quantized unit of phonon has energy hf Joules) of acoustic frequency as well as a scattered photon. This produces an optical frequency shift which varies with the scattering angle because the frequency of the sound wave varies with acoustic wavelength. For SBS, the shift in the frequency is maximum in the backward direction and zero in the forward direction, making SBS a mainly backward process.

The threshold power P_B required for SBS to occur depends on the operating wavelength (λ) and line width of the optical source. Assuming that the polarization state of the transmitted light is not maintained, one finds that the threshold power P_B required for SBS is given by

$$P_B = 4.4 \times 10^{-3} \, d^2 \, \lambda^2 \, \alpha_{dB} \Delta v \text{ (watt)} \tag{6.16}$$

where, d is the core diameter in micrometer, λ is the operating wavelength in micrometer, α_{dB} is the fiber attenuation in decibel per kilometer and Δv is the linewidth in GHz of the injection laser source.

Stimulated Raman Scattering (SRS)

SRS is similar to SBS except that a high-frequency optical phonon rather than an *acoustic phonon* is generated in the scattering process. Also, SRS can occur both the forward as well as in backward directions in optical fiber, and also may have an optical power threshold of up to three orders of magnitude higher than the Brillouin threshold in a particular optical fiber. The threshold optical power needed for SRS is given by

$$P_R = 5.9 \times 10^{-2} \, d^2 \lambda \, \alpha_{dB} \text{ (watt)} \tag{6.17}$$

where d, λ and α_{dB} are as specified for Eq. (6.16).

It is reported that both the threshold values for SRS and SBS are much above the power generally used in optical fiber communication. Thus, SBS and SRS do not contribute to attenuation in optical fiber communication.

The intrinsic loss as well as loss due to Rayleigh scattering is important that determine the overall attenuation of the optical fiber in the NIR region used for optical communication. Moreover, Rayleigh scattering depends not only on the type of material but also on the relative size of the particles with respect to the wavelength of operation. The loss due to Rayleigh scattering decreases rapidly with the increase in wavelength due to its dependence in the form of λ^{-4}. This means shorter wavelengths are scattered more as compared to longer wavelengths. It is reported that light signal with wavelength below 800 nm is unusable for optical communication is unsuitable as attenuation due to Rayleigh scattering is too high. It is also reported that the overall attenuation of a practical fiber matches closely with the predicted value of attenuation. The attenuation peak near 1400 nm (Fig. 6.4) is due to absorption by residual water molecules in the optical fiber.

(iii) Bending Loss

Any bending in a fiber-cable generates loss. Fiber-optic cable bending losses are caused by a variety of outside influences. These influences can change the physical characteristics of the cable and affect how the cable guides the light. Certain modes are affected and losses are accumulated over long distances.

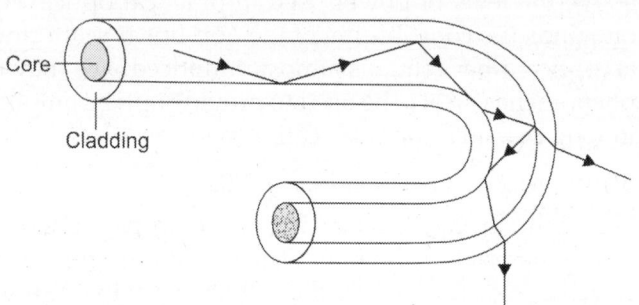

Fig. 6.5: Light propagation around a bend in an optical fiber

However, significant losses can arise from any kind of bending in a fiber cable. The cause of bending loss is easier to envisage using the ray model of light in a multimode fiber cable. When the fiber cable is straight, the ray falls within the confinement angle (θ_c) of the fiber cable. However, a bend changes the angle at which the ray hits the core cable (Fig. 6.5). If the bend is sharp enough, the ray strikes the interface at an angle outside of the confinement angle, and the ray is refracted into the cladding and then to the outside as loss. These are referred to as leaky modes, whereby the ray leaks out and the attenuation is increased.

In another class of modes, called *radiation mode*, power from these modes radiates into the cladding and increases the attenuation. In radiation mode, the electromagnetic energy is distributed in the core and cladding; however the cladding carries no light.

The bend loss, L_B for a radius R (radius of curvature) is given by

$$L_B = -10 \log_{10} \left(1 - 890 \times \frac{r_0^6}{\lambda^4 R^2} \right) \text{ for silica} \qquad (6.18)$$

The bends in optical fibers can be usually classified in two categories: (a) *microscopic bends* which have small radius of curvatures and comparable to optical fiber diameter, and (b) *macroscopic bends* which have radii of curvature much longer than the core diameter. However, both micro- and macrobending can cause significant attenuation in optical fibers.

Microbending Loss

This type of loss results due to power coupling from the guided fundamental mode of a fiber to radiation modes. This coupling takes place when the fiber axis is bent randomly in a high spatial frequency. Such bending can occur during the packing of the fiber in the cabling process (Fig. 6.6).

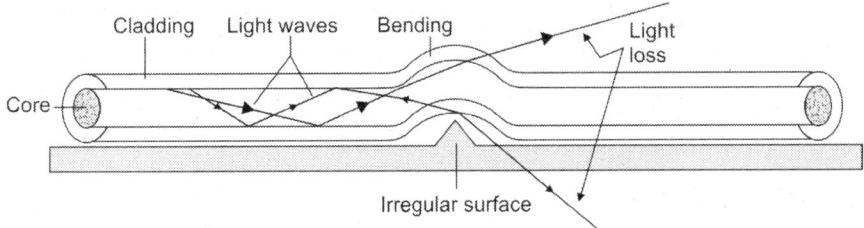

Fig. 6.6: Fiber cable microbend

Basically, when the fiber cable is installed and pressed onto an irregular surface, tiny bends can be created in the fiber cable (Fig. 6.7). One can made fibers containing microbends relatively flat by using compressible plastic jacket and applying appropriate external force.

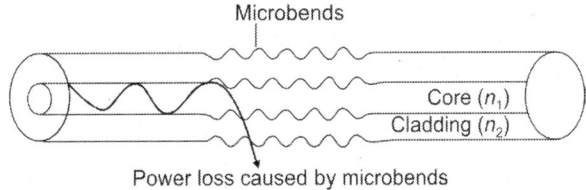

Fig. 6.7: Illustration of microbending loss from higher order mode

This method can in general significantly reduce the loss in optical fiber due to microbends. The microbending loss is reported to be as high as 1–2 dB/km.

The microbending loss of an SMF is a function of the fundamental mode spot size, r_0. Fibers with large spot sizes are extremely sensitive to microbending. It is therefore desirable to design the fiber to have as small a pot size as possible to minimize the bending loss. One can express the microbending loss by the relation

$$L_m = 2.15 \times 10^{-4} r_0^6 \lambda^{-4} L_{mn} \text{ dB/km}$$

where L_{mn} is the microbending loss of a 50 mm core multimode fiber after having an NA of 0.2.

Macrobending Loss

Macrobend, i.e. large bend in optical fibers occurs when a fiber is bent into a relatively large radius of curvature compared to the fiber diameter. Macrobends can cause a significant power loss when the radius of curvature falls below a certain critical value. These bends are formed when the fibers are wound in the form of a spool or a fiber cable roll. However, the power losses in these cases do not cause significant radiation loss provided the radius of curvature is large enough. When a fiber cable is bent uniformly to take a turn, the microbends can also be caused. Primarily the bending loss is due to radiation of energy from the fiber when the evanescent field fails to keep up pace with the part of the mode varying harmonically in the core. One can understand qualitatively this with the help of Fig. 6.8.

A *mode* is a mathematical and physical concept that describes the propagation of electromagnetic waves through an optical medium.

A mode is an allowed solution to Maxwell's equations. A mode is simply a path that a light ray can follow when travelling through a fiber cable. Currently, the number of modes supported by a fiber cable

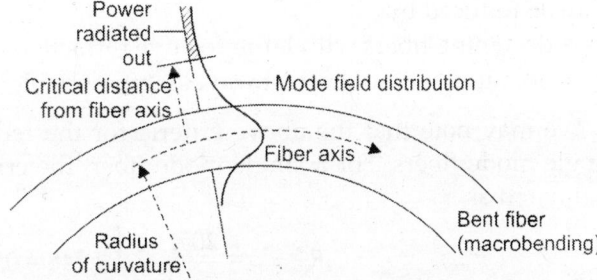

Fig. 6.8: Illustration of the radiation loss at microbending with the help of the fundamental mode field

ranges from one to hundreds of thousands. Thus, a fiber cable provides a path for one or thousands of light rays, depending on its size, design and properties.

Each mode also carried a characteristic amount of optical power. Most fiber cables today support many modes. When light is first injected into the fiber cable, a mode may carry too much or too little power, depending on the injected power of light. Over the length of the fiber cable, power transfers between modes until all modes carry their characteristics power. When a fiber cable reaches this point, it is said to have reached *steady state*, or *equilibrium mode distribution* (EMD). Achieving EMD in plastic fibers requires only a few hundred meters. For high-performance glass fiber cables, EMD often requires hundreds of kilometers.

The number of modes (N) in a fiber optic cable can be calculated from the V number $\left(V = \dfrac{2\pi d}{\lambda} (NA) \right)$ for the following cases:

(a) For single-mode-step index fiber, the number of modes (N) can be approximated by $N = V^2/2$.

(b) For a multimode step-index and graded-index fiber cable, the number of modes (N) can be approximated by $N = V^2/4$ mode which is on the outside of the band (Fig. 6.8) and required to travel faster than that on the inside so that a wavefront perpendicular to the direction of propagation is maintained. Hence, part of the mode in the cladding needs to travel faster than the velocity of light in that medium. As this is not possible, the energy associated with this part of the mode is lost through radiation.

The bending loss depends on the radius of curvature (R) and can generally be represented by empirical expression as

$$\alpha_r = c_1 \exp(-c_2 R) \tag{6.19}$$

where R is the radius of curvature of the fiber bend and c_1 and c_2 are empirical constants which are independent of R.

Large bending losses tend to occur in multimode fibers at a critical radius of curvature R_c given by

$$R_c \simeq \frac{3n_1^2 \lambda}{4\pi (n_1^2 - n_2^2)^{1/2}} \tag{6.20}$$

where n_1 and n_2 are the values of refractive index of the core and the cladding respectively and λ is the wavelength of light propagating through the fiber. When the bending is large enough that the radius of curvature (R) falls below R_c, the bending loss of the fiber tends to become very large. From Eq. (6.20), we see that potential macrobending losses may be reduced by:

• designing fibers with large relative refractive index difference;
• operating at the shortest wavelength possible.

We may note that the above criteria for the reduction of bend losses also apply to single mode fibers. For a single mode fiber, the critical radius of curvature (R_c) can be estimated as

$$R_c \simeq \frac{20\lambda}{(n_1 - n_2)^{3/2}} \left[2.748 - 0.996 \frac{\lambda}{\lambda_c} \right]^{-3} \tag{6.21}$$

where λ_c is the cutoff wavelength for the single-mode fiber.

The effective number of modes guided by a curved graded index fiber can be estimated as

$$M_{\text{eff}} = M_{\infty}\left[1 - \frac{\alpha + 2}{2\alpha\Delta}\left\{\frac{2a}{R} + \frac{3}{2n_2\,kR}\right\}\right] \tag{6.22}$$

where α denotes the grade index of the GI fiber, Δ is the index deviation and $k(= 2\pi/\lambda)$ and R is the radius of curvature of the bending. M_{∞} denotes the number of modes through a grade index straight index fiber given by

$$M_{\infty} = a^2\,k^2\,n_1^2\,\Delta\left(\frac{a}{a+2}\right) \tag{6.23}$$

(iv) Waveguide Loss

The losses due to waveguide structures arise from power leakage, bending and microbending of the fiber axis, and defects and joints between fibers. Power leakage is significant only for depressed cladding fibers.

(v) Core-Cladding Loss

In an actual or practical fiber the total loss is contributed by all kinds of dissipative and scattering mechanisms involving both the core and cladding regions of the fiber. Since the core and cladding have different indices of refraction and hence differ in composition, the core and cladding generally have different attenuation coefficients, α_1 and α_2, respectively. In the absence of mode coupling, one can express the attenuation coefficient for a mode of order (l, m) as

$$\alpha_{lm} = \alpha_1\frac{P_{\text{core}}}{P} + \alpha_2\frac{P_{\text{clad}}}{P} \tag{6.24}$$

where α_1 and α_2 are the attenuation coefficients in dB/km. The core and cladding regions, P_{core}/P and P_{clad}/P correspond to the fractional power carried by the core and cladding respectively.

Using $P_{\text{clad}} = 1 - P_{\text{core}}/P$, one can express Eq. (6.24) as

$$\alpha_{lm} = \alpha_1 + (\alpha_2 - \alpha_1)\,(P_{\text{clad}}/P) \tag{6.25}$$

For a graded index fiber, both the attenuation coefficients and modal power tend to be functions of the radial coordinate. Thus, for a graded index fiber, the loss is expected to follow the variation of the refractive index along the radius. At a distance r from the core axis the loss is

$$\alpha(r) = \alpha_1 + (\alpha_2 - \alpha_1)\,\frac{n^2(0) - n^2(r)}{n^2(0) - n_2^2} \tag{6.26}$$

where α_1 and α_2 are the axial and cladding attenuation coefficients of the GI Fiber, respectively. The overall attenuation loss encountered by a given mode is then

$$\alpha_{\text{GI}} = \frac{\int_0^{\infty}\alpha(r)\,p(r)\,r\,dr}{\int_0^{\infty}p(r)\,r\,dr} \tag{6.27}$$

where $p(r)$ is the power density of that mode at r.

(vi) Joint or Splice Loss

Ultimately, the fiber will have to be spliced together to form the final transmission link. With a fiber cable that averages 0.4–0.6 dB/km, a splice loss in excess of 0.2 dB/splice drastically reduces the unrepeated distance that can be achieved. It is, therefore, extremely important that the fiber be designed in such a way that the splice loss is minimized.

Splice loss is mainly due to the axial misalignment of the fiber core.

Splicing techniques, which rely on the alignment of the outside surface of the fibers, require extremely close tolerance on core-to-outside surface concentricity. Offsets of the order of 1 mm can produce significant splice loss. This loss is given by

$$L_s = \frac{10}{\ln 10} \left(\frac{d}{r_0} \right)^2 \text{ dB} \qquad (6.28)$$

where d is the axial misalignment of the fiber core. It is obvious that minimizing the optical loss requires trade-offs between the different sources of loss. It is advantageous to have a large spot size to minimize both Rayleigh and splicing losses, whereas minimizing bending and microbending losses requires a small spot size. In addition, as will be described in the next section, the spot size plays a significant role in the chromatic dispersion properties of SMF.

(vii) Excess Loss

There is another type of loss, called excess loss. It is defined as the ratio between the sum of all power outputs (P_1 to P_n) and input signal power. Excess loss specifies the power lost within the system. It includes dispersion, scattering, absorption, and coupling loss. Excess loss is calculated using the following formula:

$$\text{Loss (dB)} = -10 \log_{10} \left(\frac{(P_1 + P_2 + P_3 + ... + P_n)}{P_{in}} \right) \qquad (6.29)$$

Figure 6.1(b) shows fiber-optical attenuation as a function of wavelength. In the 1970s, communication systems operated in the wavelength range of 800–900 nm. At that time, fiber-optic cables exhibited a local minimum in the attenuation curve, and optical sources and photo detectors operating at this range were available. In addition, the fiber-optic cables were faster than their counterpart, the copper cabling systems. This region is referred as the *first window*.

By reducing the concentration of hydroxyl ions and metallic impurities in the fiber core material, in the 1980s manufacturers were able to fabricate fiber-optic cables with very low loss in the 1100–1600-nm region. At the same time, the demand increased for high-speed data rate transmission over long distances. Thus, the *second window* was defined, concentrated around 1310 nm. The spectral band is referred to as the long wavelength region. Due to further progress in the fabrication of fiber-optic cables and optical amplifiers, the *third window* was defined around 1550 nm.

The most important aspect of the fiber optic communication link is that many wavelengths can be sent along a fiber simultaneously, without interference, in the 1310–1625 nm spectrum. The technology of combining a number of wavelengths onto the same fiber cable is known as *wavelength division multiplexing* (WDM). Furthermore, this technology experienced advanced development by using the *dense wavelength division multiplexing* (DWDM).

6.4 MID-INFRARED AND FAR-INFRARED TRANSMISSION

In the near-infrared region of the optical spectrum, fundamental silica fiber attenuation is dominated by Rayleigh scattering and multiphonon absorption from the infrared absorption edge (Fig. 6.4). Therefore, the total loss decreases as the operational transmission wavelength increases until a crossover point is reached around a wavelength of 1.55 μm where the total fiber loss again increases because at longer wavelengths the loss is dominated by the phonon absorption edge. Since the near fundamental attenuation limits for near-infrared silicate class fibers have been achieved, more recently researchers have turned their attenuation to the mid-infrared (2 to 5 μm) and the far-infrared (8 to 12 μm) optical wavelengths.

In order to obtain lower loss fibers it is necessary to produce glasses exhibiting longer infrared cutoff wavelengths. Potentially, much lower losses can be achieved if the transmission window of the material can be extended further into the infrared by utilizing constituent atoms of higher atomic mass and if it can be drawn into fiber exhibiting suitable strength and chemical durability. The reason for this possible loss reduction is due to Rayleigh scattering which displays a λ^{-4} dependence and hence becomes much reduced as the wavelength is increased. For example, the scattering loss is reduced by a factor of 16 when the optical wavelength is doubled. Thus it may be possible to obtain losses of the order of 0.01 dB km^{-1} at a wavelength of 2.55 μm, with even lower losses at wavelengths of between 3 and 5 μm.

Candidate glass-forming systems for mid-infrared transmission are fluoride, fluoride–chloride, chalcogenide and oxide. In particular, oxide glasses such as Al_2O_3 (i.e. sapphire) offer a near equivalent transmittance range to many of the fluoride glasses and have benefits of high melting points, chemical inertness, and the ability to be readily melted and grown in air. Chalcogenide glasses, which generally comprise one or more elements Ge, Si, As and Sb, are capable of optical transmission in both the mid-infrared and far-infrared regions. A typical chalcogenide fiber glass is therefore arsenide trisulfide (As_2S_3). However, research activities into far-infrared transmission using chalcogenide glasses, halide glasses, polycrystalline halide fibers (e.g. silver and thallium) and hollow glass waveguides are primarily concerned with radiometry, infrared imaging, optical wireless, optical sensing and optical power transmission rather than telecommunications.

Research activities into ultra-low-loss fibers for long-haul repeaterless communications in the 1980s and early 1990s centered on the fluorozirconates, with zirconium fluoride (ZrF_4) as the major constituent, and fluorides of barium, lanthanum, aluminum, gadolinium, sodium, lithium and occasionally lead added as modifiers and stabilizers. Such alkali additives improve the glass stability and working characteristics. Moreover, the two most popular heavy metal fluoride glasses for fabrication into fiber are fluorozirconate and fluoroaluminate glasses. Extensive work has been undertaken on a common fluorozirconate system comprising ZrF_4–BaF_2–LaF_3–AlF_2–CaF_3–YF_3. Although ZBLAN can theoretically provide for the lowest transmission losses over the mid-infrared wavelength region, it has a significantly lower glass transition (melting) temperature than the fluoroaluminate glass and is therefore less durable when subject to both thermal and mechanical perturbations.

The fabrication of low-loss, long-length fluoride fibers presents a basic problem with reducing the extrinsic losses which remains to be resolved. In practice, however, the most critical and difficult problems are associated with the minimization of the scattering losses resulting from extrinsic factors such as defects, waveguide imperfections and radiation caused by mechanical deformation. The estimated losses of around 0.01 dB km^{-1} at a wavelength of 2.55 mm for ZrF_4-based fibers are derived from an extrapolation of the intrinsic losses due to ultraviolet and infrared absorptions together with Rayleigh scattering. Moreover, refinements of scattering loss have increased this loss value slightly to 0.024 dB km^{-1} which is still around eight times lower than that of a silica fiber. Nevertheless, practical fiber losses remain much higher, as may be observed from the attenuation spectra for the common mid- and far-infrared fibers shown in Fig. 6.9 in which the fluoride fiber (ZBLAN) is exhibiting a loss of several decibels per kilometer.

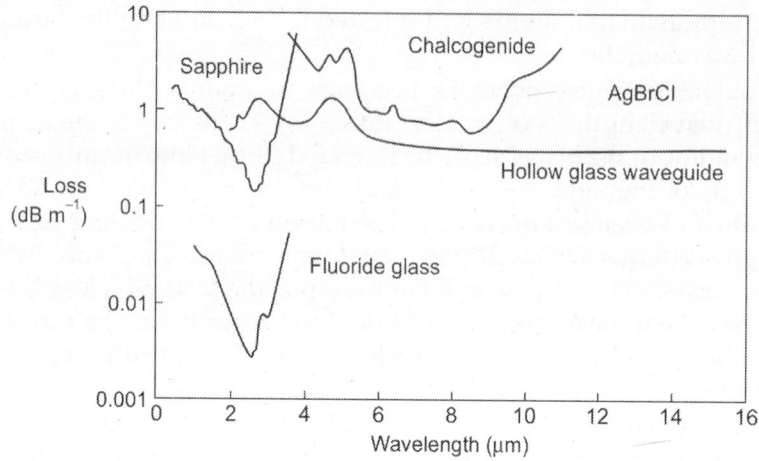

Fig. 6.9: Attenuation spectra for some common mid- and far-infrared fibers

The loss spectrum for a single-crystal sapphire fiber which also transmits in the mid-infrared is shown in Fig. 6.9. Although they have robust physical properties, including a Young's modulus six times greater as well as a thermal expansion some ten times higher than that of silica, these fibers lend themselves to optical power delivery applications, not specifically optical communications. Chalcogenide glasses which have their lowest losses over both the mid- and far-infrared ranges are very stable, durable and insensitive to moisture. Arsenic trisulfide fiber, being one of the simplest, has a spectral range from 0.7 to around 6 μm. Hence it has a cut off at long wavelength significantly before the chalcogenide fibers containing heavier elements such as Te, Ge and Se, an attenuation spectrum for the latter being incorporated in Fig. 6.9. In general, chalcogenide glass fibers have proved to be useful in areas such as optical sensing, infrared imaging and for the production of fiber infrared lasers and amplifiers.

The loss spectrum for the polycrystalline fiber AgBrCl is also shown in Fig. 6.9. Although these fibers are transmissive over the entire far-infrared wavelength region and they were initially considered to hold significant potential as ultra-low-loss fibers because their intrinsic losses were estimated to be around 10^{-3} dB m^{-1}, they are mechanically weak in comparison with silica fibers. In addition, the estimated low losses are far from being achieved, with experimental loss values being not even close to the predicted minimum as can be observed Fig. 6.9. Furthermore, polycrystalline fibers plastically deform resulting in increased transmission loss well before they fracture.

Finally, a hollow glass waveguide spectral characteristic is also shown in Fig. 6.9. This hollow glass tube with a 530 μm bore was designed for optimum response at a transmission wavelength of 10 μm. Such hollow glass waveguides have been successfully employed for infrared laser power delivery at both 2.94 μm (Er:YAG laser) and 10.6 μm (CO$_2$ laser). Concluding, the remaining limitations of high loss (in comparison with theory) and low strength have inhibited the prospect of long-distance mid-or far-infrared transmission for communications for even the most promising fluoride fibers, while a range of alternative nontelecommunication applications for the various fiber and *waveguide* types have been developed.

6.5 DISPERSION

Dispersion is caused by the expansion of light pulses as they travel through optical components. This occurs because the speed of light through the optical medium is independent on the wavelength, the propagation mode, and the optical properties of the materials along the light path. In addition to attenuation, the transmission of optical signal through an optical fiber is adversely affected by dispersion of the signal by the dielectric medium. Depending on the origin, dispersion can be broadly classified under two categories: (i) *Intramodal dispersion*, which refers to dispersion or spreading of the pulse that occurs within a particular mode and usually found in all types of fibers, and (ii) *Interamodal dispersion* is caused by the time delay between various modes to the destination point. This type of dispersion is found to be present only in a multimode fiber which supports more than one mode to carry the optical mode and the delay is caused by the time difference between the lowest and highest order modes. Since intermodal dispersion supports only one mode and hence it is not found in a single mode fiber. However, single mode fibers generally suffer from a special type of dispersion namely *Polarization Mode Dispersion* (PMD) arising out of bireferingence phenomenon.

Dispersion of the transmitted optical signal causes distortion for both digital and analog transmission along optical fibers. When considering the major implementation of optical fiber transmission which involves some form of digital modulation, then dispersion mechanisms within the fiber cause broadening of the transmitted light pulses as they travel along the channel. The phenomenon is illustrated in Fig. 6.10, where it may be observed that each pulse broadens and overlaps with its neighbors, eventually becoming indistinguishable at the receiver input. The effect is known as intersymbol interference (ISI). Thus an increasing number of errors may be encountered on the digital optical channel as the ISI becomes more pronounced. The *error rate* is also a function of the signal attenuation on the link and the subsequent *signal-to-noise ratio* (SNR) at the receiver. However, signal dispersion alone limits the maximum possible bandwidth attainable with a particular optical fiber to the point where individual symbols can no longer be distinguished.

For no overlapping of light pulses down on an optical fiber link the digital bit rate B_T must be less than the reciprocal of the broadened (through dispersion) pulse duration (2τ). Hence:

$$B_T \leq 1/2\tau \tag{6.30}$$

We have assumed that the pulse broadening due to dispersion on the channel is τ which dictates the input pulse duration which is also τ. Hence Eq. (6.30) gives a conservative estimate of the maximum bit rate that may be obtained on an optical fiber link as $1/2\tau$.

Another more accurate estimate of the maximum bit rate for an optical channel with dispersion may be obtained by considering the light pulses at the output to have a Gaussian shape with an rms width of σ. Unlike the relationship given in Eq. (6.30), this analysis allows for the existence of a certain amount of signal overlap on the channel, while avoiding any SNR penalty which occurs when ISI becomes pronounced. The maximum bit rate is given approximately by

$$B_{T \text{ (max)}} \simeq \frac{0.2}{\sigma} \text{ bit s}^{-1} \tag{6.31}$$

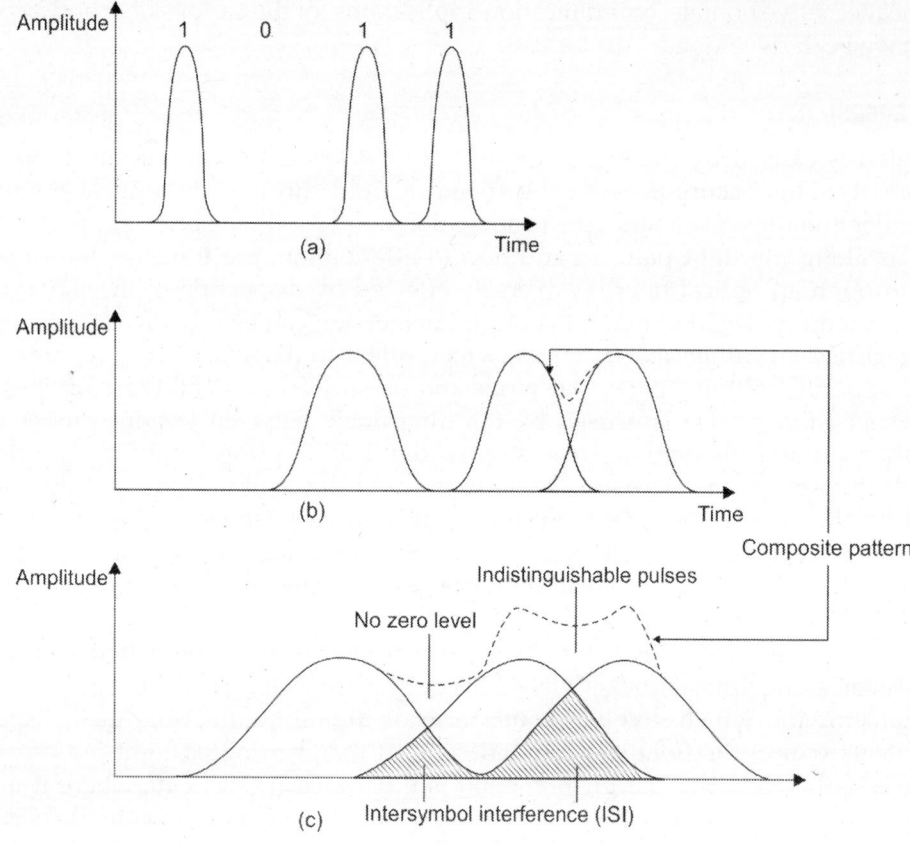

Fig. 6.10: Using the digital bit pattern 1011 of the broadening of light pulses as they are transmitted along a optical fiber: (a) fiber input (b) fiber output at a distance L_1 (c) fiber output at a distance $L_2 > L_1$.

We may note that certain sources give the constant term in the numerator of Eq. (6.31) as 0.25. Equation (6.31) gives a reasonably good approximation for other pulse shapes which may occur on the channel resulting from the various dispersive mechanisms within the fiber. Also, σ may be assumed to represent the rms impulse response for the channel.

The conversion of bit rate to bandwidth in hertz depends on the digital coding format used. For metallic conductors when a *nonreturn-to-zero code* is employed, the binary 1 level is held for the whole bit period τ. In this case there are two bit periods in one wavelength (i.e. 2 bits per second per hertz), as illustrated in Fig. 6.11(a). Hence the maximum bandwidth B is one-half the maximum data rate or:

$$B_{T\,(max)} = 2B \tag{6.32}$$

However, when a *return-to-zero code* is considered, as shown in Fig. 6.11(b), the binary 1 level is held for only part (usually half) of the bit period. For this signaling scheme the data rate is equal to the *bandwidth* in hertz (i.e. 1 bit per second per hertz) and thus $B_T = B$. The bandwidth B for metallic conductors is also usually defined by the electrical 3 dB points (i.e. the frequencies at which the electric power has dropped to one-half of its constant maximum value). However, when the 3 dB optical bandwidth of a fiber is considered it is significantly larger than the corresponding 3 dB electrical bandwidth. Hence, when the limitations in the bandwidth of a fiber due to dispersion are stated (i.e. optical bandwidth B_{opt}), it is usually with regard to a return to zero code where the bandwidth in hertz is considered equal to the digital bit rate. Within the context of

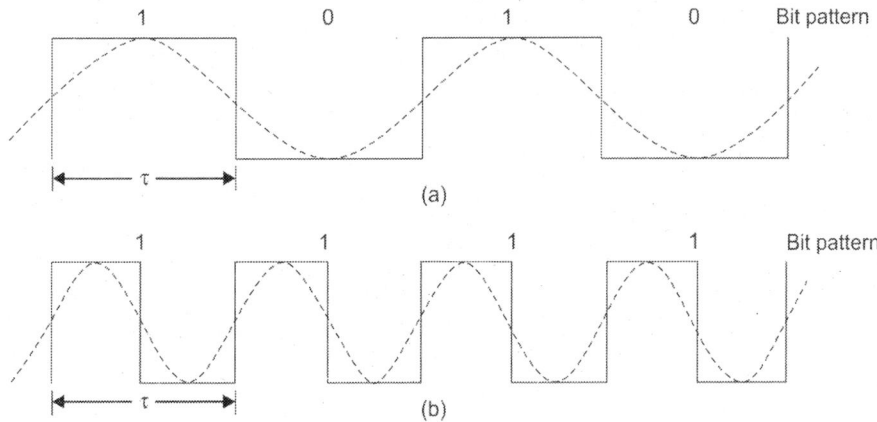

Fig. 6.11: Illustration of the relationships of the bit rate to wavelength for digital codes: (a) nonreturn-to-zero (NRZ) (b) return-to-zero (RZ)

dispersion the bandwidths expressed in this chapter will follow this general criterion unless otherwise stated. However, when electro-optic devices and optical fiber systems are considered it is more usual to state the electrical 3 dB bandwidth, this being the more useful measurement when interfacing an optical fiber link to electrical terminal equipment. Unfortunately, the terms of bandwidth measurement are not always made clear and the reader must be warned that this omission may lead to some confusion when specifying components and materials for optical fiber communication systems.

Figure 6.12 shows the three common optical fiber structures, namely *multimode step index*, *multimode graded index* and *single-mode step index*, while diagrammatically illustrating

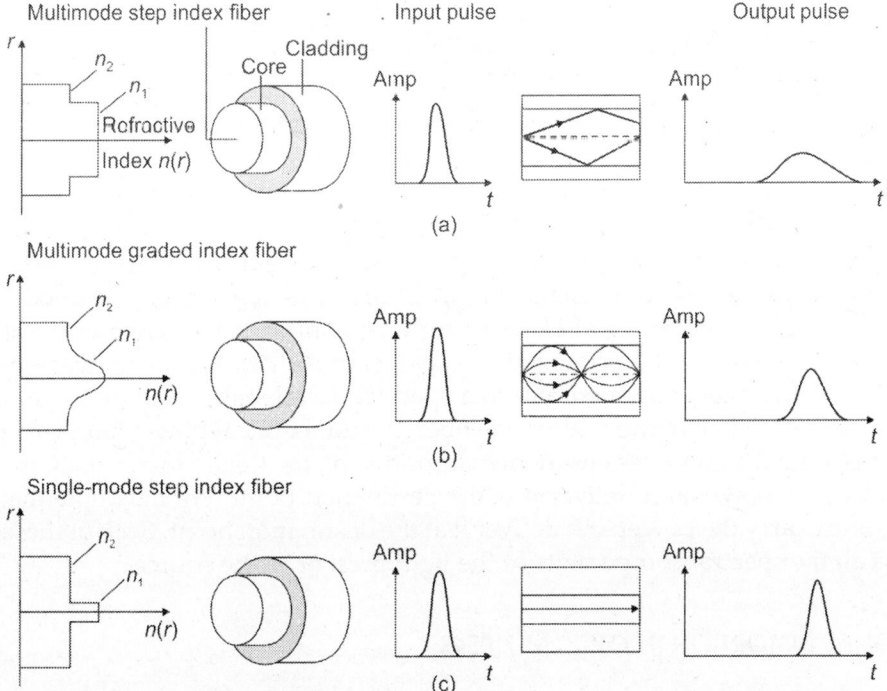

Fig. 6.12: Illustration of the pulse broadening due to intermodal dispersion in (a) multimode step index fiber (b) multimode graded index fiber (c) single-mode step index fiber

the respective pulse broadening associated with each fiber type. It may be observed that the multimode step index fiber exhibits the *greatest dispersion* of a transmitted light pulse and the multimode graded index fiber gives a considerably improved performance. Finally, the single-mode fiber gives the minimum pulse broadening and thus is capable of the greatest transmission bandwidths which are currently in the gigahertz range, whereas transmission via multimode step index fiber is usually limited to bandwidths of a few tens of megahertz. However, the amount of pulse broadening is dependent upon the distance the pulse travels within the fiber, and hence for a given optical fiber link the restriction on usable bandwidth is dictated by the distance between regenerative repeaters (i.e. the distance the light pulse travels before it is reconstituted). Thus the measurement of the dispersive properties of a particular fiber is usually stated as the pulse broadening in time over a unit length of the fiber (i.e. ns km^{-1}).

Hence, the number of optical signal pulses which may be transmitted in a given period and therefore the information-carrying capacity of the fiber, is restricted by the amount of pulse dispersion per unit length. In the absence of mode coupling or filtering, the pulse broadening increases linearly with fiber length and thus the bandwidth is inversely proportional to distance. This leads to the adoption of a more useful parameter for the information-carrying capacity of an optical fiber which is known as the *bandwidth–length product* (i.e. $B_{opt} \times L$). The typical best bandwidth-length products for the three fibers shown in Fig. 6.12 are 20 MHz km, 1 GHz km and 100 GHz km for multimode step index, multimode graded index and single-mode step index fibers respectivley.

In order to appreciate the reasons for the different amounts of pulse broadening within the various types of optical fiber, it is necessary to consider the dispersive mechanisms involved, i.e. material dispersion, waveguide dispersion, intermodal dispersion and profile dispersion.

6.5.1. Interamodal Dispersion or Chromatic Dispersion or Group Velocity Dispersion (GVD)

This refers to pulse broadening that occurs within a mode due to finite spectral width of the source.

We may note that none of the optical sources used in optical communication systems is a perfectly monochromatic source. This reveals that there will be propagation delay differences between different spectral components in the optical signal launched into the fiber from an optical source. To make it more clear, let us consider a multimode fiber in which light is launched from a LED operating at 850 nm with a spectral width of 40 nm. Obviously, LED has a peak optical emission power at 850 nm and the power emitted by the source is essentially confined within a spectral wavelength band of 40 nm ranging from 830 nm to 870 nm. In the multimode fiber, the total optical power launched into the fiber is distributed among various modes supported by the fiber. However, all the modes jointly carry the power and deliver it at the destination point. We may note that all the modes jointly carry the power and deliver it at the destination point. Each of these modes contains all the spectral components of the light present in the source.

6.6 SIGNAL DISTORTION IN OPTICAL FIBERS

Basics on group velocity: Consider a monochromatic field given by

$$E_x = A \cos (\omega t - bz) \tag{6.33}$$

where

   A is the wave amplitude,

   ω is the radial frequency, and

   β is the propagation constant along the z-direction

Setting $(\omega t - \beta z)$ constant, the wave phase velocity is given by

$$v_p = \frac{dz}{dt} = \frac{\omega}{\beta} \tag{6.34}$$

Now we consider that the propagating wave consists of two monochromatic fields of frequencies, $\omega + \delta\omega$ and $\omega - \delta\omega$, of

$$E_{x1} = A \cos\left[(\omega + \delta\omega)t - (\beta + \delta\beta)z\right] \tag{6.35}$$

$$E_{x2} = A \cos\left[(\omega - \delta\omega)t - (\beta - \delta\beta)z\right] \tag{6.36}$$

The total field is then given by

$$E_x = E_{x1} + E_{x2} = 2A \cos(\omega t - \beta z)\cos(\delta\omega t - \delta\beta z) \tag{6.37}$$

If $\omega \gg \delta\omega$, then $\cos(\omega t - \beta z)$ varies much faster than $\cos(\delta\omega t - \delta\beta z)$ as shown in Fig. 6.13. The phasor representation is given in Fig. 6.14. Now, by setting $(\delta\omega t - d\beta z)$ constant, the *group velocity* is defined as

$$v_g = \frac{d\omega}{d\beta} \rightarrow v_g^{-1} = \frac{d\beta}{d\omega} \tag{6.38}$$

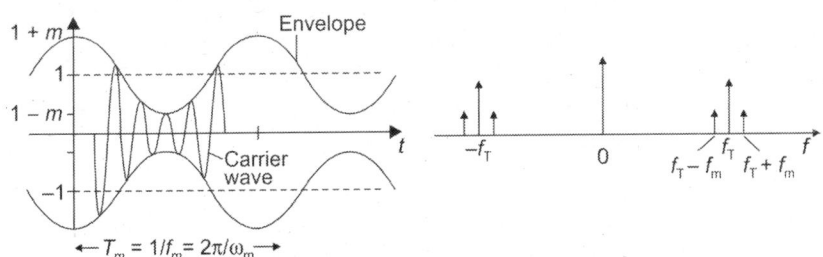

Fig. 6.13: Time signal and spectrum

The group delay t_g, per unit length (setting L at 1.0 km) is thus given as

$$t_g = \frac{L(1\,km)}{v_g} = \frac{d\beta}{d\omega} \tag{6.39}$$

The pulse spread $\Delta\tau$, per unit length due to group delay of light sources of spectral width, σ_λ (i.e. the full-width half-maximum [FWHM] of the optical spectrum of the light source), is

$$\Delta\tau = \frac{dt_g}{d\lambda}\,\sigma_\lambda, \tag{6.40}$$

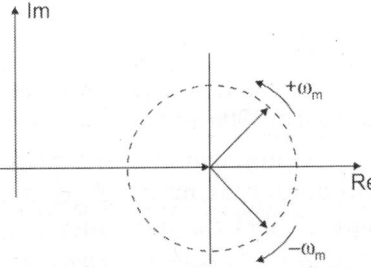

Fig. 6.14: Vector-phasor diagram of the complex envelope

i.e. the spread of the group delay due to the spread of the source wavelength in ps/km. Thus, the linewidth of the light source makes a great difference in the distortion of the optical signal transmitted through the optical fiber. The narrow the source linewidth, the less dispersed are the optical pulses. The typical linewidth of Fabry–Perot semiconductor lasers is about 1–2.0 nm, while the DFB (distributed feedback) laser exhibits a linewidth of 100 MHz.

An optical signal traveling along a fiber becomes increasingly distorted. This distortion is a consequence of intermodal delay effects and intramodal dispersion. Intermodal delay effects are significant in multimode optical fibers since each mode has a different value of group velocity at a specific frequency. Although intramodal dispersion is pulse spreading that occurs within a single mode, it is the result of the group velocity that is a function of the wavelength, λ, and is therefore referred to as chromatic dispersion.

The two main causes of intramodal dispersion are:

- *Material dispersion*, which arises from the variation of the refractive index, $n(\lambda)$, as a function of the wavelength. This causes a wavelength dependence of the group velocity of any given mode.

- *Waveguide dispersion*, which occurs because the mode propagation constant, $\beta(\lambda)$, is a function of the wavelength, λ; the core radius, a; and the refractive index difference.

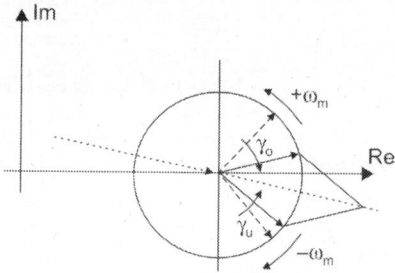

The group velocity associated with the fundamental mode is frequency dependent because of chromatic dispersion. As a result, different spectral components of the light pulse travel at different group velocities, a phenomenon referred to as *group velocity dispersion* (GVD), intramodal dispersion, or as material dispersion and waveguide dispersion. The movement of the phasors is illustrated in Fig. 6.15.

Fig. 6.15: Magnitude of the complex envelope when not sinusoidal; the envelope is subject to nonlinear distortions

6.6.1 Group Velocity Dispersion

(i) Material Dispersion

The refractive index of silica as a function of wavelength is shown in Fig. 6.16. The refractive index is plotted over the wavelength region of 1.0–2.0 μm, which is the most important range for silica-based optical communication systems, as the loss is lowest at 1300 and 1550 nm windows.

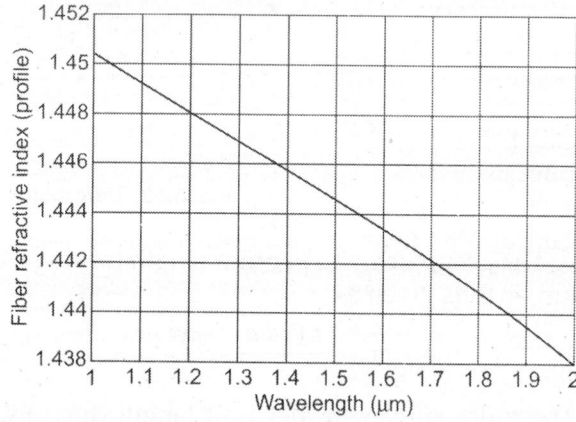

Fig. 6.16: Variation in the refractive index as a function of the optical wavelength of silica

The propagation constant, β, of the fundamental mode guided in the optical fiber can be written as

$$\beta(\lambda) = \frac{2\pi n(\lambda)}{\lambda} \tag{6.41}$$

The group delay t_{gm}, per unit length of Eq. (6.41) can be obtained from

$$t_{gm} = \frac{d\beta}{d\omega} \tag{6.42}$$

where we can use

$$d\omega = d\left(\frac{2\pi c}{\lambda}\right) = -\frac{2\pi c}{\lambda^2}\, d\lambda \tag{6.43}$$

Thus,
$$t_{gm} = -\frac{\lambda^2}{2\pi c}\frac{d\beta}{d\lambda} \tag{6.44}$$

Substituting Eq. (6.41) in Eq. (6.44), we have

$$t_{gm} = \frac{1}{c}\left[n(\lambda) - \frac{\lambda\, dn(\lambda)}{d\lambda}\right] \tag{6.45}$$

Thus, the pulse dispersion per unit length $\Delta\tau_m/\Delta\lambda$, due to the material using Eq. (6.45) for a source having an RMS spectral width, σ_λ, is

$$\Delta\tau_m = -\frac{\lambda}{c}\frac{d^2n}{d\lambda^2}\sigma_\lambda \tag{6.46}$$

If $\Delta\tau_m = M(\lambda)\sigma_\lambda$, then

$$M(\lambda) \text{ or } D_{mat}(\lambda) = -\frac{\lambda}{c}\frac{d^2n}{d\lambda^2} \tag{6.47}$$

where $M(\lambda)$ is the *material dispersion factor* or the *material dispersion parameter*; its unit is commonly expressed in ps/(nm·km).

The variation of material dispersion parameter $M(\lambda)$ or D_{mat} with wavelength is shown in Fig. 6.17. We see from the characteristic curve that it passes through zero at a wavelength of 1.27 mm. This point is *zero material dispersion* (ZMD) point. We also see that the material dispersion remain very small, maintain values close to zero for pure silica glass at a wavelength around 1300 nm. This is why, second generation optical communication was focussed at

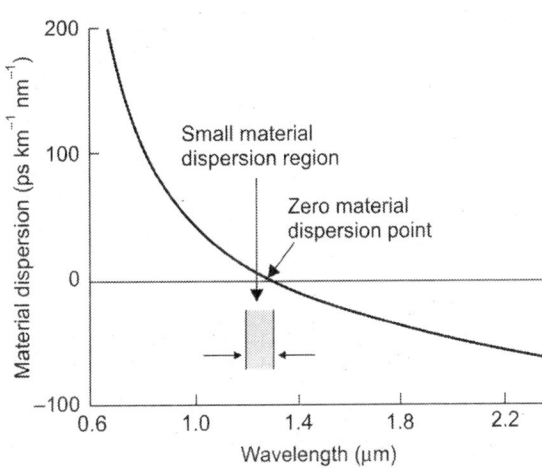

Fig. 6.17: Variation of material dispersion with wavelength for silica

this wavelength because the attenuation at this wavelength in pure silica glass is very low. It is apparent that one can reduce the material dispersion either by operating at a longer wavelength or reducing the spectral width of the source. Use of laser source in place of an LED source can reduce the material dispersion effect in optical fibers due to a smaller spectral width of the laser source.

Thus, if the refractive index can be expressed as a function of the optical wavelength, then the material dispersion can be calculated. In fact, in practice, optical material engineers have to characterize all optical properties of new materials. The refractive index, $n(\lambda)$, can usually be expressed in terms of *Sellmeier's dispersion formula* as

$$n^2(\lambda) = 1 + \sum_k \frac{G_k\lambda^2}{(\lambda^2 - \lambda_k^2)} \tag{6.48}$$

where

G_k are Sellmeier's constants

k is an integer and normally takes a value in the range of $k = 1\text{–}3$

In the later 1970s, several silica-based glass materials were manufactured and their properties were determined. The refractive indices are usually expressed using Sellmeier's coefficients. These coefficients are given in Table 6.2 for several optical fiber materials.

By using curve fitting, the refractive index of pure silica, $n(\lambda)$, can be expressed as

$$n(\lambda) = c_1 + c_2 \lambda^2 + c_3 \lambda^{-2} \tag{6.48a}$$

where $c_1 = 1.45084$
$\qquad c_2 = -0.00343 \ \mu m^{-2}$
$\qquad c_3 = 0.00292 \ \mu m^2$

Thus, from Table 6.2 and Eq. (6.48), we can use Eq. (6.47) to determine the material dispersion factor for a certain wavelength range.

For the doped core of the optical fiber, Sellmeier's expression in Eq. (6.41) can be approximated to the form in Eq. (6.42) by using the curve-fitting technique. The material dispersion factor, $M(\lambda)$, becomes zero at wavelengths around 1350 nm and about -10 psi/(nm·km) at 1550 nm. However, the attenuation at 1350 nm is about 0.4 dB/km compared with 0.2 dB/km at 1550 nm, as given in Table 6.2.

Table 6.2: Sellmeier's coefficients for several optical fiber silica-based materials with germanium doped in the core region

| Sellmeier's constant | Germanium concentration, C (mol%) | | | |
	0 (pure silica)	3.1	5.8	7.9
G_1	0.6961663	0.7028554	0.7088876	0.7136824
G_2	0.4079426	0.4146307	0.4206803	0.4254807
G_3	0.8974794	0.8974540	0.8956551	0.8964226
λ_1	0.0684043	0.0727723	0.0609053	0.0617167
λ_2	0.1162414	0.1143085	0.1254514	0.1270814
λ_3	9.896161	9.896161	9.896162	9.896161

(ii) Waveguide Dispersion

The waveguiding of fiber may also create chromatic dispersion. This results from the variation in group velocity with wavelength for a particular mode. One can identify each mode with a corresponding ray which makes a particular angle with the fiber axis. When the source of light has a finite spectral width, each of these rays will contain all the spectral components. As a result, the angle made with the fiber axis by a particular ray corresponding to a mode will also vary with the wavelength (λ). Subsequently, there will be difference between the times taken by different components leading to pulse broadening. This is called as *waveguide* dispersion.

The effect of waveguide dispersion can be approximated by assuming that the refractive index of the material is independent of the wavelength. Let us now consider the group delay, i.e. the time required for a mode to travel along a fiber of length L. This kind of dispersion depends strongly on Δ and V parameters. To estimate the results of fiber parameters, we define a *normalized propagation constant, b,* as

$$b = \frac{a^2 w^2}{V^2} = \frac{a^2(\beta^2 - k_2^2)}{a^2(k_1^2 - \beta^2 + \beta^2 - k_2^2)} = \frac{(\beta^2 - k_2^2)}{k_1^2 - k_2^2} \tag{6.49}$$

Also
$$b = 1 - \left(\frac{ua}{V}\right) = \frac{\dfrac{\beta^2}{k^2} - n_2^2}{n_1^2 - n_2^2} \tag{6.49a}$$

For small values of index difference $\Delta = (n_1 - n_2)/n_1$, Eq. (6.49) can be approximated by

$$b \cong \frac{\frac{\beta}{k} - n_2}{n_1 - n_2} \tag{6.50}$$

Solving Eq. (6.50) for β, we have

$$\beta = n_2 k (b\Delta + 1) \tag{6.50a}$$

The group delay for waveguide dispersion is then given by (per unit length)

$$t_{wg} = \frac{d\beta}{d\omega} = \frac{1}{c}\frac{d\beta}{dk} \tag{6.51}$$

$$= \frac{1}{c}\left[n_1 + n_2\Delta \frac{d(bk)}{dk}\right] = \frac{1}{c}\left[n_1 + n_2\Delta \frac{d(bV)}{dV}\right] \tag{6.52}$$

The modal propagation constant β is generally given in terms of the normalized frequency V defined as

$$V^2 = (u^2 + w^2)a^2 = \left(\frac{2\pi a}{\lambda}\right)^2 (n_1^2 - n_2^2)$$

$$= \left(\frac{2\pi a}{\lambda}\right)^2 (NA)^2 \tag{6.52a}$$

We have used the approximation

$$V = ka\,(n_1^2 - n_2^2)^{1/2} = kan_1\sqrt{2\Delta}$$

for obtaining Eq. (6.52), which is valid for small values of Δ.

The first term in Eq. (6.52) is a constant and second term represents the group delay arising from waveguide dispersion. Further, the factor $d(bV)/dV$ can be expressed as

$$\frac{d(Vb)}{dV} = b\left[1 - \frac{2J_v^2(ua)}{J_{v+1}(ua)J_{v-1}(ua)}\right] \tag{6.52b}$$

where $u^2 = k_1^2 - \beta^2$ and a is fiber radius. Figure 6.18 shows the variation of $d(bV)/dV$ with the V-number for various LP modes. We can see that, for a given value of V-number the group delay is different for different modes.

Equation (6.52) can be obtained from Eq. (6.51) by using the expression of V. Thus, the rms pulse spreading, $\Delta\tau_\omega$, due to the waveguide dispersion per unit length by a source having an optical bandwidth (or linewidth, σ_λ) is given by

$$\Delta\tau_\omega = \frac{dt_{wg}}{d\lambda}\sigma_\lambda = -\frac{n_2\Delta}{c\lambda}V\frac{d^2(Vb)}{dV^2}\sigma_\lambda \tag{6.53}$$

Taking the derivative of Eq. (6.52) and using Eq. (6.53), we get

$$t_{wg} = \frac{n_2\Delta\sigma_\lambda}{c}\left|\frac{d}{d\lambda}\left[\frac{d(Vb)}{dV}\right]\right| = \frac{Ln_2\Delta\sigma_\lambda}{c}\left|\frac{d}{dV}\left[\frac{d(Vb)}{dV}\right]\left(\frac{dV}{d\lambda}\right)\right| \tag{6.53a}$$

$$\frac{dV}{d\lambda} = \frac{d}{d\lambda}\left[a\left(\frac{2\pi}{\lambda}\right)n_2\sqrt{2\Delta}\right] = a\left(-\frac{2\pi}{\lambda^2}\right)n_2\sqrt{2\Delta} = -\frac{V}{\lambda} \tag{6.53b}$$

Substituting the value of $dV/d\lambda$ in Eq. (6.53a), we obtain

$$\Delta\tau_\omega = \frac{n_2\Delta\sigma_\lambda}{c\lambda}V\frac{d^2(Vb)}{dV^2} \tag{6.53c}$$

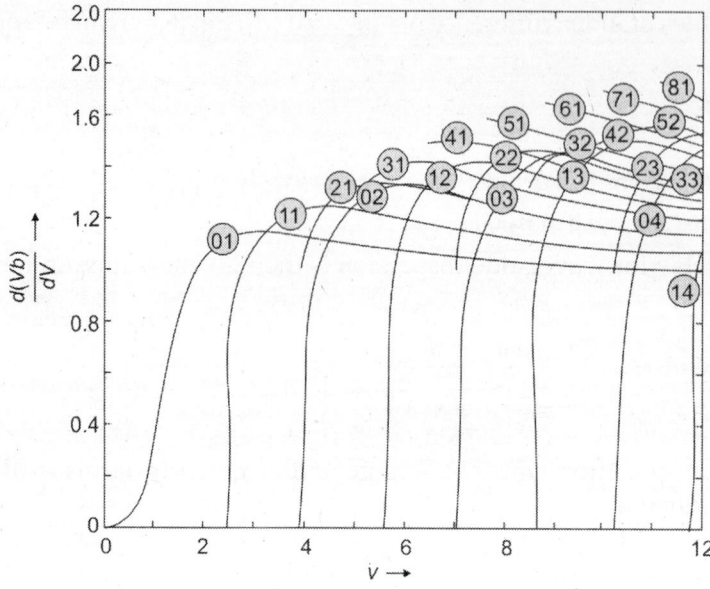

Fig. 6.18. Variation of d(Vb)/dV with V-number of the optical fiber

and the *waveguide dispersion factor or the waveguide dispersion parameter* (similar to the material dispersion factor) is then expressed as

$$D_{wg}(\lambda) = -\frac{n_2(\lambda)\Delta}{c\lambda} V \frac{d^2(Vb)}{dV^2} \tag{6.54}$$

in ps/(nm · km). In the range of $0.9 < \lambda/\lambda_c < 2.6$, the factor $V\frac{d^2(Vb)}{dV^2}$ can be approximated (to <5% error) by

$$V\frac{d^2(Vb)}{dV^2} \cong 0.080 + 0.549\,(2.834 - V)^2 \tag{6.55}$$

or, relatively, using the definition of the cutoff wavelength and the expression of the V parameters, we obtain

$$V\frac{d^2(Vb)}{dV^2} \cong 0.080 + 3.175\left(1.178 - \frac{\lambda_c}{\lambda}\right)^2 \tag{6.56}$$

Thus, from Eqs (6.56) and (6.55), we can calculate the waveguide dispersion factor and, hence, the pulse dispersion factor for a particular source spectral width, σ_λ. It is noted that the dispersion considered in this chapter is for a step-index fiber only. For a grade-index fiber, ESI parameters must be found, and the chromatic dispersion can then be calculated.

Alternative Expression for the Waveguide Dispersion Parameter, D(λ)

Alternatively, the waveguide dispersion parameter can be expressed as a function of the propagation constant, β, by using $\omega = 2\pi c/\lambda$ and Eq. (6.56); then the waveguide dispersion factor can be expressed as

$$D(\lambda) = -\frac{2\pi c}{\lambda^2}\beta_2 = -\frac{2\pi c}{\lambda^2}\frac{d\beta^2}{d\omega^2} \tag{6.57}$$

Thus, the waveguide dispersion factor is directly related to the second-order derivative of the propagation constant with respect to the optical radial frequency.

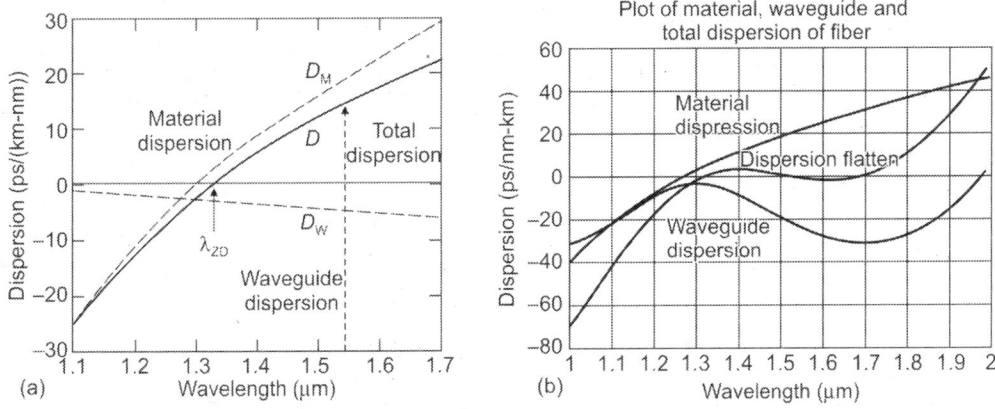

Fig. 6.19: Chromatic dispersion factors of (a) an SSMF and (b) a dispersion-flattened fiber. Plotted curves representing the material dispersion factor as a function of the optical wavelength for a silica-based optical fiber with a zero-dispersion wavelength at 1290 nm. This curve is generated as an example. For SSMF that are currently installed throughout the world, the total dispersion is around +17 ps /(nm·km) at 1550 nm and almost zero at 1310 nm

An example of a design of an optical fiber operating in the single-mode region is given in Fig. 6.19. The cladding material is pure silica. Shown in this figure are the curves of the material dispersion, the waveguide dispersion, and the total dispersion for an SMF with a nonuniform refractive index profile in the core.

A system for measurement of the relative group delay and chromatic dispersion of single mode optical fibers is shown in Fig. 6.20.

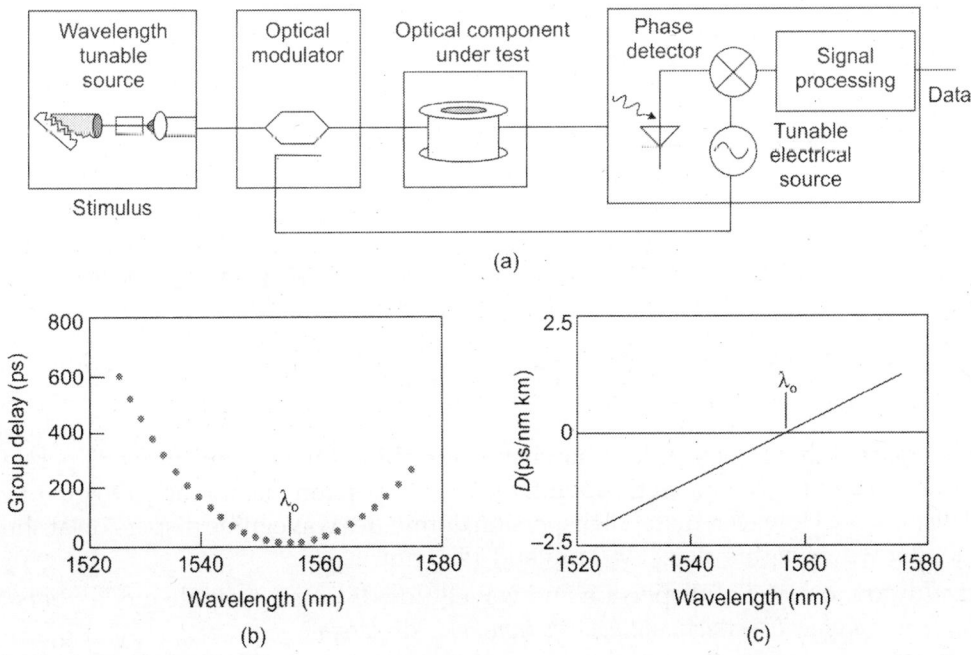

Fig. 6.20: (a) Chromatic dispersion measurement of a two-port optical device (b) relative group delay versus wavelength (c) dispersion parameter versus wavelength

6.7 WAVEGUIDE DISPERSION IN A SINGLE MODE FIBER

Equation (6.54) shows that the waveguide dispersion factor depends on the second derivative of the product of V-number and the normalized propagation constant, b, with respect to the V-number. In case of a multimode fiber, the said factor is negligibly small and as a result, the waveguide dispersion is insignificant in the case of multimode fiber as compared to material dispersion. However, in the case of a single mode fiber waveguide dispersion may become comparable to material dispersion. In order to see the behaviour of the waveguide dispersion, we consider the expression of the factor ua for the lowest order mode (the LP_{01} mode) in the normalized propagation constant. This can be approximated by

$$ua = \frac{(1+\sqrt{2})v}{1+(4+V^4)^{1/4}} \tag{6.58}$$

Substituting the value of ua from Eq. (6.58) into Eq. (6.49), we get

$$Vb(V) = V\left\{1 - \frac{(1+\sqrt{2})^2}{\left[1+(4+V^4)^{1/2}\right]^2}\right\} \tag{6.59}$$

One can obtain the second derivative of the product (Vb) with respect to V by using Eq. (6.59). Figure 6.21 shows the variations of the parameters b, $d(Vb)/dV$ and $Vd^2(Vb)/dV^2$ with the V number for the LP_{01} (HE_{11}) mode. We see that the quantity $(Vd^2(Vb)/dV^2)$ has a positive value over the entire region of single mode operation, i.e. for $0 < V \leq 2.405$ with a maximum value at $V = 1.15$. As a result waveguide dispersion, D_{wg} is negative in the entire region of single mode operation. The quantity $(Vd^2(Vb)/dV^2)$ goes to zero at $V = 3.0$ beyond the region of the true single mode operation and attains a negative value beyond this point (not shown in Fig. 6.21). For a single mode fiber with $V = 2.4$ operating at 1320 nm having $n_2 = 1.5$ and $\Delta = 0.2$ per cent, the value of $d^2(Vb)/dV^2 \approx 0.1$. One can estimate the waveguide dispersion parameter of the fiber as

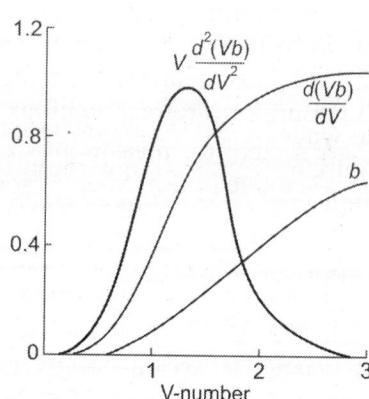

Fig. 6.21: Variation of parameters b, d(Vb)/dV and Vd²(Vb)/dV² with V-number for the lowest order mode (LP$_{01}$) in a single mode fiber

$$D_{wg} = -\frac{1}{L}\frac{n_2\Delta}{c\lambda}V\frac{d^2(Vb)}{dV^2} = -\frac{1}{10^{-3}}\times\frac{1.5\times0.002}{3\times10^8\times1320}\times2.4\times0.1$$

$$= -1.8 \text{ ps nm}^{-1}\text{ km}^{-1}$$

It is reported that for a standard nondispersion shifted fiber, waveguide dispersion is important around 1320 nm. At this point, the two dispersion factors cancel to give a zero total dispersion. However, material dispersion dominates waveguide dispersion at shorter and longer wavelengths, e.g. at 900 nm and 1550 nm.

In addition to material dispersion and waveguide dispersion, single mode fibers also suffer from: *profile dispersion and polarization mode dispersion.*

6.7.1 Profile Dispersion

This dispersion arises from the dependence of the index deviation Δ, on the operating wavelength (λ) of the light. The profile dispersion parameter is proportional to $d\Delta/d\lambda$

and the value of this dispersion is generally very small (< 0.5 ps nm^{-1} km^{-1}) and this is why usually goes unnoticed. In case of a multimode fiber, the profile dispersion is insignificant as the majority of the modes that carry the light through the fiber propagate far away from the cut-off. Thus, in a multimode fiber, the intramodal dispersion is dominated by material dispersion and waveguide dispersion only. Further, the V number of a multimode fiber is usually high and as a result the waveguide dispersion is very small as to material dispersion. However, the total dispersion in a standard single mode fiber is generally dominated by both material dispersion as well as waveguide dispersion. Considering the effect of profile dispersion, D_{pro}, one can express the total dispersion, D_{tot} of a single mode fiber as

$$D_{tot} = D_{mat} + D_{wg} + D_{pro} \qquad (6.60)$$

We have seen (Fig. 6.17) that material dispersion attends a value zero at the *zero material dispersion* (ZMD) point corresponding to $\lambda = 1.27$ μm. This means that at this wavelength, the pulse broadening due to material dispersion can be made zero. Further, the ZMD point can be shifted conveniently to a suitable wavelength by changing the constitutents of glass, e.g. by changing the concentration of GeO_2 in a pure silica from 0–15%, one finds the shifting of the ZMD point from 1.27 to 1.37 μm. However, it is reported that the overall dispersion is affected by other components such as waveguide and profile dispersion components. This means, the zero pulse-broadening point does not actually correspond to ZMD where the material dispersion component is zero. We may note that for wavelengths longer than the ZMD point, the material dispersion is positive, whereas the waveguide dispersion is negative for conventional single-mode operation region. Figure 6.22 shows the variations of material dispersion and waveguide dispersion in a single mode fiber with wavelength exhibiting ZMD point and also the wavelength, λ_0 at which the total dispersion is zero. We find that the total dispersion in a single mode fiber is approximately equal to the sum of material and waveguide dispersion, because the profile dispersion is negligible and moreover, intermodal dispersion is not present in a single mode fiber. One can easily see that there has to be a certain wavelength at which the waveguide dispersion exactly compensates the material dispersion and the total dispersion becomes zero. Further, the wavelength λ_0, at which the total first order dispersion in a single mode fiber is zero, is slightly larger than the wavelength corresponding to ZMD point. We can also see that, ZMD occurs at 1.27 μm and the waveguide dispersion component shifts this minimum dispersion point to a longer wavelength, $\lambda_0 = 1.32$ μm for minimum total dispersion. It is reported that a very low value of total intramodal dispersion in a single mode fiber which is again free from intra-modal dispersion effects, enable them to offer a very high value of

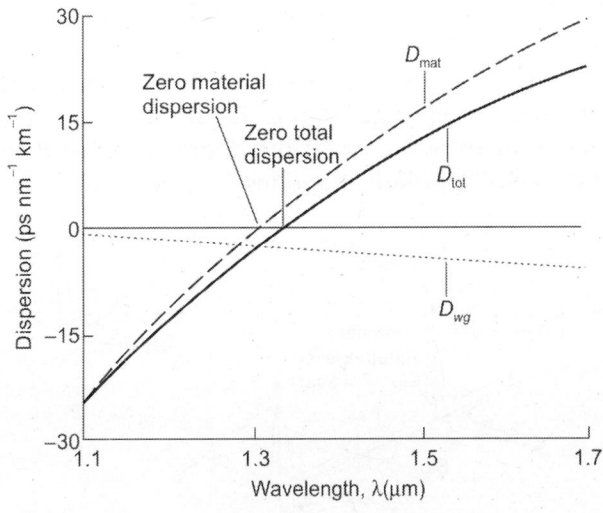

Fig. 6.22: Variations of material dispersion and waveguide dispersion in a single mode fiber with wavelength exhibiting ZMD point as well as the wavelength λ_0 at which the total dispersion is zero

bandwidth-length product (~100 GHz km^{-1}) around this wavelength. This is considered to be one of the major reasons for shifting the wavelength to this region in the second generation (2G) optical fiber communication. However, silicon fibers exhibit a moderately high value of attenuation resulting primarily from Rayleigh scattering, we may also note that material dispersion and waveguide dispersion components can be tailored by adjusting the material composition and the geometry of the fiber. As a result, one can possibly alter the value of the wavelength, λ_0, corresponding to the first order total dispersion point (Fig. 6.23). Figure 6.23 also shows that λ_0, can be selected in the range of 1.3 mm to 1.6 mm by adjusting the core diameter and index profile.

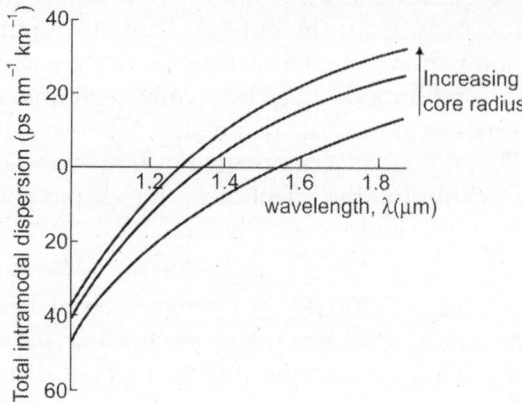

Fig. 6.23: Variation of total intramodal dispersion in a single mode fiber with wavelength λ for different values of core radius

6.7.2 Polarization Mode Dispersion (PMD)

The birefringence phenomenon affects the polarization state of the light propagating through cylindrical optical fibers. We may note that the birefringence manifests itself in the form of an additional pulse broadening component and generally termed as PMD. A small departure from the circular symmetry of the core (less than even 1% of the circularity of the core) in a single mode fiber may cause the decomposition of the fundamental HE_{11} mode into two orthogonal components, e.g. HE_{11}^{x} and HE_{11}^{y}, to support bimodal transmission. Other factors, e.g. bending, twisting, etc. of the fiber may also be responsible for birefringence. In all practical systems, usually fibers have nonperfect geometry due to one or more factors and as a result the polarization state of the fiber can only be maintained over a few meters of length of the fiber.

Figure 6.24 illustrates the propagation of the polarization components of the guide mode of the single mode fiber via the random variation of the fiber birefringence axis through a long length of fiber. Figure 6.25 shows the transmission effects of the polarization mode dispersion, that is the degradation of the eye diagram due to differential delay between the polarized modes.

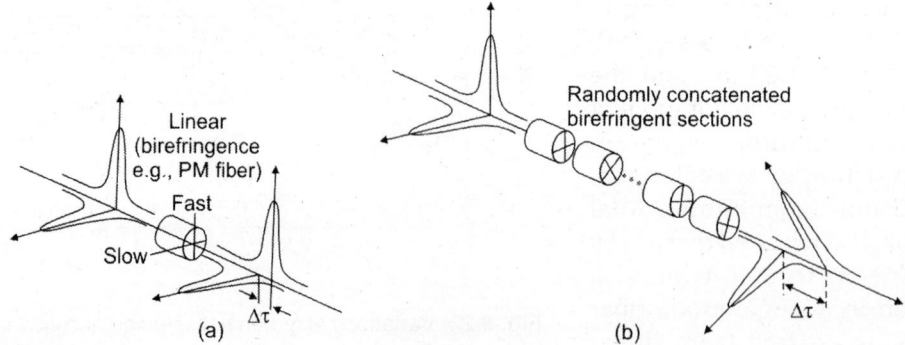

Fig. 6.24: Conceptual illustration of model of PMD (a) simple birefringence device (b) randomly concatenated birefringence

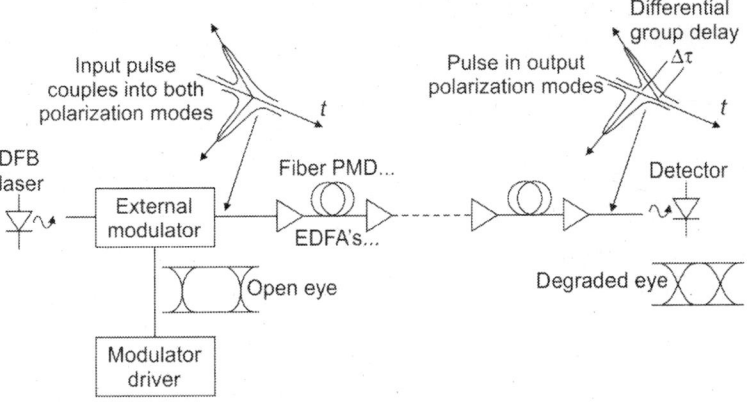

Fig. 6.25: Schematic illustration of effect of PMD in a digital optical communication system—degradation of the received eye diagram

We may note that the polarization state as such does not otherwise affect optical transmission systems that involve some kind of intensity modulation of light. For example, in IM/DD-based optical communication system the light is intensity modulated at the transmitter and it is subsequently defected with the help of a photodetector which is basically a kind of *photon counter*, i.e. insensitive to the polarization state or phase of light in the fiber. However, it is found that there are more sophisticated application including

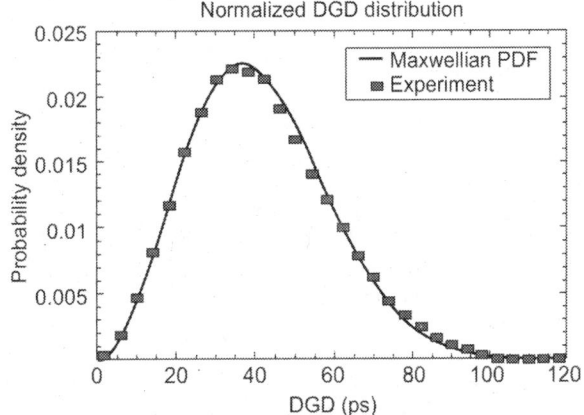

Fig. 6.26: Maxwellian distribution of a PMD random process

coherent optical communication systems where polarization state of the light is important. The delay between two principal states of polarization (PSPs) is normally negligibly small at 10 Gb/s. However, at a high bit rate and in ultra-long-haul transmission link operating over 100 Gbps/km. The instantaneous value of differential group delay (DGD), $\Delta\tau$, varies along the fiber and follows a Maxwellian distribution (Fig. 6.26). This is why in certain situations it is necessary to maintain the polarization state of the fiber over a significant length.

The Maxwellian distribution is governed by the following expression:

$$f(\Delta t) = \frac{32(\Delta\tau)^2}{\pi^2 \langle \Delta\tau \rangle^3} \exp\left\{-\frac{4(\Delta\tau)^2}{\pi \langle \Delta\tau \rangle^2}\right\} \cdot \Delta\tau \geq 0 \tag{6.61}$$

The mean DGD value, $\langle \Delta\tau \rangle$, is commonly termed *"fiber PMD"* and provided in the fiber specifications. The following expression gives an estimate of the maximum transmission limit, L_{max}, due to the PMD effect:

$$L_{max} = \frac{0.02}{\langle \Delta\tau \rangle^2 \cdot R^2} \tag{6.62}$$

where R is the bit rate. Based on Eq. (6.62), L_{max} for both old fiber vintages and contemporary fibers is obtained as follows:

- $\langle \Delta \tau \rangle$ = 1 ps/km (old fiber vintages): For a bit rate of R = 40 Gb/s, the maximum distance L_{max} = 12.5 km; for R = 10 Gb/s, L_{max} = 200 km.
- $\langle \Delta \tau \rangle$ = 0.1 ps/km (contemporary fibers for modern optical systems): For a bit rate of R = 40 Gb/s, the maximum transmission distance is L_{max} = 1,250 km; for R = 10 Gb/s, L_{max} = 20,000 km.

We now consider a uniformly birefringent fiber. Now, the light energy in the fundamental mode travels in the bimodal form supporting two components with orthogonal polarization states. The birefringence of the medium will cause the two orthogonal components to travel at a slightly different velocity. Due to this, the polarization orientation of the propagating light will rotate with distance. The two modes exhibit different group delays of τ_{gx} and τ_{gy}. The resulting delay difference, $\delta \tau_{pol}$, occuring between the two orthogonally polarized components thus gives rise to pulse broadening. One can express the delay difference as

$$\delta \tau_{pol} = |\tau_{gx} - \tau_{gy}| = \left| \frac{L}{v_{gx}} - \frac{L}{v_{gy}} \right| \tag{6.63}$$

where, v_{gx} and v_{gx} are the group velocities of the corresponding orthogonal components and L is the length of the fiber. The parameter $\delta \tau_{pol}$ denotes the *polarization mode dispersion* (PMD) of the fiber.

The group delay $\delta \tau_{pol}$ caused by the two orthogonal components lead to a pulse spreading of $(\delta \tau_{pol} L)$ over a length L of the fiber. One can use the product $(\delta \tau_{pol} L)$ as a good approximation for calculation of 3 dB bandwidth given by

$$B = \frac{0.9}{(\delta \tau_{pol} L)} \text{ Hz/km} \tag{6.64}$$

We may note that polarization mode dispersion varies randomly along the fiber length whereas chromatic dispersion remains more or less stable along the length of the fiber. The randomness of PMD is attributed to the fact the perturbations responsible for birefringence are dependent on temperature. Therefore, PMD is manifested in the form of time varying fluctuation about the mean value of the group delay, $\delta \tau_{pol}$. Equation (6.63) is strictly valid under ideal condition of a fiber with uniform stable-birefringence property. For practical applications, the PMD is often expressed in terms of mean value of the differential group delay as

$$\delta_{pol} \approx D_{PMD} \sqrt{L} \tag{6.65}$$

where, D_{PMD} is the average value of PMD measured in $\text{ps}/\sqrt{\text{km}}$. The value of D_{PMD} usually ranges between 0.1 and 1 $\text{ps}/\sqrt{\text{km}}$ and largely depends on the environmental conditions and type of installation, e.g. the value of PMD is generally large for aerial optical fiber cables as compared to buried cables. This is attributed to sudden changes of temperature and/or movements caused by the wind in the former case.

6.8 INTERMODAL DISPERSION

Pulse broadening due to intermodal dispersion (sometimes referred to simply as *modal* or *mode dispersion*) results from the propagation delay differences between modes within a multimode fiber. As the different modes which constitute a pulse in a multimode fiber travel along the channel at different group velocities, the pulse width at the output is dependent upon the transmission times of the slowest and fastest modes. This dispersion mechanism creates the fundamental difference in the overall dispersion for the three types of fiber shown in Fig. 6.12. Thus multimode step index fibers exhibit a large amount of intermodal dispersion which gives the greatest pulse broadening. However, intermodal dispersion in multimode fibers may be reduced by adoption of an optimum refractive index profile which is provided by the near-parabolic profile of most graded index fibers. Hence, the overall pulse broadening in multimode graded index fibers is far less than that obtained in multimode step index fibers (typically by a factor of 100). Thus graded index fibers used with a multimode source give a tremendous bandwidth advantage over multimode step index fibers.

Under purely single-mode operation there is no intermodal dispersion and therefore pulse broadening is solely due to the intramodal dispersion mechanisms. In theory, this is the case with single-mode step inc ex fibers where only a single mode is allowed to propagate. Hence they exhibit the least pulse broadening and have the greatest possible bandwidths, but in general are only usefully operated with single-mode sources.

The intermodal dispersion which causes pulse broadening essentially arises from the difference in time, T_{max} and T_{min}, where T_{max} is the time taken by the longest ray congruence path (most oblique ray) corresponding to highest order mode, and T_{min} is the time taken by the shortest ray congruence path (axial ray) corresponding to lowest order mode. However, this dispersion vanishes in the case single mode operation.

We may note that pulse broadening due to intermodal dispersion is most significant in the case of a step-index multimode fiber. However, this can be controlled to a great extent by using a graded-index profile. When an optical fiber is designed to have a near-parabolic refractive index profile, one finds that the pulse broadening due to intermodal dispersion is minimized. As a consequence, the bandwidth of a graded-index multimode fiber is quite larger that of a corresponding step-index multimode fiber. We may also note that single mode fibers on the otherhand do not suffer from pulse broadening arising from intermodal dispersion and this is why, they offer largest possible bandwidths which are limited by intramodal dispersion effects.

6.8.1 Pulse Broadening in a Multimode Step-Index Fiber

We consider T mode multimode step-index fiber. According to ray theory model, the fastest and slowest modes propagating in the step index fiber may be represented by the axial ray and the extreme meridional ray (which is incident at the core-cladding interface at the critical angle ϕ_c) respectively. The paths taken by these two rays in a perfectly structured step index fiber are shown in Fig. 6.27. The delay difference between these two rays when traveling in the fiber core allows estimation of the pulse broadening resulting from intermodal dispersion within the fiber. As both rays are traveling at the same velocity within the constant refractive index fiber core, then the delay difference is directly related to their respective path lengths within the fiber. Hence the time taken for the axial ray to travel along a fiber of length L gives the minimum delay time T_{min} and:

$$T_{min} = \frac{distance}{velocity} = \frac{L}{(c/n_1)} = \frac{Ln_1}{c} \tag{6.66}$$

where n_1 is the refractive index of the core and c is the velocity of light in a vacuum.

The extreme meridional ray exhibits the maximum delay time T_{Max}, where:

$$T_{max} = \frac{L/\cos\theta}{c/n_1} = \frac{Ln_1}{c\cos\theta} \tag{6.67}$$

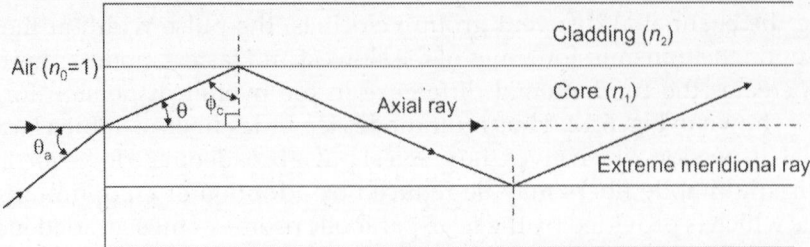

Fig. 6.27: The ray diagram of paths taken by the axial and an extreme meridional ray in a perfect multimode step index fiber

Using Snell's law of refraction at the core–cladding interface: we have

$$\sin\phi_c = \frac{n_2}{n_1} = \cos\theta \qquad (6.68)$$

where n_2 is the refractive index of the cladding. Furthermore, substituting into Eq. (6.67) for $\cos\theta$ gives:

$$T_{max} = \frac{Ln_1^2}{cn_2} \qquad (6.69)$$

The delay difference δT_s between the extreme meridional ray and the axial ray may be obtained by subtracting Eq. (6.66) from Eq. (6.69). Hence:

$$\delta T_s = T_{Max} - T_{Min} = \frac{Ln_1^2}{cn_2} - \frac{Ln_1}{c}$$

$$= \frac{Ln_1^2}{cn_2}\left(\frac{n_1 - n_2}{n_1}\right) \qquad (6.70)$$

$$\simeq \frac{Ln_1^2\Delta}{cn_2} \qquad \text{when } \Delta \ll 1 \qquad (6.71)$$

where Δ is the relative refractive index difference. However, when $\Delta \ll 1$, then the relative refractive index difference may also be given approximately by:

$$\Delta \simeq \frac{n_1 - n_2}{n_2} \qquad (6.72)$$

Hence rearranging Eq. (6.70), we obtain

$$\delta T_s = \frac{Ln_1}{c}\left(\frac{n_1 - n_2}{n_2}\right) \simeq \frac{Ln_1\Delta}{c} \qquad (6.73)$$

Also substituting for $\Delta = \frac{(NA)^2}{2n_1^2}$, we obtain

$$\delta T_s \simeq \frac{L(NA)^2}{2n_1 c} \qquad (6.74)$$

where NA is the numerical aperture for the fiber. The approximate expressions for the delay difference given in Eqs (6.73) and (6.74) are usually employed to estimate the maximum pulse broadening in time due to intermodal dispersion in multimode step index fibers. It must be noted that this simple analysis only considers pulse broadening due to meridional rays and totally ignores skew rays with acceptance angles $\theta_{as} > \theta_a$.

6.8.2 RMS Pulse Broadening

Considering the perfect step index fiber, another useful quantity with regard to intermodal dispersion on an optical fiber link is the *rms pulse broadening* resulting from this dispersion mechanism along the fiber. When the optical input to the fiber is a pulse $p_i(t)$ of unit area, as shown in Fig. 6.28, then, we have

$$\int_{-\infty}^{\infty} p_i(t)\, dt = 1$$

or

$$\int_{-\delta T_{\mathrm{mod}}/2}^{\delta T_{\mathrm{mod}}/2} pi(t)\, dt = 1 \qquad (6.75)$$

Mathematically, one can express the broadened as

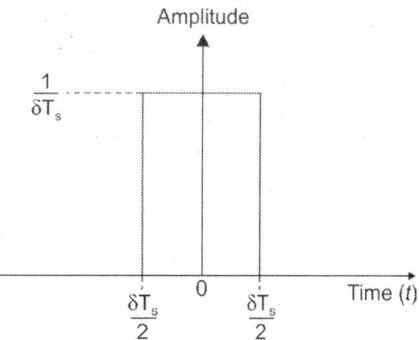

Fig. 6.28: Light input to the multimode step index fiber consisting of an ideal pulse or rectangular function with unit area, i.e. broadened rectangular pulse due to intermodal dispersion

$$p_i(t) = \frac{1}{\delta T_{\mathrm{mod}}} \quad \text{for} \quad -\frac{\delta T_{\mathrm{mod}}}{2} \le 1 \le \frac{\delta T_{\mathrm{mod}}}{2} \qquad (6.75a)$$

$$= 0 \qquad \text{otherwise} \qquad (6.75b)$$

Obviously $p_i(t)$ has a constant amplitude of $1/\delta T_s$ over the range:

$$\frac{-\delta T_s}{2} \le p(t) \le \frac{\delta T_s}{2}$$

The root mean square (rms) value of the pulse broadening at the fiber output due to intermodal dispersion for the multimode step index fiber σ_s (i.e. the standard deviation) may be given in terms of the variance σ_s^2 as

$$\sigma_s^2 = M_2 - M_1^2 \qquad (6.76)$$

where M_1 is the first temporal moment which is equivalent to the mean value of the pulse and M_2, the second temporal moment, is equivalent to the mean square value of the pulse. Hence:

$$M_1 = \int_{-\infty}^{\infty} t p_i(t)\, dt \qquad (6.77)$$

and

$$M_2 = \int_{-\infty}^{\infty} t^2 p_i(t)\, dt \qquad (6.78)$$

The mean value M_1 for the unit input pulse of Fig. 6.28 is zero, and assuming this is maintained for the output pulse, then from Eqs (6.76) and (6.78) we have

$$\sigma_s^2 = M_2 = \int_{-\infty}^{\infty} t^2 p_i(t)\, dt \qquad (6.79)$$

Integrating over the limits of the input pulse (Fig. 6.28) and substituting for $p_i(t)$ in Eq. (6.79) over this range gives:

$$\sigma_s^2 = \int_{-\delta T_s/2}^{\delta T_s/2} \frac{1}{\delta T_s} t^2\, dt$$

$$= \frac{1}{\delta T_1} \left[\frac{t^3}{3} \right]_{-\delta T_s/2}^{\delta T_s/2} = \frac{1}{3} \left(\frac{\delta T_s}{2} \right)^2 \qquad (6.80)$$

Hence substituting from Eq. (6.73) for δT_s gives:

$$\sigma_s \simeq \frac{L n_1 \Delta}{2\sqrt{3}c} \simeq \frac{L(NA)^2}{4\sqrt{3}n_1 c} \qquad (6.81)$$

Equation (6.81) permits us the estimation of the rms impulse response of a multimode step index fiber if it is assumed that intermodal dispersion dominates and there is a uniform distribution of light rays over the range $0 \leq \theta \leq \theta_a$. The pulse broadening is directly proportional to the relative refractive index difference Δ and the length of the fiber L. The latter emphasizes the bandwidth–length trade-off that exists, especially with multimode step index fibers, and which inhibits their use for wideband long-haul (between repeaters) systems. Furthermore, the pulse broadening is reduced by reduction of the relative refractive index difference Δ for the fiber. This suggests that weakly guiding fibers with small Δ are best for low-dispersion transmission. However, this is also subject to a trade-off as a reduction in Δ reduces the acceptance angle θ_a and the NA, thus worsening the launch condition.

Intermodal dispersion may be reduced by propagation mechanisms within practical fibers, e.g. there is differential attenuation of the various modes in a step index fiber. This is due to the greater field penetration of the higher order modes into the cladding of the waveguide. These slower modes therefore exhibit larger losses at any core–cladding irregularities, which tends to concentrate the transmitted optical power into the faster lower order modes. Thus the differential attenuation of modes reduces intermodal pulse broadening on a multimode optical link.

Another mechanism which reduces intermodal pulse broadening in nonperfect (i.e. practical) multimode fibers is the mode coupling or mixing. The coupling between guided modes transfers optical power from the slower to the faster modes, and vice versa. Hence, with strong coupling the optical power tends to be transmitted at an average speed, which is the mean of the various propagating modes. This reduces the intermodal dispersion on the link and makes it advantageous to encourage mode coupling within multimode fibers.

The expression for delay difference [Eq. (6.73)] for a perfect step index fiber may be modified for the fiber with mode coupling among all guided modes to

$$\delta T_{sc} \simeq \frac{n_1 \Delta}{c} (LL_c)^{1/2} \tag{6.82}$$

where L_c is a characteristic length for the fiber which is inversely proportional to the coupling strength. Hence, the delay difference increases at a slower rate proportional to $(LL_c)^{1/2}$ instead of the direct proportionality to L given in Eq. (6.73). However, the most successful technique for reducing intermodal dispersion in multimode fibers is by grading the core refractive index to follow a near-parabolic profile. This has the effect of equalizing the transmission times of the various modes. This is discussed in following section.

6.8.3 Intermodal Dispersion in a Multimode Graded-Index Fiber

Intermodal dispersion in multimode fibers can be minimized with the use of graded index fibers. Hence, multimode graded index fibers show substantial bandwidth improvement over multimode step index fibers. The reason for the improved performance of graded index fibers may be observed by considering the ray diagram for a graded index fiber shown in Fig. 6.29. The fiber shown has a parabolic index profile with a maximum at the core axis, as illustrated in Fig. 6.29(a). Analytically, the index profile is given by (with $\alpha = 2$ as):

$$n(r) = n_1[1 - 2\Delta(r/a)^2]^{1/2} \quad r < a \, (\text{core}) \tag{6.82a}$$
$$= n_1(1 - 2\Delta)^{1/2} = n_2 \quad r \geq a \, (\text{cladding})$$

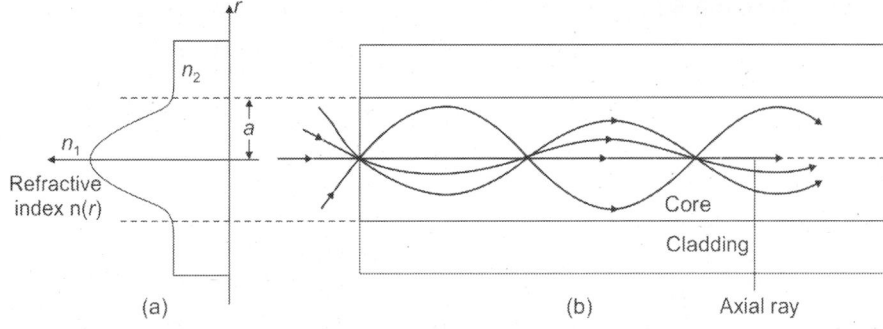

Fig. 6.29: Schematic of multimode graded index fiber: (a) parabolic refractive index profile (b) meridional ray paths within the fiber core

Figure 6.29(b) shows several meridional ray paths within the fiber core. We can observe that apart from the axial ray, the meridional rays follow sinusoidal trajectories of different path lengths which result from the index grading. However, the local group velocity is inversely proportional to the number of modes for a given value of propagation constant β can be expressed (using WKB approximation) as:

$$m = a^2 k^2 n_1^2 \Delta \frac{\alpha}{\alpha + 2} \left(\frac{k^2 n_1^2 - \beta^2}{2\Delta k^2 n_1^2} \right)^{\frac{2+\alpha}{\alpha}} \tag{6.83}$$

On rearranging the Eq. (6.83), we obtain

$$\beta = \left[k^2 n_1^2 - 2 \left(\frac{\alpha + 2}{\alpha} \frac{m}{\alpha^2} \right)^{\frac{\alpha}{\alpha + 2}} \left(k^2 n_1^2 \Delta \right)^{\frac{2}{\alpha + 2}} \right]^{1/2} \tag{6.84}$$

The propagation constant, β can also be alternatively expressed as:

$$\beta = kn_1 \left[1 - 2\Delta \left(\frac{m}{M} \right)^{\frac{\alpha}{\alpha + 2}} \right]^{1/2} \tag{6.85}$$

where, M is the total number of possible guided modes through the graded-index fiber given by

$$M = a^2 k^2 n_1^2 \Delta \left(\frac{\alpha}{\alpha + 2} \right) \tag{6.86}$$

The group delay associated with the modes propagating through a graded-index fiber can be estimated (remembering the fact that n_1 and Δ are also function of k) as:

$$\tau_g = \frac{L}{c} \frac{\partial \beta}{\partial k} \tag{6.87}$$

Taking the first derivative of the propagation constant β with respect to k and making us of Eq. (6.87), one may finally express the group delay τ_g as

$$\tau_g = \frac{L}{c} \left(\frac{kn_1}{\beta} \right) \left[\left(n_1 + k \frac{\partial n_1}{\partial k} \right) - \frac{4\Delta}{\alpha + 2} \left(\frac{m}{M} \right)^{\frac{\alpha}{\alpha + 2}} \left(\left(n_1 + k \frac{\partial n_1}{\partial k} \right) + \frac{n_1 k}{2\Delta} \frac{\partial \Delta}{\partial k} \right) \right] \tag{6.88}$$

Making the following substitutions

$$N_1 = n_1 + k\frac{\partial n_1}{\partial k} \tag{6.88a}$$

and

$$\epsilon = \frac{2n_1 k}{\left(n_1 + k\dfrac{\partial n_1}{\partial k}\right)\Delta}\frac{\partial \Delta}{\partial k} = \frac{2n_1 k}{N_1 \Delta}\frac{\partial \Delta}{\partial k} \tag{6.88b}$$

Equation (6.88) reads as

$$t_g = \frac{LN_1}{c}\left(\frac{kn_1}{\beta}\right)\left[1 - \frac{\Delta}{\alpha+2}\left(\frac{m}{M}\right)^{\frac{\alpha}{\alpha+2}}(4+\epsilon)\right] \tag{6.89}$$

Using Eq. (6.85) one may write

$$\frac{kn_1}{\beta} = \left[1 - 2\Delta\left(\frac{m}{M}\right)^{\frac{\alpha}{\alpha+2}}\right]^{-1/2} \tag{6.90}$$

Further, we may note that the core-cladding index difference $\Delta \ll 1$ and $m/M < 1$ for a given value of β lying between kn_1 and kn_2. Substituting,

$$x = \Delta\left(\frac{m}{M}\right)^{\frac{\alpha}{\alpha+2}} \ll 1 \tag{6.91}$$

Equation (6.90) can be expanded binomially to approximate as

$$\frac{kn_1}{\beta} = [1 - 2x]^{-1/2} \approx 1 + x + \frac{3x^2}{2} \tag{6.92}$$

or

$$\frac{kn_1}{\beta} \approx 1 + \Delta\left(\frac{m}{M}\right)^{\frac{\alpha}{\alpha+2}} + \frac{3}{2}\Delta^2\left(\frac{m}{M}\right)^{\frac{2\alpha}{\alpha+2}} \tag{6.93}$$

Substituting the value of (kn_1/β) from Eq. (6.93) into Eq. (6.89), the group delay is obtained as:

$$\tau_g = \frac{LN_1}{c}\left[1 + \Delta\left(\frac{m}{M}\right)^{\frac{\alpha}{\alpha+2}} + \frac{3}{2}\Delta^2\left(\frac{m}{M}\right)^{\frac{2\alpha}{\alpha+2}}\right]\left[1 - \frac{\Delta}{\alpha+2}\left(\frac{m}{M}\right)^{\frac{\alpha}{\alpha+2}}(4+\epsilon)\right] \tag{6.94}$$

$$= \frac{N_1 L}{c}\left[1 + \frac{\alpha-2-\epsilon}{\Delta+2}\Delta\left(\frac{m}{M}\right)^{\frac{\alpha}{\alpha+2}} + \frac{3\alpha-2-2\epsilon}{2(\alpha+2)}\Delta^2\left(\frac{m}{M}\right)^{\frac{2\alpha}{\alpha+2}} + O(\Delta^3)\right] \tag{6.95}$$

where, $O(\Delta^3)$ is the term containing the term Δ^3 and we can ignore it since $\Delta \ll 1$.

We can see from Eq. (6.95), that the first order term in Δ of the delay difference between the modes is zero when

$$\alpha = 2 + \epsilon \tag{6.96}$$

We see that the value of ϵ is generally very small. Therefore, we may conclude that minimum intermodal dispersion will result from the group delay between the various modes of a multimode fiber when $\alpha \approx 2$, i.e. the refractive index profile of the GI fiber is nearly parabolic.

The *rms* pulse broadening due to intermodal dispersion can be calculated only when the power carried by individual mode is known. The *rms* value of pulse spreading due to intermodal dispersion can be expressed as:

$$\sigma_{\text{modal}} = \left(\langle \tau_g^2 \rangle - \langle \tau_g \rangle^2\right)^{1/2} \tag{6.97}$$

where
$$\langle \tau_g^2 \rangle = \sum_{l,\,m} \frac{P_{lm}\,\tau_g^2(l,m)}{M} \tag{6.98}$$

and
$$\langle \tau_g \rangle = \sum_{l,\,m} \frac{P_{lm}\,\tau_g(l,m)}{M} \tag{6.99}$$

Here, P_{im} is the *optical power* contained in the mode of order (l, m) and M is the total number of modes.

Now, assuming that all modes are equally excited, i.e. each mode carries the same amount of power, i.e. this amounts of $P_{lm} = P$ for all modes irrespective of the mode order designated by (l, m). Further, if we assume that the total number of modes is very large then the summations appearing in Eqs (6.98) and (6.99) can be replaced by corresponding integrals. On the basis of the above assumptions and subsequent substitution of Eq. (6.95) into Eq. (6.97), one obtains

$$\sigma_{\text{modal}} = \frac{Ln_1\Delta}{2c}\frac{\alpha}{\alpha+1}\left(\frac{\alpha+2}{3\alpha+2}\right)^{1/2} \times \left[c_1^2 + \frac{4c_1c_2(\alpha+1)\Delta}{2\alpha+1} + \frac{16\Delta^2 c_2^2(\alpha+1)^2}{(5\alpha+2)(3\alpha+2)}\right]^{1/2} \tag{6.100}$$

where,
$$c_1 = \frac{\alpha-2-\epsilon}{\alpha+2} \tag{6.100a}$$

and
$$c_2 = \frac{3\alpha-2-2\epsilon}{2(\alpha+2)} \tag{6.100b}$$

This clearly suggests that the intermodal dispersion can be greatly reduced by making the *refractive index profile nearly parabolic* (i.e. $\alpha \approx 2$). Further, we see that when $\alpha - 2 - \epsilon$ is of the order of Δ there is a partial cancellation of the two mode dependent terms in Eq. (6.95) and the optimal value of α for minimum rms pulse broadening due to intermodal dispersion is obtained as

$$\alpha_c = 2 + \epsilon - \Delta\frac{(4+\epsilon)(3+\epsilon)}{5+2\epsilon} \tag{6.101}$$

However, it is reported that the overall pulse broadening also depends on the *chromatic* or *intramodal dispersion* which has been ignored by us in the analysis so far. In a practical measurement both intramodal and intermodal dispersion phenomena manifest in the form of the overall pulse broadening caused by the fiber. In order to obtain the optimum index profile of a GI fiber, one has to take into account the effect of intramodal dispersion, which not only depends on the transmission characteristics of the core and the cladding but also on the spectral property of the source.

The pulse broadening due to intramodal dispersion can be expressed as

$$\sigma_{\text{modal}}^2 = \left(\frac{\sigma_\lambda}{\lambda}\right)^2 \left\langle \left(\lambda\frac{d\tau_g}{d\lambda}\right)^2 \right\rangle \tag{6.102}$$

where, σ_λ is the rms spectral width of the source.

Using Eq. (6.95) and neglecting all terms containing second and higher order of the index deviation term $\Delta(<< 1)$ and terms containing negligibly small factors such as $d\Delta/d\lambda$ and $\Delta dn_1/d\lambda$, one obtains

$$\lambda\frac{d\tau_g}{d\lambda} \approx -\frac{L}{c}\lambda^2\frac{d^2 n_1}{d\lambda^2} + \frac{N_1 L\Delta}{c}\frac{a-2-\epsilon}{\alpha+2}\frac{2\alpha}{\alpha+2}\left(\frac{m}{M}\right)^{\frac{\alpha}{\alpha+2}} \tag{6.103}$$

We may note that for a GI fiber both the terms on the right hand side of the Eq. (6.102) are generally comparable when α is very different from 2. On the other hand, for a near parabolic index fiber $\alpha \approx 2$, the second term becomes negligible.

In order to evaluate the rms spreading due to intramodal dispersion, let us assume that all modes are equally excited so as to carry the same amount of power by each mode. Now, assuming that number of modes is very large in number, the summations used for computation of the average value can be conveniently replaced by integration. Substituting the value of $\lambda d\tau_g/d\lambda$ from Eq. (6.103) into Eq. (6.102), one finally obtain

$$\sigma_{\text{intramodal}} = \frac{L}{c}\frac{\sigma_\lambda}{\lambda}\left[\left(-\lambda^2\frac{d^2 n_1}{d\lambda^2}\right)^2 - N_1 c_1 \Delta\left(2\lambda^2\frac{d^2 n_1}{d\lambda^2}\frac{\alpha}{\alpha+1} - N_1 c_1 \Delta\frac{4\alpha^2}{(\alpha+2)(3\alpha+2)}\right)\right]^{1/2}$$

(6.104)

The overall rms pulse broadening, σ caused by intermodal as well as intramodal dispersion in a graded-index fiber can be estimated with the help of the following relation

$$\sigma = \left[\sigma_{\text{modal}}^2 + \sigma_{\text{intramodal}}^2\right]^{1/2}$$

(6.105)

We can now obtained the total rms pulse broadening of an α-profile, GI fiber by substituting the values of $\sigma_{\text{intermodal}}$ and $\sigma_{\text{intramodal}}$ from Eqs (6.100) and (6.104) respectively. One can be easily see that, the overall pulse broadening depends on the wavelength of operation as well as the rms spectral width of the source when intramodal dispersion is considered, i.e. the optimum value of α as predicted by considering intermodal dispersion only, may not be the same for minimizing the overall pulse broadening. Theoretical and experimental studies with titania-doped silica fiber shows that the optimum value of α indeed depends on the value of the wavelength of light as well as the rms spectral width of the source. Figure 6.30 shows the variation of the rms pulse width as a function of α for three different types of GaAs source e.g. an LED, an injection laser diode and a Distributed FeedBack (DFB) laser, all operating at 900 nm with different values of rms spectral width of 15 nm, 1 nm and 0.2 nm respectively. In Fig. 6.30 the dashed curve represents the rms pulse broadening by considering intermodal dispersion only and completely neglecting intramodal dispersion. We can also see from Fig. 6.30 that, the overall rms pulse broadening attains the minimum value for the DFB laser source which as the lowest rms spectral width. It is reported that the optimum value of α that minimizes the overall rms pulse spreading, strongly depends on the operating wavelength (λ). This can be accounted for the different dispersive properties of the core and cladding regions. However, to achieve minimum pulse broadening, i.e. maximum information capacity the radial index profile have to be modified to compensate this.

We may note that a fiber with a given refractive index profile α will exhibit different values of rms pulse spreading

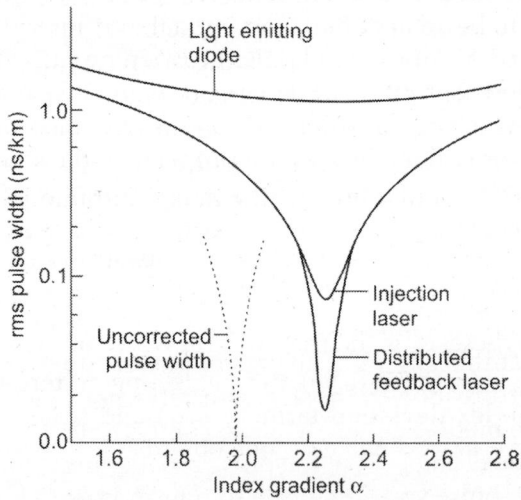

Fig. 6.30: Variation of rms pulse broadening against the index gradient α at 900 nm

which depends on the wavelength of operation. This is perhaps due to *profile dispersion effect* which arises from the compositional variation of the glass material in a graded-index fiber and finally results in different variations of refractive index with wavelength (λ) in different layers. The wavelength dependence of the optimal value of a that minimizes pulse dispersion in a GeO_2–SiO_2 fiber is shown in Fig. 6.31. We can see from the figure that the optimal value of the profile index α decreases with increase in the operating wavelength, e.g. an optical fiber having an optimal profile index parameter α_c at 0.9 nm offers a minimum pulse broadening i.e. peak bandwidth at this wavelength. For longer wavelength of operation, the index profile becomes overcompensated while at shorter wavelength the index becomes under-

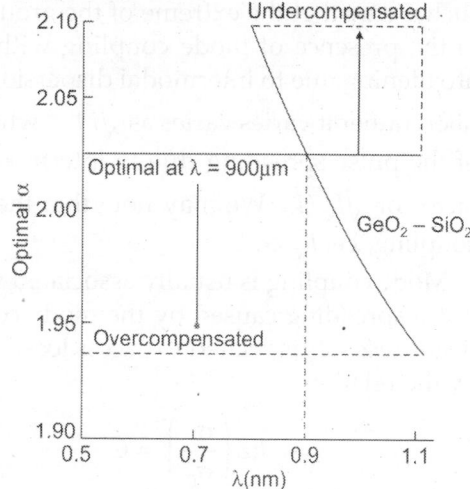

Fig. 6.31: Variation of optimal value of index profile parameter α of a GI fiber against wavelength (λ)

compensated. The multimode fibers with index profile parameter $\alpha > \alpha_c$ (optimal value corresponding to 0.9 nm) are usually considered to have undercompensated profile and these fibers tend to exhibit minimum pulse broadening or peak bandwidth at a shorter wavelength. Similarly, one finds that multimode fibers having $\alpha < \alpha_c$ (0.9 nm) may be considered to have overcompensated profile and the profile index of these fibers become optimal at a longer wavelength where they exhibit minimum pulse broadening or peak bandwidth.

6.8.4 Mode Coupling

Generally, theoretical calculation overestimates the pulse dispersion in an optical fiber. One finds that the analysis is based on a number of drastic assumptions which are in fact not valid for a practical fiber, e.g. in the theoretical calculation, one assumes that the fiber is to be ideal without any structural imperfection or undesirable index variation or any kind of deformities including macro or micro bends. Furthermore, it is also assumed that all modes are equally excited in the optical fiber. This means that every mode in the optical fiber carries the same amount of power which does not hold good for a practical fiber. Further, in actual practice the pulse dispersion is much less than the value obtained theoretically after a certain initial length of the fiber when the modes attain equilibrium. It is reported that after traversing some initial distance along the optical fiber the modes become stable and pulse dispersion increases less rapidly due to mode coupling and differential mode loss. We may note that in the initial length of the fiber immediately after launching coupling of energy from one mode to the other takes place. We may note that this kind of exchange of power from one mode to the other is initiated by random perturbations in the structure, refractive index and cabling induced microbends. However, the mode coupling tends to compensate the propagation delays associated with various modes and reduce the pulse broadening due to intermodal dispersion. The reduction in the pulse spreading due to intermodal dispersion arises due to some power originally travelling in the fast mode is eventually transferred to a slow mode and conversely a portion of the power from the slow mode gets transferred partially in the fast mode in such a way that the extreme of the group velocity spread is partly equalized. However, in the presence of mode coupling with steady state transfer of power, the rms pulse broadening due to intermodal dispersion is no longer proportional to the length L of the fiber, rather it varies varies as $\sqrt{LL_c}$, where L_c is the coupling length. Thus, the rms value of the pulse spreading due to intermodal dispersion in multimode fiber reduced by a factor of $\sqrt{L_c/L}$. We may note that the effect may be significant in the case of strong coupling, i.e. $L_c << L$.

Mode coupling is usually associated with an additional loss. The improvement in the pulse spreading caused by the mode coupling is found to be related to the loss over a distance $Z < L_c$ is related to excess loss, where hZ, where h is the loss in dB/km governed by the relation

$$hZ\left(\frac{\sigma_c}{\sigma_0}\right)^2 = C \tag{6.106}$$

where σ_0 and σ_c denotes the value of rms pulse broadening in the absence of mode coupling and in the presence of strong mode coupling respectively, hZ is the excess attenuation arising out of mode coupling and C is a constant.

We may also note that splices, connectors and other passive components in an optical fiber link may cause additional mode coupling and affect the overall performance of the system.

6.9 DISPERSION OPTIMIZATION OF SINGLE MODE FIBERS

We have read that multimode fibers are generally affected by both intramodal dispersion as well as intermodal dispersion. However, one can minimize the intermodal dispersion in a multimode fiber by making the refractive index profile graded. The graded index fiber with optimal index profile can significantly enhance the bandwidth of transmission of this fiber over its step-index counterpart. On the other hand, in a single mode fiber the intermodal dispersion is totally absent as the fiber supports only one mode and in this case the question of group delay arising from various modes does not arise. This means, single mode fibers are affected by intermodal dispersion which comprises material dispersion and waveguide dispersion. We may recall here that waveguide dispersion in a single mode fiber is relatively large as compared to that in a multimode fiber because the cladding carries a significant amount of power in the case of former while very little power is carried by cladding in the later. However, we can say that the overall dispersion of single mode fibers is much less that of multimode fibers. This is why, the single mode fibers are widely used for high-speed long-haul optical communication systems. The dispersion characteristics of single mode fibers can be tailored by changing the geometry and/or index profile of the fiber core and cladding. Now, we study various design techniques for tailoring the dispersion characterstics of single mode fibers.

6.9.1 Dispersion-Shifted Fibers (DSFs)

We have read that the single mode fibers do not suffer from intermodal dispersion. This means that the overall dispersion of single mode fiber is thus determined by the intramodal dispersion which has two components, e.g. *material dispersion* and *waveguide dispersion*. Out of these two components, the material dispersion of the fiber cannot be changed much. On the otherhand, it is found that the *waveguide dispersion* component can be significantly change by changing the refractive index profile from the conventional step-index profile to a more complex index profile. We have seen earlier (Fig. 6.21) that at wavelengths longer than the *zero material dispersion* (ZMD) point the material dispersion and waveguide dispersion components are of opposite sign. Hence, it might be possible that these two components may cancel each other at some longer wavelengths, i.e. the wavelength corresponding to zero material dispersion can be shifted to a longer wavelength to cause lowest intermodal dispersion. Moreover, since the waveguide dispersion can be tailored by using different designs, the overall dispersion can be made minimum at a desired wavelength, i.e. fibers can be designed in such a way that the minimum dispersion point is shifted to 1.55 μm. This can be done because silica fibers offer minimum loss at this wavelength and therefore, one may be benefited of the lowest attenuation as well as of lowest dispersion at this wavelength. We may note that the third generation optical communication uses single mode fibers operating at 1.55 mm wavelength with optical sources and detectors based on matured InP/InGaAs technology. The single mode fiber (SMFs) in which the minimum dispersion point is shifted to the desired wavelength are called *dispersion-shifted fibers* (DSFs).

6.9.2 Dispersion-Flattened Fibers (DFFs)

The dispersion characteristics of single mode fibers are usually modified in a way so as to exhibit a low dispersion window over the entire low-loss region ranging typically from 1.3 to 1.6 mm for silica based fibers. Further, this type of single mode fibers allows the spectral requirements of the source to be less stringent and finds applications in flexible wavelength-division multiplexing (WDM) scheme. These types of single mode fibers are called as *dispersion-flattened fibers* (DFFs).

We can see from Eq. (6.54) that the waveguide dispersion component $D_{wg}(\lambda)$ depends on the core radius (α) because V-number at a given wavelength depends on the core radius, the index deviation, Δ, and also on the shape of the refractive index profile. In principle, one can have a variety of refractive index profiles capable of tailoring the waveguide dispersion component so as to adjust the overall minimum dispersion point to the desired wavelength above the ZMD point.

Figure 6.32 illustrates the simplest technique which involves, reduction of core radius and a concomitant increase in the value of index deviation ratio Δ, of a conventional step-index profile of an optical fiber. Further, by reducing the core radius of a single mode step index fibers from 5.5 μm to 1.8 μm it is possible to shift the wavelength for zero overall-intermodal dispersion from 1.3 μm to 1.75 μm, assuming that material dispersion remains constant so that one may take a constant value. Typical material and waveguide dispersion curves for step index fibers with different sizes and material composition of the core are illustrated in Fig. 6.33, it also shows the resultant total dispersion curves.

The V number of the optical fibers have been maintained within the range: $1.5 < V < 2.4$, so that one may ensure the confinement of the fundamental mode. In order to achieve this, one will have to reduce the core radius linearly while increasing Δ as a square

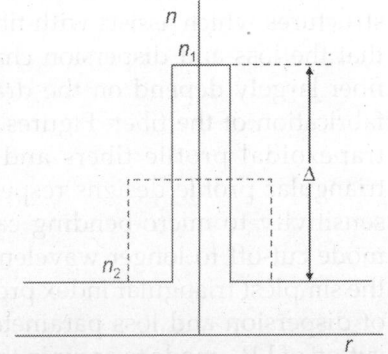

Fig. 6.32: The refractive index profile of a dispersion shifted fiber (solid line) versus the profile of a nonshifted standard fiber (dotted line) exhibiting the reduced radius of the core and increased Δn in the former case

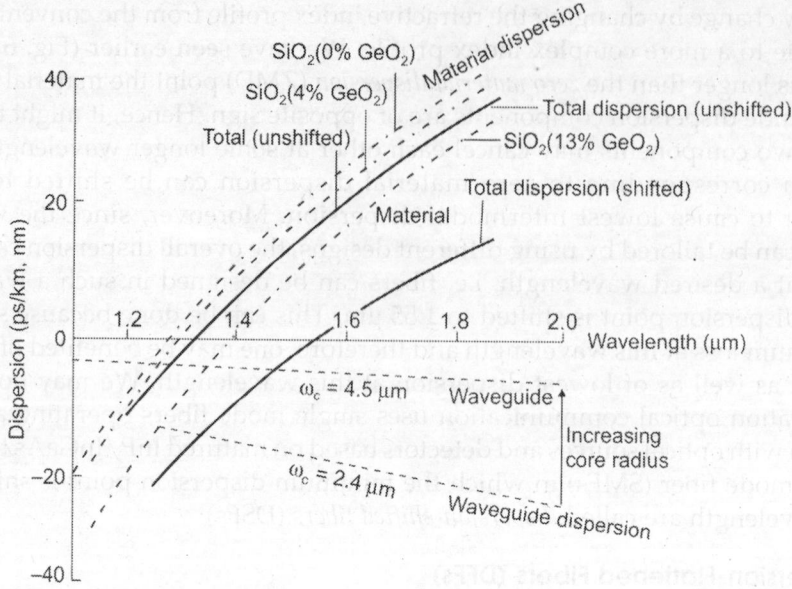

Fig. 6.33: Material, waveguide and total dispersion characteristics for conventional and dispersion-shifted step index single-mode optical fibers exhibiting variation with composite and spot size

function. One can achieve the latter by increasing the concentration of Germania in the core.

Figure 6.34 shows several of the graded refractive index structures tried for making dispersion-shifted fibers (DSFs). Figure include the triangular, trapezoidal and Gaussian refractive index profiles.

The triangular profile shown in Fig. 6.34(a) is the simplest and was the first to exhibit the same low loss (i.e. 0.24 dB/km) at wavelength of $\lambda_0 = 1.56$ mm as conventional nonshifted single mode fiber. Designs of such fiber also provide an increased MFD over equivalent step index structures which assists with fiber splicing. We may note that the loss and dispersion characteristics of the optical fiber largely depend on the drawing tension during the fabrication of the fiber. Figures 6.34(b) and (c) shows the trapezoidal profile fibers and the depressed-cladding triangular profile designs respectively, have reduced the sensitivity to micro-bending caused by shifting of LP_{11} mode cut-off to longer wavelength. It is reported that in the simplest triangular index profile fiber the optimization of dispersion and loss parameters at 1.55 μm causes the

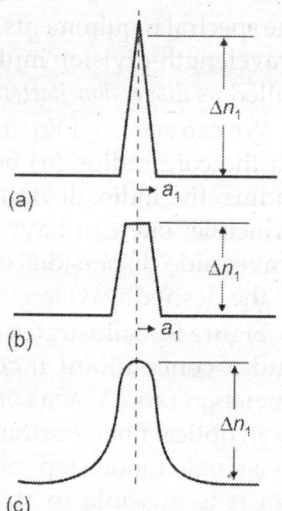

Fig. 6.34: Refractive-index profiles of dispersion-shifted graded-index fibers (a) triangular profile (b) trapezoidal profile (c) Gaussian profile

cut-off of LP_{11} mode to occur in the wavelength range 0.85–0.9 μm resulting in an enhanced sensitivity to microbending loss at 1.55 μm. To reduce the microbending loss several other graded-index profiles have also been tried earlier. These include trapezoidal profile, triangular profile with depressed cladding and Gaussian profile (Fig. 6.34). It is reported that the first single mode fiber with Gaussian profile prepared by the VAD technique exhibited a loss of 0.21 dB/km at 1.55 μm. It has also been reported that the sensitivity to micro-bending loss can be reduced to a great extent by making use of a triangular index profile incorporated in a depressed cladding index configuration (Fig. 6.34(c)). To ensure minimum leakage loss of the LP_{01} mode at 1.55 µm, the core-cladding diameter ratio was maintained above 8.5. Further, the depressed cladding triangular profile single mode fiber shifts the LP_{11} mode cut-off to 1.1 µm. However, these fibers are reported to be susceptible to increased splice loss.

To have an improvement in the micro-bending loss performance at the 1.55 µm wavelength region, several other complex index profile structures including a dual-shaped DSF have also been investigated. As shown in Fig. 6.35, said structures include triangular-profile multiple index, segmented-core triangular profile and dual shaped core. It is reported that the dual-shaped core DSF exhibits an attenuation in the tune of 0.22–0.24 dB/km at 1.55 µm with a dispersion of 0.2 ps/nm/km. These fibers are not found suitable for WDM operation, because these fibers suffer from cross-talk which occurs when multiple signals are grouped around 1.55 µm to reduce dispersion. This is why that DSFs are not longer recommended for commercial deployment.

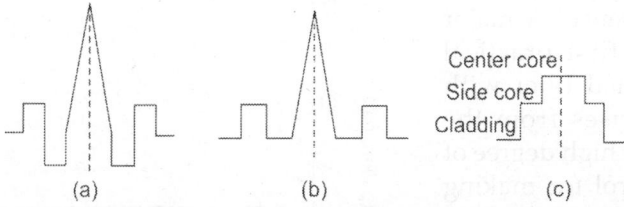

Fig. 6.35: Advanced a refractive index profiles for dispersion-shifted fibers (DSF): (a) triangular profile multiple index; (b) segmented-core triangular profile and (c) dual-shaped core design

The original "W" fiber structure was initially employed to modify the dispersion characteristics of single-mode fibers in order to give two wavelengths of zero order. Figure 6.36(a) shows a typical W fiber index profile (double clad). The relatively narrow depressed cladding region helps in modifying the waveguide dispersion to give overall intermodal dispersion curve, which turned out to give two wavelengths for zero dispersion (Fig. 6.37). Drawbacks with W-structural design included the requirement for a high degree of dimensional control so as to make reproducible DFF, completely overall fiber losses (around 0.3 dB/km), as well as a very high sensitivity to fiber bend losses. We may note that the last factor results from operation very close to the cutoff (or leakage) of the fundamental mode in the long-wavelength window in order to obtain a flat dispersion characteristics.

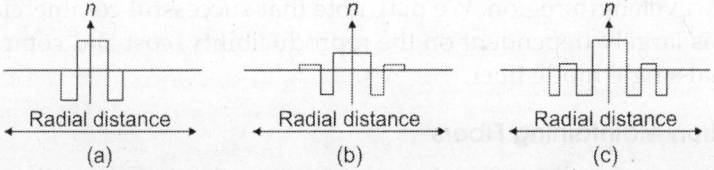

Fig. 6.36: Refractive-index profiles for dispersion-flattened fibers: (a) double clad fiber ("W " fiber) (b) Triple clad fiber and (c) quadruple fiber

In order to reduce the sensitivity to bend losses associated with the W fiber structure, the light which penetrates into the outer cladding area can be retrapped by introducing a further region of raised index into the structure. This approach has resulted in the triple clad (TC) and quadruple clad (QC) structure shown in Fig. 6.36(b) and 6.36(c) respectively.

A step index fiber with a very value of index difference and small core diameter have been studied to create waveguide dispersion that mirrors the material dispersion so as to give almost zero dispersion in 1.5–2 µm region (Fig. 6.38).

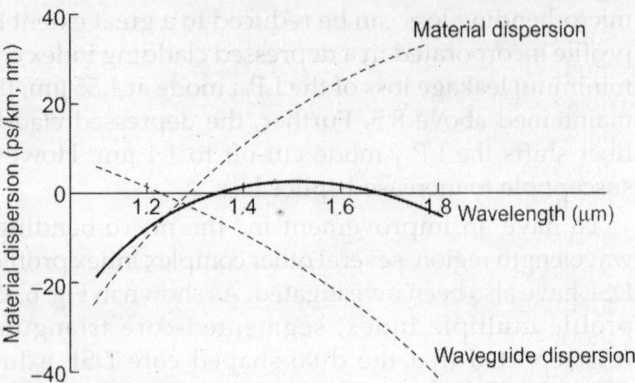

Fig. 6.37: Variation of material dispersion, waveguide dispersion, and total dispersion for a dispersion-flattened W-profile fiber with wavelength

However, this fiber suffers from excessive loss arising out of large index difference. A major limitation of the first practical dispersion-flattened fiber with "W" structure arises from the requirement of the high degree of dimensional control for making reproducible DFF in addition to relatively high overall fiber attenuation and sensitivity of such fibers to bending losses. In order to reduce the sensitivity of "W" structure dispersion-flattened fiber to bending losses "W" structure have been modified to form triple clad (TC) and quadruple clad (QC) structures

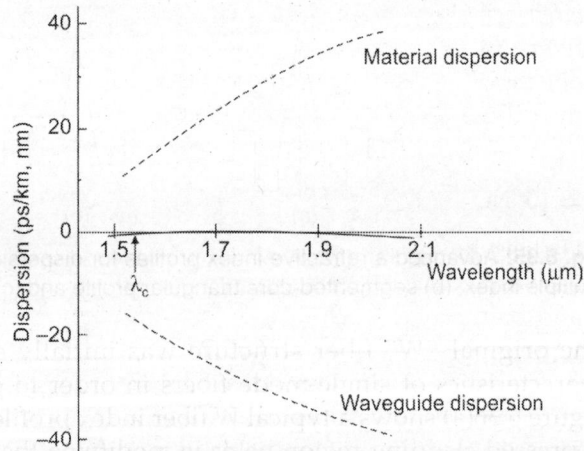

Fig. 6.38: Variation of material dispersion, waveguide dispersion with wavelength and overall dispersion

(Fig. 6.36). Recently efforts have focussed on DFFs that exhibit low-dispersion slopes in the C-band while also providing acceptably large effective core areas in order to reduce fiber nonlinear effects. A number of other structures including one involving segmented-core for single-mode dispersion-flattened have also been proposed. However, these complex DF fiber structures have low bending loss yet maintaining very low dispersion in the desired wavelength region. We may note that successful commercial deployment of these fibers is largely dependent on the reproducibility, cost and compatibility vis-a-vis conventional single mode fiber.

6.9.3 Polarization Maintaining Fibers

Single mode fibers generally suffers from *birefrigence* phenomenon. Birefrigence causes the *polarization* states of the light to change as it propagates down the fiber. Conventional photodetectors used in IM/DD systems are found to be insensitive to the polarization state of the incoming light. As a result, birefringence phenomenon does not affect conventional optical communication system. However, it may be cause of major concern in coherent optical communication systems wherein the incoming light signal is superimposed on locally generated optical signal. Moreover, the orthogonally polarized modes in the birefrigent single mode fiber may manifest in the form of polarization modal noise resulting from the interference of the two components. Similarly, the delay difference between the two orthogonal birefrigent component may also lead to *polarization mode dispersion* (PMD). In addition, it is also reported that the change of polarization state of the light may be of major concern when a single-mode fiber is used in conjuction with optical components such as *optical modulator, couplers* and various other forms of optical waveguides. However, in several situations it is necessary for a single mode fiber to maintain the state of polarization of light propagating through the optical fiber. A single mode optical fiber that maintains the state of polarization of the light propating through it is called as *polarization maintaing* (PM) *fiber*. One can classify the polarization maintained fibers in two major groups: (i) *High-birefringence* (HB) fibers and (ii) *Low-birefringence* (LB) fibers. It is reported that the conventional single mode fibers generally exhibit birefringence in the range of $B_F = 10^{-6}$ to 10^{-5}. However, a single mode needs to have B_F better than atleast 10^{-4} for maintaince of polarization. One can further classify *high-birefrigence* (HB) fibers under two categories, e.g. single polarization and two-polarization fibers. One can design a single-polarization fiber in such a way that it may allow only one mode to propagate, by imposing a cut-off condition on the other mode, by exploiting the difference in bending loss between the two modes with orthogonal polarization.

6.10 NONLINEAR EFFECTS

Usually lightwaves or photons transmitted through a fiber have little interaction with each other, and are not changed by their passage through the fiber (except for absorption and scattering). There are exceptions, however, arising from the interactions between lightwaves and the material transmitting them, which can affect optical signals. These processes are normally referred to as nonlinear effects or phenomena because their strength typically depends on the square (or some higher power) of the optical intensity. Hence nonlinear effects are weak at low powers but they can become much stronger at high optical intensities. The situation can result either when the power is increased, or when it is concentrated in a small area such as the core of a single-mode optical fiber.

Although the nonlinear effects in optical fibers are small, they accumulate as light passes through many kilometers of single-mode fiber. The small core diameters, together with the long transmission distances that may be obtained with these fibers, have enabled the occurrence of nonlinear phenomena at power levels of a few milliwatts which are well within the capability of semiconductor lasers. Furthermore, the optical power levels become much larger when wavelength division multiplexing packs many signal channels into one single-mode fiber such that the overall power level is the summation of the individual channel optical powers.

There are *two* broad categories of nonlinear effects that can be separated based on their characteristics: namely, scattering and *Kerr effects*. These fiber nonlinearities are identified in Fig. 6.39, but both these and the Kerr effects shown may also be employed in important applications for single-mode fibers including distributed in fiber

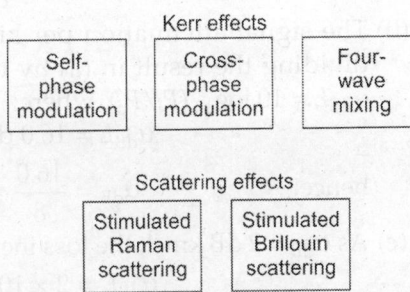

Fig. 6.39: Block schematic diagram showing the fiber nonlinear effects

amplification, wavelength conversion, multiplexing and demultiplexing, pulse regeneration, optical monitoring and optical switching. We will study in detail in the chapter.

6.11 SOLITON PROPAGATION

This results from a special case of *nonlinear dispersion compensation* in which the nonlinear chirp caused by SPM balances, and hence postpones, the temporal broadening induced by group velocity delay (GVD). Although both of these phenomena limit the propagation distance that can be achieved when acting independently, if balanced at the necessary critical pulse intensity they enable the pulse to propagate without any distortion (i.e. its shape is self-maintaining) as a soliton. In essence a soliton has two distinctive features which are potentially important for the provision of high-speed optical fiber communications: it propagates without changing shape; and the shape is unaffected, that of a soliton, after a collision with another soliton. Hence the former soliton property overcomes the dispersion limitation and avoids intersymbol interference while the collision invariance potentially provides for efficient wavelength division multiplexing.

ILLUSTRATIVE EXAMPLES

Example 1

When the mean optical power launched into an 8 km length of fiber is 120 µW, the mean optical power at the fiber output is 3 µW. Calculate:

(a) the overall signal attenuation or loss in decibels through the fiber assuming there are no connectors or splices;

(b) the signal attenuation per kilometer for the fiber.

(c) the overall signal attenuation for a 10 km optical link using the same fiber with splices at 1 km intervals, each giving an attenuation of 1 dB;

(d) the numerical input/output power ratio in (c).   **[KTU, DTU]**

Solution

(a) Using Eq. dB $= 10 \log_{10} (P_i/P_o)$, the overall signal attenuation in decibels through the fiber is:

$$\text{Signal attenuation} = 10 \log_{10} \frac{P_i}{P_o} = 10 \log_{10} \frac{120 \times 10^{-6}}{3 \times 10^{-6}}$$

$$= 10 \log_{10} 40 = 16.0 \text{ dB}$$

(b) The signal attenuation per kilometer for the fiber may be simply obtained by dividing the result in (a) by the fiber length which corresponds to it using Eq. $\alpha_{dB}L = 10 \log_{10} (P_i/P_o)$, where:

$$\alpha_{dB}L = 16.0 \text{ dB}$$

hence: $$\alpha_{dB} = \frac{16.0}{8} = 2.0 \text{ dB km}^{-1}$$

(c) As $\alpha_{dB} = 2$ dB km^{-1}, the loss incurred along 10 km of the fiber is given by:

$$\alpha_{dB}L = 2 \times 10 = 20 \text{ dB}$$

However, the link also has nine splices (at 1 km intervals) each with an attenuation of 1 dB. Therefore, the loss due to the splices is 9 dB.

Hence, the overall signal attenuation for the link is:

Signal attenuation $= 20 + 9$

$= 29$ dB

(d) To obtain a numerical value for the input/output power ratio, $P_i/P_o = 10$ (dB/10) may be used where:

$$\frac{P_i}{P_o} = 10^{29/10} = 794.3$$

Example 2

A 50 km long optical fiber link operating at 850 nm offers an average attenuation of 0.5 dB/km. An optical power of 100 μW is launched into the fiber at the input. What is the value of optical power at a distance of 30 km from the input? Also express the power in μW and in dBm. What is the output power at the end of the link? **[PTU, UTU]**

Solution

Using Eq. $\dfrac{P(0)}{P(L)} = 10^{\alpha L(dB)/10}$, we obtain

$$\frac{P(0)}{P(30\ km)} = 10^{\frac{0.5 \times 30}{10}}$$

i.e. $\qquad P(30\ km) = 10^{-1.5} \times 100\ \mu W = 3.16\ \mu W$

The power in dBm can be obtained using Eq.

$$\text{Power (in dBm)} = 10 \log \left(\frac{P}{1\text{mW}} \right)$$

Now, $\quad P(30\ km) \text{ (in dBm)} = 10 \log \left(\dfrac{3.16 \times 10^{-6}}{10^{-3}} \right) = -25\ \text{dBm}$

Alternatively, we can also express the input power in dBm as

$$P(0) \text{ (in dBm)} = 10 \log \left[\frac{100 \times 10^{-6}}{10^{-3}} \right] = -10\ \text{dBm}$$

Therefore, the power in dBm at a distance of 30 km is obtained as

$P(30\ km)$ in dBm $= -10$ dBm $- (0.5$ dB/km$)$ $(30$ km$) = -25$ dBm

The output power at the end of the link can be obtained as

$$\frac{P(0)}{P(50\ km)} = 10^{\frac{0.5 \times 50}{10}}$$

i.e. $\qquad P(50\ km) = 10^{-2.5} \times 100\ \mu W = 0.316\ \mu W$

The output power in dBm is obtained as

$P(50\ km)$ in dBm $= -10$ dBm $- (0.5$ dB/km$)$ $(50$ km$) = -35$ dBm

Example 3

Silica has an estimated fictive temperature of 1400 K with an isothermal, compressibility of 7×10^{-11} m^2 N^{-1}. The refractive index and the photoelastic coefficient for silica are 1.46 and 0.286 respectively. Determine the theoretical attenuation in decibels per kilometer due to the fundamental Rayleigh scattering in silica at optical wavelengths of 0.63, 1.00 and 1.30 mm. Given $k_B = 1.381 \times 10^{-21}$ J K^{-1}. **[UTU, DTU]**

Solution

The Rayleigh scattering cofficient may be obtained from Eq. (i) for each wavelength. However, the only variable in each case is the wavelength, and therefore the constant of proportionality of Eq. (i) applies in all cases. Hence:

$$\gamma_R = \frac{8\pi^3 n^8 p^2 \beta_c k_B T_F}{3\lambda^4} \tag{i}$$

$$= \frac{248.15 \times 20.65 \times 0.082 \times 7 \times 10^{-11} \times 1.381 \times 10^{-23} \times 1400}{3 \times \lambda^4}$$

$$= \frac{1.895 \times 10^{-28}}{\lambda^4} \, \text{m}^{-1}$$

At a wavelength of 0.63 μm; we have

$$\gamma_R = \frac{1.895 \times 10^{-28}}{0.158 \times 10^{-24}} = 1.199 \times 10^{-3} \, \text{m}^{-1}$$

The transmission loss factor for 1 kilometer of fiber may be obtained using Eq. (ii)

$$L_{km} = \exp(-\gamma_R L) = \exp(-1.199 \times 10^{-3} \times 10^3)$$

$$= 0.301 \tag{ii}$$

The attenuation due to Rayleigh scattering in decibels per kilometer may be obtained from Eq. (i) where:

$$\text{Attenuation} = 10 \log_{10} (1/L_{km}) = 10 \log_{10} 3.322$$

$$= 5.2 \, \text{dB km}^{-1}$$

At a wavelength of 1.0 μm:

$$\gamma_R = \frac{1.895 \times 10^{-28}}{10^{-24}} = 1.895 \times 10^{-4} \, \text{m}^{-1}$$

Using Eq. (ii), we obtain

$$L_{km} = \exp(-1.895 \times 10^{-4} \times 10^3) = \exp(-0.1895)$$

$$= 0.827$$

and Eq. (i), we have

Attenuation = $10 \log_{10} 1.209 = 0.8 \, \text{dB km}^{-1}$

At a wavelength of 1.30 μm:

$$\gamma_R = \frac{1.895 \times 10^{-28}}{2.856 \times 10^{-24}} = 0.664 \times 10^{-4}$$

Using Eq. (ii), we obtain

$$L_{km} = \exp(-0.664 \times 10^{-4} \times 10^3) = 0.936$$

and Eq. (i) gives

Attenuation = $10 \log_{10} 1.069 = 0.3 \, \text{dB km}^{-1}$

Example 4

A long single-mode optical fiber has an attenuation of 0.5 dB km^{-1} when operating at a wavelength of 1.3 μm. The fiber core diameter is 6 μm and the laser source bandwidth is 600 MHz. Compare the threshold optical powers for stimulated Brillouin and Raman scattering within the fiber at the wavelength specified. **[KTU, UPT]**

Solution

The threshold optical power for SBS is given by

$$P_B = 4.4 \times 10^{-3} d^2 \lambda^2 \alpha_{dB} v$$
$$= 4.4 \times 10^{-3} \times 6^2 \times 1.3^2 \times 0.5 \times 0.6$$
$$= 80.3 \text{ mW}$$

The threshold optical power for SRS may be obtained from:

$$P_R = 5.9 \times 10^{-2} d^2 \lambda \alpha_{dB}$$
$$= 5.9 \times 10^{-2} \times 6^2 \times 1.3 \times 0.5$$
$$= 1.38 \text{ mW}$$

Example 5

A silica fiber operating at 650 nm has a core refractive index of 1.46. The photoelastic coefficient and isothermal compressibility of the silica glass as 0.3 and 7×10^{-11} m^2/N respectively. Find the loss due to Rayleigh scattering in the fiber assuming the fictive temperature of glass to be 1400 K. **[UTU, DTU]**

Solution

One can estimate the Rayleigh scattering coefficient as

$$\gamma_R = \frac{8 \times (3.14)^3 (1.46)^8 \times (0.3)^2 \times 7 \times 10^{-11} \times 1.38 \times 10^{-23} \times 1400}{3 \times (650 \times 10^{-9})^4}$$
$$= 1.161 \times 10^{-3} \text{ m}^{-1}$$

The transmission loss factor over 1 km length of the fiber is obtained as

$$L = \exp(-1.161 \times 10^{-3} \times 10^{-3}) = 0.313$$

The attenuation due to Rayleigh scattering can be calculated with the help of

$$\alpha_{RS} = 10 \log (1/L)$$

$$\alpha_{RS} = 10 \log \left(\frac{1}{0.313} \right) = 5.04 \text{ dB/km}$$

Example 6

Light is launched from an injection laser diode operating at 1.55 μm to an 8/(125 μm) single mode fiber. The bandwidth of the laser source is 500 MHz. The single mode fiber offers an average loss of 0.3 dB/km. Estimate the values of threshold optical power for the cases of stimulated Brillouin scattering and stimulated Raman scattering. **[KTU, UTU]**

Solution

The threshold power required for SBS can be obtained from Eq.

$$P_B = 4.4 \times 10^{-3} d^2 \lambda^2 \alpha_{dB} \Delta v \text{ (W)}$$
$$= 4.4 \times 10^{-3} \times 8^2 \times (1.55)^2 \times 0.4 \times 0.5 \text{ W}$$
$$= 135.3 \text{ mW}$$

The threshold power required for SRS can be obtained from Eq.

$$P_R = 5.9 \times 10^{-2} d^2 \lambda \alpha_{dB} \text{ (W)}$$
$$P_R = 5.9 \times 10^{-2} \times 8^2 \times 1.55 \times 0.4 \text{ W}$$
$$= 2.34 \text{ W}$$

Example 7

Two step index fibers exhibit the following parameters:
  (a) a multimode fiber with a core refractive index of 1.500, a relative refractive index difference of 3% and an operating wavelength of 0.82 μm;
  (b) an 8 μm core diameter single-mode fiber with a core refractive index the same as (a), a relative refractive index difference of 0.3% and an operating wavelength of 1.55 μm.

Find the critical radius of curvature at which large bending losses occur in both cases.

[RTU, DTU]

Solution

(a) The relative refractive index difference is given by

$$\Delta = \frac{n_1^2 - n_2^2}{2n_1^2}$$

$$\therefore \quad n_2^2 = n_1^2 - 2\Delta n_1^2 = 2.250 - 0.06 \times 2.250$$
$$= 2.115$$

For the multimode fiber critical radius of curvature can be estimated as:

$$R_c \simeq \frac{3n_1^2 \lambda}{4\pi \, (n_1^2 - n_2^2)^{\frac{1}{2}}} = \frac{3 \times 2.250 \times 0.82 \times 10^{-6}}{4\pi \times (0.135)^{\frac{1}{2}}} \qquad \text{(i)}$$
$$= 9 \text{ mm}$$

(b) We have

$$n_2^2 = n_1^2 - 2\Delta n_1^2 = 2.250 - (0.006 \times 2.250)$$
$$= 2.237$$

The cutoff wavelength for the single-mode fiber is given by

$$\lambda_c = \frac{2\pi a n_1 (2\Delta)^{1/2}}{2.405}$$
$$= \frac{2\pi \times 4 \times 10^{-6} \times 1.500 \, (0.06)^{1/2}}{2.405}$$
$$= 1.214 \text{ μm}$$

Substituting into Eq. $R_{cs} = \dfrac{20\lambda}{(n_1 - n_2)^{3/2}} \left[2.748 - 0.996 \dfrac{\lambda}{\lambda_c} \right]^{-3}$ for the critical radius of curvature for the single-mode fiber, we obtain

$$R_{cs} \simeq \frac{20 \times 1.55 \times 10^{-6}}{(0.043)^{1/2}} \left(2.748 - \frac{0.996 \times 1.55 \times 10^{-6}}{1.214 \times 10^{-6}} \right)^{-3}$$
$$= 34 \text{ mm}$$

Example 8

A multimode graded index fiber exhibits total pulse broadening of 0.1 μs over a distance of 15 km. Calculate:

(a) the maximum possible bandwidth on the link assuming no intersymbol interference;

(b) the pulse dispersion per unit length;

(c) the bandwidth-length product for the fiber.

Solution

(a) The maximum possible optical bandwidth which is equivalent to the maximum possible bit rate (for return to zero pulses) assuming no ISI may be obtained as

$$B_{opt} = B_T = \frac{1}{2\tau} = \frac{1}{0.2 \times 10^{-6}} = 5 \text{ MHz}$$

(b) The dispersion per unit length may be acquired simply by dividing the total dispersion by the total length of the fiber. Thus, we obtain

$$\text{Dispersion} = \frac{0.1 \times 10^{-6}}{15} = 6.67 \text{ ns km}^{-1}$$

(c) The bandwidth–length product may be obtained in two ways. Firstly by simply multiply the maximum bandwidth for the fiber link by its length. Thus, we have

$$B_{opt} L = 5 \text{ MHz} \times 15 \text{ km} = 75 \text{ MHz·km}$$

Alternatively, we may obtain from the dispersion per unit length using equation

$$B_T \leq \frac{1}{2\tau}$$

We obtain

$$B_{opt} L = \frac{1}{2 \times 6.67 \times 10^{-6}} = 75 \text{ MHz·km}$$

Example 9

A 50/125 mm GI fiber with a parabolic index profile has a core refractive index of 1.458 at the centre of the core and a relative index deviation of $\Delta = 0.01$. Estimate the number of modes supported by the fiber at 850 nm. The fiber is now uniformly bent with a radius of curvature of 2 cm. Calculate the expected number of modes to be radiated out due to bending of the fiber. **[UTU, DTU]**

Solution

The number of modes in the GI fiber with parabolic index profile ($\alpha = 2$) under straight condition can be estimated using Eq. $M_\infty = a^2 k^2 \ n_1^2 \Delta \left(\dfrac{a}{a+2} \right)$ as

$$M_\infty = (25 \times 10^{-6})^2 \times \left(\frac{2 \times 3.14}{850 \times 10^{-9}} \right) \times 0.01 \times \frac{2}{2+2}$$

$$\approx 170$$

The number of modes when the fiber is bent with a radius of curvature $R = 2$ can be calculated from the following Eq.

$$M_{eff} = M_\infty \left[1 - \frac{\alpha+2}{2\alpha\Delta} \left\{ \frac{2a}{R} + \left(\frac{3}{2n_2 kR} \right)^{2/3} \right\} \right]$$

We have

$$M_{eff} = 170 \times \left[1 - \frac{2+2}{2 \times 2 \times 0.01} \left\{ \frac{2 \times 25 \times 10^{-6}}{2 \times 10^{-2}} + \left(\frac{3 \times 850 \times 10^{-9}}{2 \times 1.458 \times (1-0.01) \times 2 \times 3.14 \times 2 \times 10^{-2}} \right)^{2/3} \right\} \right]$$

$$\approx 126$$

This means that nearly 25 per cent modes will be radiated out of the fiber due to bending.

Example 10

A glass fiber exhibits material dispersion given by $|\lambda^2 (d^2n_1/d\lambda^2)|$ of 0.025. Determine the material dispersion parameter at a wavelength of 0.85 μm, and estimate the rms pulse broadening per kilometer for a good LED source with an rms spectral width of 20 nm at this wavelength.   **[KTU, RTU]**

Solution

The material dispersion parameter may be obtained from Eq.

$$M = \frac{\lambda}{c} \left| \frac{d^2n_1}{d\lambda^2} \right| = \frac{1}{c\lambda} \left| \lambda^2 \frac{d^2n_1}{d\lambda^2} \right|$$

$$= \frac{0.025}{2.998 \times 10^5 \times 850} \text{ s nm}^{-1} \text{ km}^{-1}$$

$$= 98.1 \text{ ps nm}^{-1} \text{ km}^{-1}$$

The rms pulse broadening is given by Eq.

$$\sigma_m \approx \frac{\sigma_\lambda L}{c} \left| \lambda \frac{d^2n_1}{d\lambda^2} \right|$$

Therefore in terms of the material dispersion parameter M defined by

$$\sigma_m \approx \sigma_\lambda L M$$

We obtain, the rms pulse broadening per kilometer due to material dispersion as

$$\sigma_m(1 \text{ km}) = 20 \times 1 \times 98.1 \times 10^{-12} = 1.96 \text{ ns km}^{-1}$$

Example 11

A 62.5/125 mm step-index fiber has a core and cladding refractive index values of 1.50 and 1.48 respectively at a wavelength of operation of 1330 nm. Estimate the value of the critical radius of curvature from the view point of macro-bending loss.

Solution

One can estimate the critical radius of curvature beyond which bending loss becomes very high, by using Eq.

$$R_c = \frac{3n_1^2 \lambda}{4\pi \sqrt{n_1^2 - n_2^2}}$$

We have

$$R_c = \frac{3 \times (1.5)^2 \times 1330 \times 10^{-9}}{4 \times 3.14 \times \sqrt{(1.5)^2 - (1.48)^2}} = 2.92 \text{ μm}$$

Example 12

A 6 km optical link consists of multimode step index fiber with a core refractive index of 1.5 and a relative refractive index difference of 1%. Find:

(a) the delay difference between the slowest and fastest modes at the fiber output;

(b) the rms pulse broadening due to intermodal dispersion on the link;

(c) the maximum bit rate that may be obtained without substantial errors on the link assuming only intermodal dispersion;

(d) the bandwidth–length product corresponding to (c).   **[KTU, TTU]**

Solution

(a) The delay difference is obtained as

$$\delta T_s \simeq \frac{Ln_1\Delta}{c} = \frac{6\times10^3\times1.5\times0.01}{2.998\times10^8} = 330 \text{ ns}$$

(b) The rms pulse broadening due to intermodal dispersion is obtained as

$$\sigma_s = \frac{Ln_1\Delta}{2\sqrt{3}c} = \frac{1}{2\sqrt{3}}\frac{6\times10^3\times1.5\times0.01}{2.998\times10^8} = 86.7 \text{ ns}$$

(c) The maximum bit rate may be estimated in two ways: (i) to get an idea of the maximum bit rate when assuming no pulse overlap,

$$B_{T(\text{max})} = \frac{1}{2\tau} = \frac{1}{2\delta T_s} = \frac{1}{600\times10^{-9}}$$
$$= 1.7 \text{ Mbit s}^{-1}$$

(ii) One can obtain an improved estimate using the calculate rms pulse broadening as:

$$B_{T(\text{max})} = \frac{0.2}{\sigma_s} = \frac{0.2}{86.7\times10^{-9}}$$
$$= 2.3 \text{ Mbit s}^{-1}$$

(d) Using the most accurate estimate of the maximum bit rate from (c), and assuming return to zero pulses, the bandwidth-length product is obtained as

$$B_{\text{opt}} \times L = 2.3 \text{ MHz} \times 6 \text{ km} = 13.8 \text{ MHz km}$$

Example 13

A 20 km long optical fiber exhibits an rms pulse broadening of 20 ns due to material dispersion alone, when the power is launched from an LED operating at 850 nm with a spectral width of 30 nm. Estimate the material dispersion parameter of the fiber.

[RTU, DTU]

Solution

The rms pulse broadening in terms of dispersion parameter is given by

$$\sigma_{\text{mat}} = \sigma_\lambda L D_{\text{mat}}$$

Therefore, the material dispersion is found as

$$D_{\text{mat}} = \frac{20\times10^3}{20\times30} = 100 \text{ ps km}^{-1}\text{nm}^{-1}$$

Example 14

Estimate the rms pulse broadening per kilometer for the fiber when the optical source used is an injection laser with a relative spectral width σ_λ/λ of 0.0012 at a wavelength of 0.85 μm. Comment on your result. **[DTU, UTU]**

Solution

The rms spectral width may be obtained from the relative spectral width as:

$$\sigma_\lambda = 0.0012\lambda = 0.0012 \times 0.85 \times 10^{-6}$$
$$= 1.02 \text{ nm}$$

The rms pulse broadening in terms of the material dispersion parameter can be obtained from

$$\sigma_m \simeq \sigma_\lambda L M$$

Therefore, the rms pulse broadening per kilometer due to material dispersion is:

$$\sigma_m \simeq 1.02 \times 1 \times 98.1 \times 10^{-12} = 0.10 \text{ ns km}^{-1}$$

Hence, the rms pulse broadening is reduced by a factor of around 20 (i.e. equivalent to the reduced rms spectral width of the injection laser source).

Example 15

A GI fiber with an optimal index profile has an axial refractive index $n_1 = 1.458$ and an index deviation of Δ of 1 per cent. Estimate the rms pulse broadening by assuming

$$\frac{dn_1}{d\lambda} = 0 \text{ and } \frac{d\Delta}{d\lambda} = 0$$

Compare and contrast the value with that of a corresponding step-index fiber. Comment on the bandwidth improvement in the case of GI fiber over the SI fiber. You may assume that the pulse broadening due to intramodal dispersion in negligible. **[DTU, MHTU]**

Solution

The rms pulse broadening due to intermodal dispersion in a GI fiber can be obtained from

$$\sigma_{\text{modal}} = \frac{Ln_1\Delta}{2c}\left(\frac{\alpha}{\alpha+1}\right)\left(\frac{\alpha+2}{3\alpha+2}\right)^{1/2} \times \left[c_1^2 + \frac{4c_1c_2(\alpha_1+1)\Delta}{2\alpha+1} + \frac{16\Delta^2 c_2^2(\alpha+1)^2}{(5\alpha+2)(3\alpha+2)}\right]^{1/2} \quad \text{(i)}$$

Here, $N_1 = n_1$ and $\epsilon = 0$

and using $c_1 = \dfrac{\alpha - 2 - \epsilon}{\alpha + 2}$ and $c_2 = \dfrac{3\alpha - 2 - 2\epsilon}{2(\alpha+2)}$, the optimal profile index parameter can be obtained as

$$\alpha_c = 2 - \frac{12}{5}\Delta$$

Therefore, the rms pulse spreading due to intermodal dispersion in the GI with optimal profile index (i) reduces as

$$(\sigma_{\text{modal}})_{\text{GI}} = \frac{Ln_1\Delta^2}{20\sqrt{3}c} \quad \text{(ii)}$$

Substituting the values of the given parameters, the rms pulse broadening in the case of an optimal index GI fiber is obtained as 14 ps km^{-1}.

For a corresponding SI fiber, the rms pulse spreading due to intermodal dispersion is given by

$$(\sigma_{\text{modal}})_{\text{SI}} = \frac{n_1 L \Delta}{2\sqrt{3}\, c} \tag{iii}$$

Substituting the values of the parameters, the rms pulse broadening in the case of SI fiber is obtained as 14 ns km^{-1}

Therefore, the ratio of the pulse broadening in an SI fiber to that in a GI fiber is obtained as

$$\frac{(\sigma_{\text{modal}})_{\text{SI}}}{(\sigma_{\text{modal}})_{\text{GI}}} = \frac{10}{\Delta} = \frac{10}{0.01} = 10^3$$

Example 16

A typical single-mode fiber has a zero-dispersion wavelength of 1.31 μm with a dispersion slope of 0.09 ps nm^{-2} km^{-1}. Compare the total first-order dispersion for the fiber at the wavelength of 1.28 μm and 1.55 μm. When the material dispersion and profile dispersion at the latter wavelength are 13.5 ps nm^{-1} km^{-1} and 0.4 ps nm^{-1} km^{-1}, respectively, determine the waveguide dispersion at this wavelength. **[MHTU]**

Solution

The total first-order dispersion for the fiber at the two wavelengths may be obtained from:

$$D_T(1280 \text{ nm}) = \frac{\lambda S_0}{4}\left[1 - \left(\frac{\lambda_0}{\lambda}\right)^4\right]$$

Substituting the values, we obtain

$$D_T(1280 \text{ nm}) = \frac{1280 \times 0.09 \times 10^{-12}}{4}\left[1 - \left(\frac{1310}{1280}\right)^4\right]$$

$$= -2.8 \text{ ps nm}^{-1} \text{ km}^{-1}$$

and:

$$D_T(1550 \text{ nm}) = \frac{1550 \times 0.09 \times 10^{-12}}{4}\left[1 - \left(\frac{1310}{1550}\right)^4\right]$$

$$= 17.1 \text{ ps nm}^{-1} \text{ km}^{-1}$$

The total dispersion at the 1.28 μm wavelength exhibits a negative sign due to the influence of the waveguide dispersion. Furthermore, as anticipated the total dispersion at the longer wavelength (1.55 μm) is considerably greater than that obtained near the zero-dispersion wavelength.

The waveguide dispersion for the fiber at a wavelength of 1.55 μm is obtained as

$$D_w = D_T - (D_M + D_P)$$
$$= 17.1 - (13.5 + 0.4)$$
$$= 3.2 \text{ ps nm}^{-1} \text{ km}^{-1}$$

SUMMARY

• The two most important transmission characteristics of an optical fiber are *attenuation* (or loss) and the dispersion. Attenuation limits the optical power transmitted through the fiber while dispersion restricts the bandwidth or rate at which data can be transmitted through the fiber. Both these facts play significant role in the design of optical fiber communication link.

- *Attenuation* of light signal as it propagates along a fiber is an important consideration in the design of an optical communication system, since it plays a major role in determining the maximum transmission distance between a transmitter and a receiver or an in-line amplifier. The basic attenuation mechanisms in a fiber are absorption, scattering and radiative losses of optical energy.

- *Absorption* is caused by three different mechanism: (i) absorption by atomic defects in the glass composition, (ii) extrinsic absorption by impurity atoms in the glass material, and (iii) intrinsic absorption by the basic constitutent atoms of the fiber material.

- *Electronic absorption* involves absorption of photon that results into excitation of electron from the valence band of glass to the conduction band. This absorption takes place when a photon associated with the propagating light interacts with an electron in the valence band and transfer its energy to the electron so as to excite it to a higher energy state in the conduction band. This type of absorption needs a relatively high energy photon because of the large band-gap. This absorption is significant in UV region, i.e. high frequency or small wavelength region for glass.

- Scattering losses in glass arise from microscopic variations in the material density, from compositional fluctuations, and from structural inhomogeneities or defects occuring during fiber manufacture.

- *Radiative* losses occur whenever an optical fiber undergoes a *bend* of finite radius of curvature. Fibers can be subject to two types of bends: (i) macroscopic bends having radii that are large compared with the fiber diameter, and (ii) random microscopic bends of the fiber axis that can arise when the fibers are incorporated into cables.

- *Signal distortion* is a consequence of factors such as intermodal delay, intramodal dispersion, polarization mode dispersion, and higher-order dispersion effects. These distortions can be explained by examing the behaviour of group velocities of the guided modes, where the group velocity is the speed at which energy in a particular mode travels along the fiber.

- *Intermodal delay* (or simply modal delay) appears only in multimode fibers. Modal delay is a result of each mode having a different value of the group velocity at a single frequency. From this effect one can derive an intuitive picture of the information-carrying capacity of a multimode fiber.

- *Intramodal dispersion or chromatic dispersion* is pulse spreading that takes place within a single mode. This spreading arises from the finite spectral emission width of an optical source. The phenomenon also is known as *group velocity dispersion* (GVD), since the dispersion is a result of the group velocity being a function of the wavelength. Because intramodal dispersion depends on the wavelength, its effect on signal distortion increases with the spectral width of the light source. The spectral width is the band of wavelengths over which the source emits light. This wavelength band normally is characterized by the root-mean-square (rms) spectral width σ_λ. Depending on the device structure of a LED, the spectral width is approximately 4 to 9% of a central wavelength. The two main causes of intramodal dispersion are: (i) *Material dispersion* or *chromatic dispersion* arises due to the variations of the refractive index of the core material as a function of the wavelength. (ii)*Waveguide dispersion* causes pulse spreading because only part of the optical power propagation along a fiber is confined to the core. Dispersion arises because the fraction of light power propagating in the cladding travels faster than the light confined to the core, since the index is lower in the cladding.

- *Polarization mode dispersion* results from the fact that light-signal energy at a given wavelength in a single-mode fiber actually occupies two orthogonal polarization states or modes. The effects of fiber birefringence on the polarization states of an optical signal are another source of pulse broadening. The fundamental property of an optical signal is its polarization state. Polarization refers to the electric field orientation of the light signal, which can vary significantly along the length of a fiber.

- *Modal delay*: Intramodal distortion or modal delay appears only in multimode fibers. This signal-distorting mechanism is a result of each mode having a different value of the group velocity at a single frequency.

- *Signal distortion in single-mode fibers*: For single-mode fibers, waveguide dispersion is of importance and can be of the same order of magnitude as material dispersion. The pulse spread σ_{wg} occuring over a distribution of wavelength σ_λ is given by

$$\sigma_{w\gamma} = \frac{n_2 L \Delta \sigma_\lambda}{c\lambda} V \frac{d^2(Vb)}{dV^2} = L \mid D_{wg}(\lambda) \mid \sigma_\lambda$$

where $D_{wg}(\lambda)$ is the waveguide dispersion.

- *Bending loss*: Macrobending and microbending losses are important in the design of single-mode fibers. These losses are principally evident in the 1550 nm region, and show up as a rapid increase in attenuation when the fiber is bent smaller than a certain bend radius. The lower the cutoff wavelength relative to the operating wagelength, the more susceptible single-mode fiber are to the bending.

- *Scattering losses*: These losses in glass arise from microscopic variations in the material density, from compositional fluctuations, and from structural inhomogeneities or defects occuring during fiber manfacture. Scattering losses are usually classified under two categories:

(i) *Linear scattering loss*: In linear scattering, the optical power transferred to a different mode is proportional to the power contained in the propagating mode linear scattering is further classified as

  (a) *Rayleigh scattering*: This is caused by inhomogeneities that occur on a small scale compared with the wavelength of light. Rayleigh scattering coefficient is given by

$$\gamma_R = \frac{8\pi^3}{3\lambda^4} n^\theta p^2 \beta_c kT_F$$

  where, n is the refractive index of the medium, p is the average photoelectric constant, β_c is the isothermal compressibility at a fictive temperature T_F and k is the Boltzmann's coefficient. The attenuation in decibels *per unit length* due to Rayleigh scattering can be calculated from $\alpha_{RS} = 10 \log(1/L)$, where L is the length of the fiber.

  (b) *Mie scattering*: This is the other form of linear scattering and less common in high quality fibers. Mie scattering occurs due to inhomogeneities which have comparable in size to the guided wavelength.

- *Non-linear scattering loss*: Generally, it is believed that optical fibers behave as linear waveguides in the sense that the output power increases proportionately with the increase in input optical power. However, this is not always true because non-linear effects such as non-linear scattering become dominant at high optical power levels. Non-linear scattering can be used to provide optical amplifier which find extensive application in long distance optical communication systems.

- *Stimulated Brillouin scattering* (SBS): SBS occurs from the scattering of the propagating light by thermal molecular vibrations of the material. The threshold power required for SBS to occur can be obtained as

$$P_B = 4.4 \times 10^{-3} d^2 \lambda^2 \alpha_{dB} \Delta v \text{ (watts)}$$

where d is the core diameter in micrometer, λ is the operating wavelength in micrometer, α_{dB} is the fiber attenuation in decibel per kilometer and Δv is the linewidth (in GHz) of the injection laser source.

REVIEW QUESTIONS

1. What are the two most important transmission characteristics of an optical fiber? Explain briefly their effect.
2. Explain attenuation in optical fibers. What is absorption loss mechanism in Fibers?
3. What is scattering loss in fibers? Explain linear and non-linear scattering.
4. What do you understand by bending loss in optical fibers? Explain the terms: microbending loss and macrobending loss.
5. Explain core-cladding loss.
6. How the transmission of optical signal through an optical fiber is adversely affected by dispersion of the signal by the dielectric medium? Explain intramodal dispersion and intermodal dispersion.
7. Explain material dispersion and show that material dispersion parameter of an optical fiber is a function of wavelength.
8. Explain waveguide dispersion and obtain an expression for the waveguide dispersion.
9. Write short notes on:
   (a) Pulse broadening in a multimode step-index fiber
   (b) Intermodal dispersion in a multimode graded-index fiber
   (c) Mode coupling
   (d) Dispersion-shifted and dispersion-flattened fibers
10. Discuss absorption losses in optical fibers with regard to (a) Rayleigh scattering (b) Mie scattering. **[KTU]**
11. Briefly describe linear scattering losses in optical fibers due to (a) Rayleigh scattering (b) Mie scattering. **[DTU]**
12. Compare stimulated Brillouin and stimulated Raman scattering in optical fibers, and indicate the way in which they may be avoided in optical fiber communication. **[MNTU]**
13. (a) Briefly explain the reasons for pulse broadening due to material dispersion in optical fibers. **[PTU]**
    (b) The group delay τ_g in an optical fiber is given by

$$\tau_g = \frac{1}{c}\left(n_1 - \frac{dn_1}{d\lambda}\right)$$

where c is the velocity of light in a vacuum, n is the core refractive index and λ is the wavelength of the transmitted light. Derive an expression for the rms pulse broadening due to material dispersion in an optical fiber and define the material dispersion parameter. **[KTU]**

14. The normalized propagation constant in a single-mode step index fiber is

$$b(V) \simeq \left(1.1428 - \frac{0.9960}{V}\right)^2$$

obtain a corresponding approximation for the waveguide parameter $Vd^2(VB)/dV^2$ and hence write down an expression for the waveguide dispersion in the fiber.

[UPTU]

15. Describe the phenomenon of modal noise in optical fibers and explain how it may be avoided. **[KTU, MHTU]**

16. Discuss dispersion mechanisms with regard to single-mode fibers indicating the dominating effects. Hence, describe how intramodal dispersion may be minimized within the single-mode region. **[MHTU, DTU]**

17. Explain: (a) fiber birefrigence and (b) the beat length in single mode fibers.

18. Define polarization mode dispersion (PMD) in single mode optical fibers.

Give the theory of PMD explaining the relationship between the fiber polarization beat length and correlation length.

PROBLEMS

1. Consider a 30 km long optical fiber that has an attenuation of 0.4 dB/km at 1310 nm. Find the optical output power (P_{out}) if 200 mW of the power is launched into the fiber. **[Ans. 9.0 dBm, or 12.6 mW]**

[**Hint:** $\qquad P_{in}(dBm) = 10 \log \left[\dfrac{P_{in}\,(W)}{1\,mW}\right]$

$$= 10 \left[\frac{200 \times 10^{-6}\,W}{1 \times 10^{-3}\,W}\right] = -7.0\,dBm$$

P_{out} at $z = 30$ km is

$$P_{out}\,(dBm) = 10 \log \left[\frac{P_{out}\,(W)}{1\,mW}\right]$$

$$= 10 \log \left[\frac{P_{in}\,(W)}{1\,mW}\right] = -\alpha z$$

$$= -7.0\,dBm - (0.4\,dB/km)\,(30\,km)$$

$$= -19.0\,dBm$$

$$P(30\,km) = 10^{-19.0/10}\,(1\,mW)$$

$$= 12.6 \times 10^{-3}\,mW = 12.6\,\mu W]$$

2. The mean optical power launched into an optical power link is 1.5 mW and the fiber has an attenuation of 0.5 dB/km. Show that the maximum possible link length without repeaters (assuming lossless connectors) is 57.5 km when the minimum mean optical power level required at the detector is 2 µW. **[KTU, DTU]**

3. A multimode graded index fiber has a refractive index in the core axis of 1.46 with a cladding refractive index of 1.45. The critical radius of curvature which allows large

bending losses to occur is 84 μm when the fiber is transmitting light of a particular wavelength. Show that the wavelength of the transmitted light is 0.86 μm. **[MHTU]**

4. The threshold optical powers for stimulated Brillouin and Raman scattering in a single mode fiber with a long 8 μm core diameter is found to be 190 mW and 1.70 W respectively, when using an injection laser source with a bandwidth of 1 GHz. Show that the operating wavelength of the laser and the attenuation in decibels per kilometer of the fiber at this wavelength are 1.50 μm and 0.30 dB/km respectively.

[PTU, UPTU]

5. 150 μW optical power is launched at the input of a 10 km long optical fiber link operating at 850 nm. The output power available is 5 μW. Estimate the total attenuation in dB over the link length neglecting all connector and splice losses. What is the average attenuation per km? **[DTU, UPTU]**

[**Hint:** The average attenuation of the fiber can be obtained as

$$\alpha = \frac{10}{10} \log \left(\frac{150 \times 10^{-6}}{5 \times 10^{-6}} \right) = 1.48 \text{ dB/km}$$

The total loss over the link length is

$$\alpha \times L = 1.48 \times 10 = 14.8 \text{ dB}]$$

6. A silica fiber operating at 650 nm has a core refractive index of 1.46. Compare and contrast the values of attenuation due to Rayleigh scattering at optical wavelengths of 1 μm and 1.33 μm comment on your result and assuming that the refractive index is independent of wavelength. **[KTU]**

[**Hint:** One can easily verify that at $\lambda = 1$ μm = 1000 nm the Rayleigh scattering coefficient will be scaled as

$$\gamma_R = 1.161 \times 10^{-3} \times \left(\frac{650}{1000} \right)^4 = 0.207 \times 10^{-3} \text{ m}^{-1}$$

Therefore, transmission loss factor at 1 μm is

$$L (\lambda = 1 \, \mu m) = \exp(-0.207 \times 10^{-3} \times 10^3) = 0.813$$

The attenuation due Rayleigh scattering at this wavelength would be

$$\alpha_{Rs} (\lambda = 1 \, \mu m) = 10 \log \left(\frac{1}{0.813} \right) = 0.89 \text{ dB/km}$$

For operation at $\lambda = 1.33$ μm = 1330 nm the corresponding parameters translate as

$$\gamma_R = 1.161 \times 10^{-3} \times \left(\frac{650}{1330} \right)^4 = 0.066 \times 10^{-3} \text{ m}^{-1}$$

$$L (\lambda = 1.33 \, \mu m) = \exp(-0.066 \times 10^{-3} \times 10^3) = 0.936$$

$$\alpha_{Rs} (\lambda = 1.33 \, \mu m) = 10 \log \left(\frac{1}{0.936} \right) = 0.29 \text{ dB/km}$$

We see that the loss due to Rayleigh scattering can be significantly reduced by operating at the longest possible wavelength.]

7. A multimode step index fiber has a numerical aperture of 0.3 and a core refractive index of 1.45. The material dispersion parameter for the fiber is 250 ps nm^{-1} km^{-1} which makes material dispersion the totally dominating chromatic dispersion

mechanism. Estimate (a) the total rms pulse broadening per kilometer when the fiber is used with an LED source of rms spectral width 50 nm and (b) the corresponding bandwidth-length product for the fiber. **[PTU]**

[Hint: (a) The rms pulse broadening per kilometer due to material dispersion may be obtained from

$$\sigma_m \,(1 \text{ km}) \simeq \frac{\sigma_\lambda L \lambda}{c} \left| \frac{d^2 n_1}{d\lambda^2} \right| = \sigma_\lambda LM = 50 \times 1 \times 250 \text{ ps km}^{-1}$$

$$= 12.5 \text{ ns km}^{-1}$$

The rms pulse broadening per kilometer due to intermodal dispersion for the step index fiber is given by

$$\sigma_s \,(1 \text{ km}) \simeq \frac{L(NA)^2}{4\sqrt{3} n_1 c} = \frac{10^3 \times 0.09}{4\sqrt{3} \times 1.45 \times 2.998 \times 10^8}$$

$$\doteq 29.9 \text{ ns km}^{-1}$$

The total rms pulse broadening per kilometer may be obtained using where $\sigma_c \approx \sigma_m$ as the waveguide dispersion is negligible and $\sigma_n = \sigma_s$ for the multimode step index fiber. Hence:

$$\sigma_T = (\sigma_m^2 + \sigma_s^2)^{1/2} = (12.5^2 + 29.9^2)^{1/2}$$

$$= 32.4 \text{ ns km}^{-1}$$

(b) The bandwidth-length product may be estimated from the relationship

$$B_{\text{opt}} \times L = \frac{0.2}{\sigma_T} = \frac{0.2}{32.4 \times 10^{-9}}$$

$$= 6.2 \text{ MHz km}]$$

8. Consider a single mode fiber with the following parameters.
   Core refractive index = 1.48; $\Delta = 0.1$ per cent and $\lambda = 1330$ nm. Assume the core radius of the fiber to be 4 μm. Compare and contrast the value of waveguide dispersion of the fiber with that obtained in the previous example. **[DTU]**

   [Hint: The cladding refractive index of the fiber can be estimated as

   $$n_2 = 1.48 \,(1 - 0.001) = 1.4785$$

   The V-number of the fiber is obtained as

   $$V = \frac{2 \times 3.14 \times 4 \times 10^{-6}}{1330 \times 10^{-9}} \times 1.48 \times \sqrt{2 \times 0.001} = 1.25$$

   At this V-number value the quantity

   $$V \frac{d^2(Vb)}{dV^2} \approx 1$$

   Therefore, the waveguide dispersion value of the single mode fiber can be estimated as

   $$D_{wg} = \frac{1}{L} \frac{n_2 \Delta}{c\lambda} V \frac{d^2(Vb)}{dV^2} = -\frac{1}{10^{-3}} \times \frac{1.4785 \times 0.001}{3 \times 10^8 \times 1330} \times 1.0$$

   $$= -3.7 \text{ ps km}^{-1} \text{ nm}^{-1}]$$

9. The beat length in a single-mode optical fiber is 9 cm when light from an injection laser with a spectral linewidth of 1 nm and a peak wavelength of 0.9 μm is launched

into it. Determine the modal birefringence and estimate the coherence length in this situation. Also calculate the difference between the propagation constants for the two orthogonal modes and check the result.

[**Hint:** The modal birefringence can be obtained as

$$B_F = \frac{\lambda}{L_B} = \frac{0.9 \times 10^{-6}}{0.09} = 1 \times 10^{-5}$$

Knowing B_F, we obtain the coherence length as

$$L_{bc} \simeq \frac{\lambda^2}{B_F \delta\lambda} = \frac{0.81 \times 10^{-12}}{10^{-5} \times 10^{-9}} = 81 \text{ m}$$

The difference between the propagation constant for the two orthogonal modes is given by

$$\beta_x - \beta_y = \frac{2\pi}{L_B} = \frac{2\pi}{0.09} = 69.8$$

We can check the result by using the following relation

$$\beta_x - \beta_y = \frac{2\pi B_F}{\lambda} = \frac{2\pi \times 10^{-5}}{0.9 \times 10^{-6}}$$

$$= 69.8]$$

10. A multimode step-index fiber has a numerical aperture of 0.22 and a core refractive index of 1.458. The fiber exhibits an overall intramodal dispersion of 200 ps km^{-1}. Calculate overall value of the rms pulse broadening per kilometre of the fiber when the LED source operating at 850 nm has an rms spectral width of 40 nm. Estimate the bandwidth of a 10 km link based on this fiber. **[DTU, PTU]**

[**Hint:** The rms broadening per kilometer due to material dispersion is obtained as

$$\sigma_{intra} (1 \text{ km}) = 40 \times 1 \times 200 = 8 \text{ ns km}^{-1}$$

The rms pulse broadening due to intermodal dispersion is obtained as

$$\sigma_{modal} (1 \text{ km}) = \frac{L(NA)^2}{4\sqrt{3}n_1 c} = \frac{10^3 \times 0.22}{4\sqrt{3} \times 1.458 \times 3 \times 10^8} = 15.97 \text{ ns km}^{-1}$$

The overall rms pulse broadening is obtained as

$$\sigma = \left[\sigma_{intra}^2 + \sigma_{modal}^2 \right]^{1/2} = \sqrt{8^2 + (15.97)^2}$$

For a fiber link of 10 km length, the total rms pulse broadening is

$$\sigma_T = 17.86 \times 10^{-9} \times 10 = 178.6 \text{ ns}$$

The bandwidth of the link is obtained as

$$B \simeq \frac{0.2}{178.6 \times 10^{-9}} = 1.11 \text{ MHz}]$$

11. Two polarization-maintaining fibers operating at a wavelength of 1.3 mm have beat lengths of 0.7 mm and 80 m. Determine the fiber birefringence in each case and comment on the results. **[TTU; PTU]**

[**Hint:** The modal birefringence is given by:

$$B_F = \frac{\lambda}{L_B}$$

Hence, for a beat length of 0.7 mm; we obtain

$$B_F = \frac{1.3 \times 10^{-6}}{0.7 \times 10^{-3}} = 1.86 \times 10^{-3}$$

Clearly, this typifies a high birefringence fiber.

For a beat length of 80 m; we obtain

$$B_F = \frac{1.3 \times 10^{-6}}{80} = 1.63 \times 10^{-8}$$

which indicates a low birefringence fiber.]

12. Consider a 10 km optical fiber link using a multimode step-index fiber with the following parameters:

    Core refractive index, $n_1 = 1.458$; Relative index deviation, $\Delta = 0.002$.

    Estimate the delay time difference between the axial ray and the most oblique ray. What is the value of rms pulse broadening due to intermodal dispersion? Estimate the bandwidth and the maximum bit-rate of transmission assuming RZ formatting and neglecting intramodal dispersion. **[DTU, MHTU]**

    [**Hint:** The time delay difference between the axial ray and the most oblique ray can be estimated as

    $$\delta T_{mod} = \frac{Ln_1\Delta}{c} = \frac{10 \times 10^3 \times 1.458 \times 0.002}{3 \times 10^8} = 97.2 \text{ ns}$$

    The rms pulse broadening due to intermodal dispersion can be accordingly calculated as

    $$\sigma_{mod} = \frac{Ln_1\Delta}{2\sqrt{3}c} = \frac{10 \times 10^3 \times 1.458 \times 0.002}{2\sqrt{3} \times 3 \times 10^8} \approx 28 \text{ ns}$$

    The bandwidth of transmission is obtained as

    $$B \approx \frac{0.2}{\sigma_{mod}} = \frac{0.2}{28 \times 10^{-9}} = 7.14 \text{ MHz}$$

    The maximum bit-rate can be obtained for NRZ mode as

    $$B_T = 2 \times B = 2 \times 7.14 = 14.28 \text{ Mbps}]$$

13. A 3.5 km length, of two-polarization mode PM fiber has a polarization crosstalk of −27 dB at its output end. Determine the mode coupling parameter for the fiber. **[PTU]**

    [**Hint:** We have the relation relating the mode coupling parameter h to the polarization crosstalk CT as

    $$\log_{10} \tanh(hL) = \frac{CT}{10} = -2.7$$

    Thus $\tanh(hL) = 2 \times 10^{-3}$ and $hL \approx 2 \times 10^{-3}$. Hence, we obtain

    $$h = \frac{2 \times 10^{-3}}{3.5 \times 10^{-3}} = 5.7 \times 10^{-7} \text{ m}^{-1}]$$

14. A single-mode step index fiber has a zero-dispersion wavelength of 1.29 μm and exhibits total first-order dispersion of 3.5 ps/nm/km at a wavelength of 1.32 μm. Show that the total first-order dispersion in the fiber at a wavelength of 1.54 μm is 23.6 ps/nm/km. **[RTU]**

15. A single-mode fiber maintains birefringent coherence over a length of 100 km when it is illuminated with an injection laser source with a spectral linewidth of 1.5 nm and a peak wavelength of 1.32 μm. Calculate the beat length within the fiber.

[Ans. 113.6 m]

16. A low-polarization mode PM fiber has a mode coupling parameter of 2.3×10^{-5}/m when operating at a wavelength of 1.55 μm. Show that the polarization crosstalk for the fiber at this wavelength is -16.4 dB/km. **[KTU, PTU]**

17. A low loss fiber has average loss of 3 dB/km at 900 nm. Compute the length over which: (a) power decreases by 50% (b) power decreases by 75%. **[KTU]**

[Hint: Here $\alpha = 3$ dB/km

(a) $\dfrac{P(o)}{P(z)} = 50\% = 0.5$

Now $\qquad\qquad \alpha = 10\,\dfrac{1}{z}\log\left[\dfrac{P(o)}{P(z)}\right]$

or $\qquad\qquad 3 = 10\,\dfrac{1}{z}\log\,(0.5)$

$\qquad\qquad\qquad \therefore\ z = 1$ km

(b) $\dfrac{P(0)}{P(z)} = 25\% = 0.25$

Since power decreases by 75%, we have

$$3 = 10 \times \dfrac{1}{z}\log\,(0.25)$$

$\therefore \qquad\qquad\qquad z = 2$ km.**]**

18. When mean optical power launched into an 8 km length of fiber is 12 μW, the mean optical power at the fiber output is 3 μW. Find: (a) overall signal attenuation in dB, and (b) the overall signal attenuation for a 10 km optical link using the same fiber with splices at 1 km intervals, each giving an attenuation of 1 dB. **[UPTU, PTU]**

[Hint: Here: $z = 8$ km, $P(0) = 120$ μW and $P(z) = 3$ μW

(a) $\qquad\qquad \alpha = 10\log\left[\dfrac{P(0)}{P(z)}\right] = 10\log\left(\dfrac{120}{3}\right)$

$\therefore \qquad\qquad\qquad \alpha = 16.02$ dB

(b) Overall attenuation for 10 km

We have attenuation per km

$$\alpha_{dB} = \dfrac{16.02}{z} = \dfrac{16.02}{8}$$

$$= 2\ \text{dB/km}$$

$\therefore$ Attenuation in 10 km link = 2.00 dB/km × 10 km = 20 dB

Since there will be 9 splices in 10 km at 1 km interval, hence each splice introduces attenuation of 1 dB.

Total attenuation 20 dB + 9 dB = 29 dB**]**

SHORT ANSWER QUESTIONS

1. What are the basic attenuation mechanisms in a fiber?

   Ans. (i) absorption, (ii) scattering, and (iii) radiative losses of optical energy.

2. Write the different mechanisms by which absorption is caused in fibers.

   Ans. (i) Absorption by atomic defects in the glass composition, (ii) Extrinsic absorption by impurity atoms in the glass material, and (iii) Intrinsic absorption by the constituent atoms of the fiber material.

3. Why the consideration of attenuation of a light signal propagating in a fiber is of an important consideration in the design of an optical communication system?

   Ans. Attenuation plays a major role in determining the maximum transmission distance between a transmitter and a receiver or an in-line amplifier.

4. How the power of light travelling along a fiber decreases?

   Ans. If $P(0)$ is the optical power in a fiber at the origin (at $z = 0$), then the power $P(z)$ at a distance z further down the fiber is $P(z) = P(0) e^{-\alpha_p z}$, where $\alpha_p \simeq \dfrac{1}{z} \ln \left[\dfrac{P(0)}{P(z)} \right]$ is the fiber attenuation coefficient given in units of, e.g. km^{-1}.

5. Write the units of optical signal attenuation in a fiber.

   Ans. The common procedure to express the attenuation coefficient of optical signal attenuation in a fiber is in units of decibels per kilometer, denoted by dB/km. Designating this parameter by α, we have

   $$\alpha \, (dB/km) = \frac{10}{z} \log \left[\frac{P(0)}{P(z)} \right] = 4.343 \, \alpha_p \, (km^{-1})$$

   This parameter is generally referred to as the *fiber loss* or the *fiber attenuation* and depends on several variables and it is also a function of the wavelength.

6. What is the basic reasons of atomic defects in the structure of fiber material?

   Ans. Atomic defects are imperfections in the atomic structure of the fiber material, e.g. missing molecules, high density clusters of atom groups, or oxygen defects in the glass structure.

7. What is dominant absorption factor in silica fibers?

   Ans. The presence of minute quantities of impurities in the fiber material. These impurities include OH^- (water) ions that are dissolved in the glass and transition metal ions such as iron, copper, chromium, and vanadium.

8. Explain intrinsic absorption in a fiber material.

   Ans. Intrinsic absorption is associated with the basic fiber material (e.g. pure SiO_2) and is the principal physical factor the defines the transparency window of a material over a specified spectral region. It occurs when the material is in a perfect state with no density variations, impurities, material inhomogeneities, and so on. It thus sets the fundamental lower limit on absorption for any particular material.

   Intrinsic absorption results from electronic absorption bands in the UV region and from atomic vibration bands in the near-infrared region.

9. Why scattering losses arise in glass?

   Ans. Scattering losses in glass arise from microscopic variations in the material density, from compositional fluctuations, and from structural inhomogeneities or defects occuring during fiber manufacture. Glass is composed of a randomly connected network of molecules. Such a structure naturally contains regions in which the molecular density is either higher or lower than the average density in the glass. In addition, since glass is made up of several oxides, such as SiO_2, GeO_2, and P_2O_5 compositional fluctuations can occur. These two effects give rise to refractive-index variations which occur within the glass over distances that are small compared with the wavelength. These index variations cause a Rayleigh-type scattering.

10. When the absorption effect is most significant in a fiber?

Ans. The absorption effect is most significant in a fiber when fiber is exposed to ionizing radiation in nuclear reactor, medical therapies, space missions, etc. The radiation damages the internal structure of the fiber. The damages due to radiation are proportional to the intensity of ionizing particles. This results in increasing attenuation due to atomic defects and absorbing optical energy. The total dose a material receives is expressed in rad (Si), this is the unit for measuring radiation absorbed in bulk silicon. Thus, 1 rad (Si) = 0.01 J/kg. The higher the radiation intensity more the attenuation.

11. Explain extrinsic absorption in optical fibers.

Ans. This occurs due to electronic transitions between the energy levels and also due to charge transitions from one ion to another. However, a major source of extrinsic attenuation is from transition of metal impurity ions such as iron, chromium, cobalt, and copper. These losses may be upto 1 to 10 dB/km. The effect of metallic impurities can be reduced by glass refining techniques.

There is another major extrinsic loss caused by absorption due to OH (hydroxil) ions impurities dissolved in glass. Vibrations occur at wavelengths between 2.7 and 4.2 mm and the absorption peaks occurs at 1400, 950 and 750 nm. These are first, second and third overtones respectively.

12. Write the expressions ultraviolet (UV) loss and loss in infrared (IR) region for optical fibers.

Ans. The UV loss at any wavelength is expressed as

$$\alpha_{UV} = \frac{154.2}{46.6x + 60} \times 10^{-2} \left[\exp\left(\frac{4.63}{\lambda} \right) \right]$$

where x is mole fraction of GeO_2 and λ is in dB/km. α_{UV} is in dB/km.

The loss in IR region (above 1.2 µm) is given by

$$\alpha_{IR} = 7.81 \times 10^{11} \exp\left[\frac{-48.48}{\lambda} \right]$$

The above expression is derived for GeO_2-SiO_2 glass fiber.

13. Explain Rayleigh scattering of light in optical fibers. What are Rayleigh scattering losses?

Ans. Rayleigh scattering of light in optical fibers is due to small localized changes in the refractive index of the core and cladding materials. This occurs due to following two causes during the manufacturing of the optical fiber:

(i) Due to slight fluctuations in mixing of ingradients. The random changes due to this cannot be eliminated completely.

(ii) The slight change in the density as the silica cools and solidifers. When light ray strikes such zones, rays gets scattered in all directions. The amount of scatter depends on the size of the discontinuity compared with the wavelength of the light so the shortest wavelength, i.e. highest frequency suffers most scattering.

14. Explain Rayleigh scattering losses in optical fibers and write expression for single-component glass and multi-component glasses.

Ans. Scattering losses in optical fibers due to microscopic variations in their material density and composition. A glass is composed by randomly connected network of molecules and several oxides, e.g. SiO_2, GeO_2 and P_2O_5 and these are the major cause of compositional structural fluctuation. These two effects results to variation in refractive index and Rayleigh-type scattering of light.

Scattering loss for single-component glass can be expressed by

$$\alpha_{scat} = \frac{8\pi^3}{3\lambda^4} (n^2 - 1)^2 k_B T_f \beta_T \text{ nepers} \tag{1}$$

where, n is refractive index, β_T is isothermal compressibility of the material and T_f is the temperature at which density fluctuations are frozen into the glass as it solidifies (fictive temperature. Equation (1) can also be expressed as

$$\alpha_{scat} = \frac{8\pi^3}{3\lambda^4} n^8 p^2 k_B T_f \beta_T \text{ nepers} \tag{2}$$

where p denotes photoelastic coefficient.

Scattering loss for multicomponent glasses can be expressed as

$$\alpha_{scat} = \frac{8\pi^3}{3\lambda^4} (\delta_n^2) \delta V \tag{3}$$

where δn^2 is mean-square refractive index fluctuation and δV is volume of the fiber.

15. Why overall losses in multimode fibers are more as compared to single mode fibers?

Ans. Multimode fibers have higher dopant concentrations and greater compositional fluctuations and overall losses in these fibers are more as compared to single mode fibers.

16. Explain bending loss in fibers.

Ans. A sharp bend of a fiber causes significant radiative losses and there is also possibility of mechanical failure (Fig. 6.40)

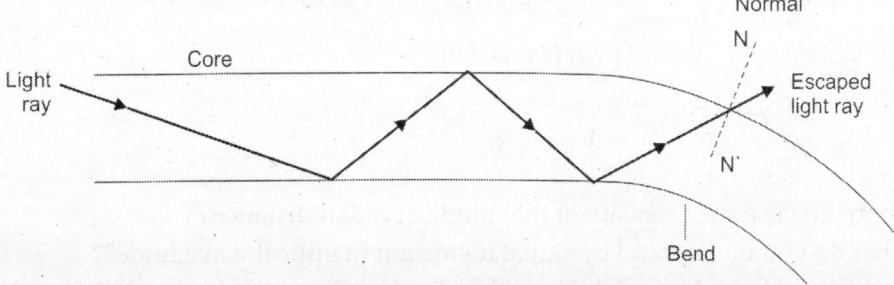

Fig. 6.40: Bending loss in a fiber

Wee see that as the core bends the normal will follow it and the ray will now find itself on the wrong side of the critical angle and will escape. This is why the sharp bends are avoided the *radiation loss* from a bend fiber depends on:

(i) The radius of curvature R

(ii) Field strength of certain critical distance x_c from the axis of the fiber where power is lost through radiation.

The higher order modes are less tightly bound to the fiber core and therefore the higher order modes radiate out of fiber firstly.

In case of the multimode fiber, the number of modes that can be guided by the curved fiber is governed by the following expression:

$$N_{eff} = N_\infty \left[1 - \left(\frac{\alpha + 2}{2\alpha\Delta} \right) \left\{ \frac{2a}{R} + \left(\frac{3}{2n_2 kR} \right)^{2/3} \right\} \right]$$

where α is graded index profile, Δ is core-cladding index difference, n_2 is refractive index of cladding, $k(= 2\pi/\lambda)$ is wave propagation constant and N_∞ is total number of modes in a straight fiber given by

$$N_\infty = \frac{\alpha}{\alpha + 2} (n_1 ka)^2 \Delta$$

17. **Explain core and cladding losses in a fiber.**

Ans. Since the core and cladding of a fiber have different indices of refraction hence they have different attenuation coefficients α_1 and α_2 respectively.

In case of a step-index fiber, the loss for a mode order (v, m) is expressed as

$$\alpha_{v, m} = \alpha_1 \frac{P_{core}}{P} + \alpha_2 \frac{P_{cladding}}{P} \tag{i}$$

For low-order modes, the relation (i) reduces to

$$\alpha_{v, m} = \alpha_1 + (\alpha_2 - \alpha_1) \frac{P_{cladding}}{P} \tag{ii}$$

where $\frac{P_{core}}{P}$ and $\frac{P_{cladding}}{P}$ represent fractional powers.

For graded index fiber, loss at radial distance r can be expressed as,

$$\alpha(r) = \alpha_1 + (\alpha_2 - \alpha_1) \frac{n^2(o) - n^2(r)}{n^2(o) - n_2^2} \tag{iii}$$

The expression for the loss for a given mode is as follows:

$$\alpha_{graded\ index} = \frac{\int\limits_0^\infty \alpha(r) P(r) r\, dr}{\int\limits_0^\infty P(r) r\, dr} \tag{iv}$$

where $P(r)$ is power density of that mode at radial distance r.

18. **What do you understand by signal distortion in optical waveguide?**

Ans. When the pulse travels along the fiber length, it gets distorted. Pulse spreading in fiber is termed as *dispersion*. Dispersion is caused by difference in the propagation times of light rays that takes different paths during the propagation. The light pulses travelling down the fiber encounter dispersion due to spreading of the pulse in time domain. Dispersion limits the information bandwidth. One can analyze the distortion effects by studying the group velocities in guided modes.

19. **Explain group delay.**

Ans. Let us consider a fiber cable carrying optical signal equally with various modes and each mode contains all the spectral components in the wavelength band. All the spectral components travel independently and they observe different *time delay* and *group delay* in the direction of propagation. The velocity at which the energy in a pulse travels along the fiber is known as group velocity,

$$V_g = \partial W / \partial \beta$$

20. **Explain material dispersion and write expression for material dispersion. What is the significance of negative sign appearing in the expression.**

Ans. Material dispersion or chromatic dispersion exist due to change in index of refraction for different wavelengths. We know that a ray of light consists of various components of different wavelengths centered at wavelength λ_0. The time delay is different for different wavelength components. This results in time dispersion of pulse at the receiving end of the fiber. The material dispersion for unit length ($L = 1$) is given by

$$D_{\text{mat}} = -\frac{\lambda}{c} \frac{d^2 n}{d\lambda^2} \tag{i}$$

where c is velocity of light and λ is central wavelength. Negative sign in (i) shows that the upperside band signal (lowest wavelength) arrives prior the power side band (highest wavelength).

21. **Explain waveguide dispersion and mention its significance.**

Ans. Waveguide dispersion is caused by the difference in the index of refraction between the core and cladding, resulting in a 'drag' effect between the core and cladding portions of the power.

Waveguide dispersion is significant only in fibers carring fewer than 5–10 modes. We may note that multimode fibers carry hundreds of modes and hence they will have almost no waveguide dispersion.

The group delay (τ_{wg}) arising due waveguide dispersion is given by

$$\tau_{wg} = \frac{L}{c} \left[n_2 + n_2 \Delta \frac{d(kb)}{dk} \right]$$

where b is normalized propagation constant, k ($= 2\pi/\lambda$) is group velocity. In terms of normalized frequency $V = ka(n_1^2 - n_2^2)^{1/2} \approx kan_2\sqrt{2\Delta}$ (for small Δ), group delay expression reads as

$$\tau_{wg} = \frac{L}{c} \left[n_2 + n_2 \Delta \frac{d(V_b)}{dV} \right]$$

The second term $\dfrac{dV_b}{dV}$ is waveguide dispersion and also mode dependent.

22. **What do you understand by higher order dispersion. Mention dispersion induced limitations?**

Ans. Higher order dispersive effects are governed by dispersion slope S given by

$$S = \frac{dD}{d\lambda} = \left(\frac{2\pi c}{\lambda^2} \right)^2 \beta_3 + \left(\frac{4\pi c}{\lambda^3} \right) \beta_2$$

where D is total dispersion and β_2 and β_3 are second and third order dispersion parameters respectively. Dispersion slope S plays an important role in designing WDM system.

The extent of pulse broadening depends on the width and the shape of input pulses. One can study the pulse broadening with the help of wave equation.

23. Explain polarization-mode dispersion (PMD).

Ans. Different frequency components of a pulse acquires different polarization states (suchas linear polarization and circular polarization). This results in pulse broadening and is known as PMD. However, PMD is a limiting factor for optical communication system at high data rates. One will have to compensate the effects of PMD.

24. Explain the effects of mode coupling.

Ans. After certain initial length, the pulse distortion increases less rapidly due to mode coupling. The energy from one mode coupling. The energy from one mode is coupled to other modes because of: structural imperfections, fiber diameter variations, refractive index variations and microbends in cable. Due to mode coupling, average propagation delay becomes less and intermodal distortion reduces. The improvement in pulse spreading by mode coupling is given by

$$hz\left(\frac{\sigma_c}{\sigma_0}\right) = C$$

where C is constant independent of all dimensional quantities and refractive indices. σ_c and σ_0 are pulse broadening under mode coupling and pulse broadening in absence of mode coupling respectively. We may note that for long fiber length's the effect of mode coupling on pulse distortion is significant.

MULTIPLE CHOICE QUESTIONS

1. The basic attenuation mechanisms in a fiber are
   (a) absorption only
   (b) scattering only
   (c) radiative losses of the optical energy only
   (d) all of the above

2. Distortion in optical fibers
   (a) limits the information carrying capacity of fiber
   (b) enhances the information carrying capacity of fiber
   (c) burn the fiber
   (d) none of the above

3. If L is the length along the fiber traversed by the light, then the attenuation or loss in the fiber can be expressed as
   (a) α (dB/km) $= \left[\dfrac{P(0)}{P(L)}\right]$
   (b) α (dB/km) $= \dfrac{10}{L}\log_{10}\left[\dfrac{P(0)}{P(L)}\right]$
   (c) α (dB/km) $= \dfrac{10}{L}\log_{10}\left[\dfrac{P(L)}{P(0)}\right]$
   (d) none of the above

4. The ultraviolet absorption near the absorption edge is governed by the empirical relation
   (a) $\alpha_{uv} = C\exp\left(\dfrac{E_0}{hv}\right)$
   (b) $\alpha_{uv} = C\exp\left(\dfrac{hv}{E_0}\right)$
   (c) $\alpha_{uv} = C\exp(hv - E_0)$
   (d) $\alpha_{uv} = C\exp(E_0 - hv)$
   (C and E_0 are empirical constants and hv is the energy of the photon)

5. The infrared absorption loss in optical fiber is given by

   (a) $\alpha_{IR} = C \exp\left(\dfrac{\lambda}{D}\right)$

   (b) $\alpha_{IR} = C \exp\left(\dfrac{D}{\lambda^2}\right)$

   (c) $\alpha_{IR} = C \exp\left(-\dfrac{D}{\lambda}\right)$

   (d) $\alpha_{IR} = C \exp\left(-\dfrac{D}{\lambda^3}\right)$

   (C and D are empirical constants)

6. For a single component glass the Rayleigh scattering coefficient (γ_R) is given by

   (a) $\gamma_R = \dfrac{8\pi^3}{\lambda^2}\, n^8 p^2 \beta_c k T_F$

   (b) $\gamma_R = \dfrac{8\pi^3}{3\lambda^2}\, n^8 p^2 \beta_c k T_F$

   (c) $\gamma_R = \dfrac{8\pi^3}{3\lambda^4}\, n^8 p^2 \beta_c k T_F$

   (d) $\gamma_R = \dfrac{8\pi^3}{3\lambda}\, n^8 p^2 \beta_c k T_F$

   ($\lambda \rightarrow$ wavelength of the propagating light, $n \rightarrow$ refractive index of the medium, $p \rightarrow$ average photoelectric constant, $\beta_c \rightarrow$ isothermal compressibility at a fictive temperature T_F)

7. The threshold power required for stimulated Brillouin scattering (SBS) in optical fibers can be obtained as

   (a) $P_B = 4.4 \times 10^{-3}\, d\lambda\, \alpha_{dB}\, \Delta v$ (watts)

   (b) $P_B = 4.4 \times 10^{-3}\, d^2\lambda^2\, \alpha_{dB}\, \Delta v$ (watts)

   (c) $P_B = 4.4 \times 10^{-3}\, d\lambda/\alpha_{dB}\, \Delta v$ (watts)

   (d) none of the above

   ($d \rightarrow$ core diameter in micrometer, $\lambda \rightarrow$ operating wavelength in micrometer, $\alpha_{dB} \rightarrow$ fiber attenuation in decibel per kilometer and $\Delta v \rightarrow$ linewidth in GHz of the injection laser).

8. The mean optical power launched into an 8 km length of optical fiber is 12 µW and the mean power at the fiber output is 3 µW. The overall signal attenuation in dB is about

   (a) 16

   (b) 8

   (c) 4

   (d) 32

   [**Hint:** $\alpha = 10 \log \dfrac{P(0)}{P(z)} = 10 \log\left(\dfrac{120}{3}\right) = 16.02$ dB]

9. Core and cladding of optical fiber have different attenuation coefficients α_1 and α_2 respectively because

   (a) they have same indices of refraction

   (b) they have different indices of refraction

   (c) they have different diameters

   (d) none of the above

10. The velocity at which the energy in a pulse travels along the fiber is known as

    (a) velocity of light

    (b) group velocity

    (c) wave velocity

    (d) none of the above

11. Material dispersion is also called as

    (a) reflection

    (b) refraction

    (c) polarization

    (d) chromatic dispersion

12. Material dispersion for unit length ($L = 1$) of the fiber is given by

(a) $D_{mat} = -\dfrac{\lambda}{c}\dfrac{d^2n}{d\lambda^2}$

(b) $D_{mat} = \dfrac{\lambda}{c}\dfrac{d^3n}{d\lambda^3}$

(c) $D_{mat} = -\dfrac{\lambda}{c}\dfrac{dn}{d\lambda}$

(d) $D_{mat} = -\left(\dfrac{\lambda}{c}\right)^2\dfrac{d^2n}{d\lambda^2}$

($c \rightarrow$ velocity of light $\lambda \rightarrow$ center velocity, $n \rightarrow$ index of refraction)

13. For a single mode fiber $n^2 = 1.48$ and $\Delta = 0.2\%$ operating at $\lambda = 1320$ nm.

If $V\dfrac{d^2(Vb)}{dV^2} = 0.26$, the waveguide dispersion in pico sec/nm/km is

(a) 1.94

(b) 3.6

(c) 5.8

(d) 4.7

14. If $\sigma_{intermodal}$ is r.m.s. pulse width due to intermodal delay distortion and $\sigma_{intramodal}$ is r.m.s. pulse with resulting from pulse broadening within each mode, then r.m.s. pulse broadening is given by

(a) $\sigma = \dfrac{\sigma_{intermodal}}{\sigma_{intramodal}}$

(b) $\sigma = \sigma_{intermodal} + \sigma_{intramodal}$

(c) $\sigma = \left(\sigma_{intermodal}^2 + \sigma_{intramodal}^2\right)^{1/2}$

(d) $\sigma = \dfrac{\sigma_{intramodal}}{\sigma_{intermodal}}$

15. The macrobending and microbending losses are significant in single mode fibers at

(a) 350 nm region

(b) 725 nm region

(c) 1175 nm region

(d) 1550 nm region

ANSWERS

1. (d)   2. (a)   3. (b)   4. (a)   5. (c)   6. (c)   7. (b)   8. (a)   9. (b)   10. (b)

11. (d)   12. (a)   13. (a)   14. (c)   15. (d)

7

Optical Sources 1—The LASER

7.1 INTRODUCTION

An optical fiber communication *transmitter* system consists of an optical source, optical interconnects and associated electronics essential for modulation of the light output in accordance with the information on intelligence signal. We may note that an optical source is the key component of *optical transmitter unit*. An optical source convert an electrical signal reliably into optical radiation (E/O conversion). There are variety of optical sources available that convert electrical energy to an optical signal (light). In view of the compatibility with the dimensions of an optical fiber, generally semiconductor optical sources, namely *light emitting diode* (LED) and *injection laser diode* (ILD) usually referred to as *Laser Diode* (LD). An optical source for use in the transmitter unit of an optical fiber communication system should ideally meet the following requirements:

(i) Size and configuration of the emitting optical source must be compatible to the size of the optical fiber .
(ii) Ideally, the light output should be highly directional for easy launching of light from the source to the fiber.
(iii) The light output (i.e. optical power) should vary linearly with the electrical input for reliable E/O conversion.
(iv) E/O conversion efficiency of optical source must be reasonably high.
(v) The emission wavelength of optical source should match with the attenuation window of the optical fiber, i.e. the wavelength at which the optical fiber offers low attenuation.
(vi) In order to reduce chromatic dispersion during propagation through the optical fiber, the spectral width of the optical source should be small.
(vii) The optical source must have a high modulation capability, i.e. large band width so that it may meet the required large information carrying capacity of the optical fiber.
(viii) The source must be capable of maintaining a stable optical output which is largely unaffected changes in ambient conditions (e.g. temperature). Optical source must also be able to couple sufficient optical power to the optical fiber so that they can travel a long distance and still deliver the required power to the detector for proper conversion of optical signal into electrical signal (O/E conversion).
(ix) The optical source should have moderately long life, comparatively cheap and highly reliable so that it may compete with conventional transmission techniques.

Interestingly, IED and ILD both meet the basic requirements of an optical source for use in optical fiber communication system. One of the major differces between LED and ILD optical sources it that the optical output from the former is *incoherent* whereas that from the latter is coherent. However, structurally, both LED and ILD consist of *pn* junction, where pn junction is made of direct band gap semiconductor-materials (most commonly III-V materials). When this *pn* junction is forward biased, electrons and holes are injected into the *p*- and *n*-regions, respectively These injected minority carriers can recombine either radiately, in which case a photon of energy hv is emitted, or non radiatively, whereupon the recombination energy is released in the form of heat which is absorbed by the lattice. The principle of operation of an LD differs significantly from that of an LED. The light from an LED results from spontaneous emission following the random radiative recombination of the carriers, whereas an ILD works on the principle of stimulated emission which dominates only under special circumstances and the optical output from ILD is coherent and highly monochromatic. This is because light in an ILD is produced in an optical resonator that ensures both *spatial* as well as well as *temporal coherence* of light emanating from the cavity. We may note that the spatial coherence ensures that the output light is highly monochromatic and temporal coherence leads that the output light beam is highly directional. On the other hand no cavity resonator is used in the case of LED and therefore, the output light beam generally exhibits a large spectral width. Moreover, the half-power beam width is also quite large because light is emitted in a hemisphere with a *cosine power distribution*. Since the total dispersion of an optical fiber depends on the rms spectral width of the optical source and hence from this point of view laser diodes are superior to LEDs. Moreover, a relatively large beam width in the case of LED makes it extremely difficult to launch power from this kind of light source to a signal mode optical fiber. This is why LEDs are generally used with multimode optical fibers. Further, incoherent light emitted from LED can couple power to a large number of modes supported by the optical fiber. Moreover, the bandwidth of an LED is also much lower as compared to that of an ILD. The transmission rate in LED-based optical fiber communication system is generally restricted to 100–200 Mbps. Also, the output power of an LED is much lower than that of an ILD. However, the output power from the LED can be improved significantly by modifying its structure. On the other side, LEDs also have several advantages over ILDs:

(i) LEDs can be used to launch power quite efficiently in low cost plastic fibers.

(ii) The use of LED with plastic fibers in short distance optical communication can cut-down substantially the overall cost of the system. No doubt, the maximum transmission rate (bps) is however, severely restricted by the limited modulation capability of the LED and also relatively large dispersion in plastic fibers.

(iii) The performance of an ILD degrades with aging.

(iv) The cost of an ILD is quite high compared to LED, and

(v) In case of ILDs a complex driver circuit is required compared to that required in the case of LEDs.

In brief, we can say that in choosing an optical source which is compatible with the optical wave guide, various characteristics of the optical fiber, such as its geometry, its attenuation as a function of wavelength, its group delay distortion (bandwidth), and its modal characteristics have to be taken into account. Further, the interplay of these factors with the optical source power, spectral width, radiation pattern, and modulation capability needs to be considered. From all these considered as discussed above, in general LEDs are used with multimode fibers, since normally it is only into a multimode fiber that the incoherent optical power from an LED can be coupled in sufficient quantities to be useful.

In order to understand the principle of operation of LEDs and ILDs, we have to acquire knowledge of some fundamental concepts of semiconductor physics. In this chapter, next few sections are devoted to the study of some selected topics on semiconductor device physics that are essential for understanding of various optoelectronic devices. Rest of chapter is devoted to the study of ILDs. LEDs are discussed in Chapter 8.

7.2 SEMICONDUCTORS

According to band theory of solids, materials may be classified into three categories from the point of view of electric conduction: (i) conductors (ii) insulators (iii) semiconductors. The sensitivity of these materials lies in the following range of values:

Conductor: 10^{-6}–10^{-4} Ω cm
Insulator: 10^{10}–10^{20} Ω cm
Semiconductor: 10^{-2}–10^{8} Ω cm

7.2.1 Energy Band Diagram

Semiconductor materials have conduction properties that lie somewhat between those of metals and insulators. As an example, we consider silicon (Si), which is located in the fourth column (group IV) of the periodic table of elements. A Si atom has four electrons in its outer shell, by which it makes covalent bonds with its neighbouring atoms in a crystal (Fig. 7.1). Such outer-shell electrons are called *valence electrons.*

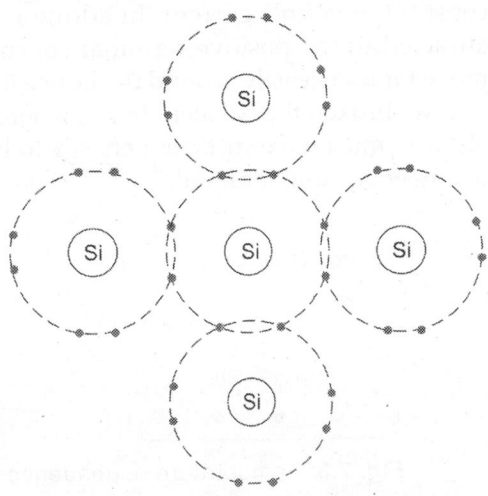

Fig. 7.1: Covalent band structure of silicon

These electrons are somewhat loosely bound. An electron can gain energy by external means, such as thermal energy, to break the covalent bond and, thereby, contribute to the *conduction band*. Further, if an electron is confined to the outermost shell of the atom, it is said to be in the *valence band* and if it is moving freely in the lattice, it is said to be in the conduction band. Strictly speaking, atoms of solid-state materials have such a strong interaction that they cannot be treated as individual entities. Valence electrons are not attached to individual atoms, instead, they belong to the system of atoms as a whole.

The conduction band and valence band are separated by an energy gap or *band gap* E_g, as shown in Fig. 7.2. For Si, the band gap is 1.1 eV. At low temperature, the chance that an electron occupies the conduction band is approximately proportional to exp $(-E_g/k_B T)$. Materials with a filled valence band and a large band gap (> 3eV) are *insulators*. Those for which the gap is small or nonexistent are *conductors* (Fig. 7.2). Semiconductors have band gaps that lie roughly in the range of 0.1 to 3 eV.

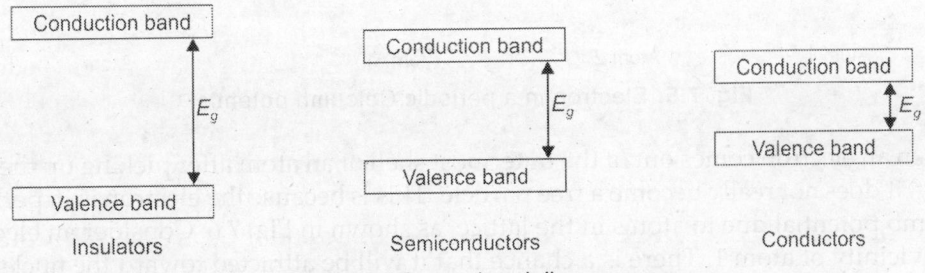

Fig. 7.2: Energy band diagrams

At very low temperature, the conduction band is nearly empty and, therefore, the valence band is nearly full, as shown in Fig. 7.3. As the temperature increases, electrons in the valence band gain energy to cross the band gap and get into the conduction band. This leads to a concentration of free electrons in the conduction band, which leaves behind equal numbers of vacancies or *holes* in the valence band. A hole refers to the absence of an electron and it acts as if it is a positive charge. Consider a semiconductor material connected to the terminals of a battery, as shown in Fig. 7.4. The electron in the leftmost region is attracted to the positive terminal of the battery and it leaves behind a hole (Fig. 7.5(a)). An electron from the neighboring atom jumps to fill the hole, thereby creating a hole as shown in Fig. 7.5(b). This process continues, and holes move in the right constituting a hole current. In addition, electrons moving freely in the lattice are also attracted to the positive terminal constituting the electron current. Free electrons can move far more easily around the lattice than holes. This is because the free electrons have already broken the covalent bond, whereas for a hole to travel through the structure, an electron must have sufficient energy to break the covalent bond each time a hole jumps to a new positive terminal.

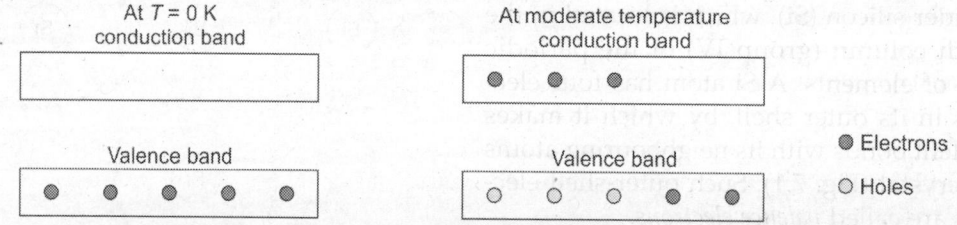

Fig. 7.3: Temperature dependence of electron density in the conduction band

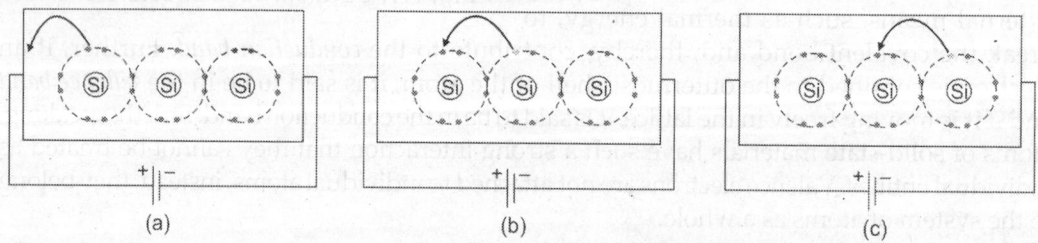

Fig. 7.4: Electron and hole current in Si

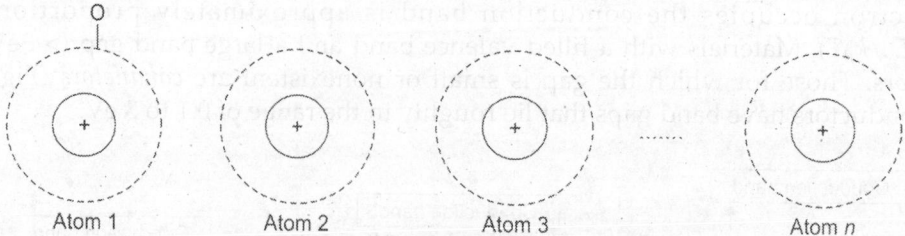

Fig. 7.5: Electron in a periodic Coloumb potential

When an electron comes out of the outermost shell of an atom after picking up thermal energy, it does not really become a free particle. This is because the electron is in periodic Coulomb potential due to atoms in the lattice, as shown in Fig. 7.6. Consider an electron in the vicinity of atom 1. There is a chance that it will be attracted toward the nucleus of

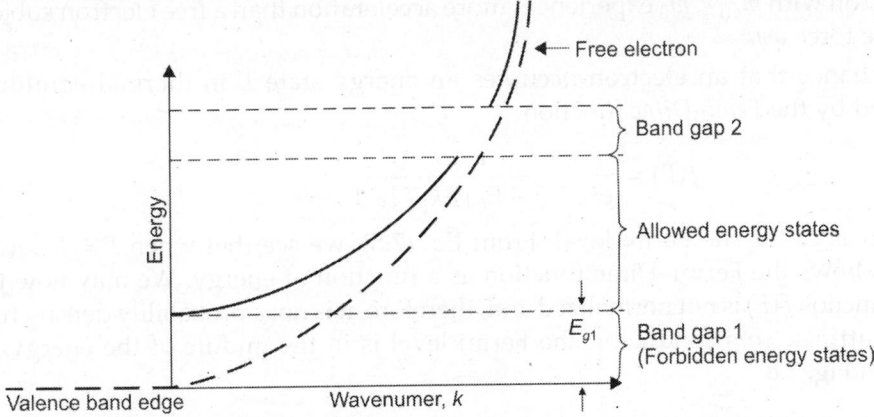

Fig. 7.6: Plot of energy vs wave number. The dotted line and solid line corresponds to the energy of a free electron and an electron in a pure semiconductor crystals, respectively

atom 2. When it is in the vicinity of atom 2, there is a chance that it will be attracted toward atom 3 or atom 1. An electron can hop on and off from atom to atom as if it were a free classical particle, but with the following difference. A free nonrelativistic particle can acquire any amount of energy and the energy states are continuous. However, for an electron in periodic potential, there is a range of energy states that are forbidden and this is called the energy band gap. The existence of a band gap can only be explained by quantum mechanics. At very low temperature, electrons have energy states corresponding to conduction bands, but are not allowed to occupy any energy states that are within the band gap, as shown in Fig. 7.6. For a free electron, the energy increases quadratically with k as given by

$$E = \frac{h^2 k^2}{2m_0} \tag{7.1}$$

when m_0 is the rest mass of an electron. Differentiating Eq. (7.1) twice, we find

$$m_0 = \frac{h^2}{d^2 E / dk^2} \tag{7.2}$$

The dotted line in Fig. 7.6 shows the plot of energy as a function of the wavenumber k, for the free electron. For an electron in a pure semiconductor crystal, the plot of energy vs wave number is shown as a solid line. We define the effective mass of an electron in the periodic potential as

$$m_{\text{eff}}(k) = \frac{k^2}{d^2 E / dk^2} \tag{7.3}$$

in the allowed range of energy states, in analogy with the case of free electrons. The effective mass can be larger or smaller than the rest mass, depending on the nature of the periodic potential. For example, for CaAs, $m_{\text{eff}} = 0.07m_0$ in the conduction band. The significance of the effective mass can be explained as follows. Suppose an electron in the pure semiconductor crystal is subjected to an external electric field intensity, ψ, then the equation of motion is given by Newton's law.

$$\frac{d(m_{\text{eff}} v)}{dt} = \text{force} = q\psi, \tag{7.4}$$

where v and q are the velocity and charge of an electron, respectively. Note that an electron in a pure semiconductor crystal behaves as if it is a free particle with effective mass m_{eff}.

An electron with $m_{eff} < m_0$ experiences more acceleration than a free electron subjected to the same force $q\psi$.

The chance that an electron occupies an energy state E in thermal equilibrium is described by the *Femi–Dirac* function

$$f(E) = \frac{1}{\exp[(E - E_F)/k_B T] + 1} \tag{7.5}$$

where E_F is called the Fermi level. From Eq. (7.5), we see that when $E = E_F$, $f(E) = 0.5$ Fig. 7.7 shows the Fermi–Dirac function as a function of energy. We may note that the Fermi function $f(E)$ is not normalized and, therefore, it is not a probability density function. For an intrinsic semiconductor, the Fermi level is in the middle of the energy gap, as shown in Fig. 7.8.

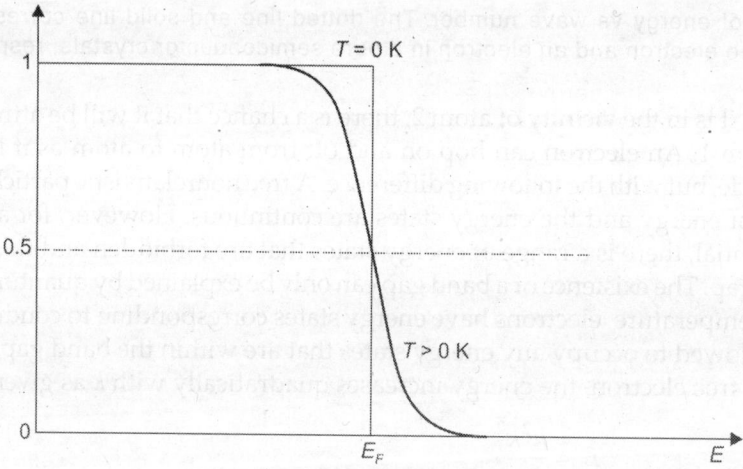

Fig. 7.7: Fermi–Dirac function

For example, at the conduction band bottom, $E_c = E_u + E_g$ and $E_F = E_u + E_g/2$, at temperature $T = 300$ K, $k_B T \approx 0.025$ eV, and with $E_g = 1$ eV.

$$f(E_c) = \frac{1}{\exp\left[\dfrac{E_g}{2k_B T}\right] + 1} \approx \exp\left[\frac{E_g}{2k_B T}\right] = \exp(-20) \tag{7.6}$$

Thus, at room temperature, the chance that an electron occupies the conduction band is very small and, therefore, the electrical conductivity of the *intrinsic semiconductor* is quite low. But the conductivity can be increased by adding impurity atoms. The basic semiconductor without doping is called an *intrinsic semiconductor* (Fig. 7.9). Doping consists of adding impurities to the crystalline structure of the semiconductor. For example, a small amount of group V elements such as arsenic can be added to silicon. Arsenic has five electrons in the outermost shell; four electron form a covalent bond with neighboring silicon atoms, as shown in Fig. 7.10, but there is one electron left over that can not take part in bonding. This fifth electron is very loosely attached and it is free to move through the crystal when an electric field is applied. Thus the number of free electron in the crystal is enhanced by doping with arsenic. Group V elements such as arsenic added to group IV elements are called *donors*, since they contribute free electrons. The resultant semiconductor material is known as an *n-type semiconductor*.

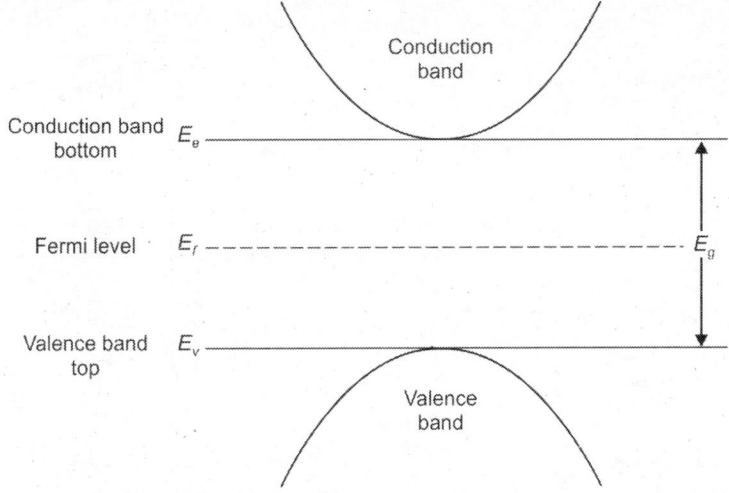

Fig. 7.8: Energy-band diagram of an intrinsic semiconductor

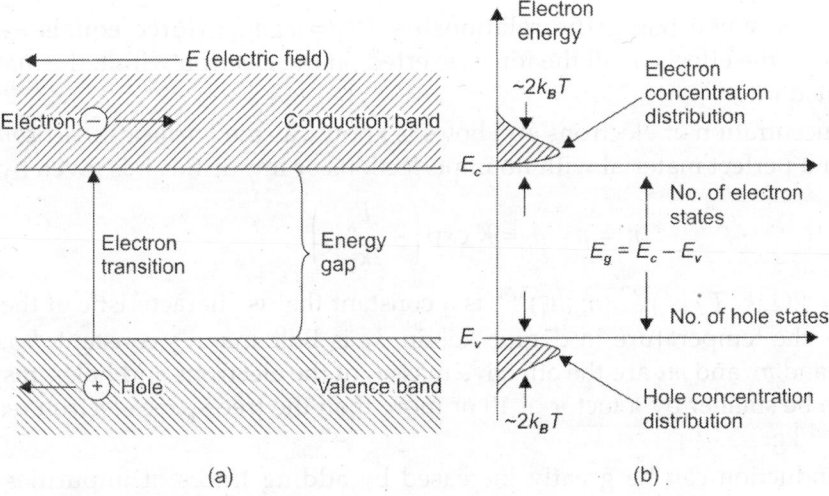

Fig. 7.9: (a) Energy level diagrams exhibiting the excitation of an electron from the valence band to the conduction band. The resultant free electrons and holes move under the influence of an external electric field E; (b) equal electron and hole concentrations in an intrinsic semiconductor created by the thermal excitation of electrons across the band gap

When a small amount of group III elements such as gallium are added to silicon, three valence electrons of gallium form a covalent bond with the neighboring three silicon atoms, while the fourth silicon atom shown in Fig. 7.11 is deprived of an electron to complete a total of eight electrons. The missing electron is a hole that can be filled by an electron that is in the neighborhood. Thus, the number of holes is increased by doping with group III elements, which are known as *acceptors*, and the resultant semiconductor is known as a *p-type semiconductor*.

When an electron propagates in a semiconductor, it interacts with the periodically arranged constituent atoms of the material and thus, experiences *external forces*. As a result, to describe its acceleration a_{crys} in a semiconductor crystal under an external force F_{ext}, its mass needs to be described by a quantum mechanical quantity m_e called the *effective*

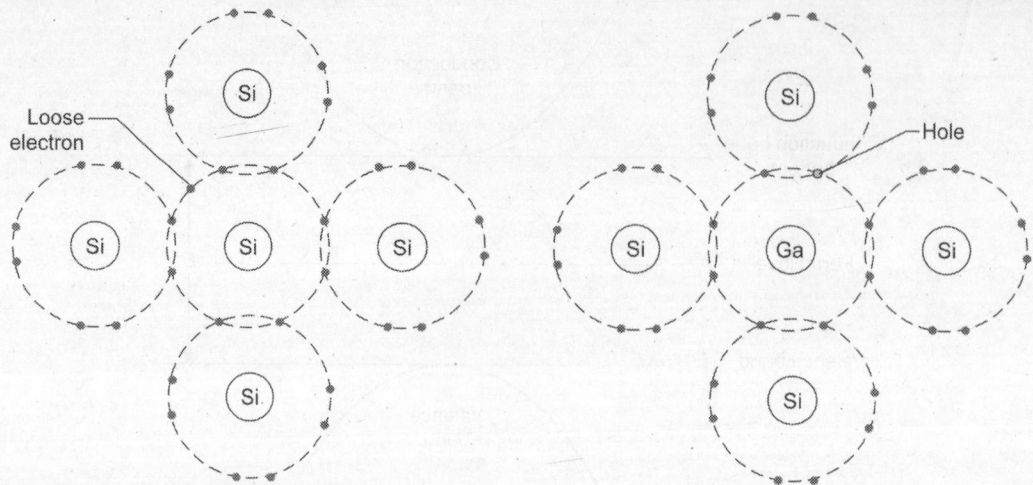

Fig. 7.10: Molecular structure of an n-type semiconductor

Fig. 7.11: Molecular structure of a p-type semiconductor

mass. That is, when using the relationship $F_{ext} = m_e a_{crys}$ (force equals mass times acceleration), the effects of all the forces exerted on the electron within the materials are incorporated into m_e.

The concentration of electrons and holes is known as the *intrinsic carrier concentration* n_i, and for a perfect material with no imperfections or impurities it is given by:

$$n = p = n_i = K \exp\left(-\frac{E_g}{2k_B T}\right) \qquad (7.7)$$

where $K = 2(2\pi k_B T / h^2)^{3/2} (m_e m_h)^{3/4}$ is a constant that is characteristic of the material. Here, T is the temperature in degree kelvin, k_B is Boltzmann's constant, h is Planck's constant, and m_e and m_h are the effective masses of the electrons and holes, respectively, which can be smaller by a factor of 10 or more than the free-space electron rest mass of 9.11×10^{-31} kg.

The conduction can be greatly increased by adding traces of impurities from the group V elements (e.g. P, As, Sb). This process is called *doping* and the doped semiconductor is called an *extrinsic material*. These elements have five electrons in the outer shell. When they replace a Si atom, four electrons are used for covalent bonding, and the fifth, loosely bound electron is available for conduction. As shown in Fig. 7.12(a), this gives rise to an occupied level, just below the conduction band, called the *donor level*. The impurities are called *donors* because they can give up an electron to the conduction band. This is reflected by the increase in the free-electron concentration in the conduction band, as shown in Fig. 7.12(b). Since in this type of material, the current is carried by (negative) electrons (because the electron concentration is much higher than that of holes), it is called *n*-type material.

The conduction can also be increased by adding group III elements, which have three electrons in the outer shell. In this case, three electrons make covalent bonds, and a hole with properties identical to that of the donor electron is created. As shown in Fig. 7.12(c), this gives rise to an unoccupied level just above the valence band. Conduction occurs when electrons are excited from the valence band to this *acceptor level* (so called because the impurity atoms have accepted electrons from the valence band). Correspondingly,

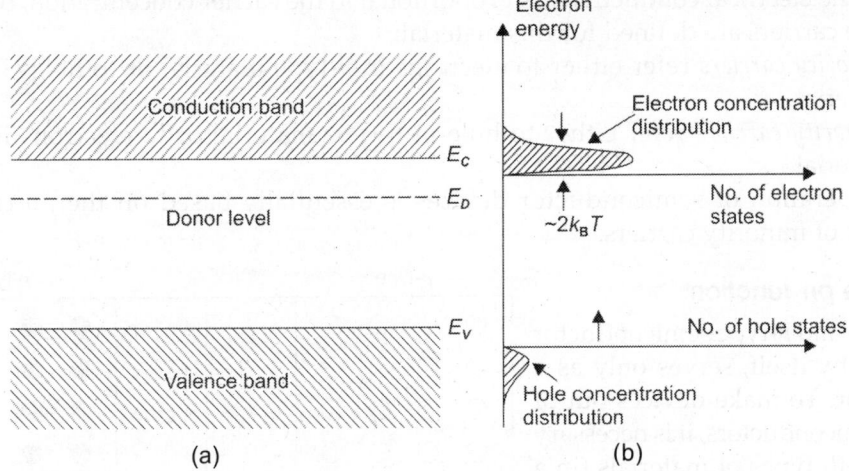

Fig. 7.12: (a) Donor level in an n-type material (b) the ionization of donor-impurities increases the electron concentration distribution in the conduction band

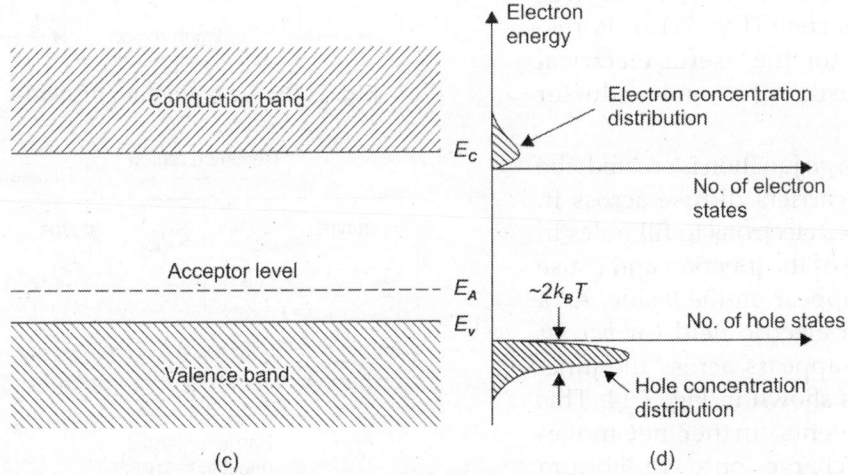

Fig. 7.12: (c) Acceptor level in a p-type material (d) the ionization of acceptor impurities increases the hole concentration distribution in the valence band

the free-hole concentration increases in the valence band, as shown in Fig. 7.12(d). This is called *p*-type material because the conduction is a result of (positive) hole flow.

Summarising a perfect material containing no impurities is called an *intrinsic material*. Because of thermal vibrations of the crystal atoms, some electrons in the valence band gain, enough energy to be excited to the conduction band. This *thermal generation process* produces free electron-hole pairs, since every electron that moves to be conduction band, leaves behind a hole. Thus, for an intrinsic material the number of electrons and holes are both equal to the intrinsic carrier density, as denoted by Eq. (7.7). In the opposite *recombination process*, a free electron releases its energy and drops into a free hole in the valence band. For an extrinsic semiconductor, the increase of one type of carrier reduces the number of the other type. In this case, the product of the two types of carriers remains constant at a given temperature. This gives rise to the *mass-action law*:

$$pn = n_i^2 \tag{7.8}$$

which is valid for both intrinsic and extrinsic materials under thermal equilibrium.

Since the electrical conductivity is proportional to the carrier concentration, two types of charge carriers are defined for this material:

(i) *Majority carriers* refer either to electrons in *n*-type material or to holes in *p*-type material.

(ii) *Minority carriers* refer either to hole in *n*-type material or to electrons in *p*-type material.

The operation of semiconductor devices is essentially based on the *injection* and *extraction* of minority carriers.

7.2.2 The *pn* Junction

Doped *n*- and *p*-type semiconductor material by itself, serves only as a conductor. To make devices out of these semiconductors, it is necessary to use both types of materials (in a single, continuous crystal structure). The junction between the two material regions, which is known as the *pn junction* (Fig. 7.13), is responsible for the useful electrical characteristics of a semiconductor device.

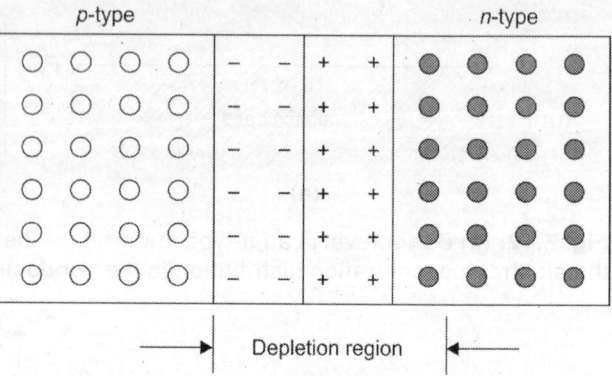

Fig. 7.13: A pn junction or diode

When a *pn* junction is created, the majority carriers diffuse across it. This causes electrons to fill holes in the *p* side of the junction and cause holes to appear on the *n* side. As a result, an electric field (or *barrier potential*) appears across the junction, as is shown in Fig. 7.14. This field prevents further net movements of charges once equilibrium has been established. The junction area now has no mobile carriers, since its electrons and holes are locked into a covalent bond structure. This region is called either the *depletion region* or the *space charge region*.

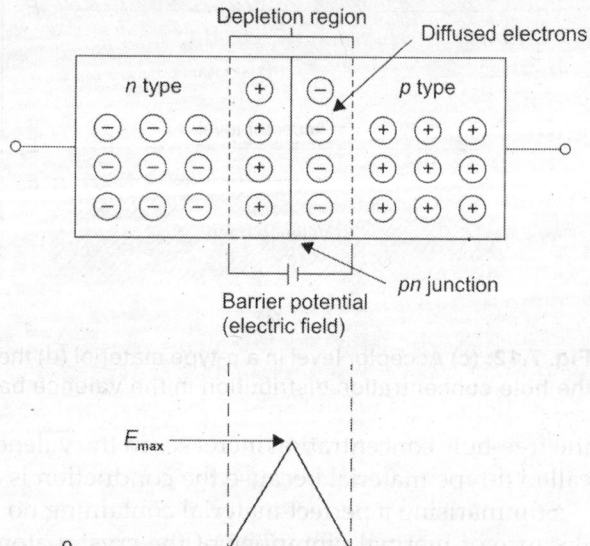

Fig. 7.14: Electron diffusion across a pn junction creates a barrier potential (electric field) in the depletion region

When an external battery is connected to the *pn* junction with its positive terminal to the *n*-type material and its negative terminal to the *p*-type material, the junction is said to be *reverse-biased*. This is shown in Fig. 7.15. As a result of the reverse bias, the width of the depletion region will increase on both the *n* side and the *p* side. This effectively increases the barrier potential and prevents any majority carriers from flowing across the junction. However, minority carriers can move with the field across the junction. The minority carrier flow is small at normal temperatures and operating voltages, but it can be significant when excess carriers are created as, for example, in an illuminated photodiode.

When the *pn* junction is *forward-biased*, as shown in Fig. 7.16, the magnitude of the barrier potential is reduced. Conduction-band electrons on the *n* side and valence-band holes on the *p* side are, thereby, allowed to diffuse across the junction. Once across, they significantly increase the minority carrier concentrations, and the excess carriers recombine with the oppositely charged majority carriers. The recombination of excess minority carriers is the mechanisms by which optical radiation is generated.

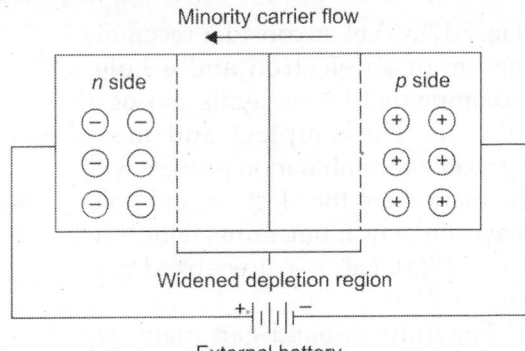

Minority carrier flow

Fig. 7.15: A reverse bias widens the depletion region, but allows minority carriers to move freely with the applied field

7.2.3 Spontaneous and Stimulated Emission at the *pn* Junction

The conduction band and valence band are similar to the excited state and ground state of the atomic system respectively. In the case of the atomic system, an atom in the ground state absorbs a photon and makes a transition to the excited state. Similarly, in a semiconductor, an electron in the valence band could jump to the conduction band by absorbing a photon if its energy exceeds the band-gap energy. As the electron moves to the conduction

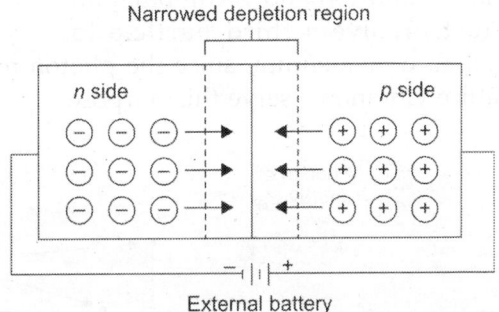

Fig. 7.16: Lowering the barrier potential with a forward bias allows majority carriers to diffuse across the junction

band, it leaves behind a hole in the valence band. In other words, a photon is annihilated to create an electron–hole pair. An electron in the conduction band is stimulated to emit a photon if a photon of the same kind is already present, and it jumps to the valence band. In other words an electron combines with a hole, releasing the difference in energy as a photon. An electron in the conduction band could jump to the valence band spontaneously, whether or not a photon is present. This occurs randomly leading to spontaneous emission.

Now let us consider the forward-biased pn junction. As electron and holes cross the junction, they combine and release the difference in energy as photons. The spontaneously generated photons act as a seed for simulated emission. As electrons are lost due to electron–hole recombination, the external voltage source injects electrons. Thus, the voltage source acts as an electrical pump to achieve population inversion.

7.2.4 Direct and Indirect Band Gap Semiconductors

In order for electron transitions to take place to or from the conduction band with the absorption or emission of a photon, respectively, both energy and momentum must be conserved. Although a photon can have considerable energy, its momentum $h\nu/c$ is very small.

Semiconductors are classified as either *direct-band-gap* or *indirect-band-gap* materials depending on the shape of the band gap as a function of the momentum k, as shown in

Fig. 7.17(a). Let us consider recombination of an electron and a hole, accompanied by the emission of a photon. The simplest and most probable recombination process will be that where the electron and hole have the same momentum value (see Fig. 7.17(a)). This is a direct-band-gap material.

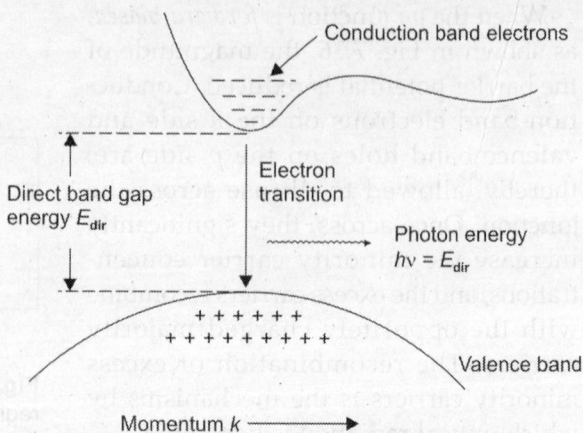

Fig. 7.17(a): Electron recombination and the associated photon emission for a direct-band gap material

For indirect-band-gap material, the conduction-band minimum and the valence-band maximum energy levels occur at different values of momentum, as shown in Fig. 7.17(b). Here, band-to-band recombination must involve a third particle to conserve momentum, since the photon momentum is very small. *Photons* (i.e., crystal lattice vibrations) serve this purpose.

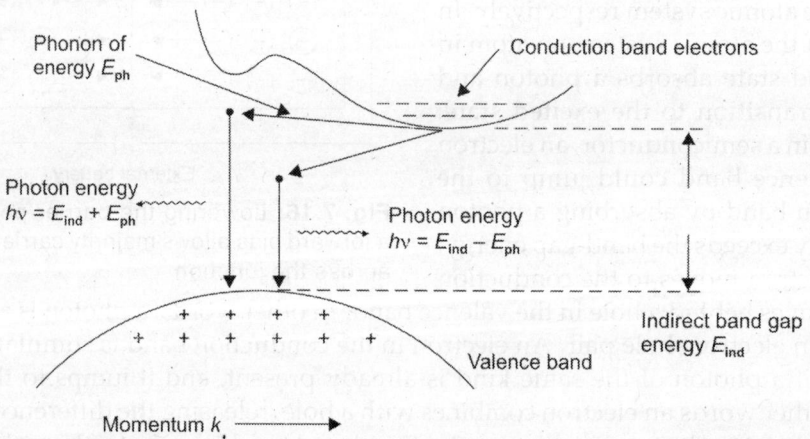

Fig. 7.17(b): Electron recombination for indirect-band-gap materials requires a photon of energy E_{ph} and momentum k_{ph}

Figure 7.18 shows a plot of energy as a function of wavenumber. Let E_g be the minimum energy required to excite an electron to the conduction band. If an electron absorbs the energy $E_1 > E_g$, the excess energy appears in the form of kinetic energy. If we assume that the energy depends on the wavenumber quadratically in the conduction band as in the case of a free particle, the energy of an electron in the conduction band is given by

$$E_1 = E_g + \frac{h^2 k_1^2}{2m_{eff,1}} \tag{7.9}$$

where $m_{eff,1}$ is the *effective mass* of an electron in the conduction band and hk_1 is the momentum. If the bottom of the conduction band is aligned with the top of the valence band as shown in Fig. 7.19, such a material is called a *direct-band gap* material. For example, GaAs and InP are direct band-gap materials. For *indirect-band gap* materials, the conduction band minimum and valence band maximum occur at different values of momentum, as shown in Fig. 7.20. Silicon and germanium are *indirect-band gap semiconductors*.

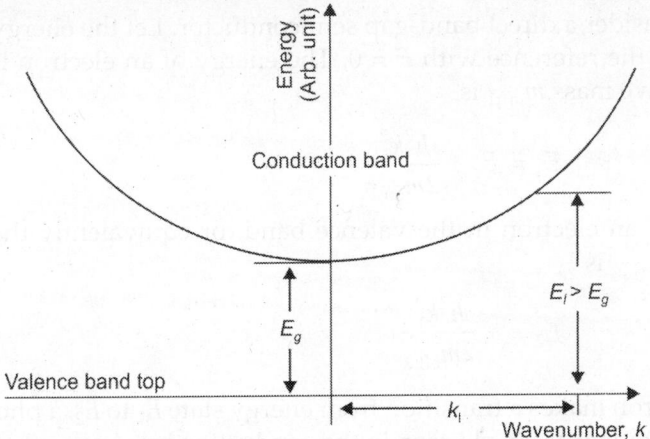

Fig. 7.18: E–k diagram assuming parabolic conduction band

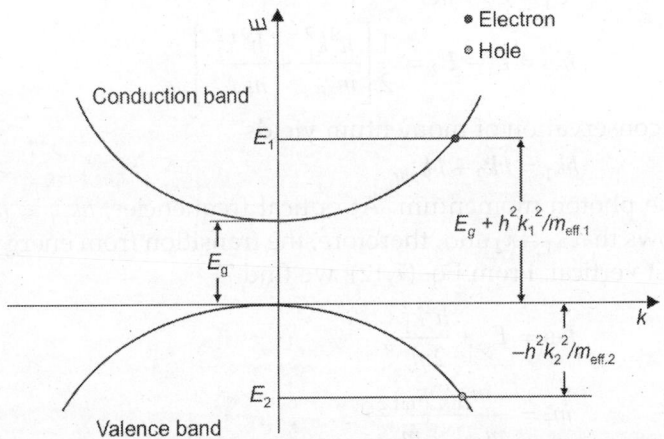

Fig. 7.19: Simplified E–k diagram for a direct band-gap material

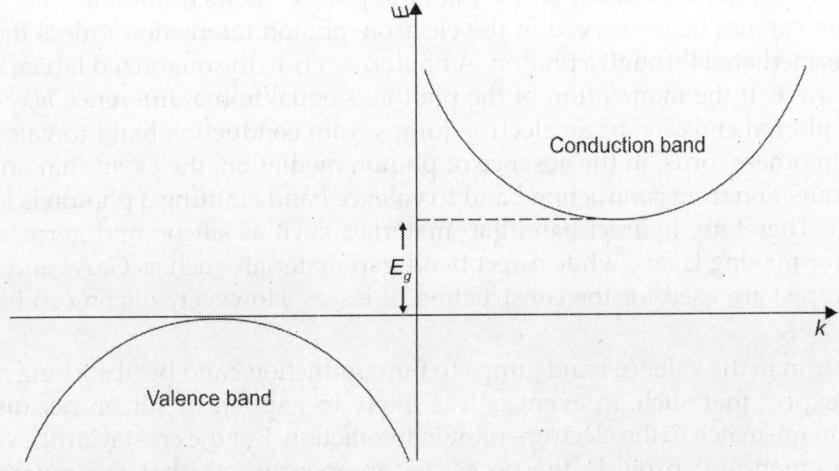

Fig. 7.20: Simplified E–k diagram for an indirect band-gap material

Let us first consider a direct band-gap semiconductor. Let the energy of the top of the valence band be the reference with $E = 0$. The energy of an electron in the conduction band with effective mass $m_{eff,1}$ is

$$E_1 = E_g + \frac{h^2 k_1^2}{2m_{eff,1}} \tag{7.10}$$

The energy of an electron in the valence band, or equivalently that of a hole with effective mass $m_{eff,2}$, is

$$E_2 = -\frac{h^2 k_1^2}{2m_{eff,2}} \tag{7.11}$$

When an electron makes a transition from energy state E_1 to E_2, a photon of energy $\hbar\omega$ is emitted. In other words, an electron in the conduction band recombines with a hole in the valence band, releasing the energy difference as a photon. The conservation of energy yields.

$$E_1 = E_2 + \hbar\omega$$

$$\hbar\omega = E_1 - E_2 = \frac{1}{2}\left[\frac{h^2 k_1^2}{m_{eff,1}} + \frac{h^2 k_2^2}{m_{eff,2}}\right] \tag{7.12}$$

Similarly, the conservation of momentum yields

$$\hbar k_1 = \hbar k_2 + \hbar k_{ph}, \tag{7.13}$$

where $\hbar k_{ph}$, is the photon momentum. At optical frequencies, $\hbar k_{ph} \ll \hbar k_j$, $j = 1.2$. From Eq. (7.13), it follows that $k_1 \cong k_2$ and, therefore, the transition from energy state E_1 to E_2 in Fig. 7.19 is almost vertical. From Eq. (7.12), we find

$$\hbar\omega = E_g + \frac{h^2 k_1^2}{2m_r}, \tag{7.14}$$

$$m_r = \frac{m_{eff,1} m_{eff,2}}{m_{eff,1} + m_{eff,2}} \tag{7.15}$$

is the *reduced effective electron mass*. For indirect band-gap materials, the momenta of electrons in the conduction band and in the valence band are different. Typically, the difference in momenta is much larger than the photon momentum and, therefore, the momentum can not be conserved in the electron–photon interaction unless the photon emission is mediated through a photon. A photon refers to the quantized lattice vibration or sound wave. If the momentum of the photon is equal to the difference $h(k_1 - k_2)$, the chance of photon emission as an electron jumps from conduction band to valence band increase. In other words, in the absence of photon mediation, the event that an electron makes a transition from conduction band to valence band emitting a photon is less likely to happen. Therefore, indirect band-gap materials such as silicon and germanium are not used for making lasers, while direct band-gap materials such as GaAs and InP (and their mixtures) are used for the construction of lasers. However, silicon can be used in *photo-detectors*.

An electron in the valence band jumps to the conduction band by absorbing a photon. We may expect that such an event is less likely to happen in silicon because of the momentum mismatch in the electron–photon interaction. But the crystal lattice vibrations (crystal momentum) provide the necessary momentum so that the momentum is conserved during the photon-absorption process. In contrast, during the photon-emission process, photon mediation is harder to come by since the free electrons in the conduction band are not bound to atoms, and, therefore, they do not vibrate within the crystal structure.

7.2.5 Compound Semiconductors

So far we have read that only direct band semiconductor materials can be used for making optical sources because electrons and holes recombine radiately and directly across the band gap without requiring the involvement of a third particle to conserve momentum. However, this radiative recombination is quite high to produce a significant level of optical emission. Further, none of the elemental semiconductors, e.g. Si or Ge are direct band gap material and therefore they cannot be used for making efficient optical source. However, there are a number of *compound semiconductors* and their alloys which are direct bandgap materials and can produce significant level of light output in the desired wavelength region for optical fiber communication. The compound semiconducting materials are also more flexible and offer several advantages over the elemental semiconductors which make them almost indispensible for making *optoelectronic devices*.

Compound semiconductors are produced by combining elements from different groups of periodic table and these materials include III-V, II-VI, IV-VI and IV, V compounds. We may note that among these materials III-V compounds and their alloys are extensively used in making optoelectronic devices and also found quite suitable for optical fiber communication. A binary III-V semiconductor compound is formed by the chemical combination of one element (say A) from Group-III with another element (say B) from Group-V of the periodic element to form the resultant compound $A_{III} B_V$. Interestingly III-V compound semiconductor has the same number of valence electrons (a total of 8 outer electrons) per atom as Si, GaAs, InP, GaP, AlAs, InSb are some examples of binary III-V compound semiconductors. We may note that Si crystallizes in the *diamond* structure forming pure covalent bands, whereas compound semiconductor such as GaAs crystallizes in the *Zinc-blends* structure by forming bonds which are predominantly covalent and partially ionic. The first synthesized III-V semiconductor binary compound is InSb, which can be synthesized easily and this has interesting electronic as well as optical properties. At 300K, the direct bandgap of InSb is 0.17 eV and it has an electron mobility of 0.8 $m^2V^{-1} m^{-1}$. This material has been extensively used for development of optoelectronic devices and far infrared (IR) applications. As stated earlier, the most important members of III-V compound semiconductor family are GaAs and InP. GaAs has a direct band gap energy of 1.42 eV at 300K and an electron mobility of 0.8 $m^2 V^{-1} m^{-1}$. These materials are extensively used for making semiconductor laser sources, Gunn diode and several other semi-conductor devices InP has a bandgap of 2.1 eV which corresponds to the wavelength in the visible region of the spectrum and has found appli-cation in visible-LEDs. We may note that GaP is an indirect bandgap material but can be doped suitably to improve its radiative transition effi-ciency. Table 7.1 summarizes some

Table 7.1: Physical parameters of some selected binary III-V semiconductor compounds

Material	Band gap energy (eV) at 300 K	Lattice constant (Å) at 298 K
GaAs	1.42	5.6532
InP	1.35	5.8697
AlAs	2.16	5.6611
GaP	2.26	5.4495
InAs	0.36	6.0584
InSb	0.17	6.479
GaSb	0.72	6.095
AlSb	1.58	5.136

important physical parameters of a few selected binary III-V semiconductor compounds.

Figure 7.21 shows the lattice constant values (in Å) of some important semiconductor compound materials plotted against their bandgap values (in eV). We can see that there exists a large number of binary III-V semiconductor compounds which fall in the category of direct bandgap and can therefore, be used for efficient emission of light at different wavelengths.

In a direct band gap material, the most probable recombination occurs across the energy band gap (in eV), the peak wavelength of emission (in micrometers) can be obtained from

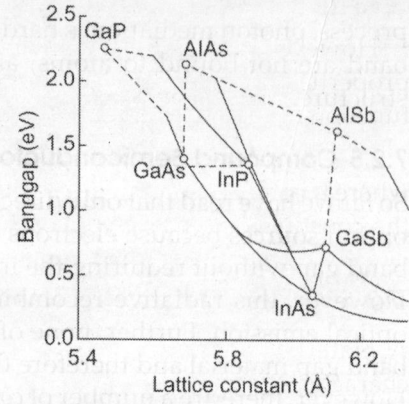

Fig. 7.21: Band gap vs lattice constant diagram for some binary III-V semiconductors

$$\lambda = \frac{hc}{Eg} = \frac{1.24}{E_g(\text{eV})} (\mu\text{m}) \tag{7.16}$$

Further, the binary compound semiconductors can easily form ternary and quaternary alloys. Basically, these alloys are solid solutions of corresponding compound semiconductors, e.g. a ternary III-V alloy can be formed by mixing GaAs and AlAs represented as $Al_x Ga_{1-x} As$; x being the mole fraction. Similarly, GaAs may form solid solution with Ga P to form $Ga_x As_{1-x} P$ in which the Group-V sublattice sites are shared by x atoms of Ga and $(1-x)$ atoms of As where as all Group-III lattice are filled with Ga atoms. The value of x in this alloy can vary from 0 to 1. $Al_x Ga_{1-x} As$ has found to be a potential material for application in a number of novel semiconductor devices while $Ga_x As_{1-x} P$ has been extensively used for developing visible LED. LEDs operating in the near-infrared region around 1.55 μm in the 3G optical fiber communication are based on $In_x Ga_{1-x} As$. In addition to these binary compound semiconductors and their ternary alloys there exist quaternary alloys containing a total of four elements from Group-III and Group V, e.g. $Ga_x In_{1-x} P_y$. This quaternary alloy contains two elements from Group III (e.g. In and Ga) and two elements from Group V (e.g., As and P). This quaternary can be obtained by dissolving P in the ternary alloy $In_x Ga_{1-x} As$ or making a solid solutions of corresponding binary crystals. We may note that there is a distinct advantage of alloying binary III-V compounds, i.e., it is possible to vary the bandgap of the resultant alloy continuously or monotonically by changing the composition. Further, one can also tailor the band structure and other optical and electronic properties by varying the mole fraction x in case of ternary and x and y in case of quaternary alloys. This particular feature of these materials (III-V Group) provides enormous flexibility in the design of optoelectronic devices (see Chapter 8) including optical sources and photodetectors (see Chapter 8) operating in the different wavelength regions.

There are many physical parameters of ternary alloys semiconductors, which can be derived from the parameters of the corresponding binaries by considering linear dependence, e.g., the lattice constant, a of a ternary alloy $A_x B_{1-x} C$ in terms of the lattice constants of the constituent binaries (AC and BC) can be expressed following Vegard's law as

$$a (A_x B_{1-x} C) = x \cdot a (AC) + (1-x) \cdot a(BC) \tag{7.17}$$

However, it is reported that the linear relationship does not hold strictly for all properties of mixed crystal alloys, e.g. the bandgap of a ternary alloy is a non-linear function of mole-fraction and one can express it as

$$E_g(A_x B_{1-x} C) = x \cdot E_g(AC) + (1-x) \cdot E_g(BC) - b \cdot x \cdot (1-x) \tag{7.18}$$

where b is called the bowing parameter which depends on the combination $(AC - BC)$ of the constitutent binary semiconductors.

7.3 SPONTANEOUS AND STIMULATED EMISSION

A material medium is composed of identical atoms or molecules, each of which is characterized by a set of discrete allowed energy states. An atom can move from one energy state to another when it receives or releases an amount of energy equal to the difference of energy between these two states. This is called *quantum transition*.

Let there are two states E_1 and E_2 of an atom. E_1 is lower energy state and E_2 is the excited state. As the constituent atoms of the medium are identical, the energy states E_1 and E_2 will be common for all atoms in the medium.

Let a monochromatic radiation of frequency (ν) be incident on the medium. In accordance with Planck's quantum theory of radiations, the radiation may be viewed as a stream of photons, each photon carrying an energy $h\nu$.

Now, if $E_2 - E_1 = h\nu$, the interaction of radiation with atom leads to the following three distinct processes in the medium: (i) *Stimulated absorption*, (ii) *Spontaneous emission* and (iii) *Stimulated emission*.

If the energy of incident photon is not equal to the energy difference between two permitted atomic levels, it passes without interacting with atoms. If it is equal to the energy difference, it is either absorbed or emitted. When more atoms are in lower energy level, it is absorbed and when there exists population inversion it is emitted with additional radiation. When atom absorbs energy, it goes in the excited state. It is called *stimulated absorption*. The excited state being unstable, atom immediately returns to lower state by radiating the energy difference. The frequency of radiation is $\nu = (E_2 - E_1)/h$, where $(E_2 - E_1)$ is the energy difference between the levels and h is Planck's constant. This process is called *spontaneous emission*. The radiation is random and incoherent. But, if there exists population inversion and a photon of correct energy is incident on excited atoms, all atoms return to lower energy level by emitting photons which are in phase with triggering photon. This process is called *stimulated emission*. Absorption, spontaneous processes and stimulated emission processes are illustrated in Fig. 7.22. The radiated (photon or) wave by this process is coherent with (triggering or) stimulating (photon or) wave. It has same frequency, direction of propagation, polarization etc. to that of triggering wave. Thus output is the amplification of input (triggering) wave. The wave needed for amplification is supplied by pumping process.

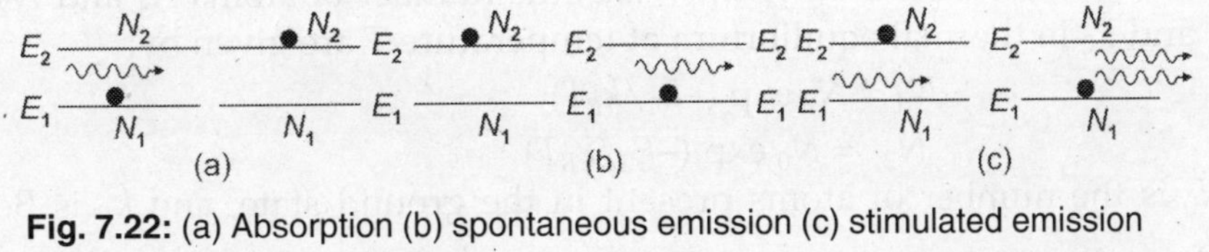

Fig. 7.22: (a) Absorption (b) spontaneous emission (c) stimulated emission

As shown in Fig. 7.22(c) that one original photon of energy $h\nu$ and other emitted photon on application of external electromagnetic radiation energy move together. The direction of propagation, phase energy and state of polarization of emitted photon is quite same as that of stimulating photon. This results in an enhancement of *coherent light*.

The probable rate of stimulated transition from excited state to lower energy state is proportional to the energy density $u(v)$ of the stimulating photon and is expressed as:

$$(P_{21})_{stimul.} = B_{21} \, u(v) \tag{7.19}$$

where B_{21} is the Einstein's constant of stimulated emission of radiation.

Now, the total probability (probable rate) of emission transition from excited state to lower energy state is summation of probable rates of spontaneous and stimulated emission:

$$P_{21} = A_{21} + B_{21} \, u(v) \tag{7.20}$$

where A_{21} is the Einstein's constant of spontaneous emission of radiation $(P_{21})_{spont.} = A_{21}$.

7.4 RELATION BETWEEN EINSTEIN'S COEFFICIENTS

Let us consider an assembly of atoms in thermal equilibrium at a particular temperature T with radiation of frequency v and energy density $u(v)$ in a two level system (TLS). Let at any instant N_1 and N_2 are the number of atoms in lower energy state E_1 and excited energy state E_2 respectively.

In state E_1, the number of atoms that absorb a quantum (photon) and rise to excited state E_2 per unit time is:

$$N_1 P_{12} = N_1 B_{12} \, u(v) \tag{7.21}$$

The number of atoms in excited state E_2 that jump to lower energy state E_1 either spontaneously or under stimulating emitting a photon per unit time is:

$$N_2 P_{21} = N_2 \, [A_{21} + B_{21} \, u(v)] \tag{7.22}$$

At thermal equilibrium between atomic system and the radiation field, the number of upward transitions should be equal to the number of downward transitions. Thus, at thermal equilibrium:

$$N_1 P_{12} = N_2 P_{21}$$

or
$$N_1 B_{12} \, u(v) = N_2 \, [A_{21} + B_{21} \, u(v)]$$
$$= N_2 A_{21} + N_2 B_{21} \, u \, (v) B_{21} \, u(v) \tag{7.23}$$

or
$$u(v) \, N_1 B_{21} - N_2 B_{21} \, u \, (v) = N_2 A_{21}$$

or
$$u(v) = \frac{N_2 A_{21}}{N_1 B_{12} - N_2 B_{21}}$$

or
$$u(v) = \frac{A_{21}}{B_{21}} \frac{1}{\left[\dfrac{N_1}{N_2} \left(\dfrac{B_{12}}{B_{21}} \right) - 1 \right]} \tag{7.24}$$

However, from *Maxwell's distribution law*, the number of atoms N_1 and N_2 in energy states E_1 and E_2 in thermal equilibrium at temperature T are given by:

$$N_1 = N_0 \exp \, (-E_1/k_B T)$$

and
$$N_2 = N_0 \exp \, (-E_2/k_B T)$$

where N_0 is the number of atoms present in the ground state, and k_B is Boltzmann's constant.

Thus, we have:
$$\frac{N_2}{N_1} = \frac{e^{-E_2/k_B T}}{e^{-E_1/k_B T}} = e^{-(E_2/E_1)/k_B T} \tag{7.24a}$$

But, $E_2 - E_1 = h\nu$, i.e. energy of emitted or absorbed photon. Then, we have:

$$\frac{N_2}{N_1} = e^{-h\nu/k_BT}$$

or
$$\frac{N_1}{N_2} = e^{-h\nu/k_BT} \qquad (7.25)$$

Using Eq. (7.25), Eq. (7.24) takes the form:

$$u(\nu) = \frac{A_{21}}{B_{21}} \frac{1}{\left[e^{h\nu/k_BT} \left(\frac{B_{12}}{B_{21}} \right) - 1 \right]} \qquad (7.26)$$

The energy density $u(\nu)$ at a particular frequency ν is given by Planck's radiation formula is:

$$u(\nu) = \frac{8\pi h\nu^3}{c^3} \frac{1}{\left[e^{h\nu/k_BT} - 1 \right]} \qquad (7.27)$$

Assuming $B_{12} = B_{21} = B$ (as per assumption of Einstein) and comparing Eq. 6.9(a) and (7.9), one obtains:

$$\frac{A_{21}}{B_{21}} = \frac{8\pi h\nu^3}{c^3} \qquad (7.28)$$

Equation (7.28) is known as *Einstein's relation* for his coefficients A and B.

We may note that the ratio of spontaneous emission and stimulated emission is proportional to ν^3. This means that the probable rate of spontaneous emission primes over stimulated emission more and more as the energy difference between the two states increases.

7.5 LASER COMPONENTS

A laser generally consists of three components: an *active medium* with energy levels that can be selectively populated, a *pump* to produce *population inversion* between some of these levels, and a *resonant electromagnetic cavity* that contains the active medium and provides feedback to maintain the coherence of electromagnetic field. In a continuously operating laser, coherent radiation will built up in the cavity to the level required to balance stimulated emission and cavity losses. The system is then said to be *lasing*, and the radiation is emitted in a direction defined by the cavity. Figure 7.23(a) shows a schematic block diagram of laser.

To achieve the population inversion a right group of atoms or molecules, which is called *active medium*, is needed. This active medium is gas or mixture of gas or crystal or semiconductor, etc. The population inversion is created by pumping process. Various techniques are used for pumping, for example, optical, pressure-temperature cycle, physical separation etc. The optical cavity is used to generate feedback. It is formed by dielectric mirrors or polished ends of crystal rod which act as reflectors. The pumping process creates population inversion. If that particular energy

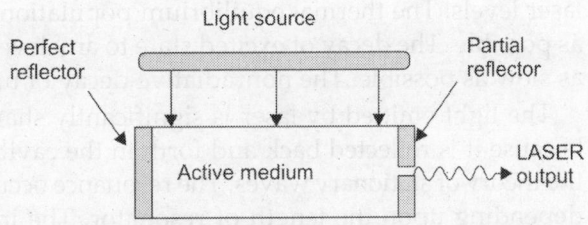

Fig. 7.23(a): Schematic block diagram of laser

state is short lived or unstable, atoms go to another lower state by way of fast decay. Generally, this state (or level) is metastable. The *metastable state* means long life state compared to other states. In general, life time of an energy state is 10^{-8} s, but for metastable (temporarily stable) state, it is 10^{-3} s or more. This is the key to the laser. In many atoms, one or more metastable states are available.

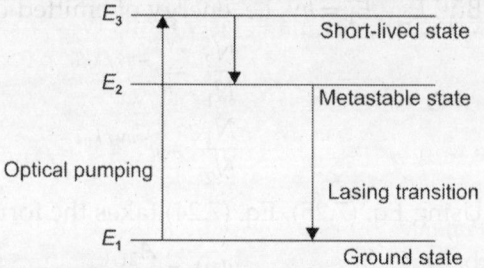

Fig. 7.23(b): Transition in a three level laser. The lasing transition takes the system from the metastable state to the ground state

After the population inversion, stimulated emission is triggered by a photon of appropriate frequency. In some cases, the first atom, making the transition from metastable state to lower state generates triggering photon. Thus, the stimulated emission produces more photons than the photons entering the system.

A material system is excited and displaced from normal thermal equilibrium by external processes such as chemical reaction, electron beam, optical field, etc. It selectively excites energy level of material, resulting in population inversion and finally in laser operation. The population inversion and its duration depends upon the relaxation rates of different

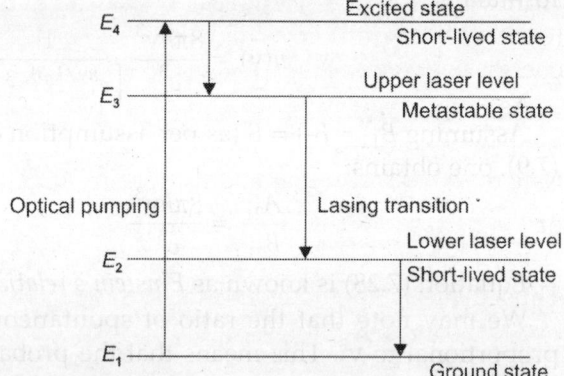

Fig. 7.23(c): Four level system. The lasing transition takes the system from the metastable state (E_3) to another short-lived (lower laser level) state (E_2). The system then returns quickly to the ground state (E_1), so the photons cannot be reabsorbed in returning the system from E_2 to E_3

energy levels, the degrees of freedom of the system and rate of stimulated emission. Consider a three-level and four-level laser system [see Figs 7.23(b) and (c)].

The pumping process excites the system from ground state to excited state. The excited state relaxes to the upper laser level. The stimulated emission (lasing action) occurs between upper and lower laser level. Finally lower laser level can either relax to the ground state or absorb the laser radiation and repopulate the upper laser level.

For ideal operation of laser, some conditions should be satisfied by the system. The relaxation rates from excited state to upper laser level and from lower laser level to ground state should be high to maintain maximum population inversion between upper to lower laser levels. The thermal equilibrium population of lower laser level should be as small as possible. The decay of excited state to any level other than upper laser level should be as slow as possible. The nonradiative decay of upper laser level should be slow.

The light emitted by laser is significantly sharper in wavelength than ordinary light because it is reflected back and forth in the cavity to form an intense pattern. We know the theory of stationary waves. The resonance occurs only for certain definite wavelengths, depending upon the length of resonator. The intense pattern is built up between two mirrors only if an exact number of waves fit between the mirrors. If there is only one wavelength that resonates, the laser gives out a single sharp line; if two or three wavelengths resonate, laser emits two or three lines.

7.6 POPULATION INVERSION

The number of active atoms occupying an energy state is called *population* of that state. Hence, N_1 and N_2 are population of E_1 (lower) and E_2 (excited) levels or states respectively.

Population inversion is the state of a system at which the population of a particular higher energy state is more than that of a specified lower energy state.

Let us consider a two level system consisting of lower energy level E_1 and higher (excited) energy level E_2. At normal condition, the number of atoms in lower level, i.e. N_1 is more (greater) than that of the atoms in excited states, i.e. N_2.

In order to produce emission from higher energy level, the population of higher (excited) level must be as high as possible. If the number of atoms (population) of higher energy level is more than that of the low energy level, then we say, it is *population inversion*.

As stated earlier, the laser beam emission takes place only when the rate of emission is greater than the rate of absorption, i.e.

Rate of (stimulated + spontaneous) emission > rate of absorption

or $A_{21}N_2 + B_{21}\, u(\nu)\, N_2 > B_{12}\, u(\nu)\, N_1$

For lasing action to be dominant, only stimulated emission is to be considered here. Thus, deleting spontaneous emission, one obtains:

$$B_{21}\, u(\nu)\, N_2 > B_{12}\, u(\nu)\, N_1$$

Taking $B_{12} = B_{21} = B$ (say), one obtains:

$$N_2 > N_1$$

Gain: The probability that a randomly chosen photon in an optical field of cross-section A will stimulate a given inverted site with a radiative cross-section σ_r as it passes through a material is σ_r/A. The radiative cross-section of the transition is proportional to the *dipole strength* of the transition and is the same for absorption and emission. If the low-energy state is degenerated, with a degeneracy of g_1, the probability of stimulated emission becomes $g_1\sigma_r/A$. The product g_1, σ_r is known as the *emission or gain cross-section* σ_g. When all of the photons in the optical field are accounted for an absorption and stimulated emission are included, then we obtain:

$$I(l) = I(o) \exp\left[(\sigma_g\rho_u - \sigma_a\rho_l)\, l\right] \tag{7.29}$$

When all the photons in an optical field of intensity I and all of the absorption sites in a material of length dl are accounted for, the intensity of an optical field passing through the material changes by:

$$dI = -I\rho_l\sigma_a\, dl$$

where $\sigma_a = g_u\sigma_r$ is known as *absorption coefficient* and g_u are identical (degenerate) high energy states. P_1 is the density of absorption sites in the material. The above equation has the solution:

$$I(l) = I(o) \exp(-\alpha l) \tag{7.29a}$$

where $I(o)$ is the intensity of the optical field as it enters the material at position $Z = o$ and $\alpha = \rho_1\sigma_a$ is the absorption coeffient of the material. When all the photons in the optical field are accounted for and absorption and stimulated emission are included, the above equation becomes Eq. (7.28).

where ρ_u is the density of inverted sites. If the material is forced out of thermal equilibrium (pumped) to a sufficient degree, so that $\sigma_g \rho_u > \sigma_a \rho_l$, stimulated emission occurs at a higher rate than absorption. The material is now said to have *gain*, with a gain coefficient:

$$g = \left[\rho_u - \left(\frac{g_u}{g_1} \right) \rho_1 \right] \sigma_g \tag{7.30}$$

The term $\rho_{\text{eff}} = \left[\rho_u - \left(\frac{g_u}{g_1} \right) \rho_1 \right]$ is referred to as the effective inversion density, and $g = \rho_{\text{eff}} \sigma_g$. When $\rho_g \rho_u = \sigma_a \rho_1$, there is no change in the intensity of an optical field passing through the material and the material is said to be in a state of *transparency*.

7.7 OPTICAL FEEDBACK

A part from population inversion, laser operation also require optical feedback. Light amplification in laser takes place when a photon interacts with an excited atom in such a way as to cause stimulated emission. The photon generated in the process joins the primary photon to cause further stimulated emission by repeated interaction with excited atoms present in the lasing medium. The photons emitted in the said process of stimulated emission are in the same phase and as a result, a kind of avalance multiplication of photons with same phase takes place. This process leads to an intense coherent beam of light. We may note that the repeated interaction of photons with the excited atom in the lasing medium is facilitated by using an optical cavity or an optical resonator. An optical resonator, in the simplest form is a pair of parallel mirrors (plane or curved) placed at the two ends, i.e., front end and rear end of the lasing medium, also called as *gain medium*. The mirrors are usually layered with optical coatings to adjust the reflectivity so as to provide optical feedback through multiple reflections at the end mirror. Thus, in general, the rear mirror is designed in a way to have high reflectivity while the front mirror is made *partially transmitting* so that laser beam output can be obtained from the front end.

In an actual system, the initial photons that trigger stimulated emission in the lasing medium are produced by stimulated emission. The photons emitted in the process are reflected back and forth by the end mirrors to interact with the excited atoms in the lasing medium* and cause more and more stimulated emissions of photons having same phase. This means the medium provides gain and optical cavity provides a kind of positive feedback that makes the laser source an oscillator rather than an amplifier. However, the gain produced by the medium due to a single pass of photons through the cavity is very small. The gain can be significantly high if the photons are allowed the have multiple passes through the medium following reflections from the end mirrors. Clearly, on an average, each photon passes through the gain medium several hundred times prior it emerges through the front mirror as one of the constituent photons in the laser beam output. We may note that the optical cavity acts like a *Fabry-Perot resonator*. Finally, a stable output from the laser medium is obtained in the form of intense monochromatic and coherent light beam when the gain of the medium exceeds the total loss in the medium arising from absorption, scattering and undesirable exist of photons through any one of the mirrors.

---

* The medium is already in a nonequilibrium condition by creating population inversion so that the stimulated emission is dominant over absorption during multiple transit of photons in the lasing medium.

We may note that the gain of the lasing medium is a function of wavelength of the light produced by stimulated emission. Oscillation in the cavity takes place in a small range of frequency where the gain exceeds the total loss in the cavity. This is the reason, why a laser source is not perfectly a monochromatic source. Nevertheless, laser can emit light in a very narrow spectral band (unlike an LED which emits light over a relatively broad spectral band) about a central wavelength determined by the mean energy level difference of the stimulated emission transitions. There are some lasers which do not make use of an optical cavity. These structures are designed so that we may produce very high gain through single pass of photons in the medium so as to produce significant *Amplified Spontaneous Emission* (ASE) without the need of feed back. Such a structure is viewed as a superluminescent light emitting diode (SLD). This does not involve optical feedback to cause oscillation and the emitted light has a low coherence and also relatively large spectral width.

7.8 CONDITIONS FOR LASER OSCILLATIONS

Consider a lossless gain medium as shown in Fig. 7.24 in which the incident light wave is amplified by stimulated emission. The optical intensity at z can be pheno-menologically described as

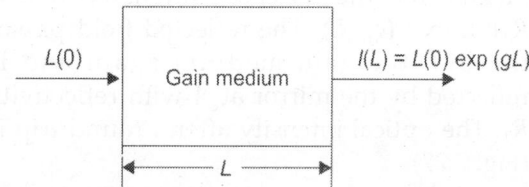

$$I(z) = I(0) \exp(gz) \qquad (7.31)$$

where g is the gain coefficient associated with stimulated emission. For the atomic

Fig. 7.24: Light amplification in a gain medium

system with two levels, an expression for g can be obtained in terms of the population densities N_1, N_2 and the Einstein coefficient B. By differentiating $I(z)$ with respect to z, Eq. (7.31) can be rewritten in differential form as

$$\frac{dI}{dz} = gI(0) \exp(gz) \qquad (7.32)$$

$$= gI \qquad (7.32a)$$

The optical field is attenuated in the gain medium due to scattering and other possible loss mechanisms similar to attenuation in optical fibers. The effect of loss is modeled as

$$I(z) = I(0) \exp(-\alpha_{int} z), \qquad (7.33)$$

where α_{int} is the coefficient of internal loss due to scattering and other loss mechanisms in the gain medium. The gain and attenuation occur simultaneously in the gain medium. So, we have

$$I(z) = I(0) \exp(g_{net} z), \qquad (7.34)$$

where $g_{net} = g - \alpha_{int}$ is the coefficient of the net gain.

A laser is an *oscillator* operating at optical frequencies. Just like an electronic oscillator, the optical oscillator (laser) has three main components: (i) amplifier, (ii) feedback, and (iii) power supply, as shown in Fig. 7.25. The atomic system we have discussed before can act as a gain medium and the light is amplified by stimulated emission. The feedback is provided by placing the gain medium between two mirrors, as shown in Fig. 7.26. The optical or electrical pumps required to achieve population inversion are the power supply.

Consider the optical wave propagating in the *Fabry–Perot* (FP) *cavity* shown in Fig. 7.26. Let $I(0)$ be the optical intensity at A. After passing through the gain medium,

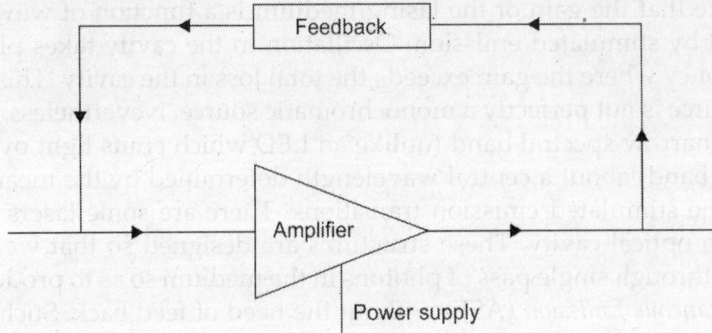

Fig. 7.25: The structure of an optical oscillator (laser) or electronic oscillator

the intensity is $I(0) \exp (g_{net} L)$, where L is the length of the cavity. The light wave is reflected by the mirror at B, whose reflectivity is R_2. This means that the reflected intensity at B is $R_2 I(0) \exp (g_{net}L)$. The reflected field passes through the gain medium again and is reflected by the mirror at A with reflectivity R_1. The optical intensity after a round trip is (Fig. 7.27).

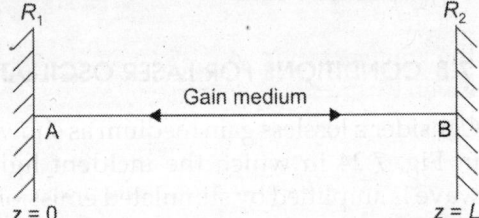

Fig. 7.26: The Fabry–Perot cavity formed by mirrors

$$I(0) \, R_1 R_2 \exp [2(g - \alpha_{int}) \, L] \tag{7.35}$$

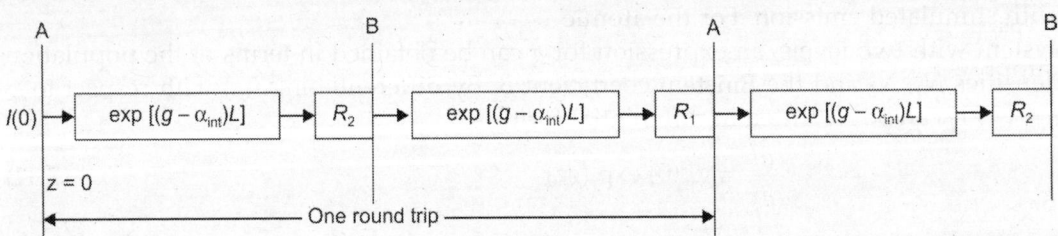

Fig. 7.27: Illustration of multiple reflections in a FP cavity

The condition for laser oscillation is that the optical intensity after one round trip should be the same as the incident intensity $I(0)$. Otherwise, after several round trips, the optical intensity in the cavity would be too low or too high. For a stable laser operation, we need

$$I(0) \, R_1 R_2 \exp [2(g - \alpha_{int}) \, L] = I(0) \tag{7.36}$$

Simplifying Eq. (7.36), we obtain

$$g = \alpha_{int} + \frac{1}{2L} \ln \left(\frac{1}{R_1 R_2} \right) \tag{7.37}$$

In Eq. (7.37), the second term represents the loss due to mirrors,

$$\alpha_{mir} = \frac{1}{2L} \ln \left(\frac{1}{R_1 R_2} \right) \tag{7.38}$$

Using Eq. (7.38) in Eq. (7.37), we find

$$g = \alpha_{int} + \alpha_{mir} = \alpha_{cav,} \tag{7.39}$$

where α_{cav} is the total cavity loss coefficient. Therefore, to have a stable laser operation, one of the essential conditions is that the total cavity loss should be equal to the gain. Suppose you are one a swing. Because of the frictional loss, the oscillations will be dampened and it will stop swinging unless you pump yourself or someone pushes you. To have sustained oscillations, the frictional loss should be balanced by the gain due to "pumping". In the case of a laser, the gain is provided by optical/electrical pumps. A monochromic wave propagating in the cavity is described by a plane wave,

$$\psi = \psi_0 \exp\left[-i(\omega t - kz)\right]. \tag{7.40}$$

The phase change due to propagation from A to B is kL. And the phase change due to a round trip is $2kL$. The second condition for laser oscillation is that the phase change due to a round trip should be an integral multiple of 2π,

$$2kL = \frac{4\pi n}{\lambda_0} L = 2m\pi, \quad m = 0, \pm 1, \pm 2, \dots \tag{7.41}$$

Otherwise, the optical field ψ at A would be different after each round trip. Here, λ_0 is the wavelength in free space and n is the refractive index of the medium. If the condition given by Eq. (7.41) is not satisfied the superposition of the field component after N round trip,

$$\psi_N = \psi_0 \exp\left(-i\omega t\right) \sum_{n=0}^{N} \exp\left(i_2 k n L\right) \tag{7.42}$$

approaches zero as $N \rightarrow \infty$. This is because sometimes the field component after a round trip may be positive and sometimes it may be negative, and the net sum goes to zero if m is not an integer. When m is an integer, the optical fields after each round trip add up coherently.

From Eq. (7.41), we see that only a discrete set of frequencies or wavelengths are supported by the cavity. They are given by

$$\lambda_m = \frac{2nL}{m}, \quad m = 1, 2, \dots, \tag{7.43}$$

or

$$f_m = \frac{mc}{2nL} \tag{7.44}$$

These frequencies correspond to the *longitudinal modes* of the cavity, and can be changed by varying the cavity length L. The laser frequency f must match one of the frequencies of the set f_m, $m = 1, 2, \dots$ The spacing Δf between longitudinal modes is constant,

$$\Delta f = fm - f_{m-1} = \frac{c}{2nL} \tag{7.45}$$

The longitudinal spacing Δf is known as the *free spectral range* (FSR). In a two-level atomic system, the gain would occur for the frequency $\omega = (E_2 - E_1)/h$. However, in practical system, these levels are not sharp; each level is a broad collection of sublevels and, therefore, the gain would occur over a range of frequencies. Figure 7.28 shows the loss and gain profiles of a FP laser. Many longitudinal modes of the FP cavity experience gain simultaneously. The mode for which the gain is equal to the loss (shown as the lasing mode) becomes the dominant mode. In theory, other modes should not reach the threshold since their gain is less than the loss of the cavity. In practice, the difference in gain between many modes of the cavity is extremely small, and one or two neighboring modes on each side of the main mode (lasing mode) carry a significant fraction of power. Such a laser is called a *multi-longitudinal-mode laser*. Figure 7.29 shows the output of a

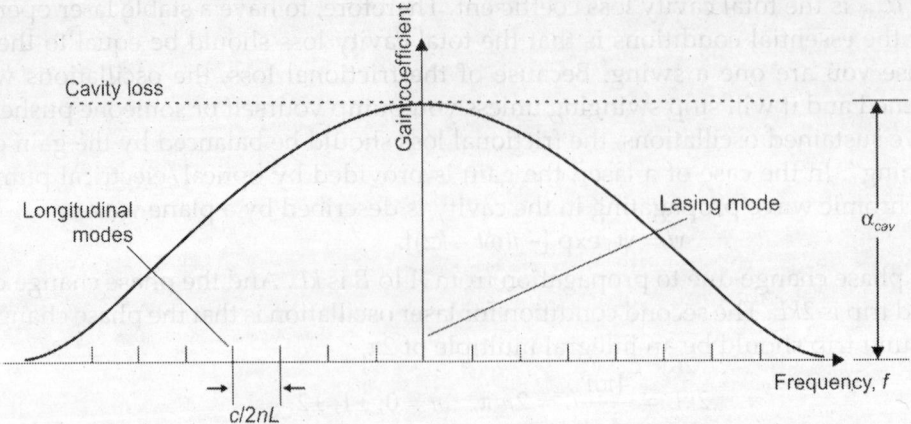

Fig. 7.28: Loss and gain profiles of a Fabry–Perot (FP) laser

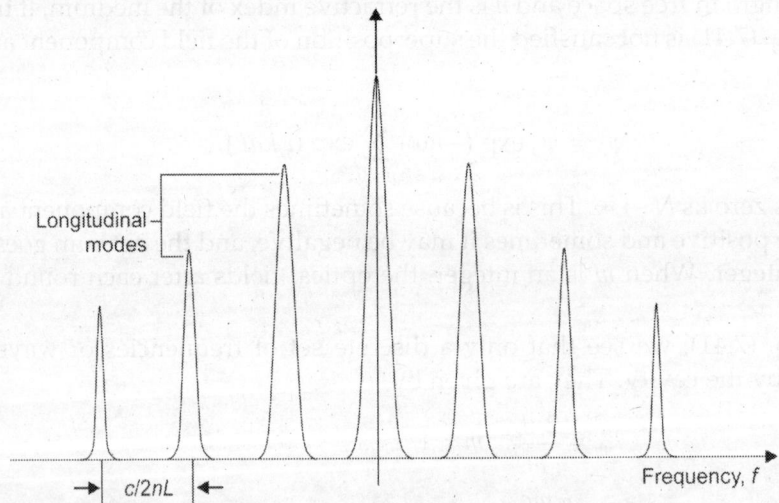

Fig. 7.29: The output spectrum of a Fabry–Perot laser

multi-longitudinal-mode laser. If a multi-longitudinal laser is used in fiber-optic communication system, each mode of the laser propagates at a slightly different group velocity in the fiber because of dispersion, which leads to intersymbol interference at the receiver. Therefore, for high-bit-rate applications, it is desirable to have a single-longitudinal-mode (SLM) laser. A distributed *Bragg grating* is used to obtain a single longitudinal mode.

Equation (7.31) provides the evolution of the optical intensity as a function of the propagation distance. Sometimes, it is desirable to find the evolution of the optical intensity as a function of time. To obtain the time rate of change of the optical intensity, we first develop an expression relating optical intensity I and energy density u. The optical intensity is power P per area S, which is perpendicular to the direction of propagation,

$$I = \frac{P}{S} \tag{7.46}$$

The power is energy ΔE per unit time,

$$P = \frac{\Delta E}{\Delta t}, \tag{7.47}$$

where Δt is a suitably chosen time interval. Combining Eqs (7.46) and (7.47), we find

$$I = \frac{\Delta E}{S \Delta t} \qquad (7.48)$$

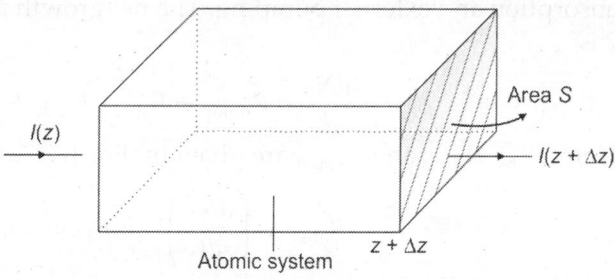

Figure 7.30 shows the optical intensity at z and $z + \Delta z$. The number of photons crossing the area S at $z + \Delta z$ over a time interval Δt is the same as the number of photons present in the volume $S \Delta z$ if

Fig. 7.30: Optical intensity incident on the atomic system of volume $S \Delta z$.

$$\Delta z = v \Delta t, \qquad (7.49)$$

where v is the speed of light in the medium. For example, if Δt is chosen as 1 ns, Δz is 0.2m assuming $v = 2 \times 10^8$ m/s. Using Eq. (7.49) in Eq. (7.47), Eq. (7.46) becomes

$$I = \frac{\Delta E v}{S \Delta z} = uv, \qquad (7.50)$$

where u is the energy density or energy per unit volume. Since $I \propto u$, Eq. (7.32) can be written as

$$\frac{du}{dz} = gu \qquad (7.51)$$

Equation (7.51) provides the rate of change of energy density as a function of the propagation distance in the gain medium. This can be converted to the time rate of change of energy density by using $dz = vdt$.

$$\frac{du}{vdt} = gu \qquad (7.52)$$

$$\frac{du}{dt} = Gu \qquad (7.53)$$

where

$$G = vg. \qquad (7.54)$$

If we include the cavity loss, Eq. (7.53) should be modified as

$$\frac{du}{dt} = (G - vz_{\text{cav}})u \qquad (7.55)$$

We may note that the cavity loss has a contribution from internal loss and mirror loss. The mirror loss is lumped, whereas the internal loss is distributed. Therefore, Eq. (7.55) becomes inaccurate for time intervals less than the transit time $2L/v$.

7.9 LASER RATE EQUATIONS

We now consider the gain rate and loss rate of photons and population densities in states 1 and 2 due to simulated emission, spontaneous emission, and various loss mechanisms. Suppose $N(t)$ is the population at t, the net rate of population growth may be modeled as

$$\frac{dN}{dt} = R_{\text{born}} + R_{\text{immigration}} + R_{\text{death}} + R_{\text{migration}} \qquad (7.56)$$

To model lasers, we follow a similar approach. Let us consider the atomic system with two levels. The population density of the excited state decreases due to stimulated emission, spontaneous emission, and nonradiative transition, while it increases due to absorption and external pumping. The net growth rate of the population density of state 2 is

$$\frac{dN_2}{dt} = R_{pump} + R_{abs} + R_{stim} + R_{spont} + R_{nr} \tag{7.57}$$

Here, R_{abs}, R_{stim}, and R_{spont} are given by Eqs (7.57a), (7.57b) and (7.57c), respectively.

$$R_{abs} = -\left(\frac{dN_1}{dt}\right)_{abs} = B_{12} \, u_s \, (\omega)/N_1 \tag{7.57a}$$

$$R_{stim} = -\left(\frac{dN_2}{dt}\right)_{stim} = B_{21} \, u_s \, (\omega)/N_2 \tag{7.57b}$$

$$R_{spont} = -\left(\frac{dN_2}{dt}\right)_{spont} = A_{21} \, N_2 \tag{7.57c}$$

R_{pump} refers to the pumping rate, which is the rate at which the population density of state 2 grows due to an external pump.

An atom in state 2 could drop down to state 1 by releasing the energy difference as translational, vibrational, or rotational energies of the atom or nearby atoms/molecules. This is known as *nonradiative transition*, since no photon is emitted as the atom makes transition from state 2 to state 1 and R_{nr} represents the rate of nonradiative transition from state 2 to state 1. It is given by

$$R_{nr} = CN_2, \tag{7.58}$$

where C is a constant similar to the Einstein coefficient A.

Using Eqs (7.57a), (7.57b), (7.57c) and (7.58d) in Eq. (7.57), we find

$$\frac{dN_2}{dt} = R_{pump} + BuN_1 - BuN_2 - (A+C)N_2 \tag{7.59}$$

The population density of the ground state increases due to simulated emission, spontaneous emission, and nonradiative transition, while it decreases due to absorption. The rate of change of the population density of the ground state is

$$\frac{dN_1}{dt} = R_{stim} + R_{spont} + R_{nr} + R_{abs}$$
$$= BuN_2 + (A+C)N_2 - BuN_1 \tag{7.60}$$

Next, let us consider the growth rate of photons. Let N_{ph} be the photon density. When an atom makes a transition from the excited state to the ground state due to stimulated emission, it emits *a* photon. If there are R_{stim} transitions per unit time per unit volume, the growth rate of photon density is also R_{stim}. The photon density in a laser cavity increases due to stimulated emission and spontaneous emission, while it decreases due to absorption and loss in the cavity. The growth rate of photon density is given by

$$\frac{dN_{ph}}{dt} = R_{stim} + R_{spont} + R_{abs} + R_{loss} \tag{7.61}$$

Here, R_{loss} refers to the loss rate of photons due to internal loss and mirror loss in the cavity. Since the energy of a photon is $\hbar\omega$, the mean number of photons present in the electromagnetic radiation of energy E is

$$n_{ph} = \frac{E}{\hbar\omega} \tag{7.62}$$

The photon density N_{ph} is the mean number of photons per unit volume and the energy density u is the mean number of photons per unit volume and the energy density u is the energy per unit volume. Therefore, they are related by

$$N_{ph} = \frac{n_{ph}}{V} = \frac{E}{\hbar \omega V} = \frac{u}{\hbar \omega} \tag{7.63}$$

The time rate of change of the energy density u in the presence of stimulated emission and loss can be obtained as

$$\frac{du}{dt} = (G - va_{cav})u \tag{7.64}$$

Since $u \propto N_{ph}$, the time rate of change of photon density is

$$\frac{dN_{ph}}{dt} = GN_{ph} - \frac{N_{ph}}{\tau_{ph}} \tag{7.65}$$

where

$$\tau_{ph} = \frac{1}{va_{cav}} \tag{7.66}$$

is the *photon lifetime*. In the absence of gain $(G = 0)$, Eq. (7.65) can be solved to yield

$$N_{ph}(t) = N_{ph}(0) \exp(-t/\tau_{ph}) \tag{7.67}$$

At $t = t_{ph}$, $N_{ph}(t) = N_{ph}(0)e^{-1}$. Thus, the photon density reduces by e over a time t_{ph}. In Eq. (7.65), G represents the net gain coefficient due to stimulated emission and absorption and, therefore, the first term on the right-hand side of Eq. (7.65) can be identified as

$$R_{stim} + R_{abs} = GN_{ph}, \tag{7.68}$$

or

$$BuN_2 - BuN_1 = GN_{ph} \tag{7.69}$$

Since $u = N_{ph}\hbar\omega$, from Eq. (7.69) we find

$$G = B(N_2 - N_1)\hbar\omega \tag{7.70}$$

In Eq. (7.65), the second term represents the loss, rate due to scattering, mirror loss, and other possible loss mechanisms,

$$R_{loss} = -\frac{N_{ph}}{\tau_{ph}} \tag{7.71}$$

Eq. (7.65) does not include the photon gain rate due to spontaneous emission. Using Eqs. (7.68), (7.71) and (7.57c) in Eq. (7.61), we obtain

$$\frac{dN_{ph}}{dt} = GN_{ph} + AN_2 - \frac{N_{ph}}{\tau_{ph}} \tag{7.72}$$

Note that when $N_2 > N_1$, population inversion is achieved, $G > 0$ [see Eq. (7.70)] and amplification of photons takes place. In other words, the energy of the atomic system is transferred to the electromagnetic wave. When $N_2 < N_1$, the electromagnetic wave is attenuated and the energy of the wave is transferred to the atomic system.

Using Eq. (7.69), Eqs (7.59) and (7.60) can be rewritten as

$$\frac{dN_2}{dt} = R_{pump} - GN_{ph} - \frac{N_2}{\tau_{21}} \tag{7.73}$$

$$\frac{dN_1}{dt} = GN_{ph} - \frac{N_2}{\tau_{21}} \tag{7.74}$$

where

$$\tau_{21} = \frac{1}{A + C} \tag{7.75}$$

is the lifetime associated with spontaneous emission and nonradiative decay from the excited state to the ground state, Eqs. (7.73) and (7.84) can be simplified further under the assumption that the population density of the ground state is negligibly small compared with the population density of the excited state. Assuming $N_1 \approx 0$, Eqs (7.73) and (7.72) become

$$\frac{dN_2}{dt} = R_{pump} - GN_{ph} - \frac{N_2}{\tau_{21}} \tag{7.76}$$

$$\frac{dN_{ph}}{dt} = R_{ph} + AN_2 - \frac{N_{ph}}{\tau_{ph}} \tag{7.77}$$

where $\qquad G = BN_2 h\omega.$ $\hfill (7.78)$

The equations describing the population densities of electrons and photons in a semiconductor laser are similar to Eqs. (7.76) and (7.77).

7.10 CHARACTERISTICS OF LASER RADIATION

Laser radiation is available both in *continuous wave mode* and in pulses. Like all other radiations, laser radiation is electromagnetic in nature. Important characteristics of laser radiations are as follows:

(i) *Coherence*: The laser radiation is highly coherent both *temporarily* and *spatially*. Coherence means that two or more waves in a radiation field bear the *same phase relationship* to each other at all times. Coherence is of two types: *spatial coherence* and *temporal coherence* or *longitudinal coherence* and *transverse coherence*.

Spatial coherence or transverse coherence means the phase relationship between waves travelling in a plane perpendicular to the direction of propagation, i.e. between waves travelling side by side. Spatial coherence requires that the waves not only are of same frequency, but they should be in phase in space. *Temporal* coherence or *longitudinal* spatial coherence applies to waves travelling the same path.

(ii) *Monochromaticity*: The laser light is nearly monochromatic. Truly speaking, no light is perfectly monochromatic, i.e. it is not characterized by spread in frequency Δv about the central frequency (or $\Delta\lambda$ in case of wavelength λ). One can define the monochromaticity of light by $\Delta v/v$. For perfect monochromaticity $\Delta v = 0$, which is not possible to attain in practice. However, the value of Δv is much smaller for laser light compared to ordinary light. For an ordinary light $\Delta v \approx 10^{10}$ Hz whereas for a laser $\Delta v \approx 500$ Hz. Thus, for ordinary light of wave length $\lambda = 6000$ Å (or frequency $v = 5 \times 10^{14}$ Hz) monochromaticity is:

$$\frac{\Delta v}{v} = \frac{10^{10} \text{ Hz}}{5 \times 10^{14} \text{ Hz}} = 2 \times 10^{-5}$$

Monochromaticity of laser light:

$$\frac{\Delta v}{v} = \frac{500 \text{Hz}}{5 \times 10^{14} \text{ Hz}} = 10^{-12}$$

Obviously, laser light is highly monochromatic compared to ordinary light.

(iii) *Directionality*: The output beam of a laser light has a well-defined wavefront and therefore, it is highly directional except for the divergence caused due to diffraction effects. The high directionality of laser light permit us to focus it into a point by passing the beam through a suitable convex lens. For example, if the focal length of the lens is

5×10^{-2} m, $\lambda = 6000$ Å, and the radius of the beam, $r = 2$ mm, then the area of the spot at the focal plane is:

$$\frac{\pi \lambda^2 f^2}{a^2} = \frac{\pi (6 \times 10^{-7} \text{ m})^2 \times (5 \times 10^{-2} \text{ m})^2}{(2 \times 10^{-3} \text{ m})^2}$$

$$= 7.1 \times 10^{-10} \text{ m}^2$$

Obviously, this is very small.

(iv) *Intensity*: The laser light beam is highly intense compared to ordinary light. Since the power of a laser is concentrated in a beam of very small diameter ($\approx$ few mm), even a small laser can deliver extremely high intensity at the focal plane of the lens. For example, if P (power) of a laser beam is 1 W, the intensity at the point is obtained as:

$$I = \frac{P}{A \text{ (area)}} = \frac{Pa^2}{\pi \lambda^2 f^2}$$

$$= \frac{1 \text{ W}}{7.0 \times 10^{-10} \text{ m}^2} = 1.4 \times 10^9 \text{ Wm}^{-2}$$

This means that even a small power of 1 W can give an intensity of 10^9 Wm^{-2}, which is quite large.

7.11 TYPES OF LASERS

Broadly, there are six different types of lasers: solid state laser, gas laser, dye laser, semiconductor laser, UV and X-ray laser and free-electron laser. In solid-state lasers, active medium is an insulating dielectric solid. These solids can be crystalline or amorphous. These lasers are used to generate a wide range of wavelength from the vaccuum ultraviolet to mid-infrared. They are capable of generating high peak powers ($\sim 10^{-14}$ W) because of long life metastable states which allow higher energy storage compared to other active media. The common examples of solid-state lasers are ruby, which is a chromium-doped Al_2O_3, titanium-doped Al_2O_3 ($Ti:Al_2O_3$), neodymium-doped yttrium aluminium garnet (Nd:YAG) and neodymium-doped glasses (Nd:glass).

In gas lasers, gas or gas mixture is capable of withstanding a large amount of power. The pointing stability and high optical quality beams are their greatest assets. Common examples are copper-vapour laser, helium-neon laser, helium-cadmium laser and carbon-dioxide laser.

The free electron lasers (FEL) are operated in far infrared and ultraviolet (below 100 nm) where atomic or molecular lasers are not readily available; and for large average power and high efficiency systems. The disadvantages of FEL are greater complexity and the cost of a particle accelerator.

The important characteristics of laser dye media are their broad wavelength tunability, wide spectral coverage and practical simplicity. Hundreds of dyes are reported to have lasing action. The examples of various dye classes are oligophenylenes, coumarins, xanthenes, merocyanines and cyanines with spectral emission from 300 nm to more than 1100 nm.

The semiconductor lasers have some special features such as compactness, high efficiency, capability for high-speed direct modulation, wide emission spectrum and high reliability. But disadvantage is that they are sensitive to temperature.

A significant percentage of today's lasers are fabricated using semi-conductor technology. Those devices are known as semiconductor lasers. In the present chapter we will restrict to the study of semiconductor lasers only.

7.12 LASER OSCILLATIONS AND RESONANT MODES

Light propagation with amplification is illustrated in Fig. 7.31. Mathematically, it is described by assuming that there is no phase change on reflection at either end (left and right). Left end is defined as $z = 0$) and right end as $z = L$. At the right facet, the forward optical wave has a fraction r_R reflected (amplitude reflection) and after reflection that fraction travels back (from right to left).

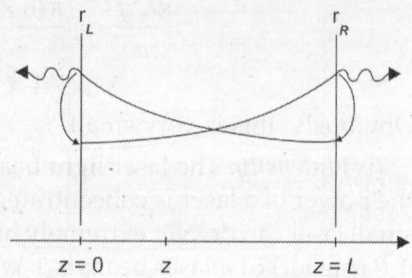

Fig. 7.31: Schematic illustration of the amplification in a Fabry–Perot (FP) semiconductor laser with homogeneously distributed gain

In order to form a stable resonance, the amplitude and phase of the wave after a single round trip must match the amplitude and phase of the starting wave. At arbitrary point z inside the cavity (Fig. 7.31), the forward wave is:

$$E_0 e^{gz} e^{-j\beta z} \tag{7.79}$$

where we have dropped $e^{i\omega t}$ term which is common and defined $g = g_m - \alpha_m$, where g_m describes gain (amplification) of the wave and α_m its losses. Also r_R and r_L are, respectively, right and left reflectivities, L length of the cavity and β propagation constant.

The wave travelling one full round will be:

$$\{E_0 e^{gz} e^{-j\beta z}\} \; \{e^{g(L-z)} e^{-j\beta(L-z)}\} \; \{r_R e^{gL} e^{-j\beta L}\} \; \{r_L e^{gz} e^{-j\beta z}\} \tag{7.80}$$

The above terms are interpreted as follows. In the first bracket, there is an original forward propagating wave which started at z, in the second bracket, there is a wave travelling from z to L, the third bracket describes a wave propagating from $z = L$ to $z = 0$, and the last one contains a wave travelling from $z = 0$ to the starting point z. At that point, the wave must match the original wave as given by Eq. (7.79). From the above, one obtains a condition for stable oscillations:

$$r_R r_L e^{2gL} e^{-2j\beta L} = 1 \tag{7.81}$$

This condition can be split into an amplitude condition:

$$r_R r_L e^{2(g_m - \alpha_m)L} = 1 \tag{7.82}$$

and phase condition:

$$e^{-2j\beta L} = 1 \tag{7.83}$$

From the amplitude condition one obtains:

$$g_m = \alpha_m + \frac{1}{2L} \ln \frac{1}{r_R r_L} \tag{7.84}$$

From the phase condition, it follows:

$$2\beta L = 2\pi n \tag{7.85}$$

where n is an integer. The last equation determines wavelengths of oscillations since:

$$\beta = \frac{2\pi}{\lambda_n} = \frac{\omega_n}{c} \tag{7.86}$$

with λ_n being the wavelength. Typical gain spectrum and location of resonator modes are shown in Fig. 7.32(a). Longitudinal modes with angular frequencies ω_{n-1}, ω_n and ω_{n+1} are shown. In time, the mode which has the largest gain will survive; the other modes will diminish (Fig. 7.32(b)).

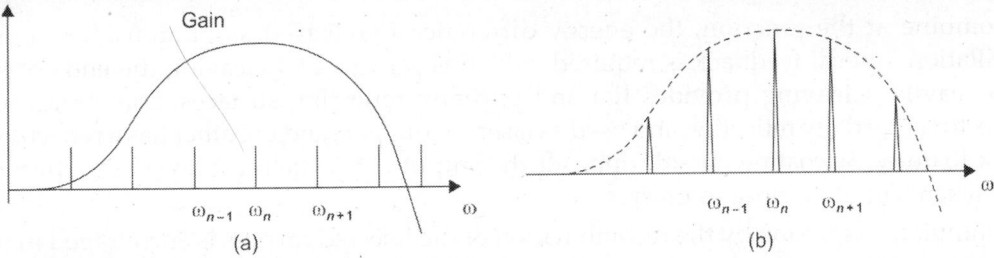

Fig. 7.32: Gain spectrum of semiconductor laser and location of longitudinal modes. ω_n are FP resonances determined from phase condition

7.13 SEMICONDUCTOR LASERS

Coherent laser radiation ranging from the infrared, through the ultraviolet regions of the spectrum has been obtained from semiconductor junction diodes.

The most common type of semiconductor used is a III-V compound. Semiconductor lasers are different from other lasers in the following aspects:

(i) Transition occurs between energy bands rather than between discrete energy levels, the emission being a result of electron transitions from the conduction to the valence bands.

(ii) The laser is very small in size, typically 50 μm × 250 μm × 50 μm.

(iii) The characteristics of the laser beam are strongly influenced by the properties of the junction material.

(iv) In *pn* junction lasers, population inversion occurs in the very narrow region about the junction. The pumping of the *pn* junction laser is accomplished by the application of a forward bias to the diode.

It is a property of semiconductors that the downward transitions of electrons recombining with holes may or may not result in the emission of option of optical energy. Based on this property, semiconductors can be classified as *indirect and direct*. This classification is related to the energy band structure, silicon and germanium are indirect types, where as most of the III-V compounds are direct. In direct types, radiative transitions take place faster than nonradiative and impurity transitions. In direct semiconductors, radiative recombination's occur faster than radiative recombinations, so that in essence, photon emission is suppressed. In fact, some radiation is emitted by almost all semiconductor *pn* junctions, but in junctions using the indirect type of semiconductors, this radiation is very inefficient.

7.13.1 Semiconductor Laser Diode or Semiconductor Injection Laser

The light emission in laser diodes is mostly by stimulated emission, whereas that in LEDs is mostly by spontaneous emission. Laser diodes can emit light at high powers (~100 mW) and also it is coherent. Because of the coherent nature of laser output, it is highly directional. The narrower angular spread of the output beam compared with a LED allows higher coupling efficiency for light coupling to single-mode fibers. An important advantage of the semiconductor laser is the narrow spectral width, which makes it a suitable optical source for WDM optical transmission systems. A semiconductor laser in its simplest form is a forward-biased pn junction. Electrons in the conduction band and holes in the valence band are separated by the hand gap and they form a two-band system similar to the atomic system discussed in Section 7.3. As electrons and holes recombine at the junction, the energy difference is released as photons. To obtain oscillation, optical feedback is required, which is achieved by cleaving the ends of the laser cavity. Cleaving provides flat and partially reflecting surfaces. Sometimes one reflector is partially reflecting and used as laser output port and the other has a reflectivity close to unity. By coating the side opposite the output with a dielectric layer, the reflection coefficient could be close to unity.

Stimulated emission by the recombination of the injected carriers is encouraged in the semiconductor injection laser [also called as the injection laser diode (ILD) or simply the injection laser] by the provision of an optical cavity in the crystal structure in order to provide the feedback of photons. ILD finds extensive application in an optical source in the transmitter module of optical fiber communication systems requiring bandwidth in excess of 200 MHz. Further, the size compatibility of semiconductor laser diode with the optical fiber make them quite attractive over other forms of laser sources. No doubt, the structure and size vary largely depending on the nature of the lasing medium (solid, liquid, gas or semiconductor). Semiconductor laser diodes are specially designed pn junctions usually realized in double hetero junction form. Configuration wise it largely resembles a double hetrostructure LED (DH–LED), where the confining layers surrounding the active layer provide carrier confinement as well as optical confinement. From the structural design point of view, laser diodes are inherent by much more complex. However, the biggest challenge in this respect is to confine the current in a small region in the lateral direction of the cavity. Further, from operational point of view laser diodes need complicated drive circuit with the provision of automatic thermal stabilization circuit due to the dependence of laser output on temperature. Laser sources are quite expensive and also prone to catastrophic degradation. However, Laser diodes have a very large bandwidth, a low spectral width, a coherent light output, large output power etc. These salient features of laser diode make it more superior to LEDs in optical fiber communication system especially for high speed and long have applications.

7.13.2 Population Inversion and Optical Feedback in a Laser Diode

Stimulated emission in a semiconductor laser diode results from radiative transitions between the distributed energy states in the conduction band to those in the valence band unlike in a gas or a solid laser where stimulated emission is caused by radiative transitions between discrete atomic or molecular levels. We have read that for the purpose of laser action creation of situation of population inversion in the lasing medium and also use of an optical resonator for providing necessary optical feedback for sustanance of oscillation are essential. One can achieve both population inversion and optical feedback in a semiconductor laser with the help of special design techniques as described below:

A semiconductor laser diode or ILD is basically a *pn* diode in which both *p* and *n* are so heavily doped that both *p* and *n* regions become degenerate. As a result Fermi level on *p*-side enters into the valence band and that on *n*-side enters into the conduction band as shown in Fig. 7.33. Figure 7.33 shows the energy band diagram prior and after formation of *pn* Junction. We know that Fermi level is a reference level, below which all states are filled up and above which are states are filled up. Fig. 7.33(a) shows the filled-in states shown by shaded lines on the *p*-side and *n*-side prior to forming the *pn* junction. After the formation of the *pn* junction, the equilibrium energy band diagram is shown in Fig. 7.33(b). Under equilibrium, the Fermi level is aligned on both sides. Shaded lines in the figure indicates the filled- in states as before. When a forward bias is applied across the *pn*-junction, the barrier height is reduced and Fig. 7.33(c) shows the respective energy band diagram. We see that under forward bias a large number of holes and electrons are injected into a narrow region near the metallurgical junction as indicated by the vertical dashed lines in the Fig. 7.33(c). One can easily verify that, in this narrow region there are a large number of filled-in states in the conduction band (higher energy level) just opposite to a large number of empty states in the valence band (lower energy level). This reveals that a population inversion is created in this region, i.e., this region forms the active region where stimulated emission takes place (shown by downward arrow in Fig. 7.33(c)).

Now, to provide a strong optical feedback, there is a necessity to create an optical resonator structure surrounding the region in which the population inversion is created by making use of a *pn*-junction which is degeneratively doped on both the sides. One can easily achieve this in a semiconductor laser diode due to the crystalline nature. Unlike in other laser sources where the Fabry–Perot resonator comprises a pair of flat and partially reflecting external mirrors, the mirror facets constructed in a laser diode just by making two parallel clefts along natural cleavage planes of the semiconductor crystal (Fig. 7.34).

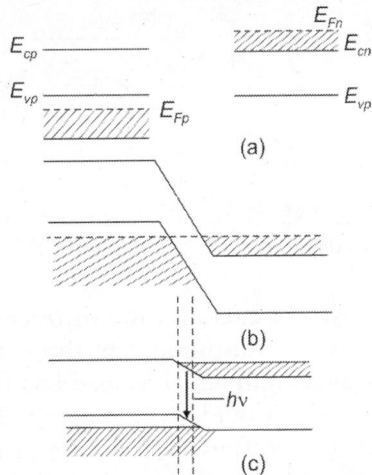

Fig. 7.33: Detailed illustration of population inversion in an semiconductor diode or ILD (a) energy band diagram of p- and n-type degenerate semiconductors prior to formation of junction (b) equilibrium energy band diagram after formation of the junction (c) pn junction under forward bias

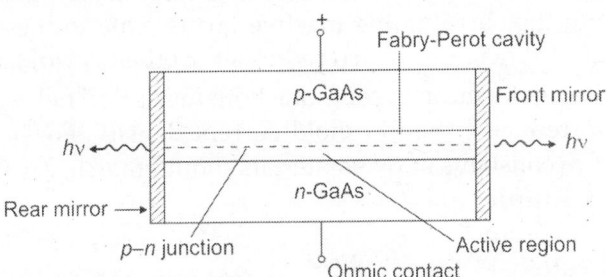

Fig. 7.34: Schematic of Fabry–Perot (FP) laser diode

We may note that those two mirrors, i.e. front and rear mirrors provide a strong optical feedback along the longitudinal direction to provide gain through repeated interaction of the emitted photon with the lasing medium such that the total gain compensates the loss. Interestingly, this feedback turns the device into an *oscillator*. We may note that a laser cavity may have a number of resonant frequencies, for each of which gain exceeds the corresponding loss. In order to reduce undesirable emission from the side walls of the cavity these sides of the cavity are usually abraded.

7.13.3 Distributed-Feedback Lasers

These lasers does not make use of Fabry–Perot (FP) cavity resonator to provide optical feedback. In these lasers the optical feedback is provided by Bragg reflectors (gratings) or periodic variations in refractive index called distributed feedback corrugations. Figure 7.35(a) shows that corrugations are incorporated along the length of the active

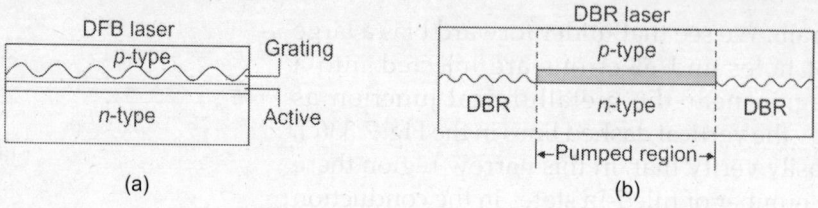

Fig. 7.35: Schematic illustration feedback based laser diode: (a) distributed feedback (DFB) diode (b) distributed Bragg reflector (DBR) laser diode

region. Generally, the diffraction grating is etched close to the *pn*-junction, i.e. active region of the diode. This Bragg grating acts more like an optical filter to select a particular wavelength which is feed back to the gain medium for lasing, obviously, in this case the grating provides the requisite feedback for lasing and as a result no separate mirror is required. These types of laser diodes are called *distributed-feedback* (DFB) laser diodes. We may note that there is also another form of distributed feedback configuration where the grating is incorporated only in the passive region unlike in the entire pumped region as in the case of DFB laser diode. This type of laser diode is called as *distributed Bragg reflector* (DBR) laser diode [Fig. 7.35(b)]. We may also note that DFB and DBR laser diodes oscillate at a single longitudinal mode unlike FP laser diode which generally oscillate at multiple longitudinal modes. Laser diodes are generally obtained in double heterostructure.

In a simple homojunction semiconductor laser, one can achieve relatively high threshold current densities because both carriers and optical confinement within the active region of device are minimum. Carriers injected into active region of device pass through it without any recombination and do not contribute to laser action. It is also seen that the optical fields leak into the surrounding inactive layers. Due to these two reasons, the threshold current density increases which reduces the efficiency of laser action.

Heterostructure provides a mean of confining both the optical fields and carriers within the active region and reducing the threshold current density. For heterostructure, it is required that the lattice constants of two materials should match, e.g. GaAs and AlGaAs. The structure of a simple GaAs-AlGa is shown in Fig. 7.36 which is called a **double heterostructure laser** because it contains two GaAs-AlGaAs interface. Since the energy bandgap of AlGaAs is greater than GaAs, therefore, there is an energy gap discontinuity between two materials. GaAs and AlGaAs are said to form a type I heterojunction in which the energy gap discontinuity is equal to the sum of the conduction and valence band edge discontinuities.

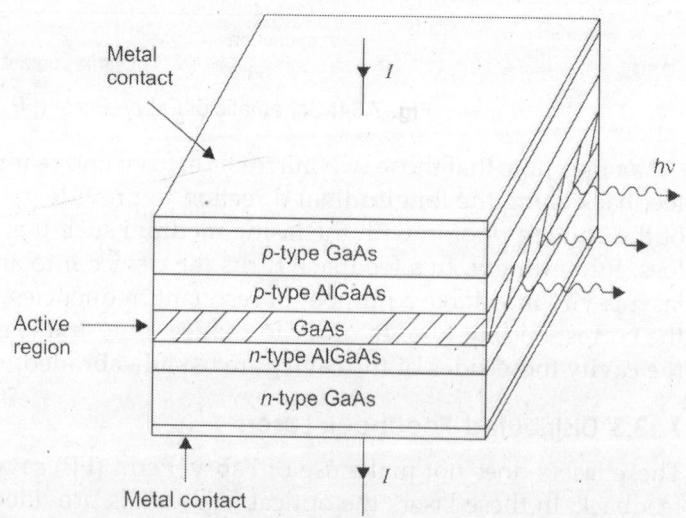

Fig. 7.36: Structure of GaAs-AlGa laser

The presence of conduction and valence band energy discontinuities in the two heterostructures act to greatly confine the injected carriers within the narrow gap GaAs layer as shown in Fig. 7.37 which ultimately can result in a radiative recombination event with the subsequent emission of a photon. Heterostructure has lower threshold current density than the homojunction laser. The double heterostructure also acts to confine the optical fields within the GaAs layer

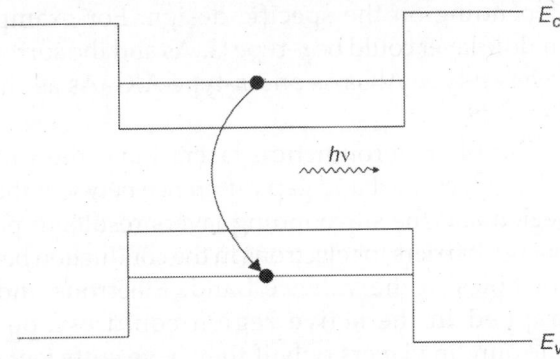

Fig. 7.37: Radiative event in GaAs layer

due to different refractive indices of the used semiconductor materials.

In the laser action photon is emitted by stimulated emission. The light bounces back and forth due to reflection from the boundaries of the device. The reflecting surfaces are produced by cleaving the crystal such that the cleaved surface provides for nearly complete reflection. Stimulated emission with the GaAs layer is triggered by reflected light. The emitted photon has the same phase as that of the stimulating light, i.e., coherence is maintained. In double heterostructure laser, the emitted light has an energy close to that of the energy gap of narrow gap material. The energy of the emitted photon thus depends on the intrinsic properties of the active medium. Now, we discuss heterostructure lasers in detail.

7.13.4 Heterojunction Lasers

The *pn* junction shown in Fig. 7.38 is called a *homo-junction*. The problem with the homojunction is that when it is forward-biased, electron-hole recombination occurs over a wide region (1 – 10 μm). Therefore, high carrier densities can not be realized.

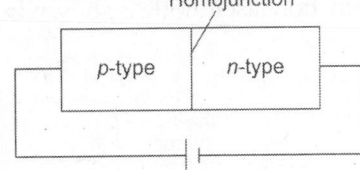

Fig. 7.38: A homojunction

A *heterojunction* is an interface between two adjoining semiconductors with different band-gap energies. In Fig. 7.39, a thin layer is sandwiched between *p*-type and *n*-type layers. The band gap of this layer is smaller than that of the *p*-type and *n*-type layers, as shown in Fig. 7.40(b). This leads to two heterojunctions and such devices are called double heterostructures. The thin layer, known as the *active region*, may or may not be doped

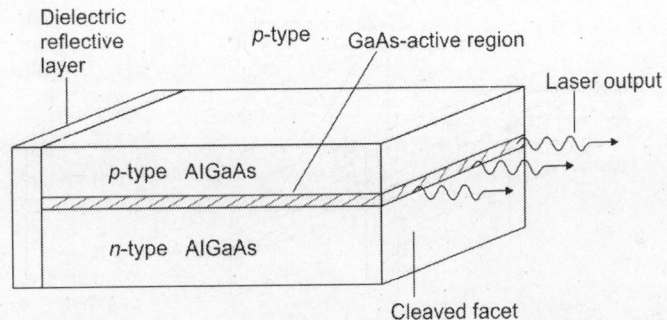

Fig. 7.39: A double-heterojunction Fabry–Perot (FP) laser diode. The cleaved end functions as a partially reflecting mirror

depending on the specific design. For example, the middle layer could be p-type GaAs and the surrounding layers p-type AlGaAs and n-type AlGaAs as shown in Fig. 7.39.

Double-heterojunction lasers have the following advantages: the band gap difference between the active region and the surrounding layers results in potential energy barriers for electrons in the conduction band and for holes in the valence band. Electrons and holes trapped in the active region could escape to the surrounding layers only if they have sufficient energy to cross the barriers. As a result, both electrons and holes are mostly confined to the active region. Because of the smaller band gap, the active region has a slightly higher refractive index. This acts as an optical waveguide and light is confined to the middle layer of the higher refractive index due to total internal reflection. Therefore, not only electrons and holes are confined to the active region, but also photons, which increases the interaction among them, and the efficiency of light generation in a double heterostructure is much higher than in the devices using homojunctions.

A typical GaAs/AlGaAs double heterostructure junction laser diode is shown in Fig. 7.40(d). A thin layer

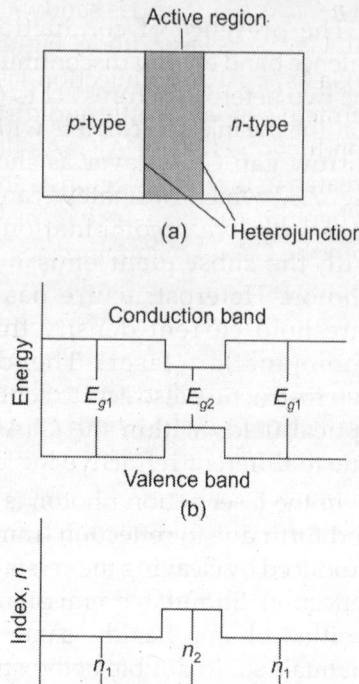

Fig. 7.40: Double heterostructure (a) heterojunctions (b) band gap (c) refractive index

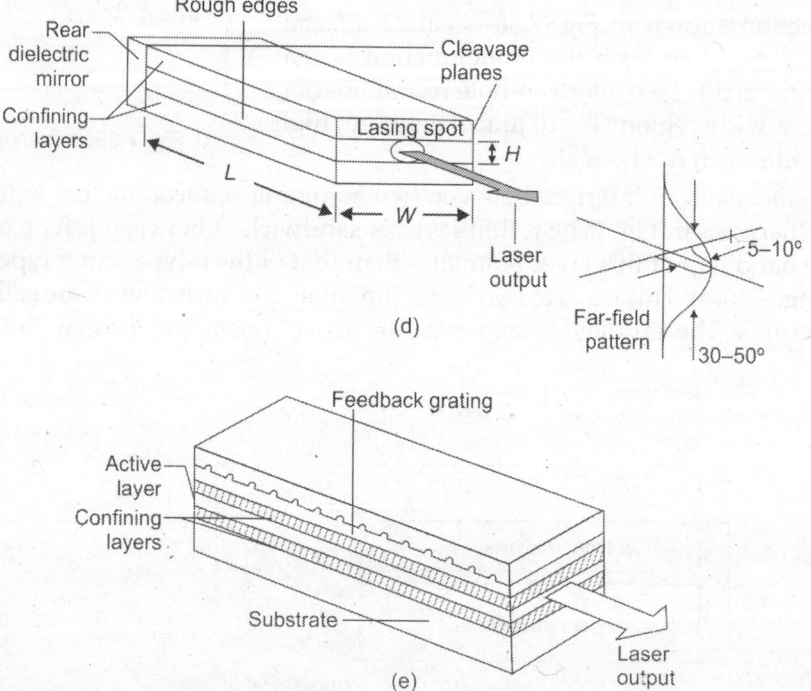

Fig. 7.40: Schematic illustration of double heterostructure injection laser diode: (d) Fabry–Perot cavity resonator laser diode (e) distributed feedback laser diode

of n-GaAs ($\sim 0.2\,\mu m$) is sandwiched between two thicker ($\sim 1\,\mu m$) layers of p- and n- type $Al_x\,Ga_{1-x}$ As laser diode. Figure 7.40(f) shows the schematic structure of the n-AlGaAs/p-GaAs/p-AlGaAs injection laser diode structure alongwith the energy band diagram, refractive index profile and distribution of photon density. We see that the bottom of the conduction band of AlGaAs lies above that of GaAs and as a result a potential well is created in the GaAs region as shown in Fig. 7.40(g) with the help of energy band diagram. When the said structure is forward-biased electrons are injected from n-AlGaAs region into the GaAs region. Further, the energy barriers on the two sides of the GaAs active region prevent the carriers from diffusing away from this region. Obviously, the carriers are forced to be confined in this region where a population inversion has already been created as evident from the energy band diagram (Fig. 7.40(g)). We see that this stimulated emission occurs in the active region and the emitted photons enter into sustained oscillation with the harp of cavity resonator or distributed feedback provided in the structure. We may also note that the double heterostructure provides confinement of photons in addition so carrier confinement. This is possible in this particular structure due to the fact that the refractive index of GaAs is more than that of AlGaAs. Obviously,

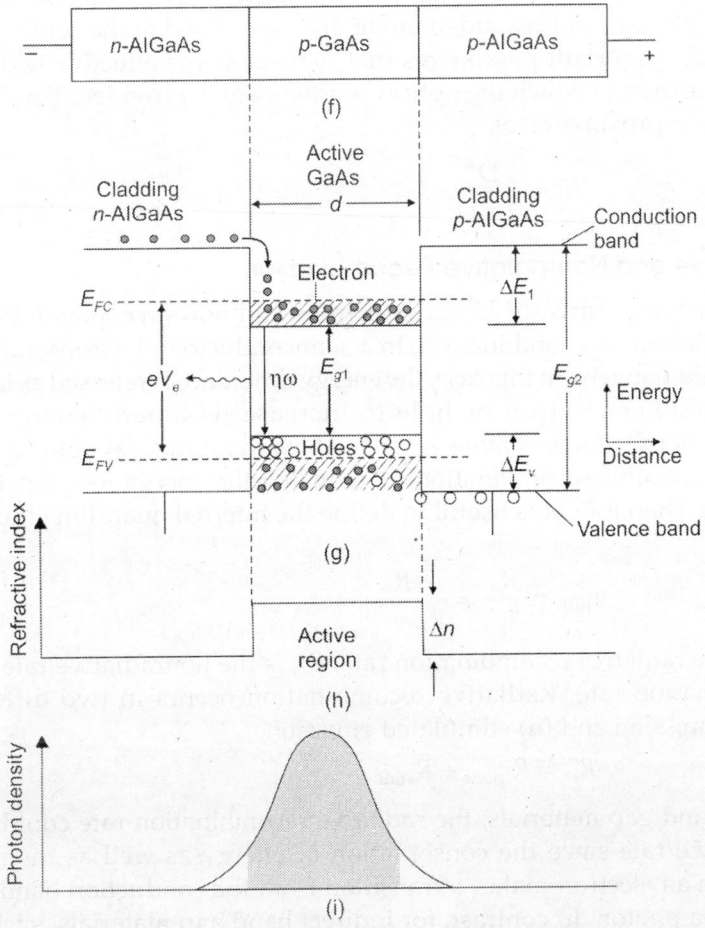

Fig. 7.40: Schematic illustration of double heterostructure AlGaAs/GaAs/AlGaAs double heterostructure laser diode: (f) schematic; (g) energy band diagram under forward bias; (h) refractive index profile (i) photon density distribution

the double heterostructure form a *three-layer waveguide* structure in the form of AlGa/GaAs/AlGaAS. Figure 4.40(h) shows the refractive index profile for the waveguide structure. We see that the photon generated in the process is essentially confined in GaAs active region in the transverse direction [Fig. 7.40(i), (**Note:** To understand the direction of confinement, one will have to consider the 3D structure of double-heterostructure) and is guided along the longitudinal direction. The confinement in the lateral direction is achieved with the help of special structural design (gain guided or index guided).]

We can see from Fig. 7.40(i) that even though the photons are essentially confined into the active region they also spread into the surrounding confining reasons. One can analyze this by considering the propagation of the emitted light in the form of electromagnetic wave through the three-dimensional (3D) waveguide structure. One can express the normalized waveguide thickness of the three-layer slab waveguide as

$$D = \left(\frac{2\pi d}{\lambda} \right) \sqrt{n_a^2 - n_c^2} \tag{7.86a}$$

where d is the thickness of the active region and n_a and n_c are respectively the refractive index for the active and cladding region respectively.

One can also define the optical confinement factor T as the fraction of the electromagnetic energy of the guided mode that is confined in the active region. We may note that it is an important parameters that represents the effective width of the active region and the extent to which the optical confinement is provided. For the fundamental mode T can be approximated as

$$T = \frac{D^2}{2 + D^2} \tag{7.86b}$$

7.13.5 Radiative and Nonradiative Recombination

When a *pn* junction is forward-biased, electrons and holes recombine to produce light. This is called radiative recombination. In a semiconductor, electrons and holes can also recombine nonradiatively. In this case, the energy difference is released as lattice vibrations or given to another electron or hole to increase its kinetic energy. This type of recombination is called *nonradiative recombination*. In a practical light source, we like to maximize the radiative recombination by reducing the energy loss due to nonradiative recombination. Therefore, it is useful to define the internal quantum efficiency of a light source as

$$\eta_{\text{int}} = \frac{R_{rr}}{R_{\text{tot}}} = \frac{R_{rr}}{R_{rr} + R_{nr}} \tag{7.87}$$

where R_{rr} is the radiative recombination rate, R_{nr} is the nonradiative rate, and R_{tot} is the total recombination rate. Radiative recombination occurs in two different ways: (i) spontaneous emission and (ii) stimulated emission,

$$R_{rr} = R_{\text{spont}} + R_{\text{stim}} \tag{7.88}$$

For direct band gap materials, the radiative recombination rate could be larger than the nonradiative rate since the conservation of energy as well as momentum can be achieved when an electron makes a transition from the conduction band to the valence band emitting a photon. In contrast, for indirect band gap materials, such as Si and Ge, the electron–hole recombination is mostly nonradiative and, therefore, the internal quantum efficiency is quite small. Typically, n_{tot} is of the order of 10^{-5} for Si and Ge.

7.13.6 Laser Rate Equations

We have developed earlier the rate equations for an atomic system with two levels. In the atomic system, the interaction takes place among the photons, the atoms in the excited level, and in the ground level. Similarly, in the semiconductor laser diode, the interaction is between the electrons in the conduction band, holes in the valence band, and photons. Therefore, Eqs (7.76) and (7.77) may be used to describe the time rate of change of electrons and photons in a cavity with N_2 being replaced by the electron density N_e,

$$\frac{dN_e}{dt} = R_{pump} + R_{stim} + R_{sp} + R_{nr}$$

$$= R_{pump} - GN_{ph} - \frac{N_e}{\tau_e} \tag{7.89}$$

$$\frac{dN_{ph}}{dt} = R_{stim} + R_{sp} + R_{loss}$$

$$= GN_{ph} + R_{sp} - \frac{N_{ph}}{\tau_{ph}} \tag{7.90}$$

Here, $\tau_e \equiv \tau_{21}$ represents the lifetime of electrons associated with spontaneous emission and nonradiative transition. We now found that $G = gu$. This result was derived under the assumption that the light is a plane wave. But in a double-heterojunction laser, the active region has a slightly higher refractive index than the surrounding layers and, therefore, it acts as a waveguide. The tails of an optical mode extend well into the surrounding regions, but they do not contribute to the photon density in the active region. Since the photon-hole recombination by photon emission depends on the photon density in the active region, we introduce a confinement factor Γ,

$$G = \Gamma gv, \tag{7.91}$$

where Γ is the ratio of optical power in the active region to total optical power carried by the mode.

Let us consider the growth of photons due to stimulated emission alone. Eqs. (7.89) and (7.90) become

$$\frac{dN_e}{dt} = -GN_{ph} \tag{7.92}$$

$$\frac{dN_{ph}}{dt} = GN_{ph} \tag{7.93}$$

Adding Eqs. (7.92) and (7.93), we find

$$\frac{d(N_e + N_{ph})}{dt} = 0 \tag{7.94}$$

or

$$N_e + N_{ph} = \text{Const.} \tag{7.95}$$

This implies that the total number of electrons and photons is conserved under these conditions. In other words, if you lose 10 electrons per unit volume per unit time by recombination, you gain 10 photons per unit volume per unit time.

Now, let us find an expression for R_{pump}. The electrons and holes are consumed by stimulated emission. Therefore, the external power supply should inject electrons continuously. The current is

$$I = \frac{n_e q}{T} \tag{7.96}$$

where n_e is the number of electrons, q is the electron charge $= 1.602 \times 10^{-19}$ C, and T is the time interval. The number of electrons crossing the active region per unit time is

$$\frac{n_e}{T} = \frac{I}{q} \qquad (7.97)$$

The above equation gives the electron pumping rate. We divide it by the volume of the active region to obtain the electron pumping rate per unit volume

$$R_{pump} = \frac{n_e}{TV} = \frac{I}{qdwL} \qquad (7.98)$$

where d, w, and L are thickness, width, and length of the active layer, respectively, as shown in Fig. 7.41. Using Eq. (7.98) in Eqs (7.89) and (7.90), we find

$$\frac{dN_e}{dt} = \frac{I}{qV} - GN_{ph} - \frac{N_e}{\tau_e} \qquad (7.99)$$

$$\frac{dN_{ph}}{dt} = GN_{ph} + R_{sp} - \frac{N_{ph}}{\tau_{ph}} \qquad (7.100)$$

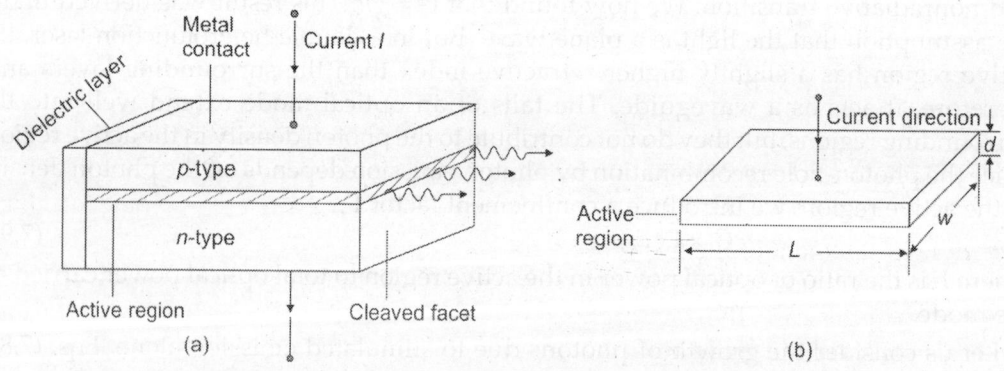

Fig. 7.41: (a) Forward-biased heterojunction laser (b) active region

In the case of an atomic system, we have derived an expression for G (see Eq. (7.78)). But in the case of a semiconductor laser, it is hard to find an exact analytical expression for the gain coefficient g. Instead, we use the following approximation

$$g = \sigma_g (N_e - N_{e0}), \qquad (7.101)$$

where σ_g and N_{e0} are parameters that depend on the specific design. σ_g is called the gain cross-section and N_{e0} is the value of the carrier density at which the gain coefficient becomes zero. Using Eq. (7.91), we find

$$G = \Gamma g v = (G_0 (N_e - N_{e0}) \qquad (7.102)$$

where

$$G_0 = \Gamma \sigma g v \qquad (7.103)$$

7.13.7 Steady-State Solutions of Rate Equations

Equations (7.99) and (7.100) describe the evolution of electron density and photon density in the active region, respectively. In general, they have to be solved numerically on a computer. However, the steady-state solution can be found analytically under some approximations. First, we ignore the spontaneous emission rate since it is much smaller than the stimulated emission are for a laser. Second, we use Eq. (7.102) for the gain, which is an approximation to the calculated/measured gain. Now, Eqs (7.99) and (7.100) become

$$\frac{dN_{ph}}{dt} = GN_{ph} - \frac{N_{ph}}{\tau_{ph}} \tag{7.104}$$

$$\frac{dN_e}{dt} = -GN_{ph} - \frac{N_e}{\tau_e} + \frac{I}{qV} \tag{7.105}$$

We assume that the current I is constant. Under steady-state conditions, the loss of photons due to cavity loss is balanced by the gain of photons due to stimulated emission. As a result, the photon density does not change as a function of time. Similarly, the loss of electrons due to radiative and nonradiative transitions is balanced by electron injection from the battery. So, the electron density does not change with time too. Therefore, under steady-state conditions, the time derivatives in Eqs. (7.104) and (7.105) can be set to zero.

$$\frac{dN_{ph}}{dt} = \frac{dN_e}{dt} = 0 \tag{7.106}$$

Form Eq. (7.104), we have

$$G\tau_{ph} = 1. \tag{7.107}$$

Using Eq. (7.102), we obtain

$$G_0(N_e - N_{e0})\,\tau_{ph} = 1 \tag{7.108}$$

$$N_e = N_{e0} + \frac{1}{G_0\tau_{ph}} \tag{7.109}$$

Form Eq. (7.104), we obtain

$$\Gamma g = \alpha_{cav} \tag{7.110}$$

which is restatement of the fact that gain should be equal to loss. If the current I is very small, there will not be enough electrons in the conduction band to achieve population inversion. In this case, the gain coefficient will be much smaller than the loss coefficient and photons will not build up. For a certain current I, the gain coefficient Γg becomes equal to the loss coefficient α_{cav} and this current is known as the threshold current, I_{th}. If $I > I_{th}$, stimulated emission could become the dominant effect and the photon density could be significant. Under steady-state conditions, there are two possibilities:

Case (i) $I = I_{th}-$. Stimulated emission is negligible and $N_{ph} \cong 0$,

$$\frac{dN_e}{dt} = -\frac{N_e}{\tau_e} + \frac{I}{qV} = 0 \tag{7.111}$$

Let $N_e = N_{e,th}$, From Eq. (7.111), we have

$$I_{th} = \frac{N_{e,th}\, qV}{\tau_e} \tag{7.112}$$

From Eq. (7.109), we have

$$N_{e,th} = N_{e0} + \frac{1}{G_0\tau_{ph}} \tag{7.113}$$

Case (ii) $I > I_{th}$. When the current exceeds the threshold current, we may expect the electron density N_e to be larger than $N_{e,th}$. However, the electron density will be clamped to $N_{e,th}$ when $I > I_{th}$. This can be explained as follows. The threshold current is the minimum current required to achieve population inversion. When $I > I_{th}$, the excess electrons in the conduction band recombine with holes and, therefore, the photon density increases while

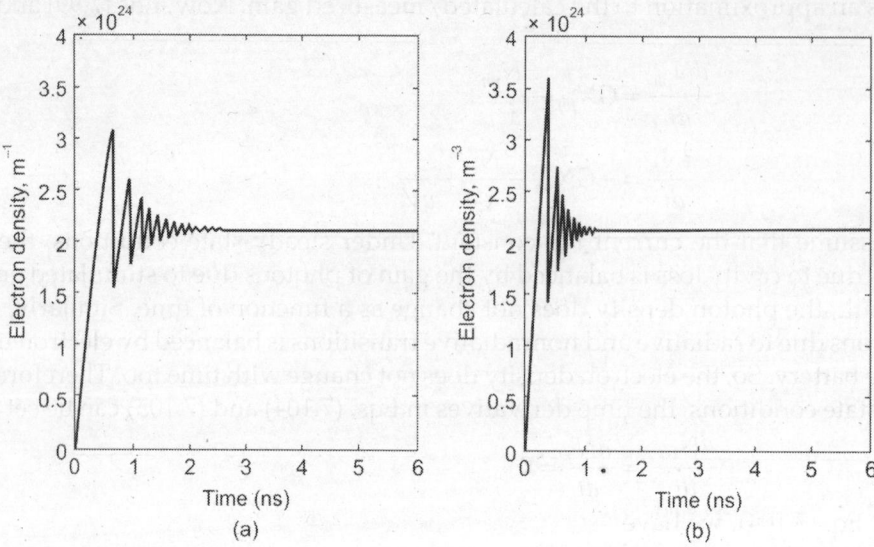

Fig. 7.42: Numerical solution of the rate equation using typical parameters of an InGaAsP laser diode: (a) I = 50 mA; (b) I = 100 mA

the electron density would maintain its value at threshold. Fig. 7.42(a) and 7.42(b) shows the numerical solution of the laser rate equations for $I = 50$ mA and 100 mA, respectively. The threshold current in this example is 9.9 mA. In Fig. 7.42(a) and 7.42(b), after $t > 5$ ns, we may consider it as steady state since N_{ph} and N_e do not change with time. Comparing Fig. 7.42(a) and 7.42(b), we find that the steady-state electron density is the same in both cases, although the bias currents are different. In fact, it is equal to $N_{e,th}$ as given by Eq. (7.43). Using Eqs (7.106) and (7.107) in Eq. (7.105), we obtain

$$\frac{N_{ph}}{\tau_{ph}} = \frac{I}{qV} - \frac{N_{e,th}}{\tau_e} \tag{7.114}$$

Using Eq. (7.112), Eq. (7.114) can be written as

$$N_{ph} = \frac{(I - I_{th})\tau_{ph}}{qV} \tag{7.115}$$

The next step is to develop an expression for the optical power generated as a function of the current. Since the energy of a photon is equal to $\hbar\omega$, the mean photon density of N_{ph} correspond to the energy density,

$$u = N_{ph}\hbar\omega \tag{7.116}$$

The relation between energy density and optical intensity is given by

$$I = uv = N_{ph}\hbar\omega v \tag{7.117}$$

Since optical intensity is power per unit area perpendicular to photon flow, the mean optical power generated can be written as

$$P_{gen} = IA = N_{ph}\hbar\omega vA, \tag{7.118}$$

where A is the effective cross-section of the mode. Using Eq. (7.115) in Eq. (7.118), we finally obtain

$$P_{gen} = \frac{(I - I_{th})\tau_{ph}\hbar wvA}{qwdL} \tag{7.119}$$

We may note that the above equation is valid only when $I > I_{th}$. If $I \le I_{th}$, $P_{gen} = 0$ under our approximations.

7.13.8 Lasing conditions and Resonant Frequencies

Let us consider a Fabry-Perot (FP) laser diode cavity. We may note that a typical FP cavity resonator is generally 250–500 μm long and 5–20 μm wide. The thickness of the cavity is generally very small (~ 0.1–0.2 μm). We can view the light within the cavity as an electromagnetic wave that sets up electromagnetic field patterns called *modes* within the cavity. These modes are either Transverse Electric (TE) mode or transverse Magnetic (TM) mode type. However, these modes are created along all three directions. The modes created along the length of the cavity are called *longitudinal modes*. The modes created along the lateral direction are called *lateral modes* and lie in the plane of *pn*-junction. The modes those are created in the direction of the thickness, i.e. perpendicular to the plane of the pn Junction constitute the *transverse* modes. Further, the longitudinal modes are related to the length of the cavity and determine the frequency spectrum of the emitted radiation. On the other hand the lateral mode decide the lateral profile of the laser beam. The transverse modes depend on the guiding properties of the structure of the three-layer waveguide comprising of the active region as well as surrounding cladding regions. We may note that these modes determine the radiation pattern as well as threshold current density of the laser diode.

We now consider the simplistic schematic of the cavity resonator shown in Fig. 7.42(c) for the determination of the lasing condition as well as resonant frequencies. The FP cavity is mode by clearing both sides of the crystal. In view of large refractive index difference between the semiconductor and the air, the

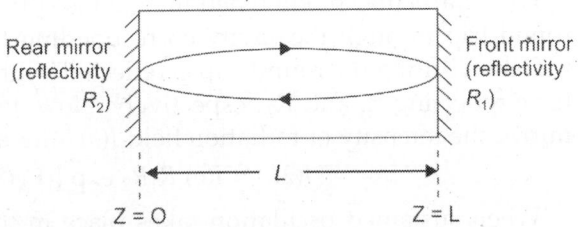

Fig. 7.42(c): Schematic illustration of a Fabry–Perot (FP) resonator cavity

cleaved edges essentially behave like mirrors. Out of these two front and rear mirrors, the reflectivity of the rear mirror is enhanced by putting additional dielectric layers whereas the front mirror is left as semi-transmitting so that laser beam can come ocet of the cavity. Now, if L is the length of the cavity, λ is the wavelength near the peak of spontaneous emission spectrum, then, one finds for the longitudinal modes

$$L = \frac{m\lambda}{2} \tag{7.120}$$

where m is an integer.

Let R_1 and R_2 be the reflectivity of front and rear mirror respectively. Let us consider that the electromagnetic wave is propagating through the cavity along the longitudinal direction (say, z-axis). Now we can express the electric field as

$$E(z, t) = I(z) \exp [j(\omega t - \beta z)] \tag{7.121}$$

where ω is angular frequency of the radiation field, β is the propagation constant and $I(z)$ is the optical field intensity.

The electromagnetic wave travelling along the axis of the cavity gets reflected back and forth multiple times by the front and rear mirrors. The optical intensity undergoes gain as well as loss during the transit in the process. The gain in the cavity arises due to the fact that medium inside the cavity is present for population inversion. Further, multiple interactions of photons associated with the radiation field propagating through the cavity results in more and more stimulated emission of radiations, i.e., causing an amplification of radiation field. On the otherhand, cavity also introduces some loss of photons that tends to reduce the intensity of radiation field. There are several factors responsible for the loss in the cavity: (i) emission of photons through any one of the facets, (ii) absorption and scattering caused by the lasing medium and (iii) absorption in the cladding regions. We may note that the lasing occurs when the gain of the cavity for a particular mode exceeds the total loss encountered by it. However, both the gain and loss of the cavity depend on the energy associated with the photons that constitute the radiation field. We may also note that as the radiation field travels along the cavity, the intensity of the radiation field increases exponentially due to gain and decreases also exponentially due to the loss with the distance z, travelled along the length of the cavity. One can express the optical field intensity at any point as

$$I(z) = I(o) \exp \left[\Gamma g(hv) - \bar{\alpha}(hv)z \right] \tag{7.122}$$

where $\bar{\alpha}$ is the absorption coefficient accounting for the average loss in the cavity per unit length, g is the gain coefficient of the cavity accounting for the gain per unit length of the cavity and Γ is the optical confinement factor which depends on the confinement of the radiation field in the transverse as well as lateral directions. The confinement f the radiation field in the lateral direction depends on the preparation of the side walls.

For a particular mode when the gain is sufficient to exceed the total loss during one round trip through the cavity corresponding to $z = 2L$, the lasing occurs. The optical radiation during the round trip is reflected by the front as well as the rear mirrors which have reflecting R_1 and R_2 respectively. Now, taking into account of the reflectivities of mirror the intensity of radiation field $I(o)$ after a complete round trip is given by

$$I(2L) = I(o) \, R_1 R_2 \exp \left[(\Gamma g(hv) - \bar{\alpha}(hv))2L \right] \tag{7.123}$$

When sustained oscillation takes place in the cavity under steady state, the lasing occurs. The condition for sustained oscillation demands that the amplitude and phase of the incident wave should be the same as those of the returned wave after a round trip. Obviously, for lasing to occurs, the following two conditions have to be satisfied:

$$I(2L) = I(o) \tag{7.124}$$

for the amplitude and

$$\exp \left[-j \, 2\beta L \right] = 1 \tag{7.125}$$

for the phase

One can obtain the threshold of the cavity gain, g_{th}, which is just sufficient to overcome the cavity loss by using Eqs. (7.124). Using Eqs (7.122) and (7.123), one obtain as

$$\Gamma g_{th} = \bar{\alpha} + \frac{1}{2L} \ln \left(\frac{1}{R_1 R_2} \right) = \bar{\alpha} + \bar{\alpha}_{end} \tag{7.126}$$

where, $\bar{\alpha}_{end}$ corresponds to end loss of the cavity and one can determine by reflectivities of the mirrors. We have $\Gamma = 1$ for 100% confinement and Eq. (7.126) reads as

$$g_{th} = \bar{\alpha} + \frac{1}{2L} \ln \left(\frac{1}{R_1} + \frac{1}{R_2} \right) \tag{7.127}$$

However, for lasing to occur, one will have to ensure that the gain of the cavity must exceed the threshold gain, i.e.

$$g \geq g_{th} \tag{7.128}$$

In the beginning, the gain of the cavity should exceed the threshold gain so that lasing may occur. This is achieved by means of strong pumping that ensures enough population inversion to provide a gain which compensates overall loss in the cavity.

As stated earlier, for an Fabry–Perot laser diode, the cleaved edge of the semiconductor crystal serve as mirrors In this case, the reflectivities R_1 and R_2 correspond to the Fresnel reflection coefficient which is decided by the refractive index of the cavity and that of the surrounding medium in which laser emits. One obtains the expression for Fresnel reflection coefficient as

$$R = \left(\frac{n_1 - n_2}{n_1 + n_2} \right)^2 \tag{7.129}$$

where n_1 and n_2 are the refractive indices of the materials on the two sides of the reflecting boundary.

In addition to semiconductor injection laser, there are some other injection laser structures: (i) gain-guided lasers (ii) index-guided lasers (iii) quantum-well lasers (iv) quantum dot lasers.

In addition to these injection lasers, there are also single-frequently injection lasers: (i) short- and couple-cavity lasers (ii) distributed feedback lasers (iii) Vertical-cavity surface emitting lasers.

We now briefly describe the basic concepts of few of these lasers.

7.14 LASER DIODE STRUCTURES AND RADIATION PATTERNS

A basic requirement for efficient operation of laser diodes is that, in addition to transverse optical and carrier confinement between heterojunction layers, the current flow must be restricted laterally to a narrow stripe along the length of the laser. Numerous novel methods of achieving this, with varying degrees of success, have been proposed, but all strive for the same goals of limiting the number of lateral modes so that lasing is confined to a single filament, stabilizing the lateral gain, and ensuring a relatively low threshold current.

Figure 7.43 shows the three basic *optical-confinement methods* used for bounding laser light in the lateral direction. In the first structure, a narrow electrode stripe (less than 8 µm wide) runs along the length of the diode. The injection of electrons and holes into

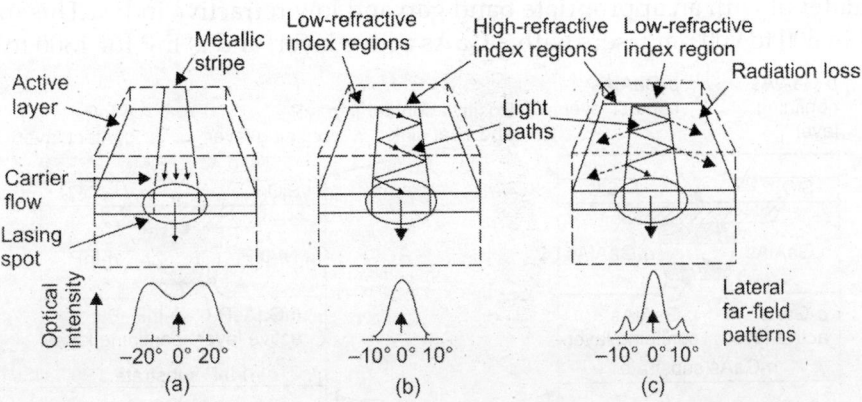

Fig. 7.43: Three fundamental structures for confining optical waves in the lateral direction: (a) in the gain-induced guide, electrons injected via a metallic stripe contact alter the index of refraction of the active layer; (b) the positive-index waveguide has a higher refractive index in the central portion of the active region; (c) the negative-index waveguide has a lower refractive index in the central portion of the active region

the device alters the refractive index of the active layer directly below the stripe. The profile of these injected carriers creates a weak, complex waveguide that confines the light laterally. This type of device is commonly referred to as a *gain-guided laser*. Although, these lasers can emit optical power exceeding 100 mW, they have strong instabilities and can have highly astigmatic, two-peaked beams as shown in Fig. 7.43(a).

More stable structures use the configurations shown in Fig. 7.43(b) and (c). Here, dielectric waveguide structures are fabricated in the lateral direction. The variations in the real refractive index of the various materials in these structures control the lateral modes in the laser. Thus, these devices are called *index-guided lasers*. If a particular index-guided laser supports only the fundamental transverse mode and the fundamental longitudinal mode, it is known as a *single-mode laser*. Such a device emits a single, well-collimated beam of light that has an intensity profile which is a bell-shaped gaussian curve.

Index-guided lasers can have either positive-index or negative-index wave-confining structures. In a *positive-index waveguide*, the central region has a higher refractive index than the outer regions. Thus, all of the guided light is reflected at the dielectric boundary, just as it is at the core-cladding interface in an optical fiber. By proper choice of the change in refractive index and the width of the higher-index region, one can make a device that supports only the fundamental lateral mode.

In a *negative-index waveguide*, the central region of the active layer has a lower refractive index than the outer regions. At the dielectric boundaries, part of the light is reflected and the rest is refracted into the surrounding material and is thus lost. This radiation loss appears in the far-field radiation pattern as narrow side lobes to the main beam, as shown in Fig. 7.43(c). Since the fundamental mode in this device has less radiation loss than any other mode, it is the first to lase. The positive-index laser is the more popular of these two structures.

Index-guided lasers can be made using any one of four fundamental structures. These are the buried heterostructure, a selectively diffused construction, a varying-thickness structure, and a bent-layer configuration. To make the *buried heterostructure* (BH) laser shown in Fig. 7.44, one etches a narrow mesa stripe (1–2 μm wide) in double-heterostructure material. The mesa is then embedded in high-resistivitry lattice-matched *n*-type material with an appropriate band gap and low refractive index. This material is GaAlAs in 800 to 900 nm lasers with a GaAs active layer, and is InP for 1300 to 1600 nm

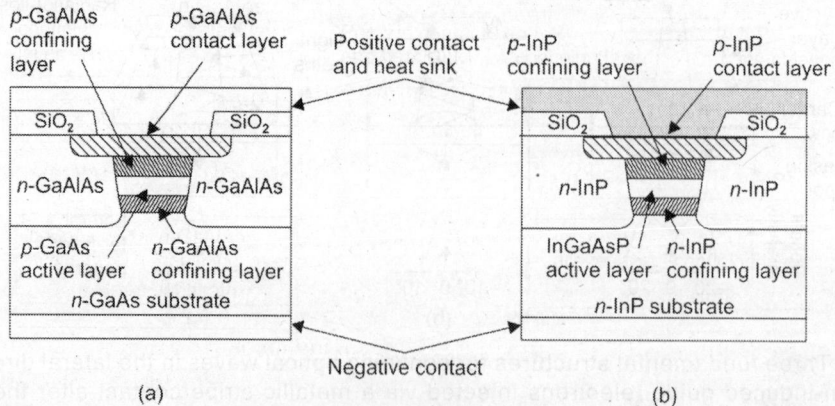

(a)   (b)

Fig. 7.44: (a) Short-wavelength (800–900 nm) GaAlAs and (b) long-wavelength (1300–1600 nm) InGaAsP buried-heterostructure laser diodes

lasers with an InGaAsP active layer. This configuration, thus strongly traps generated light in a lateral waveguide. A number of variations of this fundamental structure have been used to fabricate high-performing laser diodes.

The *selectively diffused construction* is shown in Fig. 7.44(a). Here, a chemical dopant, such as zinc for GaAlAs lasers and cadmium for InGaAsP lasers, is diffused into the active layer immediately below the metallic contact stripe. The dopant changes the refractive index of the active layer to form a lateral waveguide channel. In the *varying-thickness structure* shown in Fig. 7.44(b), a channel (or other topological configuration, such as a mesa or terrace) is etched into the substrate. Layers of crystal are then regrown into the channel using liquid-phase epitaxy. This process fills in the depressions and partially dissolves the protrusions, thereby creating variations in the thickness, the thicker area acts as a positive-index waveguide of higher-index material. In the *bent-layer structure*, a mesa is etched into the substrate as shown in Fig. 7.44(c). Semiconductor material layers are grown onto this structure using vapour-phase epitaxy to exactly replicate the mesa configuration. The active layer has a constant thickness with lateral bends. As an optical wave travels along the flat top of the mesa in the active area, the lower-index material outside of the bends confines the light along this lateral channel (Fig. 7.45).

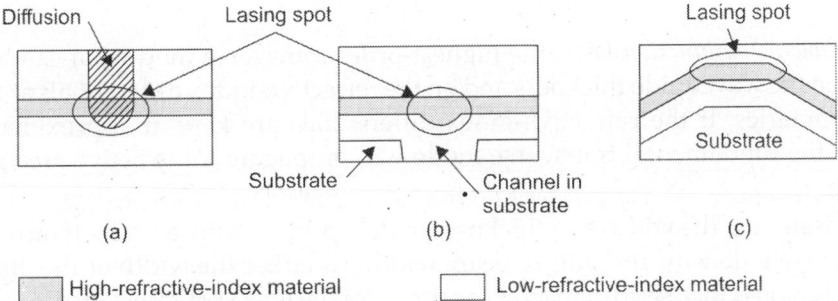

Fig. 7.45: Positive-index optical-wave-confining structure of the (a) selectively diffused (b) varying thickness, and (c) bent-layer types

In addition to confining the optical wave to a narrow lateral stripe to achieve continuous high optical output power, one also needs to restrict the drive current tightly to the active layer so more than 60 percent of the current contributes to lasing. Figure 7.46 shows the four basic *current-confinement methods*. In each method, the device architecture blocks current on both sides of the lasing region. This is achieved either by high-resistivity regions or by reverse-biased *pn* junctions, which prevent the current from flowing while the device is forward-biased under normal conditions. For structures with a continuous active layer, the current can be confined either above or below the lasing region. The diodes are forward-biased so that current travel from *p*-type to the *n*-type regions. In the *preferential-dopant diffusion* method, partially diffusing a *p*-type dopant (Zn or Cd) through an *n*-type capping layer establishes a narrow path for the current, since back-biased *pn* junctions block the current outside the diffused region. The *proton implantation method* creates regions of high resistivity, thus restricting the current to a narrow path between these regions. The *inner-stripe confinement* technique grows the lasing structure above a channel etched into planar material. Back-biased *pn* junctions restrict the current on both sides of the channel. When the active layer is discontinuous, as in a buried heterostructure, current can be blocked on both sides of the mesa by growing *pn* junctions that are reverse-biased when the device is operating. A laser diode can use more than one current-confining technique.

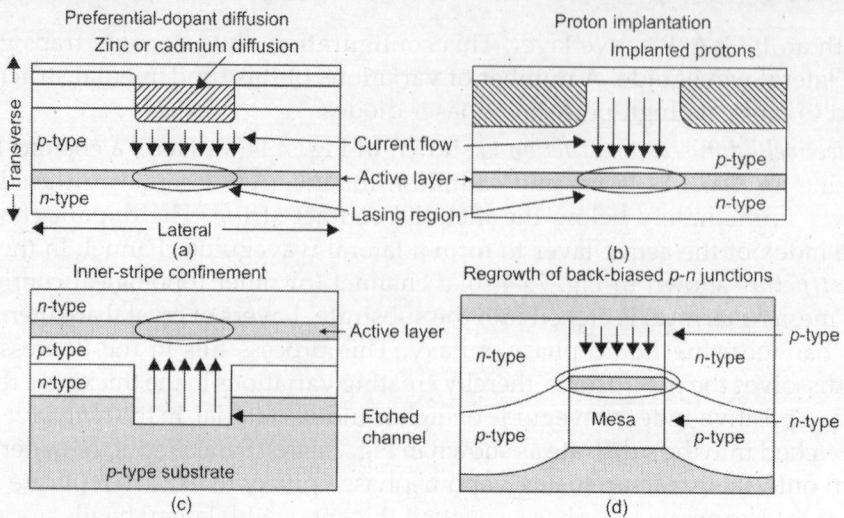

Fig. 7.46: Four basic methods for achieving current confinement in laser diodes: (a) preferential-dopant diffusion (b) proton implantation (c) inner-stripe confinement (d) regrowth of back-biased pn junctions

In a *double-heterojunction laser*, the highest-order transverse mode that can be excited depends on the waveguide thickness and on the refractive-index differentials at the waveguide boundaries. If the refractive-index differentials are kept at approximately 0.08, then only the fundamental transverse mode will propagate if the active area is thinner than 1 μm.

When designing the width and thickness of the optical cavity, a tradeoff must be made between current density and output beam width. As either the width or the thickness of the active region is increased, a narrowing occurs of the lateral or transverse beam widths, respectively, but at the expense of an increase in the threshold current density. Most positive-index waveguide devices have a lasing spot 3 μm wide by 0.6 μm high. This is significantly greater than the active-layer thickness, since about half the light travels in the confining layers. Such lasers can operate reliably only upto continuous-wave (CW) output powers of 3–5 mW. Here, the transverse and lateral half-power beam widths shown in Fig. 7.42 are about $\theta_\perp \simeq 30$–$50°$ and $\theta_\parallel \simeq 5$–$10°$, respectively.

Although, the active layer in a standard double-heterostructure laser is thin enough (1–3 μm) to confine electrons and the optical field, the electronic and optical properties remain the same as in the bulk material. This limits the achievable threshold current density, modulation speed, and linewidth of the device. *Quantum-well lasers* overcome these limitations by having an active-layer thickness around 10 nm. This changes the electronic and optical properties dramatically, because the dimensionality of the free-electron motion is reduced from three to two dimensions. As shown in Fig. 7.42, the restriction of the carrier motion normal to the active layer results in a quantization of the energy levels. The possible energy-level transitions which lead to photon emission are designated by ΔE_{ij}. Both single quantum-well (SQW) and multiple quantum-well (MQW) lasers have been fabricated. These structures contain single and multiple active regions, respectively. The layers separating the active regions are called *barrier layers*. The MQW lasers have a better optical-mode confinement, which results in a lower threshold current density. The wavelength of the output light can be changed by adjusting the laser

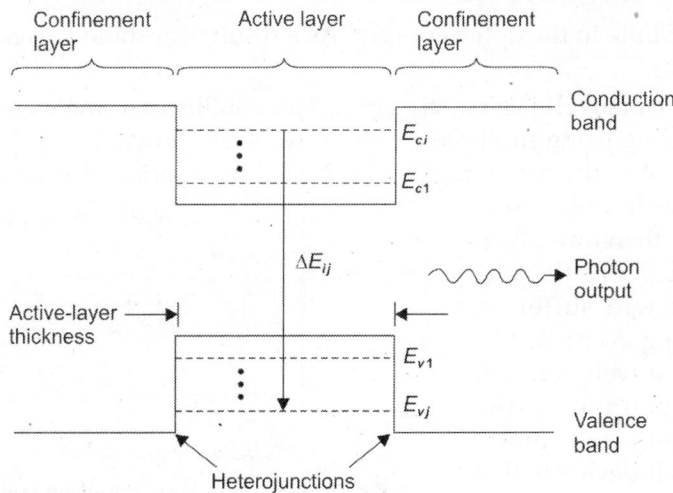

Fig. 7.47: Energy-band diagram for a quantum layer in a multiple quantum-well (MQW) laser. The parameter ΔE_{ij} represents the allowed energy-level transitions

thickness d, e.g. in an InGaAs quantum well laser, the peak output wavelength moves from 1550 nm when d = 10 nm to 1500 nm for d = 8 nm.

7.15 QUANTUM-WELL LASERS

Quantum well lasers offer an alternative to double heterostructures. In *quantum well lasers*, the energy of emitted photon can be made subsequently higher than that of the bandgap. By proper choice of well width, the energy of the emitted photon can be adjusted so that lasing can be achieved at various wavelengths using the same material. A single quantum well laser is similar in design to a double heterostructure laser except that the narrow gap. This means active region is intentionally made thin so that the spatial quantization effects occur. As we know that when the dimension of the confining region is equal to that of electron de Broglie wavelength, quantum mechanical effects occur. According to quantum mechanical theory, only certain discrete energy levels are allowed in the atom and electrons/holes can occupy only these allowed energy levels. Spatial quantization results in the production of energy levels above the conduction band minimum in a quantum well. The minimum electron and hole energies within the well are both above the conduction band and valence band minima respectively. If electron and hole recombine, the energy of the emitted photon is greater than that of the energy gap. It is found that the energy of the emitted photon is a strong function of the well width. The narrower the width, the greater the quantum state energy. This means in a very narrow width device, the energy of emitted photon is greater than that of a wider well width device. By adjusting the well width, the energy of the emitted photon can be tuned.

Limitation of quantum well lasers: The cross-section for the capture of carriers in the well is relatively small. In order to obtain a radiative recombination event, it is necessary for the injected electrons and holes to be captured within the well. To confine the carriers within the well, it is required that they must undergo an inelastic scattering event in order to lose sufficient energy. If there is no scattering events within the well width, the injected carriers will traverse the well without being captured. In other words, we can say that the injected carriers can pass directly over the well without becoming trapped and do not contribute to the optical output. As a result, threshold current density can be relatively high.

Multiple quantum well lasers: The capture probability of a single quantum well laser can be improved by using multiple quantum wells as shown in Fig. 7.48(a), the single quantum well within the active region is replaced by a series of quantum wells. Since, more quantum wells are present in the structure, therefore, there is a higher probability that the injected carrier will suffer an inelastic scattering event and be captured within a well before it can completely traverse the device. Main drawback of multiple quantum well device is that the injected electrons and holes

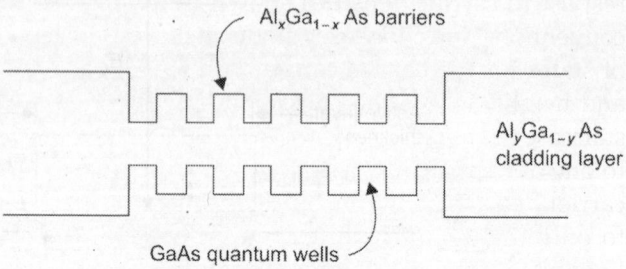

Fig. 7.48(a): Structure of multiple quantum well laser

enter the active region from opposite ends. Therefore, the electrons and holes are not necessarily captured within the same well which acts to reduce the radiative recombination rate. For this reason the multiple quantum well devices do not have the lowest threshold current density of semiconductor laser.

GRINSCH laser: The acronym stands for *graded index separate confinement heterostructures*. This has the lowest threshold current density of existing semiconductor lasers. The structure of this laser is shown in Fig. 7.48(b).

In the structure as shown in Fig. 7.48(b), a single quantum well is embedded within a graded funlike region. The graded region surrounding the quantum well provide a means by which the injected carriers can be funneled into the well. The bandgap grading induces an electric field that directs the electrons and holes into the same quantum well where they can recombine radia-

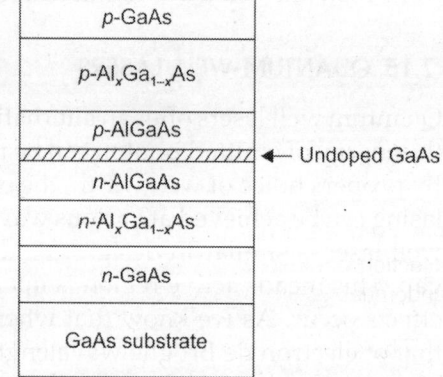

Fig. 7.48(b): Structure of GRINSCH laser

tively. As a result, fewer electrons and holes can traverse the quantum well without being trapped. Thus, the threshold current density of GRINSCH laser is relatively lower than any other lasers.

7.16 QUANTUM-DOT LASERS

More recently, quantum-well lasers have been developed in which the device contains a single discrete atomic structure or so-called *quantum dot* (QD). Quantum dots are small elements that contain a tiny droplet of free electrons forming a quantum-well structure. Hence a QD laser is also referred to as a dot-in-a-well device. They are fabricated using semiconductor crystalline materials and have typical dimensions between nanometers and a few microns. The size and shape of these structures, and therefore, the number of electrons they contain may be precisely controlled such that a QD can have anything from a single electron to several thousand electrons. Theoretical treatment of QDs indicates that they do not suffer from thermal broadening and their threshold current is also temperature insensitive. If the conventional injection laser diode is regarded as three dimensional and a quantum well (i.e. an SQW where an array of SQWs forms an MQW structure) is confined to two dimensions, then the QD structure can be considered to be zero dimensional. It should be noted, however, that the single dimensional structure forms a quantum wire or dash.

The above hierarchy is illustrated in Fig. 7.48 which identifies four different possible structure for the semiconductor laser with their corresponding energy responses with respect to carrier densities shown underneath. The three-dimensional structure of the conventional injection laser diode on the left display an exponential variation in the density of states for the charge carriers. As SQW structure exhibits two dimensions (i.e. length and height) where the corresponding energy representation is shown in Fig. 7.48 by a staircase response in the carrier density of states. However, when this structure is reduced to one dimension (i.e. length only), it displays a sharp rise and an exponential fall in the carrier density variation. Since this one-dimensional quantum-well structure is confined to only the device length, then, in general, it appears as a long wire and hence, it is known as a quantum wire. The zero-dimensional (i.e. single-point) structure shown on the right of Fig. 7.49, however, corresponds to a single QD which results in an impulse response for the variation in the charge carrier density with increasing number of carriers.

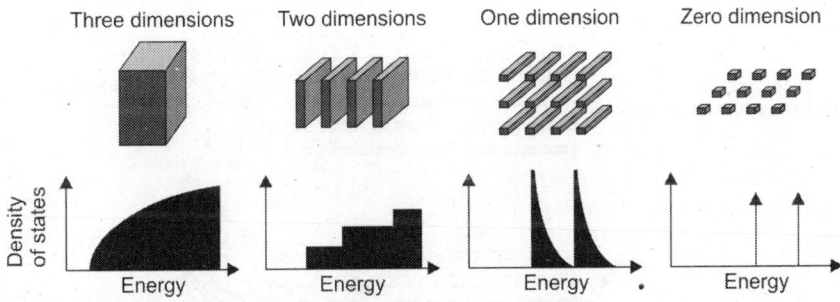

Fig. 7.49: Schematic illustration and density states for semiconductor lasers. From left to right: conventional injection laser diode; multiple quantum wells; array of quantum wires; an array of quantum dots. Shown underneath each of these illustrations is the corresponding density of states for each type of laser structure

The size and shape of the structure for a QD laser can be altered as required during the fabrication process. For example, in fabrication arrays of QDs can be formed on a GaAs substrate with different shapes being produced. Shapes such as the cube, circular disk, cylinder, pyramid or truncated pyramid can be created from self-organized crystalline growth of InGaAs material on the GaAs substrate. Each of these crystal shapes possesses different material characteristics (i.e. elasticity, stress, strain distribution, etc.) and therefore, their different shapes and sizes produce a varying impact on the operation of the QD laser (i.e. emission wavelength, polarization and operating temperature). By contrast, regularity of size and shape in an array improves the control of the QD device lasing frequency and intensity.

One of the important features of the QD laser is its *very low-threshold current density*. For example, low-threshold current densities between 6 and 20 $A \cdot cm^{-2}$ have been obtained with InAs/InGaAs QD lasers emitting at the wavelength of 1.3 μm and 1.5 μm. These low values of threshold current density make it possible to create stacked or cascaded QD structures thus providing high optical gain suitable for the short-cavity transmitters and vertical cavity surface-emitting lasers. Despite the potential benefits of QD technology, issues remain in relation to materials technology and in the design and fabrication techniques to facilitate the large-scale production of QD devices.

7.17 VERTICAL CAVITY SURFACE EMITTING LASERS (VCSELs)

In this structure, the light is emitted normal to the surface as shown in Fig. 7.50. The primary advantages of VCSELs is that the single mode operation can be achieved due to the short cavity length of the device. These devices are better suited than the edge emitting lasers to forming a two-dimensional away. Single mode operation is possible with VCSELs since the mode spacing is inversely proportional to the cavity length. Thus, the smaller the cavity length, the greater the mode spacing which leads to single mode operation. The output wavelength λ_0 is given by:

$$\lambda_0 = \lambda n' \tag{7.130}$$

where λ is wavenelgth of incident light and n' is the refractive index within the laser:

$$\text{Mode index } m = \frac{2Ln'}{\lambda_0}$$

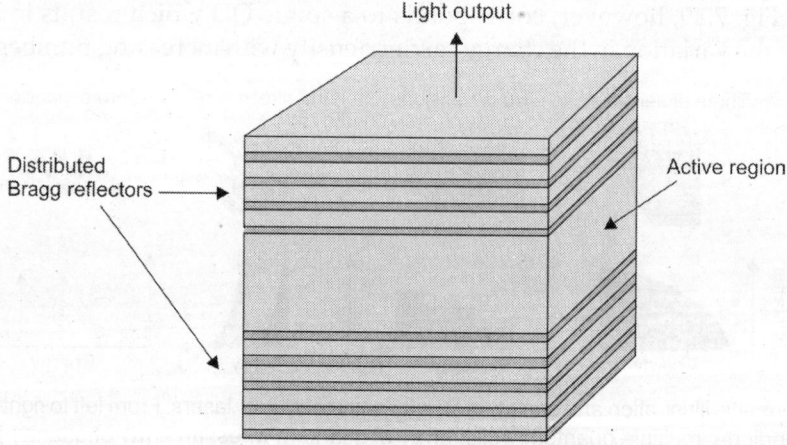

Fig. 7.50: Structure of VCSELs laser

Hence:

$$\frac{dm}{d\lambda_0} = \frac{-2Ln'}{\lambda_0^2} + \frac{2L}{\lambda_0} \frac{dn'}{d\lambda_0} \tag{7.131}$$

where $dm/d\lambda_0$ defines the mode spacing with wavelength. Solving Eq. (7.19), we have:

$$d\lambda_0 = \frac{\left(\dfrac{\lambda_0^2}{2Ln'}\right) dm}{\left[1 - \dfrac{\lambda_0^2}{n'} \dfrac{dn'}{d\lambda_0}\right]} \tag{7.132}$$

The value of dm is 1 for adjacent modes.

From Eq. (7.132), it is clear that the wavelength separation between adjacent modes is inversely proportional to the cavity length.

The major disadvantage of VCSELs is that the cavity length is short as the round trip gain of the device is low. The threshold current density of VCSELs is significantly higher than that of an edge emitting laser.

The operation of semiconductor lasers as sources of electromagnetic radiation is based on the interaction between EM radiation and the electrons and holes in semiconductors (structure of basic *pn* junction semiconductor laser is shown in Fig. 7.51). These are: *vertical cavity surface emitting lasers* (VCSELs), where light propagates perpendicularly to the main plane and in-plane laser where light propagates in the main plane (Fig. 7.52). The largest dimensions of in-plane structures is typically in the range of 250 µm (longitudnial direction), whereas the typical diameter of VCSEL cylinder is about 10 µm.

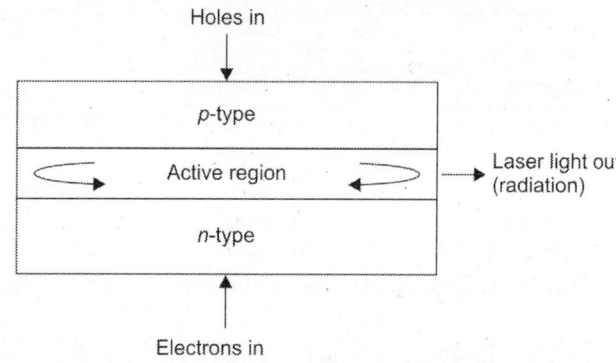

Fig. 7.51: The basic pn junction laser

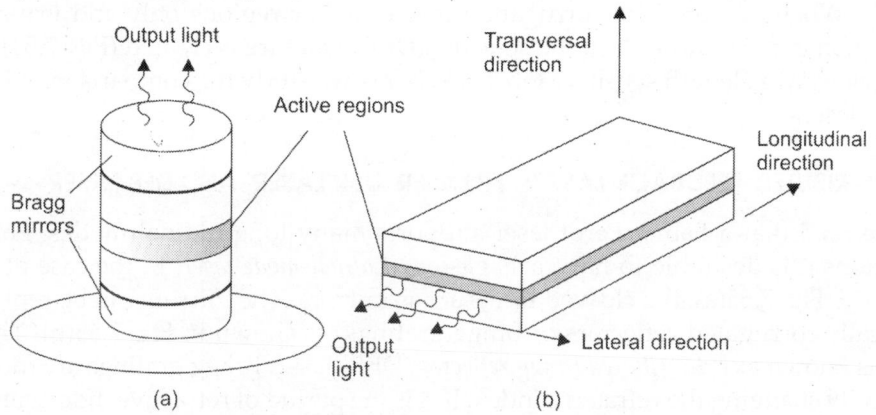

Fig. 7.52: VCSEL (left) and in-plane laser (right)

The basic semiconductor laser is just a *p-n* junction (Fig. 7.51), where cross-section along lateral-transversal directions is shown. Current flows (holes on *p*-side and electrons on *n*-side) along the transversal direction, whereas light travels along the longitudinal direction and leaves device at one or both sides.

In VCSEL, the cavity is formed by the so-called *Bragg mirrors* and an active region typically consists of several *quantum well layers* separated by barrier layers (Fig. 7.52). Bragg mirrors consists of several layers of different semiconductors which have different values of refractive index. Due to the Bragg reflection such structure shows a very large reflectivity (around 99.9%). Such large values are needed because a very short distance of propagation of light does not allow to build enough amplification when propagating between distributed mirrors.

A *three-dimensional prospective view* of some generic semiconductor lasers is shown in Fig. 7.52. The structure consists of many layers of various materials, each engaged in a different role. Those layers are responsible for the efficient transport of electrons and holes from electrodes into an active region and for confinement of carriers and photons, so they can strongly interact. Modern structures contain so-called quantum wells which form an active region and where conduction-valence band transitions are taking place. It is possible to have different types of mirrors as they also provide mode selectivity. Two basic types are illustrated in Figs 7.53 and 7.54. They are known as *distributed feedback* (DFB) and *distributed Bragg* (DBR) structures respectively.

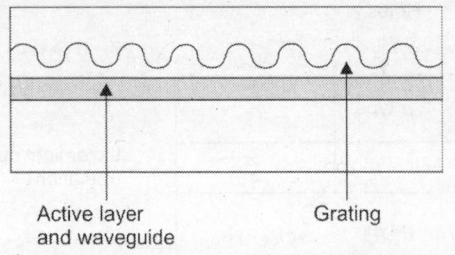

Fig. 7.53: Basic DFB laser structure

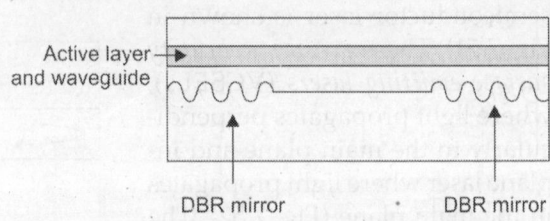

Fig. 7.54: Basic DBR laser structure

In DFB lasers, grating (corrugation) is produced in one of the cladding layers, thus creating Bragg reflections at such periodic structure. The structure causes a wavelength sensitive feedback. It should be emphasized that the grating extends over the entire laser structure. When one restricts corrugation to the mirror regions only and leaves a flat active region in the middle, then the so-called DBR structure is created (Fig. 7.54), which also provides wavelength sensitive feedback. Now, we study the comparison of FP, DBR and DFB lasers.

7.18 DISTRIBUTED-FEEDBACK LASERS: FP LASER, DBR LASER, AND DFB LASER

We have read that a Fabry–Perot laser supports many longitudinal modes. For many applications it is desirable to have a *single-longitudinal-mode laser*. In the case of Fabry–Perot lasers Fig. 7.55(a), the cleaved facets act as mirrors. The mirrors can be replaced by periodically corrugated reflectors or Bragg gratings, as shown in Fig. 7.55(b). This type of laser is known as a *distributed Bragg reflector* (DBR) laser. Bragg gratings are formed by periodically changing the refractive index. If A is the period of refractive index variations, the Bragg grating acts as a reflector with reflection maxima occurring at frequencies.

$$f_m^{\text{Bragg}} = \frac{mc}{2n \wedge}, \quad m = 1.2, \ldots \tag{7.133}$$

where n is the effective mode index. The above condition is known as the *Bragg condition*. The longitudinal modes of the cavity which do not satisfy the Bragg condition to not survive, since the cavity loss (= internal loss + Bragg reflector loss) increase substantially for those longitudinal modes. The longitudinal modes of the cavity are given by

$$f_1 = \frac{lc}{2nL}, \quad l = 0, 2, \ldots \tag{7.134}$$

As an example, if $L = 300$ μm and $n = 3.3$, the frequency separation between longitudinal modes = 0.15 THz. If the main mode frequency = 190 THz, the frequency of two neighboring modes is 189.85 THz and 190.5 THz. The reflection is the strongest for first-order gratings ($m = 1$). If we choose the grating period such that $f_m^{\text{Bragg}} = 190$ THz for

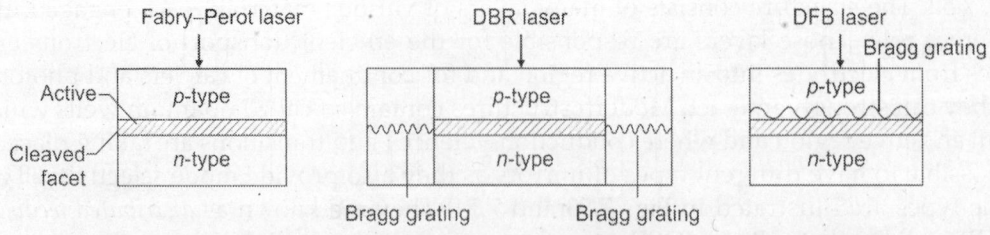

Fig. 7.55: Different laser configurations: (a) FP laser (b) DBR laser (c) DFB laser

$m = 1$, from Eq. (7.133), we find $\wedge = 0.24$ µm. The neighboring modes do not satisfy the Bragg condition given by Eq. 7.134 and, therefore, they suffer huge losses.

One drawback of the DBR is that the corrugated region is part of the cavity and it is somewhat lossy, which of the efficiency of the device. Instead, the corrugated region can be fabricated above the active region as shown in Fig. 7.55(c). Such a laser is known as a *distributed-feedback* (DFB) laser. The grating placed above the waveguide changes the effective index periodically and is equivalent to the waveguide with periodic index variation in the core region. This grating provides coupling between forward- and backward-propagating waves and maximum coupling occurs for frequencies satisfying the Bragg condition, Eq. (7.134). The advantage of a DFB laser is that the corrugated region is not part of the cavity and, therefore, cavity loss does not increase because of the grating. DFB lasers are widely used in applications such as CD players, transmites in fiber-optic communications, and computer memory readers.

7.19 ELECTRON TRANSITIONS IN SEMICONDUCTORS

We now extend the previous discussion of TLS to describe the transitions between bands in semiconductors (Fig. 7.56). We introduce:
- f_v the probability of the state of energy E_v in the valence band being filled.
- f_c the probability of the state of energy E_c in the conduction band being filled.

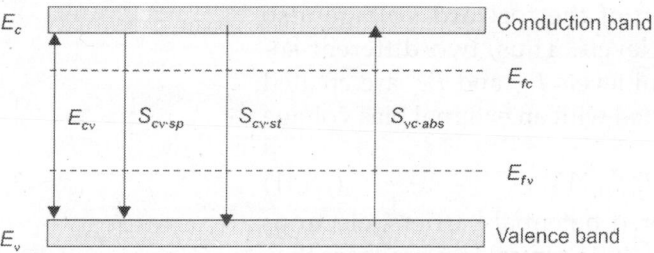

Fig. 7.56: Electron transitions between conduction and valence bands

Rates of transitions can now be determined, similarly to the TLS description. Here, we use index rotation appropriate to semiconductors, i.e. c, v instead of 1, 2. The rates are:

$$S_{\text{spon}} = S_{cv\text{-}sp} = A_{21} f_c (1 - f_v) \tag{7.135}$$

$$S_{\text{stim}} = S_{cv\text{-}st} = B_{21} f_c (1 - f_v)(E_{cv}) \tag{7.136}$$

$$S_{\text{abs}} = S_{cv\text{-}abs} = B_{12} f_v (1 - f_c)(E_{cv}) \tag{7.137}$$

Fermi-Dirac statistics are assumed for the appropriate probabilities as:

$$f_v = \frac{1}{\exp\left(\dfrac{E_v - E_{Fc}}{kT} + 1\right)} \tag{7.138}$$

$$f_c = \frac{1}{\exp\left(\dfrac{E_c - E_{Fc}}{kT} + 1\right)} \tag{7.139}$$

Here E_{Fc} and E_{Fv} are the quasi-Fermi levels for electrons and holes.

The condition for stimulated emission to exceed absorption is:

$$S_{\text{stim}} > S_{\text{abs}}$$

which gives: $\qquad B_{21} f_c = (1 - f_v) > B_{12} f_v (1 - f_c)$

Since the coefficnents B_{21} and B_{12} are equal, after substituting expressions (7.138) and (7.139), one obtains:

$$\exp\left(\frac{E_v - E_{Fv}}{kT}\right) > \exp\left(\frac{E_c - E_{Fc}}{kT}\right)$$

which can be written in the form:

$$E_{Fc} - E_{Fv} > E_c - E_v = h\nu \tag{7.140}$$

The above inequality is known as *Bernard–Duraffourg condition*.

7.20 HOMOGENEOUS *pn* JUNCTION

Figure 7.57 shows energy band diagram of *p-n* junction in thermal equilibrium and under *forward bias* condition.

Electrons at the *n*-type side do not have enough energy to climb over the potential barriers to the left. Similar situation exists for holes in the *p*-type region [Fig. 7.57(a)]. One needs to apply forward voltage to lower the potential barriers for both electrons and holes [Fig. 7.57(b)].

An application of the forward voltage also separates Fermi levels. Thus, two different so-called quasi-Fermi levels E_{Fc} and E_{Fv} are created which are connected with an external bias voltage as:

$$E_{Fc} - E_{Fv} = eV_{\text{bias}} \tag{7.141}$$

With the lowered potential barriers, electrons and holes can penetrate central region where they can recombine and produce photons. However, the confinement of both electrons and holes into the central region is very poor (there is no mechanism

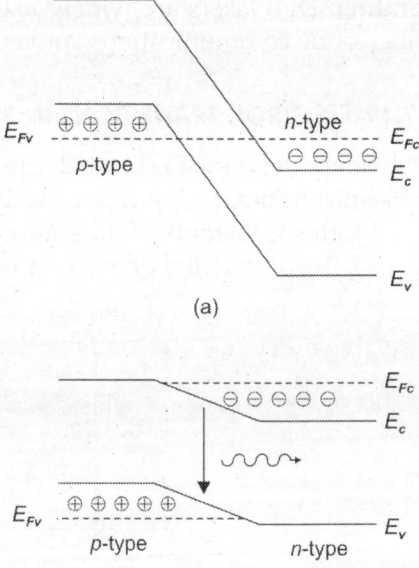

Fig. 7.57: Energy-band diagram of a p-n junction. (a) thermal equilibrium, (b) forward bias

to confine those carriers). Also, there is no confinement of photons (light) into the region where electrons and holes recombine (the region is known as an active region). Therefore, the interaction between carriers and photons is weak, which makes homojunctions a very poor light source. One must, therefore, provide some mechanism which will confine both carriers and photons into the same physical region where they will strongly interact. Such a concept is possible with the invention of heterostructures.

7.20.1 Heterostructures

A heterojunction is formed by joining dissimilar semiconductors. The basic type is formed by two heterojunctions and it is known as a *double-heterojunction* (more popular name is *double-heterostructure*).

The materials forming double heterostructures have different bandgap energies and different refractive indices. Therefore, in a natural way potential wells for both electrons and holes are created. Schematic energy-band diagram of a double-heterostructure *p-n* junction in thermal equilibrium and under forward bias conditions are shown in Fig. 7.58. The bandgap and refractive index for *InGaAsP* material (Fig. 7.59) will now be summarized.

Band Gap

For the $In_{1-x}Ga_xAs_yP_{1-y}$ system, the relation between compositions x and y which results in the lattice match to InP is:

$$y = \frac{0.1894y}{0.4184 - 0.013y} \quad (7.142)$$

In such case the bandgap is:

$$E_{gap}[eV] = 1.35 - 0.72y + 0.12y^2 \quad (7.143)$$

with the extra relations $y \approx 2.20x$ and $0 \leq x \leq 0.47$. The material for such compositions thus covers bandgaps in the range of wavelengths 0.92 µm to 1.65 µm. For example, the material $In_{0.74}Ga_{0.26}As_{0.57}P_{0.43}$ (i.e. $x = 0.26$, $y = 0.57$) has bandgap $E_g = 0.97$ eV, which corresponds to the wavelength $\lambda = 1.27$ µm.

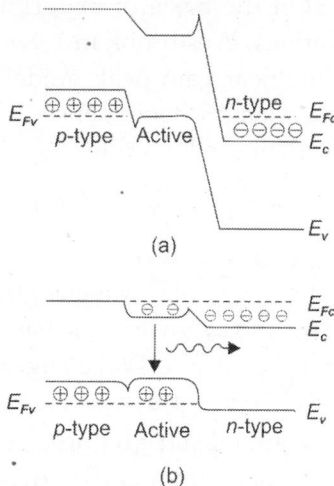

(a)

(b)

Fig. 7.58: Energy-band diagram of a double-heterostructure p-n junction. (a) Thermal equilibrium (b) forward bias

Refractive Index

As explained earlier, the dependence of refractive index as a function of wavelength is described by *Sellmeier equation*. For important telecommunication wavelengths, namely 1.3 µm and 1.55 µm, the y dependence of refractive index $In_{1-x}Ga_xAs_yP_{1-y}$ that is lattice matched to InP is shown in Table 7.2.

Table 7.2: Typical values of refractive indices for various compositions		
Wavelength (λ)	Range of y compositions	Refractive index (n)
$\lambda = 1.3$ mm	$0 \leq y \leq 0.6$	$n(y) = 3.205 + 0.34y + 0.21y^2$
$\lambda = 1.55$ mm	$0 \leq y \leq 0.9$	$n(y) = 3.166 + 0.26y + 0.09y^2$

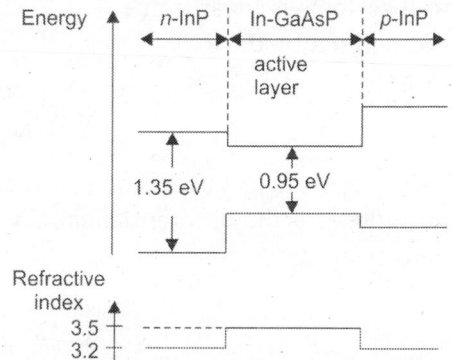

Fig. 7.59: Band structure and refractive index for InGaAsP/InP heterostructure

7.20.2 Optical Gains

For efficient and reliable numerical simulations, an exact mathematical expression of the material gain is critical. Such an expression should also be subject to an experimental verification. This problem has been investigated since the early developments of semiconductor lasers. The first step is usually the determination of gain spectra and its comparison with experiment. The simplest approach will be provided in the next section. Typical curves of gain spectra for a *four quantum well system* & comparison with experimental measurements are shown in Fig. 7.60. Mathematics involved in determining optical gain of semiconductor quantum-well structures is complex. As a result, analytic approximations of the optical gain which can be used in fast calculations were determined. From an extensive discussion, it was determined that the peak material gain for bulk materials varies linearly with carrier density.

$$g(N, \lambda) = a(\lambda) \min(N, P) - b(\lambda) \quad (7.144)$$

The parameter $a(\lambda)$ is commonly called the *differential gain*.

On the basis of experimental observations, Westbrook in 1986, 87 extended the linear gain peak model to allow for wavelength dependence. In its simplest form, it can be written as:

$$g(N, \lambda) = a(\lambda_p) \, N - b(\lambda_p) - b_a \, (\lambda - \lambda_p)^2$$

$$(7.145)$$

where λ_p is the wavelength of the peak gain and b_a governs the base width of the gain spectrum. Wavelength peak λ_p can be also carrier density dependent.

Gain (absorption) in a semiconductor is a function of carrier density n [cm^{-3}] (Fig. 7.61), which shows gain spectrum for several values of carrier concentration. When n is below *transparency density* n_{tr}, the medium absorbs optical signal. For $n > n_{tr}$, optical gain in the material exceeds loss. The dependence of the so-called *gain peak* on the carrier density for quantum well systems is logarithmic (Fig. 7.62). It is described by the expression:

$$g = g_0 \ln \frac{N}{N_{tr}}$$

$$(7.146)$$

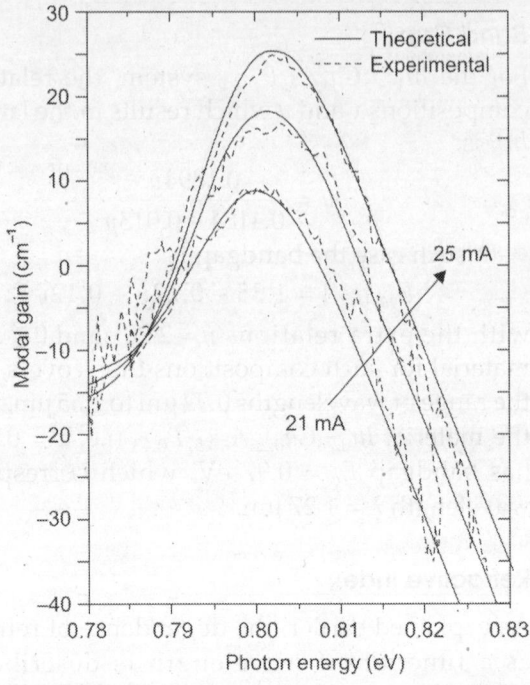

Fig. 7.60: Fitted theoretical and experimental net modal gain vs photon energy including leakage terms for three values of injected current

For modelling purposes, a linear approximation is often employed. In the above formulas g_0 is the differential gain, N_{tr} transparency carrier density and N_{th} is the carrier density at threshold.

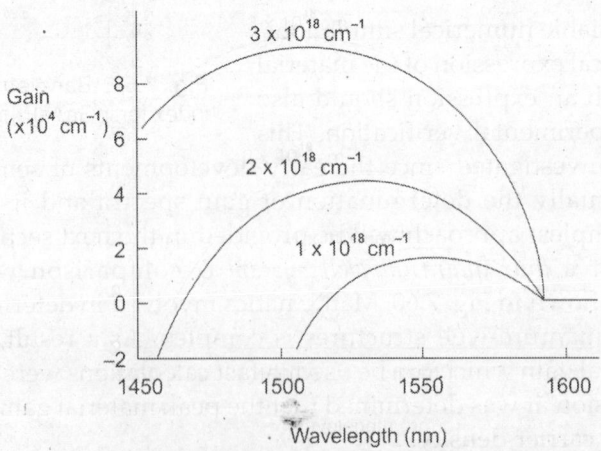

Fig. 7.61: Schematic of optical gain spectra for various carrier densities

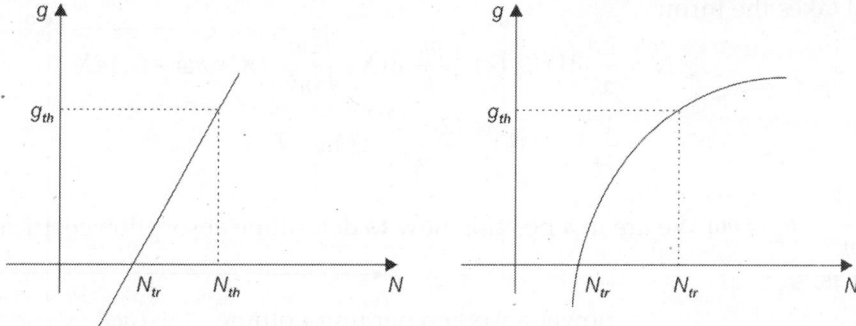

Fig. 7.62: Illustration of threshold and transparency densities for linear (left) and logarithmic (right) gain models

7.20.3 Determination of Optical Gain

The simplest approach to determine *optical gain* is based on *Fermi golden rule*. Here we derive it for $T = 0$. Transition rate between two levels a and b is:

$$W_{ab} = \frac{2\pi}{\hbar} \mid H'_{ab} \mid^2 \delta (E_b - E_a - \hbar\omega) \qquad (7.147)$$

where H'_{ab} is the matrix element describing transitions between a and b. Assume parabolic bands for both electrons and holes with the effective mass m^* taking the value of m_c^* for conduction band and m_v^* for a valence band as follows:

$$E(k) = \frac{h^2 k^2}{2m^*} \qquad (7.148)$$

From the above:

$$E_b - E_a = \frac{\hbar^2 k^2}{2} \left(\frac{1}{m_c} + \frac{1}{m_v} \right) + E_g \qquad (7.149)$$

Due to conservation of the crystal momentum in the transition, one has $k_{ln} = k_{fi}$. For a single transition at specific value of k, one therefore has:

$$W(k) = \frac{2\pi}{\hbar} \mid H'_{vc} (k)^2 \mid \delta \left(\frac{\hbar^2 k^2}{2m_r} + E_g - \hbar\omega \right) \qquad (7.150)$$

where $m_r = \dfrac{m_v m_c}{m_v + m_c}$ is reduced effective mass. If N is a total number of transitions per second in crystal volume V and $g(k) = k^2 V / \pi^2$ is number of states per unit k in volume V, the total number of transitions per second is:

$$N = \int_0^\infty W(k) \cdot g(k) \, dk$$

$$= \frac{2V}{\pi\hbar} \int_0^\infty \mid H'_{vc} (k)^2 \delta \left(\frac{\hbar^2 k^2}{2m_r} + E_g - \hbar\omega \right) k^2 dk \qquad (7.151)$$

To evaluate integral, let us introduce new variable:

$$X \equiv \frac{\hbar^2 k^2}{2m_r} + E_g - \hbar\omega$$

Integral takes the form:

$$N = \frac{2v}{\pi h} \int |H'_{vc}(k)|^2 \frac{m_r}{h} \delta(X) \sqrt{\frac{2m_v}{\hbar^2}(X + \hbar\omega - E_g)} dX$$

$$= \frac{V}{H} |H'_{vc}(k)|^2 \frac{(2m_c)^{3/2}}{\hbar^4}(\hbar\omega - E_g)^{1/2} \tag{7.152}$$

where $\frac{\hbar^2 k^2}{2m_r} + E_g = \hbar\omega$. We are in a position now to determine absorption coefficient α. It is defined as:

$$\alpha(\omega) \equiv \frac{\text{power absorbed per unit volume}}{\text{power crossing a unit area}} = \frac{N \cdot (\hbar\omega)/V}{\varepsilon_0 n E_0^2 c/2} \tag{7.153}$$

where n is refractive index, c is the velocity of light in a vacuum and E_0 is the amplitude of electric field. Use:

$$H'_{vc}(k) = \frac{eE_0 \chi_{vc}}{2}, \chi_{vc} = \langle u_{vk'} | x | u_{ck} \rangle \tag{7.154}$$

Using the above and expression for N, one finds:

$$a_0(\omega) = \frac{\omega e^2 \chi_{vc}^2 (2m_r)^{3/2}}{2\pi\varepsilon_0 n c \hbar^3}(\hbar\omega - E_g)^{1/2} = K(\hbar\omega - E_g)^{1/2} \tag{7.155}$$

Example: Estimation of K

Data for GaAs. $\hbar\omega = 1.5$ eV, $m_v = 0.46m_0$, $m_c = 0.067m_0$, $\chi_{vc} = 3.2$Å, $n = 3.64$. Those data give $K \approx 11700$ cm^{-1} (eV)$^{-1/2}$, and $\alpha_0(\omega) = 1170$ cm^{-1}.

At $T = 0$ depending on the value of $\hbar\omega$, one has the following possibilities summarized next:

$$\hbar\omega < E_g \qquad \alpha(\omega) = 0$$
$$E_g < \hbar\omega < E_{Fc} - E_{Fv} \qquad \alpha(\omega) = -\alpha_0(\omega) = -K(\hbar\omega - E_g)^{1/2} \quad \text{amplification} \tag{7.156}$$
$$E_{Fc} - E_{Fv} < \hbar\omega \qquad \alpha(\omega) = -\alpha_0(\omega) = -K(\hbar\omega - E_g)^{1/2} \quad \text{absorption}$$

7.21 RATE EQUATIONS

With all basic elements in place, we are now in a position to provide the simplest (phenomenological) description of semiconductor lasers based on rate equations. The main role in those devices is played by two subsystems: carriers (electrons and holes) and photons. They interact in the so-called **active region**, defined as part of the structure where recombining carriers contribute to useful gain and photon emission. We describe both subsystems separately, starting with carriers.

In Fig. 7.63, we schematically depict a model of a laser operating below threshold. It resembles a tank partially filled with water continuously flowing in and at the same time water leaves the tank. The water models carriers which are continuously provided by current flowing in. Not all the current at electrodes actually reaches the device (tank). Some of it is lost as so-called leakage current. Below threshold, carriers disappears through losses in the device (R_{loss}), nonradiative recombination (R_{nr}) and spontaneous emission (R_{sp}). Above threshold (Fig. 7.64), the tank is completely filled with water (in laser the situation corresponds to the so-called threshold with density (N_{th}). Its operation is mostly dominated by yet another process, namely stimulated emission (here characterized by coefficient R_{st}).

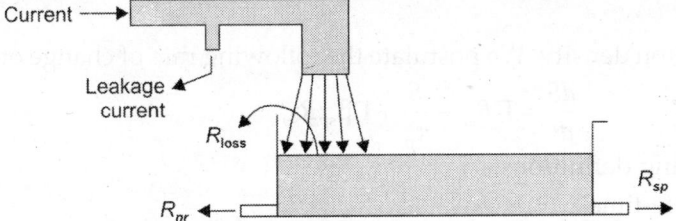

Fig. 7.63: Model of a laser operating below threshold

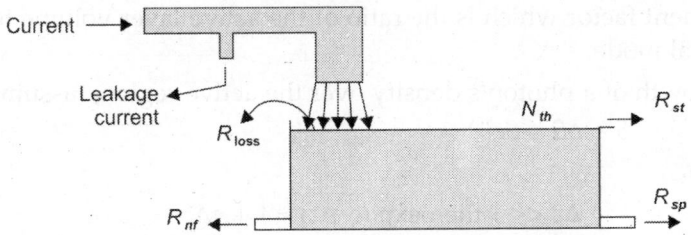

Fig. 7.64: Model of a laser operating above threshold

Now, based on the above picture, we will formulate equations describing dynamics of carriers and photons.

7.21.1 Carriers

Inside the laser, there exist two types of carriers: electrons and holes. Both are described in a similar way; however, parameters used will be different for both types.

The rate of change of carrier density is governed by:

$$\frac{dN}{dt} = G_{\text{gener}} - R_{\text{recom}} \tag{7.157}$$

where the term on right are responsible for generation and recommendation of carriers and are given by:

$$G_{\text{gener}} = \eta_i \frac{1}{q \cdot V}$$

with V being the volume of the active region, q is the electron's charge and I is the electric current. The internal efficiency n_i describes the fraction of terminal current that generates carriers in the active region. The recombination term consists of several contributions:

$$R_{\text{recom}} = R_{sp} + R_{nr} + R_l + R_{st}$$

The meaning of terms is as rollows:

R_{sp} – spontaneous recombination rate

R_{nr} – nonradiative recombination rate

R_l – carrier leakage rate

R_{st} – net stimulated recombination rate

Recombination processes are described phenomenologically as:

$$R_{\text{recom}} = \frac{N}{\tau} + v_g g(N)S \tag{7.158}$$

7.21.2 Photons

Let S be the photon density. We postulate the following rate of change of photon density:

$$\frac{dS}{dt} = \Gamma R_{st} - \frac{S}{\tau_p} + \Gamma \beta_{sp} R_{sp}$$

with the following definitions:

τ_p – photon life-time

β_{sp} – spontaneous emission factor (reciprocal of the number of optical modes)

R_{st} – stimulated recombination

Γ – confinement factor which is the ratio of the active layer volume to the volume of the optical mode.

Consider growth of a photon's density over the active region, (assume $\Gamma = 1$):

$$S + \Delta S = S e^{g \cdot \Delta z}$$

where g is gain.

If $\qquad\qquad \Delta z \ll 1$ then $\exp(g \cdot \Delta z) \approx 1 + g \Delta z$

Using the relation $\Delta z = v_g \Delta t$ (v_g – group velocity), one finds $S = S g \cdot v_g \cdot \Delta t$. Thus, the generation term can be written as:

$$\left(\frac{dS}{dt}\right)_{gen} = R_{st} = \frac{\Delta S}{\Delta t} + v_g g S$$

Finally, the rate equations used in this section are:

$$\frac{dN}{dt} = \eta_i \frac{I}{qV} - \frac{N}{\tau} - v_g g(N) S \qquad (7.159)$$

$$\frac{dS}{dt} = \Gamma v_g g(N) S - \frac{S}{\tau_p} + \Gamma \beta sp R_{sp} \qquad (7.160)$$

We have explicitly indicated that gain g depends on a carrier's concentration.

7.21.3 Rate Equation Parameters

Other important parameters which in the simple model can be taken as constants due to complicated dependencies. Those parameters are:

(i) the carrier's lifetime τ which strongly depends on carrier's density. Typical dependence is shown below:

$$\frac{1}{\tau} = A + BN + CN^2 \qquad (7.161)$$

where coefficient A describes nonradiative processes, B is responsible for spontaneous recombination and C describes *nonradiative Auger recombinations*.

(ii) photon lifetime τ_p which is:

$$\frac{1}{v_g \tau_p} = \alpha_i + \alpha_m + \Gamma g_{th} \qquad (7.162)$$

Here α_m describes mirror reflectivity:

$$\alpha_n = \frac{1}{L} \ln \frac{1}{R} \qquad (7.163)$$

and α_i account for all losses.

The meaning of all parameters appearing in rate equations and gain models is summarized in Table 7.3 along with typical values for those symbols.

Table 7.3: Basic parameters appearing in rate equation approach and their typical values

Symbol	Description	Value and unit
N	carrier density	cm^{-3}
S	photon density	cm^{-3}
I	current	mA
q	elementary charge	1.602×10^{-19}C
L	cavity length	250 µm
w	width of active region	2 µm
d	thickness of active region	80Å
h_i	fraction of the injected current I into active region	0.8
V_{active}	volume of active region	$L \cdot w \cdot d$
τ	carrier lifetime	2.71 ns
v_g	group velocity	c/n_{ref}
n_{ref}	refractive index	3.4
τ_p	photon lifetime	2.77 ps
Γ	confinement factor	0.01
β_{sp}	spontaneous emission factor	10^{-4}
a	differential gain (linear model)	5.34×10^{-16} cm^2
N_{tr}	carrier density at transparency	3.77×10^{18} cm^{-3}
I_{th}	current at threshold	1.11 mA
α_m	facet loss	45 cm^{-1}
λ_{ph}	laser wavelength	1.3 µm

In the following, rate equations will provide a starting point for analysis of dynamical properties of semiconductor lasers. Before we start detailed analysis based on rate equations, we will establish a rate equation for electric field.

7.21.4 Derivation of Rate Equation for Electric Field

The relevant equation will be derived starting from the wave equation.

$$\nabla^2 E(r, t) - \frac{1}{c^2} \frac{\partial^2}{\partial t^2} E(r, t) = \mu_0 \frac{\partial^2}{\partial t^2} P(r, t) \tag{7.164}$$

Assume the following decomposition:

$$E(r, t) = \hat{a} E_t (x, y) \sin (\beta_z z) E(t) e^{j\omega t} \tag{7.165}$$

where $\hat{a}$ is a unit vector describing polarization, β_z propagation constant in the z-direction. The transversal field $E_t (x, y)$ obeys the following equation:

$$\left(\frac{\partial^2}{\partial x^2} + \frac{\partial^2}{\partial y^2} \right) E_t (x, y) = - k_t^2 E_t (x, y) \tag{7.166}$$

It is further assumed that $E(t)$ is slowly varying compared to $e^{j\omega t}$. Substituting Eq. (7.165) into Eq. (7.164), neglecting fast-varying terms in time, one obtains:

$$\left\{ k_t^2 - \beta_z^2 - \frac{1}{c^2} \left[2j\omega \frac{\partial E(t)}{\partial t} - \omega^2 E(t) \right] \right\} a E_t (x, y) \sin (\beta_z z) e^{jwt} = \mu_0 \frac{\partial^2}{\partial t^2} P(r, t)$$

To evaluate terms on the right hand side, we need to account for a nonlocal relation between polarization and susceptibility:

$$P(r, t) = \varepsilon_0 \int \chi(r, t') E(r, t - t') dt' \qquad (7.167)$$

In the above $E(r, t - t')$ is given by Eq. (7.165). As $E(t)$ is slowly varying in time, we can expand it into Taylor series around t. The general formula for Taylor expansion of the function $f(x)$ around a is $f(x) + \dfrac{df}{dx}(x - a)$. In our case, substituting $x = t - t'$ and $a = t$, we obtain:

$$E(t - t') \approx E(t) + \frac{dE(t)}{dt}(-t')$$

Full electric field is therefore:

$$E(r, t - t') = E_t(x, y) \sin(\beta_z z) E(t - t') e^{j\omega(t - t')}$$

Substituting the last result and Taylor expansion for $E(t - t')$ into expression for polarization [Eq. (7.167)], one finally obtains the wave equation for $E(t)$:

$$\left[-\beta_0^2 + \frac{\omega^2}{c^2} \varepsilon_r(\omega) \right] E(t) - \frac{2j\omega}{c^2} \left[\varepsilon_r(\omega) + \frac{1}{2} \omega \frac{d\varepsilon_r(\omega)}{d\omega} \right] \frac{dE(t)}{dt} = 0 \qquad (7.168)$$

Here $\varepsilon_r(r, \omega) = 1 + \chi(r, \omega)$ and Fourier transform of susceptibility is (we have dropped dependence):

$$\chi(\omega) = \int dt' \chi(t') e^{-j\omega t'}$$

Susceptibility is further separated into terms which account for various physical effects as follows:

$$\chi(\omega) = 1 + \chi_b + \chi_p - j\chi_{loss}$$

where $\chi_b = \chi_b' = j\chi_b''$ is due to background $\chi_p = \chi_p' = j\chi_p''$ is induced by pump and χ_{loss} accounts for losses. The relative dielectric constant is written as (dropping argument dependencies) $\varepsilon_r = \varepsilon_r' + j\varepsilon_r''$. The real part of ε_r is approximated in terms of refractive index:

$$\varepsilon_r = (n_0 + \Delta n_p)^2 \approx n_0^2 + 2n_0 \Delta n_p$$

where n_0 is the background refractive index and Δn_p is the change induced by pump. Using the above results, ε_r takes the form:

$$\varepsilon_r = \varepsilon_r' + j\varepsilon_r'' = n_0^2 + 2n_0 \Delta n_p + j\varepsilon_r''$$
$$= 1 + \chi_b' + \chi_p' + j(\chi_b'' + \chi_p'' - \chi_{loss}) \qquad (7.169)$$

Explicitly, one has the following identifications:

$$1 + \chi_b' = n_0^2$$
$$\chi_p' = 2n_0 \Delta n_p$$
$$\chi_b'' + \chi_p'' - \chi_{loss} = \varepsilon_r''$$

Using the above relations, the term in the equation for slowly varying amplitude $E(t)$, Eq. (7.168) is:

$$\frac{\omega^2}{c^2} \varepsilon_r(\omega) - \beta_0^2 = \frac{\omega^2 - \omega_0^2}{c^2} n_0^2 + \frac{\omega^2}{c^2} \chi_p' + j \frac{\omega^2}{c^2}(\chi_b'' + \chi_p'' - \chi_{loss}) \qquad (7.170)$$

where we have used the approximate relation:

$$\beta_0 \approx \frac{\omega_0}{c} n_0$$

Imaginary parts of background and pump susceptibilities are related to gain via an experimental relation:

$$\frac{\omega}{cn_0}(\chi_b'' + \chi_p'') = \Gamma g(N)$$

where $g(N)$ is gain. Assume also:

$$\chi_{loss} = \frac{\omega}{cn_0}\alpha_{loss}$$

With the last two relations, term given by Eq. (7.170) can be expressed as:

$$\frac{\omega^2}{c^2}\varepsilon_r(\omega) - \beta_0^2 = \frac{\omega^2 - \omega_0^2}{c^2}n_0^2 + \frac{\omega^2}{c^2}2n_0\Delta n_p + j\frac{\omega n_0}{c}[\Gamma g(N) - \alpha_{loss}]$$

Using $n^2(\omega) = \varepsilon_r(\omega)$, the dispersion term in Eq. (7.168) is evaluated as:

$$\varepsilon_r(\omega) + \frac{1}{2}\omega\frac{d\varepsilon_r(\omega)}{d\omega} = n^2(\omega) + \frac{1}{2}\omega n(\omega)\frac{dn(\omega)}{d\omega} \tag{7.171}$$

$$= n(\omega) + \omega n_g(\omega)$$

where we have defined group index $n_g(\omega)$ as:

$$n_g(\omega) = n(\omega) + \omega\frac{dn(\omega)}{d\omega} \tag{7.172}$$

Using the results Eqs (7.170) and (7.171), Eq. (7.169) takes the form:

$$\frac{dE(t)}{dt} = \left\{-j(\omega - \omega_0)\frac{n_0}{n_g} - j\frac{\omega}{n_g}\Delta n_p + \frac{1}{2}v_g[\Gamma g(N) - \alpha_{loss}]\right\}E(t) \tag{7.173}$$

where we approximated $\omega^2 - \omega_0^2 = (\omega - \omega_0)(\omega - \omega_0) \simeq 2\omega(\omega - \omega_0)$ and also $\frac{n_0(\omega)}{n(\omega)} \simeq 1$ and used the relation $\frac{c}{n_g} = v_g$.

7.22 ANALYSIS BASED ON RATE EQUATIONS

Rate equation just introduced will now be used to study some *dynamical properties* of semiconductor lasers. Let us start with steady-state.

7.22.1 Steady-State Analysis

In this situation there is no change in time, i.e.:

$$\frac{dN}{dt} = \frac{dS}{dt} = 0$$

Rate equations take the form:

$$\eta_i\frac{I_0}{qV} - \frac{N_0}{\tau} - v_g g(N_0)S_0 = 0 \tag{7.174}$$

and

$$\Gamma v_g g(N_0)S_0 - \frac{S_0}{\tau_p} + \Gamma\beta_{sp}R_{sp} = 0 \tag{7.175}$$

If in the last equation, we neglect the small spontaneous emission term, we obtain an expression for a photon life-time:

$$\frac{1}{\tau_p} = \Gamma v_g g(N_0) \tag{7.176}$$

7.22.2 Small-Signal Analysis with the Linear Gain Model

When neglecting spontaneous emission and using linear gain model where gain is given by $g = a\,(N - N_{tr})$, one obtains:

$$\frac{dN}{dt} = n_i \frac{I}{qV} - \frac{N}{\tau} - v_g a\,(N - N_{tr})\,S \tag{7.177}$$

and

$$\frac{dS}{dt} = \Gamma v_g a\,(N - N_{tr})\,S - \frac{S}{\tau_p} \tag{7.178}$$

Assume that all time-dependent quantities oscillate as:

$$I = I_0 + i(\omega)e^{j\omega t}$$
$$N = N_0 + n(\omega)e^{j\omega t}$$
$$S = S_0 + s(\omega)e^{j\omega t}$$

where ω is the angular frequency of an external (small) perturbation and I_0 is the bias value of current. Here N_0 and S_0 are the solutions in the steady-state. Substitute into the first rate equation and after multiplication and neglecting second-order term $(n(\omega)s(\omega))$, one obtains:

$$j\omega n(\omega)e^{j\omega t} = \frac{n_i}{qV}[I_0 + i(\omega)e^{j\omega t}] - \frac{N_0}{\tau} - \frac{1}{\tau}n(\omega)e^{j\omega t}$$
$$-v_g a\big((N_0 - N_{tr})S_0 + (N_0 - N_{tr})s(\omega)e^{j\omega t} + S_0 n(\omega)e^{j\omega t}\big) + O(n^2)$$

Using steady-state results, expression (7.176) for photon life-time and dropping $e^{j\omega t}$ dependence, one finally obtains:

$$j\omega n(w) = \frac{n_i}{qV} i(\omega) - \frac{n(\omega)}{\tau} - \frac{s(\omega)}{\Gamma\tau_p} - v_g a S_0 n(\omega) \tag{7.179}$$

The second equation for photons is obtained in a similar way. Substituting small signal expressions, neglecting the second-order term, using the photon life-time expression and finally dropping $e^{j\omega t}$ dependence, one obtains:

$$j\omega s(\omega) = \Gamma v_g a S_0 n(\omega) \tag{7.180}$$

From the above equations, we want to determine *modulation response* which is defined as:

$$M(\omega) = \frac{s(\omega)}{i(\omega)}$$

Expressing $n(\omega)$ from Eq. (7.180) and substituting into Eq. (7.179), one obtains:

$$\frac{s(\omega)}{i(\omega)} = \frac{\dfrac{n_i}{eV}\Gamma v_g a S_0}{D(\omega)}$$

where $D(\omega)$ is given by:

$$D(\omega) = -\omega^2 + j\omega\left(\frac{1}{\tau} + v_g a S_0\right) + \frac{v_g a S_0}{\tau_p}$$

We define response function as:

$$r(\omega) = \left|\frac{s(\omega)}{i(\omega)}\right| = \frac{\dfrac{n_i}{eV}\Gamma v_g a S_0}{|D(\omega)|}$$

If we write $D(\omega) = a + jb$, we have $|D(\omega)|^2 = a^2 + b^2$. Therefore:

$$|D(\omega)|^2 = \left(\omega^2 - \frac{v_g a S_0}{\tau_p}\right) + \omega^2 \left(\frac{1}{\tau} + v_g a S_0\right)^2$$

We will see that the response function has a peak at frequency f_R. To find that frequency, we evaluate first derivative $\dfrac{\partial |D(\omega)|^2}{\tau_p}$ and set it to zero. Explicity:

$$\left.\frac{\partial |D(\omega)|^2}{\partial \omega^2}\right|_{\omega = \omega_R} = -2\left(\frac{v_g a S_0}{\tau_p} - \omega_R^2\right) - \frac{1}{2}\left(\frac{1}{\tau} + v_g a S_0\right) = 0$$

From the above:

$$\omega_R^2 = \frac{v_g a S_0}{\tau_p} - \frac{1}{2}\left(\frac{1}{\tau} + v_g a S_0\right) \tag{7.181}$$

which is known as a *relaxation-oscillation frequency* and it describes the rate at which energy is exchanged between photon system and carriers. The second term in Eq. (7.64) is usually very small and can be neglected. Relaxation-oscillation frequency is thus approximated as:

$$\omega_r = \sqrt{\frac{1}{\tau_p} \frac{S_0 v_g a}{1 + \varepsilon S_0}} \tag{7.182}$$

To estimate the typical values of the relaxation-oscillation frequency, let us assume: $L = 300 \ \mu m$, $\tau_{ph} \approx 10^{-12}$ s and $\tau \sim 4 \times 10^{-9}$ s. One finds $AP_0 \sim 10^9$ s^{-1}. So, the zeroth-order expression is a very good one.

The modulation characteristics of semiconductor lasers are shown in Fig. 7.65.

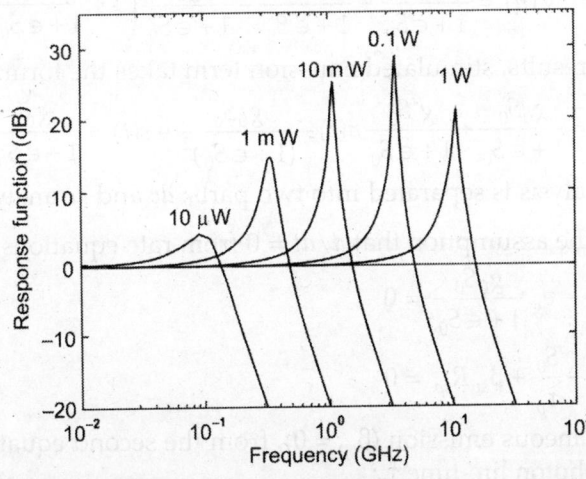

Fig. 7.65. Modulation characteristics of semiconductor lasers from small-signal analysis

7.22.3 Small-Signal Analysis with Gain Saturation

Let us remind ourselves of the rate equations which were established in the previous section:

$$\frac{dN}{dt} = n_i \frac{I}{qV} - \frac{N}{\tau} - v_g g(N)S \tag{7.183}$$

$$\frac{dS}{dt} = \Gamma v_g g(N)S - \frac{S}{\tau_p} + \beta_{sp}R_{sp} \qquad (7.184)$$

Use small-signal assumptions:

$$I(t) = I_0 + i(t)$$
$$N(t) = N_0 + n(t)$$
$$S(t) = S_0 + s(t)$$

Also, generalize the gain model to include saturation as follows:

$$g(n) = \frac{g_0 + g'(N - N_0)}{1 + \epsilon S}$$

where $g' = \left.\dfrac{\partial g}{\partial N}\right|_{N = n_0}$ is differential gain evaluated at $N = N_0$ and $g_0 = g(N_0)$. The factor $1 + \epsilon S$ introduces nonlinear gain saturation. The gain compression parameter ϵ has a small value and the term ϵS is small compared with the one even at very high optical power. The effect of this term on dc properties is small and can be neglected. However, it significantly affects dynamics of a semiconductor laser. The reason is that the laser's dynamics depends on the small difference between gain and cavity loss. This difference is only about a few percent. Therefore, even small gain compression due to ϵ produces significant effects.

One can evaluate the gain compression term as follows:

$$1 + \epsilon S\; 1 + \epsilon[S_0 + s(t)] = (1 + \epsilon S_0)\left(1 + \frac{\epsilon s(t)}{1 + \epsilon S_0}\right)$$

With the above result, gain can be approximated as:

$$g(n) = \frac{g_0}{1 + \epsilon S_0} + \frac{g'n(t)}{1 + \epsilon S_0} - \frac{g_0}{1 + \epsilon S_0}\left(1 + \frac{\epsilon s(t)}{1 + \epsilon S_0}\right) \qquad (7.185)$$

Using the above results, stimulated emission term takes the form:

$$g(n)S = \frac{g_0 S_0}{1 + \epsilon S_0} + \frac{g' S_0}{1 + \epsilon S_0}n(t) - \frac{g_0 S_0}{(1 + \epsilon S_0)^2}\epsilon s(t) + \frac{g_0}{1 + \epsilon S_0}s(t) + O(s^2) \quad (7.186)$$

The following analysis is separated into two parts: dc and ac analysis.

DC analysis: With the assumption that $d/dt = 0$ from rate equations, one obtains:

$$\eta\frac{I_0}{qV} - \frac{N_0}{\tau} - v_g\frac{g_0 S_0}{1 + \epsilon S_0} = 0$$

and $\qquad \Gamma v_g\dfrac{g_0 S_0}{1 + \epsilon S_0} - \dfrac{S_0}{\tau_p} + \beta_{sp}R_{sp} = 0$

Neglecting spontaneous emission ($\beta_{sp} = 0$), from the second equation, one obtains an expression for the photon life-time τ_p:

$$\frac{1}{\tau_p} = \Gamma v_g\frac{g_0}{1 + \epsilon S_0} \qquad (7.187)$$

AC analysis: Substituting small-signal assumptions into rate equations, and using an approximation of stimulated emission Eq. (7.186) and eliminating DC terms, one obtains:

$$\frac{dn(t)}{dt} = n_i\frac{i(t)}{qV} - \frac{n(t)}{\tau} - \frac{v_g g' S_0}{1 + \epsilon S_0}n(t) + \frac{1}{\tau_p\Gamma}\frac{S_0}{1 + \epsilon S_0}\epsilon s(t) - \frac{1}{\tau_p\Gamma}s(t)$$

$$\frac{ds(t)}{dt} = \frac{\Gamma v_g g' S_0}{1+\epsilon S_0} n(t) - \frac{1}{\tau_p} \frac{S_0}{1+\epsilon S_0} \epsilon s(t)$$

In obtaining the above equations we used Eq. (7.187). Those equations can also be written in matrix form:

$$\frac{d}{dt} \begin{bmatrix} n(t) \\ s(t) \end{bmatrix} + \begin{bmatrix} A & B \\ -C & D \end{bmatrix} \begin{bmatrix} n(t) \\ s(t) \end{bmatrix} = \begin{bmatrix} \eta_i \dfrac{n(t)}{qV} \\ 0 \end{bmatrix}$$

where $A = \dfrac{1}{\tau} + \dfrac{v_g S_0 g'}{1+\epsilon S_0}$, $B = \dfrac{1}{\tau_p \Gamma} - \dfrac{1}{\tau_p \Gamma} \dfrac{S_0}{1+\epsilon S_0} \epsilon$, $C = \dfrac{\Gamma v_g S_0 g'}{1+\epsilon S_0}$, $D = \dfrac{1}{\tau_p} \dfrac{S_0}{1+\epsilon S_0} \epsilon$

Assuming harmonic time dependence of the form $exp\,(j\omega t)$, the matrix equation is:

$$\begin{bmatrix} j\omega + A & B \\ -C & j\omega + D \end{bmatrix} \begin{bmatrix} n(t) \\ s(t) \end{bmatrix} = \begin{bmatrix} \eta_i \dfrac{i(t)}{qV} \\ 0 \end{bmatrix}$$

Solving the above system, one obtains modulation response which is expressed as:

$$\frac{s(t)}{i(t)} = \eta_i \frac{1}{qV} \frac{C}{H(\omega)}$$

where
$$H(\omega) = (j\omega + A)\,(j\omega + D) + CB$$

The function $H(\omega)$ can be written as:

$$H(\omega) = -\omega^2 + j\omega\gamma + \omega_R^2$$

Here ω_R is the relaxation-oscillation frequency and γ is the damping factor. One defines modulation response $r(\omega)$ as:

$$r(\omega) = \frac{H(\omega)}{H(0)}$$

The plot of response $r(\omega)$ is shown in Fig. 7.66 for three values of ϵ_r. The effect of gain compression parameter ϵ is clearly visible.

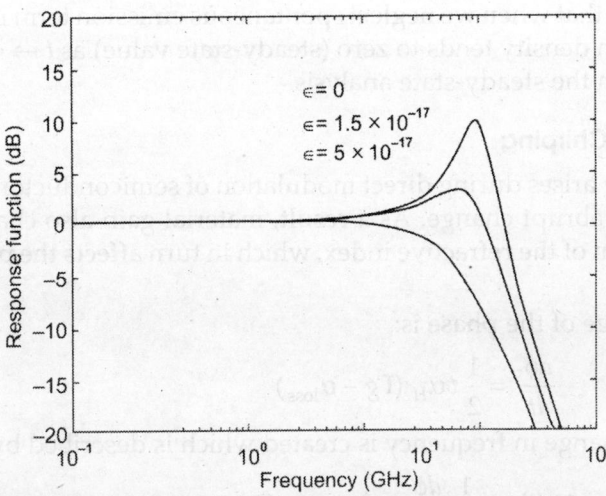

Fig. 7.66: The effect of gain compression on modulation response

7.22.4 Large-Signal Analysis for QW Lasers

Main equations for large-signal analysis without spontaneous emission are:

$$\frac{dN}{dt} = \eta_i \frac{I}{eV} - \frac{N}{\tau} - v_g g(N) \cdot S \tag{7.188}$$

$$\frac{dS}{dt} = \Gamma \cdot v_g g(N) \cdot S - \frac{S}{\tau_p} \tag{7.189}$$

All symbols have been explained previously and their values are summarized in Table 7.3.

Typical results for step current are shown in Fig. 7.67.

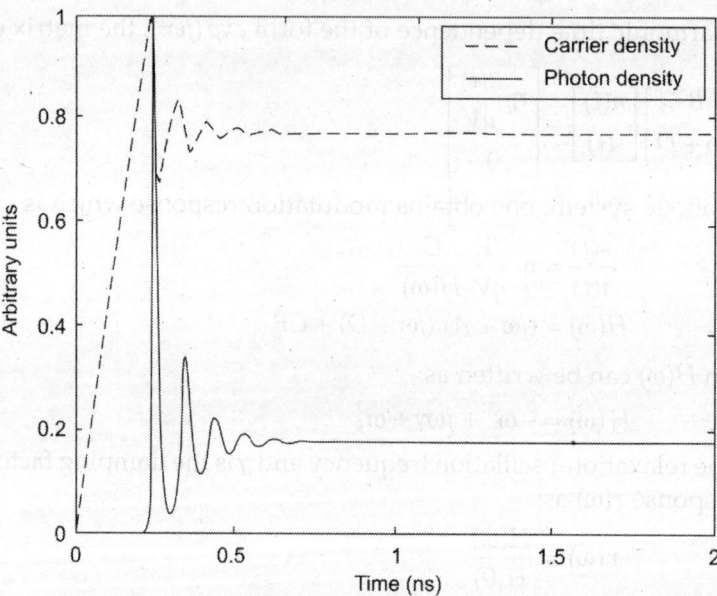

Fig. 7.67: Numerical solutions of large-signal rate equations after applying rectangular current pulse at t = 0. Normalized values of electron density N(t) and photon density S(t) are shown

One can observe that when we neglect spontaneous emission term in the rate equation for photons, photon density tends to zero (steady-state value) as $t \to \infty$, the result which is also evident from the steady-state analysis.

7.22.5 Frequency Chirping

Frequency chirping arises during direct modulation of semiconductor laser when carrier density undergoes abrupt change. As a result, material gain also changes. This change results in a variation of the refractive index, which in turn affects the phase of the electric field.

The rate of change of the phase is:

$$\frac{d\phi}{dt} = \frac{1}{2} v \alpha_H (\Gamma g - \alpha_{loss})$$

An associated change in frequency is created which is described by:

$$\Delta v(t) = \frac{1}{2\pi} \frac{d\phi}{dt} = \frac{1}{4\pi} v \alpha_{enh} (\Gamma g - \alpha_{loss}) \tag{7.189a}$$

This change in frequency is called *chirp*. During direct modulation, it results in a shift in frequency of the order of 10–20 GHz.

To eliminate chirp effect, an external modulator should be used. In such cases a laser produces constant output power and a separate modulator provides modulation.

Another way to reduce chirp is to fabricate devices with small values of line-width enhancement factor α_H.

$$\alpha_H \equiv -\frac{dn_r/dN}{dn_i/d\nu} \tag{7.189b}$$

where $n = n_r + jn_i$ (complex refractive index).

7.22.6 Equivalent Circuit Model for a Bulk Laser

Equivalent circuit models of semiconductor lasers provide further understanding of the laser properties. They are derived from rate equations. More recent works include additional effects like carrier transport or proper representation of optical gain. In the following, we outline the creation of equivalent circuit model for a bulk semiconductor laser.

For bulk lasers, rate equations are:

$$\frac{dS}{dt} = (G - \gamma)S + R_{sp} \tag{7.190}$$

$$\frac{dN}{dt} = \frac{1}{q} - \gamma_e N - G \cdot S \tag{7.191}$$

Here N, S are the total number of electrons inside the cavity and total number of photons is the lasing mode. Those are dimensionless quantities. We introduce small deviations from equilibrium as:

$$S(t) = S_0 + \delta S(t) \tag{7.192a}$$
$$N(t) = N_0 + \delta N(t) \tag{7.192b}$$

Optical gain is approximated as:

$$G = G_0 + \frac{\partial G}{\partial N}\delta N + \frac{\partial G}{\partial S}\delta S = G_0 + G_N \delta N + G_S \delta S \tag{7.193}$$

In the steady-state, one obtains:

$$0 = (G_0 - \gamma)S_0 + R_{sp,0}$$

$$0 = \frac{I_0}{q} - \gamma_e N_0 - G_0 \cdot S_0$$

Observing that spontaneous emission $R_{sp} = R_{sp}(N)$ depends on N, and performing an expansion:

$$R_{sp} = R_{sp\cdot0} + \frac{\partial R_{sp}}{\partial N}\delta N \tag{7.194}$$

one can derive small-signal equations:

$$\frac{d\delta S}{dt} = -\Gamma_S \delta S + \sigma_N \delta N \tag{7.195}$$

$$\frac{d\delta N}{dt} = -\Gamma_N \delta N + \sigma_N \delta S \tag{7.196}$$

where
$$\Gamma_S = \frac{R_{sp}}{S_0} - S_0 G_S, \quad \Gamma_N = \gamma_e + N_0 \frac{\partial \gamma_e}{\partial N} + S_0 G_N \tag{7.197}$$

and
$$\sigma_N = S_0 G_N + \frac{\partial R_{sp}}{\partial N}, \quad \sigma_S = G_0 + S_0 G_S \tag{7.198}$$

Using these equations, one creates equivalent circuit model. It is based on an observation that the small-signal rate equations are similar to the voltage and current equations of the RLC circuit. We therefore assume that electrons in a laser cavity can be represented by the charge across a capacitor and the photons are represented by the magnetic flux of an inductor. Formally one introduces the following equivalence:

$$\delta S(t) = \frac{\phi(t)}{q \cdot unit}, \ \delta N(t) = \frac{Q(t)}{q} \tag{7.199}$$

where q is an electron's charge, unit is a parameter in [H/s] to ensure proper units for the components of the electrical circuit and $\phi(t)$ is the magnetic flux in Wb. We also recall standard relations from electro-magnetism:

$$Q = C \cdot V_C \tag{7.200}$$

$$i_C = \frac{dQ}{dt} \tag{7.201}$$

$$\phi(t) = L \cdot i_L \tag{7.202}$$

$$V_L = \frac{d\phi}{dt} \tag{7.203}$$

Now, we use Eq. (7.199) and Eqs (7.200)–(7.203) to convert small-signal Eqs (7.195) and (7.196) into voltage and current relations. After simple algebra, from Eq. (7.195), one obtains:

$$V_L(t) = \Gamma_S \cdot L \cdot i_L(t) + \sigma_N \cdot C \cdot unit \cdot V_C \tag{7.204}$$

This equation can be identified with loop equation for the RLC circuit shown in Fig. 7.68. A loop equation gives:

$$V_C = V_L + V_{Rp} \tag{7.205}$$

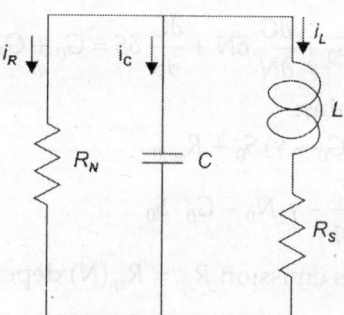

Fig. 7.68: Equivalent circuit model for a bulk laser

In order for the above equations to be identical, one makes the following identifications:

$$R_S = \Gamma_S \cdot L = \Gamma_S \cdot \frac{unit}{\sigma_S}, \quad C = \frac{1}{unit \cdot \sigma_N} \tag{7.206}$$

Similarly, from (7.196), one obtains:

$$i_C(t) = -\Gamma_N \cdot C \cdot V_C(t) - \frac{\sigma_S}{unit} \cdot L \cdot i_L(t) \tag{7.207}$$

That equation can be compared with the node equation from a circuit in Fig. 7.68:

$$i_C = -i_R - i_L \qquad (7.208)$$

For those equations to be identical, one sets:

$$R_N = \frac{1}{\Gamma_N \cdot C}, \quad \text{and} \quad L = \frac{unit}{\sigma_S} \qquad (7.209)$$

One also find the following equivalence:

$$\delta N = \frac{C \cdot V_C}{q}, \quad \text{and} \quad \delta S = \frac{L \cdot i_L}{q \cdot unit} \qquad (7.210)$$

Example 1

In a direct band-gap material, an electron in the conduction band having a crystal momentum of 7.84×10^{-26} kg·m/s makes a transition to the valence band emitting an electromagnetic wave of wavelength 0.8 μm. Calculate the band gap energy. Assume that the effective mass of an electron in the conduction band is $0.07m$ and that in the valence band is $0.5m$, where m is the electron rest mass. Assume parabolic conduction and valence band. **[PTU, KTU]**

Solution

The reduced mass m_r is related to the effective masses as

$$m = \frac{m_{eff,1} m_{eff,2}}{m_{eff,1} + m_{eff,2}}$$

$m_{eff,1} = 0.07m$, $m_{eff,2} = 0.5m$, electron mass $m = 9.109 \times 10^{-31}$ kg,

$$m_r = \frac{0.07 \times 0.5}{0.07 + 0.5} \times 9.109 \times 10^{-31} = 5.59 \times 10^{-32} \text{ kg}$$

The electron momentum is

$$\hbar k_1 = 7.84 \times 10^{-26} \text{ kg . m/s.}$$

The photon energy is

$$\hbar \omega = \hbar 2\pi \frac{c}{\lambda} = \frac{1.054 \times 10^{-34} \times 2\pi \times 3 \times 10^8}{0.8 \times 10^{-6}}$$

$$= 2.48 \times 10^{-19} \text{ J.}$$

$$E_g = \hbar\omega = \frac{\hbar^2 k_1^2}{2m_r} = 2.48 \times 10^{-19} - \frac{(7.84 \times 10^{-26})^2}{2 \times 5.59 \times 10^{-32}} \text{ J}$$

$$= 1.93 \times 10^{-19} \text{ J}$$

Example 2

Using the following parameters:

$$E_g = 1.43 \text{ eV}, \quad N_c = 4.4 \times 10^{23} \text{ m}^{-3}$$

and

$$N_p = 8.2 \times 10^{24} \text{ m}^{-3}$$

Calculate the intrinsic carrier concentration of GaAs at 300 K. **[PTU]**

Solution

At 300 K, the value of the product (kT) in eV becomes

$$kT = 1.38 \times 10^{-23} \times 300 \text{ J} = \frac{4.14 \times 10^{-21}}{1.6 \times 10^{-19}} = 0.0259 \text{ eV}$$

The intrinsic carrier concentration of GaAs at 300K can be estimated using equation

$$n_i = 2 \, (2 \times kT/h^2)^{3/2} \, (m_n^* \, m_p^*)^{3/4} \exp\left(-E_g/2kT\right)$$

or

$$n_i = \sqrt{4.4 \times 10^{23} \times 8.2 \times 10^{24}} \, \exp\left(-\frac{1.43}{2 \times 0.0259}\right) \approx 1.96 \times 10^{12} \text{ m}^{-3}$$

Example 3

A laser beam has a power of 50 mW. It has an aperture of 5×10^{-3} m and it emits light of wavelength 7200 Å. The beam is focussed with a lens of focal length 0.1 m. Show that the areal spread and the intensity of the image are 2.074×10^{-10} m^2 and 2.4×10^8 Wm^{-2} respectively.

Solution

$$d\theta = \lambda/d \qquad\qquad [\lambda = 7200 \times 10^{-10} \text{ m}]$$

or

$$d\theta = \frac{7200 \times 10^{-10}}{5 \times 10^{-3}} = 1.44 \times 10^{-4} \text{ radian} \qquad [d = 5 \times 10^{-3} \text{ m}]$$

(i)   Areal spread $= (d\theta f)^2$, Here $f = 0.1$ m.

  or $(1.44 \times 10^{-4} \times 0.1)^2 = 2.074 \times 10^{-10}$ m^2

(ii) Intensity $= \dfrac{\text{Power}}{\text{Area}} = \dfrac{\text{Power}}{\text{Area spread}} = \dfrac{50 \times 10^{-3} \text{ W}}{2.074 \times 10^{-10} \text{ m}^2}$

$$= 2.411 \times 10^8 \text{ Wm}^{-2}$$

Example 4

A laser beam has a wavelength of 8×10^{-7} m and aperture 5×10^{-3} m. The laser beam is sent to moon. The distance of the moon is 4×10^5 km from the earth's surface. Determine (i) the angular spread of the beam, and (ii) the axial spread when it reaches the moon's surface.

Solution

We have $d\theta = \lambda/d$:

(i) Angular spread, $d\theta = \dfrac{8 \times 10^{-7}}{5 \times 10^{-3}} = 1.6 \times 10^{-4}$ radiation,

$$\lambda = 8 \times 10^{-7} \text{ m}, d = 5 \times 10^{-3} \text{ m}$$

(ii) Areal spread $= (D d\theta)^2$ where $D = 4 \times 10^5$ km $= 4 \times 10^8$ m

$$= (4 \times 10^8 \times 1.6 \times 10^{-4})^2 = 4.096 \times 10^9 \text{ m}^2$$

Example 5

A laser beam of wavelength 6000 Å on earth is focussed by a lens (or mirror) of diameter 2 m on to a crater on the moon's surface. The distance of the moon from earth is 4×10^8 m. Neglecting the effect of earth's atmosphere, show that the angular spread of the spot on the moon will be 3×10^{-7} radian.

Solution

Angular spread:

$$d\theta = \frac{\lambda}{d} = \frac{6 \times 10^{-7}}{2} = 3 \times 10^{-7} \text{ radian} \qquad \lambda = 600 \times 10^{-10} \text{ m},$$

$$d = 2 \text{ m}, D = 4 \times 10^8 \text{ m}$$

Example 6

A laser beam has aperature $d = 1.8 \times 10^{-2}$ m and emits radiation of wavelength $\lambda = 5 \times 10^{-7}$ m. Calculate (i) the semi-angle of the cone of its beam (ii) the solid angle of this cone.

Solution

(i) The semi-angle of the cone of the laser beam:

$$\theta = \frac{\lambda}{d} = \frac{5 \times 10^{-7} \text{ m}}{1.8 \times 10^{-2} \text{ m}} = 2.72 \times 10^{-5} \text{ radian}$$

(ii) Solid angle of this cone:

$$\phi = \pi \frac{D^2 \theta^2}{D^2} = \pi \theta^2 = \frac{22}{7} \times (2.72 \times 10^{-5})^2 = 2.5 \times 10^{-9} \text{ steradian}$$

Example 7

The coherence length for sodium light is 2.945×10^{-2} m. The wavelength of sodium light is 5890 Å. Determine (i) the number of oscillations corresponding to coherence length, and (ii) the coherence time.

Solution

(i) Number of oscillations in coherence length L:

$$n = \frac{L}{\lambda} = \frac{2.945 \times 10^{-2}}{5890 \times 10^{-10}} = 5 \times 10^4 \quad \lambda = 5890 \times 10^{-10} \text{ m}$$

$$c = 3 \times 10^{10} \text{ m/s,}$$
$$L = 2.945 \times 10^{-2} \text{ m}$$

(ii) Coherence time $= L/c = \dfrac{2.945 \times 10^{-2}}{3 \times 10^{10}} = 9.8 \times 10^{-11}$ s

Example 8

The coherence length for sodium D_1 line is 2.5 cm. Determine (i) the spectral width of the line $\Delta\lambda$ (ii) the purity factor, Q and (iii) the coherence time τ. The wavelength of light is 6000 Å.

Solution

(i) $\Delta\lambda = \dfrac{\lambda}{2L} = \dfrac{36 \times 10^{-10}}{5}$ cm $= 7$Å $\qquad L = 2.5$ cm

$\qquad\qquad\qquad\qquad\qquad\qquad\qquad\qquad\qquad c = 3 \times 10^{10}$ cm·s^{-1}

(ii) $Q = \dfrac{\lambda}{\Delta\lambda} = \dfrac{6 \times 10^{-5}}{7 \times 10^{-8}} = 10^3$

(iii) $\tau = \dfrac{L}{c} = \dfrac{2.5}{3 \times 10^{10}} \cong 0.8 \times 10^{-10}$ s

Example 9

Light from a 2.5 mW water source of aperture diameter 1.8 cm and $l = 500$ nm is focused by a lens of focal length 20 cm. Compute: (a) the area (b) the intensity of the image:

Solution

Given

$\quad \lambda = 500$ nm $= 5 \times 10^{-7}$ m

$\quad 2a = 1.8$ m $= 0.018$

$a = 0.009$ m

$f = 20$ cm $= 0.20$ m

(a) Area of the spot at focal plane $= \dfrac{\pi \lambda^2 f^2}{a^2}$

$$= \dfrac{\pi \times (5 \times 10^{-7})^2 \times (0.20)^2}{(0.009)^2}$$

$$= 3.88 \times 10^{-10} \text{ m}^2.$$

(b) Intensity at the focus $I = \dfrac{Pa^2}{\pi^2 \lambda^2 f^2}$

$$= \dfrac{2.5 \times 10^{-3} \text{ W}}{3.88 \times 10^{-10} \text{ m}^2}$$

$$= 6.44 \times 10^6 \text{ W/m}^2$$

Example 10

Compare the approximate radiative minority carrier lifetimes in gallium arsenide and silicon when the minority carriers are electrons injected into the p-type region which has a hole concentration of 10^{18} cm^{-3}. The injected electron density is small compared with the majority carrier density. **[KTU]**

Solution

The radiative minority carrier lifetime τ_r is given by

$$\tau_r \simeq [B_r(N + P)]^{-1}$$

In the p-type region the hole concentration determines the radiative carrier lifetime as $P \gg N$. Hence:

$$\tau_r \simeq [B_r N]^{-1}$$

Thus for gallium arsenide:

$$\tau_r \simeq [7.21 \times 10^{-10} \times 10^{18}]^{-1}$$
$$= 1.39 \times 10^{-9}$$
$$= 1.39 \text{ ns}$$

For silicon:

$$\tau_r = [1.79 \times 10^{-15} \times 10^{18}]^{-1}$$
$$= 5.58 \times 10^{-4}$$
$$= 0.56 \text{ ms}$$

Thus the direct bandgap gallium arsenide has a radiative carrier lifetime factor of around 2.5×10^{-6} less than the indirect bandgap silicon.

Example 11

A GaAs injection laser has an optical cavity of length 250 μm and width 100 μm. At normal operating temperature the gain factor $\bar{\beta}$ is 21×10^{-3} A cm^{-3} and the loss coefficient $\bar{\alpha}$ per cm is 10. Determine the threshold current density and hence the threshold current for the device. It may be assumed that the cleaved mirrors are uncoated and that the current is restricted to the optical cavity. The refractive index of GaAs may be taken as 3.6. **[DTU, MHTU]**

Solution

The reflectivity for normal incidence of a plane wave on the GaAs–air interface may be obtained as

$$r_1 = r_2 = r = \left(\frac{n-1}{n+1}\right)^2 = \left(\frac{3.6-1}{3.6+1}\right)^2 = 0.32$$

The threshold current density may be obtained from

$$J_{th} = \frac{1}{\beta}\left[\bar{\alpha}\frac{1}{L}\ln\frac{1}{r}\right]$$

$$= \frac{1}{21\times 10^{-3}}\left[10 + \frac{1}{250\times 40^{-4}}\ln\frac{1}{0.32}\right]$$

$$= 2.65\times 10^3 \text{ A cm}^{-2}$$

The threshold current I_{th} is given by:

$$I_{th} = J_{th} \times \text{area of the optical cavity}$$

$$= 2.65\times 10^3 \times 250 \times 10^{-4} \simeq 663 \text{ mA}$$

Obviously, the threshold current for this device is 663 mA if the current flow is restricted to the optical cavity.

Example 12

A double-heterostructure injection laser diode with a cavity length of 400 μm offers a loss of 10^3m^{-1}. The cavity uses uncoated facets as mirrors with reflectivity of 0.33. Calculate the reduction in gain threshold when the reflectivity of the rear mirror is increased to 0.8. Assume the confinement factor to be 0.9. **[KTU, RTU]**

Solution

For the uncoated facets, we have $R_1 = R_2 = 0.33$

The threshold gain for the uncoated facets can be obtained from the relation

$$g_{th} = \frac{1}{\Gamma}\left[\bar{\alpha} + \frac{1}{2L}\ln\left(\frac{1}{R_1 R_2}\right)\right]$$

We have

$$g_{th} = \frac{1}{0.9}\left[10^3 + \frac{1}{400\times 10^{-6}}\ln\left(\frac{1}{0.33\times 0.33}\right)\right]$$

$$= 7270 \text{ m}^{-1}$$

When the reflectivity of the rear mirror is enhanced, then $R_2 = 0.8$ and $R_1 = 0.33$

Therefore, the new threshold gain requirement will be

$$g'_{th} = \frac{1}{0.9}\left[10^3 + \frac{1}{400\times 10^{-6}}\ln\left(\frac{1}{0.8\times 0.33}\right)\right]$$

$$= 4329 \text{ m}^{-1}$$

The reduction in the threshold gain becomes

$$g_u - g'_{th} = 7270 - 4329 = 2941 \text{ m}^{-1}.$$

Example 13

Compare the ratio of the threshold current densities at 20°C and 80°C for an AlGaAs injection laser with $T_0 = 160$ K and the similar ratio for an InGaAsP device with $T_0 = 55$ K.

[PTU, KTU]

Solution

The threshold current density is given by

$$J_{th} \propto \exp \frac{T}{T_0}$$

For the AlGaAs device, we have

$$J_{th}(20°C) \propto \exp \frac{293}{160} = 6.24$$

$$J_{th}(80°C) \propto \exp \frac{353}{160} = 9.08$$

Hence the ratio of the current densities is obtained as

$$\frac{J_{th}(80\,°C)}{J_{th}(20\,°C)} = \frac{9.08}{6.24} = 1.46$$

For the InGaAsP device, we have

$$J_{th}(20\,°C) \propto \exp\frac{293}{55} = 205.88$$

$$J_{th}(80\,°C) \propto \exp\frac{353}{55} = 612.89$$

Hence the ratio of the current densities is obtained as

$$\frac{J_{th}(80\,°C)}{J_{th}(20\,°C)} = \frac{612.89}{205.88} = 2.98$$

Example 14

The gain of an active cavity resonator of an injection laser diode follows Gaussian distribution. If the half-power point, $\lambda - \lambda_0 = 3$ nm, estimate the rms spectral width, σ of the source.

[KTU]

Solution

The gain characteristics of the cavity is given by

$$g(\lambda) = g(0) \exp\left[-\frac{(\lambda - \lambda_0)^2}{(2\sigma^2)}\right]$$

we have

$$g(\lambda) = \frac{1}{2}g(0) \text{ for } \lambda - \lambda_0 = 3 \text{ nm}$$

$$\therefore \qquad \frac{1}{2} = \exp\left(\frac{(3 \times 10^{-9})^2}{2\sigma^2}\right)$$

or

$$\sigma = 1.76 \text{ nm}$$

Example 15

A ruby laser emits 0.1 J pulses of light of wavelength 720 nm. How many minimum number of Cr^{+++} ions are there in ruby?

Solution

Given:
$$E = 0.1 \text{ J}$$
$$\lambda = 720 \text{ nm} = 7.2 \times 10^{-7} \text{ m}$$

The number of Cr^{+++} ions participating in laser action is given by:

$$N = \frac{E}{h\nu} = \frac{E\lambda}{hc}$$

$$= \frac{0.1 \times 7.2 \times 10^{-7}}{6.62 \times 10^{-34} \times 3 \times 10^{8}}$$

$$= 3.625 \times 10^{17}$$

Example 16

Consider an AlGaAs based heterostructure laser diode which has an optical cavity of length 200 microns. The peak radiation is at 870 nm and the refractive index of GaAs is about 3.7. What is the mode integer m of the peak radiation and the separation between the modes of the cavity? If the optical gain vs. wavelength characteristics has a FWHM wavelength width of about 6 mm, how many modes are there within the bandwidth? How many modes are there if the cavity length is 20 μm? **[B Tech]**

Solution

Figure 7.69 schematically illustrates the cavity modes, the optical gain characteristics and a typical output spectrum from a laser. The free-space wavelength λ of a cavity mode and length L are related by:

$$m \frac{\lambda}{2n} = L$$

$$\therefore \qquad m = \frac{2nL}{\lambda} = \frac{2(3.7)(200 \times 10^{-6})}{(900 \times 10^{-9})} \approx 1644.4 \approx 1644.$$

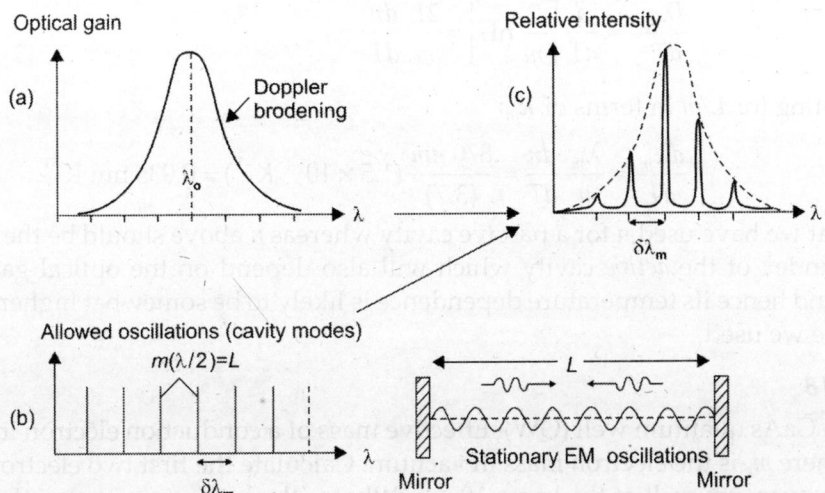

Fig. 7.69: (a) Optical gain vs wavelength characteristics (called the optical gain curve) of the lasing medium (b) allowed modes and their wavelength due to stationary EM waves within the optical cavity (c) the output spectrum (relative intensity vs wavelength) is determined by satisfying (a) and (b) simultaneously, assuming no cavity losses

The wavelength separation $\Delta\lambda_m$ between the adjacent cavity modes m and $(m + 1)$ in Fig. 7.69 is:

$$\delta\lambda_m = \frac{2nl}{m} - \frac{2nl}{m+1} \approx \frac{2nl}{m^2} = \frac{\lambda^2}{2nL}$$

Thus the separation between the modes for a given peak wavelength increases with decreasing L. When $L = 200$ μm:

$$\delta\lambda_m = \frac{(900 \times 10^{-9})^2}{2(3.7)(200 \times 10^{-6})} = 5.47 \times 10^{-10} \text{ m or } 0.5467 \text{ nm}$$

If the optical gain has a bandwidth of $\Delta\lambda_{1/2}$ as in Fig. 7.27, then there will be $\Delta\lambda_{1/2}/\Delta\lambda_m$ number of modes or (6 nm)/(0.547 nm), that is 10 modes.

When $L = 20$ μm, the separation between the modes becomes:

$$\delta\lambda_m = \frac{(900 \times 10^{-9})^2}{2(3.7)(200 \times 10^{-6})} = 5.47 \text{ nm}$$

Then $(\Delta\lambda_{1/2})/\Delta\lambda_{mi} = 1.1$ and there will be one mode that corresponds to about 900 nm. In fact m must be an integer and when $m = 1644$, $\lambda = 902.4$. It is apparent that reducing the cavity length suppresses higher modes. Note that the optical bandwidth depends on the diode current.

Example 17

Given that the refractive index n of GaAs has a temperature dependence $dn/dT \approx 1.5 \times 10^{-4}$ K^{-1} estimate the change in the emitted wavelength 870 nm per degree change in the temperature between mode hops. **[B Tech]**

Solution

Consider a particular given mode with wavelength λ_m.

$$m\left(\frac{\lambda_m}{2n}\right) = L$$

Then,

$$\frac{d\lambda_m}{dT} \approx \frac{d}{dT}\left[\frac{2}{m} nL\right] \approx \frac{2L}{m}\frac{dn}{dT}$$

Substituting for L/m in terms of λ_m:

$$\frac{d\lambda_m}{dT} \approx \frac{\lambda_m}{n}\frac{dn}{dT} = \frac{870 \text{ nm}}{(3.7)}(1.5 \times 10^{-4} \text{ K}^{-1}) = 0.035 \text{ nm K}^{-1}.$$

Note that we have used n for a passive cavity whereas n above should be the effective refractive index of the *active* cavity which will also depend on the optical gain of the medium, and hence its temperature dependence is likely to be somewhat higher than the dn/dT value we used.

Example 18

Consider a GaAs quantum well (QW). Effective mass of a conduction electron in GaAs is $0.07\ m_e$, where m_e is the electron mass in vacuum. Calculate the first two electron energy levels for a quantum well of thickness 10 nm. What is the hole energy below E_c of GaAs if the effective mass of the hole is about $0.50\ m_e$?

What is the change in the emission wavelength with respect to bulk GaAs which has an energy bandgap of 1.42 eV? **[B Tech]**

Solution

The lowest energy levels with respect to the CB edge E_c in GaAs are determined by the energy of an electron in a one-dimensional potential energy well.

$$\varepsilon_n = \frac{h^2 n^2}{8 m_h^* d^2}$$

where n is a quantum number $1, 2, ...,$ and ε_n is the electron energy with respect to E_c in GaAs or $\varepsilon_n = E_a - E_c$. Figure 7.75(b) using $d = 10 \times 10^{-9}$ m, $m_e^* = 0.07$ m, and $n = 1$ and 2, we find, $\varepsilon_1 = 0.0537$ eV and $\varepsilon_2 = 0.215$ eV respectively.

The hole energy levels below E_v in Fig. 7.70(b) are given by:

$$\varepsilon' = \frac{h^2 n^2}{8 m_h^* d^2}$$

Using $d = 10 \times 10^{-9}$ m, $m_h^* \approx 0.5\, m_e$, and $n = 1$, we find, $\varepsilon_1' = 0.0075$ eV. The wavelength of emission from bulk GaAs with $E_g = 1.42$ eV is:

$$\lambda_g = \frac{hc}{E_g} = \frac{(6.626 \times 10^{-34})(3 \times 10^8)}{(1.42)(1.602 \times 10^{-19})} = 874 \times 10^{-9} \text{ m (874 nm)}$$

Whereas from the GaAs QW, the wavelength is:

$$\lambda_{QW} = \frac{hc}{E_g + \varepsilon_1 + \varepsilon_1'} = \frac{(6.626 \times 10^{-34})(3 \times 10^8)}{(1.42 + 0.0537 + 0.0075)/(1.602 \times 10^{-19})}$$

$$= 839 \times 10^{-9} \text{ m (839 nm)}$$

The difference is $\lambda_g - \lambda_{QW} = 35$ nm.

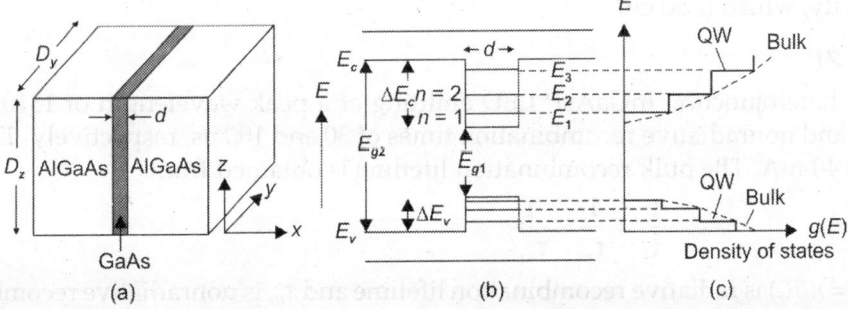

Fig. 7.70: A quantum well (QW) device. (a) Schematic illustration of a quantum well (QW) structure in which a thin layer of GaAs is sandwiched between two wider bandgap semiconductors (AlGaAs). (b) The conduction electron in the GaAs layer are confined by (DE$_c$) in the x-direction to a small length d so that their energy is quantized. (c) The density of states of a two-dimensional QW. The density of states is constant at each quantized energy level

Example 19

The reflection coefficient for a semiconductor laser are equal and have the value 0.5. The length of the cavity is 1 μm. Assuming that there are no additional loss terms, show that the gain of the laser is 6.93×10^3 cm^{-1}.

Solution

We have the gain for laser:

$$g = \alpha_i + \frac{1}{2L} \ln\left(\frac{1}{r_1 r_2}\right)$$

where α_i is the losses within the propagation medium, L is the length of the cavity and r_1 and r_2 are the reflection coefficients of the respective surface. Since there are no internal losses, means $\alpha_i = 0$. Thus, we have:

$$g = \frac{1}{2L} \ln\left(\frac{1}{r_1 r_2}\right)$$

$$= \frac{1}{2 \times 1} \ln\left(\frac{1}{0.5 \times 0.5}\right) = 6.93 \times 10^3 \text{ cm}^{-1}.$$

Example 20

An injection laser has an active cavity with losses of 30 cm^{-1} and reflectivity of each cleaved laser facet is 30%. Show that the laser gain coefficient for the cavity when it has a length of 600 μm is 50 cm^{-1}.

Solution

Here, $r_1 = r_2 = r$.

The threshold gain per unit length is given by:

$$g = \alpha + \frac{1}{L} \ln \frac{1}{r}$$

$$= 30 + \frac{1}{0.06} \ln \frac{1}{0.3}$$

$$= 50 \text{ cm}^{-1}$$

The threshold gain per unit length is equivalent to the laser gain coefficient for the active cavity, which is 50 cm^{-1}

Example 21

A double-heterojunction InGaAsP LED emitting at a peak wavelength of 1310 nm has radiative and nonradiative recombination times of 30 and 100 ns, respectively. The drive current is 40 mA. The bulk recombination lifetime is obtained from:

$$\frac{1}{\tau} = \frac{1}{\tau_r} + \frac{1}{\tau_{nr}} \tag{i}$$

where $\tau_r \ (= n/R_r)$ is radiative recombination lifetime and τ_{nr} is nonradiative recombination lifetime. Calculate τ, internal quantum efficiency (η_{int}) and internal power level.

Solution

$$\tau = \frac{\tau_r \tau_{nr}}{\tau_r + \tau_{nr}} = \frac{30 \times 100}{30 + 100} \text{ ns} = 23.1 \text{ ns}$$

The internal quantum efficiency using Eq. (i)

$$\eta_{int} = \frac{\tau}{\tau_r} = \frac{23.1}{30} = 0.77$$

This yields an internal power level of:

$$P_{int} = \eta_{int} \frac{hcI}{q\lambda}$$

$$= 0.77 \frac{(6.6256 \times 10^{-34} \text{ J} \cdot \text{s}) (3 \times 10^8 \text{ m/s}) (0.040\text{A})}{(1.602 \times 10^{-19} \text{ C}) (1.31 \times 10^{-6} \text{ m})} = 29.2 \text{ mW}$$

Example 22

A 1300 nm InGaAs semiconductor laser has the following parameters:

Active area width $w = 3$ μm

Active area thickness $d = 0.3$ μm

Length $L = 500$ μm

Electron lifetime = 1 ns (associated with spontaneous and nonradiative recombination)

Threshold electron density = 0.8×10^{24} m^{-3}

Internal cavity loss = 46 cm^{-1}

Refractive index = 3.5

Reflectivity $R_1 = R_2 = 0.65$

Under steady-state conditions, calculate (a) the photon lifetime (b) the threshold current, and (c) the current required to generate a mean photon density of 8.5×10^{21} m^{-3}.

[KTU]

Solution

(a) The photon lifetime is given by

$$\tau_p = \frac{1}{v(\alpha_{int} + \alpha_{mir})} \qquad (i)$$

$$\alpha_{int} = 46 \text{ cm}^{-1} = 46 \times 10^2 \text{ m}^{-1} \qquad (ii)$$

The mirror loss is

$$\alpha_{mir} = \frac{1}{2L} \ln\left(\frac{1}{R_1 R_2}\right)$$

$$= \frac{1}{2 \times 500 \times 10^{-6}} \ln\left(\frac{1}{0.65^2}\right)$$

$$= 8.61 \times 10^2 \text{ m}^{-1} \qquad (iii)$$

$$v = \frac{c}{n} = \frac{3 \times 10^8}{3.5} = 8.57 \times 10^7 \text{ ms} \qquad (iv)$$

Using Eqs. (ii), (iii), and (iv) in Eq. (i), we find

$$\tau_p = \frac{1}{8.57 \times 10^7 (46 \times 10^2 + 8.61 \times 10^2)} = 2.13 \text{ ps.}$$

(b) The threshold current I_{in} is related to the threshold electron density by

$$I_{th} = \frac{N_{e,th} q V}{\tau_e}$$

where V is the active volume,

$$V = wdL$$

$$= 0.3 \times 10^{-6} \times 3 \times 10^{-6} \times 500 \times 10^{-6} \text{ m}^3$$

$$= 4.5 \times 10^{-16} \text{ m}^3$$

The electron lifetime $\tau_e = 1 \times 10^{-9}$ s and $N_{e,th} = 0.8 \times 10^{24}$ m^{-3},

$$I_{th} = \frac{0.8 \times 10^{24} \times 1.602 \times 10^{-19} \times 4.5 \times 10^{-16}}{1 \times 10^{-9}} \text{ A}$$

$$= 52.7 \text{ mA.}$$

(c) The mean photon density and the current are related by

$$N_{ph} = \frac{(I - I_{th})\tau_{ph}}{qV}$$

or

$$I = I_{th} + \frac{N_{ph}qV}{qV}$$

$$= 52.7 \times 10^{-3} + \frac{8.5 \times 10^{21} \times 1.602 \times 10^{-19} \times 4.5 \times 10^{-16}}{2.13 \times 10^{-12}}$$

$$= 340.4 \text{ mA.}$$

Example 23

For an atomic system under thermal equilibrium conditions, the ratio of spontaneous emission rate to stimulated emission rate is 2×10^{14}. Find the wavelength of the light emitted. Assume that the temperature is 30°C. [DTU]

Solution

We have

$$\frac{R_{spont}}{R_{stim}} = \exp\left(\frac{\hbar\omega}{k_B T}\right) - 1$$

$$2 \times 10^{14} = \exp\left(\frac{\hbar\omega}{k_B T}\right) - 1$$

$$\approx \exp\left(\frac{\hbar\omega}{k_B T}\right)$$

With $T = 30°C = 303$ K, $k_B = 1.38 \times 10^{-23}$ J/K, and $\hbar = 1.054 \times 10^{-34}$ J·s,

$$\omega = 1.3 \times 10^{15} \text{ rad/s}$$

The wavelength is

$$\lambda = \frac{c}{f} = \frac{2\pi c}{\omega} = \frac{2\pi \times 3 \times 10^8}{1.3 \times 10^{15}} = 1.44 \ \mu\text{m.}$$

Example 24

A laser diode operating at 1.3 μm has a cavity length of 300 μm and the refractive index n of the active region is 3.5. (a) What is the frequency separation between modes? (b) What is the wavelength separation between modes? [MHTU]

Solution

(a) The frequency separation Δf is given by

$$\Delta f = f_{n+1} - f_n = \frac{c}{2nL} = \frac{3 \times 10^8}{2 \times 3.5 \times 300 \times 10^{-6}} = 142.8 \text{ GHz}$$

(b) Since

$$f = \frac{c}{\lambda}$$

we have

$$df = \frac{-c}{\lambda^2} d\lambda$$

or

$$|\Delta\lambda| = \frac{\lambda^2}{c} \Delta f = \frac{(1.3 \times 10^{-6})^2 \times (1.428 \times 10^{11})}{3 \times 10^8}$$

Example 25

In a direct band-gap material, an electron in the valence band having a crystal momentum of 9×10^{-26} kg . m/s makes a transition to the conduction band absorbing a light wave of frequency 3.94×10^{14} Hz. The band gap is 1.18 eV and the effective mass of an electron in the conduction band is 0.07 m, where m is the electron rest mass. Calculate the effective mass of the electron in the valence band.   **[GTU, DTU]**

Solution

We have
$$hf = E_g + \frac{\hbar^2 k_1^2}{2m_r} \tag{i}$$

where
$$\frac{1}{m_r} = \frac{1}{m_{eff,1}} + \frac{1}{m_{eff,2}} \tag{ii}$$

and
$$E_g = 1.18 \text{ eV} = 1.18 \times 1.602 \times 10^{-19} \text{ J} = 1.89 \times 10^{-19} \text{ J}.$$

For a direct band-gap material, $k_1 \approx k_2$. The crystal momentum $\hbar k_1 = 9 \times 10^{-26}$ kg·m/s and the energy of the photon is
$$hf = 6.626 \times 10^{-14} \times 3.94 \times 10^{14} \text{ J} = 2.61 \times 10^{-19} \text{ J}.$$

From Eq. (i), we have
$$\frac{\hbar^2 k_1^2}{2m_r} = hf - E_g = (2.61 \times 10^{-19} - 1.89 \times 10^{-19}) \text{J} = 7.2 \times 10^{-20} \text{ J}$$

$$m_r = \frac{(9 \times 10^{-26})^2}{14.4 \times 10^{-20}} = 5.62 \times 10^{-32} \text{ kg}$$

Since the electron rest mass, $m = 9.109 \times 10^{-31}$ kg, $m_{eff,1} = 0.07\text{m} = 6.37 \times 10^{-32}$ kg, using Eq. (ii), we obtain
$$\frac{1}{m_{eff,2}} = \frac{1}{m_r} - \frac{1}{m_{eff,1}} = \frac{1}{5.62 \times 10^{-32}} - \frac{1}{6.37 \times 10^{-32}} \text{kg}^{-1}$$

$$m_{eff,2} = 4.78 \times 10^{-31} \text{ kg}.$$

Example 26

A laser diode has a 320 μm cavity length, the internal loss coefficient is 10 cm^{-1}. The mirror reflectivities are 0.35 at each end. The refractive index of the active region is 3.3 under steady-state conditions. Calculate

(a) the optical gain coefficient T_g required to balance the cavity loss and
(b) the threshold electron density N_e. Assume that the gain can be modeled as $G = G_0(N_e - N_{e0})$, $G_0 = 1.73 \times 10^{-12}$ m^3/s and $N_{e0} = 3.47 \times 10^{23}$ m^{-3}.   **[DTU]**

Solution

The total cavity loss coefficient is given by
$$\alpha_{cav} = \alpha_{int} + \alpha_{mir}$$

where
$$\alpha_{mir} = \frac{1}{2L} \ln \left[\frac{1}{R_1 R_2} \right] = \frac{1}{2 \times 320 \times 10^{-6}} \ln \left[\frac{1}{0.35^2} \right] = 3.28 \times 10^3 \text{ m}^{-1}$$

The internal loss coefficient is $\alpha_{int} = 10^3$ m^{-1},
$$\alpha_{cav} = 10^3 + 3.28 \times 10^3 \text{ m}^{-1} = 4.28 \times 10^3 \text{ m}^{-1}$$

The optical gain coefficient T_g to balance the cavity loss is

$$T_g = \alpha_{cav} = 4.28 \times 10^3 \text{ m}^{-1}$$

(b) The threshold electron density is

$$N_{e,\text{th}} = N_{e,0} + \frac{1}{G_0 \tau_{ph}}$$

where

$$\tau_{ph} = \frac{1}{v \alpha_{cav}}$$

$$v = \frac{c}{n} = \frac{3 \times 10^8}{3.3} = 9.09 \times 10^7 \text{ ms}^{-1}$$

$$\tau_{ph} = \frac{1}{9.09 \times 10^7 \times 4.28 \times 10^3} = 2.57 \text{ ps}$$

$$N_{e,\text{th}} = 3.47 \times 10^{23} + \frac{1}{1.73 \times 10^{-12} \times 2.57 \times 10^{-12}} \text{ m}^{-3}$$

$$= 5.71 \times 10^{23} \text{ m}^{-3}.$$

SUMMARY

- *Semiconductors* have much higher resistivity than metals. Their temperature coefficient of resistivity (α) is both *negative* and high. They have considerably lower number density of charge carriers than metals. Semiconductors may be elemental (Si, Ge) and compound (GaAs, Cd S, etc)

- *Intrinsic semiconductors* are perfect crystals (no defects or impurities) in which the energy gap between the conduction band and valence band is from a few tenths of an eV upto 2 eV. Electrical conduction in these semiconductors occurs by means of electron-hole pairs. In an interinsic semiconductor $n_e = n_h = n_i$ where $n_e \rightarrow$ the free electron density in the conduction band, $n_h \rightarrow$ the hole density in valence band, and $n_i \rightarrow$ the interinsic carrier concentration.

- At a *given temperature* a specific number of electrons will be thermally excited into the conduction band. They leave behind an equal number of vacant states in the valence band. The action of an *applied field* causes conduction both in the conduction band and in the valence band. The conduction electrons are accelerated by the applied field and carry charge through the semiconductor. The electrons in the valence band move to occupy the adjacent vacancy and the net effect is that the vacancy moves through the material as if it were a positive charge. The vacancies are known as *holes* and are treated as positive charge carriers.

- *Extrinsic semiconductors* are those materials in which the presence of impurities (and also defects) in the crystal lattice determine the properties of semiconductor. The presence of impurities affects the conductivity significantly. The properties of the semiconductor depend on the type of impurity. These are of two two types: (i) *n*-type semiconductors, and (ii) *p*-type semi conductors.

- *p-type semiconductors*: The trivalent impurity atoms called acceptors because they create holes which can accept electrons from the nearby bonds. A semiconductor doped with acceptor type impurities is called *p*-type semiconductors and *holes* are the *majority* charge carriers and electrons are minority charge carriers in these semiconductors. Thus, $n_h \approx N_A > n_e$

- *n-type semiconductors*. The pentavalent impurity atoms are called donors because they donate electrons to the *host* crystal and the semiconductor doped with donors is called *n*-type semiconductor. In these semiconductors, electrons are the majority charge carriers and holes are minority charge carriers. Thus, $n_e \gg N_D - n_h$

- In any semiconductor, $n_e n_h = n_i^2$ and the material on the whole is electrically neutral.

- *Holes*. The vacancy or absence of electron in the bond of covalently bonded crystal is called a hole. A hole in a semiconductor serves a positive charge carrier.

- *Mobility*. The drift velocity acquired by a charge carrier in a unit electric field is called its mobility (μ). $\mu = V/E$. SI unit of μ is $m^2\,V^{-1}\,s^{-1}$.

  The mobility of an electron in the conduction band is greater than that of the hole (or electron) in the valence band.

- *Electrical conductivity of a semiconductor*. When a potential difference V is applied across a conductor of length l and area of cross-section A, then the total current I through it is given by $I = eA\,(n_e V_e + n_h V_h)$ where n_e and n_h are the electron and hole densities and V_e and V_h are their drift velocities, respectively. If $\mu_e = V_e/E$ and $\mu_h = V_h/E$ are electron and hole mobilities, respectively, then the conductivity (σ), which is reciprocal of resistivity (e), is given by

$$\sigma = \frac{1}{\rho} = e\,(n_e\,\mu_e + n_h\,\mu_h)$$

where
$$\rho = \frac{1}{e(n_e\,\mu_e + n_h\,\mu_h)}$$

- The conductivity of an intrinsic semiconductor increases exponentially with temperature as

$$\sigma = \sigma_0 \exp\left(-E_g/2k_B T\right)$$

- *p-n junction*. It is a single crystal of Ge or Si doped in such a manner that one half portion of it acts as a *p*-type semiconductor and other half functions as *n*-type semiconductor. As soon as a *p-n* junction is formed, the holes from the *p*-region diffuse into the *n*-region and electrons from *n*-region diffuse into *p*-region. This results in the development of *potential barrier* (V_B) across the junction which opposes the further diffusion of electrons and holes through the junction. The small region in the vicinity of the *p-n* junction which is depleted of free charge carriers and has immobile ions is called the *depletion region*.

  A *p-n* junction can perform various functions depending on the geometry, the bias conditions, and the doping level in each semiconductor region. Most diodes, transistors, etc., utilize the properties of one or more *p-n* junctions.

  If the materials are dissimilar, e.g. silicon and germanium, the Junction is a *hetero junction*. Normally the same material is used but doped so as to produce two different conductivity types; in this case the junction is a simple *homojunction*.

- *Forward and reverse biasing of a p-n junction*. When the positive terminal of a battery is connected to the *p*-side and the negative terminal to the *n*-side, then the *p-n* junction is said to be *forward biased*. Both electrons and holes move to wards the junction. A current, called forward current, flows across the junction. Clearly, a *p-n* junction offers a low resistance when it is forward biased.

  If the positive terminal of a battery is connected to the *n*-side and the negative terminal to the *p*-side, then *p-n* junction is said to be *reverse biased*. The majority charge carriers move away from the junction. The potential barrier offers high resistance during the reverse bias. However, due to the minority charge carriers a small current, called reverse or leakage current, flows in the opposite direction. Thus, a Junction diode has almost a unidirectional flow of current.

The forward bias current is large (mA) while the reverse bias current is small (mA) in a p-n junction diode.

. • **LASER** (**L**ight **A**mplification by **S**timulated **E**mission of **R**adiation) is a light amplifier source of near monochromatic source of radiation usually used to produce monochromatic coherent radiation in the infrared, visible, and UV regions of the electromagnetic spectrum.

The production of the laser beam depends on *stimulated emission*. The emission of photons that occur following *excitation* of electrons in a system is usually *spontaneous* and cannot be controlled. Stimulated emission is a process whereby an incoming photon of energy hv can stimulate an electron in the high energy state E_2 to jump to a lower energy state E_1, where $E_2 - E_1 = hv$. The photon resulting from this process has the same frequency $v = (E_2 - E_1)/h$, as the stimulating photon and travels in the same direction. If there are sufficient electrons in the high-energy level, both stimulating and stimulated photons can cause further stimulated emission and a narrow beam of monochromatic radiation results, the intensity of which increases exponentially. The laser beam is *coherent* (i.e. spatially and temporarily in phase) and can have a very high energy density.

A laser beam is produced by stimulated emission but can only operate efficiently if a large number of electrons are in a particular high-energy level. This condition is called *population inversion*, is a non-equilibrium condition and power has to be fed into the system to maintain the population inversion.

• **Functioning of laser:** There are three basic requirements of laser: an *active medium, population inversion*, and some sort of feedback. To achieve *population inversion* a right group of atoms or molecules, which is called *active medium* is needed. This active medium is a gas or mixture of gas or crystal or semiconductor.

• **Metastatable state:** The metastable state means long life state compared to other states. In general lifetime of an energy state is 10^{-8} s or more. This is key to the laser. In many atoms one or more metastable states are available.

• **Operation of laser:** For an ideal operation of laser, some conditions have to be satisfied by the system. The relaxation rates from excited state to upper laser level and from lower laser level to ground state should be high to maintain population inversion between upper and lower laser levels.

The *thermal equilibrium* population of laser level should be as small as possible.

The *decay of excited state* to any level other than upper laser level should be as slow as possible.

The *nonradiative decay* of upper laser level should be slow.

• **Properties of laser:**
  (i) *Monochromaticity*: The minimum frequency range for laser is 1 Hz.
  (ii) *Directionality*: Laser can travel large distance without deviation.
  (iii) *Coherence time*: $\Delta \tau = 1/\Delta v$. If $\Delta v = 1$ MHz, then $\Delta \tau = 1$ μs. This time is longer than atomic processes, which are of the order of ns. Sunlight has a bandwidth $\Delta v = 10^{14}$ Hz, hence the coherence time is very short, $\Delta \tau = 10^{-14}$ s.

(iv) *Coherence length*: The distance $\Delta L = c\Delta\tau$ is called the coherence length of the beam. If $\Delta\tau = 1\,\mu s$, the light travel $\Delta L = 3 \times 10^8\,ms^{-1} \times 1\,\mu s = 300$ m.

(v) *Spectral brightness*: The power flow per unit area, per unit bandwidth and per unit solid angle is called brightness of the source:

$$B = \frac{P}{A\,\delta v \Delta\Omega}$$

where A is the surface area (source size), Δv is the band-width and $\Delta\Omega$ is the solid angle (beam divergence). For sun $B = 10^{-12}\,W\cdot cm^{-2}\,Hz\,sr^4$.

- A typical *quantum well* device has an ultra thin, typically less than 50 nm, narrow bandgap semiconductor such as GaAs, sandwitched between two wider bandgap semiconductors, such as AlGaAs.

- The *gain coefficient* g of an active medium is defined as the fractional change in optical intensity per unit length as a light beam passes through. $g = N_{eff}\sigma_g/V_g$, where σ_g is the gain cross-section of a given inverted site, N_{eff} is effective population inversion and V_g is the volume of active medium.

- Every laser must fulfill three basic criteria: (i) Gain to provide stimulated emission (ii) Gain > loss, to sustain reflections (iii) Resonant cavity.

- The semiconductor lasers have some special features such as compactness, high efficiency, capability for high-speed direct modulation, wide emission spectrum and high reliability. However, they are sensitive to temperature.

- *Semiconductor laser* that have been well studied, such as III-V semiconductor lasers, involve strongly interacting states. In such cases, the large Bohr radii of ground state (1 S) *excitons* lead to strong overlap, as enough excitons are generated to reach the lasing threshold. Thus, the excitonic nature of the underlying recombination transition is replaced by a plasma of electrons and holes, and stimulated emission arises from recombining such electrons and holes in the plasma. This situation is naturally linked to the exciton population and to the size of excitons.

- **Exciton:** An electron in combination with a *hole* in a crystalline solid. The electron has gained sufficient energy to be in an excited state and is bound by electrostatic attraction to the positive hole. The exciton may migrate through the solid and eventually the hole and electron recombine with emission of a photon.

REVIEW QUESTIONS

1. Explain the terms: population inversion, spontaneous emission and stimulated emission.

2. Distinguish between spontaneous and stimulated emissions.

3. What are Einstein's coefficients? Derive Einstein's relation. Explain the physical significance of Einstein's coefficients?

4. Derive relation between probabilities of spontaneous and stimulated emission in terms of Einstein's coefficients.

5. Differentiate between three level and four-level systems for lasing action.

6. Describe the principle and working of a semiconductor lasers. Mention its merits and demerits.

7. Write short notes on the following: (i) Metastable state (ii) Population inversion (iii) Pumping (iv) Optical cavity (v) Gain.

8. Explain laser oscillations and obtain the expression for wavelengths of oscillations.

9. What are homogeneous and heterostructure p-n junctions? Draw their energy-band diagrams.

10. What is optical gain? How it can be determined based on Fermi's golden rule.

PROBLEMS

1. Calculate the gain constant β of a laser having the following parameters: wavelength = 650 nm, inversion density $(n_2 - n_1) = 5 \times 10^{22}/m^3$, life time for spontaneous emission 2×10^{-4} s and line width $\Delta\lambda = 15$ Å. **[Ans. 3.95]**

2. Show that for a normal optical source with temperature about 10^3 K and wavelength 6000 Å, the emission is predominantly due to the spontaneous transitions.

3. A laser beam of wave length 6000 Å, power 10 mW, and angular spread 5×10^{-5} rad is focussed by a lens of focal length 10 cm. Calculate the radius and power density of the image. What is lateral coherence width?
[Ans. (i) radius $= 2.5 \times 10^{-4}$ cm, (ii) Power density $= 5.1 \times 10^4$ W/cm^2,
(iii) lateral coherence width $= 1.2$ cm**]**

4. For sodium line, the wave length is 5890 Å and coherence time is 10^{-10} s. Show that the monochromaticity of the source is (5890 ± 0.0578) Å.

5. A transition between the energy levels E_2 and E_1 produces a light of wavelength 632.8 nm. Calculate the energy of the emitted photons. **[Ans. 1.96 eV]**

6. A semiconductor heterojunction laser is grown with GaAsP active region layer with lattice constant 0.56 nm. Assume that laser transition occurs from the bottom of conduction band involving band energy gap 1.85 eV. Determine wavelength of laser emitted. **[Ans. $\lambda = 670$ nm]**

7. The ratio of population inversion of two energy levels out of which upper one corresponds to a metastable state is 1.059×10^{-30}. Find the wavelength of light emitted at 330 K. **[Ans. $\lambda = 632$ nm]**

8. In an atomic system, the spontaneous lifetime associated with $2 \rightarrow 1$ transition is 2 ns and the energy difference between the levels is 2.4×10^{-19} J. Calculate the Einstein A and B coefficients. Assume that the velocity of light in the medium is 1.25×10^8 m/s.

[Hint: We have $A_{21} = \dfrac{1}{\tau_{sp}} = 5 \times 10^8 \text{ s}^{-1}$

The energy difference ΔE is $\Delta E = \hbar\omega$,

$\omega = \Delta E/\hbar\omega = 2.28 \times 10^{15}$ rad/s.

We have $B = \dfrac{A\pi^2 v^3}{\hbar\omega^3}$,

where $v = c/n_0$ is the velocity of light in the medium. With $v = 1.25 \times 10^8$ m/s, we obtain

$$B = \frac{5 \times 10^8 \times \pi^2 \times (1.25 \times 10^8)^3}{1.054 \times 10^{-34} \times (2.28 \times 10^{15})^3}$$

$$= 7.71 \times 10^{21} \text{ m}^3/\text{J} . \text{s}^2]$$

9. The energy levels of an atomic system are separated by 1.26×10^{-19} J. The population density in the ground state is 10^{19} cm^{-3}. Calculate (a) the wavelength of light emitted. (b) the ratio of spontaneous emission rate to stimulated emission rate, (c) the ratio of stimulated emission rate to absorption rate, and (d) the population density of the excited level. Assume that the system is in thermal equilibrium at 300 K.

[**Hint:** (a) The energy difference

$$\Delta E = \hbar \omega = \hbar 2\pi f$$
$$= hf$$

where $h = \hbar 2\pi = 6.626 \times 10^{-34}$ J $\cdot$ s and

$$f = \frac{\Delta E}{h} = \frac{1.26 \times 10^{-19}}{6.626 \times 10^{-34}} = 191 \text{ THz}$$

The wavelength of the light emitted is given by

$$\lambda = \frac{c}{f} = \frac{3 \times 10^8}{191 \times 10^{12}} = 1.56 \, \mu m$$

(b) The ratio of spontaneous emission to stimulated emission rate is given by

$$\frac{R_{spont}}{R_{stim}} = e^{\hbar \omega / k_B T} - 1 = e^{\Delta E / k_B T} - 1$$

$$k_B = 1.38 \times 10^{-23} \text{ J/K}$$
$$T = 300 \text{ K}$$

$$\frac{R_{spont}}{R_{stim}} = \exp\left(\frac{1.26 \times 10^{-19}}{1.38 \times 10^{-23} \times 300}\right) - 1$$

$$= 1.88 \times 10^{13}$$

We have
$$\frac{R_{stim}}{R_{abs}} = \frac{N_2}{N_1}$$

(c) According to Boltzmann's law,
$$N_2 = N_1 e^{-\hbar \omega / k_B T}$$

$$\frac{R_{stim}}{R_{abs}} = e^{-\hbar w / k_B T} = \exp\left(\frac{-1.26 \times 10^{-19}}{1.38 \times 10^{-23} \times 300}\right)$$

$$= 5.29 \times 10^{-14}$$

(d) The population density of the excited level is

$$N_2 = N_1 e^{-\hbar \omega / kBT}$$
$$= 5.29 \times 10^5 \text{ cm}^{-3}]$$

10. A Fabry–Perot laser has the following parameters: internal loss coefficient 50 dB/cm, $R_1 = R_2 = 0.3$, and distance between mirrors = 500 μm. Calculate the longitudinal mode spacing and the minimum gain required for laser oscillation. Assume that the refractive index $n = 3.5$.

[**Hint:** The longitudinal mode spacing Δf is given by

$$\Delta f = \frac{c}{2nL} = \frac{3 \times 10^8}{2 \times 3.5 \times 500 \times 10^{-6}} = 85.71 \text{ GHz}$$

The minimum gain required is

$$g = \alpha_{int} + \alpha_{mir}$$

$$\alpha_{mir} = \frac{1}{2L} \ln \frac{1}{R_1 R_2}$$

The internal loss is given in dB/cm. To convert this into cm^{-1}, consider, a length of 1 cm. The loss over a length of 1 cm is 50 dB,

$$P_{out} = P_{in} \exp(-\alpha_{int} \cdot 1 \text{ cm})$$

$$10 \log_{10} \frac{P_{out}}{P_{in}} = -50 \text{ dB,}$$

$$10 \log_{10} e^{-\alpha_{int} \cdot 1 cm} = -\alpha_{int} \times 1 \text{cm} \times 10 \log_{10} e = -50 \text{ dB}$$

$$\alpha_{int}(\text{cm}^{-1}) = \frac{50}{4.3429} \text{cm}^{-1} = 11.51 \text{ cm}^{-1}$$

The distance between mirrors, $L = 0.05$ cm.

$$R_1 = R_2 = 0.3,$$

$$\alpha_{mir}(\text{cm}^{-1}) = \frac{1}{2 \times 0.05} \ln \frac{1}{0.3^2}$$

$$= 24.07 \text{ cm}^{-1}$$

and

$$g = \alpha_{int} + \alpha_{mir}$$
$$= (11.51 + 24.07) \text{ cm}^{-1}$$
$$= 35.58 \text{ cm}^{-1}]$$

11. In a gain medium, under steady state conditions, the mean power is 20 mW. The area perpendicular to the direction of light propagation is 100 μm^2. The refraction index of the gain medium is 3.2. Calculate the energy density.

[**Hint:** The optical intensity I is power per unit area perpendicular to the direction of light propagation

$$I = \frac{P}{A} = \frac{20 \times 10^{-3}}{100 \times 10^{-12}} = 2 \times 10^8 \text{ W/m}^2$$

The relation between optical intensity and energy density is

$$I = uv = \frac{uc}{n}$$

The energy density is

$$u = \frac{nI}{c} = \frac{3.2 \times 2 \times 10^8}{3 \times 10^8} = 2.13 \text{ J/m}^3]$$

SHORT ANSWER QUESTIONS

1. What is a bandwidth?

Ans. In any material system, the energy levels have a finite spectral (energy) width. This results in a bandwidth for the optical transitions of the system.

Bandwidth is the difference between the upper and lower frequency limits of a band, normally measured in Hz. The band-width may be determined by effects that are common to all sites within the system, resulting in a homogeneously broadened transition, or may be determined by local variations in material properties, leading to an inhomogeneously broadened transition.

2. What is a *p-n* junction?

Ans. The region at which two semiconductors of opposite polarity (*p*-type and *n*-type) meet. A *p-n* junction can perform various functions depending on the geometry, the bias conditions, and the doping level in each semiconductor region. Most diodes transistors, etc. utilize the properties of one or more *p-n* junctions. If the materials are dissimilar, e.g. silicon and germanium, the junction is a *heterojunction*. Normally, the same material is used but doped so as to produce two different conductivity types, in this case the junction is a simple homojunction.

Under reverse bias conditions (i.e. negative bias applied to the *p*-type semiconductor) very little current flows, until *breakdown* occurs. Under forward bias conditions, carriers are attracted across the junction into the region of opposite type (where they become *minority carriers*, and a current flows in the external circuit. The forward in a homojunction increases exponentially with the voltage, i.e.:

$$I = I_0 \, (e^{-eV/k_B T} - 1)$$

where I_0 is reverse saturation current, e is electronic charge and V is applied voltage. Resistance in the material reduces the rate of rise of current through the device after a few tenths of a volt.

3. What are laser diodes?

Ans. Laser diodes are light-emitting devices, capable of emitting laser beams. One of the commonly used laser diode is the *injection laser diode* (ILD). The laser diode works exactly like an ordinary diode. The *p*-type and *n*-type materials are made of AlGaAs (aluminium gallium arsenide).

When forward biased, light is emitted at the *pn* junction. However, unlike the LED the emitted light is coherent and monochromatic. In the LED, the light emitted is scattered in all directions. In the laser diode, however, the light emitted can escape only from the end faces because the edges are roughened. In most laser diodes, one of the end faces is coated with a reflective material so that the radiation of the laser is emitted only in one direction.

The laser diode emits light when forward biased and can with-stand only relatively small reverse-biased voltages. A high reverse voltage can damage or destroy the laser diode.

Laser diodes are used primarily in fiber-optic communications. It is the only device capable of producing optical energy high enough in concentration to pass through lengthy fiber-optic cables.

4. Explain the principle and function of a Laser diode. Briefly explain its operation and mention its applications.

Ans. Laser diode: In a light emitting diode, the emitted light is incoherent. Obviously, when we require coherent light, LED is not useful. For coherent light, we use a laser beam.

Principle: A *pn* junction is manufactured with precisely defined length *L* from GaAs or GaAs combined with other materials. *L* (junction length) is related to λ (wavelength) to be emitted (Fig. 7.71(a)). The ends of the junction are polished to a mirror surface and possibly may have additional reflective coating, so that generated light may reflect back internally into the junction. One end is kept partially reflective so that light can pass through when lasing occurs.

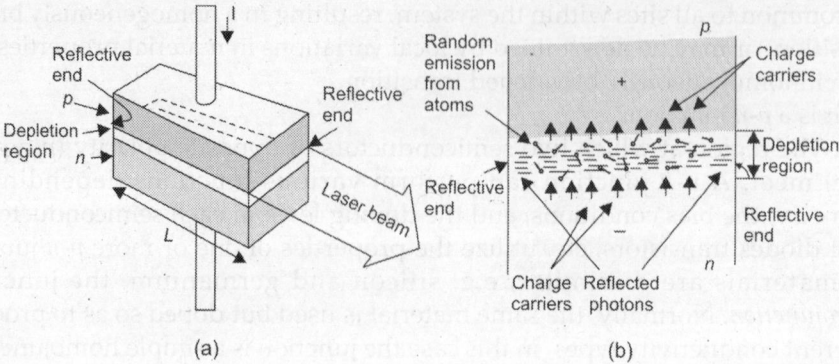

Fig. 7.71: (a) Laser diode (b) illustration of random emission and laser action within depletion region

Function: Let us consider the effect of charge carrier injection into the depletion region when the junction is forward-biased (Fig. 7.70(b)). As forward current excites the atoms that strike, first emit photons (radiant energy) of energy randomly, as electrons are raised to a high energy level and then fall back to a lower level. Consequently, several photons strike the reflective ends of the junction perpendicularly so that they are reflected back from the other end of the junction. Obviously, photons have a to-and-fro motion several times and their number goes on increasing as they cause other atoms in their path to emit photons by striking them. This activity of reflection and generation of photons causes amplification of initial reflected photons. A laser beam emerges through the partially reflected surface of the junction. GaAs laser diodes normally require high forward current levels, ranging from 10 mA to tens of amperes. At low current levels, this device emits similar as in LED. Beyond a threshold current level, light intensity increases sharply and its bandwidth decreases as lasing commences. Due to high energy density, laser beam can be quite harmful to eyes.

Laser diodes operating in a pulsed manner are called **junction laser diodes**, whereas lasers producing continuous output are called **continuous wave** (CW) laser diodes. Each type of laser emits a particular light wavelength depending upon the material and junction dimensions. Each type of laser has a threshold input current level.

Basic operation and construction: Laser diodes are light emitting devices, capable of emitting laser beams. One of the commonly used laser diodes is *injection laser diode* (ILD). A typical ILD package is shown in Fig. 7.72. The laser diode works exactly like an ordinary diode. Fig. 7.73 shows the structures of an injection laser. The *p* type and *n* type materials are made of AIGaAs.

When forward-biased, light is emitted at the *pn* junction. However, unlike in the LED, the emitted light is coherent and monochromatic. In the LED, light emitted is scattered in all directions. In the laser diode, however, light emitted can escape only from the end faces because the edges are roughened. In most laser diodes, one of the end faces is coated with a reflective material so that radiation of laser is emitted only in one direction.

The laser diode emits light when forward-biased and can

Radiant flux

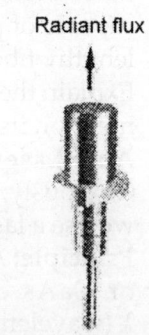

Fig. 7.72: A typical injection diode (ILD) package

withstand only relatively small reverse-biased voltages. A high reverse voltage can damage or destroy the laser diode. The symbol for laser diode is shown in Fig. 7.74. Note that light emission is shown zigzagged rather than straight, as in the symbol for an ordinary LED.

Applications of laser diode: Laser diodes are used primarily in fiber optic communications. It is the only device capable of producing optical energy high enough in concentration to pass through lengthy fiber optic cables. However, it also has some major disadvantages as compared to LEDs.

i. They cost 10 times more than LEDs.

ii. Their life expectancy is 10 times shorter than that of LEDs.

iii. They require elaborate power supplies and consume much more power than LEDs.

Laser diodes do not compete with LEDs on cost-reliability basis. Therefore, LEDs are used as much as possible in fiber optic systems and laser diodes are used only when absolutely necessary.

Some applications of laser diodes are:

i. Fixed product scanners seen in grocery stores.

ii. Handheld barcode scanners used for inventory control in warehouses.

iii. Handheld laser pointers used in presentations.

iv. Laser projection devices used by surgeons, mechanics, aviators and technicians. Laser scanners project low-power images directly onto the user's retina as an overlay in conjunction with the real-world image.

v. Land survey range-finding has been revolutionized by the use of laser diodes. Laser transmission from Total Station (reflected from a distant point) is detected, time-delay measured, and converted to an equivalent distance. Figure 7.75 shows a Leica model TC407. Total station that incorporates laser range-finding.

vi. Document printers and scanners often incorporate lasers.

vii. In construction, lasers are used to paint line and angle projection, nearly eliminating the potential for manual measurement errors.

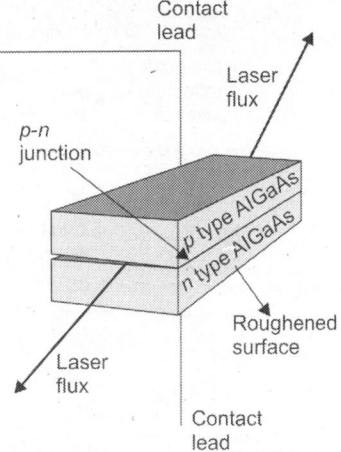

Fig. 7.73: A typical injection diode (ILD) package

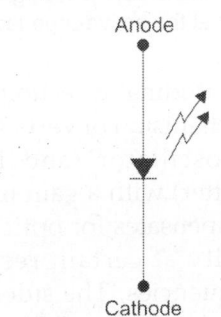

Fig. 7.74: A typical injection diode (ILD) package (symbolic representation)

5. Explain what are laser modes? Derive threshold condition.

Ans. Laser diode modes and threshold condition: The radiation in one type of laser diode configuration is generated within a Fabry–Perot resonator cavity (Fig. 7.75), as in most other types of lasers. However, this cavity is much smaller (~ 250–500 μm long, 5–15 μm wide, and 0.1–0.2 μm thick). These dimensions commonly are referred to as longitudinal, lateral, and transverse dimensions of the cavity, respectively.

As illustrated in Fig. 7.76, two flat, reflecting mirrors are directed towards each other to enclose the Fabry–Perot resonator cavity. The mirror facets are constructed by making two parallel clefts along with natural cleavage planes of the semiconductor crystal. The purpose of the mirrors is to establish a strong optical feedback in the

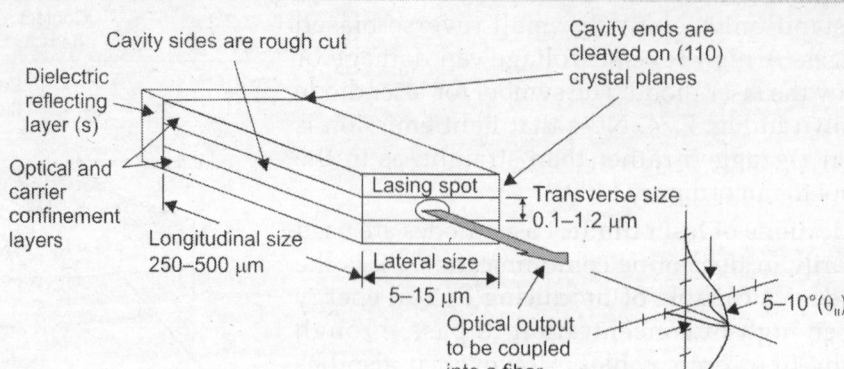

Fig. 7.75: Fabry–Perot resonator cavity for a laser diode. The cleaved crystal ends function as partially reflecting mirrors. The unused end (the rear facet) can be coated with a dielectric reflector to reduce optical loss in the cavity. The light beam emerging from the laser forms a vertical ellipse, even though the lasing spot at the active-area facet is a horizontal ellipse

longitudinal direction. The feedback mechanism converts the device into an oscillator (and hence a light emitter) with a gain mechanism that compensates for optical losses in the cavity at certain resonant optical frequencies. The sides of the cavity are simply formed by roughing the edges of the device to reduce unwanted emissions in the lateral directions.

As the light reflects back and forth within the Fabry–Perot cavity, the electric fields of the light interfere on successive round trips. Those wavelengths that are integer multiples of the cavity length interfere constructively so that their amplitudes add when they exit the device through the right-hand facet. All other wavelengths interfere destructively and thus cancel themselves out. The optical frequencies at which constructive interference occurs are the *resonant frequencies* of the cavity. Consequently, spontaneously emitted photons that have wavelengths at these resonant frequencies reinforce themselves after multiple trips through the cavity so that their optical field becomes very strong. The resonant wavelengths are called the *longitudinal modes* of the cavity, since they resonate along the length of the cavity.

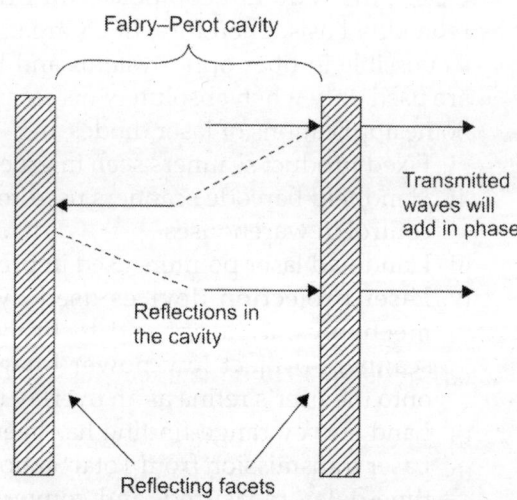

Fig. 7.76: Two parallel light-reflecting mirrored surfaces define a Fabry–Perot resonator cavity

Figure 7.77 shows the behaviour of the resonant wavelength for three values of the mirror reflectivity. The plots give the relative intensity as a function of the wavelength relative to the cavity length. As can be seen from Fig. 7.77, the width of the resonances depends on the value of the reflectivity. That is, the resonances become sharper as the reflectivity increases.

In another laser diode type, commonly referred to as the *distributed-feedback* (DFB) *laser*, the cleaved facets are not required for optical feedback. A typical DFB laser configuration is shown in Fig. 7.78. The fabrication of this device is similar to the Fabry–Perot types, except that the lasing action is obtained from Bragg reflectors (gratings) or periodic variations of the refractive index (called *distributed-feedback corrugations*), which are incorporated into the multilayer structure along the length of the diode.

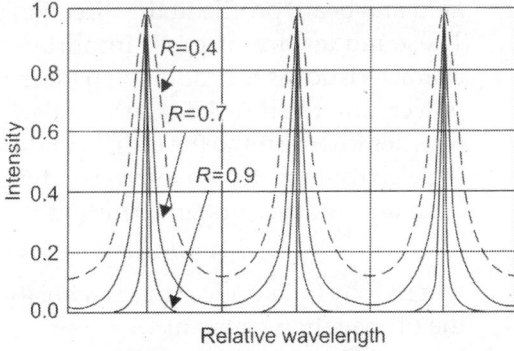

Fig. 7.77: Behaviour of the resonant wavelengths in a Fabry–Perot cavity for three values of the mirror reflectivity

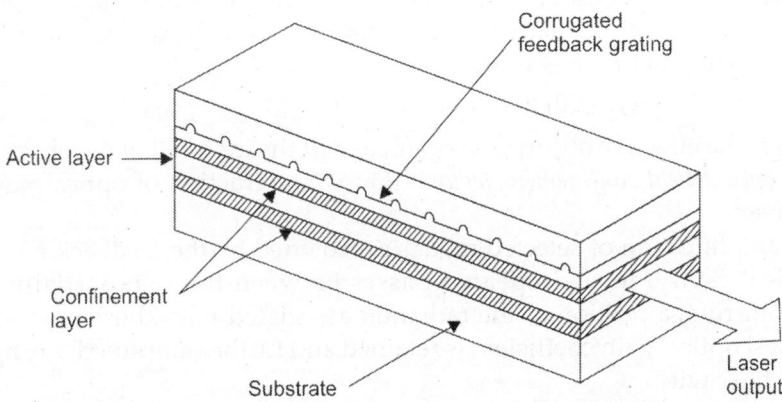

Fig. 7.78: Structure of a distributed-feedback (DFB) laser diode

In general, the full optical output is needed only from the front facet of the laser—that is, the one to be aligned with an optical fiber. In this case, a dielectric reflector can be deposited on the rear laser facet to reduce the optical loss in the cavity, to reduce the threshold current density (the point at which lasing starts), and to increase the external quantum efficiency. Reflectivities greater than 98% have been achieved with a six-layer reflector.

The optical radiation within the resonance cavity of a laser diode sets up a pattern of electric and magnetic field lines called the *modes of the cavity*. These can conveniently be separated into two independent sets of transverse electric (TE) and transverse magnetic (TM) modes. Each set of modes can be described in terms of the longitudinal, lateral, and transverse half-sinusoidal variations of the electromagnetic fields along the major axes of the cavity. The *longitudinal modes* are related to the length L of the cavity and determine the principal structure of the frequency spectrum of the emitted optical radiation. Since L is much larger than the lasing wavelength of approximately 1 µm, many longitudinal modes can exist. *Lateral modes* lie in the plane of the *pn* junction. These modes depend on the side wall preparation and the width of the cavity, and determine the shape of the lateral profile of the laser beam. *Transverse modes* are associated with the electromagnetic field and beam profile in the direction perpendicular to the plane of the *pn* junction. These modes are of great importance, since they largely determine such laser characteristics as the radiation pattern (the angular distribution of the optical output power) and the threshold current density.

In order to determine the lasing conditions and the resonant frequencies, we express the electromagnetic wave propagating in the longitudinal direction (along the axis normal to the mirrors) in terms of the electric field phasor.

$$E(z, t) = I(z) \, e^{j(\omega t - \beta z)} \tag{i}$$

where $I(z)$ is the optical field intensity, w is the optical radian frequency, and b is the propagation constant.

Lasing is the condition at which light amplification becomes possible in the laser diode. The requirement for lasing is that a population inversion be achieved. This condition can be understood by considering the fundamental relationship between the optical field intensity I, the absorption coefficient α_λ, the gain coefficient g is the Fabry–Perot cavity. The stimulated emission rate into a given mode is proportional to the intensity of the radiation in that mode. The radiation intensity at a photon energy $h\nu$ varies exponentially with the distance z that it traverses along the lasing cavity according to the relationship:

$$I(x) = I(0) \exp \{ \Gamma_g \, (h\nu) - \bar{\alpha}(h\nu) \} z \} \tag{ii}$$

where $\bar{\alpha}$ is the effective absorption coefficient of the material in the optical path and Γ is the *optical-field confinement factor*—that is, the fraction of optical power in the active layer.

Optical amplification of selected modes is provided by the feedback mechanism of the optical cavity. In the repeated passes between the two partially reflecting parallel mirrors, a portion of the radiation associated with those modes that have the highest optical gain coefficient is retained and further amplified during each trip through the cavity.

Lasing occurs when the gain of one or several guided modes is sufficient to exceed the optical loss during one roundtrip through the cavity; that is, $z = 2L$. During this roundtrip, only the fractions R_1 and R_2 of the optical radiation are reflected from the two laser ends 1 and 2, respectively, where R_1 and R_2 are the mirror reflectivities or Fresnel reflection coefficients, which are given by:

$$R = \left(\frac{n_1 - n_2}{n_1 + n_2} \right)^2 \tag{iii}$$

for the reflection of light at an interface between two materials having refractive indices n_1 and n_2. From this lasing condition, Eq. (ii) becomes:

$$I(2L) = I(0) \, R_1 R_2 \exp \{ 2L \, [\Gamma g \, (h\nu) - \alpha \, (h\nu)] \} \tag{iv}$$

For an uncoated cleaved facet the reflectivity is only about 30 percent. To reduce the loss in the cavity and to make the optical feedback stronger, the facets typically are coated with a dielectric material. This can produce a reflectivity of about 99% for the rear facet and 90% for the front facet through which the lasing light emerges.

At the lasing threshold, a steady-state oscillation takes place, and the magnitude and phase of the returned wave must be equal to those of the original wave. This yields:

$$I(2L) = I(0) \tag{v}$$

for the amplitude and

$$e^{-j2\beta L} = 1 \tag{vi}$$

for the phase. Equation (vi) gives information concerning the resonant frequencies of the Fabry–Perot cavity. From Eq. (v), one can find which modes have sufficient gain for sustained oscillation and we can find the amplitudes of these modes. The condition to just reach the lasting threshold is the point at which the optical gain is equal to the total loss α_t, in the cavity. From Eq. (v), this condition is obtained as:

$$Gg_{th} = \alpha_t = \bar{\alpha} + \frac{1}{2L} \ln\left(\frac{1}{R_1 R_2}\right) = \bar{\alpha} + \alpha_{end} \tag{vii}$$

where α_{end} is the mirror loss in the lasing cavity. Thus, for lasing to occur, we must have the gain $g \geq g_{th}$. This means that the pumping source that maintains the population inversion must be sufficiently strong to support or exceed all the energy-consuming mechanisms within the lasing cavity.

The mode that satisfies Eq. (vii) reaches threshold first. Theoretically, at the onset of this condition, all additional energy introduced into the laser should argument the growth of this particular mode. In practice, various phenomena lead to the excitation of more than one mode. Studies on the conditions of longitudinal single-mode operation have revealed that important factors are thin active regions and a high degree of temperature stability.

The relationship between optical output power and diode drive current is presented in Fig. 7.79. At low diode currents, only sponta-neous radiation is emitted. Both the spectral range and the lateral beam width of this emission are broad like that of an LED. A dramatic and sharply defined increase in the power output occurs at the lasing threshold. As this tran-sition point is approached, the spectral range and the beam width both narrow with increasing drive current. The final spectral width of approxi-mately 1 nm and the fully narrowed lateral beam width of nominally 5–10° are reached just past the threshold point. The *threshold current* I_{th} is conventionally defined by

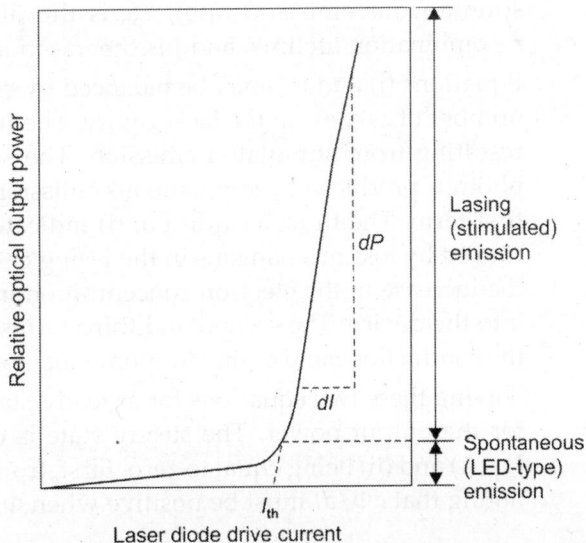

Fig. 7.79: Relationship between optical output power and laser diode drive current. Below the lasing threshold the optical output is a spontaneous LED-type emission

extrapolation of the lasing region of the power vs current curve; as shown in Fig. 7.78. At high power outputs, the slope of the curve decreases because of junction heating.

For laser structures that have strong carrier confinement, the *threshold current density* for stimulated emission J_{th} can, to a good approximation, be related to the lasing-threshold optical gain by:

$$g_{th} = \beta J_{th} \tag{viii}$$

where β is a constant that depends on the specific device construction.

6. Derive laser diode rate equation and explain their importance.

Ans. Laser diode rate equations: The relationship between optical output power and the diode drive current can be determined by examining the rate equations that govern the interaction of photons and electrons in the active region. The total carrier population is determined by carrier injection, spontaneous recombination, and stimulated emission. For a *pn* junction with a carrier-confinement region of depth *d*, the *rate equations* are given by:

$$\frac{d\Phi}{dt} = Cn\Phi + R_{sp} - \frac{\Phi}{\tau_{ph}}$$ (i)

= stimulated emission + spontaneous emission + photon gas

which governs the number of photons Φ, and

$$\frac{dn}{dt} = \frac{J}{qd} - \frac{n}{\tau_{sp}} - Cn\Phi$$ (ii)

= injection + spontaneous recombination + stimulated emission

which governs the number of *electrons n*. Here, *C* is a coefficient describing the strength of the *optical absorption and emission* interactions, R_{sp} is the rate of spontaneous emission into the lasing mode (which is much smaller than the total spontaneous-emission rate), τ_{ph} is the photon lifetime, τ_s is the spontaneous-recombination lifetime, and *J* is the injection-current density.

Equations (i) and (ii) may be balanced by considering all the factors that affect the number of carriers in the laser cavity. The first term in Eq. (i) is a source of photons resulting from stimulated emission. The second term, describing the number of photons produced by spontaneous emission, is relatively small compared with the first term. The third term in Eq. (i) indicates the decay in the number of photons caused by loss mechanisms in the lasing cavity. In Eq. (ii), the first term represents the increase in the electron concentration in the conduction band as current flows into the device. The second and third terms give the number of electrons lost from the conduction band owing to spontaneous and stimulated transitions, respectively.

Solving these two equations for a steady-state condition, one obtains an expression for the output power. The steady state is characterized by the left-hand sides of Eqs (i) and (ii) being equal to zero. First, from Eq. (ii), assuming R_{sp} is negligible and noting that $d\Phi/dt$ must be positive when Φ is small, we have:

$$Cn - \frac{1}{\tau_{ph}} \geq 0$$ (iii)

This reveals that *n* must exceed a threshold value n_{th} in order for Φ to increase. Using Eq. (iii), this threshold value can be expressed in terms of the threshold current J_{th} needed to maintain an inversion level $n = n_{th}$ in the steady state when the number of photons $\Phi = 0$:

$$\frac{n_{th}}{\phi_{sp}} = \frac{J_{th}}{qd}$$ (iv)

This expression *defines the current required to sustain an excess electron density in the laser* when spontaneous emission is the only decay mechanism.

Next, consider the photon and electron rate equations in the steady-state condition at the lasing threshold, respectively, Eqs (i) and (ii) become:

$$0 = Cn_{th}\Phi_s + R_{sp} - \frac{\Phi}{\tau_{ph}} \tag{v}$$

and
$$0 = \frac{J}{qd} - \frac{n_{th}}{\tau_{sp}} - Cn_{th}\Phi_s \tag{vi}$$

where Φ_s is the steady-state photon density. Adding Eqs (v) and (vi), using Eq. (v) for the term n_{th}/τ_{sp}, and solving for Φ_s, one obtains the number of photons per unit volume:

$$\Phi_s = \frac{\tau_{ph}}{qd}(J - J_{th}) + \tau_{ph}R_{sp} \tag{vii}$$

The first term in Eq. (7.118) is the number of photons resulting from stimulated emission. The power from these photons is generally concentrated in one or a few modes. The second term gives the spontaneously generated photons. The power resulting from these photons is not mode-selective, but is spread over all the possible modes of the volume, which are on the order of 10^8 modes.

7. Write expression for external differential quantum efficiency of a laser diode and explain.

Ans. External differential quantum efficiency: The *external differential quantum efficiency* η_{ext} is defined as the number of photons emitted per radiative electron-hole pair recombination above threshold. Under the assumption that above threshold the gain coefficient remains fixed at g_{th}, η_{ext} is obtained as:

$$\eta_{ext} = \frac{\eta_i(g_{th} - \alpha)}{g_{th}} \tag{i}$$

Here, η_i is the internal quantum efficiency. This is not a well-defined quantity in laser diodes, but most measurements show that $\eta_i \simeq 0.6$–0.7 at room temperature. Experimentally, η_{ext} is calculated from the straight-line portion of the curve for the emitted optical power P versus drive current I, one obtains:

$$\eta_{ext} = \frac{q}{E_g}\frac{dP}{dI} = 0.8056\lambda\,(\mu m)\frac{dP\,(mW)}{dI\,(mA)} \tag{ii}$$

where E_g is the band-gap energy in electron volts, dP is the incremental change in the emitted optical power in milliwatts for an incremental change dI in the drive current (in milliamperes), and λ is the emission wavelength in micrometers. For standard semiconductor lasers, external differential quantum efficiencies of 15–30% per facet are typical. High-quality devices have differential quantum efficiencies of 30–40%.

8. What are quantum-well lasers?

Ans. These lasers offer an alternative to double heterostructures. In these lasers, the energy of the emitted photon can be made subsequently higher than that of the bandgap. By proper choice of well width, the energy of the emitted photon can be adjusted so that the lasing can be achieved at various wavelength using the same material. A single quantum well laser is similar in design to a double heterostructure laser except that the narrow gap. This means that the active region is intensionally made so that the spatial quantization effects occur. Spatial quantization results in the production of energy levels above the conduction band minimum in a quantum well. The minimum electron and hole energies within the well are both above the conduction band and valence band minimum respectively. If electron and hole recombine, the energy of the emitted photon is a strong function of the well width. The narrower the width, the greater the quantum state energy. The energy of the emitted photon can be tuned by adjusting the well width.

Limitations of quantum well lasers: The cross-section for the capture of carriers in the well is relatively small. In order to obtain a radiative recombination event, there is necessity for the injected electrons and holes to be captured within the well. To confine the carriers within the well, it is desired that they should undergo an inelastic scattering event in order to lose sufficient energy. If there is no scattering events within the well, the injected carriers can pass directly over the well without getting trapped and do not contribute to the optical output. This means that the threshold current density can be relatively high.

9. Explain the resonant frequencies of a laser diode.

Ans. We have read that at the lasing threshold, a steady state oscillation takes place, and the magnitude and phase of the returned wave must be equal to those of the original wave. This yields

$$I(2L) = I(0) \tag{i}$$

for the amplitude and

$$e^{-j2\beta L} = 1 \tag{ii}$$

for the phase (see answer Q. 5)

The condition in (i) holds when:

$$2\beta L = 2\pi m \tag{iii}$$

where m is an integer. Using $\beta = 2\pi n/\lambda$ for the propagation constant, we have:

$$m = \frac{L}{\lambda/2n} = \frac{2Ln}{c} \nu \tag{iv}$$

where $c = \nu\lambda$. This states that the cavity resonates (i.e. a standing-wave pattern exists within it) when a integer number m of half-wavelengths spans the region between the mirrors.

Since in all lasers the gain is a function of frequency (or wavelength, since $c = \nu\lambda$), there will be a range of frequencies (or wavelengths) for which Eq. (iv) holds. Each of these frequencies corresponds to a mode of oscillation of the laser. Depending on the laser structure, any number of frequencies can satisfy Eqs (ii) and (iii). Thus, some lasers are *single-mode* and some are *multimode*. The relationship between gain and frequency can be assumed to have the *Gaussian form*:

$$g(\lambda) = g(0) \exp\left[-\frac{(\lambda - \lambda_0)^2}{2\sigma^2}\right] \tag{v}$$

where λ_0 is the wavelength at the center of the spectrum, σ is the spectral width of the gain, and the maximum gain $g(0)$ is proportional to the population inversion.

We now look at the frequency, or wavelength, spacing between the modes of a multimode laser. Here, we consider only the longitudinal modes. Note, however, that for each longitudinal mode there may be several transverse modes that arise from one or more reflections of the propagating wave at the sides of the resonator cavity. To find the frequency spacing, consider two successive modes of frequencies v_{m-1} and v_m represented by the integers $m-1$ and m. From Eq. (iv), one finds:

$$m - 1 = \frac{2Ln}{c} v_{m-1} \tag{vi}$$

and

$$m = \frac{2Ln}{c} v_m \tag{vii}$$

Subtracting these two equations yields:

$$1 = \frac{2Ln}{c} (v_m - v_{m-1}) = \frac{2Ln}{c} \Delta v \tag{viii}$$

from which we have the frequency spacing:

$$\Delta v = \frac{\lambda^2}{2Ln} \tag{ix}$$

This can be related to the wavelength spacing $\Delta\lambda$ through the relationship $\Delta v / v = \Delta\lambda / \lambda$, yielding:

$$\Delta\lambda = \frac{\lambda^2}{2Ln} \tag{x}$$

Thus, given Eqs (v) and (x), the output spectrum of a multimode laser follows the typical gain-versus-frequency shown in Fig. 7.80, where the exact number of modes, their heights, and their spacings depend on the laser construction.

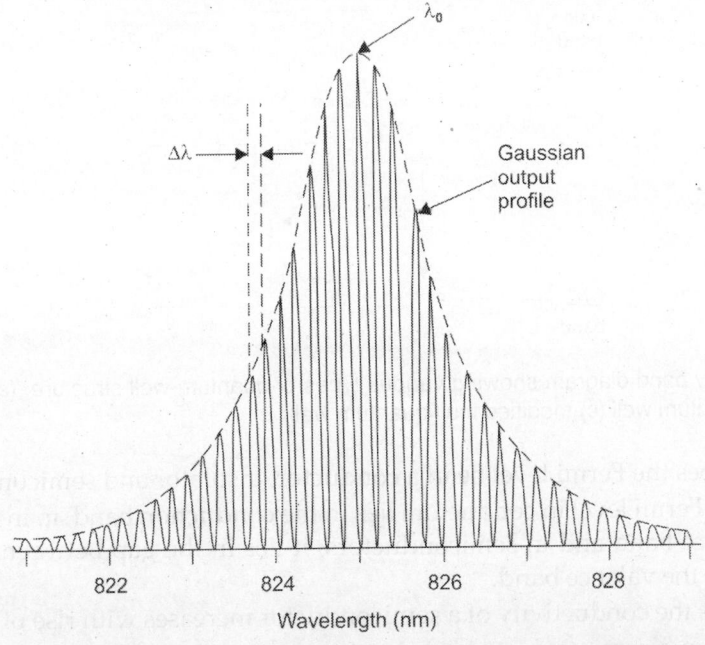

Fig. 7.80: Spectrum from a Fabry–Perot GaAlAs/GaAs laser diode

10. Explain the importance of infrared LEDs?

Ans. Infrared LEDs include GaAs LEDs which can emit light near 0.9 µm and several iii-iv compounds, e.g. quantenary $Ga_x In_{1-x} As_y P_{1-x}$ LEDs, which emit light in the range 1.1 to 1.6 µm.

Infrared LEDs find application in *optoisolators* where an input or control signal is decoupled from the output. Infrared LEDs also find application for transmission of an optical signal through an optical fiber.

11. What is major difference between LEDs and laser diodes?

Ans. The optical output from LED is *incoherent*, whereas from laser diode is coherent.

12. Draw energy level diagrams showing various types of quantum well structures.

Ans. See Fig. 7.81.

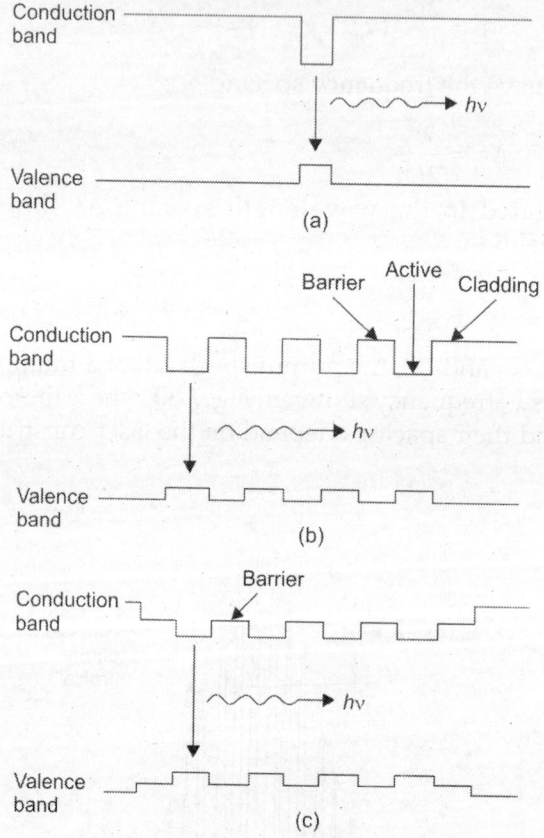

Fig. 7.81: Energy band diagram showing various types of quantum-well structure: (a) single quantum well (b) multiquantum well (c) modified multiquantum well.

13. Where does the Fermi level lie in a conductor, insulator and semiconductor?

Ans. The Fermi level in conductors lies in the conduction band, in insulator it lies in the valence band and in semiconductors, it lies in the gap between the conductor band and the valence band.

14. Why does the conductivity of a semiconductor increases with rise of temperature?

Ans. When a semiconductor is heated more and more electrons jump across the forbidden gap from valence band to conduction band where these are free to conduct electricity.

15. What are *compensated semiconductors*?

Ans. These are semiconductors in which both acceptor and donor impurities are simultaneously present, e.g. a compensated *n*-type semiconductor can be obtained by diffusing donor impurities in a p-type semiconductor such that $N_D > N_A$, where N_D is donor impurity concentration and N_A is acceptor impurity concentration. Similarly, p-type compensated semiconductor can be obtained by diffusing acceptor impurities in an n-type semiconductor such that $N_A > N_D$. When $N_D = N_D$, the semiconductor is said to be completely compensated and semiconductor behaves like an intrinsic one.

If we assume that all donors and acceptor impurity atoms are ionized at room temperature, a semiconductor doped with donor concentration of N_D and acceptor concentration of N_A in the same region one may write the charge neutrality condition as

$$N_D + p_0 = N_A + n_0 \tag{i}$$

i.e.

$$N_D + \frac{n_i^2}{n_0} = N_A + n_0 \tag{ii}$$

where n_0 and p_0 represents the electron and hole concentration under thermal equilibrium and can be expressed as

$$n_0 = N_C \exp\left[(E_F - E_C)/kT\right] \tag{iii}$$

and

$$p_0 = N_V \exp\left[(E_V - E_F)/k \cdot T\right] \tag{iv}$$

where N_C and N_V are the effective density of states in the conduction and the valence band respectively, of the semiconductor given by

$$N_C = 2\left(\frac{2\pi m_n^* kT}{h^2}\right)^{3/2} \tag{v}$$

$$N_V = 2\left(\frac{2\pi m_p^* kT}{h^2}\right)^{3/2} \tag{vi}$$

where, m_p^* and m_n^* are the hole and electron effective mass respectively.

Equation (ii) can be rearranged as a quadratic equation in terms of n_0 as

$$n_0^2 + (N_A - N_D)\, n_0 - n_i^2 \tag{vii}$$

The solution of Eq. (vii) is obtained as

$$n_0 = \frac{N_D - N_A}{2} + \sqrt{\left(\frac{N_D - N_A}{2}\right)^2 + n_i^2} \tag{viii}$$

We can easily see that when $N_D = N_A$, one finds

$$n_0 = n_i$$

We may note that both the electron and hole concentration of a semiconductor doped equally with donor and acceptor impurity are equal to the intrinsic earlier concentration similar to the case of an intrinsic semiconductor. However, the difference lies in the fact that unlike intrinsic semiconductor there exists a large number of donors and acceptor in the former material.

We may also note that when $N_D \gg N_A$, Eq. (viii) can be approximated by neglecting n_i as

$$n_0 \approx N_D$$

16. Give a brief account of optical source materials.

Ans. Optical fiber based communication system uses the *near infrared* (NIR) region of the optical spectrum (range 0.8 μm to 1.65 μm). This is because optical fibers are primarily made of silica glass and silica fibers offer minimum loss in this wavelength region. The intrinsic loss of Si fiber is quite high both in UV region and IR region (beyond 2 μm). Moreover, the emission wavelength of a semiconductor material depends on the direct energy bandgap of the material. There are many ternary and quaternary III-V semiconductor alloys of binary compounds which are *direct band gap* materials and can therefore, be used as prospective candidates for making optical sources for use in the transmitter of an optical fiber system.

The principal material used for making optical sources for operation in the 0.8 to 0.9 μm (800 – 900 nm) wavelength region of the optical spectrum is $Al_x Ga_{1-x} As$. One can use the mole fraction x to vary the bandgap of the alloy to match the desired wavelength. One can vary x in the ternary material $Al_x Ga_{1-x} As$ from 0 to 1. For $x = 0$, this material corresponds to GaAs and for $x = 1$ to AlAs. We may note that GaAs is a direct bandgap material with $E_g = 1.43$ eV while AlAs is an indirect gap material with $E_g = 2.16$ eV. Clearly, when x ivaries from 0 to 1, $Al_x Ga_{1-x} As$ ·may not be direct bandgap in nature for all values of x, i.e. there is a critical value of x (0.45 for the discussed example) below which the material is direct bandgap in nature and above. it behaves like an indirect bandgap material. One can obtain the energy bandgap and the lattice constant of the ternary alloy $Al_x Ga_{1-x} As$ from Fig. 7.82 following the line joining GaAs ($E_g = 1.43$ eV and $a = 5.64$ Å) and AlAs ($E_g = 2.16$ eV and a = 5.66 Å).

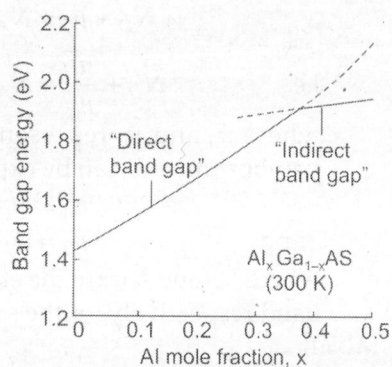

Fig. 7.82: Variation of band gap of ternary alloy $Al_x Ga_{1-x} As$ with mole fraction (x) indicating corresponding emission wavelength

One can represent the bandgap energy of the ternary alloy $Al_x Ga_{1-x} As$ with the mole fraction x between 0 to 0.37 (in the direct bandgap region) by the following relation.

$$E_g = 1.424 + 1.266x + 0.266x^2 \quad (0 < x < 0.37) \tag{i}$$

One can obtain the peak wavelength of emission by substituting the value of E_g in eV from Eq. (i) in the following relation

$$\lambda = \frac{1.24}{E_g(eV)} \text{ (μm)} \tag{ii}$$

The principal material used for making optical sources for the operating range 800–900 nm is based on $Al_x Ga_{1-x} As$. One can suitably adjust the parameter, x to achieve the appropriate bandgap necessary for peak emission in the desired wavelength. Figure 7.83 shows a typical emission spectrum of AlGaAs LED. The peak wavelength of emission corresponds to the wavelength at which the relative intensity of the emitted light is maximum. We may note that the LED emits light over a region of the spectrum centered at wavelength of peak emission (or peak power).

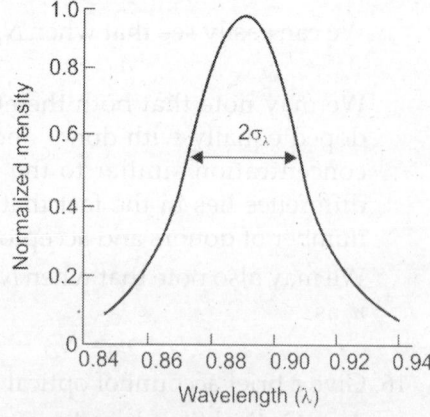

Fig. 7.83: Relative intensity of light emitted by the LED source vs wavelength (λ) of light

The spectral width of the source is generally expressed in terms of rms spectral width, σ_λ, and varies in the range of 30–100 nm depending on the quality of LED. In this considered example the spectral width of LED is shown as 33 nm.

It is reported that for application in longer wavelength region ternary InGaAs and quaternary InGaAsP grown on matured In P-based technology are quite promising the wavelength range of 0.92–1.65 μm. We have read that the quaternary material such as $Ga_x In_{1-x} As_{1-y}P_y$ is a more versatile material as the lattice constant and energy bandgap can be varied over wider ranges by varying both the mole fractions x and y. Further, the material is lattice matched to InP. For example, $In_{0.53} Ga_{0.47} As$ has a bandgap energy of 0.74 eV and is quite useful for making optical sources and photodetectors for operation at 1.55 μm using InP as the lattice matches substrate. One can obtain the appropriate composition of $In_{1-x} Ga_x As_y P_{1-y}$ For lattice matching by selecting the bandgap of the quaternary along the upper dashed line in Fig. 7.81 passing through InP point. One can obtain the energy bandgap of $Ga_x In_{1-x} As_{1-y} P_y$ composition that are lattice matched to InP from the following empirical relation.

$$E_g (In_{1-x} Ga_x As_y P_{1-y}) = 1.35 + 0.668x - 1.17y + 0.758x^2$$
$$+ 0.18y^2 - 0.069\, xy - 0.322x^2 y + 0.33xy^2 \text{ (eV)} \qquad \text{(ii)}$$

MULTIPLE CHOICE QUESTIONS

1. Laser light is considered to be coherent because it consists of:
   (a) many wavelengths
   (b) uncoordinated wavelengths
   (c) coordinated wavelengths
   (d) divergent waves

2. The relation between Einstein's A_{21} and B_{21} coefficients is:
   (a) $\dfrac{A_{21}}{B_{21}} = 1:2$
   (b) $\dfrac{A_{21}}{B_{21}} = \dfrac{8\pi h v^3}{c^3}$
   (c) $\dfrac{A_{21}}{B_{21}} = 1:1$
   (d) $\dfrac{A_{21}}{B_{21}} = \dfrac{v}{c}$

3. The ratio of the number of spontaneous to stimulated transition is:
   (a) $\dfrac{A_{21}}{B_{21}uv} = 1:1$
   (b) $\dfrac{A_{21}}{B_{21}uv} = 1:2$
   (c) $\dfrac{A_{21}}{B_{21}uv} = \exp\left(\dfrac{hv}{k_B T}\right) - 1$
   (d) $\dfrac{A_{21}}{B_{21}uv} = 8\pi \dfrac{hv^3}{c^3}$

4. When the atoms in the source go from an excited state (E_2) to a lower energy state (E_1), spontaneous emission of light takes place, the energy of the emitted photon being:
   (a) $hv_{12} = E_2 - E_1$
   (b) $hv_{12} = E_2/E_1$
   (c) $hv_{12} = E_1/E_2$
   (d) $hv_{12} = 0$

5. The order of the pumping power necessary to achieve the popula-tion inversion in a ruby is:
   (a) $10^7\,W/m^2$
   (b) $10^2\,W/m^2$
   (c) $10^{10}\,W/m^2$
   (d) $10^{16}\,W/m^2$

6. The most important characteristic of a laser is:
   (a) polarization
   (b) coherence
   (c) high intensity
   (d) directionality

7. The intensity of a laser beam does not decrease with distance in accordance with the inverse square law because:
   (a) the laser light is monochromatic
   (b) the laser light is very intense
   (c) the laser light is very directional
   (d) the laser light obeys Planck's law

8. For a laser beam $\lambda = 4400\text{Å}$ and coherence time $= 4 \times 10^{-5}$ s, the coherence length will be:
   (a) 12 km
   (b) 1.2 km
   (c) 0.12 km
   (d) 0.012 km

9. For a laser beam minimum angular divergence depends on:
   (a) wavelength λ only
   (b) diameter of mirror D only
   (c) both λ and D
   (d) alignment of mirrors only

10. The wavelengths produced by a He-Ne laser correspond to transition in:
    (a) both helium and neon
    (b) helium
    (c) neon
    (d) neither helium nor neon

11. The term 'population inversion' means:
    (a) population of the ionised state is maximum
    (b) population of the lowest state is maximum
    (c) population of the lower level is more than that of the higher level
    (d) population of the higher level is more than that of the lower level

12. A laser operates at a frequency of 3×10^{14} Hz and has an aperture of 10^{-2} m. The angular spread will be:
    (a) 10^{-2} rad
    (b) 10^{-3} rad
    (c) 10^{-4} rad
    (d) 10^{-5} rad

13. The function of He atoms in the He-Ne laser is:
    (a) to quench the neon atoms
    (b) to provide energy to the neon atoms
    (c) to make neon atoms inactive
    (d) None of the above

14. Which of the following characteristics is not associated with a laser light?
    (a) Coherence
    (b) Brightness
    (c) Polarization
    (d) Birefringes

15. In ruby laser, the rod is surrounded by a helical photographic flash lamp filled with:
    (a) cromium
    (b) aluminium
    (c) xenon
    (d) neon

16. Who invented semiconductor laser?
    (a) Albert Einstein
    (b) T.H. Maiman
    (c) Ali Javan
    (d) Robert Hall

17. Which of the following modes of operations should be used to achieve laser pulses of very high power?
    (a) Q-switched operation
    (b) Pulsed operation with free oscillation
    (c) Continuous-wave operation
    (d) All of the above

18. According to the mode of oscillation, lasers may be categorized in the following group/groups.
    (a) Continuous wave (CW) lasers
    (b) Pulsed lasers with free oscillations
    (c) Q-switched lasers
    (d) All the above

19. The temporal width of a mode-locked rhodamine 6 G dye laser emitting at 0.6 μm if $\Delta v = 10^{13}$ Hz is:
    (a) 10^{-13} s   (b) 8.4×10^{-11} s
    (c) 3.3×10^{-13} s   (d) 6.6×10^{-10} s

20. The spatial length of a mode-locked Nd^{3+} glass laser if $\Delta v = 3 \times 10^{12}$ Hz is:
    (a) 1 m   (b) 3.3 m
    (c) 5 m   (d) 0.1 mm

21. The probability of electrons to be found in the conduction band of an intrinsic semiconductor at a finite temperature
    (a) increases exponentially with increasing band gap
    (b) decreases exponentially with increasing band gap
    (c) decreases with increasing temperature
    (d) is independent of the temperature and band gap

    [**Hint:** At finite temperature, the probability of jumping an electron from valence band to conduction band decreases exponentially with the increasing band gap (E_g). Hence, correct choice (b)
    $$n = n_0 \exp\left(-E_g/kT\right)]$$

22. The electrical conductivity of a semiconductor increases when electromagnetic radiation of wavelength shorter than 2480 nm is incident on it. The band gap (in eV) for the semiconductor is
    (a) 0.9   (b) 0.7
    (c) 0.5   (d) 1.1

    [**Hint:** $E_g = hc/\lambda_{max} = \dfrac{1237.5 \text{ eVnm}}{2480 \text{ nm}} = 0.5 \text{ eV}$]

23. If the ratio of the concentration of electrons to that of holes in a semiconductor is 7/5 and the ratio of currents is 7/4, then what is the ratio of drift velocities?
    (a) 5/8   (b) 4/5
    (c) 5/4   (d) 4/7

    [**Hint:** $I = enAv_d$

    $\therefore$ $\dfrac{I_e}{I_h} = \dfrac{enAv_e}{enAv_h} = \dfrac{n_e}{n_h}\dfrac{v_e}{v_h}$

    or $\dfrac{v_e}{v_h} = \dfrac{I_e}{I_h} \times \dfrac{n_h}{n_e} = \dfrac{7}{4} \times \dfrac{5}{7} = \dfrac{5}{4}$

    Hence correct choice is (c)]

24. In the middle of the depletion layer of reverse biased *pn* junction, the
    (a) the electric field is zero   (b) potential is zero
    (c) potential is maximum   (d) electric field is maximum

[**Hint:** When a p-n Junction is reverse biased, the width of the depletion layer becomes large and so the electric field ($E = V/d$) becomes very small, nearly zero. Hence correct choice is (a)]

25. For a heavily doped n-type semiconductor, Fermi-level lies
    (a) a little below the conduction band
    (b) a little above the valence band
    (c) a little inside the valence band
    (d) at the centre of the band gap

    [**Hint:** For a heavily doped n-type semiconductor, the Fermi level lies slightly below the bottom of the conduction band. Correct choice (a)]

26. A Ge specimen is doped with Al. The concentration of acceptor atoms is $\approx 10^{21}$ atoms/m^3. Given that the intrinsic concentration of electron - hole pair is $\approx 10^{19}$/m^3, the concentration of electrons in the specimen is
    (a) $10^{17}\,\text{m}^{-3}$
    (b) $10^{15}\,\text{m}^{-3}$
    (c) $10^4\,\text{m}^{-3}$
    (d) $10^2\,\text{m}^{-3}$

    [**Hint:** Here $n_i = 10^{19}\,\text{m}^{-3}$, $n_h = 10^{21}\,\text{m}^{-3}$
    Now, $n_i^2 = n_e n_h$
    or $n_e = n_i^2/n_h = \dfrac{10^{19} \times 10^{19}}{10^{21}} = 10^{17}\,\text{m}^{-3}$
    Correct choice (a)]

ANSWERS

1. (c)   2. (b)   3. (c)   4. (a)   5. (a)   6. (b)   7. (c)   8. (a)   9. (c)   10. (c)
11. (d)   12. (c)   13. (b)   14. (d)   15. (c)   16. (d)   17. (a)   18. (d)   19. (a)   20. (a)
21. (b)   22. (c)   23. (c)   24. (a)   25. (a)   26. (a)

APPENDIX 7.1

SEMICONDUCTOR HETEROJUNCTIONS

We have studied *pn*-junctions in which the semiconductor material was homogeneous throughout the structure. Such a *pn*-junction made of the same material with different conductivities (*p* and *n*) on the two sides is referred to as a *homojunction*. When two different semiconductor materials are used to form junction, the junction is called *heterojunction*. Use of heterojunction can significantly improve the performance of a device compared to its homojunction counterpart. For example, heterojunctions provide optical and electrical confinement in injection laser diode and double heterostructure LED. In a bipolar transistor, a heterojunction at the base-emitter interface can significantly improve the emitter injection efficiency and reduce the base resistance. This is exploited in the realization of a heterojunction bipolar transistor (HBT). In a heterojunction field-effect transistor (HFET), the two-dimensional electron gas at the heterointerface can be utilized to design an ultra-fast transistor known as high-electron-mobility-transistor (HEMT) also called a *modulation-doped field-effect transistor* (MODFET) or also known as 'two-dimensional electron-gas field-effect transistor (TEGFET). These heterojunction devices are widely used for designing the pre-amplifier of an optical receiver. In a photodetector, heterojunctions are used for improving the quantum efficiency and speed of the detectors. In fact, heterojunction devices are extensively used for making optical sources and photodetectors, for optical fiber communication.

When two different materials having different values of energy bandgap and the parameters form a heterojunction, the energy band diagram experiences a discontinuity at the junction interface because of the misalignment of the conduction band and valence band on the two sides of the heterointerface. From the technological point of view, a heterojunction consists of two distinct materials having different values of lattice constant. A heterojunction is formed by chemical bonding at the heterointerface. If the values of the lattice constant of the two materials used for forming the heterojunction are very different, a large amount of misfit at the heterointerface introduces dislocations resulting in interface states. In some cases, the misfit may become so large that the device turns out to be virtually useless. We are more interested in near-perfect heterostructures, where the difference between the lattice constants of the two materials is very small. Such material combinations are called lattice-matched materials and are only used for making heterojunctions by epitaxial process. The percentage lattice mismatch can be obtained from the difference in the values of the lattice constants of the two materials. For Ge and GaAs, the percentage lattice mismatch at the heterointerface is of the order of 0.13% which is an acceptable figure. Ge-GaAs heterojunction have been studied by the several workers for making useful heterojunction devices. In a heterojunction, one side will have a band gap lower than the other side. The conductivity of the narrow band gap material is conventionally indicated by using lower case symbol (*n* or *p* as the case may be). On the other hand, the conductivity of the wider band gap material is denoted by using upper case symbol (*n* or *p* as the case may be). In a heterojunction it is not essential that the conductivity of the two materials used for making heterojunction should be different always. In a heterojunction, when the type of conductivity of the two materials is the same (both *N*-type or both *P*-type), the heterojunction is called *Isotypeheterojunction*. For example an N-Ge/N-GaAs forms an isotypehetero junction. However, when the materials on the two sides have different type of conductivity, the heterojunction is called an *anisotypeheterojunction*. Both types of heterojunctions are extensively used in optical sources and optical detectors used for optical fiber communication. The values of electron affinity (measured in terms of energy difference between the conduction band edge and the vacuum level) of the two semiconductors (with different values of bandgap) forming the heterojunction are different. As a result the energy band diagrams of the two semiconductors get differently oriented on the two

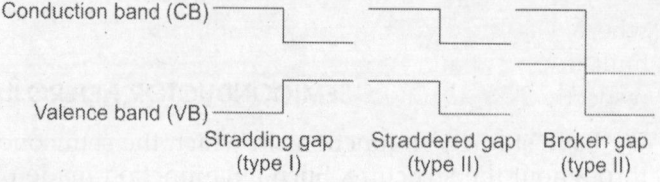

Fig. A7.1: Schematic classification of heterojunctions [types I, II and III]

sides of the heterointerface, depending on the electron affinity values of these materials. On the basis of the relative orientations, the heterojunction are generally classified under three categories (types I, II and III) as illustrated in Fig. A7.1. The energy band diagram of a heterojunction between a narrow band gap material and a wide band gap material with different type of conductivity is illustrated in Fig. A7.2. The figure shows the energy band diagrams of a typical pn-an isotypehetero junction before and after formation of the junction. The energy hand diagram of the ideal heterojunction is based on Anderson's model which neglects the presence of any interface states at the heterointerface. Practical heterojunctions do have significant interface state charges which may cause deviation in the energy band diagram from the idealized picture depicted in Fig. A7.2.

Heterojunction can be analyzed by using Anderson's model. For the heterojunction under consideration (Fig. A7.2), the following inter-relations between various parameters can be easily derived. The energy band gap difference, ΔE_g is given by

$$\Delta E_g = E_{g2} - E_{g1} \qquad (1)$$

The energy band gap difference is asymmetrically distributed between the conduction and valence band edges on the two sides, given by the following relation

$$\Delta E_g = \Delta E_c + \Delta E_v \qquad (2)$$

where, ΔE_c corresponds to conduction band edge discontinuity and ΔE_v corresponds to valence band edge discontinuity at the heterointerface. The conduction band edge discontinuity, ΔE_c at the heterointerface can be estimated from the electron affinity values of the two semiconductors for an ideal heterojunction as

$$\Delta E_c = q(\chi_2 - \chi_1) \qquad (3)$$

Now, writing

$$\delta_P = E_F - E_{v1} \qquad (4)$$

$$\delta_n = E_{i2} - E_F \qquad (5)$$

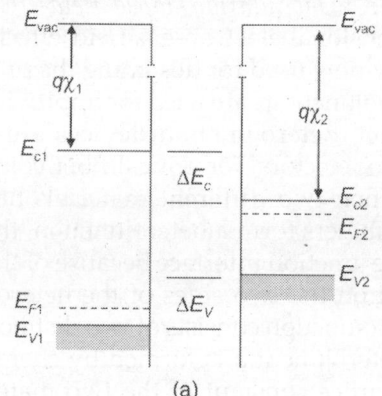

(a)

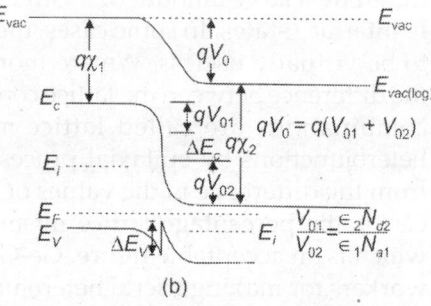

(b)

Fig. A7.2: Energy band diagram of a pn-heterojunction: (a) prior to the formation of junction (b) after formation of junction we may note that a local vacuum level is required to maintain the fact that the electron affinity is the characteristic of the material and does not change after formation of the heterojunction

the energy bandgap of the wider band gap material can be expressed as

$$E_{g1} = \delta_P + \delta_n + qV_{02} + \Delta E_c + qV_{01} \qquad (6)$$

$$= \delta_P + \delta_n + \Delta E_c + qV_0 \qquad (7)$$

where, V_0 is the total built-in potential across the heterointerface which is the sum of the built-in potential V_{01} and V_{02} created on the p-side and n-side of the heterojunction respectively, given by

$$V_0 = V_{01} + V_{02} \tag{8}$$

The band edge discontinuities or the band-offsets calculated on the basis of *Anderson's model* assume that the interface is defect free. According to Anderson's model, the conduction hand edge discontinuity of a heterojunctions can be obtained by taking the difference between the electron affinity values of the two materials. Experimentally measured values for practical heterojunctions reveal that the band offset values are very different from those predicted on the basis of Anderson's model.

One of the major advantages of binary III-V materials and their ternary and quaternary alloys is that many of these materials can form lattice matched pairs for fabrication of useful heterojunction devices. For example, GaAs and AlAs have a lattice mismatch of only 0.04%. This means that the ternary material Alx $Ga_{1-x}As$ for all compositions (different values of x) remains lattice matched almost perfectly. The GaAs/$Al_xGa_{1-x}As$ heterojunctions has been widely used for design and fabrication of near-infrared sources and photodetectors during the first generation (1G) optical fiber communication system. Similarly, $In_{0.53}Ga_{0.47}As$ ($E_g = 0.74$ eV) is lattice matched to InP ($E_g = 1.35$ eV). In GaAs/InP has been extensively used for fabrication of optical sources and photodetectors operating at 1.55 μm which is the standard for the 3G optical communication system. The ideal energy band diagrams of typical N-$Al_{0.3}Ga_{0.7}As$/n-GaAs and P-$Al_{0.3}Ga_{0.7}As$/n-GaAs heterojunctions are illustrated in Fig. A7.3.

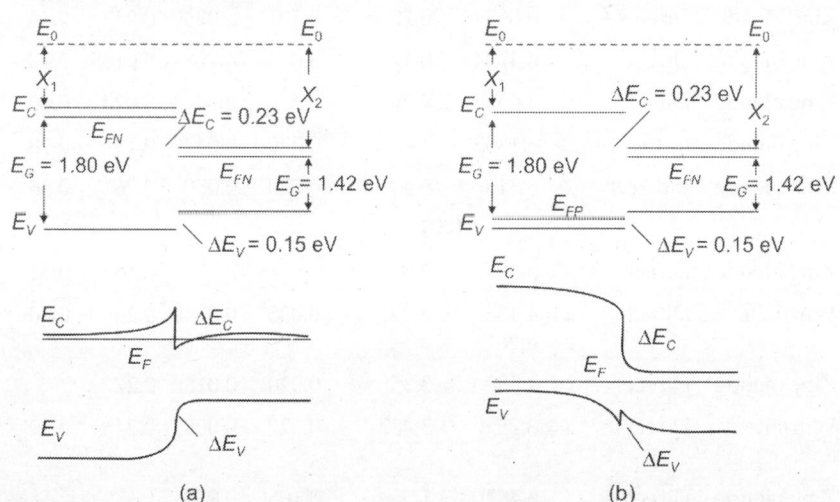

(a) (b)

Fig. A7.3: Energy band diagrams of $Al_{0.3}Ga_{0.7}As$/GaAs heterojunction: (a) N-n heterojunction; (b) pn heterojunction

Figure A7.3 is quite useful for determining the lattice matching between the binary, ternary and quaternary III-V alloys. The shaded regions help one to determine the lattice matched substrates when various binary compounds are used to make ternary and quaternary alloys. For example, it can be clearly seen that for a certain composition of $Ga_xIn_{1-x}As$ determined by the male fraction, x, the ternary material will be lattice matched to InP substrate.

APPENDIX 7.2

PARAMETERS OF SELECTED SEMICONDUCTORS AND SEMICONDUCTOR COMPOUNDS

Semicon- ductor	Crystal structure	Band	Lattice constant ($\AA$)	Band gap (300K) (eV)	Mobility $(m^2V^{-1}s^{-1})$ μ_n	μ_p	Effective mass (m_n^*/m_0)	(m_p^*/m_0)	Relative permittivity ϵ_s/ϵ_0
Elemental									
Si	Diamond	Indirect	5.43102	1.12	0.145	0.05	0.18	0.16^{lh} 0.49^{hh}	11.9
Ge	Diamond	Indirect	5.64613	0.66	0.39	0.19	0.082	0.04^{lh}	16.0
III-V Compound									
GaAs	Zinc blende	Direct	5.6533	1.42	0.8	0.04	0.063	0.076^{hh} 0.05^{lh}	12.9
AlAs	Zinc blende	Indirect	5.6605	2.36	0.018		0.11	0.22	10.1
InP	Zinc blende	Direct	5.8686	1.35	0.46	0.015	0.077	0.64	12.6
GaP	Zinc blende	Indirect	5.4512	2.26	0.011	0.0075	0.82	0.60	11.1
AlP	Zinc blende	Indirect	5.4635	2.42	0.0060	0.045	0.212	0.145	9.8
GaN	Wurtzite	Direct	$a = 3.189$ $c = 5.182$	3.44	0.0400	0.0010	0.27	0.8	10.4
GaSb	Zinc blende	Direct	6.0959	0.72	0.50	0.0850	0.042	0.40	15.7
InSb	Zinc blende	Direct	6.4794	0.17	8.0	0.125	0.0145	0.40	16.8
InAs	Zinc blende	Direct	6.0584	0.36	3.3	0.046	0.023	0.40	15.1
AlSb	Zinc blende	Indirect	6.1355	1.58	0.020	0.0420	0.12	0.98	14.4
BN	Zinc blende	Indirect	6.3157	6.4	0.020	0.050	0.26	0.36	7.1
II-VI									
CdS	Zinc blende	Direct	5.825	2.5			0.14	0.51	5.4
	Wurtizite	Direct	$a = 4.136$ $c = 6.26$	2.49	0.035	0.0040	0.20	0.70	9.1
ZnO	Zinc blende	Direct	4.580	3.35	0.020	0.018	0.27		9.0
	Wurtzite	Direct	$a = 3.25$ $c = 5.2$	3.437	0.022	0.005	0.24	0.59	
CdTe	Zinc blende	Direct	6.482	1.56	0.105	0.010			10.2
IV-IV									
SiC	Wurtzite	Indirect	$a = 3.086$ $c = 15.117$	2.996	0.040	0.005	0.60	1.0	9.66
IV-IV									
Pbs	Rock salt	Indirect	5.9363	0.41	0.060	0.070	0.25	0.25	17.0
PbTe	Rock salt	Indirect	6.4620	0.31	0.60	0.40	0.17	0.20	30.0

lh: light hole, *hh*: heavy hole.

Optical Sources 2—
The Light Emitting Diode (LED)

8.1 INTRODUCTION

We have discussed in Chapter 7, the spontaneous emission of radiations in visible and infrared regions of the spectrum from a forward-biased *pn* junction. The normally empty conduction band of the semiconductor is populated by electrons injected into it by the forward current through the junction, and light is generated when these electrons recombine with holes in the valence band to emit a photon. This is the basic mechanism by which light is emitted from an LED, but stimulated emission is not encouraged, as it is in the injection laser, by the addition of an optical cavity and mirror facets provided for feedback of photons.

The LED can therefore operate at lower current densities in comparison to the injection laser, but the emitted photons have random phases and the device is an *incoherent* optical source. Further, the energy of the emitted photons is only roughly equal to the bandgap energy of the semiconductor material, which provides a much wider spectral bandwidth (almost by a factor of 100) in comparison to the injection laser. The linewidth of an LED corresponds to a range of photon energy between 1 and 3.5 kT, where T is the absolute temperature. This gives linewidths of 30 to 40 nm for GaAs based devices operating at room temperature. Obviously, the LED supports many optical modes within its structure and this is why it is often used as a *multimode* source, although the coupling of LEDs to single-mode fibers has been pursed successfully, especially when advanced structures are employed. However, LEDs have several drawbacks as compared to injection laser. These includes:

  (i) generally lower optical power coupled into a optical fiber (microwatts)
  (ii) harmonic distortion, and
  (iii) usually lower modulation bandwidth

Nodoubt, these problems may initially appear to make the LED less attractive optical source as compared to injection laser, the LED device has a number of distinct advantages due to which it finds a prominent place in optical fiber communications:

  (i) *Simple fabrication of LED*. In LED, there are no mirror facets and in some structures no striped geometry.
  (ii) *Reduced cost*. The simpler construction of the LED leads to quite reduced cost as compared to injection laser and moreover, which is always likely to be maintained.
  (iii) *Reliability of LED*. The LED does not exhibit *catastrophic degradation* and also proved to be far less sensitive to gradual degradation as compared to the injection laser. Further, LED is also immune to *self-pulsation* and *modal noise* problems.

(iv) *LED is generally less temperature dependent.* The light output against current characteristic of LED is less affected by temperature than the corresponding characteristic for the injection laser. Moreover, the LED is not a threshold device and therefore raising the temperature does not increase the threshold current above the operating point and hence half operation.

(v) *Simple drive circuitry of LED.* This is due to the generally lower drive currents and reduced temperature dependence which makes temperature compensation circuits for LED unnecessary.

(vi) *Linear output.* Ideally, the LED exhibit linearity in light output against current characteristic, unlike the injection laser. This is found to be advantageous where analog modulation is concerned.

These advantages along with the development of high-radiance, relatively high-bandwidth devices have almost ensured that the LED remains an extensively used source for optical fiber communication.

Structures of LED fabricated using the GaAs/AlGaAs material system are well tried for operation in the shorter wavelength region. Further, there have been substantial advances in LED devices based on InGaAsP/InP material structure for use in the longer wavelength region especially around 1.3 μm. At this wavelength, the material dispersion in silica glass fibers goes through zero and thus the wider linewidth of the LED imposes a far slighter limitation on link length than does intermodal within multimode fiber. Moreover, the reduced fiber attenuation at this operating wavelength can allow longer have LED systems.

Although longer wavelength LED systems using multimode graded index optical fiber have been developed, particularly for nontelecommunication applications, activity has also been concerned with both high-speed operation and with the coupling of these InGaAsP LED to single-mode fiber. A major impetus for these strategies has been the potential deployment of such single-mode LED systems in telecommunication access network or subscriber loop. Thus, LEDs are likely to remain a significant optical fiber communication source for many system applications including operation over shorter distances with single mode fiber at transmission rates that may exceed 1 Gbit s^{-1}.

The intent of this chapter is to study photodetectors and LEDs.

8.2 PHOTOELECTRIC EFFECT

Photoelectric effect (photoeffect) is the process of emission of electrons from a metal surface when it is illuminated by high-frequency electromagnetic radiation (Fig. 8.1). The photoelectric effect is of following different forms:

8.2.1 Photoemissive Effect

When a radiation (photon) of wavelength less than a critical value is incident upon a metal surface, electrons are found to be emitted; this is called photoemissive or photoelectric effect, e.g. vacuum and gas phototubes. Kinetic energy E of emitted electrons is given by:

$$E = h\nu - e\Phi \tag{8.1}$$

The $e\Phi$ is the surface work function. No electrons will be emitted when $h\nu < e\Phi$ (or in terms of wavelength, $\lambda > hc/e\Phi$). The ratio of the number of emitted electrons to the number of absorbed photons is called *quantum yield* or *quantum efficiency*. The minimum

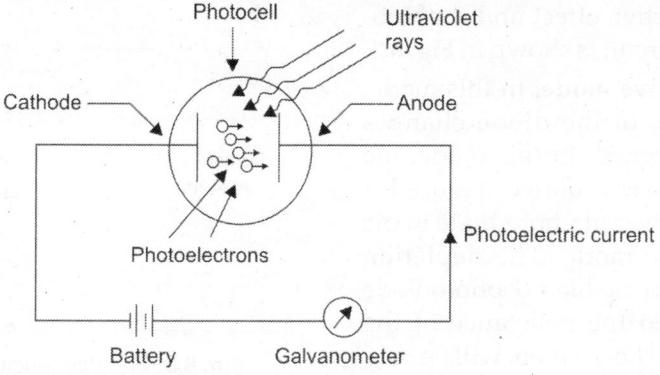

Fig. 8.1: Photoelectric effect

frequency that can cause a photoelectric effect is called *threshold frequency*, and the corresponding wavelength of light beyond which the photoelectric effect ceases is called *threshold wavelength* or *cut-off wavelength*.

8.2.2 Photoconductive Effect

An electron may be raised from the valence band to the conduction band in a semiconductor by the absorption of a photon of frequency ν provided that:

$$h\nu \geq E_g \tag{8.2}$$

where energy gap is E_g, or in terms of wavelength:

$$\lambda \leq \frac{hc}{E_g} \tag{8.3}$$

We define bandgap wavelength λ_g as the largest value of wavelength that can cause this transition, i.e.:

$$\lambda_g = \frac{hc}{E_g} \tag{8.4}$$

As long as the electron remains in the conduction band, it will cause an increase in the conductivity of the semiconductor. This is the phenomenon of *photoconductivity*. This is the basic mechanism in the working of photoconductive detectors. Figure 8.2 illustrates

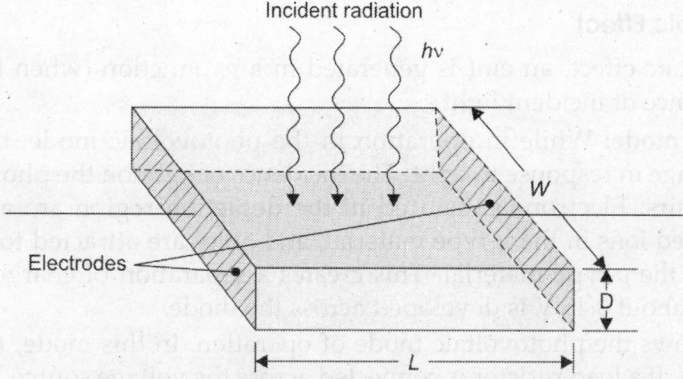

Fig. 8.2: Illustration of photoelectric effect

the photoconductive effect and a photo-conductor bias circuit is shown in Fig. 8.3.

Photoconductive mode: In this mode, the conductance of the diode changes when light is applied. In this mode, the photodiode is reverse-biased. Figure 8.4 shows a reverse-biased photodiode in the photoconductive mode. The depletion region of the reverse-biased photodiode is very wide and the resistance of the diode is high, and hence there will be only a small reverse current through it. This reverse current that flows through the diode when there is no light being applied is called *dark current* (I_o).

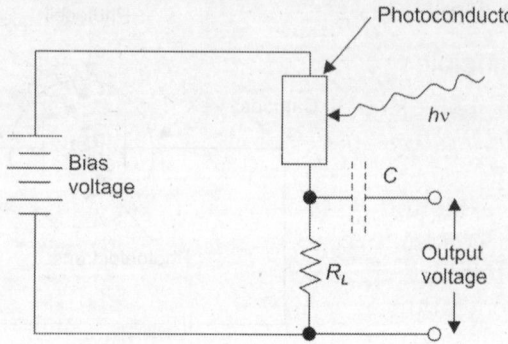

Fig. 8.3: Photoconductor bias circuit

When light is incident, electron–hole pairs are generated. Electrons are attracted to the positive bias voltage, and holes are attracted to the negative bias voltage. This movement of electrons and holes causes a considerable reverse current to flow through the photodiode. The resistance of the photodiode is extremely low when light is incident. If the intensity of light is increased, resistance decreases and therefore, reverse current increases. Current that is passed through the photodiode when light is being applied is called *light current* (I_L).

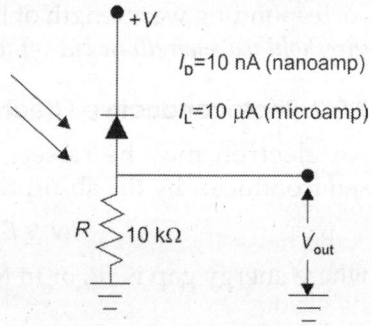

Fig. 8.4: Photoconductive mode of operation

The conductivity of the photodiode is low when there is no light incident, and conductivity increases as the intensity of light increases. Consequently, the magnitude of dark current is very much smaller than that of light current. Consider the example shown in Fig. 8.4. Assume that dark current (I_D) is dependent on the amount of current flowing in the circuit. With no light present:

$$V_{out} = I_p \times R = 10 \text{ nA} \times 10 \text{ k}\Omega = 100 \text{ }\mu\text{V}$$

With light present:

$$V_{out} = I_L \times R = 10 \text{ }\mu\text{V} \times 10 \text{ k}\Omega = 1 \text{ V}$$

8.2.3 Photovoltaic Effect

In the photovoltaic effect, an emf is generated in a *pn* junction (when reverse-biased) under the influence of incident light.

Photovoltaic mode: While in operation in the photovoltaic mode, the photodiode generates a voltage in response to light. The incidence of light on the photodiode creates electron-hole pairs. Electrons generated in the depletion region are attracted to the positively charged ions in the *n*-type material, and holes are attracted to the negatively charged ions in the *p*-type material. This creates a separation of charges, and a small voltage drop of about 0.45 V is developed across the diode.

Figure 8.5 shows the photovoltaic mode of operation. In this mode, the photodiode acts as a *solar cell*. If a load resistor is connected across the voltage source, a small current will flow from the cathode to the anode.

8.3 PHOTODETECTORS

Principle

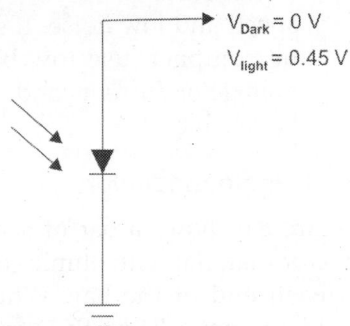

$V_{Dark} = 0 \text{ V}$

$V_{light} = 0.45 \text{ V}$

A photodetector is a device that *converts optical energy to electrical energy*. The principal mechanism responsible for this transformation is photoconductivity. This property is exhibited by all semiconductors and it is the increase in conductivity brought about by the absorption of photons. The absorption of a photon results in the generation of an electron-hole pair. The electrons and holes separate to become mobile carriers which are transported through the semiconductor under the influence of an externally applied electric field. The

Fig. 8.5: Photovoltaic mode of operation

transport of these carriers enhances the conductivity of the semiconductor. In concise terms, the three basic processes involved in this conversion are:

1. The absorption of photons and the resulting generation of carriers.
2. The transport of the generated carriers across the absorption or drift region under the influence of an applied field. Internal amplification of carriers can occur at this stage via various mechanisms. An example of a mechanism is impact ionization which occurs with the application of large electric fields.
3. Collection of carriers constituting a photocurrent which flows through an external circuitry.

Perhaps, the simplest type of photodetector is the photoconductor which is simply a slab of an intrinsic semiconductor with two contacts. The electron–hole pairs, generated by absorption of photons in the material, are collected by oppositely biased contacts to constitute a photocurrent. Other types of photodetectors are photodiodes which are based on either the *p-n* junction or the metal-semiconductor junction (also called a Schottky-barrier). A *p-i-n* (or PIN) photodiode is a reverse-biased *p-n* junction with an intrinsic layer interposed between the *p* and *n* layers. Because the depletion area is the only region supporting an electric field in a *p-n* junction, the intrinsic layer serves to increase the depletion layer width, and therefore, the photon absorption region of the device. The PIN photodiode is normally operated in a bias mode in which the device does not exhibit gain. Another type of photodetector based on a *p-n* junction is the *avalanche photodiode* (APD). APDs are operated at electric fields which are highly enough to cause impact ionization and, thereby, generate more carriers, leading to the avalanche effect. The net effect of the avalanche process is a multiplication of carriers, resulting in gain for the output photocurrent of the device. As mentioned above, another important class of photodetectors, which have recently gained prominence, are the *metal-semiconductor photodiodes* which are made from metal-semiconductor-metal (MSM), photodiodes attractive for some applications requiring monolithic integration.

As described above, there are some basic properties exhibited by all semiconductor photodetectors. These general properties can be quantified, to a certain extent, and have become figures of merit used in comparing photodetectors. The properties can be quantified in terms of quantum efficiency, responsivity, bandwidth, and noise equivalent power (NEP).

The operation of photodetector involves three steps:

- Carrier generation, i.e. the absorption of photon reate electron–hole pairs
- Carrier transport
- Interaction of current with external circuit to provide output signal. Requirements for photodetector are high sensitivity at the operating wavelengths, high response

speed and low noise. It should be compact, use low biasing voltage or currents and should be reliable.

8.3.1 Photoconductor

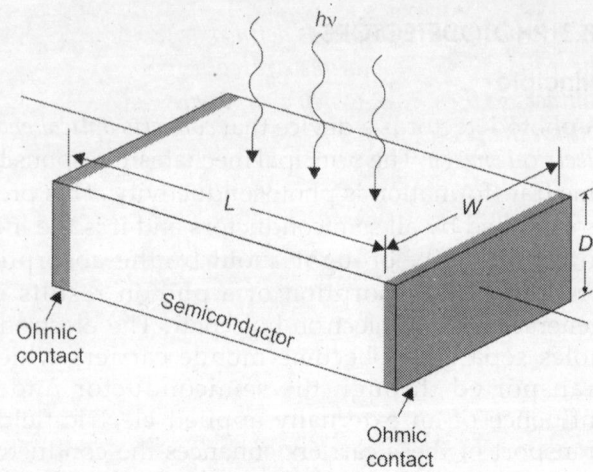

Fig. 8.6: A semiconductor bar exposed to light

Figure 8.6 shows a bar of semiconductor material with ohmic contacts at each end of the bar. When the incident light falls on the surface of the semiconductor bar (which is photoconductor) electron-hole pairs (E$_i$HP) are generated by band-to-band transition or by extrinsic transitions. This extra electron–hole pairs increase the conductivity of the material. The initial thermal-equilibrium conductivity is (before light falls):

$$\sigma_0 = q(n_0\mu_n + p_0\mu_p) \tag{8.5}$$

The increase in conductivity under illumination is mainly due to the increase in the number of carriers, and is given as:

$$\Delta\sigma = q\delta p(\mu_n + \mu_p) \tag{8.6}$$

This change in conductivity due to optical excitation is known as *photoconductivity*.

When a voltage is applied across the bar of length L, then the electric field produces current in the bar. The current density is written as:

$$J = J_0 + J_L = (\sigma_0 + \Delta\sigma)E \tag{8.7}$$

where J_0 is the current density (when no optical excitation, i.e. dark condition) and J_L is photocurrent density.

Let us assume electrons and holes are generated uniformly throughout the bar then the current due to the optical excitation is:

$$
\begin{aligned}
I_L = J_L A &= \Delta\sigma AE \\
&= \delta_p(\mu_n + \mu_p)\, A_{Eq} \\
&= G_L\tau_p(\mu_n + \mu_p)\, A_{Eq}
\end{aligned} \tag{8.8}
$$

where A is the cross-sectional area of the device. Equation (8.8) shows that photocurrent is directly proportional to the area of the device and the rate at which excess-carriers are generate.

The time required by electron to flow through the bar of the photoconductor is known as *transit time*, and is given as:

$$t_n = L/\mu_n E \tag{8.8a}$$

Substituting this value in Eq. (8.8), one finds:

$$
\begin{aligned}
I_L &= G_L\tau_p\,(\mu_n + \mu_p)\,A_q\,\frac{L}{t_n} \\
&= qAG_L\left(\frac{\tau_p}{t_n}\right)(\mu_n + \mu_p)\,\frac{L}{\mu_n} \\
&= qAG_L L\left(\frac{\tau_p}{t_n}\right)\left(1 + \frac{\mu_p}{\mu_n}\right)
\end{aligned} \tag{8.9}
$$

The *photocurrent gain is defined as the ratio of the rate at which charges are collected by the contacts to the rate at which charges are generated within the photoconductor*, i.e.:

$$\text{Gain} = \frac{I_L}{qG_L A_L} \qquad (8.10)$$

Substituting Eq. (8.9) into Eq. (8.10), one obtains:

$$\text{Gain } (g) = \frac{\tau_p}{t_n}\left(1 + \frac{\mu_p}{\mu_n}\right) \qquad (8.11)$$

If $m_p/m_n \ll 1$:

$$\text{Gain } (g) = \frac{\tau_p}{t_n} \qquad (8.12)$$

Figure 8.7 shows an InGaAs photoconductor.

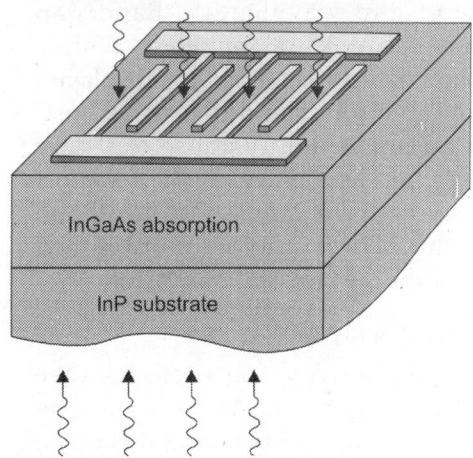

Fig. 8.7: Schematic of an InGaAs photoconductor which is illuminated on the front and back sides

8.3.2 Quantum Efficiency (η)

The quantum efficiency η of a photodetector is the number of electron–hole pairs generated per incident photon collected at the contacts. Quantum efficiency is determined by many factors. These include the fact that not all photons incident on the semiconductor will produce electron–hole pairs and that some of the photons may be reflected at the surface of the semiconductor. All these factors combine to reduce η. Quantum efficiency can therefore be given by:

$$\eta = (1 - r)\,\zeta[1 - \exp(-\alpha L)] \qquad (8.13)$$

where r is the optical power reflectance at the surface of the detector, ζ is the fraction of electron-hole pairs that actually contribute to the photo-current, α is the absorption coefficient of the detector material per centimeter, and L is the width of the detector's absorption region. By applying an antireflection coating on the detector's surface for the wavelength of operation, reflection can be reduced and, thereby, the factor $(1 - r)$ can be maximized. It is difficult to estimate the factor ζ because it depends on the quality of the material. Carriers can be lost through recombination at the surface or in the bulk of the material which reduces the photocurrent. Modern epitaxial growth methods are now capable of producing high quality materials, and therefore, for a practical estimation of quantum efficiency, ζ can be assumed as unity. The last factor $[1 - \exp(-\alpha L)]$ denotes the *fraction of the incident optical power* absorbed in bulk of the detector.

In terms of the quantities easily measured in the laboratory, quantum efficiency is given by:

$$\eta = \frac{I_p/q}{p_i/h\nu} = \frac{h\nu}{q} \cdot \frac{I_p}{p_i} \qquad (8.14)$$

where I_p is the detector photocurrent, p_i is the incident optical power, and $h\nu$ is the photon energy. The quantity η given above is known as the external quantum efficiency η_{ext}. The quantum efficiency is dependent on the absorption coefficient α which is a function of wavelength λ. Figure 8.8 shows the dependence of α on λ for some detector materials. Because only photons with energy greater than or equal to the bandgap energy E_g can be absorbed (i.e. $hc/\lambda \geq E_g$), the long-wavelength limit for a practical detector is the band gap wavelength. Band gap energies at 300 K for representative photodetector materials are displayed in Table 8.1. There is also a short-wavelength limit because α is very large at short wavelengths for most semiconductors, and consequently, all of the incident photons are absorbed near the surface of the detector.

Responsivity (R)

The responsivity, R of a detector is the photocurrent in the device divided by the input optical power and is given by:

$$R = \frac{I_p}{P_i} = \frac{nq}{h\nu} = \eta \frac{\lambda(\mu m)}{1.24} \qquad (8.15)$$

The unit of responsivity in A/W. It is seen from this expression that, for a constant η, R should increase with λ. This is illustrated in Fig. 8.9. However, because α depends on λ, there is a region between the short- and long-wavelength limits over which R increases. For photodetectors which exhibit gain, the gain factor G can be accommodated in a more general equation for responsivity given by:

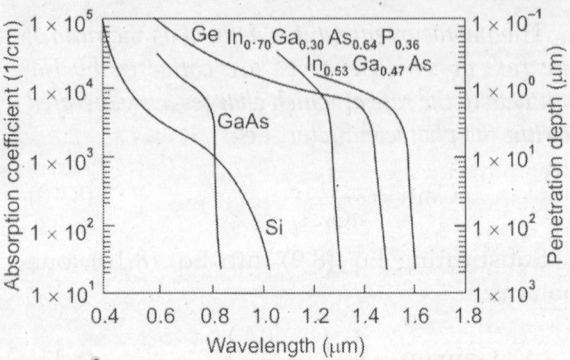

Fig. 8.8: Wavelength (λ) dependence of the optical absorption coefficients of several semiconductor materials

Table 8.1: Band gap energies (in eV) at 300 K for some photodiode materials

Material	Bandgap energy (E_g)
GaAs	1.42
GaSb	0.73
GaAs$_{0.88}$Sb$_{0.12}$	1.15
Ge	0.67
InAs	0.35
In$_{0.53}$Ga$_{0.47}$As	0.75
InP	1.35
Si	1.14

$$R = G\eta \frac{\lambda(\mu m)}{1.24} \qquad (8.16)$$

It is possible to degrade the responsivity of a detector by applying excessive incident optical power. The detector becomes saturated, thus, limiting its linear dynamic range, which is the range over which the relationship between the detector's output and the incident optical power in linear.

8.3.3 Bandwidth

The bandwidth B of a photodetector measures the shortest response time of the device. This property becomes very important when a photodetector is used in a data transmission circuit. The faster a detector can respond to a stream of optical pulses, the higher the density of the transmitted data can be. The response time of a photodetector is determined by three factors—*transit time, diffusion time*, and the *device RC time constant*.

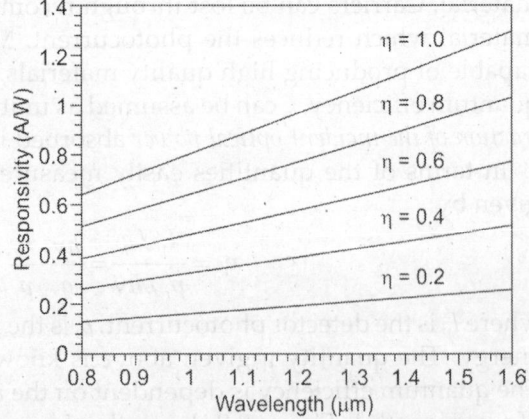

Fig. 8.9: Responsivity (R) vs wavelength (λ) for various external quantum efficiencies

Electron-hole pairs created by photons in the active region of a photo–detector move in directions opposite to the contacts for collection under an applied electric field. The carriers move by drift and diffusion. If the electric field is sufficiently large, most of the carriers travel by drift, and they reach their scattering-limited or saturation velocity in the material. The velocity of holes is usually smaller than that of electrons, therefore, the time (i.e., transit time), it takes holes to drift across the active region of the detector limits the response time of the device. If electron-hole pairs are generated uniformly throughout the material, then, a severe transit time spread between electrons and holes can occur. Diffusion time limitations can occur only at low bias where the drift field is low. Because the diffusion process is slow, it can be a severe problem even though only a small number of carriers may be involved. A judicious design of the active area of the detectors and the application of an appropriate bias can make this limitation insignificant. The last factor is the resistance R and the capacitance C of the device and its associated circuitry. This composite RC network integrates the output current of the detector and, therefore, increase the response time. Different types of photodetectors are influenced by different combinations of these limitations which set their bandwidths. However, photodetectors of a given design and material do exhibit a constant gain-bandwidth product.

8.3.4 Noise Equivalent Power (NEP)

Photodetectors are subject to several sources of noise that degrades their performance. The inherent randomness in the arrival of photons and the absorption of photons in the device save as sources of noise. Various sources of current generation exist in all photodetectors. Some of these include current due to the incoming optical signal, current due to background radiation, and the dark current that is due to surface leakage, tunneling, and thermal generation of electron-hole pairs in or around the active region. All of these currents are generated randomly and contribute to *shot noise*. The amplification process that produces gain in some detectors is the *avalanche mechanism*. This is a random effect, and, therefore, there is a gain noise associated with such detectors. Another source of noise involves the *random motion of carriers* in resistive electrical materials at finite temperatures. There are parasitic resistances intrinsic to photodetectors and also resistances in circuits in which photodetectors are utilized. An example is a receiver circuit in which a detector serves as a source of input current to a preamplifier. The noise generated by these resistive elements is called *thermal*, or *Johnson*, or *Nyquist noise*. This noise is given by:

$$\left\langle i_j^2 \right\rangle = \frac{4kT_{\text{eff}}B}{R_{\text{eff}}} \tag{8.17}$$

where R_{eff} is the parallel combination of the detector and the pre-amplifier input resistances, B is the bandwidth, and T_{eff} is the effective temperature which is related to the noise figure NF of the amplifier:

$$T_{\text{eff}} = T\left(10^{\text{NF}/10} - 1\right) \tag{8.18}$$

where T is the ambient temperature. It is, therefore, evident that, in the operation of a detector, the output signal must be above the noise level. The signal-to-noise ratio (SNR) is, therefore, an important characteristic in photodetectors, and it is related to sensitivity. The sensitivity of a photodetector is the minimum optical input power needed to achieve a given value of SNR. A measure of sensitivity is called *noise equivalent power* (NEP). NEP is the optical power (or photocurrent) required for the SNR to be unity over a 1-Hz bandwidth. Essentially, this measures when the photocurrent is exactly equal to the noise current. Thus, NEP measures the minimum detectable power in a photodetector. NEP depends on bandwidth, and, to find the optical power required to produce a SNR of unity for an entire measurement bandwidth, we have:

$$-P_i = \text{NEP} \sqrt{B}. \tag{8.19}$$

Another figure of merit also useful for determining the ultimate detection limit is *detectivity* D^* given by:

$$D^* = \frac{\sqrt{AB}}{\text{NEP}} \; (\text{cm Hz}^{1/2} \cdot \text{W}^{-1}) \tag{8.20}$$

where A is the area of the photodetector on which light is incident. As with NEP, the reference bandwidth is taken as 1 Hz. D^* is usually expressed as $D^*(\lambda, f, 1)$ where λ is the wavelength and f is the modulation frequency of the input optical signal. It must be noted that NEP and D^* are not equal to system sensitivity in actual applications because other noise sources, such as preamplifier noise, may dominate, especially in high speed (GHz) systems.

Note: The quantum efficiency of a photoconductor is given by Eq. (8.13) and the responsivity is given by Eq. (8.16), where G is the internal photocurrent gain of the device. The gain is brought about by the fact that photogenerated carriers contribute to current until they recombine. The gain is given by:

$$G = \frac{\tau}{t_{tr}} \tag{8.21}$$

where τ is the excess-carrier recombination life-time and τ_{tr} is the transit time of the majority carrier. The transit time is given by:

$$\tau_{tr} = \frac{L}{v} \tag{8.22}$$

where L is the channel length (distance between contacts) and v is the carrier velocity. It is seen from these equations that, if the recombination lifetime is greater than the majority-carrier transit time, then many carriers will travel between the contacts before recombination takes place. This is photoconductor gain, and it can be below unity or well above unity depending on various factors including semiconductor material, size of the device, and the magnitude of the applied voltage.

The bandwidth of a photoconductor is given by:

$$B = \frac{1}{2\pi\tau} \tag{8.23}$$

It is seen that, whereas a long recombination time makes for a high gain, it also reduces bandwidth. So, a trade-off between gain and bandwidth exists for photoconductors. The gain-bandwidth product of a photoconductive detector is given by:

$$GB = \frac{1}{2\pi t_{tr}} \tag{8.24}$$

where t_{tr} is a *constant for a given material and detector configuration.*

The primary contributions to noise in photoconductive detectors are made by thermal or Johnson noise and the generation-recombination noise. The thermal noise given by Eq. (8.17) results from the random motion of carriers with average energy of kT contributing to the dark current of the device. The generation-recombination noise is due to fluctuation in the generation and recombination of carriers which, in turn, leads to fluctuations in the conductivity of the device. The generation-recombination noise is given by:

$$\left\langle i_{G-R}^2 \right\rangle = \frac{4qI_0GB}{1+\omega^2\tau^2} \cdot \tag{8.25}$$

where I_0 is steady-state output photocurrent and ω is the angular modulation frequency of the input optical signal.

To describe the overall noise performance of a photoconductor, the NEP is given by:

$$\text{NEP} = \frac{8h\nu}{\eta}\left[1+\frac{kT}{qG}(1+\omega^2 r^2)\frac{G_c}{I_0}\right] \tag{8.26}$$

where G_c is the conductance of the channel. The dominant noise mechanism in a photoconductive detector is the thermal noise of the conducting channel. An increase in channel resistance is necessary to reduce thermal noise. If the thickness of the channel is reduced to increase the resistance, then quantum efficiency is reduced. To obtain the highest resistance and, hence, the lowest thermal noise achievable while maintaining high gain and quantum efficiency, it is necessary to utilize materials with the lowest carrier concentration. Thermal noise, generation-recombination noise, and dark current are high in semiconductors with smaller band gaps. Although, photoconductors can have large gains, the gain may not be enough to surmount the inherent noise limitations to make them useful in many applications.

8.4 LIGHT EMITTING DIODES (LEDs)

A LED is a *pn* junction diode of special construction. Like other semiconductor diodes, its behaviour is influenced by biasing conditions. Fig. 8.10 shows the basic operation of an LED. The *pn* junction is forward-biased when the cathode (*n* type region) is negative with respect to the anode. Under forward-bias, electrons from the *n* type region and holes in the *p* type material move towards the *pn* junction.

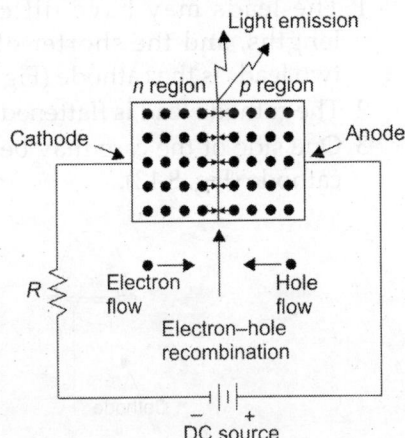

At the junction, the holes and electrons combine. Electrons are at a higher energy level than are holes. The electrons literally fall into holes as they combine, and in doing so, they release the excess amount of energy in the form of light. There is current through the LED in the forward direction, just as in the case of an ordinary diode.

When the *pn* junction is reverse-biased, the LED does not conduct and there is no release of light. Hence the LED emits light when forward-biased and does not emit light when reverse-biased. The

Fig. 8.10: Basic operation of a light emitting diode

schematic symbol of LED is shown in Fig. 8.11. The LED operates at forward voltages typically ranging from 1.2 V to 4.3 V. The reverse break-down voltage is in the range of −3 to −10 V.

The main advantages of LEDs are:

   (i) LEDs have very long life.

   (ii) LEDs are highly durable and reliable.

(iii) The efficiency of LEDs is higher than that of incandescent light bulb and can possibly exceed fluorescence bulbs.

(iv) White-light LED sources can provide significant energy saving in comparison with conventional lighting.

8.4.1 LED Construction and Working

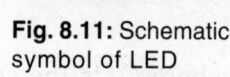

LED emits more light than an ordinary diode because ordinary diodes are made of silicon, which is opaque or impenetrable as far. Energy in ordinary diodes is, therefore, released in the form of heat.

On the other hand, LEDs are made of semiconductor materials that are semitransparent. LEDs are normally made of gallium arsenide phosphide, which emits visible red light. Gallium phosphide produces visible green light. LEDs that produce yellow and blue light are also available.

Fig. 8.11: Schematic symbol of LED

Figure 8.12 shows a LED chip and a typical LED package. The LED chip is attached to cathode and anode leads through thin wires. The plastic case serves as a lens that conducts light away from the LED and also acts as a magnifier. The entire case may be dyed or tinted with a colour that enhances the on/off contrast of the LED. LED leads are identified by one of the following three ways (Fig. 8.13):

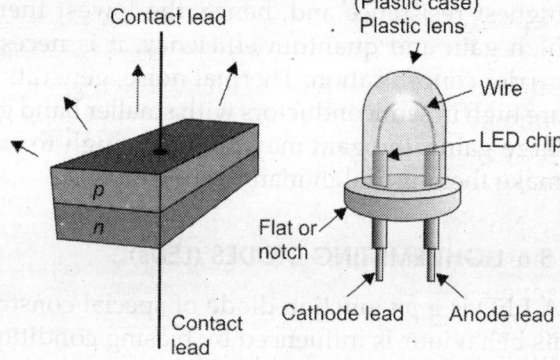

1. The leads may have different lengths, and the shorter of the two leads is the cathode (Fig. 8.13(a)).

Fig. 8.12: The LED: (a) chip (b) typical package

2. The cathode lead is flattened (Fig. 8.13(b)).
3. One side of the case may be flattened. The lead closest to the flattened side is the cathode (Fig. 8.13).

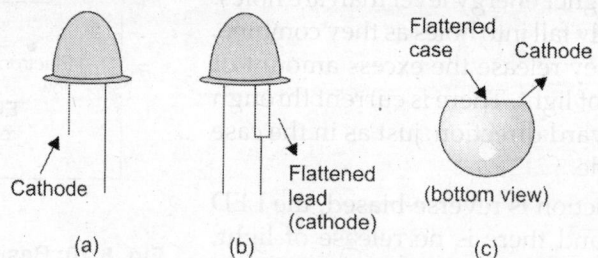

Fig. 8.13. Identification of LED leads

A cross-sectional view of a typical diffused LED is shown in Fig. 8.14.

The semiconductor material employed may be GaAs, GaAsP or GaP. Here an *n* type epitaxial layer is grown upon the substrate, and the region is created by diffusion. When the *pn* junction is forward-biased, charge carrier recombination occurs in the *p* region, so this region is kept uppermost. The *p* region, therefore, becomes the surface of the device, and the metal film anode connection must be patterned to allow most of light to be emitted

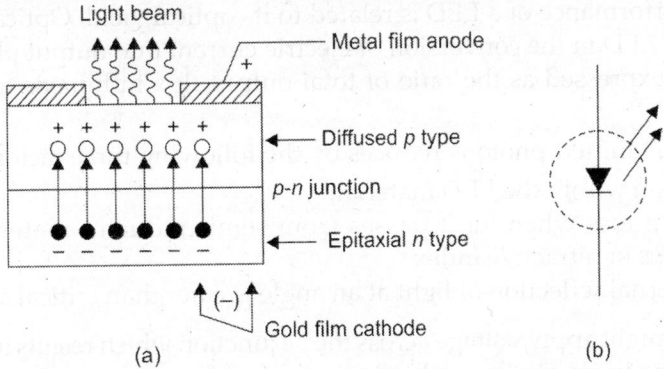

Fig. 8.14: (a) Structure of LED (b) symbol (LED)

outside it. This is done by making a connection to the outside edges of the p layer or by depositing a comb-shaped pattern in the mid-region of p material. A gold film is applied at the bottom of the substrate to reflect light as much as possible towards the upper surface of the device and to provide a cathode connection. Materials like GaAs emit infrared (invisible) radiations. However, GaAsP provides either red or yellow light, while red or green light is emitted by GaP. Its symbol is shown in Fig. 8.14(b) where the direction of arrows indicates emitted light.

Normally a single LED is used to indicate current in the circuit but generally a seven-segment display is used where seven LEDs are combined to show a numerical display [Fig. 8.15(a)]. Any desired number between 0 and 9 can be displayed. The seven segments are labelled a, b, c, d, e, f, g. We can easily follow that a display for number 2 will

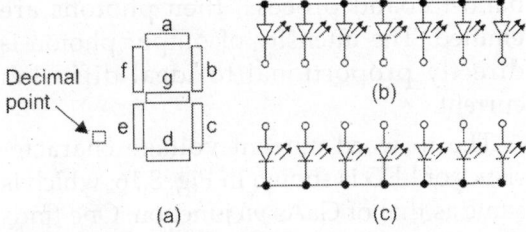

Fig. 8.15: (a) Seven-segment display (b) common anode connection (c) common cathode connection

be shown by the glow of a, b, g, e, d segments. Similarly, for a display of number 8 all the segments shall grow. In this way we have the following series:

Numerals	0	1	2	3
Display segments	a, b, c, d, e, f	b, c	a, b, g, e, d	a, b, g, c, d

The LED device is usually very small, so to enhance the lighted segments surface, solid plastic light pipes are often used. The LEDs is seven-segment display may be connected in common anode configuration (Fig. 8.15(b)) or common cathode configuration (Fig. 8.15(c)), so when selecting a display, it is important to choose the configuration.

The forward voltage for a LED is typically 1.2 V for forward current 20 mA. The relatively large amounts of current consumed by LEDs are their major disadvantage. Excluding the display, a typical electronic circuitry in LEDs may require as high as 10 mA, necessitating a bulky power supply. However, they have the big advantage of long life and ruggedness. Often LEDs are usually switched ON and OFF by means of a transistor circuit. In such cases, a resistance is connected in series with it.

With the introduction of liquid crystal diodes (LCD), its main disadvantage of requiring high current of the order of 20 mA has been offset. At present, LCDs are very popular and used mostly in measuring meters.

Luminous performance of a LED is related to its optical yield. Optical yield measures the efficiency of LED in the conversion of electric current into output photon. Luminous performance is expressed as the ratio of total output flux in lumens to input power in watts.

The quality of emitted photons reduces by the following three factors:

(i) Absorption within the LED material.

(ii) Reflection loss when light passes from semiconductor material to air due to differences in refractive index.

(iii) Total internal reflection of light at an angle greater than critical angle (θ_c).

In LEDs, one might apply voltage across the *pn* junction which results in a diode current, which in turn produces photon and light output. This inverse mechanism is termed as *injection electroluminescence*.

When a voltage is applied across *pn* junction, electron and holes are injected across the space charge region, where they became excess minority carriers. These excess minority carriers diffuse into regions of neutral semiconductor and recombine with majority carriers. If this recombination is a direct band-to-band process, then photons are emitted. The intensity of output photon is directly proportional to ideal diffusion current.

The forward current voltage characteristics of LED is shown in Fig. 8.16, which is same as that of GaAs *pn* junction. One finds that at low forward voltages, diode current is dominated by nonradiative recombination current mainly due to surface recombination near the perimeter of LED chip. Diode current is dominated by radiative diffusion current at higher voltages. At even higher

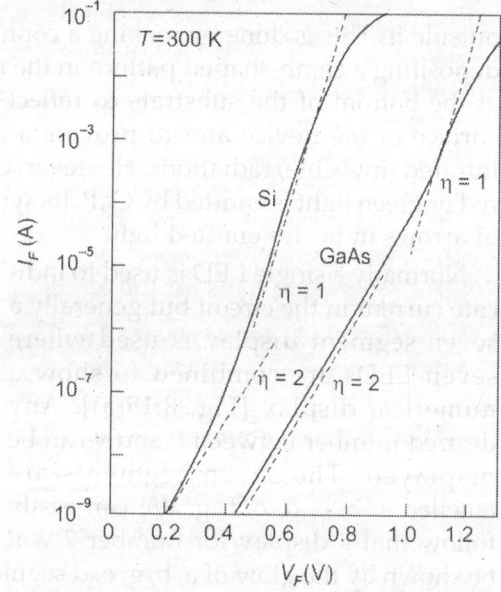

Fig. 8.16: Forward-bias current-voltage characteristic of LED

voltages, the series resistance will limit diode current. The total diode current can be expressed as the sum of saturation current due to diffusion (I_d) and saturation current due to recombination (I_r) as:

$$I = I_d \exp\left[\frac{q(V - IR_s)}{kT}\right] + I_r \exp\left[\frac{q(V - IR_s)}{2kT}\right] \qquad (8.27)$$

where R_s is device series resistance.

8.4.2 Internal and External Quantum Efficiency of an LED

The internal quantum efficiency of a LED is a function of diode that will produce luminescence and is also a function of injection efficiency as well as of percentage of radiative recombination events compared with the total number of recombination events. The internal quantum efficiency of homo junction LED is influenced by the following factors:

(i) Quality and purity of the material and substrate.

(ii) Existence of a direct energy gap spectrally matched to the desired wavelength.

The presence of traps and impurities reduce the internal quantum efficiency of an LED. The internal and external quantum efficiency bears the following relationship:

$$\eta_{ext} = \eta_{int}\, C_{ox} \tag{8.28}$$

where C_{ox} represents extraction efficiency. Extraction efficiency is defined as the fraction of generated photons that escapes from the device package and emerges from the chip.

Extraction efficiency is determined by taking care of the following issues:

(i) Absorption coefficient of the material at emission wavelength.

(ii) Radiation geometry of the LED.

(iii) Substrate.

We may note that LED is an **incoherent light source** because photons are emitted randomly from the junction in all directions and not in phase with each other. This is why, LED is less suitable for the transmission of digital information than lasers.

Recently certain organic semiconductors (e.g. 8-hydroxy-quinolinato aluminium) have been found useful for electroluminescent applications. The organic light emitting diode (OLED) is particularly useful for multicolour, large area, flat-panel display due to its attribute of low power consumption and excellent emissive quality with wide viewing angle.

For designing OLEDs, the criteria are:

(i) Ultrathin layer for low biasing voltage (typically 150 nm).

(ii) Low injection barriers.

(iii) Proper band gaps for the required colour.

There are two general types of OLED devices: those made with small organic molecules and those made with organic polymers. Low cost of OLEDs is the main advantage over standard LEDs. Since OLEDs are non-crystalline materials, they can be easily deposited. However, there are some problems with OLEDs, e.g. small lifetime of OLEDs; the organic materials used in LEDs are quite sensitive to water and oxygen, and therefore, they must be deposited on glass substrates and covered with a second sheet of glass. The usage of glass enhances the cost of manufacturing.

Applications: LEDs have replaced incandescent light bulbs as display devices. Long life expectancy, ruggedness and low power consumption have contributed to the choice of LEDs over incandescent light bulbs. Different types of liquid crystal displays have now replaced LEDs in some applications because they use much less energy than LEDs.

8.4.3 LED Structures: Homojunction and Heterojunction

As stated earlier an LED in the simplest form is basically a *pn* junction formed by using one of the direct band semiconductor of suitable bandgap which may ensure emission in the desired wavelength. Such an LED which uses the same material, e.g. GaAs on both sides with different conductivity is termed a *homojunction LED*. However, homojunction LEDs are not found useful for application in fiber optic communication system due to their poor radiance and low quantum efficiency. One can greatly improve the radiance and quantum efficiency by making use of *multiple heterojunctions*. Generally a *heterostructure LED* consists of a combination of multiple heterojunctions that secure the carriers and subsequently the emitted photon in such a way that the overall quantum efficiency and radiance of the LED is enhanced. In order to achieve a high value of radiance and high quantum efficiency, one will have to make use of suitable lattice matched materials of different bandgap values in the LED structure so as to achieve the confinement of the carriers for recombination and also confinement of photons emitted due to radiative recombination. The confinement of carriers is done in such a way that they are forced to recombine radiatively in the active region of the LED. This improves the quantum efficiency of the device significantly. Now, once the carriers recombine radiatively and generate photons, the structure of the LED have to support their confinement in such a manner that these photons do not get reabsorbed in the material. There are a variety of LED structures ranging from simple planar LED, dome LED to more complex heterostructure surface emitting LED (SLED) (Burrus type), double heterostructure edge emitting LED (ELED) and more advanced *super luminescent diode* (SLD). From the fabrication point of view, a planar LED is the simplest one. One can easily fabricate a planar LED by *Liquid Phase Epitaxy* (LPE) or *vapour phase epitaxy* (VPE) method. Figure 8.17(a) illustrates the diffusion of p-type impurity on an n-type substrate producing a planar LED. The first LED suitable for optical fiber communications was developed by Keyes and Quist in 1962 using an n-GaAs with a junction formed by doping Z_n. The LED exhibited a peak emission wavelength of 0.93 μm and a spectral width of 35 μm. Further, the LED was reported to have a modulation bandwidth in excess of 10 MHz. A GaAs LED with a hemispherical dome to enhance coupling was also fabricated in 1965 (Fig. 8.17b). The LED had a room temperature spectral width of 25 nm centered at 900 nm. At room temperature, the LED exhibited an external quantum efficiency of 7.3% and an emission rise-time of 1.6 ns at room temperature.

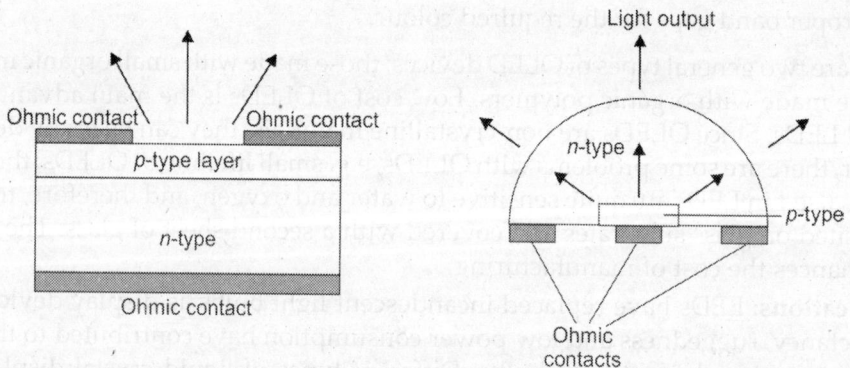

Fig. 8.17: Illustration of a simple LED structure: (a) planar LED structure (b) dome LED structure

(i) Surface Emitting LED (SLED)

In a SLED the light is emitted in the direction perpendicular to the plane of the *pn* junction. The SLEDs are usually referred to as Burrus type after the name of the inventor. Later on, a more sophisticated structure of the same design but based on heterostructure (DH) Al_xGa_{1-x} As grown on GaAs by liquid phase epitaxy (LPE) with improved efficiency and radiance by the inventor in 1971. To adjust the peak wavelength emission of the surface emitting DH-LED anywhere within 0.75 to 0.9 μm which is where silica fiber exhibit low loss, the bandgap energy of the ternary material was tailored. It was also demonstrated that the DH-LED can emit power as high as 10^6 W/m² sr for a drive current of 150 mA. One can launch approximately 2 mW power easily from this type of SLED source to a multimode fiber with a relative index difference between core and cladding of 10%. In the range of 35–40 nm lies the half-power spectral width of the source, a response time of 1–2 ns and an external quantum efficiency (η_{ext}) of 2–3%. The double heterostructrue was extensively studies in respect of different performance parameters for possible application as an optical source in fiber optic communication.

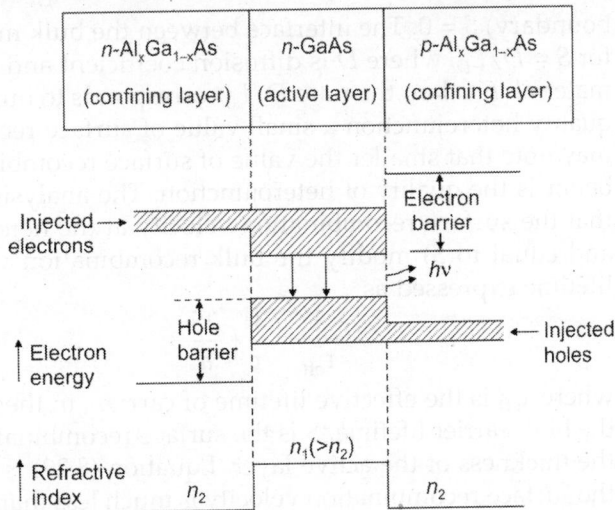

Figure 8.18 shows the schematic of a double-heterostructure $p\text{-}Al_xGa_{1-x}As/n\text{-}Al_xGa_{1-x}$ as light emitting diode (DH-LED) along-with energy band diagram. We can see that the structure consists of a lightly doped active layer made of a narrower band gap material (shown as n-GaAs in figure) sandwiched between the layers made up of a larger band-gap ternary material (shown as $Al_xGa_{1-x}As$ in figure). The binary GaAs forms heterojunction with the ternary on both sides as shown in the figure. The lightly doped

Fig. 8.18: Schematic of a double heterostructure n-Al_xGa_{1-x}As/n-GaAs/p-Al_xGa_{1-x} as LED (DH-LED) showing the energy band diagram and also illustrating the injection of carriers across the barriers along with the refractive index profile in the active and confining regions

n-GaAs region acts as a active region of the DH-LED while surrounding layers made of $Al_xGa_{1-x}As$ act as confirming regions, which help in the confinement of the carriers injected in the active region, as well as the photons subsequently emitted following the recombination of injected carriers in the active region. The confinement of the carriers is evident from the energy band diagram exhibiting the electron and hole energy barriers for the injected carriers. Moreover, the optical confinement is ensured by the difference in the refractive index between the active region and that in the confining regions (Fig. 8.19). The dual confinement of carriers as well as photons enables DH-LEDs to have high values of radiance and high quantum efficiency. There is another performance of an LED for application in optical fiber communication is the bandwidth. The bandwidth of the LED determines the modulation capability which means that the maximum frequency of the signal that can be used to modulate the intensity of the light emitted by the LED. However, the main performance parameters of the LED, e.g. quantum efficiency, radiance and bandwidth of the device are affected by the geometry as well as other device parameters such as self-absorption, heterointerface recombination velocity, doping concentration, activity layer thickness, injection current density, and carrier and optical confinement factors. Unlike in a conventional homojunction LED, it is possible to achieve higher power with the help of double heterostructure even by using a lightly doped active region in the latter case. This is because, the non-radiative recombination at the surface can be greatly reduced by making use of good quality heterointerface. We may note that the confinement of carriers enhances the injection efficiency resulting into enhanced radiative recombination caused by the recombination time by enhanced injected carrier density.

However, the performance of DH-LED depends on the quality of heterojunctions on both sides of the active regions. Usually, the quality of a heterojunction is often characterized in terms of interfacial recombination velocity or surface recombination velocity (S) at the heterointerface. For an ideal heterointerface, (a perfectly reflecting boundary) $S = 0$. The interface between the bulk material and surface material vanishes for $S = D/L_D$, where D is diffusion coefficient and L_D is the diffusion length in the bulk material. Further, the ratio D/L_0 corresponds to bulk recombination velocity. For a good quality heterojunction a small value of surface recombination velocity is desirable. We may note that smaller the value of surface recombination velocity at the heterointerface better is the quality of heterojunction. The analysis of a Burrus type DH-LED revealed that the surface recombination velocity at the heterointerface (assumed to be the same and equal to S) modify the bulk recombination velocity to an active effective carrier lifetime expressed as

$$\frac{1}{\tau_{eff}} = \frac{1}{\tau} + \frac{2S}{d} \qquad (8.29)$$

where τ_{eff} is the effective lifetime of carriers in the presence of surface combination, t is the bulk carrier lifetime, S is the surface recombination velocity at the interface and d is the thickness of the active layer. Equation (8.29) is obtained under the assumption that the surface recombination velocity is much less than the bulk recombination velocity, i.e. $SL_D/D << 1$. This can easily be verified as the effective lifetime reduces when S has a relatively high value. We may note that a reduction in the value of carrier lifetime results in a reduction of quantum efficiency and consequently a reduction of radiance and power output of the source. There is also another factor that reduces the power output of an LED is the self absorption of photons emitted due to recombination of the carriers. In order to couple power from a surface emitting LED, one will have to put the fiber $\perp^r$ to the plane of the *pn* junction which is parallel to the plane of the emitting surface. It is reported that a surface emitting Burrus type LED emits power with an isotropic emission pattern known as *lambertian pattern*. When viewed from any direction, such a source looks equally bright. However, the diminishes by a factor by a factor equal to the cosine of the viewing angle measured with respect to the normal drawn on the emitting surface. This reveals that the power emitted in a direction reduces to 50% when the viewing angle becomes 60° ($\because$ cos 60° = 1/2). Thus, the half power beam width of a surface emitting LED is 120°. Figure 8.19 shows the coupling schematic cross section of a Burrus type DH-LED with a piece of optical fiber bonded on the emitting surface.

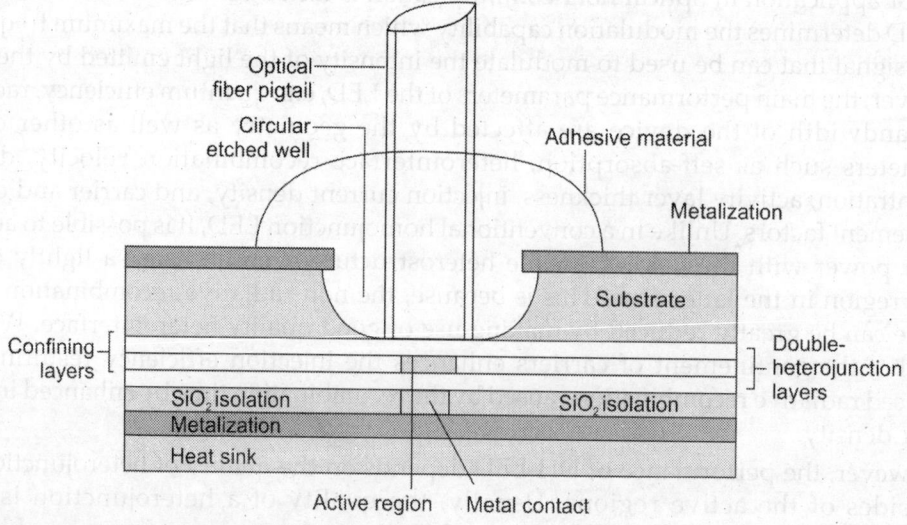

Fig. 8.19: Schematic illustration of cross-sectional view of a surface emitting DH-LED exhibiting section of the fiber connected perpendicular to the emitting surface for collecting light

It is reported that the coupling of light from noncoherent source to the optical fiber depends on the numerical aperature (NA) of the light receiving fiber. SLEDs usually suffer from the problem of lateral current spreading when the contact area is less than 25 µm. However, in such cases, the effective emission area is much less than the contact area which results in coupling loss. One can reduce the lateral current spreading by making mesa structure SLED (Fig. 8.20). One can also increase the coupling by making use of a multimode fiber with relatively large value of NA. Coupling efficiency can also be improved by making use of micro-lensing arrangement.

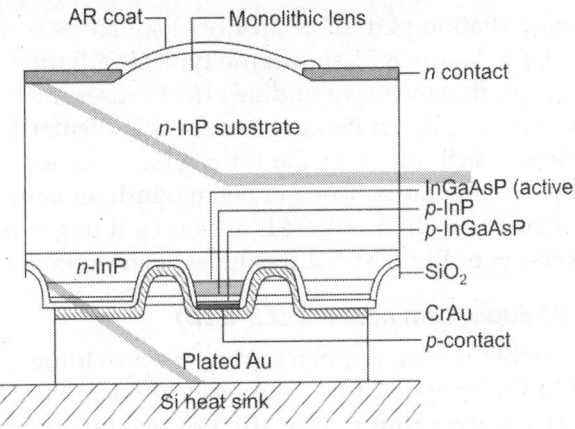

Fig. 8.20: Schematic of a Mesa etched InP/InGaAsP/InP double heterostructure surface emitting

(ii) Edge Emitting LED (ELED)

A double-heterostructure ELED uses stripe geometry similar to that uses in an injection laser diode to restrict the current spreading in the lateral direction. ELED consists of an active region which is made of a suitable material to emit light in the desired wavelength region and is switched between two guiding layers. However, both the guiding regions have the same refractive index value which is lower than the refractive index of the active region but higher than the refractive index of the surrounding material. We may note that the stripe geometry forms a complex waveguide that channelize the emitted optical toward the core of the receiving fiber whose axis is parallel to the plane of the *pn* junction (Fig. 8.21). Usually, the light is collected from one end by making the rear facet reflective. The width of the contact stripe of ELED varies in the range of 50–70 µm so as to match the diameter of standard multimode fibers of the order of 50–100 µm. However,

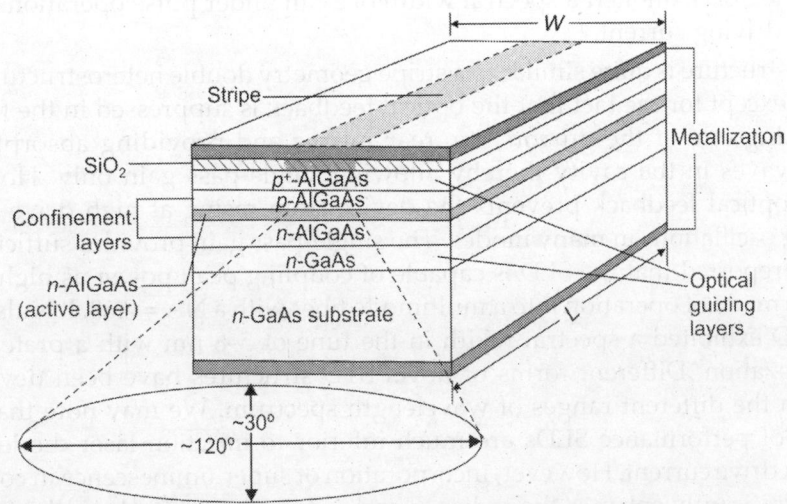

Fig. 8.21. Schematic illustration of an edge emitting LED (ELED) using stripe geometry

the radiation pattern of an ELED source is comparatively better than that of an SLED source. Figure 8.21 shows the typical radiation pattern of an GaAs/AlGaAs ELED. We can see that the waveguiding effect causes the radiation pattern of the emitted light to be more directive in the direction perpendicular to the plane of *pn* junction. A half power beam width of 30° in the transverse direction can be achieved easily in ELED. On the other hand, the half-power beam width remains 120° in the direction parallel to the plane of the *pn* junction as there is no waveguiding in the lateral direction. A variety of modified version of ELED structures have been proposed, fabricated and studied.

(iii) Super Luminescent LED (SLD)

Another device geometry which is providing significant benefits over both SLEDs and ELEDs for optical fiber communication application is the SLD. SLD offers advantages of: (a) a high output power; (b) a directional output beam; and (c) a narrow spectral line width-all of which prove useful for coupling significant optical power levels into optical fiber (in particular to single-mode fiber).

One can significantly improve the output power of an LED by making spontaneous and stimulated emission to occur simultaneously in an LED in a controlled manner, the spectral width of such a source is narrower than that of conventional LED.

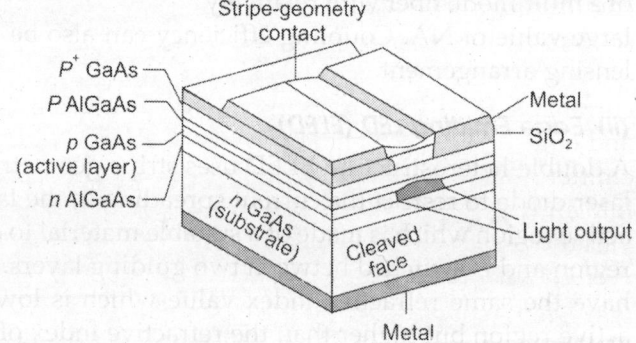

Figure 8.22 shows the structure of an SLD. We can see that structurally an SLD is similar to a stripe contact laser diode except for the fact that the stripe in the case of

Fig. 8.22. Schematic of a AlGaAs contact stripe super luminescent light emitting diode (SLD)

former device is inclined at an angle of 10° with respect to the normal to the emitting surface as to eliminate optical feedback. As a result, one finds the output light consists of a single-pass amplified spontaneous emission which is incoherent but 90% polarized. However, the SLD exhibited a spectral width of 2 nm under pulse operation mode with a very high driving current.

The SLD structure is quite similar to a stripe geometry double heterostructure injection laser diode except for the fact that the optical feedback is suppressed in the former case by eliminating one of the mirrors, i.e. rear mirror and providing absorption of the backward waves in the cavity thereby allowing single-pass gain only. However, the absence of optical feedback prevents the device from rasing at high drive current by suppressing oscillations in many modes. The single-pass gain provides sufficient output power. It is reported that the SLD is capable of coupling peak power as high as 50 mW under pulse mode of operation into a multimode fiber with a NA = 0.63. It is also reported that the SLD exhibited a spectral width in the tune of 5–8 nm with a preferential TE-mode polarization. Different forms of novel STD structures have been developed for operation in the different ranges of wavelength spectrum. We may note that from the view point of performance SLDs are much inferior to injection laser diodes and also require high drive current. However, incorporation of superluminescence in conventional LED can significantly enhance the radiance and reduce the spectral width of incoherent light emitters. The SLDs usually exhibit power around 4–5 times higher than that of

ELEDs and are commercially available for operation in different ranges of wavelength such as 1.16–1.33 μm (second attenuation window) and 1.52–1.57 μm (third attenuation window).

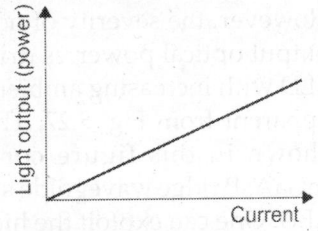

Fig. 8.23: Optical power output vs drive current characteristics of an LED

8.4.4 Characteristics of LED

The optical power vs drive current characteristics of an LED is shown in Fig. 8.23, which is linear. Intrinsically this linearity feature of an LED makes it an attractive and suitable optical source over injection laser diode for *analog* optical communication without severe impairment. The optical power at a very high value of injection drive current, tends to saturate for a variety of reasons. Further, the non-linearity also depends on the configuration of the device and is generally predominant at high radiance LED. However, the non-linearity in the output optical power vs drive current leads to harmonic as well as harmonic intermodulation distortion in analog optical communication system. As a result, one will have to use some form of linearization circuit so as to minimize distortion.

Figure 8.24 show the light output against current characteristics for typically good surface and edge emitter. We may note that the surface emitter radiates significantly more optical power into air than edge emitter. Figure 8.25 shows the variation of the output power with the drive current for a Burrus type LED. Both devices are reasonably linear at moderate drive current. This makes it suitable for direct modulation by either analog or digital signals. It is reported that the modulation bandwidths are several hundred of MHz.

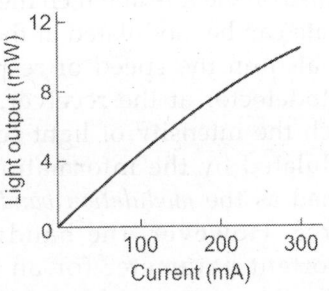

Fig. 8.24: Optical output power into air vs drive current characteristic of a typical AlGaAs surface-emitting LED

The output optical power of an LED is reported to decrease with increasing temperature. This is accounted for the reduction in the internal quantum efficiency of an LED at higher operating temperature. When a large drive current results in high radiance of the LED, the temperature of the *pn*-junction increases. The increased *pn*-junction temperature causes the output power of the LED to drop down at a given drive level. Figure 8.26 shows the variations of optical output power of LEDs with increasing junction temperature for the three basic configurations. SLED, ELED and SLD. We may note that output of the superluminescent LED is most sensitive to the variation of *pn* junction temperature as compared to surface and edge emitting LEDs. This seems to be due to the fact that the stimulated emission responsible for the operation of an SLD is adversely affected by increasing temperature.

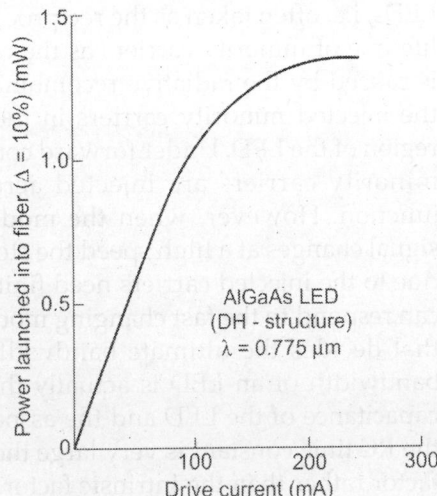

Fig. 8.25: Variation of light output power of a Burrus type DH-LED with the drive current

However, the severity of nonlinearity in the output optical power vs drive current of the SLD with increasing ambient temperature is apparent from Fig. 8.27. The characteristics shown in this figure corresponds to an InGaAsP ridge waveguide superluminescent LED. One can exploit the high output power of the SLD by operating the device at a lower temperature with the help of thermoelectric coolers. At higher operating temperature the power output vs drive current characteristics gets highly non-linear.

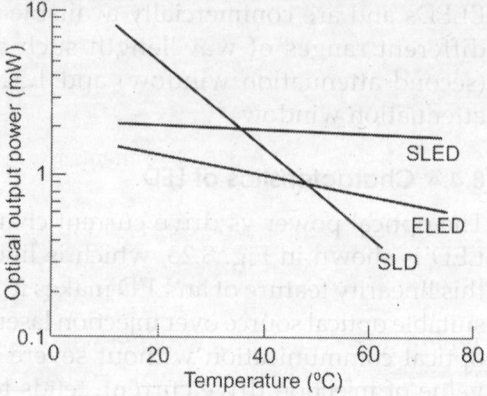

Fig. 8.26: Variation of the optical output power of three different important LED configurations, e.g. SLED, ELED and SLD operating at 1.3 μm with temperature at a constant bias current

(i) Frequency Response and Bandwidth

The speed of an optical fiber communication system depends not only on the information or data carrying capacity of the optical fiber but also on the rate at which the information or data can be modulated at the transmitter and also on the speed of response of the photodetector at the receiver. The rate at which the intensity of light source can be modulated by the information or data is termed as the *modulation bandwidth* of the source. However, the bandwidth is an important parameter for an LED for its application as a optical source in an optical fiber communication system. But the parameter is not that important for LEDs used as display devices. The bandwidth of LEDs, i.e. often taken as the reciprocal of the lifetime of minority carriers as the radiance is caused by the radiative recombination of the injected minority carriers in the active region of the LED. Under forward condition, minority carriers are injected across the junction. However, when the modulating

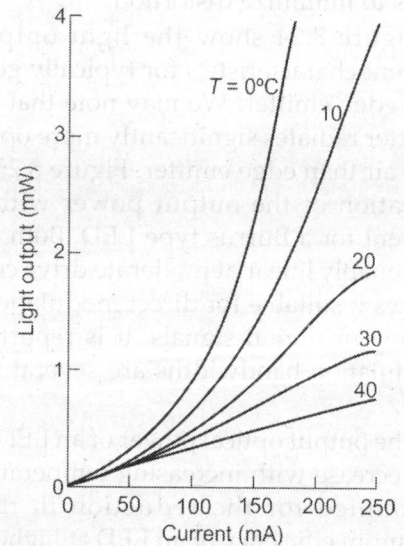

Fig. 8.27: Variation of light output of an InGaAsP ridge waveguide SLD with drive current for different ambient temperatures

signal changes at a high speed the stored minority charges can not follow it. This may be due to the injected carriers need finite time to vanish through recombination prior they can respond to the fast changing modulating signal. This may because the *intrinsic* factor that decides the ultimate bandwidth of an LED. The *extrinsic* factor that affects the bandwidth of an LED is actually the RC time constant arising out of the *pn* junction capacitance of the LED and the associated series series resistance of the circuit. Now, if the RC time constant is very large then the overall bandwidth is decided by the external factor rather than the intrinsic factor.

We now consider 1-D HJ LED structure (Fig. 8.28). One can estimate the bandwidth of an LED by assuming a small signal AC voltage ($-\exp(j\omega t)$) to be applied across the junction already biased by a DC voltage.

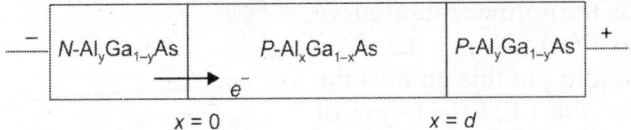

Fig. 8.28: Schematic representation of a heterojunction LED

In this case, the time dependent continuity equation can be expressed as

$$\frac{\partial(\Delta n(x, t))}{\partial t} = D_n \frac{\partial^2 \Delta n(x, t)}{\partial x^2} - \frac{\Delta n(x, t)}{\tau} \tag{8.29a}$$

where, D_n is the diffusion coefficient for electrons and τ is the mean carrier lifetime. In presence of a small signal AC voltage superimposed on the DC bias voltage, the excess carriers (Δn) will also vary in accordance with the applied AC signal. Mathematically, one can express the injected carriers as

$$\Delta n(x, t) = \Delta n(x) \exp(j\omega t) \tag{8.30}$$

Substituting Eq. (8.30) in Eq. (8.29a), one may write

$$\frac{\partial^2 \Delta n(x)}{\partial x^2} = \frac{\Delta n(x)}{L_n^2(\omega)} \tag{8.31}$$

where,

$$L_n(\omega) = \frac{\sqrt{D_n \tau}}{\sqrt{1 + j\omega\tau}} = \frac{L_n}{\sqrt{1 + j\omega\tau}} \tag{8.32}$$

The excess carrier decreases exponentially with increase in x as follows:

$$\Delta n(x) = \Delta n(0) \exp\left(-\frac{x}{L_n(\omega)}\right) \tag{8.33}$$

However, the excess carriers vanish at $x = \infty$.

Therefore, total modulated light output from the LED per unit area is obtained as

$$I(t) = \eta \int_0^\infty \Delta n(0) \exp\left(-\frac{x}{L_n(\omega)}\right) \exp(j\omega t)\, dx$$

$$= \frac{\eta \Delta n(0) L_n}{\sqrt{1 + j\omega\tau}} \exp(j\omega t) \tag{8.34}$$

where η is the quantum efficiency of the LED.

One can express the optical output power $P(\omega)$ of an LED biased by a drive current modulated at the angular frequency as

$$P(\omega) = \frac{P(o)}{\sqrt{(1 + \tau\omega)^2}} \tag{8.35}$$

where $P(o)$ corresponds to the optical power output of the LED under DC condition, i.e. without modulation.

Figure 8.29 shows the variation of the optical power output of an LED modulated by the drive current at frequency ω normalized with respect to the output of the LED in absence of modulation (i.e. DC bias current only), with the modulation frequency.

Equation (8.35) shows that the optical output power of the LED decreases with increase in the value of the angular frequency of the modulating signal. The *half-power point* which corresponds to a drop of power by 3 dB from its constant value can be obtained by locating the point on the normalization curve corresponding to $P(\omega)/P(o) = 0.5$. The frequency corresponding to this point is the 3-dB bandwidth of the LED (in terms of angular frequency) (Fig. 8.29). From Eq. (8.35) we see that for the half-power (3 dB) point

$$\frac{P(\omega)}{P(o)} = \frac{1}{2} \text{ when } (\omega\tau)^2 = 3 \qquad (8.36)$$

Designing the corresponding value of ω by ω_{3dB}, one finds

$$\omega_{3db} = \frac{\sqrt{3}}{\tau} \qquad (8.37)$$

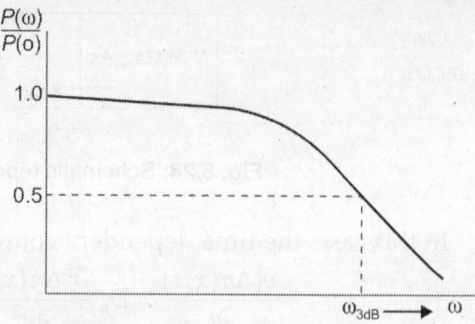

Fig. 8.29: Frequency response of an optical source exhibiting the 3-dB bandwidth

Alternatively, we can express the 3 dB bandwidth as

$$f_{3db} = \frac{\sqrt{3}}{2\pi\tau} \qquad (8.38)$$

The bandwidth calculated above is based on the consideration that bandwidth of the LED in the optical domain. Therefore, this value of bandwidth is often referred to as the optical bandwidth of the source.

(ii) Electrical Bandwidth

The bandwidth calculated above is based on the frequency response of the optical power output of the LED when the current is modulated. Further, this bandwidth corresponds to 3 dB point of emitted power of the LED in the optical domain. However, the bandwidth of the LED is usually calculated in the electrical domain. Generally, the optical power of an LED is measured with the help of an *optical power meter* which uses the optical detector at the input port. We may note that the detector is a square-law device which converts the incident optical power to an electric current. Further, the electrical current produced by the detector is proportional to the incident optical power. Now, if $I(\omega)$ is the electrical current produced by the detector in response to an intensity modulated optical power $P(\omega)$, then we have

$$I(\omega) \propto P(\omega) \qquad (8.39)$$

Further, the electrical power $P_e(\omega)$ corresponding to the electrical current $I(\omega)$ in the detector circuit is expressed as

$$P_e(\omega) = \frac{I^2(\omega)}{R} \qquad (8.40)$$

where, R is the equivalent resistance of the detector circuit.

The ratio of the output electrical power of the LED corresponding to the optical power produced by the modulated drive current, to the electrical output power produced by the LED in absence of modulation, can be obtained using Eqs (8.35), (8.39) and (8.40) as follows:

$$\frac{P_e(\omega)}{P_e(o)} = \frac{I^2(\omega)}{I^2(o)} = \frac{P^2(\omega)}{P^2(o)} = \frac{1}{1 + (\omega\tau)^2} \qquad (8.41)$$

The electrical 3 dB point corresponds to the frequency, where we have

$$P_e(\omega_{3dB}) = \frac{1}{2} P(o) \qquad (8.42)$$

One can see from Eq. (8.105) that Eq. (8.102) is satisfied when $\omega\tau = 1$, i.e. the 3 dB electrical bandwidth gets

$$f_{3dB-el} = \frac{1}{2\pi\tau} \tag{8.43}$$

We may note that at the 3 dB frequency the electrical current ratio becomes

$$\frac{I(\omega)}{I(o)} = \frac{1}{\sqrt{2}} = 0.707 \tag{8.44}$$

Thus, the bandwidth of an LED can be expressed by considering the half-power (3 dB) point of the optical power output of the LED or by estimating the half-power point in the electrical domain by converting the optical power output to the corresponding electrical power in the detector circuit. We can see that

$$f_{3dB-op} = \sqrt{3}\, f_{3dB-el} \tag{8.45}$$

We can also verify that optical 3-dB point occurs at a point where the ratio of detected modulated current to unmodulated DC current actually equals to 1/2. Figure (8.30) shows the comparison of electrical bandwidth and the optical bandwidth which corresponds to effectively 6 dB attenuation in terms of detected electrical bandwidth. We can further see that the optical bandwidth is significantly greater than the electrical bandwidth. The difference between them (in frequency terms) depends on the shape of the frequency response for the system. However, if we assume the system response to be Gaussian, then the optical bandwidth is a factor of $\sqrt{2}$ greater than the electrical bandwidth.

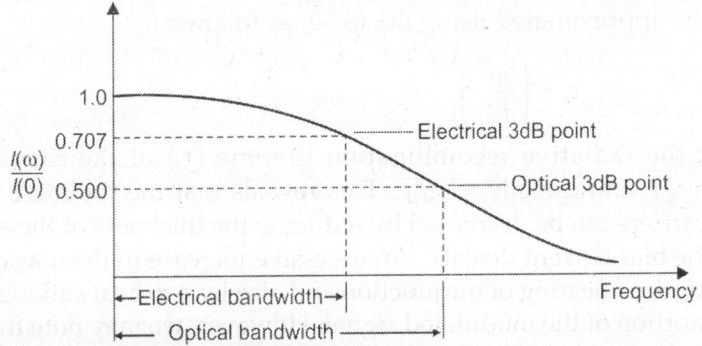

Fig. 8.30: Frequency response for an LED exhibiting the electrical bandwidth and optical bandwidths

(iii) Power Bandwidth Product

We can see that the power emitted internally by an LED is

$$P_{int} = \eta_{int}\left(\frac{I}{q}\right)\left(\frac{hc}{\lambda}\right) = \left(\frac{\tau}{\tau_r}\right)\left(\frac{I}{q}\right)\left(\frac{hc}{\lambda}\right) \tag{8.46}$$

Obviously, the power generated internally by the LED is directly proportional to the overall recombination lifetime of the minority carriers. On the other hand, the bandwidth of the LED [Eq. (8.38)] is inversely proportional to the overall recombination lifetime of the minority carriers. This means, the product of the power internally emitted by the LED and the optical bandwidth can be easily expressed as

$$\text{Power-bandwidth product} = P_{int} \times \omega_{3dB-op} = \left(\frac{\sqrt{3}}{\tau_r}\right)\left(\frac{I}{q}\right)\left(\frac{hc}{\lambda}\right) \tag{8.47}$$

We see that the power-bandwidth product of the LED is independent of the overall recombination lifetime of the carriers and depends on the radiative recombination lifetime of the carriers. The radiative recombination lifetime of minority carriers in presence of injection of minority carriers under applied forward bias can be easily expressed as

$$\tau_r = \frac{1}{B_r (n_0 + p_0 + \Delta n)} \tag{8.48}$$

Now, if the injection current density under forward bias is $J(= I/A)$ such that the current is entirely due to radiative recombination of minority carriers, then the excess carriers injected in the active region of the LED can also be expressed as

$$\Delta n = J\tau_r / qd \tag{8.49}$$

where, q is the electronic charge and d is the thickness of the active region. Substituting the value of Δn from Eq. (8.49) into Eq. (8.48), one obtains the following quadratic equation of τ_r.

$$\frac{J}{qd} B_r \tau_r^2 - B_r (n_0 + p_0) \tau_r - 1 = 0 \tag{8.50}$$

Solving Eq. (8.50) for τ_r one obtains

$$\tau_r = \frac{B_r (n_0 + p_0) + \left[B_r^2 (n_0 + p_0)^2 + 4\left(\frac{J}{qd} B_r \right) \right]^{1/2}}{2\left(\frac{J}{qd} B_r \right)} \tag{8.51}$$

Now, for a high level injection $\Delta n \gg (n_0 + p_0)$, the radiative recombination lifetime of the carrier can be approximated using Eq. (8.50) as follows:

$$\tau_r = \left(\frac{qd}{JB_r} \right)^{1/2} \tag{8.52}$$

We see that the radiative recombination lifetime (τ_r) of the carrier is inversely proportional to $\sqrt{J}$ and directly to $\sqrt{d}$. This reveals that the radiative recombination lifetime of the carriers can be decreased by reducing the thickness of the active region or by increasing the bias current density. An excessive increase in the bias current density may lead to undesired heating of the junction and also lead to heat sinking problem. This may lead to distortion of the modulated signal. However, we may note that a thin active layer thickness of a double heterostructure LED will enhance the surface recombination rate [Eq. (8.29)] and also lead to a reduction in the quantum efficiency of LED. We may note that various parameters of an LED are interrelated and have to be optimized properly for the desired application. Recent research in the field have led to successful fabrication of high radiance LED sources with surface emitting as well as edge emitting configurations. We see that the bandwidth of an LED depends on its structure. We may note that an edge emitting LED exhibits a larger bandwidth than a surface emitting LED for the same drive current. The frequency response for SLED and ELED for the same drive current is shown in Fig. 8.31. It is reported that LEDs with bandwidth as high as 1 GHz are suitable for application in high speed optical communication systems.

Neglecting the nonradiative recombination the 3 dB electrical bandwidth of the LED, one can easily approximate Eq. (8.43) as

$$f_{3dB-el} \cong \frac{1}{2\pi} \left(\frac{JB_r}{qd} \right)^{1/2} \tag{8.53}$$

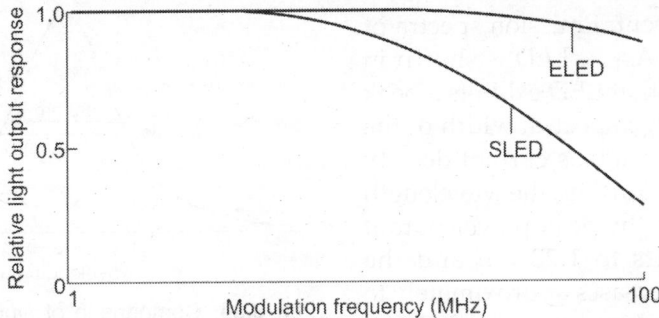

Fig. 8.31: Schematic illustration of frequency responses of LED for the surface emitter and edge emitter configuration

(iv) Output Spectrum (Spectral Response)

LED's spectral response is essentially the variation of emitted optical power from LED with wavelength. We may note that an LED is not a monochromatic source of light. Generally, the light is emitted over a finite spectral width around the peak wavelength of emission. The spectral width is measured in terms of wavelength corresponding to half maximum intensity points, i.e., full width at half power (FWHP) points. The 1G optical fiber communications was primarily focused in the wavelength range of 0.8 to 0.9 mm. The LEDs was based onGaAs/AlGaAs technology for operation in the said wavelength range. These LEDs generally exhibit

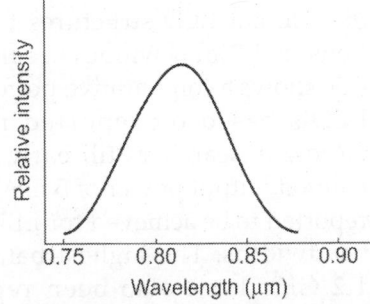

Fig. 8.32: LED output spectra, i.e. spectral response of an GaAs/AlGaAs surface emitting LED

spectral wide in the range of 25–40 nm (Fig. 8.32). On the other hand LEDs based on InP/INGaAsP and INP/InGaAs developed for operation in the longer wavelength region (1.3–1.65 µm) for the 2G and 3G optical fiber communication systems exhibiting larger spectral width ranging from 50–150 nm. We may also note that the spectral width of the source plays an important role in determining the intramodal dispersion associated with the optical fiber.

It is reported that the spectral width and peak power of emission from an LED also depends on doping concentration in the active region, the drive current and also on temperature of operation. The spectra of InGaAsP surface emitting LED for the cases of lightly as well as heavily doped active regions is shown in Fig. 8.33. The spectral width also depends on the structure of the LED, e.g. the spectral width of an edge emitting LED (ELED) is almost 1.5 times more compared to the spectral width of surface emitting LED (SLED) based on the same material combination. The spectral characteristics of an InP/InGaAsP surface emitting as well as edge emitting LEDs is shown in Fig. 8.34.

It is found that the peak wavelength of emission and the spectral response of an LED also depends

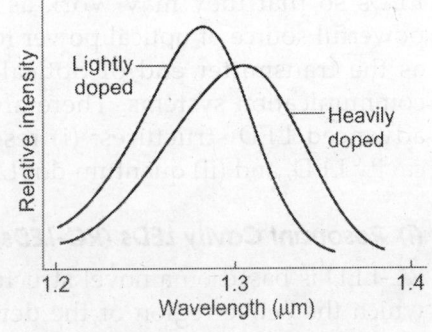

Fig. 8.33: LED output spectra, i.e. spectral responses of an InGaAsP surface emitting LED for the cases of lightly and heavily doped active regions

on the drive current. Emission spectra of an $In_{1-x} Ga_x P_z As_{1-z}$ LED is shown in Fig. 8.35. We see that LED exhibits a peak of 1.075 mm with a spectral width of the order of 56 nm for a bias current density of 1.2×10^7 Am^{-2}. Further, the wavelength corresponding to the peak power output of the LED shifts to 1.23 μm and the spectral width increases approximately to 77 nm when the bias current density is raised to 2.5×10^7 Am^{-2}. We may also note that InGaAsP/InP material system has been extensively used for the development of different LED structures for applications in 1.3 mm window region. Figure 8.36 shows a comparative performance of LED's based on reported results by various researchers till early 1980s. An emitted output power of 5 mW in air was reported to be achieved for LEDs 30 MHz bandwidths. The highest bandwidth of 1.2 GHz have also been reported by InGaAsP LED with an optical power output of 100 pW. It is also reported that for a fixed bandwidth, LEDs based on AlGaAs exhibit higher output powers than those exhibited by LEDs based on InGaAsP.

8.5 ADVANCED LED STRUCTURES

With the advent of advanced technology of III-V materials, now it is possible to tailor the characteristics of conventional LEDs so that they may work as more powerful source of optical power for use as the transmitter end of optical fiber communication systems. There are two advanced LED structures: (i) resonant cavity LED, and (ii) quantum dot LED.

(i) Resonant Cavity LEDs (RC-LEDs)

RC-LED is based on a novel structure in which the active region of the device is placed in resonant optical cavity (ROC). A quantum well is then embedded in this active cavity. As the cavity is confined to a micrometer size, the RC-LED is therefore

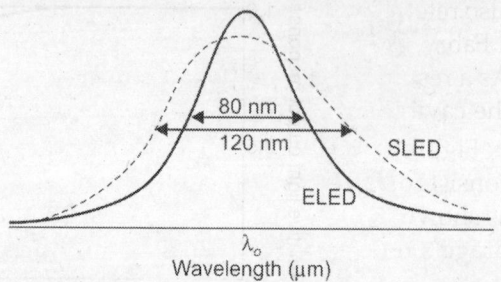

Fig. 8.34: Comparison of typical spectral output characteristics for InGaAsP surface and edge emitting LEDs operating in the 1.3 μm wavelength region

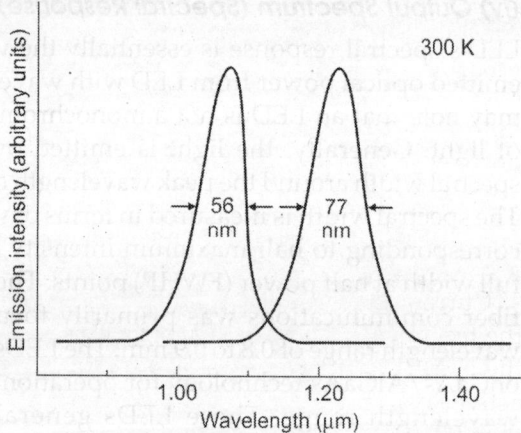

Fig. 8.35:. Emission spectra of $In_{1-x} Ga_x P_z As_{1-z}$ LED exhibiting dependence of the spectral response on the bias current density

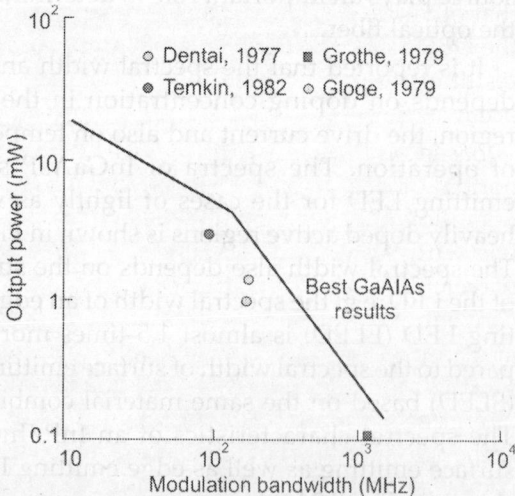

Fig. 8.36. Comparative performance for power and bandwidth of 1.3 μm LEDs based on the reported results by various researchers till early 1980s

also referred to as a *microcavity LED*. The RC-LED is based on planar technology containing a Fabry–Perot active resonant cavity between distributed Bragg reflector (DBR) mirrors. As a result, the optical power emitted from the active region is restricted to the modes of the cavity.

Figure 8.37 shows the basic structure for a RC-LED. The active region of RC-LED consists of InGaAsP/InP multi-quantum wells placed in the optical resonant cavity (ORC) as shown in Fig. 8.37. This ORC is positioned between the top and the bottom distributed Bragg's reflector (DBR) mirrors.

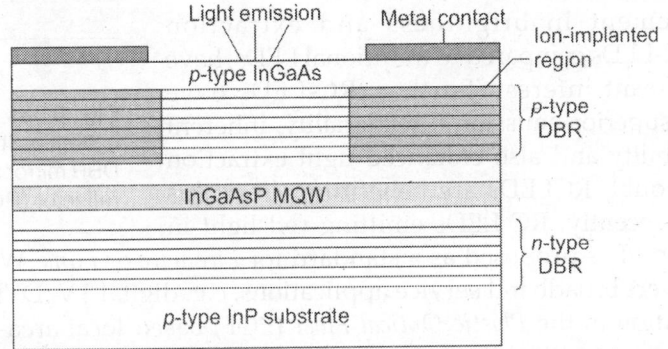

Fig. 8.37: Basic structure of resonant cavity surface-emitting LED using DBR mirrors

Current confinement is obtained through the selective ion implantation technique in the top mirror. The RC-LED structure is essentially a Fabry-Perot (FP) resonator where the optical cavity mode is in resonance amplifying the spontaneous emission from the active layer. The reflectivity of the bottom DBR mirror is kept to a maximum, i.e., higher than 90% and is achieved by incorporating more than 40 large number of gratings. The surface DBR mirror is made transparent by introducing fewer gratings, i.e. about 15, so as to create low facet reflectivity, i.e. 40% to 60% in order to allow the optical signal to exit through this mirror. Due to incorporation of the DBR mirrors these devices are usually referred to as grating-assisted RC-LEDs. Further, this RC-LED structure is just similar to that of vertical cavity surface emitting laser (VCSEL) excepting that the emitting side of the DBR mirror of the resonant cavity is semitransparent. Therefore light is emitted as a result of resonantly amplified spontaneous emission and stimulated emission does not occur.

Based on the cavity design, RC-LEDs can be constructed to emit light from either the bottom or the top surface of the device structure. Generally, RC-LEDs are fabricated for operation over a range of wavelengths between 0.85 and 0.88 µm and also at 0.65 µm for use with plastic optical fiber. However, RC-LEDs can also be fabricated for longer wavelength. Although the growth process for RC-LEDs is more complex as compared to conventional devices, their enhanced features, e.g. highly directional circular output beam and improved fiber coupling efficiency, make overcoming the fabrication problems worthwhile. Generally, external quantum efficiency of RC-LED is around 6 to 10% when operating at a wavelength of 1.3 µm or 1.55 µm due to the increased linewidth broadening at these longer wavelengths. Nevertheless, even this value of external quantum efficiency proves sufficient to provide satisfactor transmission of data at high modulation rates above 1 Gbit/s. Further, device coupling limitations associated with the planar technology used for the RC-LED can also be overcome by using an advanced resonant cavity technique known as RC²-LED. Figure 8.38 shows a basic structure for such a device which incorporates the combination of a DBR mirror and a resonant cavity to form a resonant cavity reflector. Obviously, a symmetric resonant cavity is created for the out coupling reflector instead of using a traditional DBR mirror. This structure produces a narrow radiation pattern and thus it exhibits higher output signal power which is 50% greater than that provided by conventional RC-LED designs.

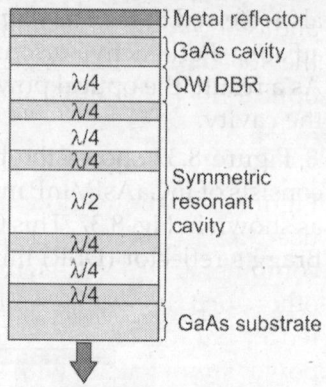

Fig. 8.38: Basic structure of bottom emitting RC²-LED using DBR mirror and resonant cavity reflector (RCR)

The enhancement in brightness and extraction efficiencies of RC-LEDs compared to traditional LEDs, have attracted significant interest. Further, RC-LEDs have spectral purity, superior emission directionality, inherent temperature stability and also enhanced light extraction efficiency. No doubt, RCLEDs are benefitting from this evolution. Very recently, RC LEDs emitting red light in combination with PF is proposed as a standard for *Fire wire* or *i.link*. We may note that this standard covers broadband service applications, e.g. digital TV, DVD, etc. RC-LEDs also find application in the *Plastic Optical Fiber* (POF)-based local-area-network (LAN) and also for in-home multimedia and automotive industries.

(ii) Quantum-Dot LED (QD-LED)

Generally quantum-dot structures are used for lasers. However, to enhance the emitted power output, one can also use quantum-dot structure in a typical RC-LED structure and the resultant device is referred to as a *quantum-dot* or *QD-LED*.

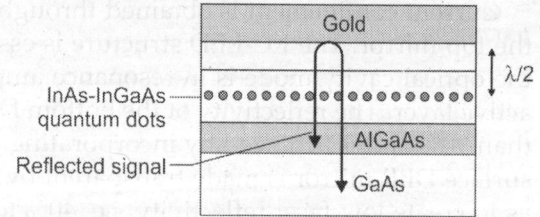

Fig. 8.39: Schematic structure of a single mirror quantum-dot LED (QD-LED)

Figure 8.39 shows a single-mirror QD-LED. In this structure of QD-LED, an active layer comprising a layer of InAs quantum-dots covered by InGaAs is positioned at a distance from a gold coated mirror on the device surface. The active region consists of a single layer of quantum dots. In order to confine the injected carriers an additional layer of AlGaAs is incorporated between the GaAs substrate and the active region. The quantum-dot layer is placed at half the emission wavelength distance so as to maximize the output light power. The optical signal reflected by the mirror constructively interferes with the radiation emitted downwards from the active layer and thereby causes the optical signal power emerging from the bottom (substrate side) to increase by fourfold.

QD-LEDs with 10 mW output power when operating at wave-lengths of 1.30 mm and 1.55 mm have also been successfully fabricated.

(iii) Organic Light Emitting Diode (OLED)

This uses a layer of an organic compound film having emissive electroluminescence properties. This kind of emissive properties is exhibited by a host of organic polymers. In OLED, the organic semiconductor layer is placed between two electrodes, out of which one electrode is made transparent (ITO) to deliver the emitted light output. Generally, OLEDs are used in digital display devices, e.g. television screens, computer monitors and other portable system, e.g. mobile phones, handhold game consoles, etc. However, the speed of OLEDs is generally very poor and hence OLEDs don't find application in optical fiber communication.

8.5.1 LED Indicator Circuits

Figure 8.40 shows how a LED can be used as a power level indicator in a computer, CD player, stereo amplifier or other such devices. The LED is connected in parallel to the system's internal power supply along with series resistor R_s. When the power switch is on, the diode is forward-biased and emits a light.

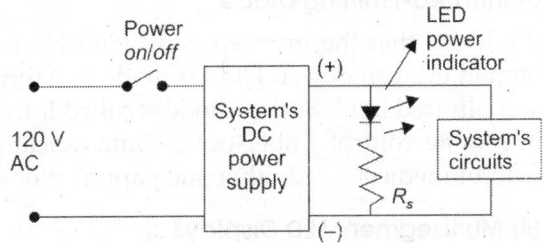

Fig. 8.40: LED power indicator

Series resistor R_s limits current to the LED and is often referred to as a *current limiter*. Most LEDs have a forward-biased voltage drop between 1.2 V and 2.5 V although high intensity LEDs can have higher-biased voltage drops. Note that this is much higher than for a normal silicon diode (0.7 V) or germanium diode (0.3 V). The resistance value and wattage rating of R_s can be calculated using Ohm's law. R_s value is found by subtracting the LED's voltage drop from the source and then dividing by the LED's desired current. To find wattage rating for R_s, simply apply the power formula $P = I^2R$.

Example

What is the resistance and wattage rating of a limiting resistor in a 12 V DC circuit for a LED that requires 2 V forward-bias with 20 mA current rating?

Solution

$$R_s = \frac{V_S - V_D}{I_D} = \frac{12 \text{ V} - 2 \text{ V}}{20 \text{ mA}} = 500\,\Omega$$

and

$$P = I^2R = (20 \text{ mA})^2 \times 500\,\Omega = 200 \text{ mW}$$

Therefore, a standard-size 0.25 watt (= 250 mW) resistor is required:

8.5.2 Multicolour LEDs

Multicolour LEDs are available that will:
  (i) emit one colour when supply voltage is one polarity.
  (ii) emit a second colour when polarity is reversed.
  (iii) emit a third colour when bias polarity is rapidly switched.

Figure 8.41 shows the schematic of multicolour LEDs. Multicolour LEDs are usually two LEDs connected in antiparallel. That is, the anode of each diode is connected to the cathode of the other. Each LED can emit light only when forward-biased. Thus, when voltage of either polarity is applied, one LED is forward-biased and emits its native colour.

The most commonly used are red and green in colour. The green LED is normally used to indicate whether something is

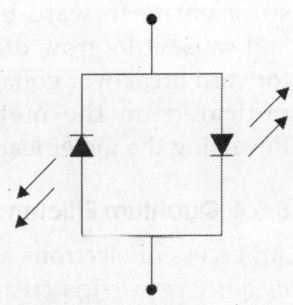

Fig. 8.41: Multicolour LEDs

functioning properly, and the red LED is used to indicate that there is a problem. If a multicolour LED is rapidly switched between two polarities, the red/green LED appears to produce a third colour (yellow).

(i) Infrared-Emitting Diode

We know that the infrared band (30 THz to 400 THz) falls below the frequencies the human eye can detect. Diodes made of gallium arsenide release energy by way of heat and infrared light. Such a diode is called infrared-emitting diode (IRED). IREDs are used in remote controls, fiber-optic communication, discriminating organic solvents in the field of medicine and other such applications.

(ii) Multisegment LED Displays

LEDS are widely used in multisegment displays. Figure 8.42 shows the most commonly used multisegment display. Its seven segments are labelled a, b, c, d, e, f and g. The LED labelled *dp* is used to display the decimal point. By lighting a combination of different LEDs, any number from 0 to 9 can be displayed.

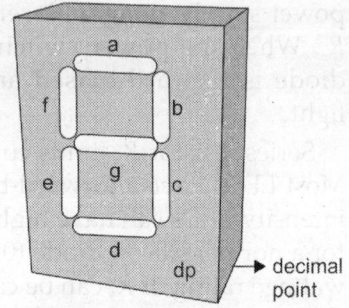

The seven-segment display cannot be used effectively to display the alphabet, and thus other multisegment displays have been developed. The 16-segment display is illustrated in Fig. 8.43, and the 5 × 7 dotmatrix display is shown in Fig. 8.44.

Numerals	0	1	2	3
Segments turned ON	a b c d e f	b c	a b d e g	a b c d g

Fig. 8.42: Seven-segment display

8.5.3 LED Testing

LEDs are usually damaged by excessive current flowing through them. Such LEDs can be identified by discolouration on their casing, due to the burned junction. The LED can be tested with a DMM (digital multimeter). In the diode check position, the DMM supplies about 2.5 V at very low current.

If at this setting the cathode of LED is connected to the negative lead of DMM and the anode of LED is connected to the positive lead of DMM, the supplied 2.5 V should be sufficient to forward-bias the LED and cause it to grow dimly, and the forward breakover voltage should be indicated on the meter display.

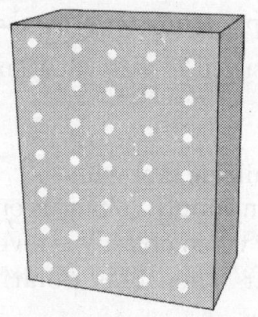

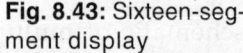

Fig. 8.43: Sixteen-segment display

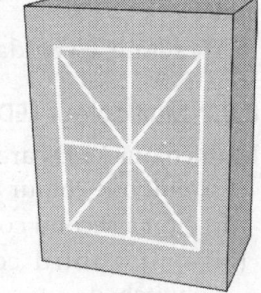

Fig. 8.44: 5 × 7 dotmatrix

Reversing the meter leads should, as in conventional dioded, read open (∞).

8.5.4 Quantum Efficiency and LED Power

An excess of electrons and holes in *p*- and *n*-type material, respectively (referred to as *minority carriers*) is created in a semiconductor light source by carrier injection at the device contacts. The excess densities of electrons n and holes p are equal, since the injected carriers are formed and recombine in pairs in accordance with the requirement for charge neutrality in the crystal. When carrier injection stops, the carrier density returns to the equilibrium value. In general, the excess carrier density decays exponentially with time according to the relation:

$$n = n_0 e^{-t/\tau} \tag{8.54}$$

where n_0 is the initial injected excess electron density and the time constant τ is the carrier lifetime. This lifetime is one of the most important operating parameters of an electro-optic device. Its value can range from milliseconds to fractions of a nanosecond depending on material composition and device defects.

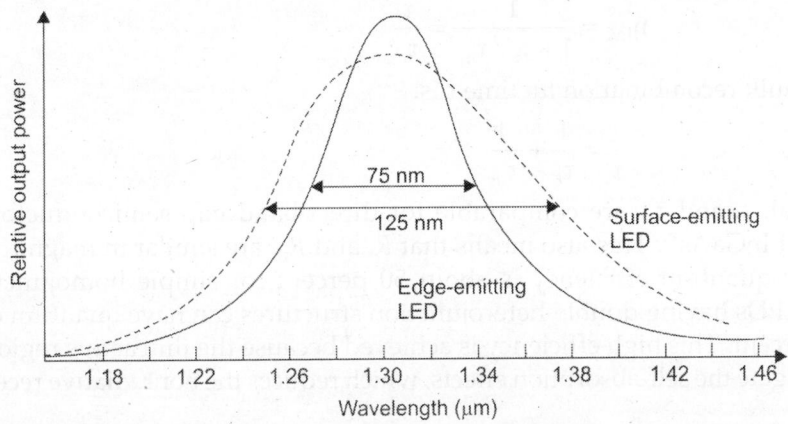

Fig. 8.45: Typical spectral patterns for edge-emitting and surface-emitting LEDs at 1310 nm. The patterns broaden with increasing wavelength and are wider for surface emitters

The excess carriers can recombine either radiatively or nonradiatively. In radiative recombination, a photon of energy $h\nu$, which is approximately equal to the bandgap energy, is emitted. Nonradiative recombination effects include optical absorption in the active region (self-absorption), carrier recombination at the heterostructure interfaces, and the Auger process in which the energy released during an electron-hole recombination is transferred to another carrier in the form of kinetic energy (Fig. 8.45).

When there is a constant current flow into a LED, an equilibrium condition is established. That is, the excess density of electrons n and holes p is equal since the injected carriers are created and recombined in pairs such that charge neutrality is maintained within the device. The total rate at which carriers are generated is the sum of the externally supplied and the thermally generates rates. The externally supplied rate is given by J/qd, where J is the current density in A/cm², q is the electron charge, and d is the thickness of the recombination region. The thermal generation rate is given by n/τ. Hence, the rate equation for carrier recombination in a LED can be written as:

$$\frac{dn}{dt} = \frac{J}{qd} - \frac{n}{\tau} \tag{8.55}$$

The equilibrium condition is found by setting Eq. (8.89) equal to zero, yielding:

$$n = \frac{J\tau}{qd} \tag{8.56}$$

This relationship reveals the steady-state electron density in the active region when a constant current is flowing through it.

The *internal quantum efficiency* in the active region is the fraction of the electron-hole pairs that recombine radiatively. If the radiative recombination rate is R_r and the nonradiative recombination rate is R_{nr}, then the internal quantum efficiency η_{int} is the ratio of the radiative recombination rate to the total recombination rate:

$$\eta_{int} = \frac{R_r}{R_r + R_{nr}} \tag{8.57}$$

For exponential decay of excess carriers, the radiative recombination lifetime is $\tau_r = n/R_r$ and the nonradiative recombination lifetime is $\tau_{nr} = n/R_{nr}$. Thus, the internal quantum efficiency can be expressed as:

$$\eta_{int} = \frac{1}{1 + \tau_r/\tau_{nr}} = \frac{\tau}{\tau_r} \tag{8.58}$$

where the bulk recombination lifetime t is:

$$\frac{1}{\tau} = \frac{1}{\tau_r} + \frac{1}{\tau_{nr}} \tag{8.59}$$

In general, τ_r and τ_{nr} are comparable for direct-band gap semiconductors, such as GaAlAs and InGaAsP. This also means that R_r and R_{nr} are similar in magnitude, so that the internal quantum efficiency is about 50 percent for simple homojunction LEDs. However, LEDs having double-heterojunction structures can have quantum efficiencies of 60–80 percent. This high efficiency is achieved because the thin active regions of these devices mitigate the self-absorption effects, which reduces the nonradiative recombination rate.

If the current injected into the LED is I, then the total number of recombinations per second is:

$$R_r + R_{nr} = I/q \tag{8.60}$$

Substituting Eq. (8.94) into Eq. (8.91), then yields $R_r = \eta_{int}I/q$. Noting that R_r is the total number of photons generated per second and that each photon has an energy $h\nu$, then the optical power generated internally to the LED is:

$$P_{int} = \eta_{int}\frac{I}{q}h\nu = \eta_{int}\frac{hcI}{q\lambda} \tag{8.61}$$

Assuming the outside medium is air and letting $n_1 = n$, we have $T(0) = 4n/(n+1)^2$. The external quantum efficiency is then approximately given by:

$$\eta_{int} \approx \frac{1}{n(n+1)^2} \tag{8.62}$$

From this, it follows that the optical power emitted from the LED (Fig. 8.47) is:

$$P = \eta_{ext}P_{int} \approx \frac{P_{int}}{n(n+1)} \tag{8.63}$$

We may note that not all internally generated photons will exit the device. To find the emitted power, one needs to consider the *external quantum efficiency* η_{ext}. This is defined as the ratio of the photons emitted from the LED to the number of internally generated photons. To find the external quantum efficiency, we need to take into account reflection effects at the surface of the LED. As shown in Fig. 8.46, at the interface of a material boundary only that fraction of light falling within a cone defined by the critical angle ϕ_c = $\pi/2 - \theta_c$ will cross the interface. We have that $\phi_c = \sin^{-1}(n_2/n_1)$. Here, n_1 is the refractive index of the semiconductor material and n_2 is the refractive index of the outside material,

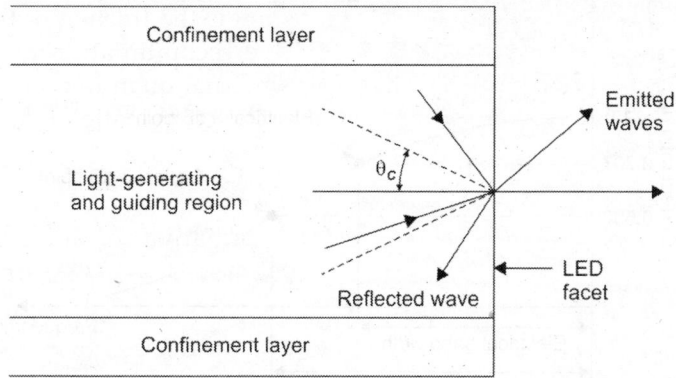

Fig. 8.46: Only light falling within a cone defined by the critical angle will be emitted from an optical source

which nominally is air with $n_2 = 1.0$. The external quantum efficiency can then be calculated from the expression:

$$\eta_{ext} = \frac{1}{4\pi} \int_0^\phi T(\phi)\,(2\pi \sin \phi)\, d\phi \qquad (8.64)$$

where $T(\phi)$ is the *Fresnel transmission coefficient* or *Fresnel transmissivity*. This factor depends on the incidence angle ϕ, but, for simplicity, we can use the expression for normal incidence, which is:

$$T(0) = \frac{4n_1 n_2}{(n_1 + n_2)^2} \qquad (8.65)$$

Assuming the outside medium is air letting $n_1 = n$, we have $T(0) = 4n/(n+1)^2$. The external quantum efficiency is then approximately given by:

$$\eta_{ext} \approx \frac{1}{n(n+1)^2} \qquad (8.66)$$

From this, it follows that the optical power emitted from the LED is:

$$P = \eta_{ext} P_{int} \approx \frac{P_{int}}{n(n+1)^2} \qquad (8.67)$$

8.5.5 Modulation of an LED

The *response time* or *frequency response* of an optical source dictates how fast an electrical input drive signal can vary the light output level. The following three factors largely determine the response time: the doping level in the active region, the injected carrier lifetime t_i in the recombination region, and the parasitic capacitance of the LED. If the drive current is modulated at a frequency ω, the optical output power of the device will vary as:

$$P(\omega) = P_o \,[1 + (\omega \tau_i)^2]^{1/2} \qquad (8.68)$$

where P_o is the power emitted at zero modulation frequency. The parasitic capacitance can cause a delay of the carrier injection into the active junction, and consequently, could delay the optical output. This delay is negligible if a small, constant forward bias is applied to the diode. Under this condition, Eq. (8.68) is valid and modulation response is limited only by the carrier recombination time.

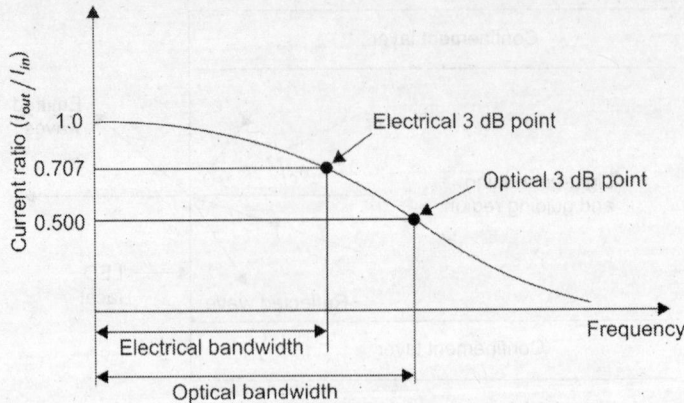

Fig. 8.47: Frequency response of an optical source showing the electrical and optical 3 dB bandwidth points

The modulation bandwidth of an LED can be defined in either electrical or optical terms. Normally, electrical terms are used since the bandwidth is actually determined via the associated electrical circuitry. Thus, the modulation bandwidth is defined as the point where the electrical signal power, designated by $p(\omega)$, has dropped to half its constant value resulting from the modulated portion of the optical signal. This is the electrical 3 dB point; that is, the frequency at which the output electrical power is reduced by 3 dB with respect to the input electrical power, as shown in Fig. 8.47.

Since an optical source exhibits a linear relationship between light power and current, currents rather than voltages (which are used in electrical systems) are compared in optical systems. Thus, since $p(\omega) = I^2(\omega)/R$, the ratio of the output electrical power at the frequency w to the power at zero modulation is:

$$\text{Ratio}_{\text{elec}} = 10 \log \left[\frac{p(\omega)}{p(o)} \right] = 10 \log \left[\frac{I^2(\omega)}{I^2(o)} \right] \tag{8.69}$$

where $I(\omega)$ is the electrical current in the detection circuitry. The electrical 3 dB point occurs at that frequency point where the detected electrical power $p(\omega) = p(o)/2$. This happens when:

$$\frac{I^2(\omega)}{I^2(o)} = \frac{1}{2} \tag{8.70}$$

or $I(\omega)/I(0) = 1/\sqrt{2} = 0.707$.

We may note that sometimes, the modulation bandwidth of an LED is given in terms of the 3 dB bandwidth of the modulated optical power $P(\omega)$; that is, it is specified at the frequency where $P(\omega) = P_o/2$. In this case, the 3 dB bandwidth is determined from the ratio of the optical power at frequency ω to the unmodulated value of the optical power. Since the detected current is directly proportional to the optical power, this ratio is:

$$\text{Ratio}_{\text{optical}} = 10 \log \left[\frac{P(\omega)}{P(o)} \right] = 10 \log \left[\frac{I(\omega)}{I(o)} \right] \tag{8.71}$$

The optical 3 dB point occurs at that frequency where the ratio of the currents is equal to 1/2. As shown in Fig. 8.49, this gives an inflated value of the modulation bandwidth, which corresponds to an electrical power attenuation of 6 dB.

Example 1

Calculate the ratio of rates of spontaneous and stimulated emission for a tungsten filament lamp operating at a temperature of 2000 K. Take average frequency = 5×10^{14} Hz.

Solution

$$R = \exp\left(\frac{h\nu}{kT}\right) - 1$$

$$R = \exp\left(\frac{6.6 \times 10^{-34} \times 5 \times 10^{14}}{1.38 \times 10^{-23} \times 2000}\right) - 1$$

or $$= e^{12} - 1 = 1.5 \times 10^{5}.$$

Example 2

Estimate the relative populations of two energy levels such that a transition from higher to lower will give a visible radiation.

Solution

Average wavelength of visible radiation = 550 nm

$$\therefore \quad E_2 - E_1 = \frac{hc}{\lambda} = \frac{6.6 \times 10^{-34} \times 3 \times 10^{8}}{550 \times 10^{-9}}$$

$$= 3.6 \times 10^{-19} \, J = 2.25 \, eV$$

Assuming room temperature = 300 K and $g_1 = g_2$, we have:

$$\frac{N_2}{N_1} = \exp\left[\frac{-3.6 \times 10^{-19}}{1.38 \times 10^{-23} \times 300}\right]$$

$$\approx e^{-87} = 10^{-37}.$$

Example 3

A single crystal of silicon sample having width of 0.3 μm is illuminated with a monochromatic light of energy 3 eV. The incident power is 10 MW. Calculate: (i) total energy absorbed by material per second (ii) the rate of excess thermal energy dissipated to the lattice (iii) the number of photons per second given off from the recombination of intrinsic transition. Given α = 4×10^4/cm. **[B Tech]**

Solution

(i) Energy absorbed/sec is equal to:

$$\phi_o \left[1 - \exp\left(4 \times 10^4 \times 0.3 \times 10^{-4}\right)\right] = 10^{-12} \left(1 - \exp\left(4 \times 10^4 \times 0.3 \times 10^{-4}\right)\right)$$
$$= 10^{-2} \left[1 - e^{1.2}\right] = 6.3 \, mW$$

(ii) The portion of each photon energy that is converted into heat is obtained as:

$$\frac{h\nu - E_g}{h\nu} = \frac{3 - 1.12}{3} = 62\%$$

Obviously, the amount of energy dissipated/sec to lattice is 62% × 6.3 = 3.9 mW.

(iii) Number of photons/sec from recombination is:

$$\frac{2.4}{1.6 \times 10^{-19} \times 1.12} = 1.3 \times 10^{16} \, photon/sec$$

$\therefore$ Recombination radiation $= 6.3 - 3.9$

$$= 2.4 \text{ mW}.$$

Example 4

An InGaAsP surface emitter has an activation energy of 1 eV with a constant of proportionality (β_0) of 1.84×10^7 h^{-1}. Estimate the CW operating lifetime for the LED with a constant junction temperature of 17°C, if it is assumed that the device is no longer useful when its optical output power has diminished to 0.67 of its original value.

[DTU, MHTU]

Solution

Initially, we have to obtain the degradation rate β_r. Thus from equation

$$\beta_r = \beta_0 \exp (-E_a/kT)$$

$$= 1.84 \times 10^7 \exp \left(\frac{-1 \times 1.602 \times 10^{-19}}{1.38 \times 10^{-23} \times 290} \right)$$

$$= 1.84 \times 10^7 \exp (-40)$$

$$= 7.82 \times 10^{-11} \text{ h}^{-1}$$

Now, using $\qquad \dfrac{P_e(t)}{P_{\text{out}}} = \exp(-\beta_r t) = 0.67.$

$$\therefore \ \beta_r t = -\ln 0.67$$

and: $\qquad t = \dfrac{\ln 0.67}{7.82 \times 10^{-11}} = \dfrac{0.40}{7.82 \times 10^{-11}}$

$$= 5.1 \times 10^9 \text{ h}$$

Example 5

The minority carrier recombination lifetime for an LED is 5 ns. When a constant d.c. drive current is applied to the device the optical output power is 300 µW. Determine the optical output power when the device is modulated with an rms drive current corresponding to the d.c. drive current at frequencies of (a) 20 MHz (b) 100 MHz.

You may assume that parasitic capacitance is negligible. Further, determine the 3 dB optical bandwidth for the device and estimate the 3 dB electrical bandwidth assuming a Gaussian response.

[KTU]

Solution

(a) The optical output power at 20 MHz is:

$$P_e(20 \text{ MHz}) = \frac{P_{dc}}{[1 + (\omega \tau_i)^2]^{1/2}}$$

$$= \frac{300 \times 10^{-6}}{[1 + (2\pi \times 20 \times 10^6 \times 5 \times 10^{-9})^2]^{1/2}}$$

$$= \frac{300 \times 10^{-6}}{[1.39]^{1/2}}$$

$$= 254.2 \text{ µW}$$

(b) We have

$$P_e(100 \text{ MHz}) = \frac{300 \times 10^{-6}}{[1 + (2\pi \times 100 \times 10^6 \times 5 \times 10^{-9})^2]^{1/2}}$$

$$= \frac{300 \times 10^{-6}}{[10.87]^{1/2}}$$

$$= 90.9 \text{ }\mu\text{W}$$

Clearly, this example illustrates the reduction in the LED optical output power as the device is driven at higher modulating frequencies. It is therefore apparent that there is a somewhat limited bandwidth over which the device may be usefully utilized.

Now, we determine the optical 3 dB bandwidth. The high-frequency 3 dB point occurs when $P_c(\omega)/P_{dc} = 1/2$. Hence,

$$\frac{1}{[1 + (\omega\tau_i)^2]^{1/2}} = \frac{1}{2}$$

and $1 + (\omega\tau_i)^2 = 4$. Therefore $\omega\tau_i = \sqrt{3}$, and:

$$f = \frac{\sqrt{3}}{2\pi\tau} = \frac{\sqrt{3}}{\pi \times 10^{-8}} = 55.1 \text{ MHz}$$

Clearly, the 3 dB optical bandwidth B_{opt} is 55.1 MHz as the device, similar to all LEDs, operates down to DC level.

Assuming a Gaussian frequency response, the 3 dB electrical bandwidth B will be:

$$B = \frac{55.1}{\sqrt{2}} = 39.0 \text{ MHz}$$

Thus the corresponding electrical bandwidth is 39 MHz. However, we may note that parasitic capacitance may reduce the modulation bandwidth below this value.

Example 6

The reflection coefficients for a semiconductor laser are equal and have the value 0.5. The length of cavity is 1 μm. Assume that there are no additional loss terms. Calculate the gain of the laser. **[B Tech]**

Solution

No internal loss means $d_i = 0$; we have:

$$g = \frac{1}{2L} \ln\left(\frac{1}{r_1 r_2}\right)$$

$$= \frac{1}{2 \times 1} \ln\left(\frac{1}{0.5 \times 0.5}\right)$$

$$= 6.93 \times 10^3 /\text{cm}$$

Example 7

A cadmium sulphide photodetector is irradiated over a receiving area of 4×10^{-6} m^2 by a light of wavelength 0.4×10^{-6} m and intensity 200 Wm^{-2}. Assuming that each quantum generates an electron-hole pair, calculate the number of pairs generated per second.

[B Tech]

Solution

Here: $\lambda = 0.4 \times 10^{-6}$ m,

Area of the crystal $= 4 \times 10^{-6}$ m^2,

Intensity of light $= 200$ Wm^{-2}

Now, the number of photons $= \dfrac{\text{Intensity}}{h\nu} \times \text{Area}$

$$= \frac{200 \times 4 \times 10^{-6} \lambda}{hc}$$

$$= \frac{200 \times 4 \times 10^{-6} \times 0.4 \times 10^{-6}}{6.626 \times 10^{-34} \times 3 \times 10^{8}}$$

$$= 1.609 \times 10^{15}$$

As each quantum of energy will generate an electron–hole pair and hence the number of pairs generated per second $= 1.6 \times 10^{15}$.

Example 8

A photodiode has a quantum efficiency of 70% when photons with energy 2.2×10^{-19} J are incident on it. Calculate: (a) operating wavelength of photodiode (b) the incident power required to obtain a photocurrent of 0.2 mA when the diode is operating in the above condition. **[B Tech]**

Solution

(a) $\qquad E = h\nu = \dfrac{hc}{\lambda}$ or $\lambda = \dfrac{hc}{E}$

$\therefore \quad \lambda = \dfrac{6.62 \times 10^{-34} \times 3 \times 10^{8}}{2.2 \times 10^{-19}}$

$\qquad = 0.9\ \mu\text{m}$

$\qquad \eta = 70\%$ of photoenergy $= 0.70$

$\qquad E = 2.2 \times 10^{-19}$ J

$\qquad I_p = 0.2$ mA

and $\nu = \dfrac{c}{\lambda} = \dfrac{3 \times 10^{8}}{0.9 \times 10^{-6}}$

$\qquad = 3.33 \times 10^{14}$ Hz

(b) $R = \dfrac{\eta e}{h\nu} = \dfrac{\eta e \lambda}{hc} = \dfrac{\eta e}{h\nu}$ $\qquad (\because c = \nu\lambda)$

$\qquad = \dfrac{0.70 \times 1.6 \times 10^{-19}}{6.62 \times 10^{-34} \times 3.33 \times 10^{14}}$

$\qquad = 0.51$ AW^{-1}

$\qquad R_o = \dfrac{I_p}{P_o}$ or $R_o = \dfrac{I_p}{P} = \dfrac{2.0 \times 10^{-6}}{0.51} = 3.92\ \mu\text{W}$

Example 9

3×10^{11} photons each with a wavelength of 0.85 are incident on a photodiode. On an average 1.5×10^{11} electrons are collected at the terminals of the device. Calculate: (i) Quantum efficiency (η), and (ii) responsivity (R) of the photodiode at the wavelength of 0.85 mm.   [B Tech]

Solution

(i) $\eta = \dfrac{r_e}{r_p} = \dfrac{\text{number of hole pairs generated}}{\text{number of incident photon}}$

$= \dfrac{1.5 \times 10^{11}}{3 \times 10^{11}} = 0.5$

(ii) Responsivity, $R = \eta \dfrac{e\lambda}{hc}$

$= \dfrac{0.5 \times 1.6 \times 10^{-19} \times 0.85 \times 10^{-6}}{6.62 \times 10^{-34} \times 3 \times 10^{8}} = 0.34 \ \text{AW}^{-1}$

Example 10

Compare the electrical and optical bandwidths for an optical fiber communication system and develop a relationship between them.   [KTU, PTU]

Solution

To obtain a simple relationship between the two bandwidths it is necessary to compare the electrical current through the system. Current rather than voltage (which is generally used in electrical systems) is compared as both the optical source and optical detector may be considered to have a linear relationship between light and current.

Electrical bandwidth: The ratio of the electric output power to the electric input power in decibels RE_{dB} is given by:

$$RE_{dB} = 10 \log_{10} \frac{\text{electric power out (at the detector)}}{\text{electric power in (at the source)}}$$

$$= 10 \log_{10} \frac{I_{out}^2 / R_{out}}{I_{in}^2 / R_{in}}$$

$$\propto 10 \log_{10} \left[\frac{I_{out}}{I_{in}} \right]^2$$

Now, the electrical 3 dB points occur when the ratio of electric powers shown above is $1/2$. Hence, we find that this must occur when:

$$\left[\frac{I_{out}}{I_{in}} \right]^2 = \frac{1}{2} \quad \text{or} \quad \frac{I_{out}}{I_{in}} = \frac{1}{\sqrt{2}}$$

Thus in the electrical regime the bandwidth may be defined by the frequency when the output current has dropped to $1/\sqrt{2}$ or 0.707 of the input current to the system.

Optical bandwidth: The ratio of the optical output power to the optical input power in decibels RO_{dB} is given by:

$$RO_{dB} = 10 \log_{10} \frac{\text{optical power out (received at detector)}}{\text{optical power in (transmitted at source)}} \propto 10 \log_{10} \frac{I_{out}}{I_{in}}$$

(due to the linear light/current relationships of the source and detector). Hence the optical 3 dB points occur when the ratio of the currents is equal to 1/2, and:

$$\frac{I_{out}}{I_{in}} = \frac{1}{2}$$

Obviously, in the optical regime the bandwidth is defined by the frequencies at which the output current has dropped to 1/2 or 0.5 of the input current to the system. This corresponds to an electric power attenuation of 6 dB.

Example 11

$GaAs_{0.88}Sb_{0.12}$ is a direct band gap semiconductor and has a band gap energy of 1.115 eV. Determine the critical wavelength above which an intrinsic photodetector from this material can be operated. **[B Tech]**

Solution

The critical wavelength is given by:

$$\frac{hc}{\lambda_c} = E_g$$

or

$$\lambda_c = \frac{hc}{E_g}$$

$$h = 6.62 \times 10^{-34}$$
$$c = 3 \times 10^8 \text{ m/s}$$
$$E_g = 1.15 \times 1.6 \times 10^{-19} \text{ V}$$

or

$$\lambda_c = \frac{6.62 \times 10^{-34} \times 3 \times 10^8}{1.15 \times 1.6 \times 10^{-19}}$$

$$= 1.06 \text{ mm} = 1060 \text{ nm}$$

Example 12

Photons of wavelength 0.90 µm are incident on a *pn* photodiode at a rate of 5×10^{10} s^{-1} and, on an average, the electrons are collected at the terminals of the diode at the rate of 2×10^{10} s^{-1}. Calculate the quantum efficiency (η) and the responsibility (R) of the diode at this wavelength. **[B Tech]**

Solution

$$\eta = \frac{r_e}{r_p} = \frac{2 \times 10^{10}}{5 \times 10^{10}} = 0.40$$

Here:

$\lambda = 0.90 \text{ µm} = 0.90 \times 10^{-6}$ m

Rate of electron $(r_e) = 2 \times 10^{10}$ s^{-1}

Rate of photons $(r_p) = 5 \times 10^{10}$ s^{-1}

$$R = \frac{\eta e \lambda}{hc} = \frac{0.40 \times 1.6 \times 10^{-19} \times 0.90 \times 10^{-6}}{6.626 \times 10^{-34} \times 3 \times 10^8} = 0.29 \text{ AW}^{-1}$$

Example 13

A *pn* photodiode has a quantum efficiency of 70% for photon of energy 1.52×10^{-19} J. Calculate (i) the wavelength at which the diode is operating and (ii) the optical power required to achieve a photocurrent of 3 μA when the wavelength of the incident photons is that calculated in part (i). **[B Tech]**

Solution

(i) Photon energy, $E = h\nu = \dfrac{hc}{\lambda}$

or $\qquad \lambda = \dfrac{hc}{E} = \dfrac{6.626 \times 10^{-34} \times 3 \times 10^8}{1.52 \times 10^{-19}}$

$\qquad\qquad = 1.30 \times 10^{-6}\,\text{m} = 1.30\,\mu\text{m}$

(ii) $\qquad R = \dfrac{\eta e}{h\nu} = \dfrac{0.70 \times 1.6 \times 10^{-19}}{1.52 \times 10^{-19}} = 0.736\,\text{AW}^{-1}$

$\qquad \therefore \quad R = \dfrac{I_p}{P_{in}} \quad\text{or}\quad P_{in} = \dfrac{I_p}{R} = \dfrac{3 \times 10^{-6}}{0.736} = 0.736\,\text{AW}^{-1}$

or $\quad P_{in} = 4.07 \times 10^{-6}\,\text{W} = 4.07\,\mu\text{W}$.

Example 14

A silicon RAPD (reach through avalanche photodiode), operating at a wavelength of 0.80 μm, exhibits a quantum efficiency of 90%, a multiplication factor of 800, and a dark current of 2 nA. Calculate the rate at which photons should be incident on the device so that the output current (after avalanche gain) is greater than the dark current. **[B Tech]**

Solution

We have, $\qquad I = I_p M = P_{in}\,RM = P_{in}\left(\dfrac{\eta e\lambda}{hc}\right)M = \left(\dfrac{P_{in}}{hc/\lambda}\right)\eta e M$

$\qquad\qquad = [(\text{photon rate})\,e]\,\eta M = \dfrac{2 \times 10^{-9}}{1.6 \times 10^{-19} \times 0.90 \times 800}$

$\qquad\qquad = 1.736 \times 10^{7}\,\text{s}^{-1}$

Thus, for $I > 2$ nA, photon rate $\approx 1.74 \times 10^{7}\,\text{s}^{-1}$.

Example 15

The recombination processes in an LED working at 1650 nm are governed by radiative recombination with mean lifetime of 10 ns while the nonradiative recombination dominated by SRH and Auger processes with mean lifetime values of 20 ns and 100 ns respectively. Estimate the internal quantum efficiency of the LED. **[PTU, KTU]**

Solution

The effective lifetime of the carrier can be estimated with the help of following relation as

$$\frac{1}{\tau} = \frac{1}{\tau_r} + \frac{1}{\tau_{nr}} = \frac{1}{\tau_r} + \frac{1}{\tau_{SRH}} + \frac{1}{\tau_{AU}}$$

$$= \left(\frac{1}{10} + \frac{1}{20} + \frac{1}{100}\right)\text{ns}^{-1}$$

or $\qquad\qquad \tau = \dfrac{100}{16} = 6.25\,\text{ns}$

The internal quantum efficiency is obtained as

$$\eta_{int} = \frac{6.25}{10} = 62.5\%$$

Example 16

The carrier recombination lifetime for a double heterostructure LED (DH-LED) at room temperature is 20 ns. The surface recombination velocity of the carriers at each heterointerface is $S = 100$ m/s and the thickness of the active region is 1.0 mm. Estimate the optical bandwidth of the DH-LED. **[MHTU, DTU]**

Solution

The effective lifetime of the carriers for the DH-LED can be estimated as

$$\frac{1}{\tau_{eff}} = \frac{1}{\tau} + \frac{2S}{d} = \frac{1}{20 \times 10^{-9}} + \frac{2 \times 100}{1.0 \times 10^{-6}} = 0.5 \times 10^8 + 2 \times 10^8 = 2.5 \times 10^8$$

The effective carrier lifetime for the DH-LED is thus obtained as

$$\tau_{eff} = \frac{1}{2.5 \times 10^8} = 4 \text{ ns}$$

The 3-dB optical bandwidth of the DH-LED can be estimated as follows:

$$f_{3dB-op} = \frac{\sqrt{3}}{2\pi \times 4 \times 10^{-9}} = 68.93 \text{ MHz}$$

Example 17

The carrier recombination life-time for an LED operating at 50 mA DC drive current is 1 ns. Find the values of electrical and optical bandwidth of the LED. **[MPTU, RTU]**

Solution

The electrical bandwidth of the LED can be calculated as

$$f_{3dB-el} = \frac{1}{2\pi\tau}$$

$$f_{3dB-el} = \frac{1}{2\pi \times 1 \times 10^{-9}} = \frac{10^8}{6.28} = 159.23 \text{ MHz}$$

The optical bandwidth of the LED is equivalently,

$$f_{3dB-op} = \sqrt{3} f_{3dB-el} = 275.8 \text{ MHz}$$

Example 18

A Fabry-Perot laser diode with a 400 mm long cavity uses GaAs as the material in the active region with uncoated facets. The cavity offers an average loss of 1000 m^{-1} at the operating wavelength. Estimate the value of the threshold gain assuming the refractive index of GaAs to be 3.6. **[DTU, KTU]**

Solution

The reflectivities of the uncoated facets can be estimated as

$$R = [(n_1 - n_2)/(n_1 + n_2)]^2$$

Here $R_1 = R_2 = R$

$\therefore$ $R_1 = R_2 = \left(\frac{3.6-1}{3.6+1}\right)^2 = 0.32$

The threshold gain can be estimated as

$$\Gamma_{g_{th}} = \bar{\alpha} + \frac{1}{2L} \ln\left(\frac{1}{R_1 R_2}\right)$$

$$= 1000 + \frac{1}{400 \times 10^{-6}} \ln\left(\frac{1}{0.32 \times 0.32}\right) = 6697.17 \text{ m}^{-1}$$

Example 19

A Fabry–Perot injection laser diode with an active cavity of length 500 μm is operating at 850 nm. Calculate the wavelength separation between the successive modes in the cavity assuming the refractive index of the cavity to be 3.6. **[MHTU]**

Solution

The wavelength separation between the successive modes of the injection laser diode can be calculated as

$$\Delta\lambda = \frac{\lambda^2}{2nL} = \frac{(850 \times 10^{-9})^2}{2 \times 3.6 \times 500 \times 10^{-6}}$$

$$= 0.2 \text{ nm}$$

Example 20

A FP injection laser diode operating at 850 nm has a cavity width of 20 μm. Find the divergence angle of the emitted beam in the lateral and transverse directions of the cavity assuming the thickness of the active region to be 2 μm.

Solution

The angular beam divergence of the laser diode in the transverse direction is obtained as

$$\theta_\perp = 2\sin^{-1}\left(\frac{\lambda}{H}\right) = 2\sin^{-1}\left(\frac{850 \times 10^{-9}}{2 \times 10^{-6}}\right) = 50°.3$$

The angular beam divergence in the direction transverse to the plane of the *pn*-junction is obtained as

$$\theta_{||} = \sin^{-1}\left(\frac{850 \times 10^{-9}}{20 \times 10^{-6}}\right) = 4°.8$$

Example 21

A planar LED is fabricated from gallium arsenide which has a refractive index of 3.6.

(a) Calculate the optical power emitted into air as a percentage of the internal optical power for the device when the transmission factor at the crystal-air interface is 0.68.

(b) When the optical power generated internally is 50% of the electric power supplied, determine the external power efficiency. **[PTU, KTU]**

Solution

(a) For the optical power emitted in which the refractive index n for air is 1, we have

$$P_e \simeq \frac{P_{int}Fn^2}{4n_x^2} = \frac{P_{int}0.68 \times 1}{4(3.6)^2} = 0.013P_{int}$$

Hence the power emitted is only 1.3% of the optical power generated internally.

(b) The external power efficiency is given by

$$\eta_{ep} = \frac{P_c}{P} \times 100 = 0.013 \frac{P_{int}}{P} \times 100$$

Also, the optical power generated internally $P_{int} = 0.5P$.

Hence:

$$\eta_{ep} = \frac{0.013 P_{int}}{2P_{int}} \times 100 = 0.65\%$$

SUMMARY

1. The phenomenon of emission of electrons from a metal surface under the effect of light radiations is termed a photoelectric effect. The minimum frequency of light that can cause photoelectric effect is called threshold frequency.

2. A photoconductive cell is a two-terminal semiconductor device, whose resistance decreases with the intensity of light falling on it, and as a result free electrons are available. It is also called light (photo) *dependent resistance* (LDR).

3. An LED is a specially fabricated semiconductor *pn* junction diode that emits monochromatic light when forward-biased. LED has voltage drop-rating of about 2 V and current rating of about 20 mA.

4. The internal quantum efficiency of an LED is the fraction of diode current that will produce luminescence.

5. The external quantum efficiency of an LED is defined as the ratio of the number of photons emitted from the device per incident injected electron.

6. The brightness of light emitted by an LED depends upon current flowing through it.

7. LEDs have replaced small incandescent light bulbs as display devices. The long life expectancy, ruggedness, and much lower power consumption have contributed to the choice of LEDs over incandescent light bulbs. Some of the applications of LEDs are seven-segment display, polarity tester, and continuity tester.

8. An optocoupler or optoisolator is an arrangement of coupling (or isolating) a light emitting source from a light dependent device (light detector) through a transparent insulating medium.

9. An LCD consists of a thin film (about 15 μm) of a conductive crystal in liquid form. Normally the crystal is transparent. However, when energized by an AC source in the presence of light, it changes to provide black-tone or gray readout.

REVIEW QUESTIONS

1. What is optical light spectrum?
   (a) Frequency and wavelength
   (b) Visible versus invisible
   (c) Infrared and ultraviolet

2. The infrared band is given as 30 to 400 THz. What is its value in terms of wavelength?

3. Mention the difference between coherent and incoherent light.

4. Discuss the operation of LED.
   (a) How does it emit light? (b) When does it emit light.

5. A certain piece of equipment shows a green light when it is working properly and red light when it is not working properly. The light appears to come from the same device. How might this work?

6. A particular fiber-optic application will use a very long length of fiber-optic cable. Would this application use an LED or a laser diode? Why?

7. A certain control circuit is being used to control the operation of a high-power motor starter. The motor starter generates enormous amounts of noise that might interfere with the control system. Discuss how the circuit might be designed to isolate noise from the control.

8. What is an LED? Explain the modulation of an LED?

9. You wish to operate a door opener with a light source. Draw a block diagram to show how this might be done.

10. What is an LCD? Write its applications, make a comparison of LCD and LED.

11. Mention where the liquid crystal diode is practically used?

12. Show that when the simple bias circuit (Fig. 8.48) is used with a photoconductive detector to detect small signal levels, then maximum voltage output signals across R_L are obtained when R_L is equal to detector resistance R_D.

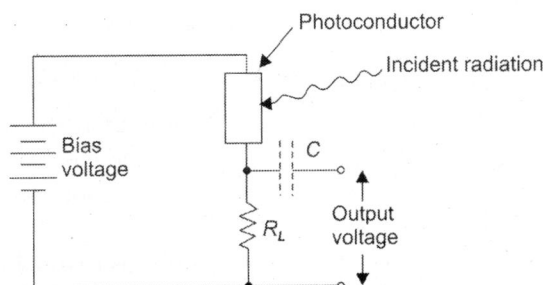

Fig. 8.48: Photoconductor bias circuit. The photoconductor is placed in a series circuit comprising a voltage source, a load resistor R_L, and the photoconductor. Changes in the resistance of photoconductor cause changes in voltage appearing across R_L. If only the AC component of this voltage is required, then a blocking capacitor C may be placed as shown

13. Show that gain G of a photoconductive detector can be written as $Ge = \tau_c / \tau_d$ where t_c is minority carrier lifetime, and τ_d is given by:

$$\frac{1}{\tau_d} = \frac{1}{\tau_n} + \frac{1}{\tau_p}$$

τ_n and τ_p being the times taken for electrons and holes to drift across the photodetector.

14. Show the responsivity of a photodiode detector can be written as:

$$R(f) = \frac{R(o)}{(1 + 4\pi^2 f^2 C^2 R_L^2)}$$

where C is diode capacitance and R_L load resistance.

15. Give a brief account of optical source materials used in optical fiber communication system.

16. Explain LED power and efficiency and show that the internal quantum efficiency of the LED can be expressed as

$$\eta_{int} = \tau/\tau_r$$

where τ is the effective lifetime of the carrier and τ_r is mean lifetime for radiative carriers. Also show that the optical power generated internally to the LED is given by

$$P_{int} = \eta_{int} \frac{hc}{q\lambda} I$$

where I is the drive current flows through the device under steady state.

17. Explain external quantum efficiency of an LED and show that the optical power available outside the LED is

$$P_{emitted} = \eta_{ext} P_{int}$$

where η_{ext} is the external quantum efficiency of the LED and P_{int} is the optical power generated internally to the LED.

18. Describe homojunction and heterojunction LED structures. How the surface recombination velocity at the heterointerfaces (assumed to be same and equal to S) modify the bulk recombination velocity?

19. What are super-luminescent LEDs? Describe its working?

20. What are LED characteristics? Explain special features LEDs based on LED characteristics which make them an attractive optical source over injection laser diode for analog optical communication?

21. Show that the optical output power $P(\omega)$ of an LED biased by a drive current modulated at an angular frequency ω can be expressed as $P(\omega) = \dfrac{P(0)}{\sqrt{1+(\tau\omega)^2}}$.

PROBLEMS

1. A photocell cathode is coated with materials having a work function of 3.5 eV. A photocell is irradiated of frequency 4×10^{15} Hz. Calculate the velocity of emitted electrons. **[Ans.** 2.08×10^6 ms^{-1}**]**

2. The electrical conductivity of a semiconductor increases when electromagnetic radiation of wavelength shorter than 2480 nm is incident on it. Calculate the bandgap of the semiconductor. **[Ans.** $\Delta E_g = 0.5$ eV**]**

3. A *pn* photodiode has a quantum efficiency of 50% at $\lambda = 0.90$ μm. Calculate (a) its responsivity at this wavelength, (b) if the mean photocurrent is 10^{-6} A, then the optical power received, and (c) the corresponding photons received at this wavelength. **[Ans.** (a) 0.362 AW^{-1}, (b) 2.76 mW, (c) 1.25×10^{13} s^{-1}**]**

4. In a photocell, a copper surface was irradiated by light of wavelength 1849Å, the stopping potential was found to be 2.72 eV. Show that the maximum energy (I_{max}) of photoelectrons is 2.72 eV.

5. Find the current through LED in the circuit shown (Fig. 8.49). Assume that voltage drop across the LED is 2 V. **[Ans.** $I_F = 5.91$ mA**]**

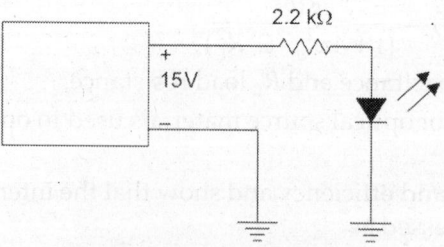

2.2 kΩ

+ 15V

Fig. 8.49: LED circuit

6. Calculate the responsivity of an ideal photodiode at the following wavelengths:
   (a) 1.55 μm (b) 1.30 μm (c) 0.85 μm.   **[B Tech]**

   [Ans. (a) 1.248 AW^{-1}, (b) 1.046 AW^{-1}, (c) 0.684 AW^{-1}]

7. The quantum efficiency of an APD is 50% at 1.3 μm. It produces an output current of 8 μA, after avalanche gain when illuminated with optical power of 0.4 μW at this wavelength. Show that the multiplication factor of the diode is 38.

8. The responsivity of a typical photodiode is 0.40 AW^{-1} for a He–Ne laser source (λ = 632.8 nm). If the active area of the photodiode is 2 mm^2, calculate the output photocurrent when the incident flux is 100 λW/mm^2?   **[Ans. 80 μA]**

9. Estimate the external quantum efficiency of a GaAs LED operating at 0.86 mm and emitting light in the surrounding medium of air. Assume the relative permittivity of GaAs to be 12.9.   **[PTU]**

   [**Hint:** The refractive index of GaAs is obtained as

   $$n = \sqrt{12.9} \approx 3.6$$

   The external quantum efficiency of the LED can be estimated as

   $$\eta_{\text{ext}} = \frac{1}{n(n+1)^2}$$

   Here n = 3.6,

   $$\therefore \ \eta_{\text{ext}} = \frac{1}{3.6 \times (1+3.6)^2} \approx 1.31\% \ ]$$

10. The values of radiative and nonradiative carrier life-time for an LED are 10 ns and 100 ns respectively. The LED emits an optical power of 100 μW at a constant bias current. Estimate the value of the optical power output of the LED when it is modulated with an rms drive current corresponding to the DC drive current at a frequency of 10 MHz. What is the bandwidth of the LED?

                                                                    [KTU]

    [**Hint:** The mean carrier lifetime in this case is obtained as

    $$\frac{1}{\tau} = \frac{1}{\tau_r} + \frac{1}{\tau_{nr}} = \frac{1}{10 \times 10^{-9}} + \frac{1}{100 \times 10^{-9}}$$

    The effective lifetime of the carrier,

    $$\tau = \frac{10 \times 100 \times 10^{-18}}{110 \times 10^{-9}} = 9.09 \text{ ns}$$

    The optical output power from the LED when biased by a drive current at 10 MHz is obtained as

    $$P(10 \text{ MHz}) = \frac{100 \times 10^{-6}}{\sqrt{1 + (2\pi \times 10 \times 10^6 \times 9.09 \times 10^{-9})^2}}$$

    $$= 75.75 \text{ μW}$$

The optical bandwidth of the LED is obtained as

$$f_{3dB-op} = \frac{\sqrt{3}}{2\pi \times 9.09 \times 10^{-9}} = 30.34 \text{ MHz}$$

The electrical bandwidth of the LED is obtained as

$$f_{3dB-el} = \frac{1}{2\pi \times 9.09 \times 10^{-9}} = 17.51 \text{ MHz}]$$

11. A double heterojunction LED with negligible surface recombination at the heterointerfaces has an active region of thickness 0.3 μm operating at 0.85 μm wavelength region. Estimate the optical bandwidth of the LED when the drive current is neglecting the nonradiative recombination. Assume the radiative recombination coefficient $B_r = 10^{-12}$ m^3/s. The drive current of LED without modulation is 0.5×10^5 A/m^2. **[MPTU]**

[**Hint:** The radiative recombination lifetime of the carriers for the LED is obtained as

$$\tau_r = \left(\frac{qd}{JB_r} \right)^{\frac{1}{2}} = \left(\frac{1.6 \times 10^{-19} \times 0.3 \times 10^{-6}}{0.5 \times 10^5 \times 10^{-14}} \right)^{\frac{1}{2}}$$

$$= 9.7 \text{ ns}$$

Now, neglecting the nonradiative and surface recombination, the overall recombination lifetime of the carriers for the LED can be easily approximated as

$$\tau \approx \tau_r$$

The optical bandwidth of the LED is found as

$$f_{3dB-op} = \frac{\sqrt{3}}{2\pi \times 9.7 \times 10^{-9}} = 28.43 \text{ MHz}]$$

12. The radiative and nonradiative recombination lifetimes of the minority carriers in the active region of a double heterojunction LED are 60 ns and 100 ns respectively. Determine the total carrier recombination lifetime and the power internally generated within the device when the peak emission wavelength is 0.87 μm at a drive current of 40 mA. **[KTU]**

[**Hint:** The total carrier recombination lifetime can be obtained as

$$\tau = \frac{\tau_r \tau_{nr}}{\tau_r + \tau_{nr}} = \frac{60 \times 100}{60 + 100} \text{ ns} = 37.5 \text{ ns}$$

To calculate the internal power generated, it is necessary to obtain the internal quantum efficiency of the device. Thus, we have

$$\eta_{int} = \frac{\tau}{\tau_r} = \frac{37.5}{60} = 0.625$$

Now,
$$P_{int} = \eta_{int} \frac{hci}{e\lambda} = \frac{0.625 \times 6.626 \times 10^{-34} \times 2.998 \times 10^8 \times 40 \times 10^{-3}}{1.602 \times 10^{-19} \times 0.87 \times 10^{-6}}$$

$$= 35.6 \text{ mW}]$$

13. The carrier recombination lifetime for an LED is 20 ns. The LED emits an optical power of 200 μW when biased with a constant DC current. Estimate the optical output power when the LED is modulated by an rms drive current corresponding to the DC drive current at a frequency of 100 MHz.   **[DTU, RTU]**

[**Hint:** We can obtain the optical power output of the LED when modulated by the drive current at 100 MHz as

$$P(100 \text{ MHz}) = \frac{200 \times 10^{-6}}{\sqrt{1 + (2\pi \times 100 \times 10^6 \times 20 \times 10^{-9})^2}}$$

$$= 15.88 \text{ μW}]$$

SHORT ANSWER QUESTIONS

1. Do all optoelectronic devices produce light, either visible or invisible?
   Ans. No.
2. Is an LED a specially fabricated *pn* junction diode that works in forward-bias?
   Ans. Yes.
3. Do laser diodes find application in compact disk players and laser printers?
   Ans. Yes.
4. Can a photovoltaic cell be used to measure the intensity of illumination?
   Ans. Yes.
5. What is a photovoltaic cell?
   Ans. This is a device that converts light directly into electric energy.
6. What is a autocoupler?
   Ans. This is an assembly in a single package that contains a light emitting diode and a photosensitive device.
7. What do you understand by photodiode sensitivity?
   Ans. It is the ratio of photocurrent output (in amperes) to radiant energy (in watts) and expressed in amps/watts.
8. What is a laser diode?
   Ans. A laser diode is a heavily doped *pn* junction diode.
9. What is photoemissive or photoelectric effect?
   Ans. When radiation with a wavelength less than a critical value is incident upon a particular metal (sodium, potassium, etc.) surface, electrons are found to be emitted, this is called photo-emissive or photoelectric effect.
10. What is a solar cell?
    Ans. The solar cell is basically a *pn* junction detector operated under conditions such that it can deliver power into an external load. It is used to convert light energy to electrical energy and thereby serves as a DC voltage source.
11. What is a phototransistor?
    Ans. A phototransistor is a light detecting device, which is also called a photo-sensor.
12. Why there has been interest in the development of white LEDs for general illumination?
    Ans. LEDs are three times as efficient as incandescent lamps and can last ten times longer. A white LED requires LEDs of red, green and blue colours.

13. **What is the advantage of using heterojunction LEDs?**

Ans. Since a photon emitted to a radiative recombination process of direct bandgap material in one part of the device and reabsorbed prior to it reaches the surface, one obvious choice is to put the *pn* junction close to the surface to avoid reabsorption. However, the presence of surface states, producing non-radiative recombination channels, can result in a reduction in radiative efficiency of the device. To solve this problem, heterojunction is used instead of avoiding reabsorption. A commonly used heterojunction is that of GaAs and AlGaAs. A heterojunction LED is designed in such a way that recombination occurs on the narrow gap semiconductor. Light is subsequently emitted through the AlGaAs window into the external environment. The band gap of AlGaAs is greater than that of GaAs and therefore, most of the light will transmit through the AlGaAs without being absorbed.

14. **Explain the importance of infrared LEDs.**

Ans. Under infrared LEDs fall GaAs LEDs which can emit light of wavelength near 0.9 μm and many III–IV compounds such as quaternary $Ga_x In_{1-x} As_y P_{1-y}$ LEDs, which emit light from 1.1 to 1.6 μm. Infrared LEDs have an important application in opto-isolators where an input or control signal is decoupled from the output. Infrared LEDs also find application for transmission of optical signal through an optical fiber.

15. **When LEDs are best suited for optical fiber communication system?**

Ans. LEDs are best suited for optical power communication system when the power requirement of the source is more than a few tens of microwatt and the desired bit rate is in the range of 100–200 Mbps. However, the structure of an LED largely depends on the desired application, e.g. the structure of an LED intended for use as a display device may vary widely from that of an LED intended to be used in optical communication

16. **Write expression for recombination rate of LED under steady-state condition with a constant bias current flowing through it and define internal quantum efficiency of LED.**

Ans. Under steady-state condition, with a constant bias current flowing through the LED, the recombination rate which corresponds to the number of carriers recombining per unit volume per second is given by

$$r = \frac{\Delta n}{\tau} = \frac{J}{qd} \qquad \text{(i)}$$

where q is the electronic charge, J is the bias current density flowing through the diode and d is the thickness of the recombination region (active region) of the LED.

The recombination may either be *radiative* or *nonradiative* in nature. Thus, the total recombination rate, r given by Eq. (i) comprises the contribution of both the radiative (r_r) as well as the non-radiative, (r_{nr}) rates. Thus Eq. (i) reads as

$$r = r_r + r_{nr} = \frac{J}{qd} \qquad \text{(ii)}$$

where
$$r_r = \frac{\Delta n}{\tau_r} \qquad \text{(iii)}$$

and
$$r_{nr} = \frac{\Delta n}{\tau_{nr}} \qquad \text{(iv)}$$

Here, τ_r and τ_{nr} corresponds to mean lifetime of carriers for radiative and non-radiative recombination respectively. We may note that each radiative recombination is associated with emission of a photon with energy equal to the bandgap energy of the material and each nonradiative recombination is responsible for a loss of an electron-hole pair and subsequent release of heat, which is absorbed by the lattice leading the *quantized latice vibration* or emission of a *phonon*. As regards the electroluminescence, any nonradiative recombination is viewed as a loss responsible for lowering the efficiency of the LED. We may note that the *internal quantum efficiency* (η_{int}) of an LED is a measure of the ability of the device to convert electron-hole pairs to photon, i.e., it is a measure of the ability of the LED to convert the electrical energy to optical energy (E/O conversion). Thus, one can view η_{int} of the LED as the fraction of the total recombination that occurs relatively. We can write

$$\eta_{int} = \frac{r_r}{r} = \frac{r_r}{r_r + r_{nr}} \tag{v}$$

Substituting the values of r_r and r_{nr} from Eqs (iii) and (iv) in Eq. (v), one obtains

$$\eta_{int} = \frac{\Delta n / \tau_r}{\Delta n / \tau_r + \Delta n / \tau_{nr}} \tag{vi}$$

or

$$\eta_{int} = \frac{1/\tau_r}{1/\tau_r + 1/\tau_{nr}} = \frac{\tau}{\tau_r} \tag{vii}$$

where, τ is the effective time of the carrier given by

$$\frac{1}{\tau} = \frac{1}{\tau_r} + \frac{1}{\tau_{nr}} \tag{viii}$$

The *direct band gap* semiconductors suchas AlGaAs and InGaAsP which are widely used for making LEDs in the near-infrared region (NIR) for application in optical fiber communication systems have nearly equal values of lifetime of carriers for radiative as well as non-radiative recombination. As a result, the effective-lifetime of carriers becomes half the value of the lifetime for radiative recombination (τ_r). This is why, LEDs based on these materials exhibit values of internal quantum efficiency of about 50% only. However, the internal quantum efficiency of a simple LED can be enhanced in the range of 60–80% by making use of double hetero-structures. The specially designed structure helps to reduce the non-radiative recombination through self-absorption. However, such structures under certain conditions may be dominated by surface recombination at the heterointerfaces which are non-radiative in nature and may also lead to reduction in the quantum efficiency of the LED. We may note that internal quantum efficiency accounts for the photons which are generated internally in respect of the number of carriers recombining internally. The actual number of photons emitted out of the device is always is always less than the number of internally generated photon. The external quantum efficiency is defined as the ratio of photons emitted out of the LED to the number of internally generated photons. It is also defined as the number of photons emitted out of LED to the total number of carrier recombination.

When an LED is forward biased, a drive current I flows through the device under steady-state, the total recombination rate per second can be defined as

$$R = R_r + R_{nr} = \frac{I}{q} \tag{ix}$$

where R_r and R_{nr} denotes the total radiative recombination rate and total non-radiative recombination rate per second. Now, the internal quantum efficiency can be alternatively defined in terms of R_r and R_{nr} as

$$\eta_{int} = \frac{R_r}{R_r + R_{nr}} = \frac{R_r}{R} \tag{x}$$

Eqs. (ix) and (x) yields

$$R_r = \eta_{int}\left(\frac{I}{q}\right) \tag{xi}$$

We may note that R_r which corresponds to the total radiative recombination rate, also corresponds to the total number of photons emitted internally per unit time per second. Further, the energy associated with each emitted photon is hn, the optical power generated internally to the LED can be obtained as

$$P_{int} = R_r\,(h\nu) = \eta_{int}\left(\frac{I}{q}\right)$$

$$= \eta_{int}\frac{hc}{q\lambda}I \tag{xii}$$

Obviously, P_{int} is directly proportional to the drive current, I flowing through the device. Further, the power actually emitted by the LED is less than P_{int} because of a number of factors which lowers down the value of the available power from an LED. We may note that the LED output power also follows a similar relationship except for the fact that η_{int} is replaced by a new factor called the external quantum efficiency (η_{ext}) which is the overall quantum efficiently for the device.

The power emitted by an LED clearly depends on the radiative recombination. To improve the quantum efficiency of an LED, one will have to make the radiative recombinations dominate over the nonradiative recombination lifetime so that radiative recombinations dominate over the nonradiative recombination. We may note that the value of non-radiative recombination lifetime depends on the properties of the defects which create energy levels in the forbidden bandgap of the material. Further, the energy released out of recombination of carriers at these levels is dissipated by phonons. Moreover, for heavily doped regions and narrow bandgap semiconductor, another form of non-radiative recombination called *Auger recombination* may become significant. The other form of non-radiative recombination in LED arises from surface recombination at the heterointerfaces in *double heterostructures*.

17. Explain Shockley–Read–Hall (SRH) Recombination.

Ans. Non-radiative recombination is dominated by SRH occuring via recombination centres created by traps/defect. The non-radiative SRH lifetime of carriers is expressed as

$$\tau_{SRH} = \frac{1}{N_T\,\sigma\,V_{th}} \tag{i}$$

where, σ is the capture cross section of the particular type of carrier (electron or hole) N_T is the trap density of the corresponding type of carriers and V_{th} is the carrier thermal velocity given by

$$V_{th} = \sqrt{\frac{3\,kT}{m^*_{n,\,p}}} \tag{ii}$$

where, k is Boltzmann's constant, T is the absolute temperature and $m^*_{n,\,p}$ is the effective mass of the carrier (electron/hole).

18. Explain Auger recombination.

Ans. Auger recombination process is nonradiative bulk recombination process which is generally dominant in heavily doped semiconductors and narrow-band semiconductors. The Auger process involves three carriers for completing the recombination. In this process, the excess energy released by recombination of an electron-hole pair is transferred by Coulombic collisions as kinetic energy of a third carrier, which is raised in energy deep into the respective band. The carrier finally returns back to the bottom of the band by releasing the energy in the form of thermal vibration. There are different forms of Auger recombination processes, e.g. Auger recombination in one case may involve two conduction band electrons and one heavy hole. In this recombination process, one conduction band electron transfers its energy to another electron in the conduction band which moves up in the band and then the first electron drops down to the valence band to recombine with a hole. This way the other Auger recombination processes may involve one conduction band electron and two holes in the valence band (any one of the heavy-hole, light-hole or a hole from the spin-split off band). The carrier lifetime for the Auger process can be expressed as

$$\tau_{AU} = \frac{n}{R_{AU}} = \frac{1}{Cn^2} \qquad \text{(i)}$$

where, C is the Auger recombination coefficient which is a fundamental characteristic of the material, n is the majority carrier concentration and R_{AU} is the rate of Auger recombination given by

$$R_{AU} = Cn^3 \qquad \text{(ii)}$$

When both the nonradiative recombinations are present, the overall nonradiative lifetime of the carrier can be expressed as

$$\frac{1}{\tau_{nr}} - \frac{1}{\tau_{SRH}} + \frac{1}{\tau_{AU}} \qquad \text{(iii)}$$

19. What is radiative recombination?

Ans. Radiative recombination involves direct transition of an electron in the conduction band to valence band where it recombines with a hole. In this process the balance energy following each recombination is released in the form of a photon light and the momentum is conserved. The radiative recombination lifetime can be expressed as

$$\tau_r = \frac{1}{B_r(n_0 + p_0)} \qquad \text{(i)}$$

where, B_r is the coefficient for band-to-band recombination, n_0 and p_0 are the equilibrium electron and hole concentrations respectively. In presence of excess carrier injection, the radiative recombination lifetime can be obtained as

$$\tau_r = \frac{1}{B_r(n_0 + p_0 + \Delta n)} \qquad \text{(ii)}$$

where, Δn is the excess injected carrier density.

20. Explain external quantum efficiency of an LED and show that

$$P_{\text{emitted}} = \eta_{\text{ext}} P_{\text{int}}$$

Ans. All photons generated internally in an LED will not be able to exit the device and finally contribute to the power emitted by the device. Let us consider the schematic of the LED. We can see that the light generated within the LED strikes the LED surface from inside. The surface of the LED is the interface between the emitting region of the LED and the surrounding medium in which the light is finally emitted. The former has a larger refractive index than that of the surrounding medium. Therefore, at the interface there would be a critical angle ϕ_c (with respect to the normal drawn on the interface at the point of incidence) such that the light incident at the interface at an angle larger than Φ_c would be reflected back into the emitting region. The light falling at the interface making an angle less than Φ_c, as shown in Fig. 8.50, would be refracted out of the LED to contribute to the emitted power. It can be easily seen from Fig. 8.50 that only the fraction of light falling within a cone subtending an angle at the vertex equal to the critical angle Φ_c $(= \pi/2 - \theta_c)$ will manage to escape out of the LED to contribute to the external power. Applying Snell's law at the interface, between the LED material emitting light having refractive index of n_1 and the outside medium having refractive index, n_2 $(< n_1)$, one finds

$$\phi_c = \sin^{-1}\left(\frac{n_2}{n_1}\right) \tag{i}$$

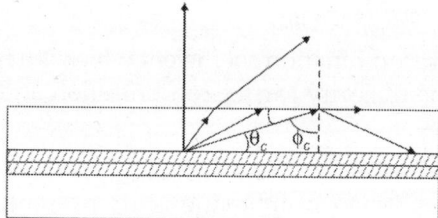

Fig. 8.50: Light emitted out of an LED through refraction exhibiting that light falling beyond the critical angle Φ_c with respect to the normal is reflected back

The outside medium is generally air ($n^2 = 1$). However, in optical fiber communication application the source is generally cemented to a small portion of a fiber called *pigtail* or *flylead* with the help of some transparent adhesive made up of some index matching fluid to reduce the Fresnel loss. The external quantum efficiency of the LED is given by

$$\eta_{ext} = \frac{1}{4\pi} \int_0^{\Phi_c} T(\phi)\,(2\pi \sin \phi)\, d\phi \tag{ii}$$

where, $T(\Phi)$ is the *Fresnel transmission coefficient* which is a function of the angle of incidence. For normal incidence, the Fresnel transmission coefficient can be expressed as

$$T(0) = \frac{4n_1 n_2}{(n_1 + n_2)^2} \tag{iii}$$

Consider the surrounding medium to be air ($n_2 = 1$) and assuming $n_1 = 1$, one finds

$$T(0) = \frac{4n}{(n+1)^2} \tag{iv}$$

The external quantum efficiency (η_{ext}) under this condition can be approximated by using Eq. (ii) as

$$\eta_{ext} \approx \frac{1}{n(n+1)^2} \qquad \text{(v)}$$

The optical power actually available outside the LED can be expressed as

$$P_{emitted} = \eta_{ext} P_{int} \qquad \text{(vi)}$$

21. When LEDs best suited for optical fiber communication system?

    Ans. When the power requirement of the source is not more than a few tens of microwatt and the desired bit rate is in the range of 100 – 200 Mbps.

22. Write the expression for internal quantum efficiency in terms of recombination rate and the optical power generated internally to the LED.

    Ans. The internal quantum efficiency in terms of recombination rate ratio of an LED is

    $$\eta_{int} = \frac{R_r}{R_r + R_{nr}} = \frac{R_r}{R}$$

    where R_r and R_{nr} corresponds to total radiative recombination rate and total non-radiative recombination rate per second respectively. $R = R_r + R_{nr}$ is the total non-radiative recombination rate per second.

    The optical power generated to the LED is given as

    $$P_{int} = R_r\,(h\nu) = \eta_{int}\frac{hc}{q\lambda}I$$

    where I is the drive current flows through the device under steady state when an LED is forward biased.

    The power emitted by an LED depends on the radiative recombination.

23. How one can improve the quantum efficiency of an LED?

    Ans. In order to improve the quantum efficiency of an LED it is necessary to make the radiative recombination lifetime much smaller than the non-radiative recombination lifetime so that radiative recombination dominate over the non-radiative recombination.

24. How optical power actually available outside the LED ($P_{emitted}$) is related to optical power generated internally (P_{int})?

    Ans. $P_{emitted} = \eta_{ext} P_{int}$ where external quantum efficiency (η_{ext}) is given as

    $$\eta_{ext} \approx \frac{1}{n(n+1)^2}$$

    where n is the refractive index of LED material and it is assumed that the surrounding medium is air.

25. What are homojunction and heterojunction LED structures?

    Ans. An LED in the simplest form is essentially a *pn* junction formed by using one of the direct bandgap semiconductor of suitable bandgap that ensures emission in the desired wavelength. Such an LED which uses same material (say, GaAs) on both sides with different conductivity is called *homojunction* LED. These type of LEDs are not useful for application in fiber optical communication system in view of their poor radiance and low quantum efficiency.

    A *heterostructure LED* generally consists of a combination of multiple heterojunctions that secure the carriers and subsequently the emitted photon in such a way that overall quantum efficiency and radiance of the LED is increased. In order to achieve a high value of radiance and high quantum efficiency is necessary to make use of suitable lattice matched materials of different bandgap values in the LED structure.

26. What are surface emitting LEDs (SLEDs)?

Ans. In a SLED the light is emitted in direction perpendicular to the plane of the *pn*-junction.

27. What is an edge emitting LED (ELED)?

Ans. A double heterostructure ELED uses stripe geometry similar to that used in injection laser diode to restrict the current spreading in the lateral direction. It consists of an active region which is made of a suitable material to emit light in the desired wavelength region and is sandwitched between two guiding layers. Both the guiding regions have the same refractive index value which is lower than the refractive index of the active region but higher than the refractive index of the surrounding material.

28. What is modulation bandwidth?

Ans. The speed of an optical communication system depends not only on the information or data carrying capacity of the fiber but also on the rate at which the information or data can be modulated at the transmitter and the speed of response of the photoconductor at the receiver. The rate at which the intensity of light source can be modulated by the information or data is known as the *modulation bandwidth*.

29. What is electrical bandwidth of an LED?

Ans. The optical power of an LED is usually measured with the help of an optical power meter which uses an optical detector at the input parts. The detector is a square-law device which converts the incident optical power to an electric current. The electrical current produced by the detector is proportional to the incident optical power. Now, if $I(\omega)$ is the electrical current produced by the detector in response to an intensity modulated optical power $P(\omega)$, then

$$I(\omega) \propto P(\omega)$$

The electrical power $P_e(\omega)$ corresponding to $I(\omega)$ in the detector circuit is given by

$$P_e(\omega) = \frac{I^2(\omega)}{R}$$

where R is the equivalent resistance of the detector circuit.

The electrical 3-dB point corresponds to the frequency where

$$P_e(\omega_{3dB}) = \frac{1}{2} P(0)$$

where $P(0)$ corresponds to the optical power output of the LED under DC condition (without modulation).

The 3 dB electrical bandwidth is obtained as

$$f_{3dB-el} = \frac{1}{2\pi\tau}$$

where τ is the bulk carrier lifetime.

We further find that

$$f_{3dB-op} = \sqrt{3}\, f_{3dB-el}$$

30. What are resonant cavity LEDs?

Ans. A resonant cavity LED is based on a novel structure in which the active region of the device is placed in a resonant optical cavity. As a consequence, the optical power emitted from the active region is restricted to the modes of the cavity. RC-LED is based on planar technology. It consists of a Fabry–Perot active resonant cavity between distributed Bragg reflector (DBR) mirrors. Since the cavity size is of the order of a micrometer, the RC-LED is generally referred to as a microcavity LED.

31. What are Quantum Dot-LEDs?

Ans. It is possible to use quantum-dot structure in a typical RC-LED structure to enhance the emitted power output. This resultant device is called as a Quantum Dot or QD LED. QD-LEDs without put optical power as high as 10 mW have been reported for operation in the wavelength regions of 1.30 μm and 1.55 μm.

32. The carrier recombination lifetime for an LED is 10 ns. Estimate the optical bandwidth of the LED.

Ans. The optical bandwidth of the LED can be obtained as

$$f_{3dB-op} = \frac{\sqrt{3}}{2\pi \times 10 \times 10^{-9}} = 275.8 \text{ MHz}$$

MULTIPLE CHOICE QUESTIONS

1. The densities of electrons and holes are same in:
   (a) a *p-n* junction in equilibrium
   (b) a forward biased *p-n* junction
   (c) an extrinsic semiconductor
   (d) an intrinsic semiconductor

2. Which of the following material is not suitable for making an LED?
   (a) GaAlAs   (b) Silicon
   (c) GaAs   (d) InGaAsP

3. To make an efficient LED, the material should be:
   (a) a metal   (b) an insulator
   (c) an indirect band gap type semiconductor
   (d) a direct band gap type semiconductor

4. An LED with an external quantum efficiency of 0.012 is coupled to an optical fiber having NA = 0.15 (with air between them). The overall source-fiber coupling efficiency is:
   (a) 3.2×10^{-4} (b) 1.8×10^{-4}
   (c) 1.1×10^{-4} (d) 2.7×10^{-4}

5. In a *p-n* homojunction, the majority concentration are almost equal to the dopant concentrations at:
   (a) high temperature   (b) absolute zero temperature
   (c) normal temperature   (d) all temperatures

6. In an LED, which of the following factors affects severely the efficiency of the diode and also cannot be eliminated in principle?
   (a) Back emission   (b) Total internal reflection
   (c) Absorption   (d) Fresnel reflection

7. The internal quantum efficiency (η_{int}) of an LED is given by:

(a) $\eta_{int} = \dfrac{1}{1 + \tau_{rr}\tau_{nr}}$

(b) $\eta_{int} = \dfrac{1}{\tau_{rr} + \tau_{nr}}$

(c) $\eta_{int} = \dfrac{1}{1 + \dfrac{\tau_{rr}}{\tau_{nr}}}$

(d) $\eta_{int} = \dfrac{\tau_{nr}}{\tau_{rr}}$

8. For LEDs, the overall source-fiber coupling efficiency (η_T) is given by:

(a) $\eta_T = n_{ext}\dfrac{(NA)^2}{n_a^2}$

(b) $\eta_T = \dfrac{n_a}{n_{ext}}(NA)^2$

(c) $\eta_T = \dfrac{n_{ext}}{n_a^2}(NA)$

(d) $\eta_T = \dfrac{n_{ext}}{n_a^2}(NA)^{1/2}$

9. Which of the following pairs are suitable for making a heterojunction?
   (a) GaAs and GaAlAs
   (b) Si and GaAs
   (c) Si and Ge
   (d) GaAs and AlAs

10. A photodetector is a device that converts:
    (a) heat energy to optical energy
    (b) sound energy to electrical energy
    (c) optical energy to electrical energy
    (d) mechanical energy to electrical energy

11. The principal mechanism of converting optical energy to electrical energy in a photodetector is:
    (a) photoconductivity
    (b) photovoltaics
    (c) polarization
    (d) photoelasticity

12. A *p-n* junction photodiode is:
    (a) forward biased
    (b) a very fast photodetector
    (c) embedded in an opaque capsule
    (d) dependent on thermally generated minority carriers

13. A *pn* junction that radiates energy as light instead of heat is called as:
    (a) Zener diode
    (b) LED
    (c) photocell
    (d) photodiode

14. Internal quantum efficiency of an LED (η_{itr}) is given by
    (a) $\eta_{int} = \tau/\tau_r$
    (b) $\eta_{int} = \tau_r/\tau$
    (c) $\eta_{int} = \sqrt{\tau_r/\tau}$
    (d) none of the above

    ($\tau \to$ overall carrier recombination lifetime and $\tau_r \to$ mean life time of carriers for radiative recombination)

15. When an LED is forward biased and a drive current I flows through the device under steady-state, the optical power generated internally to the LED is related to its internal quantum efficiency (η_{int}) as

    (a) $P_{int} = \eta_{int} I$

    (b) $P_{int} = \eta_{int}\dfrac{hc}{q\lambda}I$

    (c) $P_{int} = \eta_{int} I \Big/ \dfrac{hc}{q\lambda}$

    (d) $P_{int} = \sqrt{\eta_{int}}$

16. If C is the Auger recombination coefficient and n is the majority carrier concentration, then the rate of Auger recombination (R_{AU}) is given by

(a) $R_{AU} = Cn$

(b) $R_{AU} = Cn^2$

(c) $R_{AU} = Cn^3$

(d) $R_{AU} = C\sqrt{n}$

17. The optical power actually available outside the LED ($P_{emitted}$) and the optical power generated internally (P_{int}) to the LED are related as

(a) $P_{emitted} = \eta_{ext} P_{int}$

(b) $P_{emitted} = \sqrt{\eta_{ext}} \, P_{int}$

(c) $P_{emitted} = \eta_{ext}^2 P_{int}$

(d) $P_{emitted} = \eta_{ext}^3 P_{int}$

18. The optical power versus drive current characteristic of an LED exhibit

(a) linearity feature

(b) parabolic feature

(c) circular feature

(d) none of the above

19. The output of the superluminescent LED is most sensitive to the variation of

(a) junction density

(b) junction frequency

(c) junction temperature

(d) none of the above

20. The SLDs (super luminescent LEDs) generally exhibit power around

(a) 2-3 times higher than that of ELEDs (edge-emitting LED)

(b) 4-5 times higher than that of ELEDs

(c) 7-8 times higher than that of ELEDs

(d) none of the above

ANSWERS

1. (d)   2. (b)   3. (d)   4. (d)   5. (c)   6. (b)   7. (c)   8. (a)   9. (a)   10. (c)

11. (a)   12. (b)   13. (b)   14. (b)   15. (b)   16. (c)   17. (a)   18. (a)   19. (c)   20. (b)

9

Optical Receivers

9.1 INTRODUCTION

Optical receivers are the essential and important parts of optical communication system. An optical receiver converts an optical signal, transmitted through an optical fiber cable into an electrical signal suitable for a receiving device installed at the other end of the communication system. The conversion process in the receiver is performed by two essential parts: a *detector* and an *electronic signal processor*. The detector converts the optical signal into an electrical signal. The electronic signal processor converts the raw detector signal into a form *decipherable* by the receiving device, e.g. a telephone, camera, or scanner.

A block diagram of an optical detector is shown in Fig. 9.1.

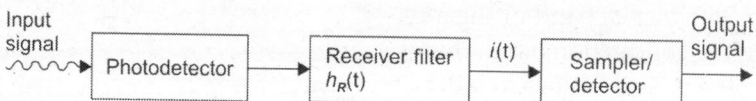

Fig. 9.1: Block diagram of an ideal optical receiver

The receiver consists of a photodetector which converts the optical signal into electrical current. A good light detector should generate a large photocurrent at a given incident light power. They should also respond fast to the input changes and add minimal noise to the output signal. This last requirement is of crucial importance since the received signal is typically very weak. In digital optical communication system the detection process is often conducted with a PIN photodiode.

There are generally two types of detection: *direct detection* (also called *incoherent detection*) and *coherent detection*.

Direct detection detects only the intensity of the incident light. It is used mainly for intensity or amplitude modulation schemes. It can only detect an amplitude modulated (AM) signal.

Coherent detection can detect both the power and phase of the incident light. It is, therefore, used when phase modulation (PM) or frequency modulation (FM) is preferred. Coherent detection is also important in applications such as WDM.

The coherent detection requires a local oscillator to coherently down-convert the modulated signal from optical frequency to intermediate frequency (IF). The incoherent detection which dominates in currently deployed systems is based on square-law envelope detection of the optical signals.

After detection, the electrical current is often amplified (not shown in Fig. 9.1) and then passes through an electrical filter which is normally of the Bessel type. At that point, electrical eye diagrams are typically observed for the assessment of signal quality. Next, sampling of electrically filtered received signal is performed. The received electrical signal is corrupted with noise of various origins. The noise sources will be discussed in the following sections.

Performance evaluation of an optical transmission system is done by evaluating optical signal-to-noise ratio, eye opening and bit error rate (BER) which is the ultimate indicator of the system's performance.

As stated above, the function of the optical receiver is to pick up an optical signal and convert it into an electrical signal suitable for a receiving device at the end of the communication line. Optical signals can be data, video, or audio. Optical detectors perform this conversion of an optical signal into an electrical signal. This is why *optical receivers are sometimes called optical detectors*. Optical detectors perform the opposite function of optical transmitters, such as light-emitting diodes (LEDs), and semiconductor lasers.

The detector requirements in optical fiber communication system are very similar to those of optoelectronic sources, i.e. they should have *very high sensitivity* at operating wavelengths, *high fidelity, fast response, high reliability, low noise* and *low cost*. Moreover, the size of the detector should be comparable with that of fiber employed in the link. These requirements are easily met by detectors made of semiconducting materials.

The most common type of optical detector is the *semiconductor photodiode*, which produces current in response to incident light. Detectors operate based on the principle of the semiconductor diode (*p-n* junction). An incident photon striking the diode gives an electron in the valence band of the atom. If the photon has sufficient energy to move the electron to the conduction band, this creates a free-moving electron and a hole. If the creation of these carriers occurs in a depleted region, the charge carriers (electrons and holes) will quickly separate and create a current. As they reach the edge of the depleted area, the electrical forces diminish and current cases.

Figure 9.2 shows one application of an optical receiver as conversion of an optical signal into a digital form. The incoming optical signal is converted to an electronic signal using a photodetector, such as a *p-i-n* (PIN) photodiode or an avalanche photodiode (APD). The signal is then amplified by a preamplifier, and passed through a bandpass filter that removes unwanted wavelengths. Further amplification, with a gain feedback control circuit, provides stable signal levels for the rest of the process. This control circuit controls the bias current, and thus the sensitivity of the photodiode.

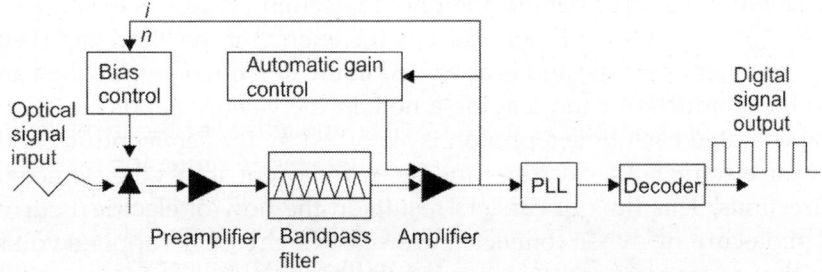

Fig. 9.2: Optical signal conversion process

A phase-locked loop (PLL) recovers the data bit stream and the timing information. The stream of bits needs to be decoded, from the coding used on the line, into its data format coding. This decoding process varies, depending on the encoding, and is occasionally integrated with the PLL, depending on the code in use.

9.2 PRINCIPLE OF OPTOELECTRONIC DETECTION

Figure 9.3 shows a reverse-biased *p-n* junction. A bias voltage V is applied to the *p-n* junction. Electrons diffuse away from the *n*-region into the *p*-region, leaving behind positively-charged ionized atoms called *donors*.

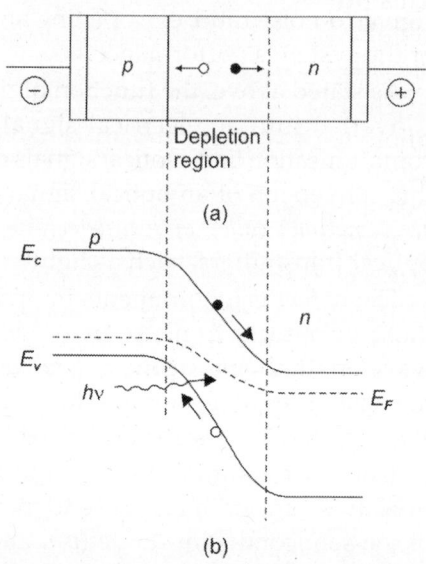

In the *p*-region, these electrons recombine with the abundant holes. Similarly, holes diffuse away from the *p*-region, leaving behind negatively-charged ionized atoms (called *acceptors*). In the *n*-region, the holes recombine with the abundant mobile electrons.

This diffuse process cannot continue indefinitely, however, because it causes a disruption of the charge balance in the two regions. As a result, a narrow region on both sides of the junction becomes almost totally depleted of mobile charge carriers (electrons and holes). This region is called the *depletion region*. This region has a built-in electric field E_o, due to the acceptors and donors beyond its edges. This occurs even without an applied voltage.

Fig. 9.3: (a) A reverse-biased p-n junction and depletion region (b) energy band diagram showing carrier generation and their drift

When a photon of energy greater than the band gap of the semiconductor material (i.e. $h\nu \geq E_g$) is incident on or near the depletion region of the device, it excites an electron from the valence band into the conduction band. The vacancy of an electron creates a hole in the valence band. Electrons and holes so generated experience a strong electric field and drift rapidly towards the n and p sides, respectively. The resulting flow of current is proportional to the number of incident photons. Such a reverse-biased *p-n* junction, therefore, acts as a photodetector and is normally referred to as a *p-n* photodiode.

The fundamental principle behind the photodetection process is *optical absorption*. If the energy ($h\nu$) of an incident photon exceeds the energy of the band gap (between the conduction and valence bands) and is absorbed in the depletion region, then an electron moves upto the conduction band leaving a hole in the valence band. Thus an electron-hole pair is generated each time a photon is absorbed by the semiconductor. Under the influence of the electric field, electrons and holes are swept across the semiconductor in opposite directions. This flow of carriers results in the flow of electrical current called "generated photocurrent" when connected to an electric circuit. An applied voltage serves to speed up the carrier movement, increasing the current.

The fraction of light absorbed by the photodiode depends on:

(i) Wavelength (λ) of the light, determined by the photon energy ($\varepsilon = h\nu = hc/\lambda$).

(ii) The thickness of the absorption material (depletion region width or depletion layer thickness).

9.3 OPTICAL RECEIVER

The main characteristics of optical receiver are:

9.3.1 Sensitivity

This property is a measure of the minimum level of optical power P_{sens} at the receiver required for a reliable operation. Specifically, one expects that the BER is smaller than a specified level. Typically, that level is established to be equal to 10^{-9}.

The receiver sensitivity is a function of both the *signal* and also the *noise* parameters of photodetector and a preamplifier. It is a measure of the operating limit of the optical receiver, which, however, rarely operates close to that limit. There always exists a possibility of degradation of the system (temperature, ageing, etc.), so a typical margin (normally 3–6 dB).

Receiver sensitivity is a fundamental parameter of an optical receiver. It is directly responsible for the spacing between two points in any optical link, e.g. between transmitter and receiver or between repeaters.

9.3.2 Dynamic Range

It (expressed in dB) is the difference betwen the maximum allowable power and minimum power determined by receiver sensitivity. The maximum allowable power on the receiver is determined by nonlinearity and saturation.

Large dynamic range is important because it allows for more flexibility in the design of an optical network. The design of every network should take into account the wide range of possible changes of received optical powers due to change in temperature, ageing or various types of losses (in the fiber, connectors, etc.)

9.3.3 Bit-Rate Transparency

It refers to the ability of the optical receiver to operate over a range of bit rates. It describes the ability of the same receiver to be used for several networks operating at different bit rates.

9.3.4 Bit-Pattern Independency

This is the property of an optical receiver determining its operation for various data formats. The main constraint is imposed by non-return-to-zero (NRZ) code.

9.3.5 Optical Receiver Configuration

Figure 9.4 shows the block diagram of a typical optical receiver of a *digital optical* communication system. We can see from figure that the first two blocks consisting of the photodetector and low-noise pre-amplifier constitute the front-end of the receiver. This first-end of the receiver is followed by an equalizer, which remove the distortion by the nonlinearity of the front-end and the dispersive effects in the fiber medium. The function

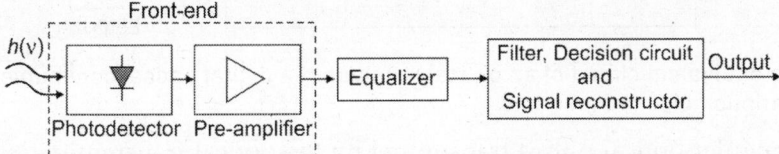

Fig. 9.4: Block diagram of a typical optical receiver of a digital optical communication system

of the filter is to maximize the signal-to-noise ratio while preserving the essential features of the signal. The function of the decision circuit is to compare the signal at the input with pre-decided threshold to identify the received signal as "1" or "0". The bits ("1" or "0") are subsequently given the required pulse shape by the signal reconstructor circuit so that it can deliver the final signal output. However, in the ideal situation, in the absence of noise, the output signal electrical pulses would be a replica of the optical pulses transmitted by the optical transmitter. In practice the reproduced signal at the receiver output differ from the transmitted signal due to various noise components which try to multilate the transmitted signal.

We may note that in a digital optical communication the error is measured in terms of bit-error rate. Sensitivity is an important figure of merit of the receiver and it corresponds to the minimum optical power that must be received by the receiver so as to reproduce the signal with the given bit rate. Further, the bit-error rate in a digital optical communication system is related to the signal to noise ratio. Now, for an analog optical communication system in which the signal is in the analog form, the sensitivity is measured in terms of signal-to-noise ratio rather than bit error rate. We may note that the overall signal-to-noise ratio of the receiver is effectively decided by the signal-to-noise ratio at the output of the front-end stage shown by dotted line box in Fig. 9.4. The desired signal-to-noise ratio have to be maintained in the front-end stage when the signal is weak because there is absolutely no way to improve the signal-to-noise ratio after the front-end stage. This means that the front-end of the receiver in a way decides the overall sensitivity of an optical receiver. Clearly, we have to give more emphasis to the study of the front-end of an optical receiver. Figure 9.5 shows the equivalent circuit of the receiver front end. In Fig. 9.5, i_p corresponds to the photogenerated signal current, C_d denotes the capacitance of the photodetector, R_b denotes the bias resistance of the photodetector generally considered as the load resistance and R_a and C_a denotes the input resistance and input capacitance of the following amplifier stage respectively. $\langle i_s^2 \rangle$ and $\langle i_T^2 \rangle$ in Fig. 9.5 correspond to the mean square value of shot noise current and mean square value of the thermal noise current in the circuit respectively. In Fig. 9.5, the input amplifier noise arising out of the thermal noise associated with the amplifier resistance, R_a, is represented as i_{amp}, whereas thermal noise associated with the amplifier channel noise is represented by $e_n(t)$. Further, the noise introduced by the amplifier stage depends largely on the configuration of the amplifier and also on the detailed noise analysis of the front-end of a digital optical communication receiver. In order to enhance the receiver sensitivity, it is necessary to reduce the noise components shown in Fig. 9.5. We can realize the front-end of an optical receiver comprising a photodetector and pre amplifier in three basic forms, e.g. low impedance (LZ), high impedance (HZ) and transimpedance (TZ) configuration.

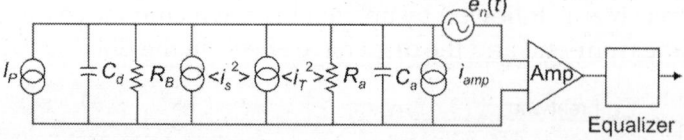

Fig. 9.5: The equivalent circuit of an optical receiver of a digital optical communication system exhibiting various noise components

The rectangular optical pulses transmitted by the optical transmitter are received by the receiver in a digital optical communication system in the form of distorted binary pulses. Thus, the received optical power can be represent as a train of binary pulses expressed as follows:

$$P_{op}(t) = \sum_{n=-\infty}^{\infty} b_n h_p(t - nT_b) \tag{9.1}$$

where, $P_{op}(t)$ is the optical power received by the receiver, b_n denotes the amplitude of the nth digit of the received pulse, T_b is the bit period and $h_p(t)$ corresponds to the shape of the received pulse. For a normalized pulse, one finds

$$\int_{-\infty}^{\infty} h_p(t)\, dt = 1 \tag{9.2}$$

and in that case b_n corresponds to the energy of the nth pulse.

Photodetector convert the received optical power into output photocurrent. One can obtain the mean output detector current as

$$\langle i(t) \rangle = \frac{\eta q}{h\nu} M P_{op}(t) \tag{9.3}$$

where, M is the multiplication gain of the amplifier. We may note that $M = 1$ for a p-i-n photodetector. Using Eq. (9.1), Eq. (9.3) reads as

$$\langle i(t) \rangle = R_o M \sum_{-\infty}^{\infty} b_n h_p (t - nT_b) \tag{9.4}$$

where $R_o = \eta q / h\nu$ is the sensitivity of the photodetector. We may note that the output current of the photodetector is subsequently amplified by the pre-amplifier to produce a mean voltage at the output of the equalizer. However, the equalizer output voltage is subsequently compared with a pre-decided threshold to decide for "1" or "0".

(i) Frequency Domain Representation

One finds it conveniets to calculate the mean voltage at the output of the equalizer by using frequency domain representation with the help of Fourier transforms. One can obtain the mean voltage at the equalizer output from the mean photodetector output current at the time domain with the help of convolution. The mean voltage at the equalizer output can be expressed as

$$\langle V_{out}(t) \rangle = A R_o M P_{op}(t)^* h_B^*(t)\, h_{eq}^{(t)} \tag{9.5}$$

where $h_B(t)$ denotes the impulse response of the bias circuit comprising the photodetector bias resistance, R_b; R_a is the amplifier input resistance, C_d is the photodetector capacitance, C_a is the amplifier input capacitance and $h_{eq}(t)$ is the impulse response of the equalizer circuit.

Let us assume that the form of the mean voltage at the equalizer output is analogous to Eq. (9.1), we may write

$$\langle V_{out}(t) \rangle = \sum_{n=-\infty}^{\infty} b_n h_{out}(t - nT_b) \tag{9.6}$$

where, $h_{out}(t)$ is the pulse shape produced at the output of the equalizer.

Now, comparing Eqs (9.6) and (9.5) in conjunction with Eq. (9.1), one obtains

$$h_{out}(t) = A R_0 M h_p(t) * h_B(t) * h_{eq}(t) \tag{9.7}$$

Taking Fourier transform on both sides of Eq. (9.5), one finds

$$H_{out}(f) = A R_0 M H_p(f)\, H_B(f)\, H_{eq}(f) \tag{9.8}$$

where $H_{out}(f)$, $H_p(f)$, $H_B(f)$ and $H_{eq}(f)$ are the Fourier transforms of $h_{out}(t)$, $h_p(t)$, $h_B(t)$ and $h_{eq}(t)$ respectively. From Fig. 9.5 the transfer function $H_B(f)$ of the photodetector bias circuit which is essentially the Fourier transform of the impulse response of the circuit is given by the following expression

$$H_B(f) = \cfrac{1}{\cfrac{1}{R_T} + \cfrac{1}{1/j2\pi fC_T}} = \frac{R_T}{1 + j2\pi R_T C_T} \qquad (9.9)$$

where

$$\frac{1}{R_T} = \frac{1}{R_b} + \frac{1}{R_a}, \qquad (9.10)$$

and

$$C_T = C_a + C_d \qquad (9.11)$$

(ii) Low Impedance (LZ) Front-end

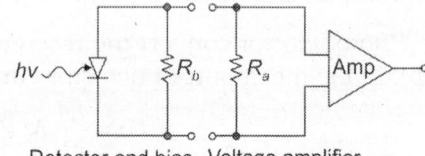

Detector and bias   Voltage amplifier

Fig. 9.6: Front-end configuration of low impedance configuration

Low impedance configuration is the simplest form of receiver front end. This configuration consists of a pre-amplifier with a low value of input impedance (~50 Ω) which is matched with a low value of the photodetector bias resistance (R_b) (Fig. 9.6). We see that the bias resistance of the photodetector is modified by the input resistance of the following stage amplifier. The effective resistance is found as

$$R_T = \frac{R_b R_a}{R_b + R_a} \qquad (9.12)$$

We may note that the most important features of an optical receiver front-end are the bandwidth and total noise introduced by this section. One can obtain the bandwidth of the LZ front-end from the effective RC time constant of the receiver front end. Now, if C_T is the overall capacitance of the front end [Eq. (9.11)], the bandwidth (B) of the front end is obtained as

$$B = \frac{1}{2\pi R_T C_T} \qquad (9.13)$$

Since the values of R_b and R_a are small in the LZ-end configuration and hence the available bandwidth is very high.

One can estimate the mean-square value of the thermal noise generated by the front-end as

$$\langle i_T^2 \rangle = 4kT\left(\frac{1}{R_T}\right)B \qquad (9.14)$$

Equation (9.14) reveals that the thermal noise produced by the front-end in the LZ configuration is very high as R_T is smaller than both R_b and R_a which have low values.

Thus, a low-impedance (LZ) receiver front-end offers a high value of bandwidth but a low value of sensitivity due to enhanced thermal noise current.

(iii) High-impedance (HZ) Front-end

A HZ receiver front-end *configuration* makes use of a high value of *photodetector-bias* resistance, which is matched with the high value of input impedance of suitable pre-amplifier stage (Fig. 9.7). We can see that the high value of the effective resistance eventually reduces the value of the mean square value of the thermal noise component of the front-end. However, a high value of the effective resistance enhances the RC time constant and at the same time reduces the bandwidth of the HZ front-end configuration.

Since the output of the photoconductor in this configuration is effectively integrated over a large time constant, the signal gets distorted and for restoration of the signal at the later stage a heavy equalization is needed (Fig. 9.7). Perhaps this is significant drawback of the configuration.

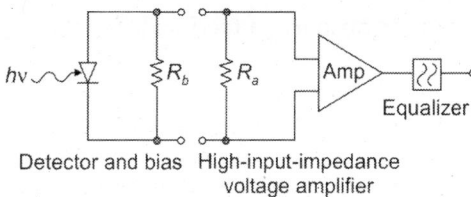

Detector and bias   High-input-impedance
voltage amplifier

Fig. 9.7: High-impedance (HZ) front-end configuration emphasizing the requirement of post-amplification equalization

This configuration exhibits better sensitivity in view of a reduce thermal noise current but a smaller bandwidth accompanied by the requirement of heavy equalization.

(iv) Transimpedance (TZ) Front-end

We have read that LZ front-end offers a large bandwidth and a relatively low sensitivity while the HZ front-end offers a smaller bandwidth without equalization and a relatively better sensitivity. However, the main advantage of the HZ configuration is the improvement in the sensitivity over the simplistic LZ configuration. TZ configuration is a compromise between the two extreme configuration, which is essentially similar to an HZ front-end configuration with a negative feedback (Fig. 9.8). We can see that a negative feedback reduces the high input impedance of the amplifier and the TZ configuration circuit essentially works as a current mode amplifier in which the detected photocurrent is translated into a voltage at the output of the amplifier (Fig. 9.8).

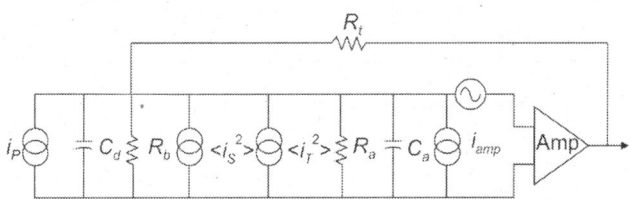

Fig. 9.8: A transimpedance (TZ) front-end circuit

For the computation of the current-to-voltage transfer function, the equivalent circuit of the TZ-front-end is shown in Fig. 9.9. In this equivalent circuit, the pre-amplifier is considered to be a differential amplifier operating in the inverted mode with a gain $-G$.

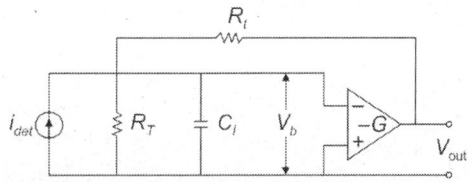

Fig. 9.9: A schematic of equivalent circuit for calculation of the current to voltage transfer function

Applying KCL at the node connected to the inverting input of the differential amplifier, one may write

$$i_{\text{det}} + \frac{V_{\text{out}} - V_{\text{in}}}{R_f} = V_{\text{in}}\left(\frac{1}{R_T} + j2\pi f C_T\right) \qquad (9.15)$$

where the effective values of resistance, R_T and capacitance, C_T are given by

$$R_T = \frac{R_a R_b}{R_b + R_a}$$

and

$$C_T = C_a + C_b \qquad (9.15a)$$

In the absence of feedback resistance, the amplifier is in open-loop and Eq. (9.15) reads as

$$i_{det} = V_{in} \left(\frac{1}{R_T} + j2\pi f C_T \right) \tag{9.16}$$

Now, the open-loop gain of the differential amplifier can be expressed as

$$-G = \frac{V_{out}}{V_{in}} \tag{9.17}$$

Using Eqs. (9.14) and (9.15), one obtains

$$i_{det} = \frac{-V_{out}}{G} \left(\frac{1}{R_T} + j2\pi f C_T \right) \tag{9.18}$$

where, f is the frequency of the input signal.

One can express the open-loop transfer function of the front-end configuration without feedback

$$H_{OL}(f) = \frac{-V_{out}}{i_{det}} = \frac{-GR_T}{1 + j2\pi f R_T C_T} VA^{-1} \tag{9.19}$$

In the absence of feedback (e.g. LZ, HZ cases) the bandwidth without equalization is determined by Eq. (9.13).

In the presence of feedback (closed loop), use of Eqs. (9.15) and (9.17) yields

$$i_{det} = -V_{out} \left(\frac{1}{R_f} + \frac{1}{GR_f} + \frac{1}{GR_T} + \frac{j2\pi f C_T}{G} \right) \tag{9.20}$$

Now, the closed-loop transfer function of the transimpedance (TZ) front-end can be expressed as

$$H_{CL}(f) = \frac{V_{out}}{i_{det}} = \frac{-R_f}{1 + \frac{1}{G} + \frac{R_f}{GR_T} + \frac{j2\pi f R_T C_T}{G}} \tag{9.21}$$

That is,

$$H_{CL}(f) = \frac{-R_f \Big/ \left(1 + \frac{1}{G} + \frac{R_f}{GR_T} \right)}{1 + \frac{j2\pi f R_T C_T}{1 + G + \frac{R_f}{R_T}}} \tag{9.21}$$

The open loop gain of the amplifier is generally high such that

$$G \gg 1 + \frac{R_f}{R_T} \tag{9.22}$$

Under the above condition the closed-loop transfer function of the TZ front-end can be approximated as

$$H_{CL}(f) \approx \frac{-R_f}{1 + \frac{j2\pi f R_T C_T}{G}} VA^{-1} \tag{9.23}$$

We may not that the closed-loop transfer function of a transimpedance (TZ) front-end configuration corresponds to gain which is measured in ohms.

The closed-loop transfer function of transimpedance front-end can be expressed as

$$H_{CL}(f) \approx \frac{-R_f}{1 + j\left(\dfrac{f}{B}\right)} VA^{-1} \qquad (9.24)$$

where B is the bandwidth of the transimpedance (TZ) front-end given by

$$B = \frac{G}{2\pi R_T C_T} \qquad (9.25)$$

We may note that the bandwidth of a TZ front-end without equalization can be made much larger as compared to that obtain in front-end configurations without feedback. Further, the gain of the amplifier can be adjusted to increase the bandwidth.

A TZ configuration is essentially a HZ configuration that uses negative feedback in order to improve the bandwidth of the system without equalization. However, the increase in bandwidth is obtained at the expen₃e of an enhanced thermal noise component arising out of the extra feedback resistance, R_f. One can see that when $R_f \ll R_T$, the thermal noise introduced by the feedback resistance dominates over the other thermal noise components and the former tends to dictate the overall sensitivity of the receiver front-end. Further, when the feedback resistance R_f has a comparatively larger value, the thermal noise current introduced by the feedback resistance becomes low. However, when $R_f = R_T$, the sensitivity of a TZ front-end approaches that of HZ front end. Obviously, a large value of feedback resistance may lead to instability problem.

(v) Pre-amplifier

These are based on active components, e.g. transistors. In principle, one can used both the forms of transistors e.g. BJT and FET for designing the pre-amplifier stage. We have read that the pre-amplifier is desired to have a low-noise characteristics since the photodetector converts the incoming optical signal to a weak electrical signal which is subjected to different noise components. This reveals that, a FET which offers low noise as compared to its bipolar counterpart, i.e. BJT, turns out to be more attractive for designing the pre-amplifier of an optical receiver. Moreover, when the gate of an FET is reversed biased, the input impedance of an FET

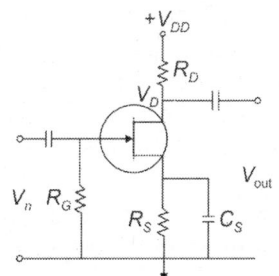

Fig. 9.10: Circuit for common source configuration of an FET based pre-amplifier

amplifier (Fig. 9.10) is extremely high. The low noise as well as low value input capacitance of an Si FET makes it quite attractive for application in optical receiver front end. We may note that FET based amplifier usually offer much less gain as compared to that offered by its bipolar counterpart. The common source (grounded source) FET amplifier (Fig. 9.10) offers quite high impedance and hence can be used to realize a high impedance (HZ) receiver front-end by making use of quite large bias resistance. However, in this form of configuration, eventhough the thermal noise current reduces to a great extent, but its bandwidth is marginalized without equalization. We can improve the bandwidth by making use of an equalization circuit at a later stage. However, the current gain of an Si FET generally drops to unit at 25 MHz.

(vi) FET Based Receiver Front-ends

The high frequency limitation of junction field effect transistor (JFET) restricted its application in high speed optical communication systems. However, high performance microwave FET based on Schottky gate configuration became quite popular for use as pre-amplifier in an optical receiver front end. The Schottky gate FETs generally known as metal-semiconductor-field-effect transistors (MESFETs) were primarily based on GaAs material in view of its high electron mobility as compared to Si. Further, the Schottky contact enables the device to be operated at a very high speed. At microwave frequency (~GHz) the high gain alongwith a relatively low-noise made GaAs based MESFET as an attractive component for designing the pre-amplifier of high-speed optical receivers. Further, MESFET biased receiver front-end generally contain a *p-i-n* photodetector or an APD as the preceding photodetector stage. Usually, the *p-i-n* photodetector and the MESFET pre-amplifier are realized in the form of hybrid IC (integrated circuit) using thick film technology. The hybrid IC is called a PIN FET. The thick film substrate reduces the stray capacitance value. We may note that the early PIN FET structures were mostly focused in the 0.8–0.9 µm window. Nowadays, PIN FET based receivers operating at longer wavelength have been reported.

In FET based photoreceivers, the preamplifier is made of a FET, e.g. JFET. In this device, the metal semiconductor field effect (MSFE) is around 1.3 µm. Figure 9.11 shows a typical circuit of a PIN FET hybrid receiver designed in the NZ configuration. We can see that the HZ stage integrates the signal and the integrated output after pulse shaping with the help of a suitable filter is allowed to pass through an equalizer (which is a differentiator in this case) prior decision making. Further, the receiver is reported to be capable of handling transmission rate of 140 Mbps. A PIN FET receiver which exhibit a sensitivity of −44.2 dBm at a bit rate error (BER) of 10^{-9} has been demonstrated.

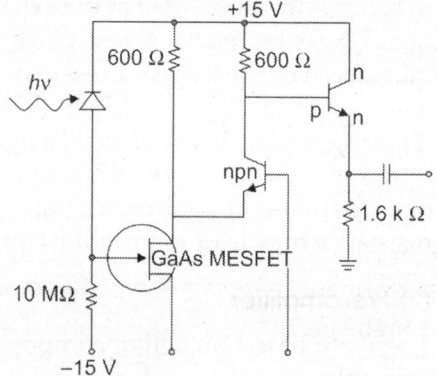

Fig. 9.11: A typical circuit diagram of a PIN FET hybrid receiver

Figure 9.12 shows a circuit of a PIN FET based high-speed optical receiver front-end designed in the transimpedance configuration. In this circuit design, the receiver front-end makes use of a GaAs MESFET followed by two complimentary microwave BJTs.

A negative feedback is provided from the output to the gate of a MESFET to convert it into a transimpedance amplifier. It is reported that the receiver can handle transmission rate of 274 MBps without any equalization. The receiver's sensitivity is reported as −35 dBm at a BER of 10^{-9}. In order to improve the sensity of the receiver, in some cases a basic pin detector has been replaced by avalanche photodetector. Further, a variety of transistors, e.g. FET and HBT have been used for designing a photodetector so that it may serve as the receiver suitable for operation in the longer wavelength region, i.e. 1.3 µm to 1.55 µm. It is also reported that use of monolithic integration into place of hybrid integration can enhance the performance of optical receiver in various wavelength regions of operation. Figure 9.13 shows a circuit schematic of the PINFET opto electronic

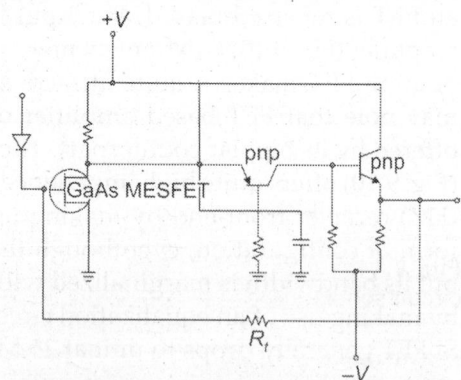

Fig. 9.12: A schematic circuit diagram of a PIN FET hybrid receiver front-end configured in TZ mode

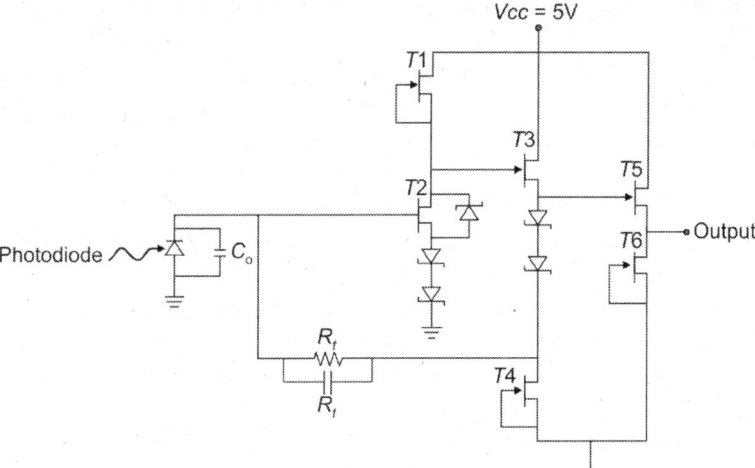

Fig. 9.13: Circuit schematic of a planar p-i-n photodetector/GaAs pre-amplifier OEIC receiver front-end

integrated circuit (OEIC) receiver front end. The OEIC receiver chip comprises Be-implanted GaAs *p-i-n* photodetector integrated with a transimpedance preamplifier containing six GaAs depletion mode MESFET and five Schottky diodes particularly fabricated by selective implantation in a semi-insulating substrate. This enhances the performance to a great extent as compared to its hybrid counterpart.

A high-sensitivity with wide dynamic range *p-i-n* photodiode and MOSFET pre-amplifier photoreceiver for 1.55 μm wavelength region at low bit rate employing an optically coupled feedback rather than conventional feed resistor was also reported (Fig. 9.14). The sensitivity of photoreceiver reported to be –63.8 dBm at a speed of 1.5 Mb/s for a BER of 10^{-7}. It is reported that the use of optical feedback eliminates the thermal noise component associated with the feedback resistor of a conventional TZ configuration.

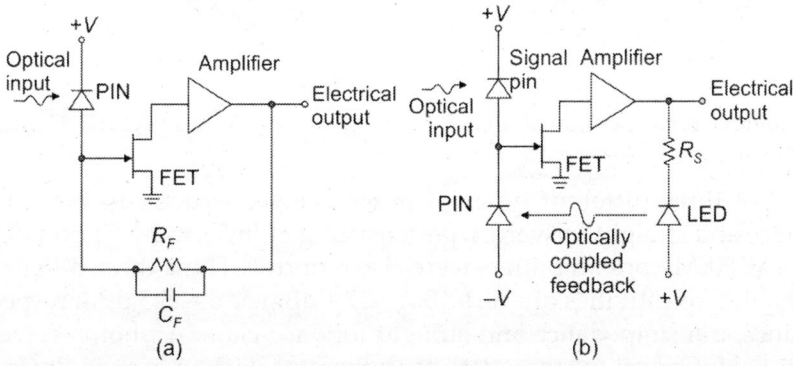

Fig. 9.14: Circuit schematic of transimpedance optical receiver front-end (a) Conventional circuit schematic (b) proposed optical-feedback transimpedance photoreceiver; front-end

An APD/FET photoreceiver for operation at a bitrate of 8 Gb/s with sensitivity of –25.8 dBm at a bit-error-rate of 10^{-9} for operation in the 1.3–1.5 μm wavelength region was reported. The receiver exhibited a gain bandwidth product of 60 GHz for InGaAs/ InGaAsP/InP heterojunction avalanche photodiode followed by hybrid GaAs MESFET pre amplifier. Further, this photoreceiver consists of separate absorption, grading and multiplication avalanched photodiode (SAGM-APD) with GaAs preamplifier. The gain bandwidth product of SAGM-APD was reported to be 140 GHz for 2 µm wide multiplication layer. SAGM-PAD photodetector exhibited a speed of 8 Gb/s with a sensitivity of –37 dBm for a BER of 10^{-9} for the said gain band width. Later, a delta-doped avalanche photodiode for high bit rate light receiver was reported.

9.3.5.1 Heterojunction Field Transistor (HFET) Based Photoreceivers

To improve the speed of photoreceivers, the preamplifier should used high speed devices, e.g. HFET, i.e. modulation doped field transistor (MODFET) also known as high electron mobility transistor (HEMT). Based on this, good number of photoreceivers have been tested and studied by several researchers. For the HFET based photoreceivers, the photodetector can be p-i-n photodiode, APD or MSM photodetector.

Figure 9.15 shows the schematic cross-section of the p-i-n/HEMT OEIC front-end. For 1 µm gate length, the transconductance of the HEMT preamplifier was reported to be 270 MS/mm. The receiver exhibited a sensitivity of –23.7 dBm with a speed of 2 Gb/s for the NRZ random signal. The photoreceiver based on InGaAs/InP exhibited a sensitivity of –32.7 dBm with a speed of 560 Mb/s. A high impedance HEMT pre-amplifier based photoreceiver with p-i-n photodiode as the front-end of the receiver, which exhibited a sensitivity of –30.4 dBm with a speed of 1.6 Gbps was also reported.

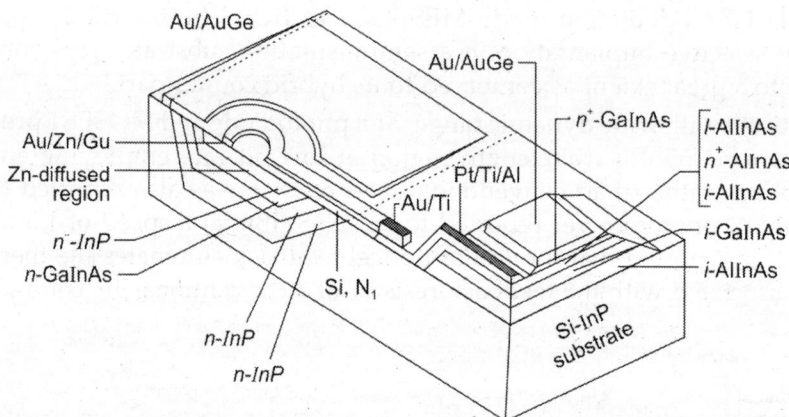

Fig. 9.15: Schematic cross section of an InP-GaInAsp-i-n/AlInAs/GaInAs HEMT OEIC receiver front-end

Fabrication of three different types of photoreceiver structures: high impedance, transimpedance and straight forward type consisting of InGaAs p-i-n photodetector and InAlAs/InGaAs HEMT pre-amplifiers were also reported. These three different types of receivers exhibited sensitivities of –30.4 dBm, –27.1 dBm and –25.5 dBm respectively for high impedance, transimpedance and straight forward class. A photoreceive based on Be-ion implanted InGaAs p-i-n photodetector integrated with an InAlAs/InGa As HEMT grown by MOVPE was reported. Figure 9.16 shows the cross-sectional view of the p-i-n/HEMT receiver front-end. The 3-dB bandwidth of the receiver was measured to be 8 GHz. The receiver also exhibited a good eye-pattern definition of 10 Gb/s NRZ optical signal. The sensitivity of this receiver was reported to be –16.5 dBm.

A monolithic OEIC optical receiver based on p-i-n/HEMT for long wavelength application at 12 GB/s for low-noise study of the performance was also reported. In this case, the monolithic integration was achieved using stacked layer structure and growing

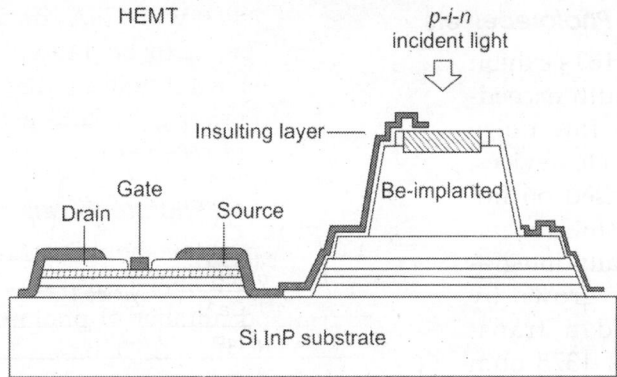

Fig. 9.16: Schematic cross-sectional view of monolithic OEIC *p-i-n*/HEMT receiver front-end

the *p-i-n* structure on a pre-grown HEMT structure. Figure 9.17 shows the circuit. The sensitivity of the receiver was reported to be –17.7 dBm at 10 Gb/s and –15.8 dBm at 12 Gb/s at a BER of 10^{-9}.

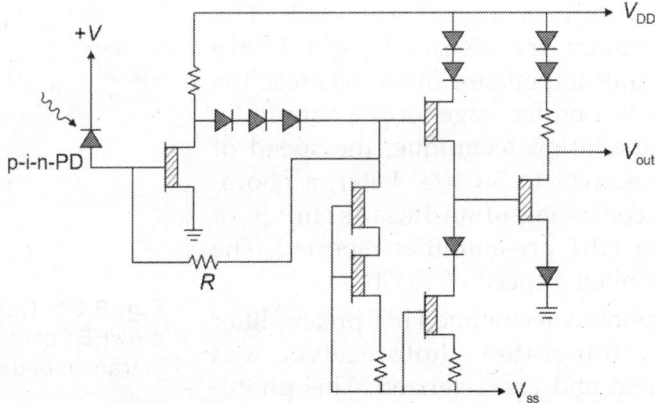

Fig. 9.17: The circuit diagram of a monolithically integrated p-i-n/HEMT optical receiver

A photoreceiver consisting of MSM photodiode, a transimpedance amplifier and three limiting amplifier stages for high speed optical fiber link was also proposed. Figure 9.18 shows the schematic cross-section of the InGaAs MSM integrated with AlGaAs/GaAs HEMT. The IC was fabricated using a 0.2 µm gate length HEMT with a cut off frequency of 60 GHz. The bandwidth of this photoreceiver was reported to be 16 GHz. To this receiver, a high transimpedance gain of 14 kW at 10 Gb/s bit-rate was achieved. Further, this photoreceiver was designed for the use in 1.3–1.55 µm wavelength application. A monolithic fabricated pseudomorphic InGaAs/AlGaAs MOSFET-APD receiver was also reported. This photoreceiver exhibited a gain of 8 dB at 1 GHz bandwidth. For high speed application a 10 Gb/s hybrid APD-HEMT photoreceiver was reported. This employed a lossless tuned noise-matching technique between an APD and HEMT amplifier stages for high sensitivity and a transimpedance feedback scheme for a wide dynamic range. For this photoreceiver, a sensitivity of –29.4 dBm at a speed of 10 Gb/s was reported.

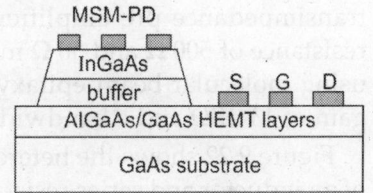

Fig. 9.18: Schematic of cross-sectional view of an MSM/HEMT optical receiver front-end

9.3.5.2 HBT Based Photoreceivers

It is reported that HBTs exhibit very large bandwidth exceeding 100 GHz and low noise capabilities as discrete devices, especially those based on InP substrates. An InP/InGaAs p-i-n HBT monolithically integrated photoreceiver grown by MOVPE exhibited a transimpedance gain of 1375 ohm and a dynamic range of 25 dB. Figure 9.19 shows the cross-sectional view of p-i-n/HBT structure. It is reported that a

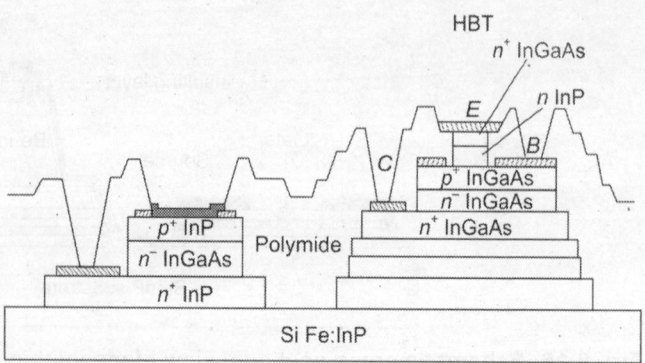

Fig. 9.19: Schematic cross-sectional view of the post-fabricated p-i-n/HBT integrated photoreceiver front-end

sensitivity of –26.1 dBm at a speed of 1 Gb/s is achievable. Figure 9.20 shows the circuit schematic of the monolithic photoreceiver front end. The heterojunction bipolar transistors T_1 and T_2 are connected in the transimpedance mode whereas the third HBT T_3 acts as a buffer stage for the output. By improving the fabrication technique, the speed of p-i-n/HBT photoreceiver to 5 Gb/s. Later, a photodetector module consisting of an InGaAs/InP p-i-n photodetector and HBT pre-amplifier reported. The photoreceiver exhibited a speed of 10 Gb/s.

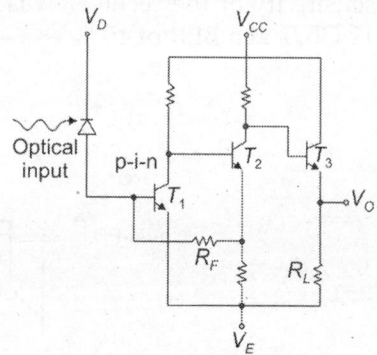

Fig. 9.20: Circuit diagram of a p-i-n/HBT photoreceiver front-end in transimpedance configuration

Based on p-i-n photodetector and HBT preamplifier a monolithically integrated photoreceiver was designed, fabricated and characterized. This photo-receiver had a three-stage transimpedance amplifier with a feedback resistance of 550 Ω. Figure 9.21 shows the schematic cross-section of the p-i-n/HBT after fabrication alongwith the circuit. The photoreceiver demonstrated a transimpedance gain of 46 dBΩ and a 3 dB bandwidth of 20 GHz.

9.3.5.3 Other Photoreceivers

There are also other photoreceivers based on pre-amplifiers described above Si based integrated NMOS photoreceiver involving p-i-n photodetector and NMOSFET pre-amplifier is reported to exhibit a bandwidth of 30 MHz. This photoreceiver shows an eye diagram at 400 Mb/s. A photodetector consisting of p^+-n-n^+ photodiode and transimpedance pre amplifier based on three stages SiGe/Si HBTs with a feedback resistance of 500 Ω and 50 Ω matching resistance and other passive elements was grown using molecular beam epitaxy (MBE). This photoreceiver exhibited a transimpedance gain of 43 dBΩ and a bandwidth of 5.5 GHz.

Figure 9.22 shows the heterojunction photo-transistor (HPT) based receiver consisted of an inductor and series resistance. This receiver exhibited an ultrabroadband operation with 3 dB bandwidth with 0.43–121 GHz and over 11 dB gain as compared to a photodiode with identical quantum efficiency. This was used in the front-end of the photoreceiver and HBT as the pre-amplifier. Later on, monolithically integrated receivers based on

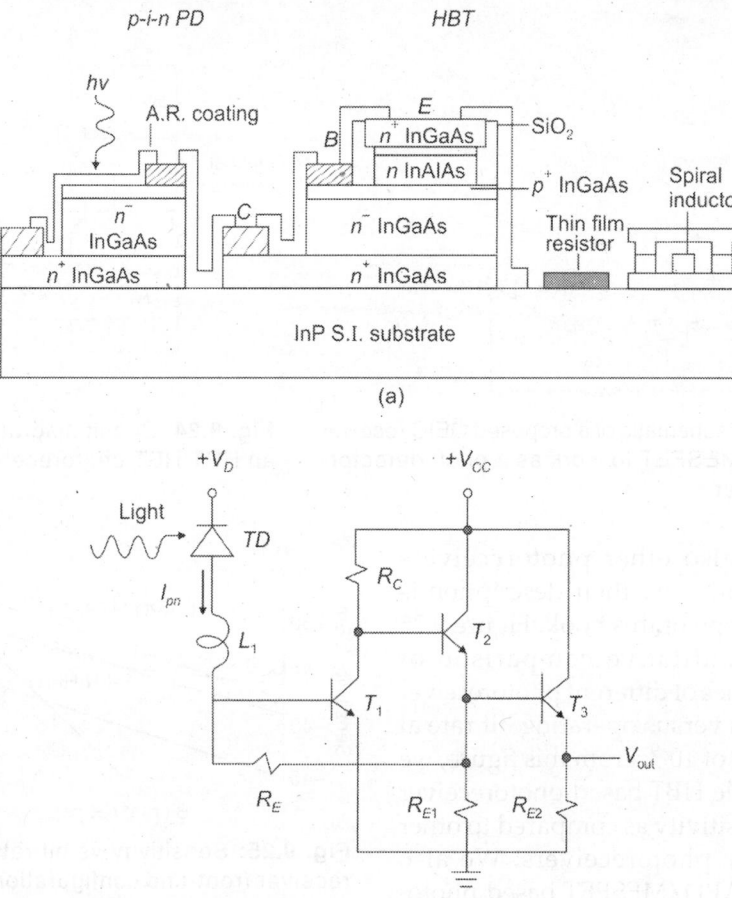

(a)

(b)

Fig. 9.21: Schematic of *p-i-n*/HBT OEIC receiver front-end: (a) cross-sectional view after fabrication (b) schematic circuit diagram in the transimpedance configuration

HPT were reported. Out of these two types of receivers, the first receiver consisted of only HPT while the second receiver consisted of an HPT followed by an HBT pre-amplifier. HPT/HBT receiver exhibited bandwidth of 12 GHz and had a ultra-wideband operation from 8.5–20.5 GHz with over 20 dB gain.

Figure 9.23 shows the schematic circuit diagram of a novel OEIC based photodetector-cum pre amplifier. The sensitivity of OEIC receiver designed in the transimpedance mode was estimated for an InGaAs based MESFET

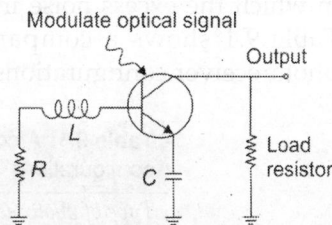

Fig. 9.22: Schematic of circuit diagram of a single HPT based photoreceiver

for operation in 1.6 μm wavelength region. This OEIC proposed receiver was claimed to exhibit a wider bandwidth, higher sensitivity and wider dynamic range at a speed of 20 Gb/s as compared to OEIC receiver based on conventional photodetectors.

Figure 9.24 shows an schematic diagram of proposed HPT/HBT optical receiver front-end based on InP/InGaAs to design a novel OEIC photoreceiver front-end for operation at 1.55 μm. The reported results of the analysis revealed that this receiver has a high transimpedance gain in excess of 60 dBΩ, a large bandwidth of nearly 30 GHz and also a reasonably high sensitivity of the order of −34.8 dBm at a Ber of 10^{-9}.

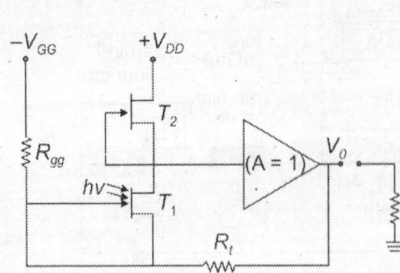

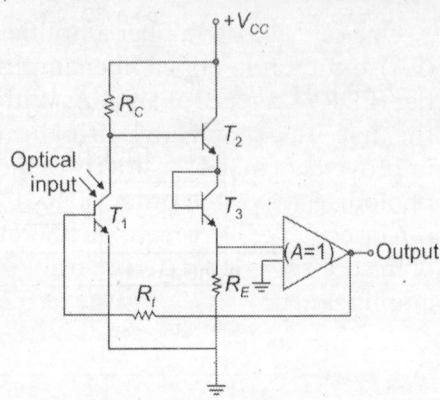

Fig. 9.23: Circuit schematic of a proposed OEIC receiver using a single MESFET to work as a photodetector-cum-preamplifier

Fig. 9.24: Circuit diagram of proposed an HPT/HBT photoreceiver front-end

There are also other photoreceivers reported recently and their description is beyond the scope of this book. Figure 9.25 depicts a quantitative comparison of sensitivity values of different photoreceiver configurations versus operating bit rate at a bit-error rate of 10^{-9}. From this figure, we see that a single HBT based photoreceiver has a high sensitivity as compared to other contemporary photoreceivers. We also note that the APD/MESFET based photo-

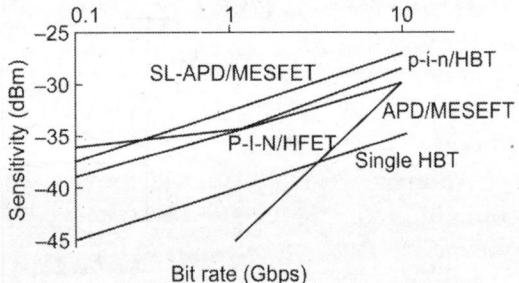

Fig. 9.25: Sensitivity vs bit rate for different receiver front-end configuration

receiver has a better sensitivity as compared to the single HBT based receiver at 1 Gbps. However, we see that the sensitivity of APD/MESFET based receiver degrades very fast beyond 1 Gb/s. This is reported to be due to inherent drawback of APD based receivers in which the excess noise increases rapidly at higher bit-rate of operation (> 1 Gbps). Table 9.1 shows a comparison of sensitivity values of BER of 10-9 for different photoreceiver configurations for operating bit rates of 1 Gbps and 20 Gbps.

Table 9.1: A comparison of sensitivity values for different receiver configurations

Type of photoreceiver	Sensitivity (dBm) at	
	1 Gbps	10 Gbps
APD/MESFET	−45.41	−29.58
SL-APD/MESFET	−32.25	−27.00
p-i-n/HFET	−34.31	−29.76
p-i-n/HBT	−34.48	−28.62
Single MESFET	–	−44.00
Single HBT	−40.05	−34.77

One can achieve further improvement in the sensitivity of photodetector at a given bit rate of operation by using in-built semiconductor laser amplifier (SLA) based preamplifier (Fig. 9.26).

One can also use a fiber amplifier (FA), e.g. Erbium doped fiber amplifier (EDFA) in place of an SLA. With the use of optical amplifier, an improvement in the sensitivity of the photodetector of the order of 10 dB

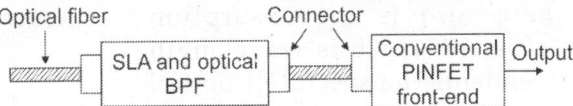

Fig. 9.26: Schematic block diagram of an SLA based optical receiver

can be achieved. However, further improvement in the sensitivity by increasing the gain of the optical amplifier is not feable due to the increased noise associated with the optical amplifier at a very high value of the gain.

9.4 PHOTODETECTORS

At the end of travel through an optical fiber, the optical signal reaches a photodetector (PD), where it is converted into an electrical signal. In PD photon of energy $h\nu$ is absorbed and produces photocurrent i_p:

$$i_p = \eta \frac{P}{h\nu} e \tag{9.26}$$

where P is the power of the incoming light, η is the quantum efficiency, h is Planck's constant and $\nu = c/\lambda$ is the frequency of the absorbed light. PD is similar to a semiconductor diode polarized in the reverse direction. Therefore, PD can be *modelled as a current source.*

Another very popular detector is a *human eye.* It is the most popular natural detector of light but it has several disadvantages: *it is slow, has bad sensitivity for low-level signals, has no natural connection to electronic amplifiers* and its *spectral response is limited* to the 0.4–0.7 μm range.

Artificial (human made) optical detectors are based on two physical mechanisms: external photoelectric effect and internal photoelectric effect. In the external photoelectric effect, electrons are removed from the metal surface of electrode known as a cathode by absorbing energy from incident light. Then, under an electric field due to the potential difference between both electrodes, they travel to another electrode known as an anode, thus producing electrical current. Vacuum photodiodes and photomultiplier tubes operate on that principle.

Main choices for photodetectors are the *p-i-n* (*p*-type intrinsic *n*-type) photodiode and avalanche photodiode (APD). APD provides gain which increases system sensitivity but introduces more noise.

In internal photoelectric effect, physical processes take place inside semiconductor junction devices. There, free carriers (electrons and holes) are generated by absorption of incoming photons, and as a result an electrical current is produced. These devices can be viewed as the inverse of a light emitting diode (LED).

9.5 PRINCIPLES OF PHOTODETECTION

Photodetection using semiconductors is possible because of optical absorption. When light is incident on the semiconductor surface, it may or may not be absorbed depending on the wavelength.

Absorbed optical power is described as:

$$\frac{dp}{dx} = \alpha(\lambda) P \tag{9.27}$$

where $\alpha(\lambda)$ is the absorption coefficient which is wavelength dependent. The spectra of optical absorption for several semiconductors and semiconductor compounds which are commonly used is shown in Fig. 9.27. As can be seen the absorption coefficient $\alpha(\lambda)$ strongly depends on wavelength.

We now consider a photodiode. Photodiode absorbs photons of a specific wavelength to produce electron-hole pairs and thus a photocurrent depends on the absorption coefficient $\alpha(\lambda)$ (hereafter α).

We assume that the total optical power incident on the photodiode is P_{in} and the Fresnel reflection coefficient at the air-semiconductor

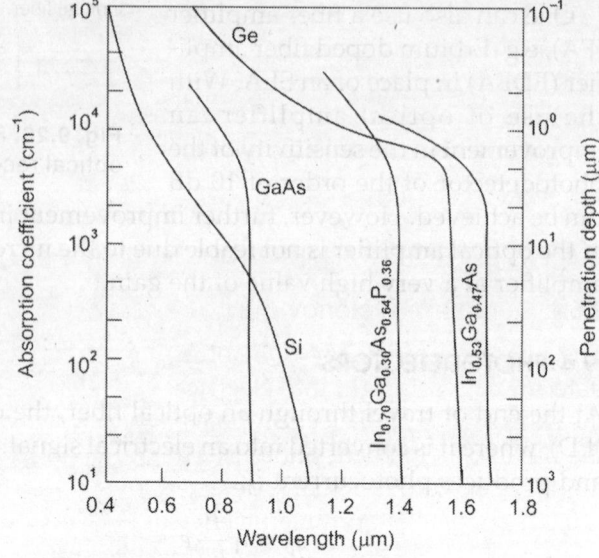

Fig. 9.27: Wavelength dependence of the absorption coefficient a for some semiconductors

interface is R. Then the optical power entering the semiconductor will be, $P = P_{in} (1 - R)$. If d is the absorption region of the semiconductor, then the power absorbed by the semiconductor can be obtained by integrating Eq. (9.27) (in accordance with Beer's law), we have:

$$P_{abs} (d) = P_{in} (1 - R) [1 - \exp (-\alpha d)] \tag{9.28}$$

Let us assume that the incident light is monochromatic and energy of each photon in $h\nu$. Then the rate of photon absorption will be given by:

$$\frac{P_{abs} (d)}{h\nu} = \frac{P_{in} (1 - R)}{h\nu} [1 - \exp (-\alpha d)]$$

$$= \frac{P}{h\nu} [1 - \exp (-\alpha d)] \tag{9.29}$$

Incident light penetrates the semiconductor surface and generates electrical current I_p (rate of flow of charge carriers) is given by:

$$I_p = \frac{P_e}{h\nu} [1 - \exp (-\alpha d)] \tag{9.30}$$

where e is electronic charge. Here, we have assumed that (i) the semiconductor is an intrinsic absorper, i.e. the absorption of photons excites the electrons from the valence band directly to the conduction band (ii) each photon produces an electron-hole pair (iii) all charge carriers are collected at the electrodes.

A schematic of a photodetector is shown in Fig. 9.28.

We may note that the intensity of the optical signal at the receiver is very low, the detector has to meet high performance specifications:

(i) The conversion efficiency should be high at the operating wavelength.

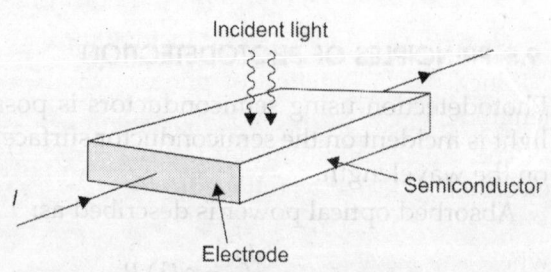

Fig. 9.28: Schematic of a photodetector

(ii) The speed of response should be high enough to ensure that signal distortion does not occur.

(iii) The detection process introduce the minimum amount of noise.

(iv) The detector size should be compatible with the fiber dimensions.

(v) It must be possible to operate continuously over a wide range of temperature for several years.

9.6 PROPERTIES OF SEMICONDUCTOR PHOTODETECTORS

9.6.1 Quantum Efficiency (η)

The quantum efficiency (QE) of a photodetector is a measure of how effectively the detector converts light into electrical current. QE denoted by η, is defined as the ratio of the flux of generated electron-hole pairs (EHPs) that contribute to the detector current, to the flux of the incident photons. The quantum efficiency of a detector is the ratio of the number of photons actually detected, to the number of incident photons. The QE range is $0 \leq \eta \geq 1$. The quantum efficiency of the photodiode is defined as:

$$\eta = \frac{\text{Number of free EHP generated and collected}}{\text{Number of incident photons}} = \frac{r_e}{r_p} \tag{9.31}$$

Since QE is a function of photon energy, the QE is calculated at a particular photon energy. The measured photocurrent (I_{ph}) in the external circuit is due to the flow of electrons to the terminals of the photodiode. The number of electrons collected at the terminal per second is I_{ph}/e, where e is the charge of an electron. For incident optical power P_o, the number of incident photons arriving per second is P_o/hv. Thus, the QE (η) can also be defined as:

$$\eta = \frac{I_{ph}/e}{P_o/hv} \tag{9.32}$$

One of the major factors which determines η is the absorption coefficient (α) of semiconductor material used within the photodetector. η is generally less than unity as not all of the incident photons are absor-bed to create electron-hole (e-h) pairs. η is often quoted as a percentage, e.g. 75% is equivalent to 75 electrons collected per 100 incident photons. Further, in common with α, η is also a function of photon wavelength and must, therefore, only be quoted for a specific wavelength.

9.6.2 Responsivity (R)

The responsivity (R) of a photodetector is defined as the ratio of the photocurrent (I_{ph}) flowing in the device, to the incident optical power (P_o). Responsivity is measured in amps per watt. Thus:

$$R = \frac{\text{Photocurrent}}{\text{Incident optical power}} = \frac{I_{ph}}{P_o} = \frac{I_p}{P_o} \, (\text{AW}^{-1}) \tag{9.33}$$

Since R is a function of photon wavelength, R is calculated at a particular wavelength λ.

The output photocurrent (I_{ph} or I_p) may be expressed in terms of the rate, r_e of the electrons collected as follows:

$$I_p = e \, r_e \tag{9.34}$$

where e is the electronic charge. Combining Eqs (9.31) and (9.34), one obtains:

$$I_p = e \, \eta \, r_p \tag{9.35}$$

The rate of incident photon is given by:

$$r_p = \frac{\text{Incident optical power}}{\text{Energy of the photon}} = \frac{P_{in}}{h\nu} \qquad (9.36)$$

Thus,

$$I_p = \frac{\eta e P_{in}}{h\nu} \qquad (9.37)$$

Substituting for I_p from Eq. (9.37) in Eq. (9.33), we get expression for R in terms of η as follows:

$$R = \eta \frac{e}{h\nu} = \eta \frac{e\lambda}{hc} \qquad (9.38)$$

Also given in Eq. (9.32) and Eq. (9.38), the efficiency and responsivity depend on wavelength, R is also called the *spectral responsivity* or *radiant sensitivity*. The R vs λ characteristics represent the spectral response of the photodiode. Spectral response curves are generally provided by the manufacturer. The spectral response characteristics for various quantum efficiencies are shown in Fig. 9.29, and can be calculated using Eq. (9.38). The outer area of the detector has a higher responsivity than the centre area, which can cause problems when aligning the fiber cable to the detector.

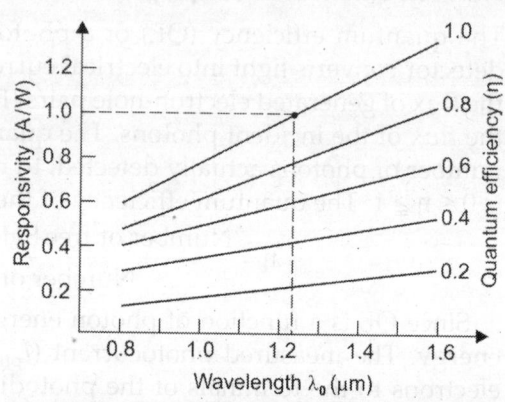

Fig. 9.29: Responsivity vs wavelength for various quantum efficiencies

Equation (9.38) also shows that the responsivity (R) is directly proportional to η at a particular wavelength and in the ideal case, when $\eta = 1$, R is directly proportional to λ (Fig. 9.29). This means that ions responsivity is a linear function of wavelength.

In case of a practical diode, as the wavelength of the incident photon becomes longer, its energy becomes smaller than that required for exciting the electron from the valence band to the conduction band. The responsivity (R), thus falls of the cut-off wavelength (λ_c) as shown in Fig. 9.30(b).

We may note that responsivity gives transfer characteristics of detector, i.e. photocurrent per unit incident optical power.

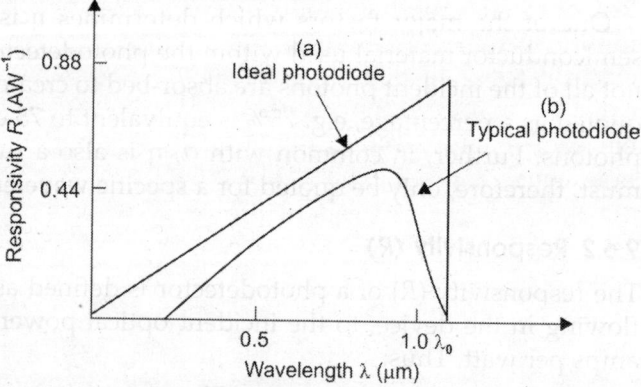

Fig. 9.30: Responsivity (R) as a function of wavelength (λ) for (a) an ideal Si photodiode and (b) a practical Si diode

Typical responsivities of *p-i-n* photodiodes are as follows:
- Silicon pin photodiode at 900 nm → 0.65 AW⁻¹
- Germanium pin photodiode at 1.3 μm → 0.45 AW⁻¹
- In GaAs pin photodiode at 1.3 μm → 0.9 AW⁻¹

In most photodiodes the quantum efficiency (η) is independent of the power level falling on the detector at a given photon energy. This means that ideal responsivity (R) is a linear function of the optical power, i.e. the photocurrent I_p is directly proportional to the optical power P_i incident upon the photodetector, so that R is constant at a given wavelength. However, η is not a constant at all wavelengths, since, it varies according to photon energy ($h\nu$). Consequently, R is a function of λ and of the photodiode material.

9.6.3 Long-Wavelength Cut-off

It is essential when considering the intrinsic absorption process that the energy of incident photons be greater than or equal to the band gap energy E_g of the material used to fabricate the photoconductor. Therefore, the photon energy:

$$\frac{hc}{\lambda} \geq E_g \tag{9.39}$$

giving:

$$\lambda \leq \frac{hc}{E_g} \tag{9.40}$$

Thus, the threshold for detection, commonly known as the long-wavelength cutoff point λ_c, above which photons are simply not absorbed by the semiconductor, given by:

$$\lambda_c = \frac{hc}{E_g} \tag{9.41}$$

The expression given in Eq. (9.41) allows the calculation of the longest wavelength of light to give photodetection for the various semiconductor material used in the fabrication of detectors.

We may note that the above criterion is only applicable to intrinsic photodetectors. Extrinsic semiconductors violate the condition given by Eq. (9.41), but are not currently used in optical fiber communication.

9.6.4 Response Time

Response time is defined as the time needed for the photodiode to respond to an optical input by producing photocurrent. When light incident on the photodiode generates an electron-hole pair in a photo-detector material, an electrical charge is generated in an external circuit, as shown in Fig. 9.31. This electrical charge, due to the electron and hole, equals $2e$ (e is the charge of an electron).

The charge delivered to the external circuit, by the movement of carriers in the photodetector material, is not provided instantaneously. The charge is delivered over an extended period. It is as if the motion of the charged carriers in the material draws charge slowly away from the wire on one side of the device and then pushes it slowly into the wire at the other side. In this way, each charge passing through the external circuit is spread out in time. This phenomenon is called *transit-time spread*. It is an important limiting factor for the speed of operation of all semiconductor photodetectors.

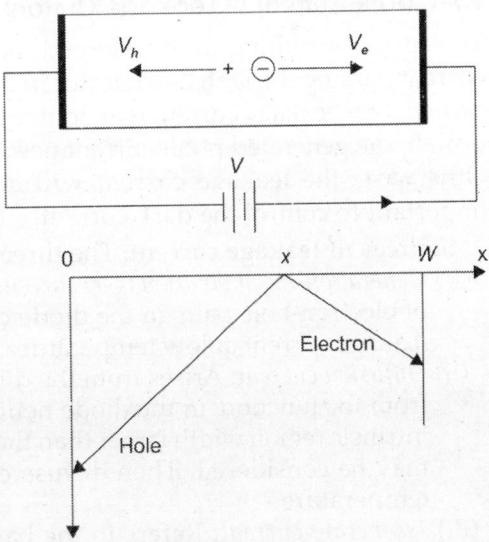

Fig. 9.31: Generated electron-hole pair at position x

Consider an electron-hole pair generated (by photon absorption, for example) at position x in a semiconductor material. The semiconductor material has width W, to which a voltage V is applied, as shown in Fig. 9.31. When an electron-hole pair is generated at position x, the hole moves to the left with velocity v_h, and the electron moves to the right with velocity v_e. This movement terminates when the carriers reach the edge of the material. The current (i) in the external circuit, generated by this movement, is given by:

$$i(t) = \frac{Q}{W} v(t)$$

(9.42)

where t is the time

Q is the total charge of the photogenerated electrons

If the voltage is increased, the electron velocity increases, and thus current increases. This means that for an input light pulse, the output current pulse will have a faster response time, for a higher applied voltage.

Response time can be affected by dark current, noise, responsivity linearity, back-reflection, and detector edge effect. Edge effect occurs because detectors only provide a fast response in their centre area.

9.6.5 Sensitivity

A photodetector is a device that converts photon energy into an electrical signal. A photodetector usually detects the energy of some photons better than others. Detection sensitivity is a function of the photon's energy being detected. The sensitivity is usually given as a function of the wavelength and expressed as the quantum efficiency. A high sensitivity allows a low level of light to be detected.

9.7 PERFORMANCE PARAMETERS OF PHOTODETECTORS

Main parameters which determine characteristics of photodetector are: dark current, spectral response, quantum efficiency, noise, detectivity, linearity and dynamic range, speed and frequency range. We have:

9.7.1 Dark Current or Leakage Current

The current resulting from absorbed incident light is called *generated photocurrent*. The current passing through the detector in the absence of light is called *dark current* or *leakage current*. Low leakage current is an important measure of device quality. If the dark current is high, the generated photocurrent needs to be larger, in order to provide a good signal. Otherwise, the leakage current will dominate the detector current. Therefore, it is important to control the dark current.

Sources of leakage current: The three fundamental sources of leakage current are:
(i) *Generation-recombination (g-r) current*: Arises from the generation and recombination of electron-hole pairs in the diode depletion region. The *g-r* current dominates the leakage current at low temperature.
(ii) *Diffusion current*: Arises from the diffusion of the minority carriers, toward or away from the junction, in the diode neutral region. In the case of p^+-n junction with the intrinsic region width larger than the hole diffusion length, the intrinsic region alone may be considered. Then diffuse current dominates the leakage current at high temperature.
(iii) *Tunneling current*: Refers to the band-to-band tunneling in the presence of high electric fields. A high field reduces the effective band gap barrier, allowing carriers to cross the band gap.

Typical values of dark current for popular semiconductors are shown in Table 9.2.

9.7.2 Quantum Efficiency

See Section 9.6.

9.7.3 Responsivity (R)

See Section 9.6.

9.7.4 Speed of Response

It determines how photodetector responds to an optical signal. Fig. 9.32 shows a typical response to a pulse.

Speed of response is determined by the RC time constant. In terms of parameters of previously introduced equivalent circuit, the *rise time* τ_r is given by:

$$\tau_r = 2.19 \cdot R_L \cdot C_j \qquad (9.43)$$

The evaluation of τ_r is left as an exercise. Time response is directly related to the frequency response. The 3 dB bandwidth is given by:

$$f_{s-\text{dB}} = \frac{1}{2\pi R_L C_j} \qquad (9.44)$$

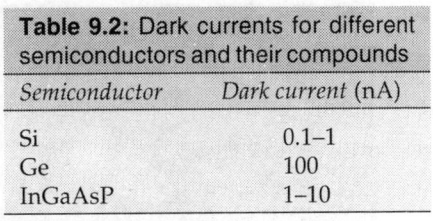

Table 9.2: Dark currents for different semiconductors and their compounds

Semiconductor	Dark current (nA)
Si	0.1–1
Ge	100
InGaAsP	1–10

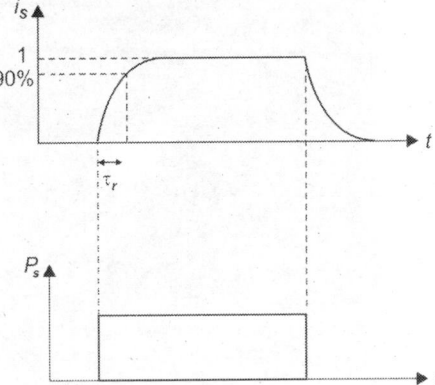

Fig. 9.32: Typical response of a photodetector to a square-pulse signal

9.8 TYPES OF OPTICAL DETECTORS

There are many types of optical detectors including the phototransistor, photovoltaic, metal-semiconductor-metal (MSM), *pin* photodiode, and avalanche photodiode (APD). These detectors are explained in the following sections.

9.8.1 Phototransistors

Phototransistors are the simplest type of photodetector. The basic operating principle of a phototransistor is shown in Fig. 9.33. The device consists of an *n-p-n* junction, in which *n* is the emitter, *p* is the base, and the other *n* is the collector. The base terminal is normally open, and there is a voltage applied between the collector and emitter terminals (just as in the normal operation of common bipolar junction transistor (BJT).

A large space charge layer (SCL) forms between the base and collector. The SCL region is called the absorption region. The operation of this device begins when an incident photon is absorbed in the SCL, and generates an electron-hole pair. The electrical field E_o drifts the electron and hole in opposite directions. Phototransistors operate as a photodetector that amplifies the photocurrent. An applied voltage V will increase E to become E_o plus V. When the drifting electron reaches the collector, it gets collected (and thereby neutralized) by the power supply (applied voltage). On the other hand, when the hole enters the neutral base region, it can only be neutralized by injecting a large number of electrons into the base. It forces a large number of electrons to be injected from the emitter.

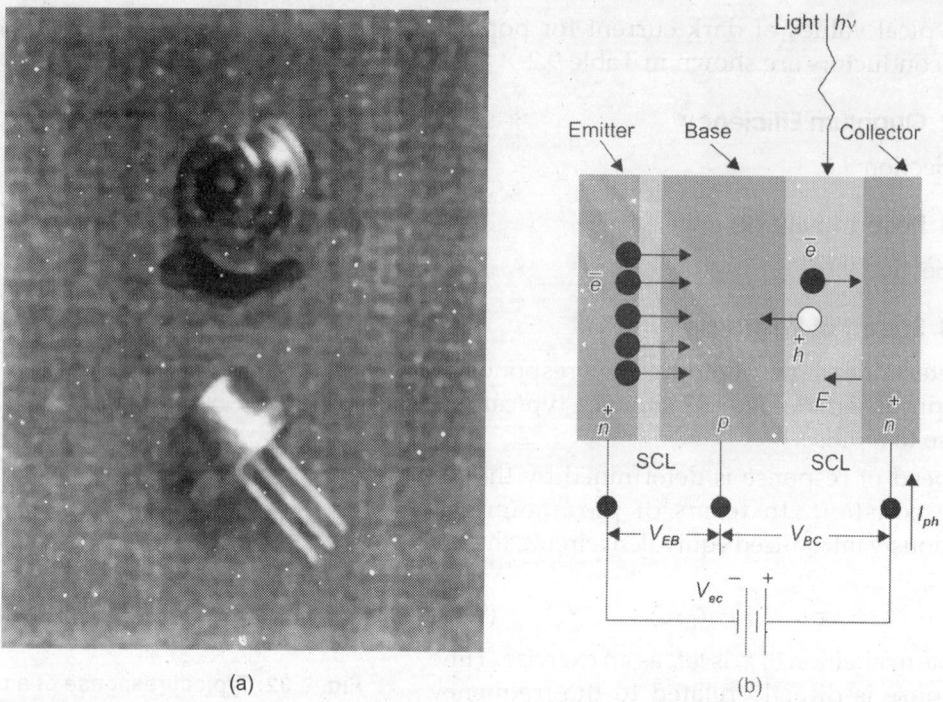

Fig. 9.33: Phototransistor

Normally, the electron recombination time in the base is very long, compared with the time it takes for electrons to diffuse across the base. The means that only a small fraction of electrons injected from the emitter can recombine with holes in the base. Thus, the emitter has to inject a large number of electrons to neutralize this extra hole in the base. These electrons diffuse across the base and reach the collector, and thereby, create a photocurrent, which is amplified compared to the original electron. Thus, phototransistors have photocurrent gain.

9.8.2 Photovoltaics

Photovoltaic panels, or solar cells, convert the incident solar radiation, through the photovoltaic effect, into electrical current. The basic principle behind this effect relies on the small energy gap between the valence and conduction bands of the photovoltaic material. When light photons incident on a photovoltaic have enough energy to excite electrons from the valence to the conduction band, the resulting accumulation of charge leads to a flow of current.

Figure 9.34 shows a typical solar panel and its cross-section. Consider a p-n junction with a very narrow and more heavily doped n-region. Solar radiation is incident on the thin n-side. The electrodes attached to the n-side must allow illumination to enter the cell and at the same time have a small series resistance. The electrodes are deposited on the n-side to form an array of finger electrodes on the surface. A thin anti-reflection coating on the surface reduces reflections and allows more light to enter the cells.

The width (W) of the depletion region or the space charge layer (SCL) extends primary into the p-side. Most photons are absorbed within the n-region and depletion region. Thus, short and medium wavelengths are absorbed. The generated electron-hole pairs

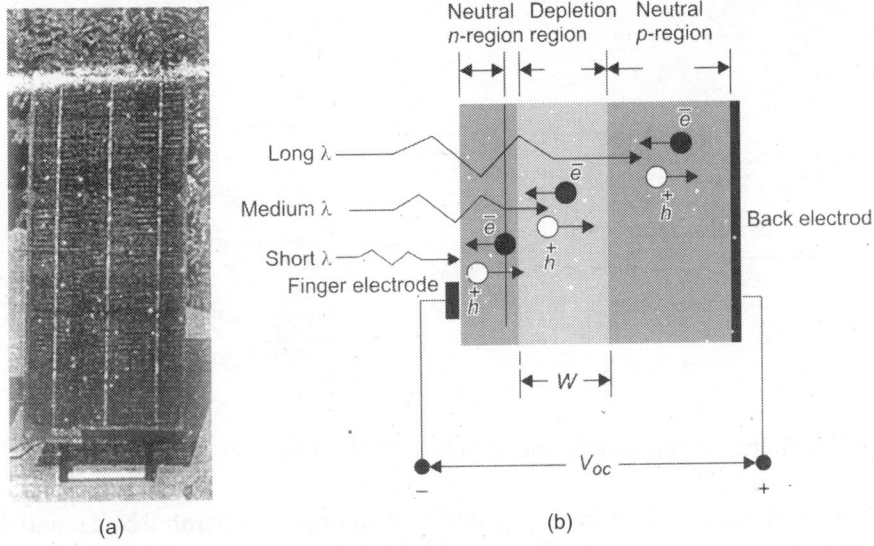

Fig. 9.34: Photovoltaic panel

are swept away by the built-in field E_o in the depletion layer. This creates an open circuit voltage V_{oc} between the electrodes. If an external load is connected, a photo-current results.

The efficiency of a solar cell is one of its most important characteristics; it allows the device to be accessed economically, in comparison to other energy conversion devices. The solar cell efficiency refers to the fraction of incident light energy converted to electrical energy. This conversion efficiency depends on the semiconductor material properties, the device structure, and the incident light wavelength spectrum, which is mostly solar radiation. The efficiency of a solar cell decreases with increasing temperature. Therefore, the temperature of solar cells must be controlled for maximum efficiency.

Most solar cells are silicon based; silicon based semiconductor fabrication is a very developed technology, enabling cost effective devices for energy production in remote applications. A solar cell fabricated by making a *p-n* junction in the same crystal is called *homojunction*. A silicon homojunction solar cell is called a *single crystal passivated emitter rear locally diffused* (PERLD) *cell*. It has higher efficiency than other types of semiconductor solar cells.

9.8.3 Metal-Semiconductor-Metal (MSM) Detectors

Metal-semiconductor-metal (MSM) detectors are probably the fastest and simplest optical detector to fabricate. The basic idea is to create a Shottky barrier, which forces the material at the surface to be depleted. This barrier is created by contacting a metal to the semiconductor surface. Fig. 9.35(a) shows the cross-section of a metal area. Fig. 9.35(b) shows top view of MSM structure and its cross-sectional view is shown in Fig. 9.35(c). The

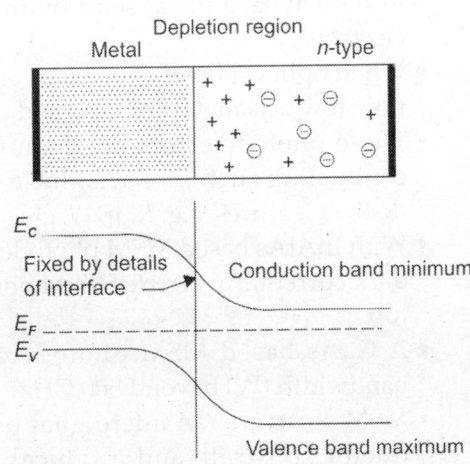

Fig. 9.35: (a) Shottky barrier and energy diagram

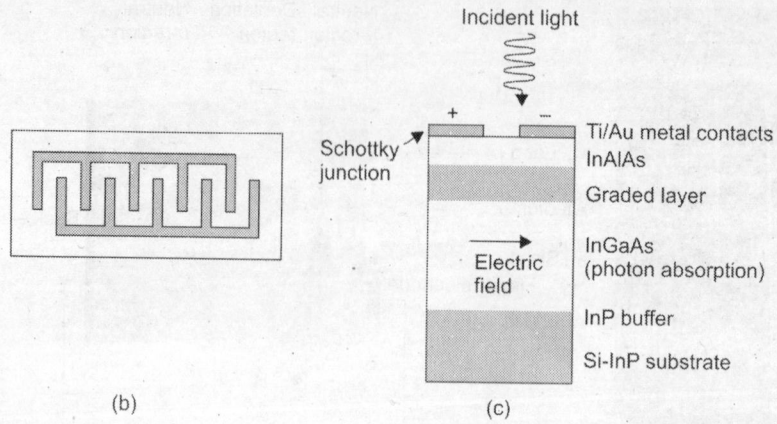

Fig. 9.35: (b) Top view of the structure of MSM (c) and its cross-section

barriers are often in the form of inter-digitated metal fingers separated by a small distance, typically on the order of microns. The metal is usually opaque to the incoming light; the remainder of the surface area absorbs the light. All the depletion layers are connected together. Any absorbed light generates electron-hole pairs, which are quickly swept out to the contacts. Full-width at half maximum (FWHM) pulses are measured in picoseconds for such structures, since the response time is so quick.

When using the MSM for the detection of 1300–1500 nm ranges, the MSM suffers from following two serious drawbacks:

(i) Shottky barriers on indium phosphate (InP) tend to have high dark current, and therefore, low receiver sensitivity.

(ii) Low quantum efficiency results, because the metal fingers prevent some of the incoming light from reaching the absorption layer.

Salient Features of MSM Photodetectors

- MSM photodetector uses a sandwitched semiconductor between two metals. The middle semionductor layer acts as optical absorbing layer. A Schottky barrier is formed at each metal semiconductor interface (junction), which prevents flow of electrons.

- When optical power is incident on it, *e-h* pairs generated through photoabsorption flow towards metal contacts and causes photocurrent.

- These photodetectors are manufactured using different combinations of semi-conductors such as GaAs, InGaAs, InP, InAlAs. Each MSM photodetector has distinct features, e.g. R, η, W, etc.

- With InAlAs based MSM photodetector, 92% η can be achieved at 1.3 μm with low dark current. An *inverted* MSM photodetector shows high R when illuminated from top.

- A GaAs based MSM photodetector with travelling wave structure gives a bandwidth (W) beyond 500 GHz.

- MSM structure (an interdigital pattern of metal fingers deposited on a semicon-ductor substrate and a typical *p-i-n* detector) shows several improvements compared to traditional designs, e.g. sensitivity. Most of the improvements result from the lateral design.

9.8.4 *pn* Photodiode

Figure 9.36(a) shows the simplest structure of a *p-n* photodiode. Incident photons of energy (say *hv*) are absorbed not only inside the depletion region but also outside it [Fig. 9.36(b)]. Photons absorbed within the depletion region generate electron-hole (*e-h*) pairs. Due to built-in strong electric field [Fig. 9.36(c)], electrons and holes generated within this region get accelerated in opposite directions, and thereby, drift to the *n*-side and *p*-side respectively. The resulting flow of photocurrent constitutes the response of the photodiode to the incident optical power. The response time is governed by the transit time τ_{drift} in accordance with the relation:

$$\tau_{\text{drift}} = \frac{W}{V_{\text{drift}}} \quad (9.45)$$

where *W* is the width of the depletion region and V_{drift} is the average drift velocity. τ_{drift} is of the order of 100 ps, which is small enough for the photodiode to operate upto a bit rate of about 1 G bits/s. The depletion layers width *W* of a *p-n* photodiode is given by:

$$W = \left[\frac{2\varepsilon}{e} (V_{bi} + V_o) \left(\frac{1}{N_a} + \frac{1}{N_d} \right) \right]^{1/2} \quad (9.46)$$

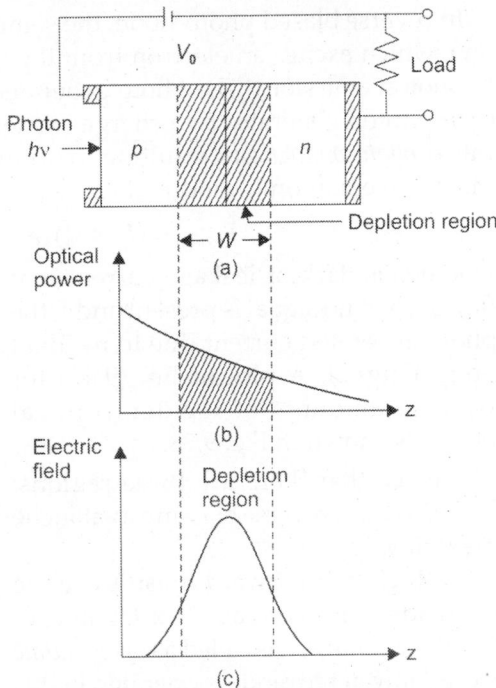

Fig. 9.36: (a) Schematic structure of a pn photodiode and the associated depletion region under reverse bias (b) variation of optical power within the diode (c) variation of electric field inside the diode

Here ε is the dielectric constant, V_{bl} is built in voltage and depends on semiconductor, V_o is the applied bias voltage, and N_a and N_d are the acceptor and donor concentrations respectively used to fabricate the *p-n* junction. V_{drift} depends on the bias voltage but attains a saturation value depending on the semiconductor of the *p-n* diode.

Incident photons are absorbed outside the depletion region also [Fig. 9.36(b)]. The electrons generated in the *p*-side have to diffuse to the depletion region boundary, prior to they can drift (under the built in electric field) to the *n*-side. In a similar way, holes generated in the *n*-side have to diffuse to the depletion region boundary for their drift towards the *p*-side. However, the diffusion process is inherently slow, and therefore, the presence of a diffusive component may distort the temporal response of a photodiode (Fig. 9.37).

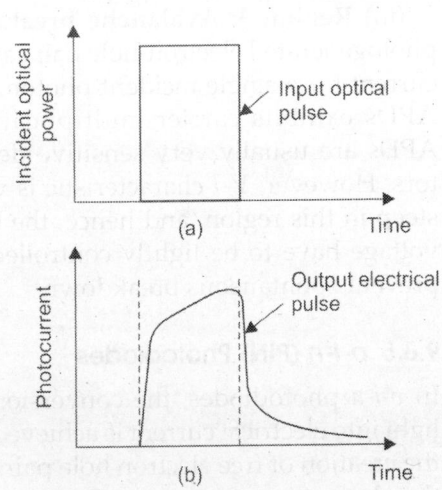

Fig. 9.37: Schematic response of a typical p-n photodiode to a rectangular optical pulse when both drift and diffusion contribute to the photocurrent

In reverse biased photodiode, the semiconductor material absorbs a photon of energy (hv), which excites an electron from the valence band to the conduction band (opposite to photon emission). The photo generated electron leaves behind it a hole (h), and thus, each photon generates two charge carriers. This enhances the material conductivity, so called *photoconductivity* resulting in an increase in the diode current (I_{diode}). Obviously, the diode equation is modified as:

$$I_{diode} = (I_d + I_s)(e^{V_q/nkT} - 1) \tag{9.47}$$

where I_d is dark or leakage current that flows when no signal is present and I_s the photo generated current due to incident optical signal. A plot of Eq. (9.47) for varying amounts of incident optical power is shown in Fig. 9.38.

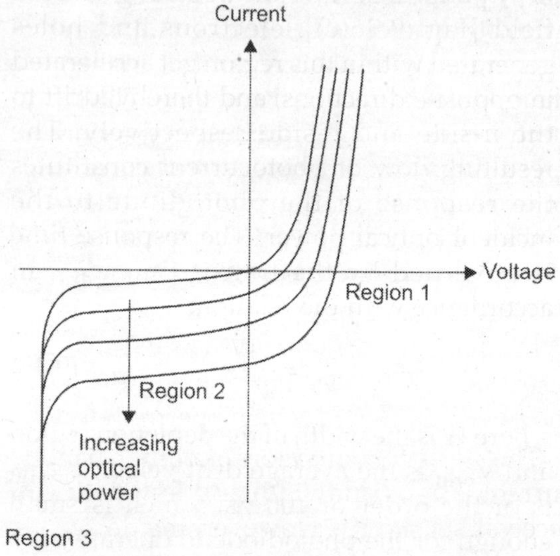

We see that there are three regions: Fowards bias, reverse bias and avalanche breakdown.

(i) **Region 1: Forward bias:** A change in incident power causes a change in terminal voltage, it is called as *photovoltaic mode*. Now, if the diode is operated in this mode, the frequency response of the diode is poor and this is why photovoltaic operation is rarely used in optical links.

(ii) **Region 2: Reverse bias:** We see that a change in optical power produces a proportional change in diode current and it is called as *photoconductive mode* of operation which most optical detector use. Under these conditions, the exponential term in Eq. (9.47) becomes insignificant and one obtains the reverse bias current as:

$$I_{diode} = (I_d + I_s) \tag{9.48}$$

Fig. 9.38: *V-I* characteristics of photodiode

(iii) **Region 3: Avalanche breakdown:** When photodiode biased in this region, a photogenerated electron-hole pair causes avalanche break-down, resulting in large diode current for a single incident photon. *Avalanche photodiode* (APD) operate in this region. APDs exhibits carrier multiplication. APDs are usually very sensitive detectors. However, V-I characteristic is very steep in this region, and hence, the bias voltage have to be tightly controlled to prevent spontaneous breakdown.

9.8.5 *p-i-n* (PIN) Photodiodes

In *p-i-n* photodiodes, the conversion of light into electrical current is achieved by the creation of free electron hole pairs by the absorption of photons. This absorption process creates electrons in the conduction band and holes in the valence band. Figure 9.39 shows the simplified

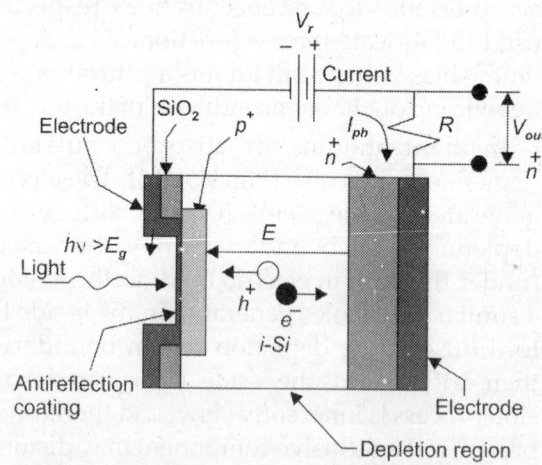

Fig. 9.39: A *p-i-n* junction photodiode

structure of a typical p-i-n junction photodiode. The structure of the photodiode is the p^+-intrinsic-n^+ junction. The intrinsic silicon (i-Si) layer has much less doping than both the p^+ and n^+ regions, and it is much wider than these regions. At long wavelengths, where penetration depth is large, the photons can be absorbed in the wide depletion region. Thus, the width depends on the particular wavelength used in the application. In contrast, a p-n junction has a narrow depletion region and fewer photons are absorbed.

When the structure is formed, holes diffuse from the p^+ side, and electrons from the n^+ side, into the i-Si layer, also called the depletion region. In this region, they recombine (with other holes and electrons) and disappear. This leaves behind a thin layer of exposed, negatively-charged acceptor ions in the p^+ side, and a thin layer of exposed, positively-charged donor ions in the n^+ side. The two charges are separated and create the built-in electric field E in the i-Si layer. An exterior voltage increases E, which increase the response speed. While the photogenerated carriers are drifting through the i-Si layer, they create an external photocurrent, when a voltage is applied. The photo-current can be detected as the voltage across a small external resistor R, as shown in Fig. 9.39. A larger thickness of the i-Si layer increases QE, but slows the response time since carriers have further to travel.

In some photodiodes, such as pyroelectric detectors, the energy conversion generates heat, which increases the temperature of the detector. The temperature increase changes the polarization and relative permittivity of the photodiode.

The p-i-n photodetectors offer high bandwidth, high quantum efficiency, and low dark current. High bandwidth and low dark current are important characteristics for good receiver sensitivity. However, the device has no gap, which places a lower limit on the sensitivity achievable, before dark current becomes significant. The p-i-n photo-detectors are small devices with small capacitance, thus can detect high-speed signals with high sensitivity. The most important applications of the photodiodes are in optical communications.

A double heterostructure (Fig. 9.40) improves the performance of p-i-n photodiode. In this structure, the middle i-region of a material with lower bandgap is sandwiched between p- and n-type materials of higher bandgap, so that incident light is absorbed only in i-region (Fig. 9.40). The bandgap of InP is 1.35 eV and hence, transparent to light for $\lambda > 0.2$ μm, whereas the bandgap of lattice matched InGaAs is about 0.75 eV, which corres-ponds to λ_c of 1.65 μm. This means that the intrinsic layer of InGaAs absorbs strongly in the wavelength range 1.3–1.6 μm. In heterostructure, the diffusive component of the photocurrent is completely eliminated, because the incident photons are absorbed only within the depletion region. Heterostructure p-i-n photodiodes

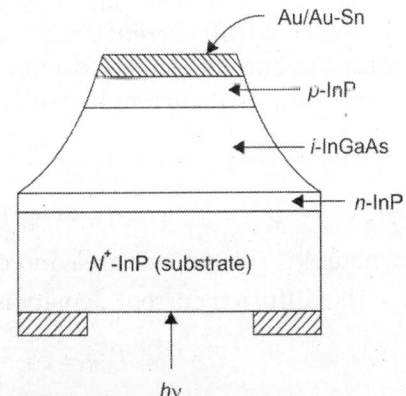

Fig. 9.40: Schematic of double hetero-structure of p-i-n photodiode using InGaA/InP

are very useful for fiber-optic communication systems operating in the range 1.3–1.6 μm.

Salient features of p-i-n photodiodes

(i) In the absence of light, p-i-n photodiodes behave electrically just like an ordinary rectifier diode. When forward biased, they conduct large amount of current.

(ii) *p-i-n* detectors can be operated in two modes: *photovoltaic* and *photoconductive*. In photovoltaic mode, no bias is applied to the detector. In this mode, the detector works very slow, and output of the detector is approximately *logarithmic* to the input level. In practice, fiber optic receivers never usethis mode.

In *photoconductive mode*, the detector is reverse biased. In this case, the output is a current that is very linear with the input light power.

(iii) The intrinsic region somewhat improves the sensitivity of the *p-i-n* photodetector. It does not provide internal gain. The combination of different semiconductors operating at different wavelength permits the selection of material capable of responding to the desired operating wavelength. Table 9.3 summarizes the characteristics of common *p-i-n* photodiodes.

Table 9.3: Characteristics of common p-i-n photodiodes

S. No.	Parameters	Symbols	Unit	Si	Ge	InGaAs
1.	Wavelength	λ	μm	0.4–1.1	0.8–1.8	1.0–1.7
2.	Responsivity	R	A/W	0.4–0.6	0.5–0.7	0.6–0.9
3.	Quantum efficiency	η	%	75–90	50–55	60–70
4.	Dark current	I_d	nA	1–10	50–500	1–20
5.	Rise time	T_r	nS	0.5–1	0.1–0.5	0.02–0.5
6.	Bandwidth	B	GHz	0.3–0.6	0.5–3	1–10
7.	Bias voltage	V_b	V	50–100	5–10	5–6

Depletion Layer Photocurrent

Figure 9.41 shows a reverse biased *p-i-n* photodiode and electric field distribution under reverse bias. The total current density through depletion layer is:

$$J_{\text{total}} = J_{\text{drift}} + J_{\text{diffusion}} \qquad (9.49)$$
$$(J_{\text{tot}}) \qquad (J_{\text{dr}}) \qquad (J_{\text{diff}})$$

where, J_{dr} is drift current density due to carriers generated in depletion region and J_{diff} is diffusion current density due to carriers generated outside depletion region. One can express the drift current density as:

$$J_{\text{dr}} = \frac{I_p}{A}$$

or
$$J_{\text{dr}} = e\phi_o \left(1 - e^{\alpha W}\right) \qquad (9.50)$$

where A is photodiode area and ϕ_o is incident photon flux per unit area.

The diffusion current density is given as:

$$J_{\text{diff}} = e\phi_o \frac{\alpha L_p}{1 + \alpha L_p} e^{-\alpha W} + eP_{\text{no}} \frac{D_p}{L_p} \qquad (9.51)$$

where D_p is hole diffusion coefficient, P_{no} is equilibrium hole density. Substituting (9.50) and (9.51) in (9.49), one obtains:

$$J_{\text{tot}} = e\phi_o \left[1 + \frac{\alpha W}{1 + \alpha L_p}\right] + eP_{\text{no}} \frac{D_p}{L_p} \qquad (9.52)$$

Response Time

Response time of a photodiode depends upon the following factors:

(a) Transit time of photocarriers within the depletion region.

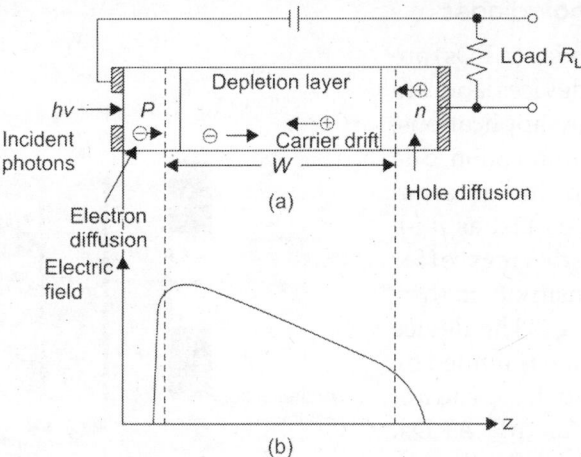

Fig. 9.41: (a) Schematic structure of a reverse biased p-i-n photodiode (b) Electric-field distribution inside the device under reverse bias

(b) Diffusion of photocarriers outside the depletion region.

(c) RC time constant of diode and external circuit.

The transit time (t_d) is given by:

$$t_d = \frac{W}{V_d} \tag{9.53}$$

The diffusion process is slow and diffusion times are less than carrier drift time. One can calculate the effect of diffusion by considering the photodiode response time. Figure 9.42 shows the response time of photodiode which is not fully depleted.

If R_T is the combination of the load and amplifier input resistance and C_T is the sum of the photodiode and amplifier capacitances, the detector behaves like a simple RC low-pass filter with a passband given by:

$$B = \frac{1}{2\pi R_T C_T} \tag{9.54}$$

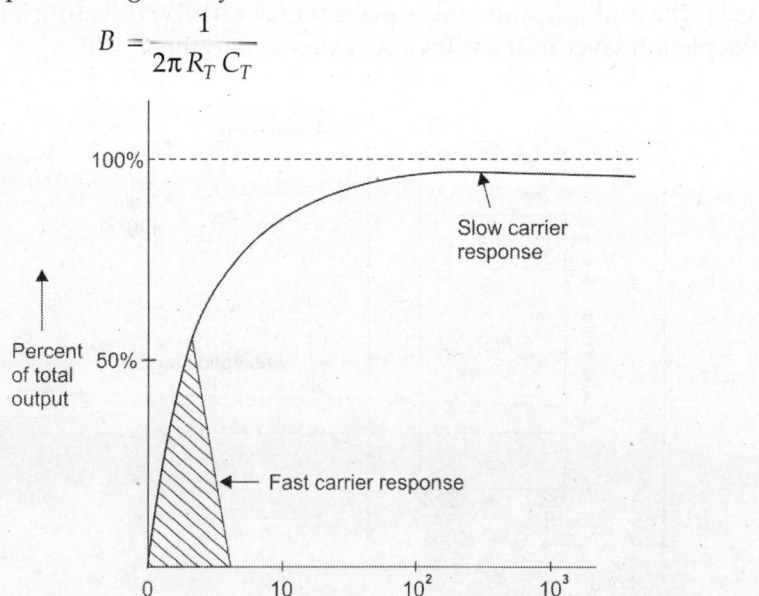

Fig. 9.42: Response time of photodiode not fully depleted

9.8.6 Avalanche Photodiodes

Avalanche photodiodes (APDs) are high performance devices and are widely used in many applications, such as optical communication, due to their high speed and internal gain. Although not as fast as *p-i-n* photodiodes, the devices offer superior receiver sensitivity in their own bandwidth range. The device bandwidth at high gain is limited by the gain-bandwidth product (GBW), for InGaAs-InP APDs. However, there are difficulties in fabricating the device; this process requires stringent process control. For this reason, commercial high performance APDs cost more than similar photodetectors.

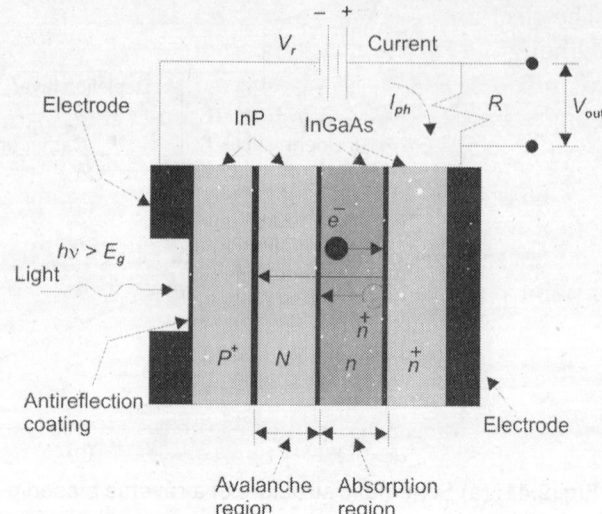

Fig. 9.43(a): Avalanche photodiode

Figure 9.43 shows the cross-section of the structure of an InGaAs-InP avalanche photodiode with separate absorption and multiplication (SAM) regions. The InP multiplication (avalanche) layer has a wider bandgap than InGaAs absorption layer. The *p*-type and *n*-type multiplication (avalanche) layer has a wider bandgap than InGaAs absorption layer. The *p*-type and *n*-type doping of InP is indicated by capital letters, *P* and *N*. Fig. 9.43(b) shows the configuration for achieving carrier multiplication with little excess noise and is called a *reach through avalanche photodiode* (RAPD).

The main depletion layer forms between the P^+-InP and the N-InP layers and is within the N-InP [Fig. 9.43(a)]. The electric field is greatest in this N-InP layer, this is, therefore, where avalanche multiplication takes place [Fig. 9.43(b)]. With sufficient reverse voltage bias, the depletion layer in the *n*-InGaAs extends into the N-InP layer.

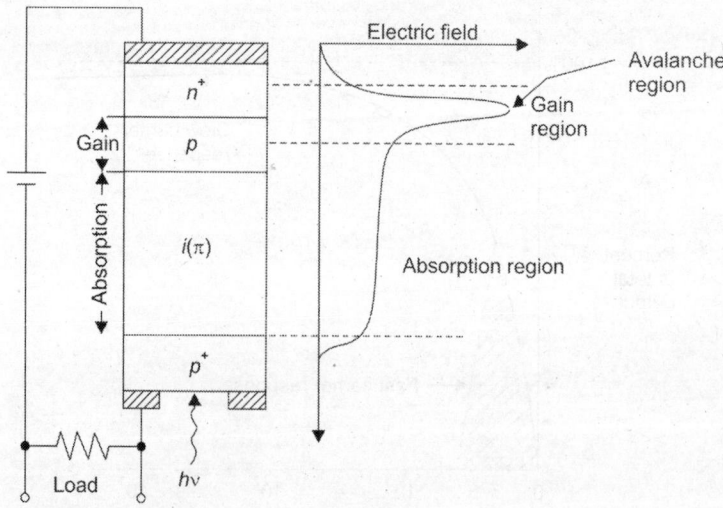

Fig. 9.43(b): Schematic configuration of RAPD and the variation of electric field in the depletion and multiplication regions

The electric field in the n-InGaAs depletion layer is not as great as that in the N-Initial Although long wavelength photons are incident on the InP side, they are not absorbed by InP, since the photon energy is less than the band gap energy of InP (E_g = 1.35 eV). Long wavelength photons pass through the InP layer and are absorbed in the n-InGaAs layers.

The electric field E in the n-InGaAs layer drifts the holes to the multiplication region, where impact ionization multiplies the carriers. The impact ionization, from the physics point of view, is the mechanism that creates the internal current gain. Primary electrons and/or holes (carriers) are generated through the absorption of photons. Carriers can acquire large amounts of energy from a high E field, when the device has a strong reverse-voltage bias. This can be translated into high-speed motion. When a collision between a carrier and the lattice occurs, the energy from the carrier can be transferred to the lattice. Sufficient energy can be absorbed by the lattice for an electron to be promoted from the valence to the conduction band, creating an electron-hole pair. This process is called "impact ionization". These new carriers are swept out by E and can acquire high energy, causing further electron-hole pairs to be created. The entire process in which many carriers are created from one initial carrier is called "avalanche multiplication".

Salient features of APD

- APD uses the avalanche breakdown phenomena for its operation. The APD has its internal gain which increases its responsivity (R).
- When APD is biased close to breakdown, it will result in reverse leakage current. This is why, APDs are usually biased just below breakdown, with the bias voltage being tightly controlled.
- The multiplication (M) for all carriers generated in the photodiode is given as:

$$M = \frac{I_M}{I_P}$$

where I_M is average value of total multiplied output current, and I_P is primary unmultiplied photocurrent.

- Responsivity of APD is given by:

$$R_{APD} = \frac{\eta e}{h\nu} M = \frac{ne\lambda}{hc} M \quad (\because \nu = c/\lambda) \tag{9.55}$$

$$\therefore \qquad R_{APD} = R_o M \tag{9.56}$$

where $R_o = \dfrac{ne\lambda}{hc}$ is unity gain responsivity.

Characteristics of common APD are given in Table 9.4.

A comparison of p-i-n and APD photodetectors is given in Table 9.5.

9.9 PHOTODETECTOR NOISE

Typical optical signals arriving at the receiver front end are very weak. They are, therefore, significantly affected by various noise sources.

There are several physical processes which contribute to noise. For example, the APD generates noise in the avalanche process and optical amplifiers produce noise due to amplified spontaneous emission (ASE). In addition, there is always a *quantum noise* which exists in all devices and sets a fundamental lower limit on noise power.

Table 9.4: Characteristics of common APDs

S. No.	Parameters	Symbols	Unit	Si	Ge	InGaAs
1.	Wavelength	λ	μm	0.4–1.1	0.8–1.8	1.0–1.7
2.	Responsivity	R_{APD}	A/W	80–130	3–30	5–20
3.	APD gain	M	–	100–500	50–200	10–40
4.	k-factor	kA	–	0.02–0.05	0.7–1.0	0.5–0.7
5.	Dark current	I_d	nA	0.1–1	50–500	1–5
6.	Rise time	T_r	ns	0.1–2	0.5–0.8	0.1–0.5
7.	Bandwidth	B	GHz	0.02–1	0.4–0.7	1–10
8.	Bias voltage	V_b	V	200–250	20–40	20–30

Table 9.5: Comparison of *p-i-n* and APD photodetectors

p-i-n detectors	APD detectors
• Fast	Not as fast
• High bandwidth, upto 40 GHZ at quantum efficiency > 80%	Significantly less bandwidth
• Low dark current	High dark current
• No gain, which leds to lower sensitivity	Built in gain, which extends the sensitivity to lower levels of received light
• Conversion efficiency (responsivity) from 0.5 to 1.0 A/W	Conversion efficiency (responsivity) from 0.5 to 100.0 A/W
• Less expensive	More expensive
• Sensitivity less (0–12 dB)	More sensitivity (5 to 15 dB)
• Low reverse biasing voltage (5 to 10 V)	High reverse bias voltage (20 to 40 V)
• Wavelength region 300 to 1100 nm	Wavelength region 400–100 nm
• S/N ratio poor	S/N ratio better
• Simple detector circuit	More complex detector circuit

The working parameter characteristizing the photodetector is the signal-to-noise ratio (SNR), which is defined as:

$$\frac{S}{N} = \frac{\text{signal power from photocurrent}}{\text{photodetector noise power + amplifier noise power}} \tag{9.57}$$

Equation (9.59) clearly reveals that to achieve high S/N, (i) the photo-detector should have high quantum efficiency and low noise so that it generate large signal power, and (ii) the amplifier noise must be kept low. The sensitivity of a detector is defined as the power necessary to generate a photocurrent equal in magnitude to the *rms* value at the total noise current. Noise appears as random fluctuations in a signal. A typical measure of noise is associated with the variance or the mean square deviation of signal s, defined as:

$$a_s^2 = (s - \overline{s})^2 = s^2 - \overline{s}^2$$

The mean value (average) of s is defined as:

$$\overline{s} = \sum_s p(s)s$$

where $p(s)$ is the probability of the measured signal having a value s and the sum is evaluated over all possible values obtained from measuring the signal.

Noise in a signal s can be represented by random variable s_n:

$$s_n = s - \bar{s}$$

If in the device (or system), there are two or more simultaneously present noise sources $s_{n1}, s_{n2}, \ldots$ which are independent, their combined effect is found by adding their mean square values (or their powers):

$$\overline{s_n^2} = \overline{s_{n1}^2} + \overline{s_{n2}^2} + \ldots$$

In terms of the above quantities, the SNR is expressed as:

$$\text{SNR} = \frac{\overline{s^2}}{\overline{s_n^2}} = \frac{\overline{s^2}}{\sigma_s^2} \quad \text{or} \quad \text{SNR} = 10 \log \frac{\overline{s^2}}{\sigma_s^2} \text{ [dB]} \tag{9.58}$$

Main types of noise arising in a photodetector are as follows:

9.9.1 Shot Noise

Shot noise is due to random distribution of electrons generated in the photodetector. It is associated with the quantum nature of photons arriving at the photodetector which generates carriers. Photons arrive at the photodetector randomly in time due to their quantum-mechanical nature. Their randomness is described by Poisson statistics. The resulting expression for shot noise of current in the photodetector is:

$$\overline{i_s^2} = 2eB\overline{i_s} \tag{9.59}$$

where e is the electron charge, B is the bandwidth and $\overline{i_s}$ is the average value of signal current.

9.9.2 Thermal Noise

Thermal noise or *Johnson noise* is due to the random motion of electrons in the resistor R. It is modelled as a Gaussian random process with zero mean and autocorrelation function given by:

$$\frac{4k_B T}{R} \delta(\tau) \tag{9.60}$$

where $\delta(\tau)$ is the Dirac delta function. Thermal noise powder in a bandwidth B is:

$$p_{s \cdot th} = 3k_B T \, B \tag{9.61}$$

where $k_B = 1.38 \times 10^{-23}$ J/K is the Boltzmann's constant and T is the absolute temperature. Thermal noise can be expressed as a current source:

$$\overline{i_{s.th}^2} = \frac{4k_B T}{R} B \equiv I_T^2 \, B \tag{9.62}$$

Here I_T is the parameter used to specify standard deviation in units of $\text{pA}/\sqrt{\text{Hz}}$. Its typical value is $1\text{pA}/\sqrt{\text{Hz}}$.

Now, we can write a current generated by a *p-n* or *p-i-n* photodiode in response to an instantaneous optical signal as:

$$I(t) = <i_p(t)> + i_s(t) + i_d(t) + i_T(t) \tag{9.63}$$

where $\langle i_p(r) \rangle = I_p = RP_{\text{in}}$ is the average photocurrent, and $i_s(t)$, $i_d(t)$, and $i_T(t)$ are the current fluctuations related to *shot noise*, *dark current noise*, and *thermal noise*, respectively.

Quantum or shot noise arises

$$\langle i_s^2(t) \rangle = 2eI_p \, \Delta f \, M^2 F(M) \tag{9.64}$$

where $F(M)$ is excess noise factor related to the random nature of an avalanche process and Δf is the effective noise bandwidth. Experimentally, it has been reported that $F(M) = M^x$, where x depends on the material and varies from 0 to 1. For p-n and p-i-n photodiodes, $F(M)$ and M are unity.

The excess noise factor, $F(M)$, which is a function of multiplication gain M is defined as the ratio of the mean-square gain divided by the square of the mean gain, given by

$$F(M) = \frac{\langle m^2 \rangle}{M^2} \qquad (9.65)$$

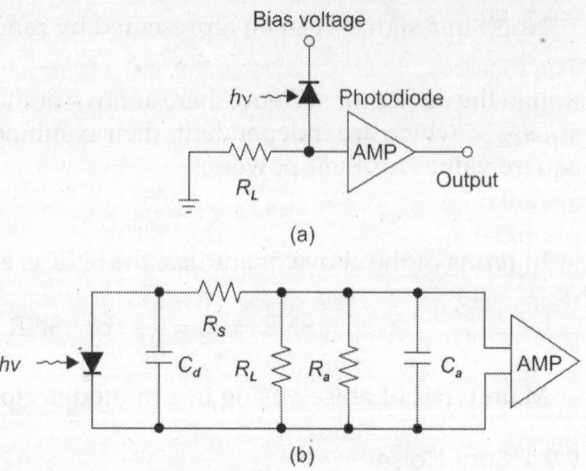

Fig. 9.44: (a) A schematic of simplest model of an optical receiver (b) equivalent circuit

The excess-noise factor, $F(M)$, depends on the ionization rate ratio and the type of carrier (hole or electron) initiating the ionization. One can express the excess noise factor for electron initiated ionization in terms of multiplication gain, M as

$$F(M) = kM + \left(2 - \frac{1}{M}\right)(1 - k) \qquad (9.65a)$$

Dark current or leakage current is a reverse leakage current that continues to flow through the device when no light is incident on the photodetector. Normally, it arises from the electrons or holes which are thermally generated near the p-n junction of a photodiode. In an APD, these carriers get multiplied by the avalanche gain mechanism. Thus, the mean square value of the dark current is given by:

$$\overline{i_d^2(t)} = \langle i_d^2(t) \rangle = 2eI_d M^2 F(M)\, \Delta f \qquad (9.66)$$

where I_d is the average primary dark current (before multiplication) of the detector.

Thermal (or *Johnson*) noise is a random fluctuation in current due to the thermally induced random motion of electrons in a conductor. The load resistance R_L adds such fluctuations to the current generated by the photodiode. The mean square value of this current is given by:

$$\langle i_T^2 \rangle = \frac{4kT}{R_L}\, \Delta f \qquad (9.67)$$

where k is Boltzmann's constant and T is the absolute temperature of the load resistor.

The noise power associated with the amplifier following the detector will depend on the active elements of the amplifier circuit. For the present discussion, let us assume that its mean square noise current is $\langle i_{\text{amp}}^2 \rangle$.

In general, therefore, the signal to noise ratio (S/N) of an optical receiver may be written as:

$$\frac{S}{N} = \frac{\langle i_p^2 \rangle M^2}{2e(I_p + I_d)\, \Delta f\, M^2 F(M) + \dfrac{2kT\Delta f}{R_L} + \langle i_{\text{amp}}^2 \rangle} \qquad (9.68)$$

When p-n and p-i-n photodiodes are used in the receiver, M and $F(M)$ become unity.

9.9.3 Quantum Noise

The mechanism of photodetection by a conventional photodetector is mainly based on the theory of interaction of light with matter, where the former is considered to be a stream of discrete particles called quanta, i.e. photons with energy $E = hv$. The absorption of a photon in the photodetector creates a pair of electron-hole. The discrete nature of arrival of photon and their subsequent creation of pairs of electron-hole randomly in the photodetector give rise to a form of noise called *quantum noise*. However, this noise actually originates from the very mechanism of the photodetection process. We may note that this process of the arrival of photons at the receiver is statistical in the primary photogenerated current arising due to random arrival of photons at the photodetector is a time varying Poisson's process. Now, if the photodetector detects on an average $\overline{N}$ number of photons then the probability $P(n)$ of detecting n number of photons in time period τ is governed by Poisson's distribution as

$$P(n) = \frac{\overline{N}^n}{n!} \exp(-\overline{N}) \tag{9.69}$$

We may note that there is an uncertainty associated with the number of electrons and holes actually generated in the detector by a given optical power incident on the receiver for a fixed duration. Further, this randomness in the total number of electron-hole pairs generated by the incident radiation is the source of this form of shot-noise termed *quantum-noise*.

In Eq. (9.69), $\overline{N}$ is actually the mean value and also corresponds to the variance of the distribution function. However, the special characteristic of Poisson's distribution is that the mean and the variance of the distribution function are the same. The rate of generation of electron-hole pairs by the incident photons, R, is given by

$$R = \eta \frac{P_{op}}{hv} \text{ per second} \tag{9.69a}$$

where, η is the efficiency of the photodetector.

Now, if the detector receives an optical radiation $P(t)$ over a period τ, the average number of electron-hole pairs during the period can be expressed as follows:

$$\overline{N} = \frac{\eta}{hv} \int_0^\tau P(t)\, dt = \frac{\eta E}{hv} \tag{9.69b}$$

where, E denotes the total optical energy received by the photodetector over the duration τ.

9.9.4 Quantum Limit

We have read that the quantum noise arises from the fundamental mechanism of operation of a photodetector. Now, if we ignore the presence of all other forms of noise in an optical detector system, we are left with the quantum noise which sets the fundamental lower limit of a photodetector system. Further, to appreciate the actual meaning of quantum limit, we consider a digital optical communication system transmitting light in the form of optical pulses, such that, the presence of optical pulse in a given bit period corresponds to the bit "1" and absence of light during a given bit period corresponds to bit "0". Let us now consider an ideal situation where there is no dark current produced by the photodetector and also there i no other form of noise. In such a situation, in the absence of light no current will be produced by the photodetector and even a single electron-hole pair produced by the light in the detector can be detected. This means, under such a situation, an error can only occur when light pulse is present and no electron-hole pair is produced by the photodetector to cause a flow of current in the external load. We can obtain the probability that no electron-hole pair is produced in presence of a light pulse from Eq. (9.69a) as

$$P(0/1) = P(0) = \exp(-\overline{N}) \tag{9.69c}$$

where, $P(0/1)$ corresponds to the probability that the received bit is interpreted as a "0" given that the bit "1" is being transmitted. However, this probability equals the probability that no electron-hole pair is produced in presence of a light pulse.

We may note that Eq. (9.69c) is valid under the ideal condition that no electron-hole pair is produced in the dark and also there is no other component of noise present in the receiver circuit. Further, Eq. (9.69) permits one to compute the ultimate limit called quantum limit in the *digital optical communication system*. Now, we can define the quantum limit as the minimum energy of light pulse required to maintain a given Bit Error Rate (BER).

9.10 RECEIVER ANALYSIS

This involves detection of signals with noise. In optical systems the information is transmitted using light which consists of photons (Fig. 9.68). Due to their statistical nature, the transmitted information will always show random fluctuations. Those fluctuations determine the lowest limit on transmitted power. In addition, there exist other noise contributions which originate from various processes. Some of them have already been discussed.

Digital signal under consideration operates at a bit rate B. The time slot (or bit interval) T is:

$$T = 1/B$$

and it is the inverse of the bit rate. The input data sequence in the communication system is denoted by $\{b_k\}$. The optical power $p(t)$ falling on the photodetector is the sequence of pulses and it is written as:

$$p(t) = \sum_{k=-\infty}^{k=+\infty} b_k \, h_p \, (t - k \cdot T) \tag{9.70}$$

where k is a parameter denoting the k-th time slot and $h_p(t)$ represents the pulse shape of an isolated optical pulse at the photodetector input.

It is assumed that:

$$\frac{1}{T} \int_{-\infty}^{+\infty} h_p(t) \, dt = 1 \tag{9.71}$$

so that b_k represents the received optical power in the k-th time slot.

Equation (9.70) is based on the assumption that the system consisting of transmitter and optical fiber is a linear one and time-invariant. b_k in Eq. (9.70) can take two values b_0 and b_1, which correspond to logical values in the k-th time slot being zero or one. In an ideal case, one would expect the b_0 to be zero so no optical power is transmitted for the logical zero. However, semiconductor lasers always operate at the nonzero bias current, so there is always some small optical power transmitted.

9.11 BER OF AN IDEAL OPTICAL RECEIVER

There are several ways to measure *bit error rate* (BER), that is the rate of error occurrence in a digital data stream. It is equal to number of errors occurring over some time interval divided by total number of pulses (both ones and zeros).

The simplest method to define BER is:

$$\text{BER} = \frac{N_e}{N_p} = \frac{N_e}{B \cdot t} \tag{9.72}$$

where N_e is the number of errors appearing over time interval t, N_p is the number of pulses transmitted during that interval, $B = 1/T$ is the bit rate and T is the bit interval or bit period.

The required BER for high-speed optical communication systems today is typically 10^{-12}, which means that on average one bit error is allowed for every terabit of data transmitted. BER depends on the various signal-to-noise ratio (SNR) of the fiber system, like the receiver noise level.

Direct optical detection is a process of determining the presence or absence of light during a bit interval. No light is interpreted as logical zero; some of the light present signals is logical one.

In a real life, the detection process is not so simple because of the random nature of photons arriving at the receiver. Their arrival is modelled as a Poisson random process. The random process, in time arrivals of photons at the photodetector is shown in Fig. 9.45.

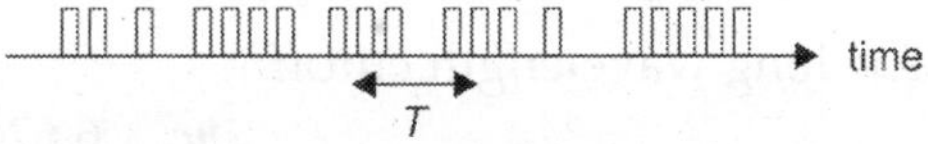

Fig. 9.45: Random arrivals of photons at photodetector are described by the Poisson process. Each photon is represented by a box and they all have the same amplitude

For an ideal optical receiver, we will assume that there are no noise sources in the system. The average number of photons arriving at the photodetector, with $h\nu_c$ being the energy of a single photon, is thus:

$$N = \frac{p(t)}{h\nu_c} \tag{9.73}$$

where $p(t)$ is power of light signal, h is Planck's constant and ν_c is the carrier frequency. The output power impinging on the photodetector is expressed by Eq. (9.70)

A simple expression for BER for ideal receiver (not noise) can be obtained as follows:

The probability that n photons are received during a bit interval T is:

$$e^{-\frac{N}{S}} \frac{\left(\frac{N}{B}\right)^n}{n!}$$

where N is the average number of photons given by Eq. (9.46). Probability of not receiving any photons ($n = 0$) is $\exp(-N/B)$. Assume equal probabilities of receiving zero and one. The BER of an ideal receiver is thus:

$$\text{BER} = \frac{1}{2}e^{-N/B} \equiv \frac{1}{2}e^{-M} \tag{9.74}$$

where $M = \dfrac{N}{B} = \dfrac{p}{h\nu_c B}$ represents the average number of photons received during one bit.

Equation (9.74) represents BER for an ideal receiver and it is called the *quantum limit*. To get a typical bit rate of 10^{-12}, the average number of photons is $M = 27$ per one bit.

Example 1

When 3×10^{11} photons each with a wavelength of 0.85 μm are incident on a photodiode, on an average 1.2×10^{11} electrons are collected at the terminals of the device. Calculate the quantum efficiency (η) and the responsivity (R) of the photodiode at 0.85 μm.

Solution

$$\eta = \frac{\text{Number of electrons collected}}{\text{Number of incident photons}} = \frac{1.2 \times 10^{11}}{3 \times 10^{11}} = 0.4$$

Thus, η of the photodiode at 0.85 μm is 40%.

$$R = \frac{\eta e \lambda}{hc} = \frac{0.4 \times 1.602 \times 10^{-19} \times 0.85 \times 10^{-6}}{6.626 \times 10^{-34} \times 3 \times 10^{8}} = 0.274 \text{ AW}^{-1}$$

Thus, R of the photodiode at 0.85 μm is 0.27 AW^{-1}.

Example 2

GaAs has a bandgap energy (E_g) of 1.43 eV at 300 K. Determine the wavelength (λ_c) above which an intrinsic photodetector fabricated from this material will cease to operate.

Solution

The long wavelength cutoff:

$$\lambda_c = \frac{hc}{E_g} = \frac{6.626 \times 10^{-34} \times 3 \times 10^{8}}{1.43 \times 1.602 \times 10^{-19}} = 0.867 \text{ μm}$$

Obviously, GaAs photoconductor will cease to operate above 0.867 μm.

Example 3

A p-n photodiode has a quantum efficiency (η) of 70% for photons of energy 1.52×10^{-19} J. Calculate (a) the wavelength at which the diode is operating, and (b) the optical power required to achieve a photocurrent of 3 μA when the wavelength of incident photons is that calculated in part (a). **[B Tech]**

Solution

(a) The photon energy

$$E = h\nu = \frac{hc}{\lambda}$$

Therefore, $\lambda = \dfrac{hc}{E} = \dfrac{6.626 \times 10^{-34} \times 3 \times 10^{8}}{1.52 \times 10^{-19}} = 1.30 \times 10^{-6} \text{ m}$

$$= 1.30 \text{ μm}$$

(b) $R = \dfrac{\eta e}{h\nu} = \dfrac{0.70 \times 1.6 \times 10^{-19}}{1.52 \times 10^{-19}} = 0.736 \text{ AW}^{-1}$

Since $R = \dfrac{I_p}{P_{in}}$, $P_{in} = \dfrac{I_p}{R} = \dfrac{3 \times 10^{-6}}{0.736}$

or $\quad P_{in} = 4.07 \times 10^{-6} \text{ W} = 4.07 \text{ μW}$.

Example 4

A photodiode has a quantum efficiency (η) of 65% when photons of energy 1.5×10^{-19} J are incident upon it. Calculate: (a) at what wave-length is the photodiode operating?

(b) the incident optical power required to obtain a photocurrent of 2.5 µA when the photodiode is operating as stated above. **[B Tech]**

Solution

We have:

Photon energy $h\nu = hc/\lambda$

$\therefore$ $$\lambda = \frac{hc}{E} = \frac{6.626 \times 10^{-34} \times 3 \times 10^8}{1.5 \times 10^{-19}} = 1.32 \text{ µm}$$

Thus, the photodiode is operating at a wavelength of 1.32 µm.

Responsivity $$R = \frac{\eta e}{h\nu} = \frac{0.65 \times 1.602 \times 10^{-19}}{1.5 \times 10^{-19}} = 0.964 \text{ AW}^{-1}$$

We have $$R = \frac{I_o}{P_o}$$

$\therefore$ $$P_o = \frac{I_o}{R} = \frac{2.5 \times 10^{-6}}{0.694} = 3.60 \text{ µW}$$

Clearly, the incident optical power required is 3.60 µW.

Example 5

Photons of wavelength 0.90 µm are incident on a *p-n* photodiode at a rate of 5×10^{10} s^{-1} and, on an average, the electrons are collected at the terminals of the diode at the rate of 2×10^{10} s^{-1}. Calculate (a) the quantum efficiency (η), and (b) the responsivity (R) of the diode at this wavelength. **[B Tech]**

Solution

(a) $$\eta = \frac{2 \times 10^{10}}{5 \times 10^{10}} = 0.40$$

(b) $$R = \frac{\eta e \lambda}{hc} = \frac{0.40 \times 1.6 \times 10^{-19} \times 0.90 \times 10^{-6}}{6.626 \times 10^{-34} \times 3 \times 10^8} = 0.29 \text{ AW}^{-1}$$

Example 6

A *p-i-n* photodiode has an intrinsic region with a width of 20 µm and a radius of 500 µm in which the drift velocity of electrons is 10^5 ms^{-1}. When the permittivity of the device material is 10.5×10^{-13} F cm^{-1}, calculate: (a) the drift time of the carriers across the depletion region; (b) the junction capacitance of the photodiode. **[B Tech]**

Solution

We have the drift time for the carriers across the depletion region for the photodiode:

$$t_{\text{drift}} = \frac{W}{V_d} = \frac{20 \times 10^{-6}}{1 \times 10^5} = 2 \times 10^{-10} \text{ s}$$

Thus, the drift time for the carriers across the depletion region is 200 ps.

The junction capacitance:

$$C_j = \frac{\varepsilon_s A}{W} = \frac{10.5 \times 10^{-13} \times 0.79 \times 10^{-6}}{20 \times 10^{-6}} = 0.41 \times 10^{-13} = 4 \text{ pF.}$$

Here, $$A = \pi r^2 = 3.14 \times (500 \times 10^{-6})^2 \approx 0.79 \times 10^{-6} \text{ m}^2$$

Example 7

A *p-i-n* photodiode, on an average, generates one electron-hole pair per two incident photons at a wavelength of 0.85 µm. Assuming all the photo-generated electrons are collected, calculate (a) the quantum efficiency of the diode: (b) the maximum possible band gap energy (in eV) of the semiconductor, assuming the incident wavelength to be a long-wavelength cut-off; and (c) the mean output photocurrent when the incident optical power is 10 µW.

Solution

(a) $\eta = \dfrac{1}{2} = 0.5 = 50\%$

(b) $E_g = \dfrac{hc}{\lambda_c} = \dfrac{6.626 \times 10^{-34} \times 3 \times 10^8}{0.85 \times 10^{-6}} = 2.33 \times 10^{-19}\ \text{J} = 1.46\ \text{eV}$

(c) $I_P = RP_{in} = \dfrac{\eta e}{h\nu} P_{in} = \dfrac{0.5 \times 1.6 \times 10^{-19}}{2.33 \times 10^{-19}} \times 10 \times 10^{-6} = 3.43 \times 10^{-6}\ \text{A}$

$\quad\quad = 3.43\ \mu\text{A}$

Example 8

The carrier velocity in a silicon photodiode with a 25 µm depletion layer width is $3 \times 10^4\ \text{ms}^{-1}$. Calculate the maximum response time for the device. **[B Tech]**

Solution

The maximum 3 dB bandwidth for the photodiode may be obtained from:

$$B_m = \frac{V_d}{2\pi w} = \frac{3 \times 10^4}{2\pi \times 25 \times 10^{-6}} = 1.91 \times 10^8\ \text{Hz}$$

Maximum response time for the device $= \dfrac{1}{B_m} = \dfrac{1}{1.91 \times 10^8} = 5.2\ \text{ns}$

Example 9

A germanium *p-i-n* photodiode with an active area dimensions of 100×50 µm has a quantum efficiency (η) of 60% when operating at a wavelength 1.2 µm. The measured dark current is 10 nA. Calculate the noise equivalent power and specific directivity of the device. Assume that dark current is the main source of noise. **[B Tech]**

Solution

We have, the noise equivalent power.

Here:

$I_B = 10\ \text{nA} = 10 \times 10^{-9}\ \text{A}$

$\eta = 0.6$

$\lambda = 1.2 \times 10^{-6}\ \text{m}$

$\text{NEP} = \dfrac{hc\,(2eI_D)^{1/2}}{\eta e \lambda}$

$\quad = \dfrac{6.62 \times 10^{-34} \times 3 \times 10^8\ (2 \times 1.6 \times 10^{-19} \times 10 \times 10^{-9})^{1/2}}{0.6 \times 1.6 \times 10^{-19} \times 1.2 \times 10^{-6}} = 9.8 \times 10^{-14}\ \text{W}$

Specific directivity:

$$D^* = DA^{1/2} = \frac{\eta e \lambda}{hc \left(\dfrac{2eI_D}{A} \right)^{1/2}} = \frac{A^{1/2}}{\text{NEP}}$$

$$= \frac{(100 \times 10^{-6} \times 50 \times 10^{-6})^{1/2}}{9.8 \times 10^{-14}} = 7 \times 10^8 \text{ mHz}^{1/2} \cdot \text{W}^{-1}$$

Example 10

A silicon RAPD, operating at a wavelength of 0.80 μm, exhibits a quantum efficiency of 90%, a multiplication factor of 800, and a dark current of 2 nA. Calculate the rate at which photons should be incident on the device so that the output current (after avalanche gain) is greater than the dark current. **[B Tech]**

Solution

$$I = I_P M = P_{in} R M = P_{in} \left(\frac{\eta e \lambda}{hc} \right) M = \left(\frac{P_{in}}{hc/\lambda} \right) \eta e M = [(\text{photon rate}) e] \eta M$$

For $I = 2$ nA:

$$\text{Photon rate} = \frac{I}{e\eta M} = \frac{2 \times 10^{-9}}{1.6 \times 10^{-19} \times 0.90 \times 800} = 1736 \times 10^7 \text{ s}^{-1}$$

For $\quad I > 2$ nA:

$$\text{Photon rate} \approx 1.74 \times 10^7 \text{ s}^{-1}$$

Example 11

In a 100 ns pulse, 6×10^6 photons at a wavelength of 1300 nm fall on an InGaAs photodetector. On an average, 5.4×10^6 electron-hole (e-h) pairs are generated. Calculate the quantum efficiency (η). **[MSc (Ele)]**

Solution

$$\eta = \frac{\text{number of } e\text{-}h \text{ pairs generated}}{\text{number of incident photons}} = \frac{5.4 \times 10^6}{6 \times 10^6} = 0.90$$

Thus, at 1300 nm, $\eta = 90\%$.

Example 12

The quantum efficiency (η) for the wavelength range 1300 nm $< \lambda <$ 1600 nm for InGaAs is around 90%. Calculate the responsivity (R) and cutoff wavelength. **[B Tech]**

Solution

$$R = \frac{\eta e}{h\nu} = \frac{\eta e \lambda}{hc} = \frac{(0.90 \times 1.6 \times 10^{-19}) \lambda}{(6.62 \times 10^{-34})(3 \times 10^8)} = 7.25 \times 10^5 \lambda$$

At 1300 nm, we have:

$$R = 7.25 \times 10^5 \left(\frac{\text{AW}}{\text{m}} \right) (1.30 \times 10^{-6} \text{ m}) = 0.92 \text{ AW}^{-1}$$

At wavelength higher than 1600 nm, the photon energy is not sufficient to excite an electron from the valence band to the conduction band, e.g. $In_{0.53}Ga_{0.47}As$ has an energy gap $E_g = 0.73$ eV. Thus, the cutoff wavelength is:

$$\lambda_c = \frac{1.24}{E_g} = \frac{1.24}{0.73} = 1.73 \text{ μm}$$

We may note that at wavelength less than 1100 nm, the photons are absorbed very close to the photodetector surface, where the combination rate of the generated electron-hole pairs is very short. The responsivity (R) thus decreases rapidly for smaller wavelengths, since many of the generated carriers do not contribute to the photocurrent.

Example 13

An APD has a quantum efficiency (η) of 40% and 1.3 μm. When illuminated with optical power of 0.3 μW at this wavelength, it produces an output photocurrent of 6 μA, after avalanche gain. Calculate the multiplication factor (M) of the diode.　　　**[B Tech]**

Solution

$$M = \frac{I}{I_P} = \frac{I}{P_{in}R} = \frac{I}{P_{in}\left(\dfrac{\eta e\lambda}{hc}\right)} = \frac{I\,(hc)}{P_{in}\,(\eta e\lambda)}$$

$$= \frac{6\times10^{-6}\times(6.626\times10^{-34}\times3\times10^{8})}{0.3\times10^{-6}\times(0.4\times1.6\times10^{-19}\times1.3\times10^{-6})} = 47.6.$$

Example 14

A silicon avalanche photodiode has a quantum efficiency of 65% at a wavelength of 900 nm. Suppose 0.5 μW of optical power produces a multiplied photocurrent of 10 μA. Find the multiplication M.

Solution

We have the primary photocurrent

$$I_p = R\,P_{in} = \frac{\eta e}{h\nu}P_{in} = \frac{\eta e\lambda}{hc}P_{in}$$

$$= \frac{(0.65)\,(1.6\times10^{-19})\,(9\times10^{-7})}{(6.62\times10^{-34})\,(3\times10^{8})}\times5\times10^{-7} = 0.235\,\mu A$$

$\therefore$ Multiplication factor: $M = \dfrac{I_M}{I_p} = \dfrac{10\,\mu A}{0.235\,\mu A} = 43$

This means that the primary photocurrent is multiplied by a factor of 43.

Example 15

An InGaAs p-i-n photodiode has the following parameters at a wavelength of 1300 nm: $I_D = 4$ nA, $\eta = 0.90$, $R_L = 1000\,\Omega$ and the surface leakage current is negligible. The incident optical power is 300 nW (-35 dBm), and the receiver bandwidth is 20 MHz. Calculate the various noise terms of the receiver.

Solution

We have:　　　　$I_p = R\,P_{in} = \dfrac{\eta e}{h\nu}P_{in} = \dfrac{\eta e\lambda}{hc}P_{in}$

Substituting　　　$I_p = \dfrac{(0.90)\,(1.6\times10^{-19})\,(1.3\times10^{-6})}{(6.62\times10^{-34})\,(3\times10^{8})}\times3\times10^{-7} = 0.282\,\mu A$

Mean square shot noise current for p-i-n photodiode is given by:

$$\langle I_{shot}^2\rangle = 2eI_pBe = 2\times1.6\times10^{-19}\times0.282\times10^{-6}\times20\times10^{6} = 1.80\times10^{-18}\text{ A}^2$$

or　　　$\langle I_{shot}^2\rangle^{1/2} = 1.34\text{ mA}$

Mean square dark current:

$$\langle I_{DB}^2 \rangle = 2eI_D B$$
$$= 2 \times 1.6 \times 10^{-19} \times 4 \times 10^{-9} \times 20 \times 10^6 = 2.56 \times 10^{-20} \text{ A}^2$$

$$\therefore \qquad \langle I_{DB}^2 \rangle^{1/2} = 0.16 \text{ nA}$$

Mean square thermal noise current: We have:

$$\langle I_T^2 \rangle = \frac{4k_B T}{R_L} B = \frac{4 \times 1.38 \times 10^{-23} \times 293 \text{ K} \times 20 \times 10^6}{1 \text{ k}\Omega}$$
$$= 323 \times 10^{-18} \text{ A}^2$$

$$\therefore \qquad \langle I_T^2 \rangle^{1/2} = 18 \text{ nA}$$

We see that for this receiver, the *rms* thermal noise current is about 14 times greater than the *rms* shot noise current and about 100 times greater than *rms* dark current.

Example 16

A low-impedance (LZ) optical receiver front-end uses a photodetector bias resistance of 50 Ω which to matched to the following stage amplifier with the same value of input resistance. The input capacitance of the photodetector is 5 pF whereas the input capacitance of the amplifier is only 3 pF. Show that the values of the bandwidth and the mean-square value of the thermal noise component of the receiver end are 796.18 MHz and 5.27×10^{-13} A^2 respectively. **[DTU, KTU]**

Solution

We have

Bias resistance, $R_b = 50$ Ω

Input resistance of the amplifier = 50 Ω

Now, the effective resistance

$$R_T = \frac{50 \times 50}{50 + 50} = 25 \text{ }\Omega$$

The overall capacitance of the front end is

$$C_T = 5 \text{ pF} + 3 \text{ pF} = 8 \text{ pF}$$

Now, the bandwidth of the given LZ front-end

$$B = \frac{1}{2\pi R_T C_T}$$
$$= \frac{1}{2 \times 3.14 \times 25 \times 8 \times 10^{-12}} = 796.18 \text{ MHz}$$

The mean value of the thermal noise current generated by LZ front-end

$$\langle i_T^2 \rangle = 4kT \left(\frac{1}{R_T} \right) B$$
$$= 4 \times 1.38 \times 10^{-23} \times 300 \times \frac{1}{25} \times 796.18 \times 10^6 \text{ A}^2 \text{ Hz}^{-1}$$
$$= 5.27 \times 10^{-13} \text{ A}^2 \text{ Hz}^{-1}$$

Example 17

A high-impedance (HZ) optical receiver front-end uses a photodetector bias resistance of 5 MΩ which is matched to the stage amplifier having the same value of input resistance.

Given, the input capacitance of the photodetector is 4 pF while the input capacitance of the amplifier is 6 pF. Find the values of the bandwidth and the mean square value of the thermal noise component per unit bandwidth of the receiver front end.

[MHTU, MPTU]

Solution

Given, bias resistance and the input resistance of the amplifier

$$R_b = 5 \text{ M}\Omega \text{ and } R_b = 5 \text{ M}\Omega$$

Now, the effective resistance

$$R_T = \frac{R_b \, R_a}{R_b + R_a} = \frac{5 \times 5}{5 + 5} = 2.5 \text{ M}\Omega$$

The overall capacitance of the front-end is

$$C_T = 4 \text{ pF} + 6 \text{ pF} = 10 \text{ pF}$$

We can now estimate the bandwidth of the given HZ front-end without equalization as

$$B = \frac{1}{2\pi R_T C_T}$$

$$= \frac{1}{2 \times 3.14 \times 2.5 \times 10^6 \times 8 \times 10^{-12}} = 6.34 \text{ kHz}$$

One can improve the bandwidth of HZ front-end configuration by using equalizer circuit following the pre-amplifier.

Now, the mean square value of the thermal noise current generated by the HZ front-end can be obtained as

$$\langle i_T^2 \rangle = 4 \, kT \left(\frac{1}{R_T} \right) B$$

$$= 4 \times 1.38 \times 10^{-23} \times 300 \times 10^{-6} \text{ A}^2 \text{ Hz}^{-1}$$

$$= 6.624 \times 10^{-27} \text{ A}^2 \text{ Hz}^{-1}$$

SUMMARY

- In an optical fiber system, it is required to convert the optical signals at the receiver end back into electrical signal. This task is performed by an optical receiver system. Optical receiver converts optical energy into electrical signal, amplify the signal and process it.
- The important blocks of an optical receiver are:
  (i) Photodetector/front end
  (ii) Amplifier/linear channel
  (iii) Signal processing circuitary/data recovery.
- The aim of a receiver is the recovery of the transmitted data. This process involves two steps:
  (i) the recovery of bit clock
  (ii) the recovery of transmitted bit within each bit interval.
- A good light detector should generate a large photocurrent at a given incident light power. They should also respond fast to the input changes and add minimal noise to the output signal. This last requirement is of crucial importance since the received

signal is typically very weak. In digital optical communication systems, the detection process is often conducted with a PIN photodiode.

- There are generally two types of detection: direct detection (also called incoherent detection) and coherent detection.

- *Direct detection* detects only the *intensity* of the incident light. It is used mainly for intensity or amplitude modulation schemes. It can only detect an amplitude modulated (AM) signal.

- *Coherent detection* can detect both the power and phase of the incident light. It is, therefore, used when phase modulation (PM) or frequency modulation (FM) is preferred. Coherent detection is also important in applications such as WDM.

- The *coherent detection* requires a local oscillator to coherently down-convert the modulated signal from optical frequency to intermediate frequency.

- The *incoherent detection* which dominates in currently deployed systems is based on square-law envelope detection of the optical signals.

- A reverse biased *p-n junction* is used for conversion of the optical signals at the receiver end back into electrical signals. An incidence photon of energy ($h\nu$) greater than the band gap of the semiconductor creates an electron-hole pair. The two charge carriers are swept in opposite directions by the applied bias, and photocurrent flows in the external circuit.

- The photocurrent (I_p) depends on the absorption coefficient (α) of the semiconductor for incident wavelength. The relation between I_p and α is:

$$I_p = \frac{P_{in}\,(1-R)\,e}{h\nu}\,[1 - \exp(-\alpha d)]$$

where P_{in} is power incident on the photodiode, R is Fresnel reflection coefficient at the air-semiconductor interface, d is the width of the absorption region.

- The *quantum efficiency* (η) of a device is the ratio of the rate of electrons collected at the diode terminals to the rate of photons incident on it. η is related to the responsivity (R) of the detector by the relation:

$$R = \frac{\eta e}{h\nu} = \frac{\eta e \lambda}{hc}$$

- The absorption of photon of energy ($h\nu$) is possible only when its energy is greater than or equal to the energy gap (E_g) of the semiconductor, i.e. $hc/\lambda \geq E_g$. Therefore, there is a long wavelength cutoff λ_c, above which photons are not absorbed by the semiconductor. λ_c is given by:

$$\lambda_c\,(\mu m) = \frac{hc}{E_g} = \frac{1.24}{E_g\,(eV)}$$

- Photodiodes are of three types: (i) *p-n*, (ii) *p-i-n*, and (iii) Avalanche photodiodes. The first two diodes produce current without gain, whereas the third one produces current with gain. One can use photoconductivity detectors for long wavelength operations.

- Main characteristics of optical receivers are:

  (i) *Receiver sensitivity*: This property is a measure of the minimum level of optical power P_{sens} at the receiver required for a reliable operation.

(ii) *Dynamic range*: Dynamic range (in dB) is the difference between the maximum allowable power and minimum power determined by receiver sensitivity.

(iii) *Bit-rate transparency*: This refers to the ability of the optical receiver to operate over a range of bit rates.

(iv) *Bit-pattern independency*: This determines the operation of an optical receiver for various data formats. The main constraint is imposed by non-return-to-zero (NRZ) code.

- Performance evaluation of an optical transmission system is done by evaluating optical signal-to-noise ratio, eye opening and bit error rate (BER) which is the ultimate indicator.

REVIEW QUESTIONS

1. Explain the principle and working of optical receivers.

2. Explain the detection process in a *p-n* photodiode. Compare the device with *p-i-n* photodiode.

3. Explain the quantum efficiency (η) and responsivity (R) of a photodiode. Derive the relation between η and R.

4. Draw the layer diagram and explain the operation of *p-i-n* diode. Draw diagrams for three practical photodiodes and show that the detector current is given by:

$$I_p = \frac{eP_o}{\eta f} [1 - \exp(-\alpha(\lambda) W)(1 - R_f)$$

where R_f is reflectivity, W is the width of the depletion layer, η is quantum efficiency and P_o is optical power.

5. What is the difference between *p-n* diode, *p-i-n* diode and an APO? Can we make these types of photodiodes using the same semiconductor?

6. Define the quantum efficiency (η) of photodiode and show that:

$$\eta = \frac{I_p}{P_o} \frac{h\nu}{e} [1 - \exp\{(-\alpha(\lambda) W)\}] (1 - R_f)$$

Also define responsivity (R) and show that:

$$R = \eta \frac{e}{h\nu} = \frac{e}{h\nu} (1 - R_f)[1 - \exp\{(-\alpha(\lambda) W)\}]$$

where I_p is average photocurrent, P_o is optical power, R_f is effect of reflectivity, $\alpha(\lambda)$ is absorption coefficient at the opening wavelength and W is width of depletion layer.

7. Explain, why the responsivity (R) vs wavelength (λ) curve for a practical Si diode deviate from an ideal curve? How, one can improve the quantum efficiency of such a diode?

8. Describe with the help of a relevant diagram the operation of a silicon RAPD and explain how it differs from a *p-i-n* photodiode. Outline the advantages and drawbacks of RAPD as detector in optical fiber communication.

9. The avalanche photodiode and photoconducting detector both provide gain. Compare their merits for their use in optical fiber communication and other applications.

10. Describe the different types of noise encountered in a photodetector.

PROBLEMS

1. Calculate the cutoff wavelength for Si and Ge *p-i-n* photodiodes. Their bandgap energies are 1.1 eV and 0.67 eV respectively.

   [**Hint.** $\lambda_c = \dfrac{hc}{E_g} = \dfrac{1.24}{E_g \ (eV)}$

   $h = 6.62 \times 10^{-34}$

   $c = 3 \times 10^8$

   (i) For Si, $\lambda_c = \dfrac{6.62 \times 10^{-34} \times 3 \times 10^8}{1.1 \times 10^{-19}} = 1.8 \times 10^{-6}$ m $= 1.8\ \mu$m

   (ii) For Ge, $\lambda_c = \dfrac{6.62 \times 10^{-34} \times 3 \times 10^8}{0.67 \times 10^{-19}} = 2.96 \times 10^{-6}$ m $= 2.96\ \mu$m]

2. A *p-i-n* photodiode is fabricated by GaAs which has bandgap energy 1.43 eV at 300 K. Calculate its upper cutoff wavelength.

   [**Hind.** $\lambda_c = \dfrac{hc}{E_g} = \dfrac{6.62 \times 10^{-34} \times 3 \times 10^8}{1.43 \times 10^{-19}} = 1.33 \times 10^{-6}$ m $= 1.33$ m]

3. A *p-n* photodiode has a quantum efficiency (η) = 50% at $\lambda = 0.90\ \mu$m. Calculate (a) its responsivity (R) at this wavelength, (b) the optical power received for mean photocurrent 10^{-6}A, and (c) the corresponding number of photon received at this wavelength. **[B Tech]**

   [**Ans.** (a) 0.36 AW^{-1}, (b) 2.76 μW, (c) $\eta_p = 1.25 \times 10^{13}$ s^{-1}]

4. A pulse of 85 ns emits 6×10^6 photons at 1300 nm wavelength from an InGaAs photoconductor. Average number of *e-h* pairs generated are 5.4×10^6. Calculate quantum efficiency (η) of the detector. **(MSc (Ele)**

   [**Hint.** $\eta = \dfrac{\text{Number of } e-h \text{ pairs generated}}{\text{Number of incident photons}}$

   $= \dfrac{5.4 \times 10^6}{6 \times 10^6} = 0.9 = 90\%$]

5. Calculate the responsivity of an ideal *p-n* photodiode at the following wavelengths: (a) 0.85 μm, (b) 1.35 μm, and (c) 1.55 μm. **[BSc (Ele)]**

   [**Ans.** (a) 0.684 AW^{-1}, (b) 1.046 AW^{-1}, (c) 1.248 AW^{-1}]

6. Photons having energy 1.53×10^{-19} J are incident on a photodiode having responsivity (R) = 0.65 AW^{-1}. If output power (P_o) = 10 μW, calculate the generated photocurrent. **[B Tech]**

   [**Hint.** $R = \dfrac{I_P}{P_o}$ or $I_P = RP_o = 0.65 \times 10 = 6.5\ \mu$A]

7. The quantum efficiency (η) of an APD is 50% at 1.3 μm. When this APD is illuminated with optical power of 0.4 μW, this wavelength, it produces an output photocurrent of 0.8 μA, after avalanch gain. Show that the multiplication factor of diode is 30.

8. Compute the bandwidth (W) of a photodetectors having parameters as: (a) photodiode capacitance = 3 pF (ii) amplifier capacitance = 4 pF (iii) load resistance (R_L) = 50 Ω (iv) amplifier input resistance = 1 MΩ.

[**Hint.** Total capacitance of photodiode and amplifier:

$$C_T = 3 + 4 = 7 \text{ pF}$$

Combination of load resistance and amplifier input resistance:

$$R_L = 50 \ \Omega \ || \ 1 \ \text{M}\Omega \approx 50 \ \Omega$$

Bandwidth of photodetector:

$$W = \frac{1}{2\pi R_L C_T} = \frac{1}{2 \times 3.14 \times 50 \times 7 \times 10^{-12}} = 454.95 \text{ MHz}]$$

9. A typical photodiode has a responsivity $(R) = 0.40 \text{ AW}^{-1}$ for a He-Ne laser source $(\lambda = 632.8 \text{ nm})$. The active area of the photo-diode is 2 mm^2. If the incident flux is 100 μW/mm^2, calculate the output photocurrent. [**Ans.** 80 μA]

10. The maximum 3 dB bandwidth permitted by an InGaAs photo-conducting detector is 450 MHz when the electron transit time in the device is 6 ps. Calculate (a) the gain G, and (b) the output photo-current when an optical power of 5 μW at a wavelength of 1.30 μm is incident on it, assuming quantum efficiency of 75%.

[**Hint.** We know that the current response in the photoconductor decays exponentially with time once the incident optical pulse is removed. The time constant of this decay is equal to the slow carrier transit time t_s. Therefore, the maximum 3 dB bandwidth (Δf_m) of the device will be given by:

$$(\Delta f)_m = \frac{1}{2\pi t_s} = \frac{1}{2\pi t_f G} \qquad \left(\because G = \frac{t_s}{t_f} \right)$$

(a) $G = \dfrac{1}{2\pi t_f (\Delta f)_m} = \dfrac{1}{2\pi \times 6 \times 10^{-12} \times 450 \times 10^6} = 58.94$

(b) $I = G I_p = \dfrac{G \eta P_{in} e \lambda}{hc}$

$$= \frac{58.94 \times 0.75 \times 5 \times 10^{-6} \times 1.6 \times 10^{-19} \times 1.3 \times 10^{-6}}{6.626 \times 10^{-34} \times 3 \times 10^8}$$

$$= 232.1 \ \mu\text{A} = 2.321 \times 10^{-4} \text{ A}]$$

11. A given APD has a quantum efficiency (η) of 65% at wavelength of 900 nm. If a 0.5 μW of optical power produced a multiplied photo-current of 10 μA, calculate the multiplication factor (m).

[**Hint.** $R = \dfrac{\eta e \lambda}{hc} = \dfrac{0.65 \times 1.6 \times 10^{-19} \times 900 \times 10^{-9}}{6.62 \times 10^{-34} \times 3 \times 10^8} = 0.47 \text{ AW}^{-1}$

Photocurrent, $I_p = P_{in} \times R = 0.5 \times 10^{-6} \times 0.4705 = 0.235 \ \mu$A

Multiplication factor $(M) = \dfrac{I_M}{I_p} = \dfrac{10 \times 10^{-6}}{0.235 \times 10^{-6}} = 42.55]$

12. An InGaAs p-i-n photodiode is operating at room temperature (300 K) at a wavelength of 1.3 μm. Its quantum efficiency (η) is 70% and the incident optical power is 500 nW. Take the primary dark current I_d of the device is 5 nA, R_L is a kΩ, and the effective bandwidth is 25 MHz. Calculate (a) the rms values of shot noise current, dark current, and thermal noise current (b) S/N at the input end of an amplifier of the receiver. [**B Tech**]

[Hint.

(a) $I_P = RP_{in} = \dfrac{\eta e \lambda}{hc} P_{in}$

$$I_P = \dfrac{0.70 \times 1.6 \times 10^{-19} \times 1.3 \times 10^{-6}}{6.626 \times 10^{34} \times 3 \times 10^{8}} \times 500 \times 10^{-9}$$

$\qquad = 3.663 \times 10^{-7} \text{ A} = 0.3662 \text{ } \mu A$

$\langle i_s^2 \rangle = 2e I_p (\Delta f) M^2 F(M)$

$\qquad = 2 \times 1.6 \times 10^{-19} \times 3.662 \times 10^{-7} \times 25 \times 10^{6} \times 1 \times 1$

$\qquad = 293.03 \times 10^{-20} \text{ A}^2$

$\langle i_s^2 \rangle^{1/2} = 17.15 \times 10^{-10} \text{ A} = 1.715 \text{ nA}$

$\langle i_s^2 \rangle^{1/2} = 2e I_d (\Delta f)$ (M and $F(M)$ are unity)

$\qquad = 2 \times 1.6 \times 10^{-19} \times 5 \times 10^{-19} \times 25 \times 10^{6}$

$\qquad = 400 \times 10^{-22} \text{ A}^2 = 4 \times 10^{-20} \text{ A}^2$

$\langle i_d^2 \rangle^{1/2} = 20 \times 10^{-11} \text{ A} = 0.2 \text{ nA}$

$\langle i_T^2 \rangle = \dfrac{4kT(\Delta f)}{R_L} = \dfrac{4 \times 1.38 \times 10^{-23} (J/K) \times 300(K)}{1,000} \times 25 \times 10^{6}$

$\qquad = 414 \times 10^{-18} \text{ A}^2$

(b) Sum of mean square noise current $= 41698.16 \times 10^{-20} \text{ A}^2$

$\qquad\qquad\qquad\qquad\qquad\qquad\qquad = 4.17 \times 10^{-16} \text{ A}^2$

and $I_p^2 = 1.352 \times 10^{-13} \text{ A}^2$

$\dfrac{S}{N} = \dfrac{1.352 \times 10^{-13}}{4.17 \times 10^{-16}} = 0.324 \times 10^{3} = 324]$

13. To maintain a bit-error rate a fiber optic link operating at 870 nm is required. Find the theoretical quantum limit of the receiver system in terms of quantum efficiency of the photodetector and also the energy of the incident photon. Show that the minimum optical power required to maintain the above bit-error-rate is $\approx 57 \text{ pW}$ ($= -72.45$ dBm) assuming that the system uses a binary signaling operating at 500 Mbps and quantum efficiency of photodetector is 100%.   **[PTU, MHTU]**

[Hint: One can decide the probability of error by the BER to be maintained by the system. Thus, we have

$$P(0) = \exp(-\overline{N}) = BER = 10^{-9}$$

or $\qquad \overline{N} = 20.7$

Obviously, around 20.7 number of photons are required to detect a binary "1" in digital binary "1" in digital binary signaling with a bit error rate of 10^{-9}.

The minimum pulse energy $E = E_{min}$ (say) corresponding to the quantum limit can be obtained as

$$20.7 = \dfrac{\eta E_{min}}{h\nu}$$

or $\qquad E_{min} = 20.7 \left(\dfrac{hc}{\lambda \eta} \right)$ $\qquad\qquad\qquad\qquad\qquad$ (i)

Now, for binary signaling with a bit period of τ and average power P_0, the energy can be expressed as

$$E_{min} = P_0\tau \tag{ii}$$

Using Eqs (i) and (ii), the average power for binary signaling can be obtained as

$$P_0 = 20.7\left(\frac{hc}{\lambda\tau\eta}\right) \tag{iii}$$

The bit period is related to the bit-rate, B can be obtained by assuming equal number of "0" and "1" bits as

$$\frac{B}{2} = \frac{1}{\tau} \tag{iv}$$

Now, using the above relationship, the average power can be obtained as

$$P_0 = 20.7\left(\frac{hcB}{2\lambda\eta}\right) \tag{v}$$

Here, $\lambda = 870$ nm, $B = 500$ MHz and $\eta = 1$

Substituting these values in (v), we obtain

$$P_0 = 20.7\left(\frac{6.62\times10^{-34}\times3\times10^8\times500\times10^6}{2\times870\times10^{-9}\times1}\right) \approx 57 \text{ pW}$$

In terms of dBm, one can estimate the average power as

$$= 10\log_{10}\frac{57\times10^{-12}}{10^{-3}}$$

$$= 10\log_{10}(57\times10^{-9})$$

$$= 17.55 - 90 = -72.45 \text{ dBm}]$$

SHORT ANSWER QUESTIONS

1. What is an optical receiver?

   Ans. An optical receiver is an essential part of an optical fiber communication system. An optical receiver converts an optical signal, transmitted through an optical fiber cable into an electrical signal suitable for a receiving device installed at the other end of the communication system. The conversion process in the receiver is performed by two essential parts: (i) *photodetector*, and (ii) an *electronic signal processor*.

2. What is the function of a photodetector?

   Ans. The photodetector senses the luminescent power falling upon it and converts the variation of this optical power into a correspondingly varying electric current.

3. How many types of photodetectors are in existence?

   Ans. Several different types of photodetectors are in existence. Among these are photomultipliers, pyroelectric detectors, and semi-conductor based photoconductors, phototransistors, and photodiodes.

4. What is the function of electronic signal processor?

   Ans. The electronic signal processor converts the raw detector signal into a form decipherable by the receiving device, such as a telephone, camera, or a scanner.

5. Of the semiconductor-based photodetectors, which is used almost exclusively for fiber optic systems and why?

Ans. Photodiode is used almost exclusively for fiber optic communication system because of its small size, suitable material, high sensitivity, and fast response time.

6. For efficient operation should a detector have a high or low responsivity?

   Ans. High.

7. Which two types of photodiodes are used in fiber optic communication?

   Ans. (i) *p-i-n* photodiode (ii) Avalanche photodiode (APD).

8. What is photocurrent?

   Ans. The current produced when photons are incident on the active area of the detector.

9. What is responsivity?

   Ans. The ratio of optical detector's output photocurrent in amperes to the incident power in watts.

$$R = \frac{I_p \, (A)}{P_{in} \, (W)} \, (\text{in Aw}^{-1})$$

10. How are *p-i-n* photodiodes usually biased?

    Ans. Usually reverse-biased.

11. What is dark current or leakage current?

    Ans. The leakage current that continuous to flow through a photodetector when there is no incident light.

12. Whether dark current increase or decrease as the temperature of photodiode increases?

    Ans. Increases.

13. How upper wavelength cutoff (λ_c) is related to band gap energy?

    Ans. $\lambda_c \, (\mu m) = \dfrac{h_c}{E_g} = \dfrac{1.24}{E_g \, (eV)}$

14. On what factors the fraction of light absorbed by the photodiode depends.

    Ans. (i) Wavelength (λ) of the light, determined by the photon energy ($\varepsilon = h\nu = hc/\lambda$). (ii) The thickness of the absorption material (depletion region width or depletion layer thickness).

15. Why it is important to control the dark current below a certain value?

    Ans. Low leakage current is an important measure of device quality. If the dark current is high, the generated photocurrent needs to be larger, in order to provide a good signal. Otherwise, the leakage current will dominate the detector current. This is why, it is important to control the dark current below the dark current.

16. Should the capacitance of photodetector be small or large? Explain why?

    Ans. Small. This prevents RC time constant from limiting the response time.

17. What is quantum efficiency (η) of a device?

    Ans. The ratio of the rate of electrons collected at the diode terminals to the rate of photons incident on it is called the quantum efficiency of a device.

18. How the quantum efficiency (η) of a device is related to its responsivity (R).

    Ans. $R = \dfrac{\eta e \lambda}{hc} = \dfrac{\eta e}{h\nu}$

19. What are the sources of leakage current?

    Ans. 1. *Generation-recombination current*: Arises from the generation and recombination of electron-hole pair in the diode depletion region. 2. *Diffusion current*: Arises from the diffusion on the minority carriers towards or away from the junction, in the diode neutral region. 3. *Tunneling current*: Refers to the band-to-band tunneling in the presence of high electric field.

20. How the gain of APD can be increased?

   Ans. By increasing reverse-bias voltage.

21. What are the main types of noises in receiver?

   Ans. (i) Thermal noise (ii) dark current noise (iii) quantum noise.

22. The sensitivity of receiver is decided by which parameter?

   Ans. Noise.

23. What is response time?

   Ans. Response time is defined as the time needed for the photodiode to respond to an optical input by producing photocurrent.

24. What are phototransistors?

   Ans. These are simplex type of photodetectors. The device consists of an *n-p-n* transistor. A large *space charge layer* (SCL) is formed between the base and collector. The SCL region is called the absorption region. Phototransistors operate as a photodetector that amplifies the photocurrent.

25. What are metal-semiconductor-metal (MSM) detectors?

   Ans. MSM detectors are probably the fastest and simplest optical detector to fabricate. The basic idea is to create a Shottky barrier, which forces the material at the surface to be depleted.

26. What factors limit the speed of response of a photodiode?

   Ans. (i) Drift time of carriers through the depletion region:

$$t_{drift} = \frac{\text{Depletion layers width }(W)}{\text{Drift velocity }(v_d)}$$

(ii) Diffusion time of carriers generated outside the depletion region:

$$t_{drift} = \frac{d^2}{2D_c}$$

where d is distance for carriers to diffuse and D_c is the minority carriers diffusion time.

(iii) Time constant incurred by the capacitance of the photodiode with its load. The junction capacitance C_j is given by:

$$C_j = \frac{\varepsilon_s A}{W}$$

$\varepsilon_s \rightarrow$ permittivity of semiconductor, A $\rightarrow$ diode junction area and W $\rightarrow$ depletion layer width.

27. What are important requirements of an optical detector?

   Ans. (i) High responsivity (R) (ii) high quantum efficiency (η) (iii) least response time (iv) zero dark current.

28. What is 'bulk dark' current?

   Ans. The flow of current through a detector in the absence of light.

29. Explain, how long wavelength cutoff related to photodiode?

   Ans. Photodiode of long cutoff wavelength can emit optical power in wide range that is used for a fiber optic communication.

MULTIPLE CHOICE QUESTIONS

1. If r_e is the rate of electrons collected at the detector terminals and r_p is the rate of photons on the device, then quantum efficiency (η) of a optoelectronic detector is:

   (a) $\eta = \sqrt{\dfrac{r_e}{r_p}}$

   (b) $\eta = \dfrac{r_e}{r_p}$

   (c) $\eta = \dfrac{r_e^2}{r_p^2}$

   (d) $\eta = \left(\dfrac{r_e}{r_p}\right)^{1/3}$

2. If I_p is the output photocurrent in amperes and P_{in} is the incident optical power in watts, then:

   (a) $R = \dfrac{I_p(A)}{P_{in}(W)}$

   (b) $R = \sqrt{\dfrac{I_p(A)}{P_{in}(W)}}$

   (c) $R = \dfrac{P_{in}(W)}{I_p(A)}$

   (d) $R = \dfrac{P_{in}^2(W)}{I_p(A)}$

3. The cutoff wavelength (λ_c) for intrinsic absorption process bears a following relation between bandgap energy (E_g) of the material and energy of incident photons ($h\nu = hc/\lambda$):

   (a) $\lambda_c = \dfrac{h\nu}{E_g}$

   (b) $\lambda_c = \dfrac{h\lambda}{E_g}$

   (c) $\lambda_c = \dfrac{hc}{E_g}$

   (d) $\lambda_c = \dfrac{h}{E_g}$

4. The performance parameters of a photodetector are:
   (a) responsivity (R) only
   (b) quantum efficiency (η) only
   (c) response time and dark current only
   (d) All of the above

5. The photodiode which produce current with gain is:
   (a) p-n
   (b) p-i-n
   (c) Avalanche photodiode (APD)
   (d) p-n and p-i-n

6. The photodiodes produce current with gain are:
   (a) p-n, p-i-n and APD
   (b) p-n diode only
   (c) p-i-n diode only
   (d) p-n and p-i-n both

7. In a fiber-optic communication system, it is required to convert the optical signals at the receiver end into electrical signals. This task is performed by:
   (a) detector
   (b) transmitter
   (c) optic connector
   (d) none of the above

8. Practically, in order to create an electron-hole pair in a p-n diode, the energy of the incident photon should be:
   (a) less than E_g
   (b) equal to E_g
   (c) greater than E_g
   (d) much greater than E_g

9. The responsivity of a given p-i-n diode is 0.5 AW^{-1} for a wavelength of 1 μm. What is the output photocurrent when optical power of 0.2 μW at this wavelength is incident on it?
   (a) 0.1 μA
   (b) 1 μA
   (c) 10 μA
   (d) 1 A

10. Which of the following is an inherent property of an optical signal and cannot be eliminated even in principle?
    (a) Thermal noise
    (b) Shot noise
    (c) Environmental noise
    (d) Background noise

11 A photoconducting detector can be constructed from:
    (a) an intrinsic semiconductor
    (b) an extrinsic semiconductor
    (c) polycrystalline material
    (d) All of the above

12. Given the germanium (Ge) has a bandgap of 09.67 eV, what is the maximum wavelength that will be absorbed by it?
    (a) 7,080 nm
    (b) 4,560 nm
    (c) 1,850 nm
    (d) 1,100 nm

13. The highest wavelength that silicon (Si) can absorb is 1.12 μm. What is the approximate band gap of Si?
    (a) 1.1 eV
    (b) 1.4 eV
    (c) 1.74 eV
    (d) 2.3 eV

14. Which one of the following material is more suitable for making a *p-n* diode?
    (a) A direct band gap semiconductor
    (b) An indirect band gap semiconductor
    (c) A metal
    (d) An insulator

15. A *p-n* photodiode, on an average, generates one electron-hole pair per five incident photons at a wavelength of 0.90 μm. Assuming all the photogenerated electrons are collected, what is the quantum efficiency of the diode?
    (a) 20%
    (b) 60%
    (c) 40%
    (d) 50%

16. Photons of wavelength 0.85 μm are incident on a *p-i-n* photo-diode at the rate of 4 × 10^{10} s^{-1} and, on an average, electrons are collected at the terminals of the diode at the rate of 2 × 10^{10} s^{-1}. What is the responsivity of the diode at this wavelength?
    (a) 0.15 AW^{-1}
    (b) 0.23 AW^{-1}
    (c) 0.34 AW^{-1}
    (d) 0.50 AW^{-1}

17. Which of the following detectors give amplified output?
    (a) *p-n* photodiode
    (b) *p-i-n* photodiode
    (c) Avalanche photodiode
    (d) Photovoltaic detector

18. A photodiode has a quantum efficiency (η) of 65% when photons of energy 1.5 × 10^{-19} J are incident upon it, the photodiode is operating at wavelength (λ).
    (a) 1.32 μm
    (b) 0.66 μm
    (c) 2.64 μm
    (d) 0.33 μm

[**Hint.** $\eta = \dfrac{\text{No. of electrons collected}}{\text{No. of incident photons}}$

$= \dfrac{1.2 \times 10^{11}}{3 \times 10^{11}} = 0.4$]

19. When 3 × 10^{11} photons each with a wavelength of 0.85 μm are incident on a photodiode, on an average 1.2 × 10^{11} electrons are collected at the terminals of the device. The quantum efficiency of photodiode at 0.85 μm is:

(a) 0.8
(b) 0.4
(c) 0.6
(d) 0.3

[Hint. $R = \dfrac{ne\lambda}{hc} = \dfrac{0.4 \times 1.6 \times 10^{-19} \times 0.85 \times 10^{-6}}{6.62 \times 10^{-34} \times 3 \times 10^{8}} = 0.27\ \text{AW}^{-1}$]

20. In Q. No. 19, the responsivity of photodiode is:
    (a) 0.624 AW^{-1}
    (b) 0.424AW^{-1}
    (c) 0.274 AW^{-1}
    (d) 0.324 AW^{-1}

[Hint. $R = \dfrac{ne\lambda}{hc} = \dfrac{0.4 \times 1.6 \times 10^{-19} \times 0.85 \times 10^{-6}}{6.62 \times 10^{-34} \times 3 \times 10^{8}} = 0.27\ \text{AW}^{-1}$]

ANSWERS

1. (b)   2. (a)   3. (c)   4. (d)   5. (c)   6. (d)   7. (a)   8. (c)   9. (a)   10. (b)
11. (d)   12. (c)   13. (a)   14. (b)   15. (a)   16. (c)   17. (c)   18. (a)   19. (b)   20. (c)

10

Optical and Photonic Components—Optical Amplifiers

10.1 INTRODUCTION

An *optical amplifier* (OA) is a device that amplifies the optical signal directly, without converting it to an electrical signal and then to an optical signal again. OAs are used for amplifying a weak signal in order to increase the distance, the signal can be transmitted down the transmission lines. In comparison, repeaters and generators convert the signal to electrical form, regenerate or amplify the signal, and then convert it to optical form again. The conversion of the signal from one form to another is a complex process, subject to high losses, slow speed, and more costlier than simple optical amplifiers.

An optical amplifier operates solely in the optical domain, i.e. it takes in a weak optical signal from one segment of the link, amplifies it optically to produce a strong optical signal (without recourse to photon-to-electron conversion and *vice versa*), and couples it to the next segment of the link. Obviously, such devices offer several advantages over regenerators, e.g. (i) they are insensitive to data rate or signal format, and (ii) they have large gain widths. Clearly, a single OA can simultaneously amplify many WDM signals, propagating through the same fiber. On the other hand, if the system employs regenerators, it will need a regenerator for each wavelength. A major disadvantage of the present OAs is that they cannot regenerate signals, i.e. they cannot clean up noise or compensate for dispersion. However, if one can take appropriate steps to reduce noise or compensate for dispersion, such OAs are much simpler, less expensive and widely applicable. This clearly reveals that OAs have become essential components in high performance, long-hand and multichannel fiber optic communication systems.

Some of the basic applications of OAs are listed below:
(a) as in-line amplifiers for power boosting
(b) as per-amplifiers to increase the received power at the receiver
(c) as power amplifiers to increase transmitted power
(d) as a power booster in a local area network.

The main types of optical amplifiers are:
- erbium doped fiber amplifiers (EDFAs),
- Raman and Brillouin amplifiers, and
- semiconductor optical amplifiers (SOAs).

The operation and characteristics of all types of amplifiers are:
1. population inversion is created, which means that more systems (atoms, molecules) are in a high energy state than in a lower one,
2. the incoming pulse of signal induce stimulated emission,
3. amplifiers saturate above a certain signal power, and
4. amplifiers add noise to the signal.

The general characteristics of EDFA and SOA are compared in Table 10.1.

Table 10.1: Some properties of EDFA and SOA

Properties of amplifiers	EDFA	SOA
Active medium	Er^{3+} ion in silica	Electron-hole in semiconductors
Typical length	Few meters	500 μm
Pumping	Optical	Electrical
Gain spectrum	1.5–1.6 μm	1.3–1.5 μm
Gain bandwidth	24–35 nm	100 nm
Relaxation time	0.1–1 ms	< 10–100 ps
Maximum gain	3–50 dB	25–30 dB
Saturation power	> 10 dBm	0–10 dBm
Crosstalk	–	For bit rate 10 GHz
Polarization	Insensitive	Sensitive
Noise figure	3–4 dB	6–8 dB
Insertion loss	< 1 dB	4–6 dB
Optics	Pump laser diode couplers, fiber splice	Antireflection coatings, fiber-waveguide coupling
Integration	No	Yes

These technologies and applications are discussed in the following sections.

10.2 SEMICONDUCTOR OPTICAL AMPLIFIERS

The functional applications of *semiconductor optical amplifiers* (SOAs) were first studied in the early 1990s. Since then, the diversity and scope of such applications have been steadily growing. SOAs are another common type of in-line amplifiers that are developed to support *dense wavelength division multiplexing* (DWDM) and to expand to the other wavelength bands supported by fiber optics. They have many applications in optical fiber communication, switching, and signal processing systems.

SOAs are based on the same technology as basic-semiconductor Fabry–Perot diodes, but they have anti-reflection (AR) coating at the endfaces. Fabry–Perot laser diodes are generally presented in the laser theory. The structure of the SOAs is much the same as the diode, with two stacked slabs of specially designed semiconductor material, with another material between them that forms the active layer, as shown in Fig. 10.1(a). The schematic diagram of an SOA is shown in Fig. 10.1(b) and Fig. 10.1(c) shows SOA in an amplifier configuration. An electrical current is passed through the device in order to excite electrons to high-state level. The electrons then fall back to the non-excited ground state, emitting photons by stimulated emission. An incoming optical signal stimulates emission of photons at its own wavelength. This is accomplished by blocking the cavity reflectors using an antireflection (AR) coating on both end faces. Fiber optic cables are attached to both ends. As explained in EDFAs, optical

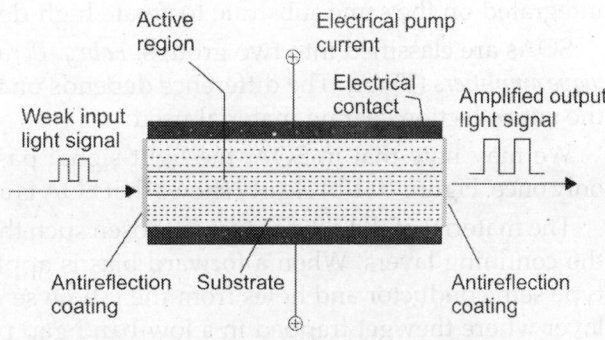

Fig. 10.1(a): Semiconductor optical amplifier (SOA)

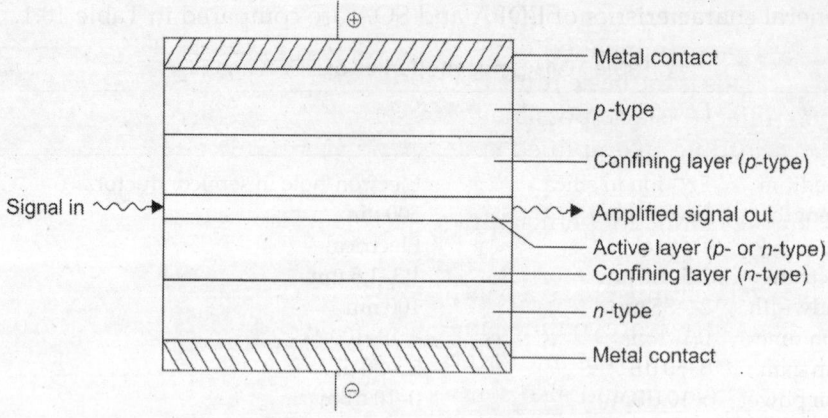

Fig. 10.1(b): Schematic diagram of an SOA

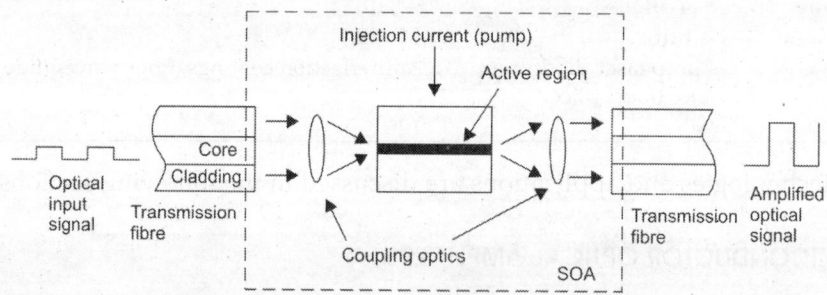

Fig. 10.1(c): SOA in amplifier configuration

isolators are commonly used at both ends of the SOA to prevent light signals from returning back. Depending on the material of the active layer, they operate from 1310 to 1550 nm in telecommunication systems.

SOAs are typically constructed in a small package. In addition, they transmit bi-directionally, making the reduced size of the device an advantage over EDFAs. They can be integrated with optical devices, such as semiconductor lasers, modulators, and DWDM. But the actual performance is still not compatible with EDFAs. They have high noise, less gain, medium polarization dependence, and high optical gain non-linearity with fast transient time. High nonlinearity makes the SOAs attractive for optical signal processing, such as all-optic switching, wavelength conversion and regeneration, time demultiplexing, clock recovery, and pattern recognition. A number of SOA chips can be integrated on the same substrate to create high-density switching matrices.

SOAs are classified into two groups: *Fabry–Perot cavity amplifiers* (EPA) and *travelling wave amplifiers* (TWA). The difference depends on the efficiency of the reflection value of the antireflection coating material used.

We may note that in SOA, the light signal passes through the amplifying medium only once. Figure 10.1(b) clearly shows that SOA is a familiar double-heterostructure (DH).

The material of the active layer is chosen such that it has a band gap lower than that of the confining layers. When a forward bias is applied to this DH, electrons from the *n*-type semiconductor and holes from the *p*-type semiconductor travel towards the active layer where they get trapped in a low-band gap potential well. If the biasing current is large enough, large concentrations of electrons and holes built up in the active layer, leading to *population inversion*. Signal photons passing through the active layer can stimulate radiative recombination of electrons and holes, resulting in the amplification of signal power. This is the basic principle underlying the functioning of this structure as an optical amplifier. It is also possible that the carriers (electrons and holes) recombine spontaneously, leading to amplified spontaneous emission (ASE), or even decay non-radiatively.

In order that a DH functions efficiently as an OA, at least following requirements have to be met:

(i) The active layer must have a band gap lower than that of the surrounding layers so that the carriers are confined in this layer and population inversion is achieved. This implies that the lifetime of the carriers should also be sufficiently long.

(ii) The active layer should also confine the light passing through the structure. Its lower band gap with respect to the confining layers implies a large refractive index of this layer, leading to waveguiding within this region.

(iii) The energy of signal photons should match with that of the inverted active layer in order to achieve optical gain. Further amplification should be independent of the polarization of the signal beam.

(iv) The signal beam must be coupled efficiently into and out of the SOA chip, usually to a single-mode optical fiber. This implies that the SOA should function as a single-mode waveguide with a circular beam waist matching the mode field diameter of the single-mode fiber.

(v) Finally, the optical feed-back have to be suppressed. This means that all measures must be taken to reduce optical reflections at the facets of the active layer to less than 0.01%.

Basic parameters of SOA are summarized in Table 10.2.

Table 10.2: Basic parameters of SOA		
Description	*Symbol*	*Value*
Differential gain	a	2.7×10^{-16} cm^2
Gain coefficient	a_2	0.15 cm^{-1} nm^{-2}
Gain coefficient	a_3	2.7×10^{-17} nm·cm^{-3}
Transparency density	n_o	1.1×10^{18} cm^{-3}
Amplifier length	L	350 μm
Density at threshold	n_{th}	1.8×10^{18} cm^{-3}

10.2.1 General Properties of Optical Amplifiers

Amplification in optical amplifiers is through stimulated emission (the same as in lasers). One can, therefore, consider similar characteristic parameters, like gain and its spectrum, bandwidth, etc. We will discuss them in some detail.

10.2.2 Gain Spectrum and Bandwidth

The model gain, one typically starts with a homogeneously broadened two-level system. Local gain coefficient for such system is:

$$g(v, P) = \frac{g_0}{1 = \frac{(v - v_0)^2}{\Delta v_0^2} + \frac{P}{P_{sat}}} \tag{10.1}$$

where g_0 is the *peak value of the unsaturated gain*, v_0 atomic transition frequency, Δv_0 3 dB local gain bandwidth, P_{sat} saturation power and P and v are optical power and frequency of the amplified signal.

Local gain can also be expressed as:

$$g(\omega, P) = \frac{g_0}{1 + (\omega - \omega_0)^2 T_2^2 + P/P_{sat}} \tag{10.2}$$

where $\omega = 2\pi v$ is the angular frequency and T_2 is known as dipole relaxation time.

For small signal power one can consider a unsaturated regime defined as $P \ll P_{sat}$. In this limit local gain is:

$$g(\omega) = \frac{g_0}{1 + (\omega - \omega_0)^2 T_2^2} \tag{10.3}$$

The following conclusions can be derived from the above equation:

(i) maximum gain corresponds to transitions with angular frequency $\omega = \omega_0$,
(ii) for $\omega \neq \omega_0$ gain spectrum is described by Lorentzian profile,
(iii) local gain bandwidth, which is defined as the *full width at half maximum* (FWHM), is:

$$\Delta\omega_0 = \frac{2}{T_2} \tag{10.4}$$

Local gain bandwidth $\Delta\omega_0$ is defined by points in frequency where local gain takes half the value at the maximum. In terms of frequency it can be written as:

$$\Delta v_0 = \frac{\Delta\omega_0}{2\pi} = \frac{1}{\pi T_2} \tag{10.5}$$

Let $P(z)$ be be the optical power at a distance z from the input end. Its change is described as:

$$\frac{dP(z)}{dz} = g(v, P) \cdot P(z) \tag{10.6}$$

Assume a linear device (here for power levels $P \ll P_{sat}$), where local gain is independent of the signal power. Integration of the above equation gives:

$$P(z) = P(0) \, e^{g \cdot z} \tag{10.7}$$

where $P(0) = P_{in}$ is the signal input power. Linear amplifier gain is defined as:

$$G = \frac{P(L)}{P(0)} \tag{10.8}$$

where $P(L) = P_{out}$ is the output power. From the above solution, one obtains:

$$G = \frac{P(L)}{P(0)} = e^{gL} = \exp\left[1 = \frac{g_0 \cdot L}{\dfrac{(v - v_0)^2}{\Delta v_0^2}} \right] \tag{10.9}$$

$$= \exp\left[g_0 L - \left(\frac{P(L) - P(0)}{P_{sat}} \right) \right]$$

where P_{sat} is saturation power.

If $P(L) \gg P(0)$ and the small signal gain of the amplifier is expressed by $G_0 = \exp(g_0 L)$, one may write to a good approximation:

$$\log G = \log G_0 - \frac{P(L)}{P(0)} \tag{10.9a}$$

Amplifier bandwidth B_0 is evaluated using the above solution. It is defined by two frequency points where power drops by 50%, i.e. $P_{3dB} = \frac{1}{2} P_{max}(L)$, which translates into $G_{3dB} = \frac{1}{2} G_{max}$. Here G_{max} is the maximum value of gain evaluated at $v = v_0$. One can determine following from Eq. 11.9(a).

$$\ln(G_0/2) = \ln G_0 - \frac{(P_{sat})_{3dB}}{P_{sat}} \tag{10.9b}$$

or

$$(P_{sat})_{3dB} = \ln(2)\, P_{sat} = \ln(2)\frac{hv\, A}{\Gamma \sigma_g\, \tau_c} \tag{10.9c}$$

where Γ is confinement factor, τ_0 being life time, hv is photon energy, A is cross-section area of active region and σ_g is gain cross-section.

In detail:

$$\exp\left[\frac{g_0 \cdot L}{1 + \dfrac{B_0^2}{\Delta v_0^2}}\right] = \frac{1}{2}\exp\left[\frac{g_0 \cdot L}{1 + \dfrac{0}{\Delta v_0^2}}\right] = \frac{1}{2}\exp(g_0 \cdot L)$$

where we have introduced 3 dB bandwidth B_0 as $B_0 = v - v_0$. By the straightforward algebra, from the above relation, one finds:

$$B_0 = \Delta v_0 \sqrt{\frac{\ln 2}{g_0 L - \ln 2}} \tag{10.10}$$

Macroscopic bandwidth of the amplifier B_0 is smaller than the local gain bandwidth Δv_0.

10.2.3 Gain Saturation

Let us now analyse the gain when signal power has large value and saturation effects are becoming important. Assume that $\omega = \omega_0$. Substituting Eq. (10.2) into (10.6), one obtains:

$$\frac{dP}{dz} = \frac{g_0 P}{1 + P/P_{sat}} \tag{10.11}$$

We introduce new variable $u = P/P_{sat}$ and use separation of variables method to integrate the above equation. One obtains:

$$\int_{u_{in}}^{u_{out}} \frac{1+u}{u}\, du = \int_0^L g_0 dz$$

where $u_{in} = P_{in}/P_{sat}$, $u_{out} = P_{out}/P_{sat}$ and P_{in}, P_{out} are input and output powers, respectively, L is the length of an amplifier. Gain G is defined as:

$$G = \frac{P_{out}}{P_{in}} \tag{10.12}$$

One obtains:

$$G = G_0 \exp\left(-\frac{G-1}{G}\frac{P_{out}}{P_{sat}}\right) \tag{10.13}$$

where $G_0 = \exp(g_0 \cdot L)$.

Figure 10.2 shows saturation gain dependence from Eq. (10.13).

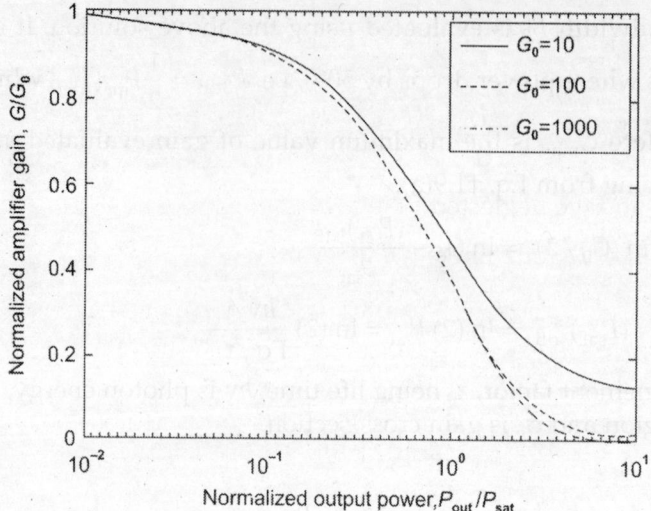

Fig. 10.2: Saturated normalized amplifier gain G/G_0 as a function of the normalized output power for three values of the unsaturated amplifier gain G_0

10.2.4 Amplifier Noise

Signal-to-noise ratio (SNR) of optical amplifiers is degraded because spontaneous emission adds to the signal during its amplification. Amplifier noise figure F_n is defined as:

$$F_n = \frac{(SNR)_{in}}{(SNR)_{out}} \tag{10.14}$$

SNR refers to the electrical power generated when the signal is converted to electric current by using a photodetector. We model F_n by considering an ideal detector limited only by a shot noise:

$$(SNR)_{in} = \frac{\langle I \rangle^2}{\sigma_s^2} \tag{10.15}$$

where $\langle I \rangle = RP_{in}$ is the average photocurrent, $R = q/h\nu$ is the responsivity of an ideal detector with unit quantum efficiency $\sigma_s^2 = 2q\,(RP_{in})\Delta f$ is the variance from shot noise and Δf is the detector bandwidth. At the output, we should add spontaneous emission to the receiver noise.

$$S_{sp}(\nu) = (G-1)\,n_{sp}h\nu \tag{10.16}$$

Here, S_{sp} is the spectral density of the noise induced by spontaneous emission, ν is optical frequency and n_{sp} is the spontaneous-emission factor or population inversion factor. The value of n_{sp} is $n_{sp} = 1$ for amplifiers with complete population inversion (all atoms in the upper state) and $n_{sp} > 1$ for incomplete population inversion.

For a two-level system:

$$n_{sp} = \frac{N_2}{N_2 - N_1} \tag{10.17}$$

where N_1 and N_2 are the atomic populations in the lower and upper states, respectively.

Total variance of the shot noise plus spontaneous emission noise is thus:

$$\sigma^2 = 2q\,(RGP_{in})\,\Delta f + 4\,(GRP_{in})(RS_{sp})\,\Delta f \tag{10.18}$$

All other contributions to the receiver noise are neglected. At the output, the SNR of the amplified signal is:

$$(SNR)_{out} = \frac{\langle I \rangle^2}{\sigma^2} = \frac{(RGP_{in})^2}{\sigma^2} \approx \frac{GP_{in}}{4S_{sp}\Delta f} \tag{10.19}$$

assuming $G \gg 1$ and we neglected first term in (10.18).

Using definition of F_n, one finds:

$$F_n = 2n_{sp} \frac{G-1}{G} \approx 2n_{sp} \tag{10.20}$$

It shows that even for an ideal amplifier ($n_{sp} = 1$), amplified signal is degraded by a factor of 2 (3 dB). In practice, F_n is in the range 6–8 dB.

SOA is very similar to a semiconductor laser. There are two categories of SOA (Fig. 10.3): (a) *Fabry-Perot* (FP) *amplifier* (b) *travelling-wave amplifier* (TWA). The FP amplifier displays high gain but has a non-uniform gain spectrum, whereas TWA has broadband gain but requires very low facet reflectivities. The FP amplifier has large reflectivities at both ends which results in resonant amplification, and also has large gain at the wavelength corresponding to longitudinal modes of the FP cavity.

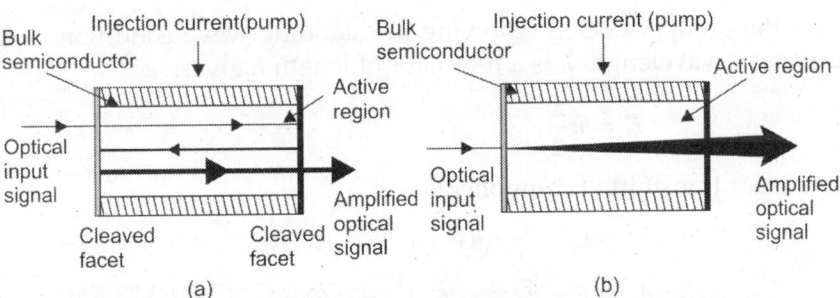

Fig. 10.3: Types of SOA: Fabry–Perot (left) and travelling-wave (right)

TWA has very small reflectivities, achieved by AR (antireflection) coating; its gain spectrum is broad but small ripples exist in gain spectrum, resulting from residual facet reflectivity. It is more suitable for system applications but the gain must be polarization independent. The phenomenological expression for gain of SOA is written as:

$$g_m = a\,(n - n_0) - a_2\,(\lambda - \lambda_p)^2 \tag{10.21}$$

and the wavelength peak values as:

$$\lambda_p = \lambda_0 + a_3\,(n - n_0) \tag{10.22}$$

Typical values of the parameters which appear in the above relations are given in Table 10.2.

From the previous equations, the 3 dB gain bandwidth is determined as:

$$2\Delta\lambda = 2\sqrt{\frac{a(n - n_0)}{2n_2}}$$

Substituting typical values from Table 10.2, one obtains SOA bandwidth equal to 54 nm.

10.2.5 Gain Formula for SOA with Facet Reflectivities

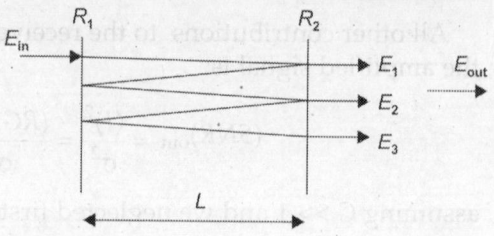

Fig. 10.4: Basic model of a Fabry–Perot amplifier

Consider a typical *Fabry–Perot ethalon* with a gain medium in-between (Fig. 10.4). Total output electric field E_{out} consists of all transmitted contributions:

$$E_{\text{out}} = E_1 + E_2 + E_3 + \ldots$$

Here R_1 and R_2 are coefficients of internal reflections for electric field, and $1 - R_1$ and $1 - R_2$ corresponding coefficients of transmission. The single-pass gain G_s for field is:

$$G_s = e^{\Gamma(g-a)\cdot L} \tag{10.23}$$

where Γ is optical confinement factor, g is gain coefficient and α are internal losses. The longitudinal propagation constant β_2 is:

$$\beta_z = k_0 \cdot n_g \tag{10.24}$$

where $k_0 = \dfrac{2\pi}{\lambda}$ and n_g effective group index:

$$n_g = \frac{c}{v_g} \tag{10.25}$$

Here v_g is the group velocity. Applying the standing wave condition to an electromagnetic wave of wavelength λ is a resonator of length L gives:

$$L = m\frac{\lambda}{2} \tag{10.26}$$

Expressions for transmitted components are:

$$E_1 = E_0 e^{-j\beta_2 L} \sqrt{G_s} \sqrt{1-R_1} \sqrt{1-R_2}$$

$$E_2 = E_0 e^{-j\beta_2 \cdot 3L} \left(\sqrt{G_s}\right)^3 \sqrt{1-R_1} \sqrt{1-R_2} \sqrt{R_1} \sqrt{1-R_2}$$

$$E_3 = E_0 e^{-j\beta_2 \cdot 5L} \left(\sqrt{G_s}\right)^5 \sqrt{1-R_1}\, R_2 R_1 \sqrt{1-R_2}$$

Total field, which is determined as a sum of all the above components, is therefore:

$$E_{\text{out}} = E_0 \sqrt{(1-R_1)(1-R_2)G_s}\, e^{-j\beta_2 L}\{1 + G_s\sqrt{R_1 R_2}\, e^{-j\beta_2 \cdot 2L} + G_s^2 R_1 R_2 e^{-j\beta_2 \cdot 4L} + \ldots\}$$

Summing geometrical series, one finally obtains:

$$E_{\text{out}} = \frac{\sqrt{1-R_1} \sqrt{1-R_2}\, G_s E_0 e^{-j\beta_2 L}}{1 - G_s\sqrt{R_1 R_2}\, e^{-2j\beta\cdot L}}$$

Finally, gain of SOA with facet reflectivities R_1 and R_2 is:

$$G = \frac{(1-R_1)(1-R_2)G_s}{\left(1-\sqrt{R_1 R_2}\, G_s\right)^2 + 4\sqrt{R_1 R_2}\, G_s \sin^2 \phi} \tag{10.27}$$

Phase shift ϕ is obtained by assuming that the phase of the incident wave is taken as zero. The relation for phase change ϕ at the output is thus:

$$\phi = \frac{2\pi}{\lambda} L \tag{10.28}$$

Using Eq. (10.25), one can write the above relation for frequency as:

$$\nu = \phi \frac{v_g}{2\pi L} \tag{10.29}$$

The above relation can be interpreted on gain spectrum graph as shown in Fig. 10.5, where frequency ν_0 corresponds to gain peak G_{max}, which is obtained when $\sin \phi = 0$, or $\phi = k\pi$. Using an expression for phase (10.28), one finds its value corresponding to ν_0 (using relation $1/\lambda_0 = \nu_0/v_g$):

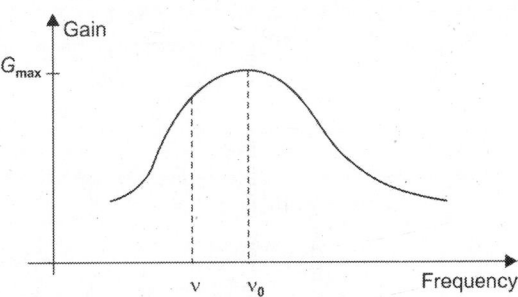

Fig. 10.5: Gain spectra showing frequency corresponding to gain peak

$$\phi = \frac{2\pi}{\lambda_0} L = \frac{2\pi}{v_g} \nu_0 L$$

or $\qquad \nu_0 = \frac{v_g}{2L} \cdot k = \frac{v_g}{2L}$

assuming $k = 1$. The difference in frequencies $\nu - \nu_0$ is determined as:

$$\nu - \nu_0 = \frac{v_g}{2\pi L} \phi - \frac{v_g}{2L} = \frac{v_g}{2L} \left(\frac{\phi}{\pi} - 1 \right)$$

or $\qquad \dfrac{2\pi (\nu - \nu_0) L}{v_g} = \pi \left(\dfrac{\phi}{\pi} - 1 \right) = \phi - \pi$

Finally:

$$\phi = \frac{2\pi (\nu - \nu_0) L}{v_g} \tag{10.30}$$

where we have neglected π since $\sin \pi = 0$.

10.2.6 The Effect of Facet Reflectivities

An uncoated SOA has facet reflectivities (due to FP reflections) determined by taking the values of refractive indices of a typical semiconductor and the air and is approximately equal to 0.32. Even with the AR coatings, there are some residual reflectivities which result in the appearance of the so-called gain ripples (Fig. 10.6).

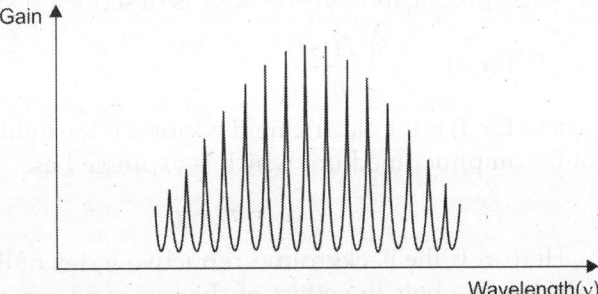

Fig. 10.6: Typical gain spectra of Fabry–Perot amplifier showing gain ripples

Ripples are superimposed on gain spectrum. The peak-to-valley ratio between the resonant and non-resonant gains is known as the *amplifier gain ripple* G_r. From Eq. (10.27), one obtains:

$$G_r = \frac{1 + G_s \sqrt{R_1 R_2}}{1 - G_s \sqrt{R_1 R_2}} \tag{10.31}$$

where G_s is the *single-pass amplifier gain*.

For an ideal TWA both R_1 and R_2 are zero. In this case, $G_r = 1$, i.e., no ripple occurs at the cavity mode frequencies. The quantity G_r is plotted in Fig. 10.7 as a function of reflectivity (R) (assuming that $R_1 = R_2$) for two values of gain. One observes that gain ripple increases with increasing gain and also increasing facet reflectivity.

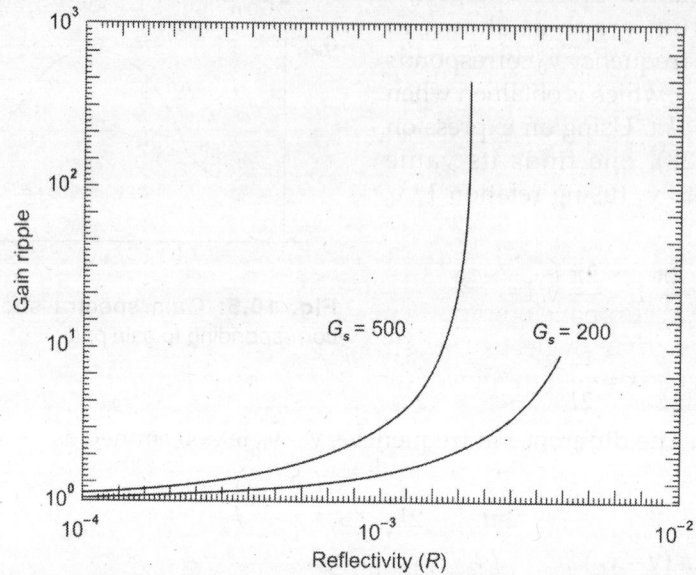

Fig. 10.7: Gain ripple as a function of reflectivity for two values of gain

10.2.7 SOA Rate Equations for Pulse Propagation

Let us discuss basic rate equations describing pulse propagation in SOA. Discussion involves electromagnetic field and carriers. We start with the development of electromagnetic equation.

Pulse propagation inside SOA is described by the wave equation:

$$\nabla^2 E(r, t) - \frac{\varepsilon}{c^2} \frac{\partial^2 E(r, t)}{\partial t^2} = 0 \tag{10.32}$$

where $E(r, t)$ is the electric field vector, c is the light velocity and ε is the dielectric constant of the amplifier medium which is expressed as:

$$e = n_b^2 + \chi \tag{10.33}$$

Here n_b is the background refractive index of the semiconductor and susceptibility χ which represents the effect of charges inside an active region in the phenomenological model is:

$$\chi = -\frac{cn}{w_0} (\alpha_H + i) g(n) \tag{10.34}$$

where n is the effective mode index, α_H is the linewidth enhancement factor (Henry factor) and $g(n)$ is the optical gain approximated here (for bulk devices) as:

$$g(n) = a(n - n_0) \tag{10.35}$$

where a is differential gain, n is the injected carrier density and n_0 is the carrier density at transparency.

In the following, we assume a travelling wave semiconductor wave amplifier which supports single mode propagation with a perpendicular electric profile described by $F(x, y)$. The electric field $E(r, t)$, which obeys wave equation [Eq. (10.32)] is expressed as:

$$E(r, t) = \hat{n} \frac{1}{2} \{F(x, y) A(z, t) e^{i(k_0 z - \omega_0 t)}\} \tag{10.36}$$

when $\hat{n}$ is the polarization vector, $k_0 = n\omega_0/c$ and $A(z, t)$ is the slowly varying amplitude of the propagating wave. We introduce the following notation:

$$\nabla^2 = \nabla_\perp^2 + \frac{\partial^2}{\partial z^2}, \quad \text{where } \nabla_\perp^2 = \frac{\partial^2}{\partial x^2} + \frac{\partial^2}{\partial y^2}$$

and evaluate derivatives:

$$\nabla^2 E \sim (\nabla_\perp^2 F) A e^{ik_0 z} + F \frac{\partial^2 A}{\partial z^2} e^{ik_0 z} + 2F \frac{\partial A}{\partial z} ik_0 e^{ik_0 z} + FA(ik_0)^2 e^{ik_0 z} \tag{10.37}$$

In the slowly varying envelope approximation (SVEA), the term with second derivative with respect to z and r is neglected. Substituting (10.37) into (10.32), applying SVEA with respect to z and t and integrating over the transverse direction gives:

$$\nabla_\perp^2 F + \frac{\omega_0^2}{c^2} (n_b^2 - n^2) F = 0 \tag{10.38}$$

and

$$\frac{\partial A}{\partial z} + \frac{1}{v_g} \frac{\partial A}{\partial t} = \frac{i\omega_0 \Gamma}{2cn} \chi A - \frac{1}{2} \alpha_{\text{loss}} A \tag{10.39}$$

where we have accounted for losses described by α_{loss}. The group velocity is defined as c/n_g and group index n_g is:

$$n_g = n + \omega_0 \frac{\partial n}{\partial \omega} \tag{10.40}$$

The confinement factor Γ is:

$$\Gamma = \frac{\int_0^\omega dx \int_0^d dy |F(x, y)|^2}{\int_{-\infty}^{+\infty} dx \int_{-\infty}^{+\infty} dy |F(x, y)|^2} \tag{10.41}$$

where ω and d are the width and thickness of the amplifier active region. At this stage, one simplifies Eq. (10.39) by introducing transformation to a reference frame moving with pulse as:

$$\tau = t - \frac{z}{v_g}$$

$$z' = z$$

In the new reference frame (Eq. 11.39) takes the form:

$$\frac{\partial A}{\partial z} = \frac{i\omega_0 \Gamma}{2cn} \chi A - \frac{1}{2} \alpha_{\text{loss}} A \tag{10.42}$$

Rate equation for carrier density n is in the following form:

$$\frac{dn}{dt} = \frac{1}{qV} - \frac{n}{\tau_c} - \frac{\Gamma g(n)}{h\omega_0 \sigma_m} |A|^2 \tag{10.43}$$

where l is the injection current, V is the active volume, q is the electron charge, τ_c is the carrier lifetime and σ_m is the cross-section of the active region. In the new reference frame, the above equation is:

$$\frac{dn}{d\tau} = \frac{1}{qV} - \frac{n}{\tau_c} - \frac{\Gamma g(n)}{h\omega_0 \sigma_m} |A|^2 \tag{10.44}$$

Slowly varying amplitude $A(z, t)$ of the propagating wave is expressed as:

$$A = \sqrt{P}\, e^{i\phi} \tag{10.45}$$

where $P(z, \tau)$ and $\phi(z, \tau)$ are the instantaneous power and the phase of the propagating pulse. Using the above equations, one obtains:

$$\frac{\partial A}{\partial z} = \frac{1}{2}(1 + i\alpha_H)\, g \cdot A \tag{10.46}$$

$$\frac{dg}{d\tau} = \frac{g - g_0}{\tau_c} - \frac{gP}{E_{sat}} \tag{10.47}$$

$$\frac{\partial P}{\partial z} = (g - \alpha_{loss})\, P \tag{10.48}$$

$$\frac{\partial \phi}{\partial z} = \frac{1}{2}\alpha_H g \tag{10.49}$$

The quantity E_{sat} is defined as $E_{sat} = \tau_c P_s$, where P_s is the saturation power of the amplifier:

$$P_s = \frac{h\omega_0 \sigma_m}{a\Gamma\tau_c} \tag{10.50}$$

In the above g_0 is the small signal gain:

$$g_0 = \Gamma a \left(\frac{I\tau_c}{eV} - n_0 \right) \tag{10.51}$$

Finally, the cross section σ_m of the active region is $\sigma_m = wd$.

10.2.8 Pulse Amplification

Using previously defined equations, let us now analyse pulse propagation assuming zero losses, i.e. $\alpha_{loss} = 0$, and also assuming that $\tau_p \ll \tau_c$, where τ_p is the width of the input pulse. Under this approximation pulse is so short that gain has no time to recover. Observing that $\tau_c = 0.2$–0.3 ns for typical SOA, this approximation works for τ_p equal to about 50 ps. Under the above approximations, one can obtain the analytical solution of the amplifier equations. One first integrates Eq. (10.49) to obtain output power as:

$$P_{out}(\tau) = P_{in}(\tau)\, e^{h(\tau)} \equiv P_{in}(\tau)\, G(\tau) \tag{10.52}$$

where $P_{in}(\tau)$ is the input power, and

$$h(\tau) = \int_0^L g(z, \tau)\, dz \tag{10.53}$$

Quantity $h(\tau)$ is known as the *total integrated net gain*. Replacing the last term in Eq. (10.47) using (10.48) gives:

$$\frac{dg}{d\tau} = \frac{g_0 - g}{\tau_c} - \frac{1}{E_{sat}}\frac{dP}{dz}$$

Integrating the above over amplifier length and using (10.52) gives:

$$\frac{dh(\tau)}{d\tau} = \frac{g_0 L - h(\tau)}{\tau_c} - \frac{1}{E_{sat}} P_{in}(\tau)\, [G(\tau) - 1] \tag{10.54}$$

The solution of the previous equation is:

$$G(\tau) = e^{h(\tau)} = \frac{G_0}{G_0 - (G_0 - 1)\exp\left[-E_0(\tau)/E_{sat}\right]} \tag{10.55}$$

where G_0 is the unsaturated gain of the amplifier and the quantity $E_0(t)$ is given by:

$$E_0(\tau) = \int_{-\infty}^{t} P_{in}(\tau')\tau' \tag{10.56}$$

$E_0(\tau)$ represents the fraction of the pulse energy contained in the leading part of the pulse to $\tau' \leq \tau$.

The above solution shows that due to time dependence of the gain, different parts of input pulse experience different amplification which leads to a modification of pulse shape after being amplified by SOA.

In the following, we will restrict our analysis to the Gaussian input pulse:

$$P_{in}(\tau) = P_0 \exp(-\tau^2) \tag{10.57}$$

For the Gaussian input pulse, the expression for the quantity $E_0(\tau)$ can be found in a closed form as:

$$E_0(\tau) = P_0\tau_0 \frac{1}{2} \sqrt{\pi} \left[1 + erf(\tau)\right] \tag{10.58}$$

where $er f(\tau)$ is the error function defined as:

$$erf(\tau) = \frac{2}{\sqrt{\pi}} \int_{\tau}^{\infty} e^{-x^2} dx \tag{10.59}$$

We have also used the following property of error function:

$$1 - er f(\tau) = \frac{2}{\sqrt{\pi}} \int_{\tau}^{\infty} e^{-x^2} dx \tag{10.60}$$

Fig. 10.8 shows pulse shape for several values of unsaturated gain G_0. One can ecomes asymmetric, i.e. its leading edge is sharper compared to its trailing edge.

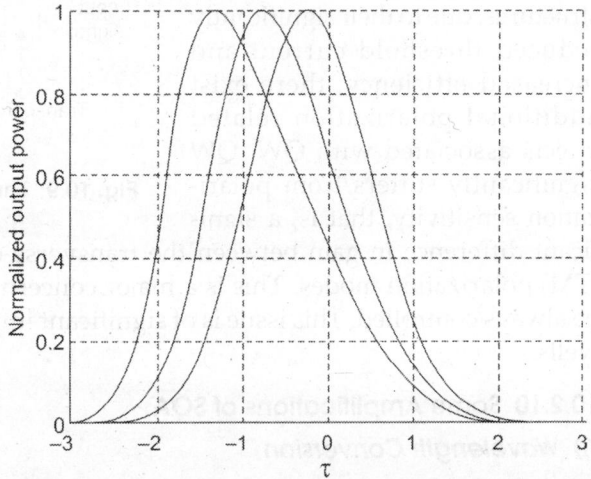

Fig. 10.8: Output pulse shapes for several values of the unsaturated gain G_0 = 10, 100, 1000 (increasing values to the left)

10.2.9 Design of SOA

Let us now briefly describe the main effects which must be considered when designing SOA with proper characteristics. Out of many issues related to the design of SOA, one should briefly concentrate here on two: *suppression of cavity resonances* and *polarization insensitivity*.

(i) Suppression of Cavity Resonance

To fabricate a travelling wave SOA, the Fabry-Perot cavity resonances must be suppressed. To accomplish this, the reflectivities at both facets must be reduced. Three approaches were used to achieve this goal (Fig. 10.9): (a) to put anti-reflection (AR) coating at both facets (b) to tilt the active region, and (c) to use transparent window regions.

AR coating only works for a particular wavelength and it is not suitable for a wide bandwidth. The analysis shows that this appropriate combination of the previously discussed methods, it is possible to obtain an effective facet reflectivity of less than 10^{-4}. Multilayer coatings can broaden wavelength range where there is low reflectivity.

(ii) Polarization Insensitive Structures

The state of polarization of an electric field during propagation in optical fiber changes randomly. Therefore, after propagation, when signal is ready for amplification (say, in SOA), its state of polarization is unknown. For amplifications of such signals, it is therefore, desirable that SOA has polarization independent amplification. The main factor responsible for polarization sensitivity is the difference between confinement factors for TE and TM modes. Proper design of polarization insensitivities SOA involves several techniques.

Additionally, in modern SOAs which are based on quantum well (QW) designs instead of bulk structures, due to their significantly reduced threshold current and increased efficiency, there exist additional polarization related effects associated with QW. QW significantly suffers from polari-zation sensitivity, that is, a signi-

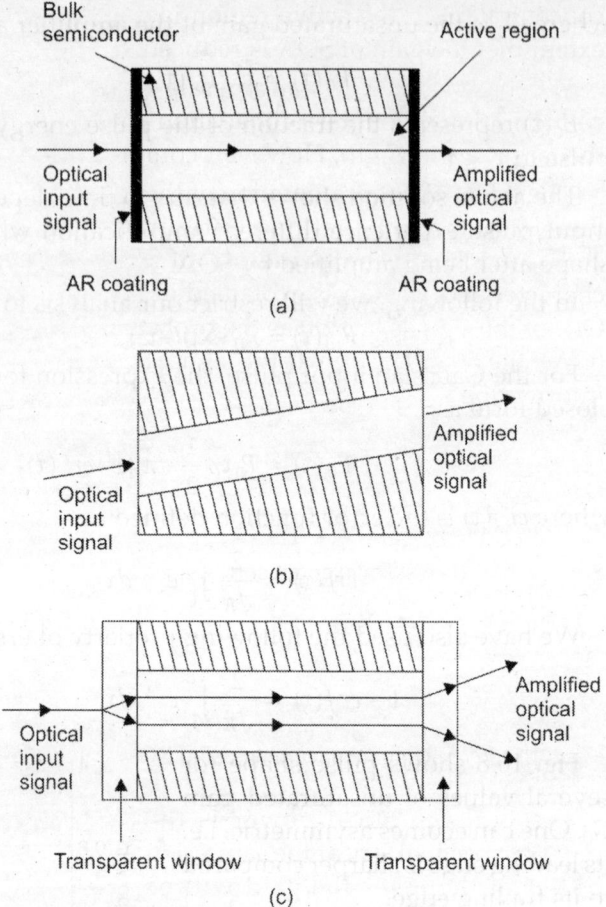

Fig. 10.9: Three main ways to make travelling wave SOA

ficant difference in gain between the transverse-electric (TE) and transverse-magnetic (TM) polarization modes. This is a major concern as the polarization of a signal cannot be always controlled. This issue is of significant importance for SOA built using quantum wells.

10.2.10 Some Amplifications of SOA

(i) Wavelength Conversion

One of the important applications of SOA is for wavelength conversion (WC). Three main methods of WC have been analysed: *cross-gain modulation* (XGM), *cross-phase modulation* (XPM) and *four-wave mixing* (FWM). XGM will be discussed in detail in the following section.

Other methods include those based on the nonlinear optical loop mirror (NOLM) with the nonlinearity achieved by using fiber or SOA.

Cross-gain modulation

The reduction of gain, known as gain saturation, typically occurs for input powers of the order of 100 μW or higher. To understand this effect, one must remember that the amplification in SOA is the result of stimulated emission. The rate of stimulated emission in turn depends on the optical input power. At high optical injection, the carrier concentration in the active region is depleted through stimulated emission to such an extent that the gain of SOA is reduced.

WC based on XGM can operate in either copropagation or counter-propagation configurations. Counter-propagation configuration does not require optical filtering of the target wavelength. However, counter-propagation suffers from speed limitations.

The schematic representation of the XGM used as wavelength conversion is shown in Fig. 10.10 (copropagation configuration) and in Fig. 10.11 (counter-propagation configuration). The principle of wavelength conversion employing nonlinear characteristics of SOA is explained in Fig. 10.12. Two optical signals enter a single SOA. One of the signals known as the probe beam) at wavelength λ_{CW} is injected continuously (CW); the other (known as the signal beam) injected at wavelength λ_S is carrying digital information.

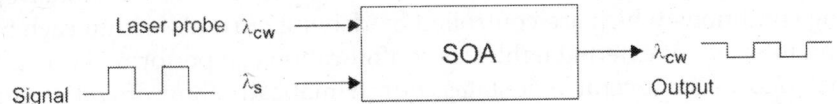

Fig. 10.10: Wavelength conversion using XGM in SOA in copropagation configuration

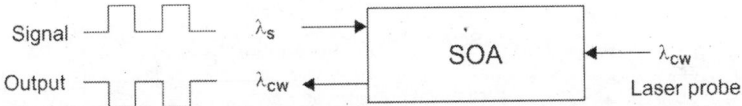

Fig. 10.11: Wavelength conversion using XGM in SOA in a counter-propagation configuration

If the peak optical power is the modulated signal is near the saturation power of the SOA, the gain will be modulated synchronously with the power. When the data signal is at high level (a logical **one**), the gain is depleted and vice versa. This gain modulation is imposed on the unmodulated (CW) input probe beam. Thus, an inverted replica of the input data is created at the probe beam wavelength. This form of wavelength conversion is one of the simplest all-optical wavelength conversion mechanisms available today.

Very fast wavelength conversion can be achieved with speeds in the order of 40 Gbs^{-1} with a small bit error

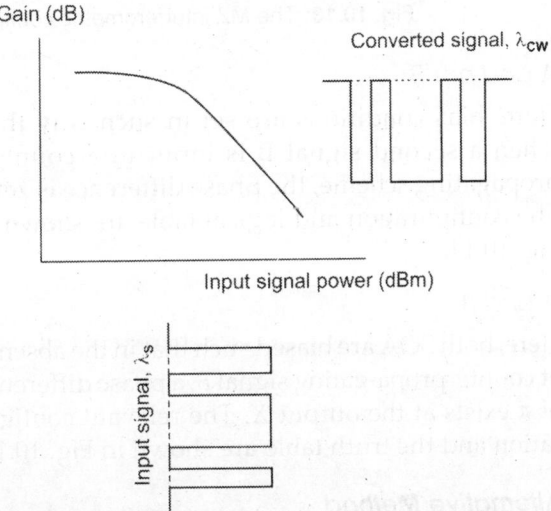

Fig. 10.12: Principle of wavelength conversion in SOA using XGM

ratio penalty. Previously, it was thought that the speed of WC is limited by the intrinsic carrier lifetime, which is around 0.5 ns. This is because the effective carrier lifetime can be decreased by the use of high optical injection to values as low as 10 ps.

Another effect associated with pulse propagation in long SOA (>1 mm) is that *pulse distortion* of the input data due to gain saturation effects can tend to sharpen the leading edge of the data pulse at the probe wavelength.

(ii) All-optical Logic Based on Interferometric Principles

For the future high-speed optical networks, several all-optical signal processing functionalities will be required to avoid cumbersome and power consuming electro-optic conversion. The central role in this process is played by all-optical high-speed logic gates.

In recent years several schemes of implementation have been investigated. Some of these schemes exploit gain saturation of SOA, and the other methods employ the interferometric configurations.

Optical logic devices are constructed using the *Mach-Zehnder interferometer (MZI)* (Fig. 10.13) for an introduction to the notation and symbols $\Delta\phi$ is the phase difference between signals propagating in the upper and lower arms of MZI. Each arm of the interferometer contains SOA where the effect of cross-phase modulation (XPM) is utilized to change phase of the transmitted light. The XPM effect is based on the physical effect of the dependence of refractive index on the carrier density in the active region. Depending on operating conditions which are controlled by driving currents within each SOA and direction and intensity of external light, this configuration can perform like an all-optical gain. In what follows, for several logic states, we schematically show operating conditions of MZI, the resulting phase difference and the equivalent logical table.

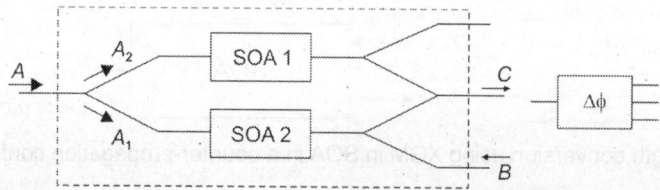

Fig. 10.13: The MZ interferometric configuration and its equivalent symbol

A and not B

Here, bias conditions are set in such way that, when a second signal B is input in a counter-propagating scheme, the phase difference is zero. The configuration and logical table are shown in Fig. 10.14.

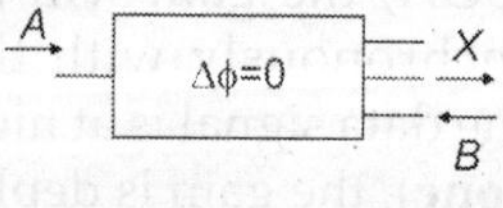

A	B	X
0	0	0
0	1	0
1	0	1
1	1	0

Fig. 10.14: Block diagram of A not B and truth table

A and B

Here, both SOA are biased such that in the absence of counterpropa-gating signal B, a phase difference of π exists at the output X. The relevant configuration and the truth table are shown in Fig. 10.15.

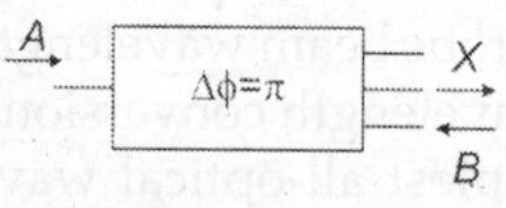

A	B	X
0	0	0
0	1	0
1	0	0
1	1	1

Fig. 10.15: Block diagram of A and B and truth table

Alternative Method

Optical gain

Let us consider the schematic structure of an SOA, shown in Fig. 10.1(b). The optical signal power P propagating through such an amplifier may be described by:

$$\frac{dP}{dz} = gP - \alpha_{eff}\, P \qquad (10.61)$$

where g is the gain coefficient (per unit length) and α_{eff} is the effective loss coefficient (per unit length). If N is the carrier concentration (per unit volume), N_u is the carrier concentration (per unit volume) at transparency (i.e. when the gain is unity), σ_g is the gain cross-section (also known as differential gain coefficient and normally expressed as dg/dN), and Γ is the confinement factor, the gain coefficient can be expressed as:

$$g = \Gamma \sigma_g (N - N_{tr}) \qquad (10.62)$$

The rate equation can be written by considering various physical phenomena through which the carrier population N changes with the injection current I and the signal power P. Thus,

$$\frac{dN}{dt} = \frac{I}{eV} - \frac{N}{\tau_c} - \frac{gP}{h\nu A} \qquad (10.63)$$

The first term on the right-hand side of Eq. (10.63) gives the total number of carriers (per unit volume) pumped into the active region by the injection current I. Here, e is the electronic charge and V is the volume of the active region. The second term describes the carrier loss (per unit volume) through nonradiative processes, τ_c being the carrier lifetime. The third term gives the carrier loss (per unit volume) through the stimulated emission process. Here, $h\nu$ is the photon energy and A is the cross-sectional area of the active region.

Under steady-state conditions, $dN/dt = 0$ and the solution for N may be obtained. Setting the left-hand side (LHS) of Eq. (10.63) to be zero and solving for N, we get:

$$N = \frac{I\tau_c}{eV} - \frac{gP\tau_c}{h\nu A} \qquad (10.64)$$

Substituting this value of N in Eq. (10.62) gives:

$$g = \frac{\Gamma \sigma_g \left[\dfrac{I\tau_c}{eV} - N_{tr} \right]}{\left[1 + \dfrac{\dfrac{P}{h\nu A}}{\Gamma \sigma_g \tau_c} \right]} \qquad (10.65)$$

It the signal power P is small, the second term in the denominator of Eq. (10.65) may be neglected, and hence, a small-signal gain coefficient g_0 is obtained, which is expressed by the following relation:

$$g_0 = \Gamma \sigma_g \left[\frac{I\tau_c}{eV} - N_{tr} \right]$$

The term $(h\nu A/\Gamma \sigma_g \tau_c)$ gives the saturation power P_{sat} of the amplifier. Thus, in terms of g_0 and P_{sat}, Eq. (10.65) may be written as:

$$g = \frac{g_0}{(1 + P/P_{sat})} \qquad (10.66)$$

Substituting the value of g from Eq. (10.66) in Eq. ((10.61), one obtains:

$$\frac{dP}{dz} = \frac{g_0}{\left(1 + \dfrac{P}{P_{sat}} \right)} P - \alpha_{eff} P \qquad (10.67)$$

Neglecting α_{eff} and integrating Eq. (10.67), one obtains:

$$\int_{P = P_{in}}^{P_{out}} \frac{dP}{\left[\dfrac{P}{1 + P/P_{sat}} \right]} = \int_{z=0}^{L} g_0 \, dz$$

where P_{in} and P_{out} are the input and output signal powers, respectively, and L is the length of the active region. Solving this, one obtains:

$$\int_{P=P_{in}}^{P_{out}} \frac{dP}{P} + \frac{1}{P_{sat}} \int_{P_{in}}^{P_{out}} dP = g_0 \int_0^L dz$$

or

$$[\ln P_{out} - \ln P_{in}] + \frac{1}{P_{sat}} [P_{out} - P_{in}] = g_0 L$$

or

$$\left[\ln \frac{P_{out}}{P_{in}} \right] = g_0 L - \left(\frac{P_{out} - P_{in}}{P_{sat}} \right) \tag{10.68}$$

Therefore, the amplifier gain G may be expressed as:

$$G = \frac{P_{out}}{P_{in}} = \exp \left[g_0 L - \left(\frac{P_{out} - P_{in}}{P_{sat}} \right) \right] \tag{10.69}$$

If $P_{out} \gg P_{in}$ and the small-signal gain of the amplifier is expressed by $G_0 = \exp(g_0 L)$, we may write to a good approximation:

$$\ln G = \ln G_0 - \frac{P_{out}}{P_{sat}} \tag{10.70}$$

The 3 dB saturation power $(P_{sat})_{3dB}$ is defined as the output power P_{out} at which the amplifier gain G has dropped to $G_0/2$. By putting $G = G_0/2$ and $P_{out} = (P_{sat})_{3dB}$, we can determine the following from Eq. (10.70):

$$\ln (G_0/2) = \ln G_0 - \frac{(P_{sat})_{3dB}}{P_{sat}}$$

or

$$(P_{sat})_{3dB} = \ln (2) P_{sat} = \ln(2) \frac{h\nu A}{\Gamma \sigma_g \tau_c} \tag{10.71}$$

Thus amplifier saturation is governed by the material properties σ_g and τ_c.

Effect of Reflections

The performance of amplifier can severely affected by the optical reflections at the facets of active region, especially when the single pass gain is high. At high signal powers, the reflections at the facet create a Fabry–Perot type of resonator, which may lead to oscillations in the amplifier gain versus wavelength curve. This is termed as *gain ripple*.

If we assume that the reflections at the facets are independent of wavelength, then one can obtain the equation governing the transmitted optical power $P(L)$ relative to the input power $P(O)$. This leads to a well-known expression for a Fabry–Perot resonator (FPR) with optical gain:

$$\frac{P(L)}{P(O)} = G = \frac{(1 - R_1)(1 - R_2) G_s}{(1 - G_s \sqrt{R_1 R_2})^2 + 4 G_s \sqrt{R_1 R_2} \sin^2 \phi} \tag{10.72}$$

where R_1 and R_2 are input and output reflectivities, G is the real (i.e. measured) gain, G_s is the single pass gain, and ϕ is the phase shift that the light wave L of the amplifier once (i.e., the single-pass phase shift). We have:

$$\phi = \frac{2\pi n (\nu - \nu_o) L}{c} \tag{10.73}$$

where n is the refractive index of the active region material, ν is the incident signal frequency, ν_o is the frequency of the resonant mode of the amplifier, and c is the speed of light in vacuum ($= 3 \times 10^8$ m·s^{-1}).

Using Eqs (10.72) and (10.73), one may calculate the 3 dB spectral bandwidth $\Delta v = 2(v - v_o)$ of a single longitudinal mode of a *Fabry–Perot amplifier* (FPA). One obtains:

$$\Delta v = \frac{c}{\pi n L} \sin^{-1} \frac{1 - G_s \sqrt{R_1 R_2}}{(4 G_s \sqrt{R_1 R_2})^{1/2}} \qquad (10.74)$$

We may note that the 3dB spectral bandwidth of a single-pass amplifier (with $R_1 = R_2 = 0$), also known as pure *travelling wave amplifier* (TWA), is determined by the full gain width of the amplifier medium itself (Fig. 10.16). For near TWAs, the pass band comprises peaks and troughs whose relative amplitudes are governed by R_1 and R_2, the single pass gain and input signal power. One can define the *peak-trough* ratio of the pass band ripple, ΔG as the difference between the resonant FPA and nonresonant TWA signal gain (Fig. 10.16). ΔG is given by:

$$\Delta G = \left(\frac{1 + G_s \sqrt{R_1 R_2}}{1 - G_s \sqrt{R_1 R_2}} \right)^2 \qquad (10.75)$$

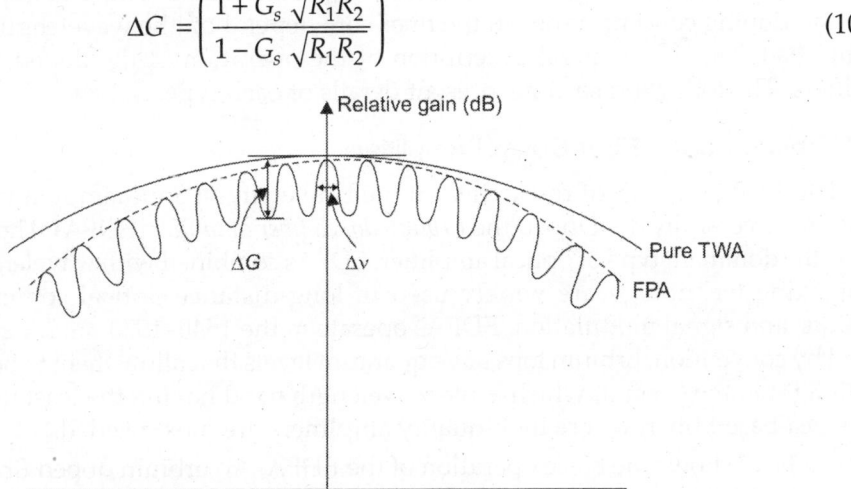

Fig. 10.16: Schematic passband characteristics of pure TWA and FPA showing large ripples in the latter case

Limitations

The theory of SOA discussed so far is valid under the assumption of continuous wave (CW) operation. However, optical signal carrying information through optical fibers are modulated in time. If one assumes that the signals are intensity-modulated, then according to Eq. (10.9b), the gain will adjust itself to the changing signal intensity, but only as long as the carriers can respond to the time-varying signal. However, in the case of an SOA, the carrier lifetime is of the order of 0.1 ns, hence, the gain recovery time is short with respect to the rate of the order of gigahertz. Therefore, different levels of signal intensity (e.g., 0's and 1's in a digital signal) will experience different optical gains, leading to signal distortion. This effect gets significant when the SOA is operating close to saturation conditions. This poses an upper limit on the maximum amplifier output power. Moreover, in many applications, it is required that the gain be independent of the polarization of the input signal wave, but the semiconductor active layers are, in general, sensitive to polarization. In a multichannel operation, it is ideally expected that each channel should be amplified by the same amount and there is no crosstalk. In practice, however, the presence of several non-linear phenomena in SOAs leads to interchannel crosstalk, an undesirable feature. In spite of these drawbacks, SOAs have found application in wavelength conversion and fast-switching in WDM networks.

The said drawbacks of SOAs led to the developments of *rare-earth doped fiber amplifiers*, and *Raman fiber optical amplifiers*. These are discussed in subsequent sections.

10.3 RARE EARTH DOPED FIBER AMPLIFIERS

Doped fiber optical amplifiers are made from optical fiber whose core is doped with atoms of an element that can be excited by an external pump light to a state where stimulated emission can occur. Pump light from an external laser source is steadily pumped in one end or both ends of the fiber. The pump light is guided along the fiber length where it excites the doped atoms of the core. The core also guides the input light signal and the amplified light resulting from stimulated emission. The doped material types and doping concentrations in the fiber core depend on the wavelengths of light to be amplified. This is a general description of the operation of the doped fiber optical amplifiers. The following sections present details of each type.

10.3.1 Erbium-Doped Fiber Optical Amplifiers

In the late 1980s, a group of researchers at the University of Southampton in the United Kingdom successfully developed the *Erbium doped fiber amplifier* (EDFA). The EDFA then became the dominant type of optical amplifier. EDFAs combined with wavelength division multiplexing technology are widely used in long-distance optical communications, networks, and signal modulation. EDFAs operate in the 1540–1570 nm range, called the C-band by convention. Erbium ions have quantum levels that allow them to be stimulated to emit light in the C-band, which is the wavelength band having the least power loss in most silica-based fiber, where high-quality amplifiers are most needed.

Figure 11.17 shows the basic operation of the EDFA. An erbium doped fiber amplifier consists of a 10–30 meter length of optical fiber, the core of which is doped with a rare-earth element of erbium (Er^{3+}). The fiber is pumped with a laser light at 980 or 1480 nm to raise the erbium ions to a high energy state. When an erbium ion is in a high energy state, an incident photon of input light signal can stimulate the erbium ions to give up some of its energy in the form of light and return to a lower energy state, which is more stable. This operation is called stimulated emission, and is generally presented in light production and laser theory.

The pump laser power supplies the optical energy for the amplifier. The pumped laser light is mixed with the input light signal via a coupler at the input fiber cable. The mixed light is guided into the fiber section with erbium ions included in the core. A

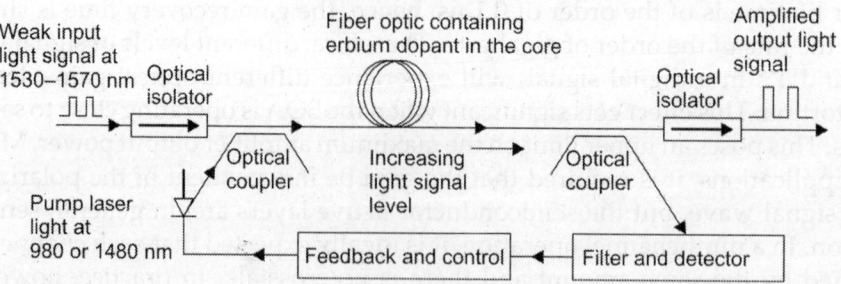

Fig. 10.17: Schematic of erbium-doped fiber optical amplifier (basic operation)

photon of the laser excites the erbium ion to its higher-energy state. When the photon of the input light signal meets the excited erbium atom, the erbium atom gives up some energy in the form of a photon and returns to its lower-energy state. The new photon is in exactly the same phase and direction at the light signal that is being amplified. Thus, the light signal is amplified along the fiber core in a forward direction of travel only. Figure 10.17 also shows the need to have a pump laser beam along the length of a fiber to provide the energy for EDFAs. This design requires power and optics, such as couplers and filters.

EDFAs also have gain that varies with a signal's wavelength, which creates problems in many WDM applications. This can be solved by using special optical passive filters that are designed to compensate for the gain variation of the EDFA.

Pumping power can be applied in a forward direction, as shown in Fig. 10.17, backward from the output end, or in both directions. Optical isolators are commonly used at the output end or both ends of the EDFA, to prevent the pump power signal and light signal from returning back down the fiber, or unwanted reflections that may affect laser stability.

As explained above, the pump laser light is supplied using a coupler at the inlet of the fiber cable, as shown in Fig. 10.17. Pump laser light can be pumped in the direction and/ or opposite direction of the light signal. The pump signal can be coupled in various locations in the amplification system, as shown in Fig. 10.18, it also shows that the pump power can be (a) at the end of the fiber cable using a coupler, or (b) coupled on both ends. Figure 10.18 shows a design for the remote pumping of the power, used where the pump laser is a long distance from the amplifier, such as in undersea systems.

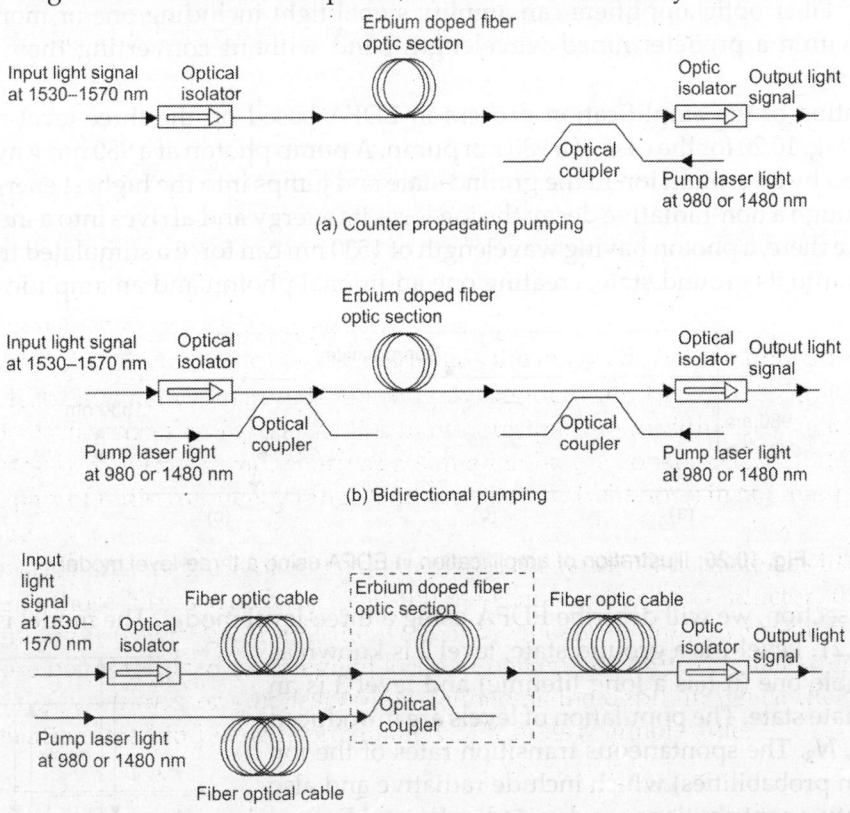

Fig. 10.18: Erbium-doped fiber optical amplifier basic operation

EDFAs have a number of main technical characteristics, such as efficient pumping, wavelength selection, minimal polarization sensitivity, low insertion loss, low distortion and interchannel crosstalk, high power output, low noise, very high sensitivity, low power consumption, and low cost.

An optical fiber amplifier consists of an optical fiber where amplification takes place which is doped with a rare-earth element, and a pumping light supply system for supplying pumping light to the optical fiber for amplification (Fig. 10.19). The pumping light supply system usually includes a semiconductor laser and an optical coupler for guiding the pumping light into the optical fiber for amplification.

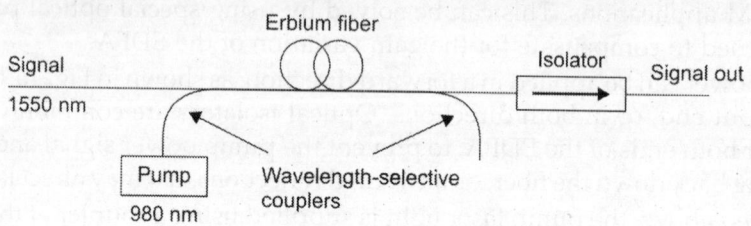

Fig. 10.19: Schematic of EDFA

Erbium-doped amplifiers are made by doping a segment of the fiber with erbium and then exciting the erbium atoms to a high energy level through the introduction of pumping light. The energy is transferred gradually to signal light passing through the fiber segment during excitation, resulting in an amplification of the signal light upon exit from the amplifier. Fiber optic amplifiers can amplify signal light including one or more wavelengths within a predetermined wavelength band without converting them into an electrical signal.

Illustration of the amplification process in EDFA based on the three-level model is shown in Fig. 10.20 for the case of a 980 nm pump. A pump photon at a 980 nm wavelength is absorbed by an erbium ion in the ground state and jumps into the highest energy level. Then, through a non-radiative decay the ion loses its energy and arrives into a metastable state. Once there, a photon having wavelength of 1530 nm can force a stimulated transition of the ion into its ground state, creating one additional photon and an amplification.

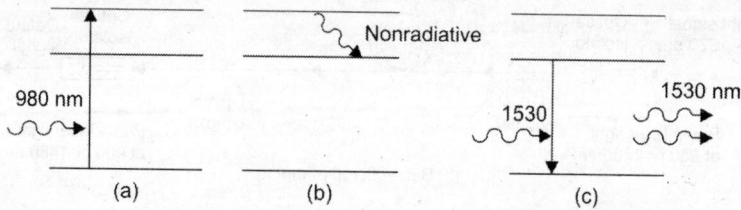

Fig. 10.20: Illustration of amplification in EDFA using a three-level model

In this section, we will describe EDFA using a three-level model. The model is shown in Fig. 10.21. Level 1 is a ground state, level 2 is known as a metastable one (it has a long lifetime) and level 3 is an intermediate state. The population of levels are introduced as N_1, N_2, N_3. The spontaneous transition rates of the ion (transition probabilities) which include radiative and also non-radiative contributions are denoted as Γ_{32} and Γ_{21} and correspond to transitions between levels $3 \rightarrow 2$ and $2 \rightarrow 1$, respectively. σ_p is the pump absorption cross section and

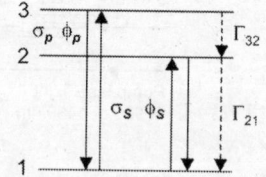

Fig. 10.21: Illustration of notation for a three-level system

σ_s is the signal emission cross section. The incident light intensity fluxes of pump and signal are denoted by ϕ_p and ϕ_s, respectively. They are defined as number of photons per unit time per unit area.

This three-level model represents energy level structure of Er^+ which is involved in the amplification process. To obtain amplification, we need a population inversion between levels 1 and 2. Here, we only cosnider a one-dimensional model where we assume that the pump and signal intensities and also distribution of Er ions are constant in the transverse direction.

Based on the above observations, the rate equations for the changes of populations for all levels are postulated as:

$$\frac{dN_1}{dt} = \Gamma_{21}N_2 - (N_1 - N_3)\sigma_p\phi_p + (N_2 - N_1)\sigma_s\phi_s \tag{10.76}$$

$$\frac{dN_2}{dt} = -\Gamma_{21}N_2 + \Gamma_{32}N_3 - (N_2 - N_1)\sigma_s\phi_s \tag{10.77}$$

$$\frac{dN_3}{dt} = -\Gamma_{32}N_3 + (N_1 - N_3)\sigma_p\phi_p \tag{10.78}$$

10.3.2 Steady-State Analysis

In the steady-state conditions:

$$\frac{dN_1}{dt} = \frac{dN_2}{dt} = \frac{dN_3}{dt} = 0 \tag{10.79}$$

Also, total population N is assumed to be constant:

$$N = N_1 + N_2 + N_3 \tag{10.80}$$

From Eq. (10.78), one obtains:

$$N_3 = N_1 \frac{1}{1 - \dfrac{\Gamma_{32}}{\sigma_p\phi_p}} \tag{10.81}$$

In what follows, we will assume fast decay from level 3 to level 2; i.e. decay from level 3 is dominant compared to pump rate. Mathematically, the assumption corresponds to the following condition $\Gamma_{32} \gg \sigma_p\phi_p$. Lifetime of level 3, τ_{32} is related to transition probability as $\tau_{32} = 1/\Gamma_{32}$. In this limit, there is almost no population of level 3, and therefore, $N_3 \approx 0$. With those assumptions the system can be effectively considered as consisting of two levels only which are described by the following equations:

$$\frac{\sigma_p\phi_p + \sigma_s\phi_s}{\Gamma_{21} + \sigma_s\phi_s} N_1 - N_2 = 0 \tag{10.82}$$

$$N_1 + N_2 = N \tag{10.83}$$

One obtains the solution for population inversion as:

$$N_2 - N_1 = N \frac{\sigma_p\phi_p - \Gamma_{21}}{\Gamma_{21} + 2\sigma_s\phi_s + \sigma_p\phi_p} \tag{10.84}$$

10.3.3 Effective Two-Level Approach

Keeping the above assumptions, i.e. $\Gamma_{32} \gg \sigma_p\phi_p$ which allows us to neglect level 3, from Eq. (10.83), one has:

$$\frac{dN_1}{dt} = -\frac{dN_2}{dt}$$

If is, therefore, enough to consider only one equation, say for N_2; the other population N_1 can be found from $N_1 = N - N_2$. We postulate the following equations:

$$\frac{dN_2}{dt} = -\Gamma_{21}N_2 + [\sigma_s^{(a)}N_1 - \sigma_s^{(e)}N_2]\phi_s - [\sigma_p^{(e)}N_2 - \sigma_p^{(a)}N_1]\phi_p \quad (10.85)$$

$$\frac{dN_1}{dt} = -\Gamma_{21}N_2 + [\sigma_s^{(e)}N_2 - \sigma_s^{(a)}N_1]\phi_s - [\sigma_p^{(a)}N_1 - \sigma_p^{(e)}N_2]\phi_p \quad (10.86)$$

where $\sigma_s^{(a)}, \sigma_s^{(e)}, \sigma_p^{(e)}$ represent signal and pumping cross sections for absorption and emission, respectively. Assume steady-state and from Eq. (10.85) determine N_2.

$$N_2 = N\frac{\sigma_s^{(a)}\phi_s + \sigma_p^{(a)}\phi_p}{\frac{1}{\tau} + \left[\sigma_s^{(a)} + \sigma_s^{(e)}\right]\phi_s + \left[\sigma_p^{(a)} + \sigma_p^{(e)}\right]\phi_p}.$$

where we have introduced $\tau = 1/G_{21}$. Further, introduce signal I_s and pump I_p intensities as:

$$\phi_s = \frac{I_s}{h\nu_s}, \quad \phi_p = \frac{I_p}{h\nu_p}$$

where h is the Planck constant and ν_s, ν_p are frequencies of the signal and pump, respectively. This allows us to write:

$$N_2 = N\frac{\tau\frac{\sigma_s^{(a)}}{h\nu_s}I_s(z) + \tau\frac{\sigma_p^{(a)}}{h\nu_p}I_p(z)}{\tau\frac{\sigma_s^{(a)} + \sigma_s^{(e)}}{h\nu_s}I_s(z) + \tau\frac{\sigma_p^{(a)} + \sigma_p^{(e)}}{h\nu_p}I_p(z) + 1}$$

We further assume that N is independent of distance along fiber z. The variation of signal and pump intensities is described as:

$$\frac{dI_s(z)}{dz} = \left[\sigma_s^{(e)}N_2 - \sigma_s^{(a)}N_1\right]I_s(z)$$

$$\frac{dI_p(z)}{dz} = \left[\sigma_p^{(e)}N_2 - \sigma_p^{(a)}N_1\right]I_p(z)$$

Typical parameter of a low-noise in-line EDFA is given in Table 10.3.

Table 10.3: Typical parameters of a low-noise in-line EDFA			
Parameter	Symbol	Value	Unit
Signal mode area	πw^2	1.3×10^{-11}	m^2
Erbium concentration	N_{tot}	5.4×10^{24}	m^{-3}
Signal overlapping integral	Γ_s	0.4	–
Pump overlapping integral	Γ_s	0.4	–
Signal emission cross section	S_{se}	5.3×10^{-25}	m^2
Signal absorption cross section	S_{sa}	3.5×10^{-25}	m^2
Pump absorption cross section	S_p	3.2×10^{-25}	m^2
Signal local saturation power	P_{ss}	1.3	mW
Pump local saturation power	P_{sp}	1.6	mW

10.3.4 Gain Characteristics of Erbium-Doped Fiber Amplifiers

We outline a basic approach to evaluate the performance of EDFA. Neglecting amplified spontaneous emission (ASE) and assuming copropagation configuration, the equations describing the steady-state are:

$$\frac{dI_s(z)}{dz} = 2\pi\Gamma_s \left\{ \sigma_{se} N_{me}(z) I_s(z) - \sigma_{sa} N_{gr}(z) I_s(z) \right\} \tag{10.87}$$

$$\frac{dI_p(z)}{dz} = 2\pi\Gamma_p \sigma_{sa} N_{gr}(z) I_p(z) \tag{10.88}$$

$$N_{me}(z) = N_{tot} \frac{I_s(z)/I_{ss} + I_p(z)/I_{sp}}{1 = I_p(z)/I_{sp} + 2I_s(z)/I_{ss}} \tag{10.89}$$

$$N_{me}(z) + N_{gr}(z) = N_{tot} \tag{10.90}$$

In the previous equation $N_{gr}(z)$ is the population of the ground state, $N_{me}(z)$ is the population of the metastable state, $I_p(z)$ is the intensity of the pump wave propagating at the wavelength λ_p and $I_s(z)$ is the intensity of the signal wave propagating at the wavelength λ_s in the positive z-direction.

Finally, the overall *amplifier gain G* is obtained using the following relation:

$$G = \frac{I_s(L)}{I_s(0)} \tag{10.91}$$

where L is the doped fiber length.

10.3.5 Typical EDFA Characteristics

The variation of gain with fiber length summarized in Fig. 10.22 for different values of pump power. Constant signal input power of 10 µW and constant erbium doping density have been assumed. Gain was evaluated for four different pump power levels equal to 3, 5, 7 and 9 mW. As it is shown, gain increases up to a certain fiber's length and then begins to decrease after reaching a maximum point.

The optimum fiber length (the one which corresponds to a maximum gain) is a few metres and it increases with the pump power. The reason for the decrease in gain is insufficient population inversion due to excessive pump depletion.

Figure 11.23 shows the variation of gain with pump power for three different values of fiber lengths of 5, 10 and 15 m and a constant signal input power equal to 1 mW. Constant *Er* doping density was also assumed. As it is seen, gain of the EDFA increases with the increasing pump power and then saturates after a certain level of pump power. The pump saturation effect occurs for input powers in the range 3–6 mW.

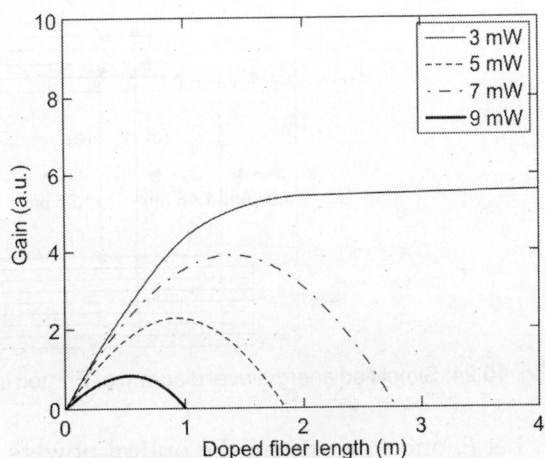

Fig. 10.22: Variation of gain vs fiber length for four different values of pump power

10.3.6 Alternative Model of EDFA

The energy bands of an Er^{3+} ion in a silica matrix, shown in Fig. 10.24, can be approximately described as a non-degenerate three-level system, provided the transition is characterized by different absorption and emission cross-section. Let us assume that the core of the erbium-doped silica fiber has erbium ion density of N_t and that the fiber is single-moded at both pump wavelength ($\lambda_p = 0.98$ μm) and signal wavelength ($\lambda_s = 1.55$ μm). Further, assume that the population density (number of ions per unit volume) of Er^{3+} ion in the ground state $^4I_{15/2}$ (with energy E_1) is N_1 and that

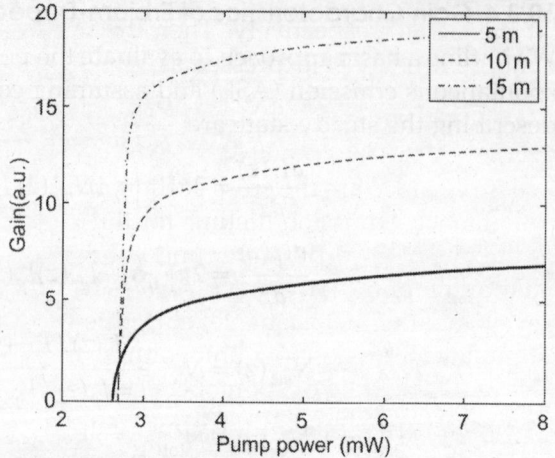

Fig. 10.23: Variation of gain vs pump power for three different values of fiber length

in the upper amplifier level (metastable level) $^4I_{13/2}$ (with energy E_2) is N_2. Pumping this system by $\lambda_p = 0.98$ μm takes the ground-state Er^{3+} ions from E_1 to the pump level $^4I_{11/2}$ (with energy E_3), from which the ions rapidly relax to the metastable level (energy E_2). Since the relaxation rate of the pump level is very fast, we may assume that this top level (energy E_3) remains almost empty. Thus, one may write:

$$N_1 + N_2 = N_1 \qquad (10.92)$$

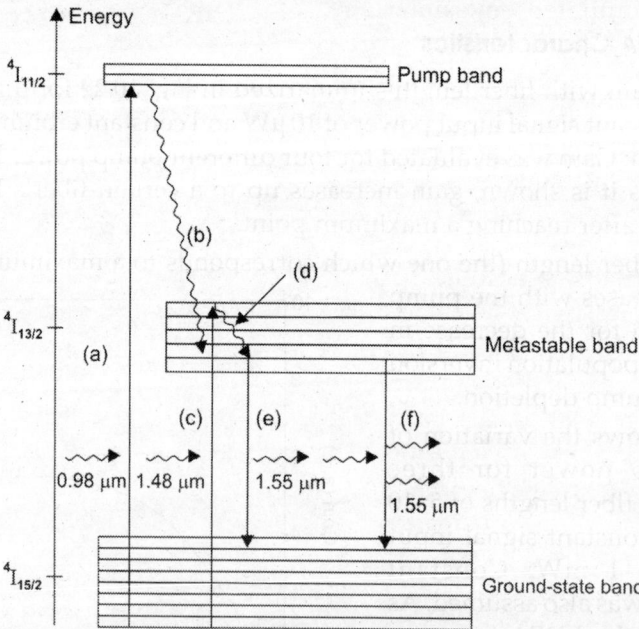

Fig. 10.24: Simplified energy-level diagram of Er^{3+} ion in silica fiber exhibiting various possible transitions

Let P_p and P_s represent the optical powers for the pump and signal waves, and σ_{pa}, σ_{sa}, and σ_{se} denote the absorption cross section at the pump frequency ($\nu_p = c/\lambda_p$), absorption cross section at the signal frequency ($\nu_s = c/\lambda_s$), and the emission cross-section at the signal, respectively. Then the rate of change of population of the ground level (energy E_1) may be expressed as:

$$\frac{dN_1}{dt} = -\frac{\sigma_{pa} P_p}{a_p h v_p} N_1 - \frac{\sigma_{sa} P_s}{a_s h v_s} N_1 + \frac{\sigma_{se} P_s}{a_s h v_s} N_2 + \frac{N_2}{\tau_{sp}} \qquad (10.93)$$

where a_p and a_s are the cross-sectional areas of the fiber modes for λ_p and λ_s, and τ_{sp} is the spontaneous emission lifetime for the transition from E_2 to E_1. Further, $(\sigma_{pa} P_p/a_p h v_p) N_1$ is the rate of absorption per unit volume from the ground level E_1 to the pump level E_3 due to the pump at v_p $(\sigma_{sa} P_s/a_s h v_s)$, N_1 is the rate of absorption per unit volume from level E_1 to the metastable level E_2 due to the signal at v_s, $(\sigma_{pa} P_s/a_s h v_s)$, N_2 is the rate of stimulated emission (per unit volume) from level E_2 to level E_1 due to the signal at v_s, and (N_2/τ_{sp}) is the rate of spontaneous emission (per unit volume) from level E_2 to level E_1.

Similarly, the rate for the upper amplifier level N_2 may be written as:

$$\frac{dN_2}{dt} = \frac{\sigma_{pa} P_p}{a_p h v_p} N_1 + \frac{\sigma_{sa} P_s}{a_s h v_s} N_1 - \frac{\sigma_{se} P_s}{a_s h v_s} N_2 - \frac{N_2}{\tau_{sp}} \qquad (10.94)$$

Equations (10.93) and (10.94) can be reduced to the following compact forms:

$$\frac{dN_1}{dt} = \frac{-\sigma_{pa} P_p}{a_p h v_p} N_1 + \frac{P_s}{a_s h v_s} [\sigma_{se} N_2 - \sigma_{se} N_1] + \frac{N_2}{\tau_{sp}} \qquad (10.95)$$

and

$$\frac{dN_2}{dt} = \frac{\sigma_{pa} P_p}{a_p h v_p} N_1 + \frac{P_s}{a_s h v_s} [\sigma_{sa} N_1 - \sigma_{se} N_1] - \frac{N_2}{\tau_{sp}} \qquad (10.96)$$

The pump power P_p and the signal power P_s vary along the length of the amplifier due to absorption, stimulated emission, and spontaneous emission. If we neglect the contribution of spontaneous emission, the variation of P_s and P_p along the amplifier length z is given by:

$$\frac{dP_s}{dz} = \Gamma_s (\sigma_{se} N_2 - \sigma_{sa} N_1) P_s - \alpha P_s \qquad (10.97)$$

$$\pm \frac{dP_p}{dz} = \Gamma_p (-\sigma_{pa} N_1) P_p - \alpha' P_p \qquad (10.98)$$

where α and α' take into account fiber losses at the signal and pump wavelengths, respectively. Such losses can be neglected for small amplifier lengths.

The confinement factors Γ_s and Γ_p take into account the fact that the doped region within the core provides the gain for the entire fiber mode. The $\pm$ sign in the LHS of Eq. (10.98) indicates the direction of propagation of the pump wave (positive for the forward direction and negative for the backward direction).

For lumped amplifiers, the fiber length is small (10–30 m) and hence, both the absorption coefficients α and α' can be assumed to be zero. Because N_1 and N_2 are related through Eq. (10.92), one only need to solve either Eq. (10.95) or Eq. (10.96). Let us consider Eq. (10.96). Under steady-state conditions, we have:

$$\frac{dN_2}{dt} = 0$$

$$\therefore \qquad N_2(z) = -\frac{\tau_{sp}}{a_d h v_s} \frac{dP_s}{dz} - \frac{\tau_{sp}}{a_d h v_p} \frac{dP_p}{dz} \qquad (10.99)$$

assuming pump propagation in the forward direction. Hence $a_d = \Gamma_s a_s = \Gamma_p a_p$ is the cross-sectional area of the doped portion of the fiber core. Substituting $N_2(z)$ from Eq. (10.99) into Eqs (10.97) and (10.98) and integrating over the fiber length, one can get the pump power P_p and signal power P_s in the analytical form at the output end of the doped fiber.

The total gain G for an EDTA of length L can be obtained using the expression:

$$G = \Gamma_s \exp\left[\int_0^L (\sigma_{se} N_2 - \sigma_{sa} N_1)\,dz\right] \tag{10.100}$$

where $N_1 = N_1 - N_2$ and N_2 is given Eq. (10.47). The variation of gain with fiber length L and the pump power are same as shown in Figs 10.22 and 10.23 respectively.

In the above analysis, we have assumed that the pump and signal beams are continuous waves. However, in practice, the EDFA is pumped by cw ILD and the signal is in the form of pulses of 1's and 0's, whose duration is inversely proportional to the bit rate. Fortunately, owing to a relatively longer lifetime of the excited state (≈ 10 ms) for Er^{3+} ions, the gain does not vary from pulse to pulse.

10.3.7 Other Rare Earth Doped Fiber Optical Amplifiers

(a) Praseodymium-doped Fluoride Optical Amplifiers

EDFAs have shifted the optical telecommunication emphasis towards the third transmission window, called long wavelength band in the 1510–1600 nm range. There is still great interest in 1300 nm in O-band amplifiers. This is mainly because a substantial part of the fiber optic network worldwide is designed for operation in the second transmission window of about 1310 nm. Praseodymium-doped fluoride fiber amplifiers (PDFFAs) can provide substantial gain in this region. However, to compete with EDFAs, the quantum efficiency of the 1310 nm transition of Pr^{3+} should be increased. Low-photon-energy glass hosts are needed for this purpose. Other alternatives are directed towards gallium-lanthanum-sulfide (GLS) and gallium-sulfide-iodide (GSI) glasses.

(b) Neodymium-doped Optical Amplifiers

Neodymium (Nd)-doped optical amplifiers amplify in the 1310 nm band. Nd will amplify over the 1310–1360 nm range when doped into Fluoro-zirconate (ZBLAN) glass and over the 1360–1400 nm range when doped into silica. The most efficient pump wavelengths are at 795 and 810 nm.

(c) Telluride-based, Erbium-doped Fiber Optical Amplifiers

Telluride-based, Erbium-doped optical amplifiers offer the potential optical bandwidth of over 76 nm in the 1532–1608 nm band, thus increasing the potential bandwidth of an Erbium doped optical amplifier from 30 to over 110 nm.

(d) Thulium-doped Optical Amplifiers

Thulium-doped optical amplifiers amplify between about 1450–1500 nm in the S-band.

(e) Other Doped Fiber Optical Amplifiers

Other fiber optical amplifiers use doping materials, such as ytterbium (Yb). The host fiber material can be silica, a fluoride-based glass, or a multi-component glass. Some plastic fiber amplifiers are under research and development. Modern plastics have characteristics similar to doped glass.

10.4 RAMAN FIBER OPTICAL AMPLIFIERS OR FIBER RAMAN AMPLIFIERS (FRA)

Raman optical amplifiers differ in principle from EDFAs. They utilize *stimulated Raman scattering* (SRS) to create optical gain. Stimulated Raman scattering occurs when light waves interact with molecular vibrations in a material having a solid lattice structure. In Raman scattering, the molecule absorbs the light, then quickly re-emits a photon with energy equal to the original photon, plus or minus the energy of a molecular vibration mode. This has the effect of both scattering light and shifting its wavelength.

When a fiber transmits two suitably spaced wavelengths, stimulated Raman scattering can transfer energy from one wavelength to the other. In this case, one wavelength excites the molecular vibration; then light of the second wavelength stimulates the molecule to emit energy at the second wavelength.

Figure 10.25 shows the topology of a typical Raman optical amplifier. The pump laser and circulator comprise the two key elements of the Raman optical amplifier. The pump laser, in this case, has a wavelength of 1535 nm. Raman amplifiers work in the 1550 nm window. The circulator provides a convenient means of injecting light backwards into the transmission fiber with minimal optical loss. The pump laser is coupled into the transmission fiber either in the same direction as the transmission signal, which is called "co-directional pumping", or is coupled into the transmission fiber in the opposite direction, which is called "contra-directional pumping". Contradirectional pumping is more common because codirectional pumping has the problem of optical nonlinearity (nonlinear amplification)). In contradirectional pumping, the attenuation of the pump light is so small that it travels a great distance, several kilometers along the transmission fiber. It also keeps pump photons from reaching the receiver, where they could interfere with reception of the desired signal.

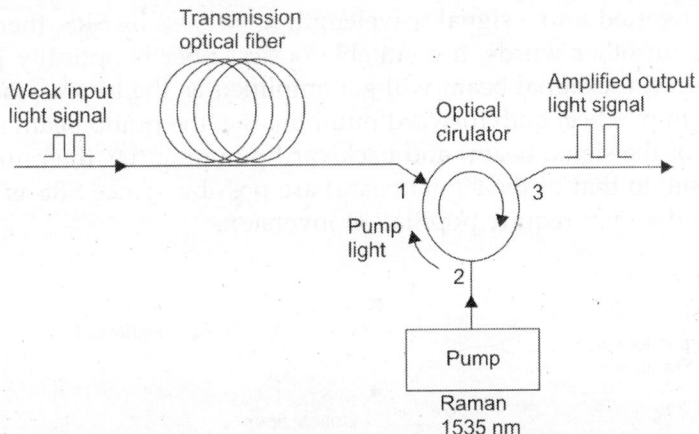

Fig. 10.25: Raman optical amplifier

Optical isolators are commonly used at both ends of the Raman amplifier to prevent pump power and light signal from returning back down in the fiber or unwanted reflections that may affect laser stability. Raman amplifiers are used as pre-amplifiers, power amplifiers, and distributed amplifiers in digital and analogue transmissions in communication systems.

Figure 11.26 shows another technique for pumping light into Raman amplifiers. The amplification bandwidth can be extended, by using multiple pump light sources along with a wavelength division multiplexor (WDM). This can be done by using more than two pump light sources, producing a broadband amplifier over bands of more than 100 nm, for example in the range of 1500–1600 nm.

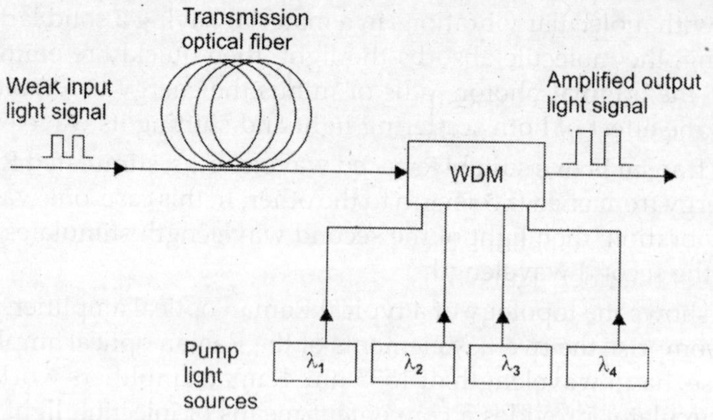

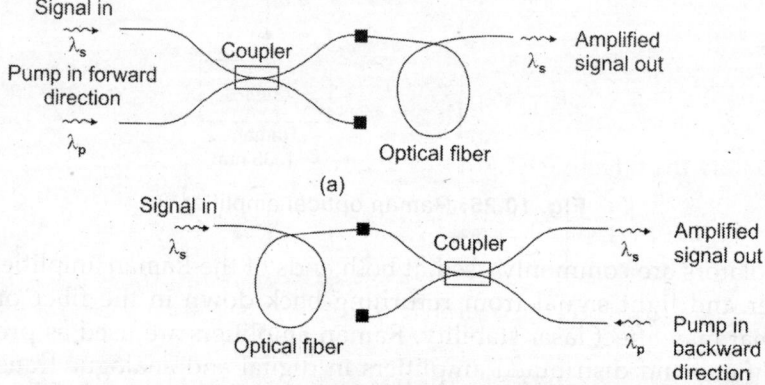

Fig. 10.26: Raman optical amplifier with multiple pump light sources

Raman amplifiers have a number of main technical characteristics, such as efficient pumping, simplicity, wider wavelength coverage, minimal polarization sensitivity, low insertion loss, high gain, low noise, fast reaction to changes of the pump power, low power consumption, and low cost. These amplifiers are used in long-haul and ultra-haul DWDM transmission systems.

The basic configuration of an FRA is shown in Fig. 10.27. Both the pump beam at a frequency v_p and the input signal beam at frequency v_s are injected into a specific optical fiber serving as an optical amplifier, through an optical coupler. The pump wavelength λ_p ($= c/v_p$) is converted into a signal wavelength λ_s ($= c/v_s$) by SRS, thereby increasing the power at λ_s. In other words, if a suitable optical fiber is optically pumped by an appropriate source, the signal beam will get amplified as the two beams co-propagate along the fiber. In practice, both forward pumping (i.e. the pump beam in the direction of propagation of the signal beam) and backward pumping (i.e. the pump beam in the direction opposite to that of the signal beam) are possible. Since SRS is not a resonant phenomenon, it does not require population inversion.

Fig. 10.27: Basic configuration of an FRA with (a) forward pumping (b) backward pumping

In the case of a forward pumping, the variation of pump and signal powers along the FRA for small-signal amplification may be studied by solving the following two equations:

$$\frac{dP_s}{dz} = -\alpha_s P_s + \left(\frac{g_R}{a_p}\right) P_p P_s \qquad (10.101)$$

and
$$\frac{dP_s}{dz} = -\alpha_s P_s \qquad (10.102)$$

where α_s and α_p represent fiber losses (per unit length) at the signal and pump frequencies v_s and v_p, respectively, P_s and P_p are the signal and pump powers, respectively, that vary along the length z of the fiber, g_R is the Raman gain coefficient, and α_p is the cross-sectional area of the pump beam inside the fiber.

Solving Eq. (10.102), one obtains the expression for pump power $P_p(z)$ at any point z along the length of the fiber. Thus

$$\int_{P_{p,\,in}}^{P_{p(z)}} \frac{dP_p}{P_p} = -\alpha_p \int_0^z dz$$

or
$$P_p(z) = P_{p,\,in} \exp(-\alpha_p z) \qquad (10.103)$$

where $P_{p,\,in}$ is the input pump power (at $z = 0$). Substituting for P_p in Eq. (10.101) from Eq. (10.103), one obtains:

$$\frac{dP_s}{dz} = -\alpha_s P_s + \left(\frac{g_R}{a_p}\right) P_s P_{p,\,in} \exp(-\alpha_p z)$$

$$= \left[-\alpha_s P_s + \left(\frac{g_R}{a_p}\right) P_s P_{p,\,in} \exp(-\alpha_p z)\right] P_s \qquad (10.104)$$

If we assume that the signal power at the input end of the FRA is $P_{s,\,in}$ and that at the output end of the total fiber length L is $P_s(L)$, solving Eq. (10.104), we have:

$$\int_{P_{s,\,in}}^{P_s(L)} \frac{dP_s}{P_s} = \int_0^L \left[-\alpha_s + \left(\frac{g_R}{a_p}\right) P_{p,\,in} \exp) - \alpha_p z\right] dz$$

or
$$\ln\left[\frac{P_s(L)}{P_{s,\,in}}\right] = \left[\frac{g_R}{a_p} P_{p,\,in} \frac{(1 - e^{-\alpha_p L})}{\alpha_p} - \alpha_s L\right]$$

or
$$P_s(L) = P_{s,\,in} \exp\left[\frac{g_R}{a_p} P_{p,\,in} \frac{(1 - e^{-\alpha_p L})}{\alpha_p} \alpha_s L\right]$$

$$= P_{s,\,in} \exp\left[\frac{g_R}{a_p} P_{p,\,in} L_{eff} - \alpha_s L\right] \qquad (10.105)$$

where L_{eff} is called the effective length of the fiber and is given by:

$$L_{eff} = \left[\frac{1 - \exp(-\alpha_p L)}{\alpha_p}\right] \qquad (10.106)$$

If $\alpha_p L \gg 1$, $L_{eff} \approx 1/\alpha_p$. Thus the overall net gain, for small-signal amplification, will be given by:

$$G_{FRA} = \frac{P_s(L)}{P_{s,\,in}} = \exp\left[\frac{g_R}{a_p} P_{p,\,in} L_{eff} - \alpha_s L\right] \qquad (10.107)$$

This can also be written as:

$$G_{FRA} = \exp[(g_0 - \alpha_s)L] \qquad (10.108)$$

where
$$g_0 = \frac{g_R P_{p,\,in} L_{eff}}{a_p L} \qquad (10.109)$$

Gain (in dB) may be obtained as follows:

$$\text{Gain (dB)} = 10 \log_{10} (G_{FRA}) = 4.343 \, [g_0 - \alpha_s)L] \qquad (10.110)$$

In this case of backward pumping, for small-signal amplification, Eq. (10.101) for signal variation will be modified. Therein, dP_s/dz will be replaced by $-dP_s/dz$. Other things will remain the same. In this case the gain of the amplifier can be shown to be given by:

$$G_{FRA} = \frac{P_{s,\, in}}{P_s(L)} = \exp\left[(g_0 - \alpha_s)L\right] \qquad (10.111)$$

where the symbols have their usual meaning.

For *fiber Raman amplifiers* used either in the forward or backward configuration, gains exceeding 20 dB have been achieved experimentally in a silica fiber, which in principle exhibits a broad spectral bandwidth of upto 50 nm with suitable doping. Such a broad bandwidth is attractive for WDM-based system applications. The main drawback with the FRA is that it requires high power lasers for pumping.

10.5 PLANER WAVEGUIDE OPTICAL AMPLIFIERS

Rare-earth-doped planar waveguide optical amplifiers are becoming increasingly important and provide compact and inexpensive alternatives to fiber amplifiers. In addition, planar technology is quite suitable for *optical integration* and will be essential to the development of fully integrated advanced optical devices.

10.6 LINEAR OPTICAL AMPLIFIERS

The design of the linear optical amplifier is similar to that of the semi-conductor optical amplifier. The device has an active waveguide gain region; the input and output fibers are aligned to this waveguide. Unlike a semiconductor optical amplifier, the linear optical amplifier also features an integrated orthogonal laser that shares the gain region of the waveguide, as shown in Fig. 10.28. This laser makes the amplifier gain linear. It also acts as an ultra-fast optical feedback circuit that responds to changes in the network. During the operation, the multiple wavelength signals to be amplified pass horizontally through the device, directly through the path

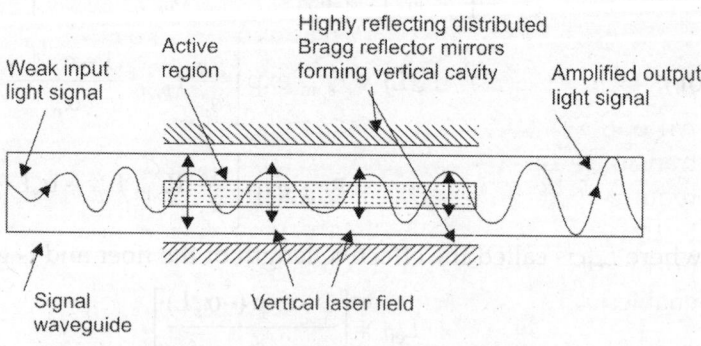

Fig. 10.28: Linear optical amplifier

of the laser, which is pumping photons of light vertically in the same device. The linear optical amplifiers are designed to be small and low cost. They are used in high data telecommunication systems.

10.7 BASIC APPLICATIONS OF OPTICAL AMPLIFIERS

Optical amplifiers (OAs) are used to boost signals over long distances in network systems. A schematic diagram illustrating the components of a basic communication system is shown in Fig. 10.29.

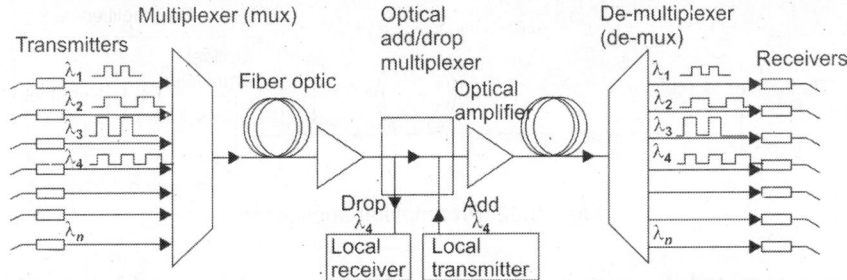

Fig. 10.29: A schematic diagram of basic communication system

The characteristics and advantages of the OAs have led to many applications. OAs can be used to boost signal power after multiplexing, or prior to multiplexing, or at any point in modern optical networks. OAs are ideal for metro and long-hour dense multiplexing (DWDM) as well as single wavelength applications. The optical design, coupled with sophisticated control circuitry, permit these OAs to provide constant gain even with signals being added to the network, such as λ_4.

(i) In-line Optical Amplifiers

An optical amplifier is used as a in-line amplifier allowing signals to be amplified within the optical signal path, as shown in Fig. 10.30. Optical amplifiers can compensate for transmission loss and thus increase the distance between the transmitters and receivers. This application enables the signal to travel through lines hundreds of kilometres long.

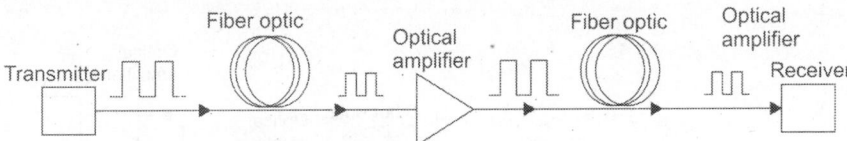

Fig. 10.30: In-line optical amplifier

(ii) Postamplifier

An optical amplifier is used as a postamplifier when placed immediately after the transmitter, as shown in Fig. 10.31. An optical amplifier will boost the light signal to the required power level at the beginning of a fiber line. This arrangement enables the signal to travel hundreds of kilometres down the fiber cable. A common application of the post-amplification technique, together with an optical preamplifier at the receiving end, enables continuous underwater transmission distances up to a few kilometers.

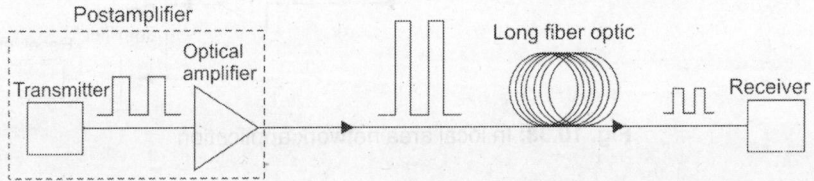

Fig. 10.31: Postamplifier application

(iii) Preamplifier

An optical amplifier is used as a preamplifier when placed immediately before the receiver, as shown in Fig. 10.32. An OA will boost the light signal to the required power level

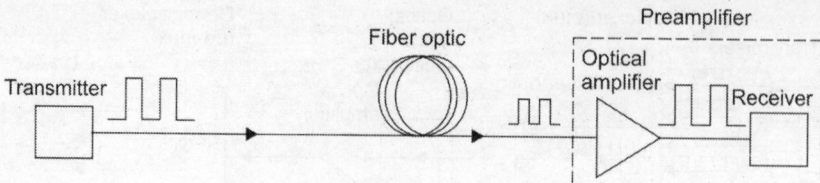

Fig. 10.32: Preamplifier application

before being received by an optical receiver. The preamplifier enables the signal to be processed directly by the receiver. The preamplification technique is commonly used before optical herodyne detectors or avalanche photodiodes.

(iv) Local Area Network

Optical amplifiers are used to boost signals in local area networks, when placed in subcentres within the transmission lines and branches, as shown in Fig. 10.33. This type of arrangement also enables optical amplifiers to have the characteristics suitable for analogue transmission. The video content multiplexed by head-end equipment is converted from optical/electrical transmission into the 1550 nm band-wavelength optical video signal that is suitable for optical communication. The optical video signals are optically amplified to compensate the losses of splitting and transmission. We may note that the signals repeatedly undergo amplification, splitting and transmission.

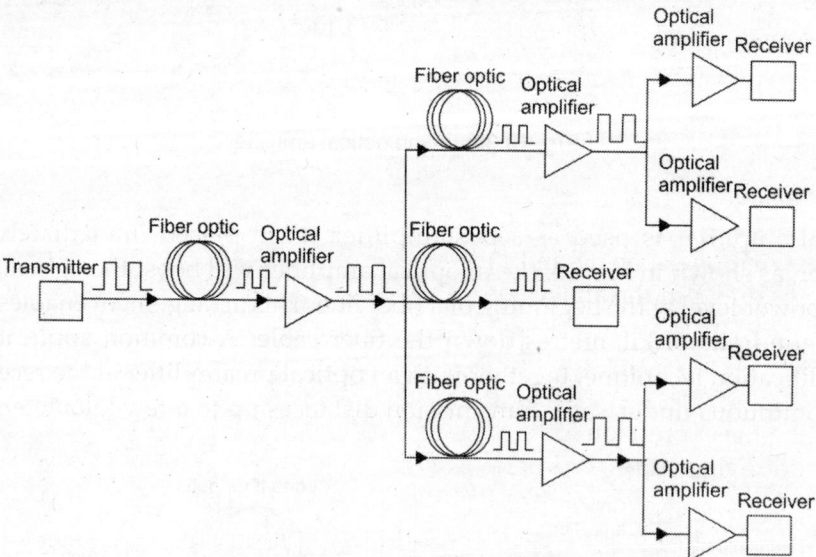

Fig. 10.33: In local area network application

Example 1

Consider an InGaAsP SOP with amplifier width (W) = 5 µm and thickness (d) = 0.5 µm. Given that group velocity (v_g) = 2 × 10⁸ m·s⁻¹, if a 1.0 µW optical signal at 1500 nm enters the device, then calculate the photon density.

Solution

We have:

$$N_{ph} = \frac{P_s}{v_g \, (h\nu)\,(Wd)}$$

$$= \frac{1 \times 10^{-6} \text{ W}}{(2 \times 10^8 \text{ ms}^{-1}) \dfrac{(6.626 \times 10^{-34} \text{ Js}) \times 3 \times 10^8 \text{ m} \cdot \text{s}^{-1}}{1.55 \times 10^{-6} \text{ m}} (5\,\mu m)(0.5\,\mu m)}$$

$$= 1.56 \times 10^6 \text{ photons m}^{-3}$$

Here

$P_s = 1 \times 10^{-6}$ W

$v_g = 2 \times 10^8$ m·s^{-1}

$\nu = \dfrac{c}{\lambda} = \dfrac{3 \times 10^8 \text{ m} \cdot \text{s}^{-1}}{1.55 \times 10^{-6} \text{ m}}$

$W = 5\,\mu m$

$d = 0.5\,\mu m$

Example 2

A SOA has uncoated facet reflectivities of 30% and a single-pass gain of 5 dB. The device has an active region of length 320 μm, a mode spacing of 1 nm, and a peak gain wavelength of 1.55 μm. Calculate the refractive index of the active region and the spectral bandwidth of the amplifier.   **[B Tech, MSc (Ele)]**

Solution

The refractive index n of the active region at the peak gain wavelength λ is given by:

$$n = \frac{\lambda^2}{2(\delta\lambda)L}$$

where $\delta\lambda$ is the mode spacing and L is the length of the active region. Substituting the values of λ, $\delta\lambda$ and L in the above equation, one obtains:

$$n = \frac{\left(1.55 \times 10^{-6}\right)^2}{2 \times 1 \times 10^{-9} \times 320 \times 10^{-6}} = 3.75$$

Now, using the expression for the 3 dB spectral bandwidth of the amplifier as follows and substituting the values, one obtains:

$$\Delta\nu = \frac{c}{\pi n L} \sin^{-1} \frac{1 - G_s \sqrt{R_1 R_2}}{(4G_s \sqrt{R_1 R_2})^{1/2}}$$

$$= \frac{3 \times 10^8 \text{ (m} \cdot \text{s}^{-1})}{\pi \times 3.75 \times 320 \times 10^{-6} \text{ m}} \sin^{-1} \left[\frac{1 - 3.16 \sqrt{0.30 \times 0.30}}{(4 \times 3.16 \sqrt{0.30 \times 0.30})^{1/2}} \right]$$

(5 dB gain is equivalent to 3.16)

$$= 2.125 \times 10^9 \text{ Hz}$$

$$= 2.125 \text{ GHz}$$

Example 3

Consider an EDFA being pumped at 980 nm with 30 mW pump power. If the gain at 1550 nm is 20 dB, then calculate the maximum input and output powers.   **[B Tech]**

Solution

Here, $\dfrac{\lambda_p}{\lambda_s} = \dfrac{980}{1550}$, $P_{p,\,in} = 30$ mW, $G = 100$

We have input signal power:

$$P_{s,\,in} \le \frac{(\lambda_p / \lambda_s)\, P_{p,\,in}}{G - 1} \le \frac{(980/1550)\,(300\text{ mW})}{100 - 1} = 190\;\mu W$$

$$P_{s,\,out} \le P_{s,\,in} + \frac{\lambda_p}{\lambda_s}\, P_{p,\,in} = 190\;\mu W + 0.03\,(30\text{ mW})$$

$$= 190\;\mu W + 0.03\,(30\text{ mW}) = 19.1\text{ mW} = 12.8\text{ dB}\cdot m$$

Example 4

Consider an EDFA which is used as a power amplifier with a 10 dB gain. Assume the amplifier input is 0-dB m level from a laser diode transmitter. If the pump wavelength is 980 nm, then calculate the least pump power for a 10dB m output at 1540 nm.

[MSc (Ele)]

Solution

We have: $P_{p,\,in} \ge \dfrac{\lambda_s}{\lambda_p}\,(P_{s,\,out} - P_{s,\,in}) = \dfrac{1540}{980}\,(10\text{ mW} - 1\text{mW}) = 14\text{ mW}.$

Example 5

Consider a typical EDFA with the following parameters: doping concentration 6×10^{24} m^{-3}, signal wavelength $\lambda_s = 1.536$ μm, absorption cross section at λ_s, $\sigma_{sa} = 4.644 \times 10^{-25}$ m^2, emission cross section at λ_s, $\sigma_{sc} = 4.644 \times 10^{-25}$ m^2, lifetime for spontaneous emission, $\tau_{sp} = 1.2 \times 10^{-2}$ s, length of the doped fiber $L = 7$ m, and $\Gamma_s = 0.80$. Assume that (N_2/N_1) is nearly constant over the length of the EDFA and is equal to 0.70. (In actual practice, N_1 and N_2 vary with z). Calculate the small-signal gain of EDFA and the maximum possible achievable gain.   **[B Tech]**

Solution

The total gain G for a lumped EDFA of length L can be obtained using following expression for total gain:

$$G = \Gamma_s \exp\left[\int_0^L (\sigma_{se} N_2 - \sigma_{sa} N_1)\, dz\right]$$

where Γ_s is confinement factor taking into account the fact that the doped region within the core provides the gain for the entire mode fiber. σ_{se} and σ_{sa} represent the absorption cross-section at the pump frequency ($v_p = c/\lambda_p$) and absorption cross section at the signal frequency ($v_s = c/\lambda_s$) respectively. N_1 and N_2 represent the population density of Er^{3+} ion in the ground state and that in the upper amplifier level (metastable level) respectively. With the above assumptions, simple mathematical manipulation of this equation gives:

$$G = \Gamma_s \exp\left[\sigma_{sa} N_t \left\{\left(\frac{\sigma_{se}}{\sigma_{sa}} + 1\right)\frac{N_2}{N_t} - 1\right\} L\right]$$

Here N_1 has been replaced by $N_t - N_2$. Thus, one finds:

$$\left[G = 0.80 \exp (4.644 \times 10^{-25} \text{ m}^2)(6 \times 10^{24} \text{ m}^{-3}) \times \left\{ \left(\frac{4.644 \times 10^{-25}}{4.644 \times 10^{-25}} + 1 \right) \times 0.70 - 1 \right\} \times 7 \text{ m} \right]$$

or $G = 0.80 \exp 97.80) = 1956 = 32.9 \text{ dB}$

In the above expression for G, if we substitute $N_2 = N_t$ and $\Gamma_s = 1$, we get the expression for maximum possible achievable gain:

$$G_{max} = \exp (s_{se} N_t L)$$

Substituting the values of relevant parameters, one obtains for the present case:

$$G_{max} = \exp [(4.644 \times 10^{-25} \text{ m}^2) \times (6 \times 10^{24} \text{ m}^{-3}) \times 7 \text{ (m)}]$$
$$= 2.9568 \times 10^8 = 84.70 \text{ dB}$$

Indeed this value of G_{max} is quite high. A more realistic estimate of G_{max} can be obtained using the principle of conservation of energy. Thus, if $P_{s,\,in}$ and $P_{s,\,out}$ are the signal powers at the input and output ends of the erbium-doped fiber at the signal wavelength λ_s, and $P_{p,\,in}$ is the input pump power at wavelength λ_p, the following inequality should hold true:

$$P_{s,\,out} \le P_{s,\,in} + \frac{\lambda_p}{\lambda_s} P_{p,\,in}$$

Assuming that there is no spontaneous emission, the gain may be written as:

$$G = \frac{P_{s,\,out}}{P_{s,\,in}} \le 1 + \frac{\lambda_p}{\lambda_s} \frac{P_{p,\,in}}{P_{s,\,in}}$$

This yields: $\qquad G_{max} = 1 + \dfrac{\lambda_p}{\lambda_s} \dfrac{P_{p,\,in}}{P_{s,\,in}}$

Example 6

Consider an optical transmission path containing N cascaded optical amplifiers each having a 30 dB gain. If a fiber has a loss of 0.2 dB/km, then the span between optical amplifiers is 150 km if there are no other system impairments. A 900 km link require five amplifiers. Calculate the noise penalty factor over the total path. **[MSc (Ele)]**

Solution

We have: $\qquad F_{path}(G) = \dfrac{1}{G} \left(\dfrac{G-1}{\log G} \right)^2$

Substituting the values, one obtains:

$$10 \log F_{path}(G) = 10 \log \left[\frac{1}{1000} \left(\frac{1000 - 1}{\log 1000} \right)^2 \right] = 10 \log 20.9 = 13.2 \text{ dB}$$

Now, if we reduce the gain to 20 dB, then the impairment free transmission distance is 100 km for which one need eight amplifiers. Now, the noise penalty factor is obtained as:

$$10 \log F_{path}(G) = 10 \log \left[\frac{1}{100} \left(\frac{100 - 1}{\log 100} \right)^2 \right] = 10 \log 4.62 = 6.6 \text{ dB}$$

Example 7

A fiber Raman amplifier has a length of 2 km. The attenuation coefficients α_s and α_p for signal and pump wavelengths for this fiber are 0.15 and 0.20 dB/km, respectively. Assume that $a_p = 60\ \mu m^2$ and $g_R = 5 \times 10^{-14}$ m/W. The amplifier is pumped by a laser of 1 W power. If the input signal power is 1 μW, calculate (a) the output signal power for forward pumping, and (b) the overall gain in dB.

Solution

In the case of forward pumping, we can use the following relation:

$$P_s(L) = P_{s,\,in}\ \exp\left[\frac{g_R}{a_p}P_{p,\,in}\left\{\frac{1-\exp(-\alpha_p L)}{\alpha_p}\right\}-\alpha_s L\right]$$

$$P_{s,\,in} = 1\ \mu W = 1 \times 10^{-6}\ W,\ P_{p,\,in} = 1\ W$$

$$g_R = 5 \times 10^{-14}\ mW^{-1},\ a_p = 60\ \mu m^2 = 60 \times 10^{-12}\ m^2$$

$$L = 2\ km = 2000\ m,\ a_s = 0.15\ dB/km\ (= 3.39 \times 10^{-5}\ m^{-1})$$

$$\alpha_p = 0.20\ dB/km\ (= 4.50 \times 10^{-5}\ m^{-1})$$

$$P_s(L) = 1 \times 10^{-6}\ (W)\exp\left[\frac{5 \times 10^{-14}\ mW^{-1}}{6 \times 10^{-1}\ m^2} \times 1\ (W)\right.$$

$$\left. \times\left\{\frac{1-\exp(-3.40 \times 10^{-5}\ (m^{-1}) \times 2000(m)}{4.5 \times 10^{-5}\ m^{-1}}\right\}-3.39 \times 10^{-5}(m^{-1}) \times 2000(m)\right]$$

Therefore, the net gain of the amplifier will be:

$$G_{FRA} = \frac{4.582}{1\ \mu W} = 4.582$$

Gain (in dB) = $10\log_{10} G_{FRA} = 10\log_{10}(4.582) = 6.61$ dB.

Example 8

A Fabry-Perot amplifier (FPA) has uncoated facets with reflectivities of 20% each. The single-pass gain of the cavity is 6.02 dB and the mode spacing is 1 nm and the peak gain wavelength of the amplifier is 1550 nm. Taking refractive index of the cavity 3.7, calculate the length of the cavity and 3 dB bandwidth of the amplifier. **[PTU, DTU]**

Solution

We have the relation for the length of the cavity

$$L = \frac{\lambda^2}{2n\,\Delta\lambda} = \frac{(1550 \times 10^{-9})^2}{2 \times 3.6 \times 10^{-9}} = 325\ \mu m$$

Now, gain of the cavity (in terms of ratio)

$$G_s = \text{antilog}(0.602) = 4$$

The 3 dB bandwidth of FPA is given by

$$B = \frac{c}{\pi n L}\sin^{-1}\left[\frac{1}{2}\left(\frac{(1-R_1)(1-R_2)}{\sqrt{R_1 R_2}\ G}\right)\right]$$

where R_1 and R_2 are the reflectivities of the front and rear facets respectively and G is the gain of the cavity. Substituting the values, we obtain

$$B = \frac{3 \times 10^8}{3.14 \times 3.7 \times 325 \times 10^{-6}} \sin^{-1} \left[\frac{1}{2} \times \frac{1 - \sqrt{0.2 \times 0.2 \times 4}}{(\sqrt{0.2 \times 0.2} \times 4)^{1/2}} \right]$$

$$= 7.94 \times 10^{10} \sin^{-1} \left[\frac{0.2}{2 \times (0.2 \times 4)^{1/2}} \right]$$

$$= 7.94 \times 10^{10} \times 0.112 = 8.89 \text{ GHz}$$

Example 9

Consider a planar waveguide with step-index profile. The refractive index of central waveguide region is 1.52 and that of the surrounding region is 1.48 at the operating wavelength of 900 nm. Find the maximum thickness of the guiding slab so that the waveguide supports only the fundamental TE mode. **[MHTU, KTU]**

Solution

To support only the fundamental mode, the thickness of the guiding layer for single-mode operation can be obtained from the following relation

$$h < \frac{\lambda}{2(n_1 - n_2)^{1/2}}$$

Substituting the values, we obtain

$$h < \frac{900 \times 10^{-9}}{2[(1.52)^2 - (1.48)^2]^{1/2}} < 1.3 \ \mu\text{m}$$

Clearly, the thickness of the guiding slab should not be more than 1.3 μm.

Example 10

A transverse electro-optic modulator uses a KD*P Pockels cell of length 5 cm and width 0.5 cm. A light beam of wavelength of 550 nm is to pass through the material. Assuming the electro-optic coefficient of KD*P crystal to be 26.5×10^{-12} m V^{-1} at the operating wavelength and taking the refractive index of KD*P cell as 1.51, calculate the half-wave voltage of the modulator. **[RTU, MHTU]**

Solution

In this case, the half-wave voltage corresponds to the voltage required to be applied in the transverse direction so as to create a phase difference of π in the lightwave passing through the cell. The desired relation for V_π is

$$V_\pi = \frac{\pi d}{rn^3 L} = \frac{550 \times 10^{-9} \times 0.5 \times 10^{-2}}{26.5 \times 10^{-12} \times (1.51)^3 \times 5 \times 10^{-2}} = 602.8 \text{ V}$$

Example 11

An asymmetrical ZnS planar waveguide structure has a planar film of refractive index $n_1 = 2.35$ sandwitched between a substrate with a refractive index of n_2 at the bottom and a cover layer of refractive index on the top such that $n_1 > n_2 \geq n_3$ ($n_2 = n_3 = 1$) at the operating wavelength of 650 nm. Taking the refractive index of the substrate as 1.5, estimate the range of value of the thickness of the ZnS in order to support at least one guiding mode. **[KTU, PTU]**

Solution

We have for single mode operation, h the number of modes, m supported by the waveguide at a given wavelength

$$h \geq \frac{\left(m + \dfrac{1}{2}\right)\lambda}{2(n_1^2 - n_2^2)^{1/2}}$$

Here $m = 0$ and $m = 1$, i.e. h of the film must lie between the values $m = 0$ and $m = 1$. Thus, we have

$$h = \frac{3\lambda}{4(n_1^2 - n_2^2)^{1/2}} = \frac{3 \times 650 \times 10^{-9}}{4[(2.35)^2 - (1.5)^2]^{1/2}} = 0.27\ \mu m$$

Now, for $m = 0$, the thickness value is obtained as

$$h = \frac{\lambda}{4(n_1^2 - n_2^2)^{1/2}} = \frac{650 \times 10^{-9}}{4[(2.35)^2 - (1.5)^2]^{1/2}} = 0.09\ \mu m$$

Clearly, for single mode operation the thickness of guiding film must lie between $0.09\ mm \leq h \leq 0.27\ \mu m$.

SUMMARY

- The optical signal gets attenuated as it propagates along the fiber in a fiber-optic communication system. Therefore, signal strength have to be restored at appropriate points along the link. This can be achieved using either an amplifier or a regenerator. A regenerator requires conversion of the optical signal into the electrical domain and reconversion again into the optical domain. The use of regenerators is limited to some specific systems.

- An optical amplifier is a laser without feedback. An optical amplifier operates solely in the optical domain. Most amplifiers amplify incident light through stimulated emission. Optical gain is achieved when the amplifier is pumped optically or electrically to achieve *population inversion*.

- Optical amplification depends on:
  (i) Frequency (or wavelength) of incident signal.
  (ii) Local beam intensity.

- In an optical amplifier, the external pump source energy is absorbed by the electrons in the active medium. The electrons shifts to the higher energy level producing population inversion. Photons of incoming signal triggers these excited electrons to lower energy level through a stimulated emission process, producing amplified optical signal.

- Types of optical amplifiers:
  (a) *Doped fiber amplifiers* (DFA); (i) In these amplifiers, active medium is created by erbium (Er), ytterbium (Yb), neodymium (Nd), and praseodymium (Pr), (ii) these amplifiers can pump device at several different wavelength, (iii) coupling loss is low, and (iv) there is constant gain which is provided either by rare-earth dopants or stimulated Raman scattering.
  (b) *Semiconductor optical amplifiers* (SOA): These amplifiers utilize stimulated emission from injected carriers. In these amplifiers active medium consists of alloy semiconductor (P, Ga, In, As). SOA works in both low attenuation

windows, i.e. 1300 nm and 1550 nm. The 3 dB bandwidth is about 70 nm because of very broad gain spectrum. SOA consumes less power and has fewer components.

  – SOAs are mainly of two types: (i) Fabry–Perot amplifier (FPA) (ii) travelling wave amplifier (TWA).
  – SOA has rapid gain response 1 ps to 0.1 ns.

(c) *Raman fiber optical amplifiers* (RFOA): These amplifiers differ in principle from Erbium-doped fiber optical amplifiers (EDFOA). They utilize stimulated Raman scattering (SRS) to create optical gain. SRS occurs when light waves interact with molecular vibrations in a material having a solid lattice structure.

- Light signal in an SOA passes through the active layer of the forward-biased semiconductor DH and in the process gets amplified. The amplifier gain (G) is given by:

$$G = \frac{P_{\text{out}}}{P_{\text{in}}} = \exp\left[g_o L - \frac{P_{\text{out}} - P_{\text{in}}}{P_{\text{sat}}} \right]$$

where P_{sat} is saturation power of amplifier, g is the gain coefficient (per unit length), P_{in} and P_{out} are the input and output powers respectively, and L is the length of the active region.

- At the facets of the active region, the optical reflections can severely affect the performance of the amplifier, especially when the single pass gain is high. Moreover, several nonlinear phenomena in SOAs, lead to interchannel crosstalk in multichannel operation.

- An EDFA operates on the principle of optical pumping of an Er^{3+} ion in silica fiber by either a 0.98 μm or a 1.48 μm source and stimulated emission at 1.55 μm, which is the low-attenuation window of silica based fibers. EDFAs combined with WDM technology are widely used in long-distance optical communi-cations, networks, and signal modulation. The gain of EDFA depends on several factors, e.g. doping concentration, fiber length, pump power, etc. EDFAs are widely used in multichannel systems.

- FRA utilize stimulated Raman scattering (SRS) to create optical gain. Herein, the pump energy at λ_p is transferred to the signal energy at λ_s in a non-resonant process to provide gain at λ_s. The overall gain for small signal amplification is given by:

$$G_{\text{FRA}} = \exp\left[(g_o - \alpha_s) L \right]$$

where α_s represents fiber losses per unit lengths at the signal, frequency v_s, L is total fiber length, and:

$$g_o = \frac{g_R \, P_{p, \text{in}} \, L_{\text{eff}}}{a_p \, L}$$

where $L_{\text{eff}} \approx 1/\alpha_p$, where α_p resent fiber losses at the pump frequencies v_p and L_{eff} is called the effective length of the fiber, and g_R is the Raman gain coefficient.

- FRA have a number of main technical characteristics, e.g. efficient pumping, simplicity, wider wavelength coverage, minimal polarization sensitivity, low insertion loss, high gain, low noise, fast reaction to changes of the pump power, low power consumption, and low cost. FRA are used in long-haul and ultra-haul DWDM transmission systems.

- The design of the *linear optical amplifier* is similar to that of the semiconductor optical amplifier. The device has an active waveguide gain region; the input and output fibers are aligned to this waveguide. They are used in high data rate telecommunication systems.
- Optical amplifiers (OAs) are used to boost signals transmitted over long distances in network systems. OAs are ideal for metro and long-haul dense wavelength multiplexing (DWDM) as well as single wavelength applications. The optical design, coupled with sophisticated control circuitry, allows these OAs to provide constant gain even with signals being added to the network.

REVIEW QUESTIONS

1. Explain the principle of the optical amplifiers. Write their characteristics and important applications.
2. Describe the basic operation of EDTA. Mention its main technical characteristics.
3. Derive an expression for amplifier gain of SOA. Mention limitations of SOA.
4. Derive an expression for total gain G fo an EDTA of length L.
5. Explain the principle of FRA. Distinguish between the amplification processes in (a) EDFA (b) FRA.
6. What requirements should be met so that semiconductor DH functions efficiently as an optical amplifier?
7. Derive an expression for gain ripple G_r of an SOA.
8. Using steady-state amplifier equations and appropriate approxi-mation, derive an analytical expression for an optimum length of fiber which gives maximum amplication for EDFA.
9. Distinguish between pure non-resonant TWA and resonant FPA signal gain.
10. The power conversion efficiency (PCE) of an EDFA is defined as:

$$PCE = \frac{P_{s,\,out} - P_{s,\,in}}{P_{p,\,in}}$$

Show that PCE is less than unity and the maximum value of its quantum conversion efficiency (QCE), which is defined by:

$$QCE = \frac{\lambda_s}{\lambda_p}\,(PCE)$$

is unity.

11. Explain the origin of gain saturation in FRAs. Derive an expression (approximate) for the saturated amplifier gain.
12. Write the flexibilities available in FRAs that are not available in SOAs and EDFAs.
13. Briefly mention the application of optical amplifiers.
14. Write the limitations of SOAs.

PROBLEMS

1. Taking the following parameters for a 1300 nm InGaAsP SOA:

W	active area width	3 μm
d	active area thickness	0.3 μm
L	amplifier length	500 μm

T	confinement factor	0.3
τ_r	time constant	1 ns
a	gain coefficient	$2 \times 10^{-20} \text{ m}^2$
n_{th}	threshold density	$1.0 \times 10^{24} \text{ m}^{-3}$

(a) Calculate the pumping rate if a 100 mA bias current is applied to the device.

(b) Calculate the zero signal gain.

[Ans. (a) 1.39×10^{33} (electron/m^3), (b) 2340 m^{-1} = 23.4 cm^{-1}]

[Hint:

(a) $R_p(t) = \dfrac{J(t)}{qd} = \dfrac{1}{qdWL}$

$= \dfrac{0.1 \, A}{(1.6 \times 10^{-19} C)(0.3 \, \mu m)(3 \, \mu m)(500 \, \mu m)}$

$= 1.39 \times 10^{33}$ (electrons/m^3)/s

(b) $g_o = a\tau_r \left(\dfrac{J}{qd} - \dfrac{n_{th}}{\tau_r} \right) = 0.3 \, (2.0 \times 10^{-20} \text{ m}^2)(1 \text{ ns})$

$\times \left(1.39 \times 10^{33} \text{ m}^{-3}\text{s}^{-1} - \dfrac{1.0 \times 10^{24} \text{ m}^3}{1.0 \text{ ns}} \right)$

$= 2340 \text{ m}^{-1} = 23.4 \text{ cm}^{-1}$]

2. To achieve a bit error rate (BER) = 10^{-9}, the factor Q specifying the receiver performance is 6. Calculate the optical signal-to-noise ratio (OSNR). Comment on your result. **[Ans.** OSNR (BER = 10^{-9}) ≈ 13.5 dB]

[Hint: OSNR $= \dfrac{1}{2}Q(Q + \sqrt{2})$

or   OSNR = (BER = 10^{-9})

$= 0.5(6)(6 + \sqrt{2})$

$= 22.24 \approx 13.5 \text{ dB}$

This reveals that if an OSA measures an OSNR ≤ 13.5 dB, then the corresponding error rate are equal to or higher than BER = 10^{-9}.]

3. An EDFA being pumped at 0.98 μm is being used as a power of 0 dB·m at λ_s = 1.55 μm, the output of amplifier is 20 dB·m. Show that the gain of the amplifier is 20 dB and input pump power required to achieve this gain is 156.6 mW.

4. A typical InGaAsP SOA is operating at 1.3 μm with the following parameters:
active region thickness = 0.5 mm
active region length = 200 mm
confinement factor (Γ) = 0.4
Time constant (τ_c) = 1 ns
σ_g (gain cross section or differential gain coeffiient = dg/dN) = 3×10^{-20} m^2
N_{tr} (carrier concentration per unit volume) = 1.0×10^{24} m^{-3}
Bias current (I) = 100 mA
Calculate (i) P_{sat}, (ii) the zero-signal gain coefficient, and (iii) the zero signal net gain.
[Ans. (i) 31.85 mW (ii) 3000 m^{-1} (iii) 1.82]

5. A SOA has single-pass gain of 10 dB. Calculate the peak-trough ratio of the passband ripple if the facet reflectivities are (i) 0.01%, (ii) 1%.
[Ans. (i) 1.004 (ii) 1.4938]

6. An EDFA being pumped at 0.98 μm with 30 mW pump power. The signal wavelength is 1.55 μm. Using the following data:
   - cross-sectional area of the fully doper fiber cone = 8.50 μm^2
   - doping concentration = 5×10^{24} m^{-3}
   - pump absorption cross-section = 2.17×10^{-25} m^2
   - signal absorption cross-section = 2.57×10^{-25} m^2
   - signal emission cross section = 3.41×10^{-25} m^2
   - input signal power = 200 μW

   and assuming that the fiber modes for λ_p and λ_s are fully confined, calculate (a) the rate of absorption per unit volume from the Er^{3+} level E_1 to level E_3 due to pump at λ_p (assuming $N_2 \approx 0$); and (b) the rate of absorption per unit volume from level E_1 to the metastable level E_2 and the rate of stimulated emission per unit volume from level E_2 to level E_1, both due to the signal at λ_s (assuming $N_2 \approx N_1$).
   [**Ans.** (a) 1.888×10^{28} m^{-3} s^{-1}, (b) 1.178×10^{26} m^{-3} s^{-1}, 1.5640×10^{26} m^{-3} s^{-1}]

SHORT ANSWER QUESTIONS

1. How the development of optical amplifiers revolutionized communication system?
   Ans. Optical amplifiers had an important impact similar to the invention of laser in early 1960s. Both devices contributed to the development of communication systems and other applications, such as lower pump optical power, single pixel multicolour displays, and light emitting devices.
2. How a regenerator is an optoelectronic device?
   Ans. Yes, a regenerator is an optoelectronic device. It amplifies and cleans up the optical signal in three steps: (i) The first step is to convert an optical signal into an electrical signal and then amplify it electronically, (ii) In the second step, to clean up the signal pulses using re-timing and pulse-shaping circuits, and (iii) In the third step, to reconvert the amplified electrical signal into an optical signal. This signal is then coupled into the next segment of the optical fiber.
3. What is an optical amplifier (OA)?
   Ans. An OA is an in-line optical device that amplifies the optical signal directly, without converting it to an electrical signal and then to an optical signal again. An OA operates solely in the optical domain, i.e. it takes in a weak optical signal from one segment of the link, amplifies it optically to produce a strong optical signal (without recourse to photon-to-electron conversion and vice versa), and couples it to the next segment of the link, or the OA is ideally a transparent box which provides gain and is also insensitive to the bit rate, modulation format, power and wavelengths of the signal(s) passing through it. The signals remain in optical form during amplification. Much of the most relevant recent advances in OAs (i.e. long distance NRZ and soliton systems, and wide area and broadcast multi-channel systems) can be traced to the incorporation of OAs.
4. How many types of optical amplifiers are there?
   Ans. There are mainly two classes of amplifiers, namely (i) semiconductor optical amplifiers, which utilize stimulated emission from injected carriers, and (ii) fiber optical amplifiers, in which the gain is provided by either rare-earth dopants or stimulated Raman scattering.
5. What is planar waveguide optical amplifiers?
   Ans. Rare-earth-doped planar waveguide optical amplifiers provide compact and inexpensive alternatives to fiber amplifiers. Moreover, planar technology is quite

suitable for optical integration and will be essential to the development of fully integrated advanced optical devices.

6. What is EDFA?

Ans. EDFA is a length of glass fiber which has been doped with the rare-earth metal Erbium ions. These ions act as an active medium with the potential to experience inversion of carriers and emit spontaneous and stimulated emission of light near a desirable signal wavelength. To produce the amplifier gain medium, the silica fiber core of a standard single-mode fiber is doped with Erbium ions.

7. What are semiconductor optical amplifiers (SOA)?

Ans. SOA is nothing more than a semiconductor laser, with or without facet reflections (the anti-reflection coating reduces the reflections). An electrical current inverts the medium, e.g. electrons are transferred from the valence to the conduction band, which produces spontaneous emission (fluorescence) and the potential for stimulated emission if external optical field is present. The stimulated emission yields the signal gain.

8. Why EDFAs have been used in multi-channel WDM systems?

Ans. EDFAs have been used in multi-channel WDM systems to compensate for (i) fiber attenuation losses in transmission, (ii) component excess losses, and (iii) optical network splitting losses.

9. What material properties govern the amplifier saturation in semiconductor optical amplifiers?

Ans. (i) gain cross section (σ_g) (ii) carrier life time (τ_c).

10. Give some examples of rare-earth elements which can be dissolved in glass to make optical amplifiers.

Ans. A number of SOA chips can be integrated on the same substrate to create high-density switching matrices.

11. How high-density switching matrices can be created using SOA chips?

Ans. Neodymium, praseodymium, holonium, and erbium. However, the laser transition in erbium-doped glass occurs at a wavelength that is very close to the wavelength of minimum attenuation of glass fibers, and this gives erbium special importance.

12. Mention important features of OAs.

Ans. (i) OAs are bidirectional and offer enough linearity for simultaneously amplifying signals in a multiplexed form without any cross-talk.

(ii) OAs can provide amplification to any optical signal irrespective of the modulation format and bit rate of transmission.

These features of OAs make them ideal choice in low dispersion long-haul communication link for boosting optical signal level without making use of regenerative repeaters.

13. What are fiber amplifiers?

Ans. These are generally viewed as passive components in the sense that the optical power decreases as the light propagates down the fiber. Obviously, the power available at the output end (P_{out}) of the fiber is less than that of the input (P_{in}). We can express the loss or attenuation of the fiber as $\alpha(dB) = 10\log_{10}(P_{in}/P_{out})$.

14. Explain the concept of photonic integrated circuits (PICs) and also mention the factors responsible for the limited growth of integrated optics (IOs).

Ans. PICs also known as integrated optics involve integration of planar light wave components on a single substrate to perform a variety of complex optical functions. The motivation behind IOs basically originated from the microelectronic circuits technology in the form of IC chip. Further, the IC technology of electronic components registered dramatic development resulting in the evolution of VLSI involving billions of transistors on a single chip. However, IO could not grow that way as was envisaged during its inception in early years due to following reasons:

(i) IO require optical interconnects to connect various optical components on the chip. We cannot reduce the dimension of the optical waveguide much below the operating wavelength.

(ii) In comparison to electronic components, the design of optical components is quite complex.

(iii) The size of the optical components unlike electronic components cannot be scaled down below a certain limit.

(iv) Technologically, the integration of planar optical devices with vertical structures is quite challenging, e.g. integration of an optical amplifier with a directional coupler is much more complex than integrating electronic amplifiers based on transistors in electronic ICs.

15. Write names of materials which are used for making planar waveguides for IC applications.

Ans. The principal materials used for making electro-optic IO devices are lithium niobate (LaNbO$_3$), Lithium tantalite (LiTaO$_3$), Zinc oxide (ZnO), Zinc sulphide (ZnS), titanium oxide (TiO$_2$), etc. Among iii-v semiconductors, GaAs, InP, GaSb, InAs, and their ternary are quaternary alloys are widely used for making optical waveguides. In addition, a large number of organic polymers are used for IO applications.

16. What are electro-optic modulators (EOMs)?

Ans. EOM is an IO device in which the electro-optic effect of an electro-optic material is exploited to modulate a beam of light in respect of phase, frequency, amplitude, or polarization of the beam. Modulation bandwidth in excess of gigahertz can be obtained by making use of a laser beam.

MULTIPLE CHOICE QUESTIONS

1. An optical amplifier operates:
   (a) solely in the optical domain
   (b) solely in the ultraviolet domain
   (c) solely in the infrared region
   (d) none of the above

2. Semiconductor optical amplifiers utilize:
   (a) stimulated Raman scattering
   (b) stimulated emission from injected carriers
   (c) spontaneous emission from injected carriers
   (d) None of the above

3. The amplifier gain (G) for SOA may be expressed as:

   (a) $G = \dfrac{P_{out}}{P_{in}} = \exp\left[g_o L - \left(\dfrac{1 - P_{in}}{P_{sat}}\right)\right]$

   (b) $G = \dfrac{P_{out}}{P_{in}} = \exp\left[g_o L - \dfrac{P_{in}}{P_{sat}}\right]$

   (c) $G = \dfrac{P_{out}}{P_{in}} = \exp\left[g_o L - \dfrac{1}{P_{sat}}\right]$

   (d) $G = \dfrac{P_{out}}{P_{in}} = \exp\left[g_o L - \dfrac{P_{out} - P_{in}}{P_{sat}}\right]$

4. Which of the following optical amplifiers is most suited for multichannel bidirectional operation?
   (a) SOA   (b) EDFA
   (c) FRA   (d) None of these

5. Optical amplifiers can be used as:
   (a) in-line amplifiers to compensate for loss
   (b) power amplifiers to follow transmitter
   (c) pre-amplifiers to precede the receiver
   (d) All of the above

6. Erbium-doped fiber amplifiers operate at the following windows:
   (a) low-dispersion window (around 1.30 µm)
   (b) low-attenuation window (around 1.55 µm)
   (c) both the windows
   (d) none of these

7. The structure of a semiconductor optical amplifier differs from a semiconductor laser in the following aspect:
   (a) the reflectivity of the end facets of the active region in the SOA is zero
   (b) the reflectivity of the end facets of the active region is 100%
   (c) the SOA is pumped electrically   (d) there is no difference

8. An SOA differs from an EDFA in the following manner:
   (a) an SOA operates in the electrical domain while the EDFA operates in the optical domain
   (b) an SOA is pumped electrically while the EDFA amplifies 1.55 µm
   (c) an SOA amplifies 1.30 µm while the EDFA amplifies 1.55 µm
   (d) there is no difference

9. Gain in EDFA depends on the following factors:
   (a) doping concentration   (b) length of the doped fiber
   (c) pump power   (d) all of these

10. The power conversion efficiency (PCE) of an EDFA defined as $\mathrm{PCE} = \dfrac{P_{s,\,out} - P_{s,\,in}}{P_{p,\,in}}$ is:

    (a) equal to 1   (b) less than 1
    (c) greater than 1   (d) infinite

11. The difference between a regenerator and an optical amplifier is:
    (a) a regenerator amplifies as well as restores the signal
    (b) an optical amplifier compensate for transmission loss
    (c) a regenerator converts the optical signal into the electrical domain for amplification and then reconverts it into the optical domain, whereas an optical amplifier operates only in the optical domain
    (d) there is no difference between the two

12. The most suitable wavelength for pumping an EDFA is:
    (a) 0.85 µm   (b) 0.98 µm
    (c) 1.30 µm   (d) 1.55 µm

13. In what way does an EDFA differ from a fiber Raman amplifier?
    (a) An EDFA requires population inversion while the FRA does not
    (b) An FRA operates on the principle of stimulated Raman scattering
    (c) An EDFA operates on the principle of stimulated emission
    (d) There is no difference

14. In what way are EDFA and FRA similar?
    (a) Both of them operate in the all-optical domain
    (b) Both of them can be used around the 1.55 μm window
    (c) Both of them can be employed for multichannel operation
    (d) All of the above

15. A Raman optical amplifier is based on a nonlinear effect called:
    (a) spontaneous Raman scattering   (b) stimulated Raman scattering
    (c) Rayleigh scattering   (d) none of the above

16. In a long transmission system, optical amplifiers are needed to periodically restore the power level after it has decreased due to:
    (a) attenuation in the fiber   (b) reflection in the fiber
    (c) absorption in the fiber   (d) None of the above

17. The most popular fiber amplifier makes use of silica fiber doped with erbium. Such a fiber amplifier is known as
    (a) Raman optical amplifier   (b) Raman and Brillouin fiber amplifier
    (c) planar waveguide   (d) erbium doped fiber amplifier

18. A symmetrical planar waveguide supports only one TE and TM mode when the V-number becomes
    (a) $V = \dfrac{\pi h}{\lambda} (n_1 - n_2) < \pi/2$ (b) $V = \dfrac{\pi h}{\lambda} (n_1^2 - n_2^2)^{1/2} < \pi/2$

    (c) $V = \dfrac{\pi h}{\lambda} (n_1^2 + n_2^2)^{1/2} > \pi/2$ (d) $V = \dfrac{\pi h}{\lambda} (n_1^2 - n_2^2)^{1/3} < \pi/2$

19. For a symmetrical waveguide structure with a central guiding region of thickness h the number of modes, m supported by the waveguide at a given length can be estimated using the relation
    (a) $h \geq \dfrac{\left(m + \dfrac{1}{2}\right) h}{2(n_1^2 - n_2^2)^{1/2}}$ (b) $h \geq \dfrac{m\lambda/2}{2(n_1^2 - n_2^2)^{1/2}}$

    (c) $h \geq \dfrac{m\lambda/4}{2(n_1^2 - n_2^2)^{1/3}}$ (d) $h \geq \dfrac{m\lambda/8}{2(n_1^2 - n_2^2)^{1/2}}$

20. The refractive index of an electro-optic material can be expressed as the function of the applied electric field, E using Taylor's series about $E = 0$ as $n(E) = n + a_1$, $E + \dfrac{1}{2} a_2 E^2 + \dots$ This equation can be expressed in terms of electro-optic coefficients r and ξ which depend on the direction of electric field and
    $$n(E) = n - \frac{1}{2} rn^3 E - \frac{1}{2} \xi n^3 E^2 + \dots$$
    For certain materials, the third on the right-hand side is negligible and the equation can be approximated as $n(E) = n - \dfrac{1}{2} rn^3 E$. The corresponding material is called
    (a) Pockels medium   (b) Raman active material
    (c) Ruby   (d) Kerr medium

ANSWERS

1. (a)	2. (b)	3. (d)	4. (b)	5. (d)	6. (b)	7. (a)	8. (b)	9. (d)	10. (b)
11. (c)	12. (b)	13. (a)	14. (d)	15. (b)	16. (a)	17. (d)	18. (b)	19. (a)	20. (a)

APPENDIX

OPTICAL SWITCHES

A10.1 INTRODUCITON

There are many optical networks which integrate optical switches into their design. *Opto-mechanical switches* redirect optical signals from one port to another by moving an optical fiber tube assembly or an optical component, such as a mirror or prism. There are several types of optical switches incorporated into networks. However, in practice, most optical switches are still operated mechanically and controlled by an electronic control circuit. Speed is a crucial parameter in network applications, since a high-speed data transmission of tenths of milli-seconds is required. In few years, we expect that dynamic optical routing will require much faster speeds. However, more technology exists for optical switches than any other functional component within the optical network. Efforts through research are there for developing optical switches to increase the number of outputs, and to reduce size, cost and switching time. Presently, optical switches include many types, e.g., *opto-mechanical switches, thermo-optic switches, electro-optic switches, micro-electro-mechanical switches* (MEMSs), and *micro-opto-mechanical switches* (MOMSs). Development of new types of optical switches are in the research and development ranges.

Opto-mechanical and electro-mechanical switches are the oldest type of optical switches and most widely deployed at this time. These devices achieve switching of moving fiber or other optical components by means of stepper motors or relay arms. This causes them to have relatively slow switching time; however, their reliability is excellent and they offer low insertion and crossmark losses.

This chapter presents a few optical switch designs, i.e. four cases in building opto-mechanical switches using a movable mirror or prism to switch between the input and output ports for use in communication systems.

A10.2 OPTO-MECHANICAL SWITCHES

Figure A10.1 illustrates common switch configuration. The input signal comes through the input fiber cable on the left side of the switch. A mechanical slider moves that fiber up and down, latching into one of the two output fiber cables on the right side of the switch. In OFF/ON positions, the switch directs light from the input fiber into one of the two outputs. This arrangement is called "1 × 2 switch configuration". As input at port 1, the signal can be switched to either port 2 or port 3.

For the following definitions, assume the switch is configured to couple to port 2. The insertion loss L_{IL} (in decibels) is defined by Eq. (A10.1). Insertion loss depends on fiber cable alignment at the input and output ports. Low insertion loss value can be obtained on switches with good mechanical alignment. A good switch provides similar values of insertion loss for all switch positions.

$$L_{IL} = -10 \times \log_{10} \frac{P_2}{P_1} \quad \text{(A10.1)}$$

where, P_1 is the power going into port 1 and P_2 is the power exiting from port 2.

Crosstalk loss L_{CT} is one of the important losses, which should be considered in opto-mechanical switches. Crosstalk loss is a measure of how well the uncoupled port is isolated. The crosstalk loss L_{CT} (in decibels) is

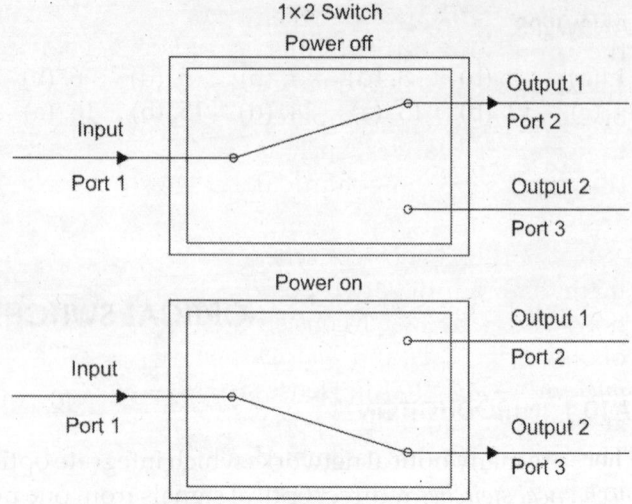

Fig. A10.1: A typical 1 × 2 switch configuration

defined by Eq. (A10.2). Crosstalk loss values depend on the particular design of the switch.

$$L_{CT} = -10 \times \log_{10} \frac{P_3}{P_1} \quad \text{(A10.2)}$$

where, P_1 is the power going into port 1 and P_3 is the power exiting from port 3.

There are other important optical parameters that need to be specified for each switch type. These parameters include: *polarization dependent loss* (PDL), *return loss* (RL), and the *Etalon effect*. The PDL is defined as the maximum difference in insertion loss between any two-polarization states. It is caused by mechanical stress and temperature variation on optical components or fiber cables. This causes changes in the birefringence and a gradient of index of refraction (n) of the optical material. The RL is defined as the light reflected back into the input path. It is caused by scattering and reflection from optical surfaces like mirrors, lenses, and connectors or from defects, such as cracks and scratches. The back reflection is equal to the RL with a negative quantity. Elaton effect is defined as light resonance (ripple) at a certain wavelength. It is caused by reflection of light from parallel optical surfaces and interference between the signals. All the above losses are measured in decibels (dB). Special optical parameters can be specified by the customers.

Another important parameter of the optical switches is the repeatability—achieving the same insertion loss each time the switch is returned to the same position. Switching speed is also another important specification of a switch. The switching speed is defined as how fast the switch can charge the signal from one port to the other. It is an important factor in some switch applications in communication systems.

Figure A10.2 shows a schematic diagram of a mechanical switch configuration with two inputs and two outputs. The inputs are located on the one side and the outputs on the other side of the switch. This configuration is called a 2 × 2 switch. The signal enters port 1 and port 4, and exists from port 2 and port 3, respectively. This case is called the *bypass state*, in the OFF position. When the latching mechanism changes position between port 2 and port 3, signal enters port 1 and exists port 3 and from port 4 to port 2. This case is called the *operate state*, in the ON position.

Opto-mechanical switches collimate the optical beam from each input and output fiber and move these collimated beams around inside the switch. This creates low optical loss, and allows distance between the input and output fiber. These switches have more bulky components compared to newer alternatives, such as the micro-optomechanical switches.

Figure A10.3 shows a schematic diagram of a two-position switch. The switch consists of a *sliding prism* and *quarter pitch graded index* (GRIN) lenses at the input and output ports. The components are assembled in a packaging base and sealed with a lid. Each GRIN lens is connected to the fiber tube assembly using an epoxy. Figure A10.3 illustrates the OFF/ON positions of a 1 × 2

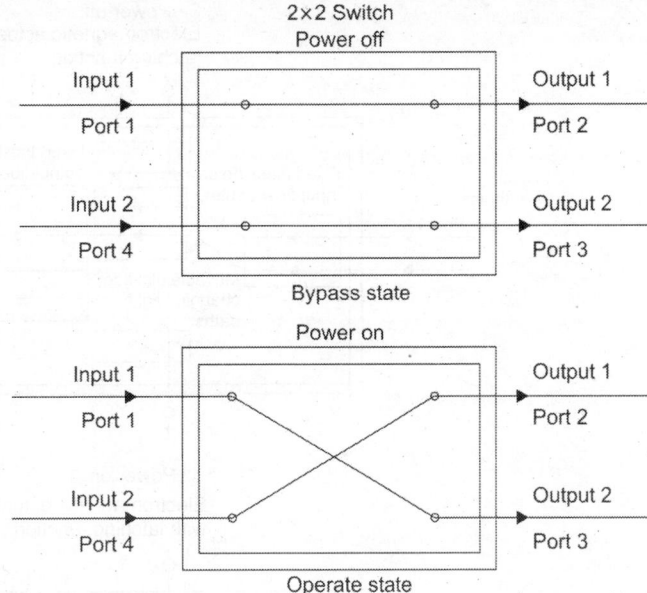

Fig. A10.2: A typical 2 × 2 switch configuration

switch. As explained above, the GRIN lens collimates the divergence beam exiting from the input fiber. The right angle prism deflects the light by total internal reflection (TRIN)

at its two slanting surfaces. The GRIN lens refocuses the collimated beam onto a fiber cable at one of the output ports. To direct the signal from port 1 to port 3, the prism slides to a new position, as shown in Fig. A10.3 in the OFF position. Figure A10.3 also shows the signal directed between port 1 and port 2, in the ON position, when the prism changes position.

Opto-mechanical switches drive optical fiber networks mechanically. They can switch between light paths at high speed and with low insertion loss. They are widely used in rapidly developing areas of the fiber-optic field, such as optical cross connection and wavelength multiplexing. Figure A10.4 shows the design of a 2 × 4 opto-mechanical switch. The switch uses an electromagnetic actuator with a latching function to drive a movable block to change the light path between the ports. Figure A10.4 shows the switch in the OFF position. The light passes through from port 1 and port 2 to

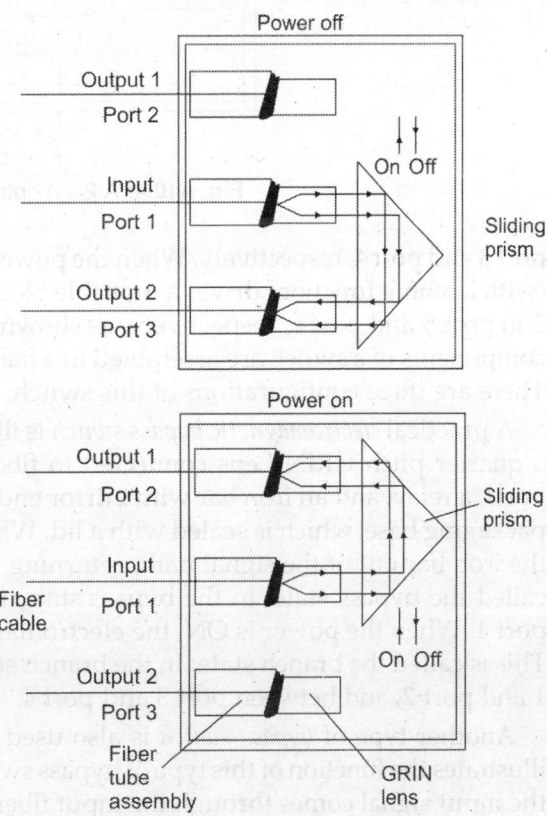

Fig. A10.3: A 1 × 2 optomechanical switch

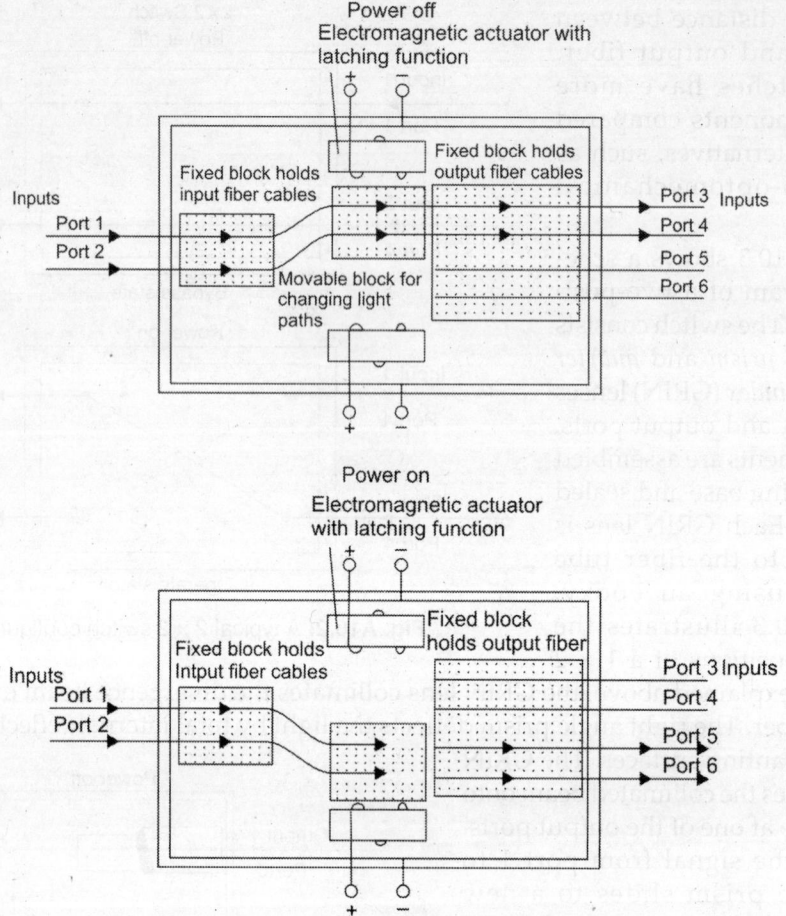

Fig. A10.4: A 2 × 4 opto-mechanical switch

port 3 and port 4, respectively. When the power is turned ON, an electromagnetic actuator (with latching function) drives a movable block to change light path from port 1 and port 2 to port 5 and port 6, respectively, as shown in Fig. A10.4. The optical and mechanical components of a switch are assembled in a packaging box with minimal alignment work. There are three configurations of this switch: 1 × 2, 2 × 2, and 2 × 4.

A practical *electromagnetic bypass switch* is illustrated in Fig. A10.5. The switch contains a quarter pitch GRIN Lens connected to fiber tube assembly at the input and output ports, a relay, and an iron bar with mirror end faces. The components are assembled in a packaging base, which is sealed with a lid. When the power is turned OFF, a spring pulls the iron bar out of the signal path, returning the switch to the bypass condition. This is called the bypass state. In the bypass state, the signal passes directly from port 1 and port 4. When the power is ON, the electromagnet is activated and the iron bar is raised. This is called the branch state. In the branch state, mirrors direct the signal between port 1 and port 2, and between port 3 and port 4.

Another type of *bypass switch* is also used in communication network. Figure A10.6 illustrates the function of this type of bypass switch. When the power is in the OFF position, the input signal comes through the input fiber cable on port 1 on the left side and leaves through the output port 4 on the right side of the switch. This is called the bypass state.

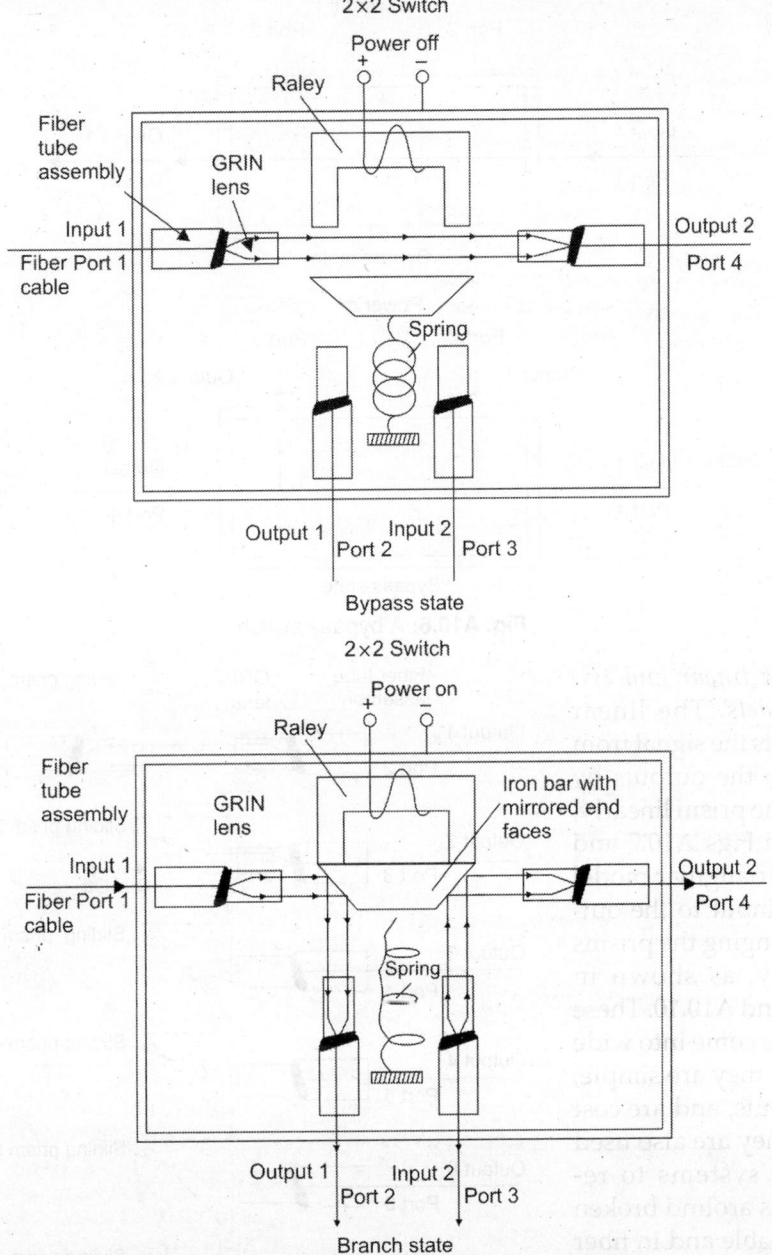

Fig. A10.5: An electromagnetic bypass switch

When the power is ON, a mechanical slider moves two fiber connections to the up position, latching into two output fiber cables at port 2 and port 3 on the side of the switch. In this position, the input signals from port 1 and port 4 are launched into port 2 and port 3, respectively. This position is called *branch state*. As input at port 1, the signal can be directed to either port 4 or port 2. Also, an input signal at port 4 can be directed to output port 3.

Now, we present new switch designs of a 1 × 8 latching switch configuration using prisms. These switches are commercially available in the market. There are two types of

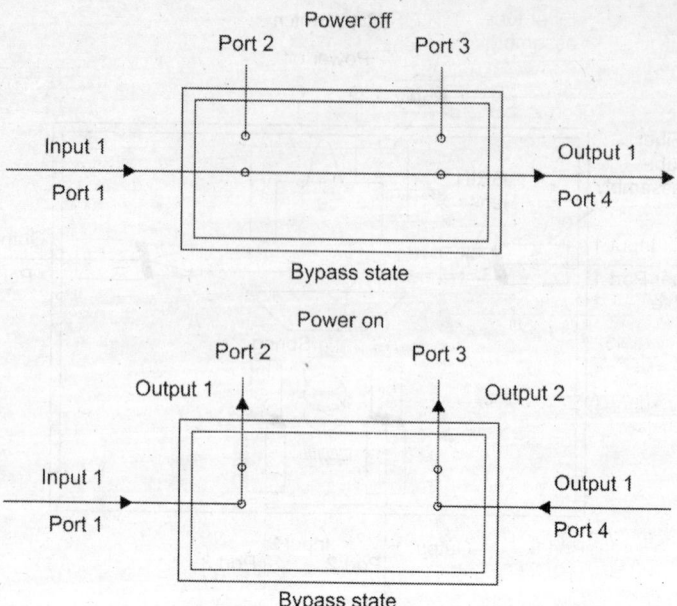

Fig. A10.6: A bypass switch

models: *the linear and triangular models.* The linear model directs the signal from the input to the outputs by arranging the prism linearly, as shown in Figs A10.7 and A10.8. The triangular model directs the input to the outputs by arranging the prisms triangularly, as shown in Figs A10.9 and A10.10. These models have come into wide use because they are simple, offer 8 outputs, and are cost effective. They are also used in back-up systems to re-route signals around broken fiber optic cable and in fiber optical instruments.

Figure A10.7 illustrates a schematic diagram for one configuration of a *linear model of a 1 × 8 latching switch.* The common element of this type of opto-mechanical switch is that their operation involves mechanical sliding motion of prisms in OFF/ ON positions to direct the

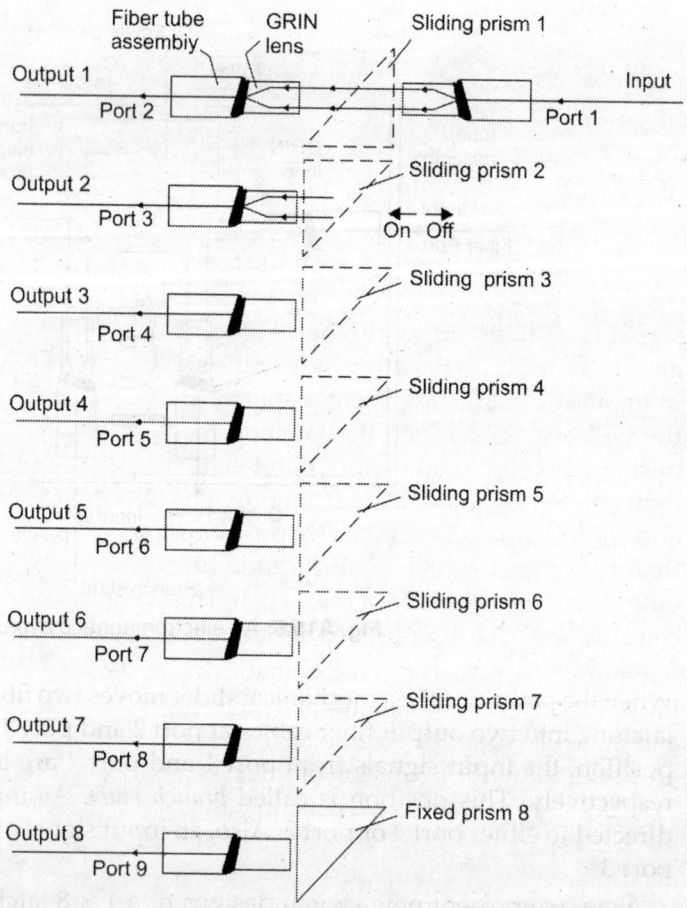

Fig. A10.7: Schematic configuration of the one type of linear model of a 1 × 8 latching switch

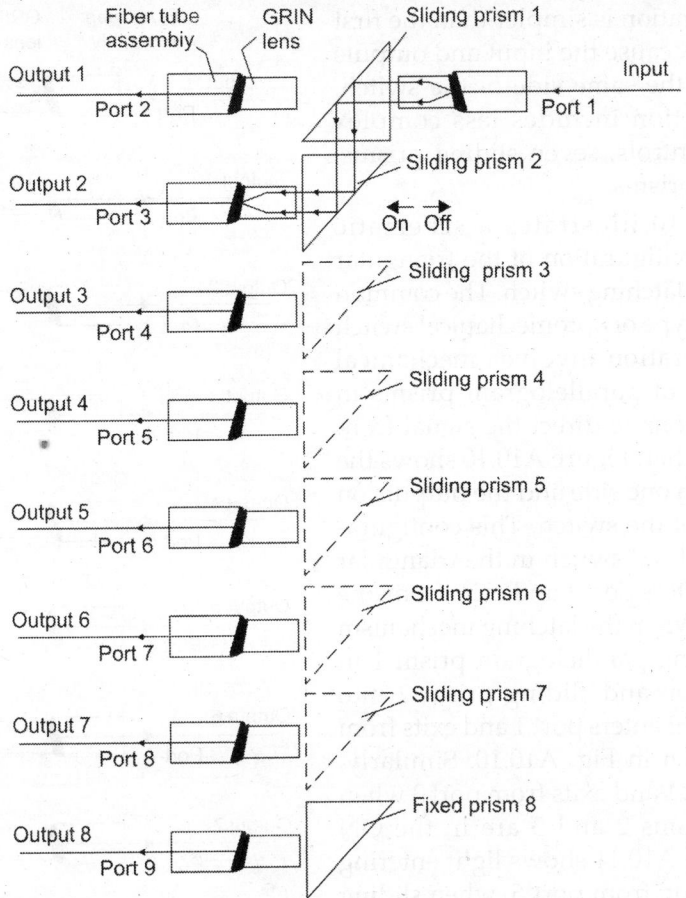

Fig. A10.8: Signal from port 1 to port 3 in the linear model of a 1 × 8 latching switch

signal from one port to another. Figure A10.7 shows the input located on the one side and the outputs on the other side of the switch. This configuration is called a 1 × 8 switch in the linear model. Light enters port 1 and exits from port 2 when sliding prism 1 is in the OFF position. When the latching mechanism places the sliding prisms 1 and 2 in position, the light enters port 1 and exits from port 3, as shown in Fig. A10.8. Similarly, light enters port 1 and exits from port 4, when the sliding prism 2 is in the OFF position and sliding prism 3 is in the ON position. This switch configuration is more complicated than the second switch configuration because the input is located on one side and the outputs on the other side of the switch. This configuration includes a complex mechanism, controls, seven sliding prisms, and one fixed prism.

Figure A10.9 illustrates a schematic diagram of the second type of configuration of the linear model of a 1 × 8 latching switch. This configuration is different because the input and the outputs are located on the same side of the switch, as shown in Fig. A10.9. Prisms are also used in the operation of this type of switch configuration. Light enters port 1 and exits from port 2 when fixed prism 1 and sliding prism 2 are in position. When the latching mechanism places the sliding prism 2 in the OFF position and sliding prism 3 in the ON position, the light enters port 1 and exits from port 3. Similarly, light enters port 1 and exits from port 4 when the sliding prism 3 is in the OFF position and sliding prism 4 is in the ON position. The same procedure is used for the signal exiting from other ports. This switch configuration is simpler than the first configuration because the input and outputs are located on the same side of the switch. This configuration includes less complex mechanism, controls, seven sliding prisms, and two fixed prisms.

Figure A10.10 illustrates a schematic diagram of a configuration of the triangular model of a 1 × 8 latching switch. The common element of this type of optomechanical switch is that the operation involves mechanical sliding motion of parallelogram prisms in OFF/ON positions to direct the signal from one port to another. Figure A10.10 shows the input located on one side and the outputs on the other side of the switch. This configuration is called a 1 × 8 switch in the triangular model. Light enters port 1 and exits from one of the outputs. When the latching mechanism places the sliding parallelogram prism 1 in the OFF position and sliding prism 2 into position, the light enters port 1 and exits from port 4, as shown in Fig. A10.10. Similarly, light enters port 1 and exits from port 3 when the sliding prisms 2 and 3 are in the ON position. Figure A10.11 shows light entering port 1 and exiting from port 5, when sliding prism 1 is in the OFF position. This switch configuration is more complicated than the linear model because the input is located on one side, and the outputs on the other side of the switch. Seven sliding parallelogram prisms with additional mechanisms and

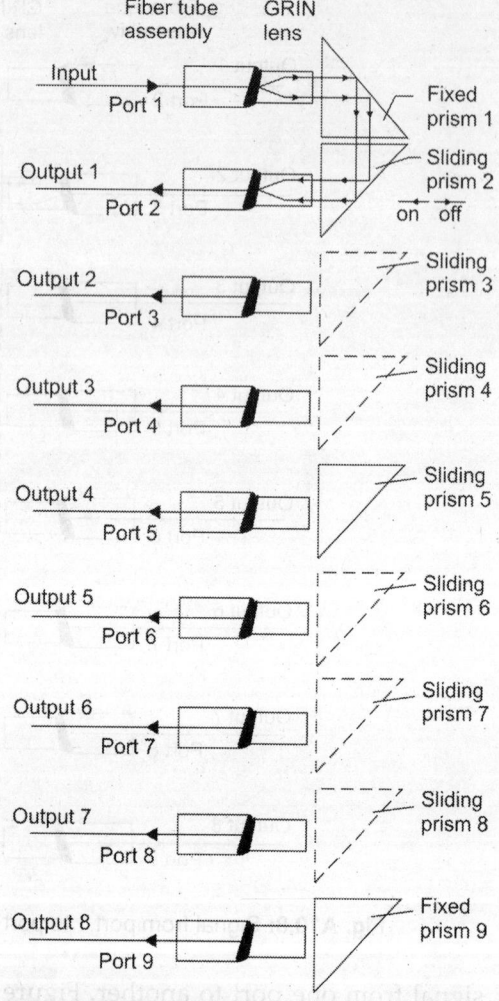

Fig. A10.9: Schematic of second configuration of the linear model of a 1 × 8 latching switch

controls form this configuration. Both models have difficulty achieving precise alignment and low losses during the manufacturing processes.

Many other modern opto-mechanical switches are used in telecommunication networks management, monitoring, restoration, and protection. They have excellent optical performance and the high reliability necessary for network applications. They feature low insertion loss, high RL and channel isolation, excellent repeatability, and fast switching speeds. The switches are available in single-mode and multi-mode, and cover wide wavelength ranges. They are available in 1× 1, 1 × 2, and 2 × 2 configurations. The switching mechanism is latching and remains in its selected states following a loss of power. The switch consists of a quarter pitch GRIN lens glued to a double bore fiber tube assembly, relay, and mirror mounted on a shaft. The components are assembled inside a packaging base box and covered by a lid. Figure A10.12 illustrates a schematic diagram of a 2 × 2 switch. This figure illustrates the switch in the OFF/ON positions. When the power is off, light transmits from port 1 to port 2 and port 4 to port 3. This configuration is called the *transmission state*. When the power is ON, the mirror is in position, the light

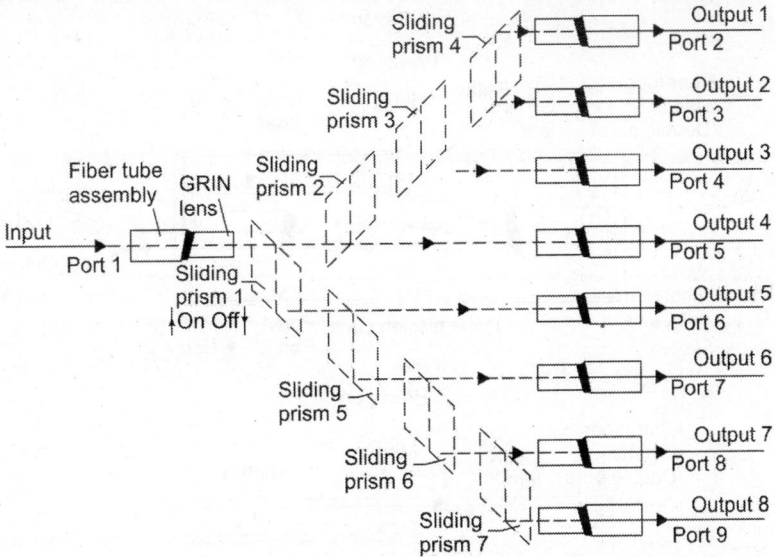

Fig. A10.10: Schematic of the triangular model of a 1 × 8 latching switch

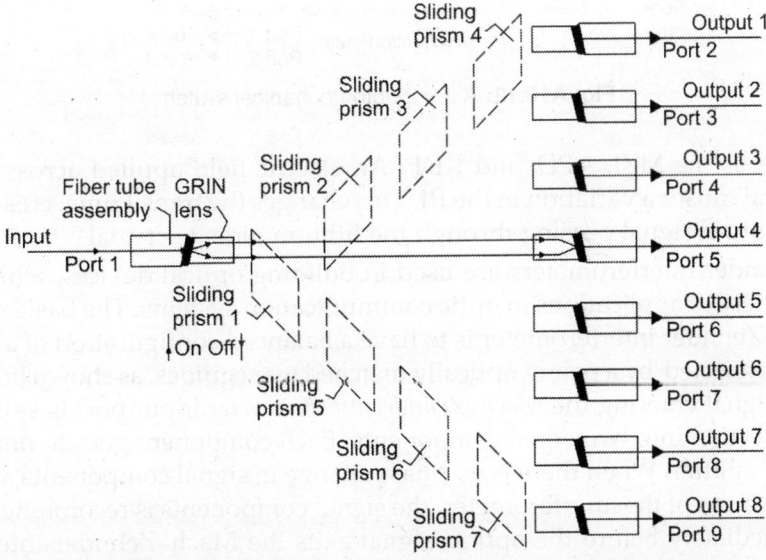

Fig. A10.11: Signal from port 1 to port 5 in a 1 × 8 latching switch

is reflected by the mirror, light exits port 1 and reflects to port 4 and similarly, port 2 reflects to port 3. This state is called the *reflection state*.

A10.3 ELECTRO-OPTIC SWITCHES

Switches with no moving parts can be built by using some of the passive devices, such as Mach–Zehnder interferometers (MZIs) and couplers. Some optical materials, such as lithium niobate crystal (LiNiO$_3$), Avalanche photo diode (APD) (NH$_4$H$_2$PO$_4$), and KDP (KH$_2$PO$_4$) exhibit an electro-optic effect. The index of refraction (RI) of the optical material changes in the presence of an electric field. These optical materials are used in building

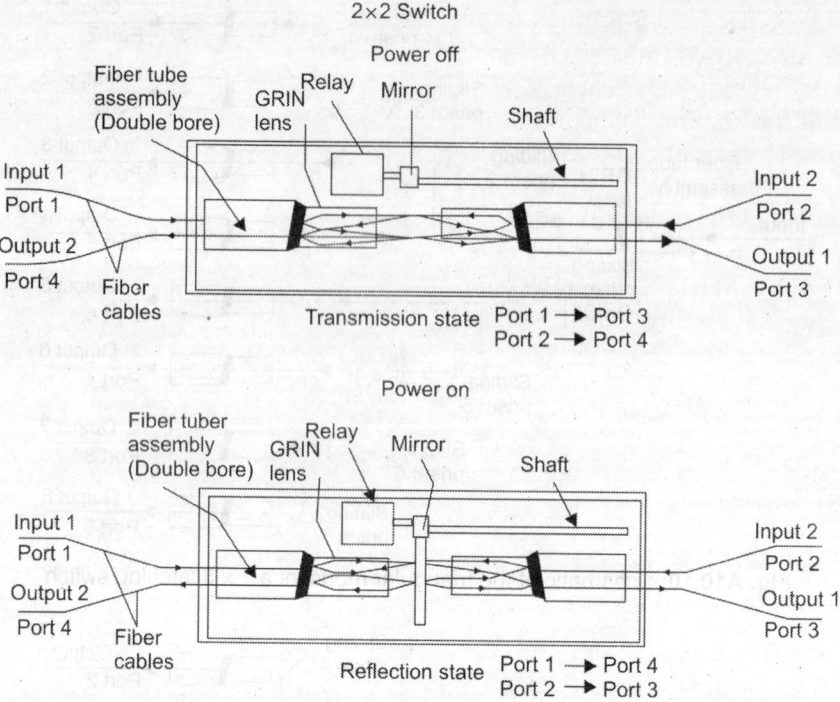

Fig. A10.12: A 2 × 2 optomechanical switch

devices, such as the MZI, APD, and KDP. An electric field applied across the lithium niobate crystal causes a variation in the RI. This changes the transit time, creating a phase shift of the optical signal passing through the lithium niobate crystal.

Mach–Zehnder interferometers are used in building optical devices, which are used in a wide variety of applications in optic communication systems. The basic requirement of the Mach–Zehnder interferometer is to have a balanced configuration of a splitter and a combiner connected by a pair of optically matched waveguides, as shown in Fig. A10.13. The optical signal entering the *Mach–Zehnder interferometer* input port is split through a "Y" splitter section into two equal components. Each component goes to one of the two arms of the Y splitter. When there is no phase change in signal components after passing through both arms of the interferometer, the signal components is recombined at the "Y" coupler immediately before the optical signal exits the Mach–Zehnder interferometer. The recombination of the two signal components takes place as constructive interference between two components and regenerates the original optical signal. In this case, the Mach–Zehnder interferometer acts as a passive device.

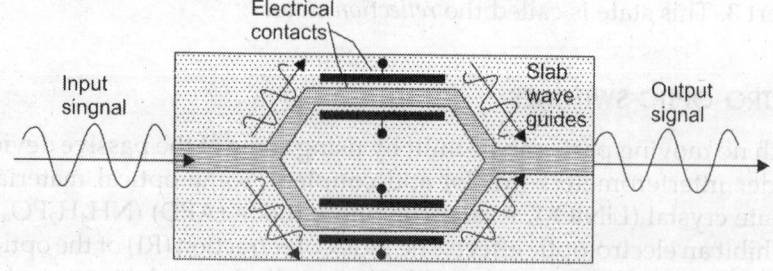

Fig. A10.13: Mach-Zehnder interferometer acts as a passive device

When an electric field is applied to one arm of the Mach–Zehnder Interferometer, the RI changes and causes 180° shift in the phase of the signal component, due to the change in optical path length of this arm. As shown in Fig. A10.14, when there is a difference in phase at the destination "Y" coupler, the signal components will be out of phase with one another. The signal components recombination will be lost because the components will cancel each other in destructive interference. If the phase difference is a full 180°, then the output will be zero. In other words, applying the electric field to one of the arms of the Mach–Zehnder interferometer will make the phase shift one of the signal components. The Mach–Zehnder interferometer acts as an active device, when an external electric voltage is applied causing the switching.

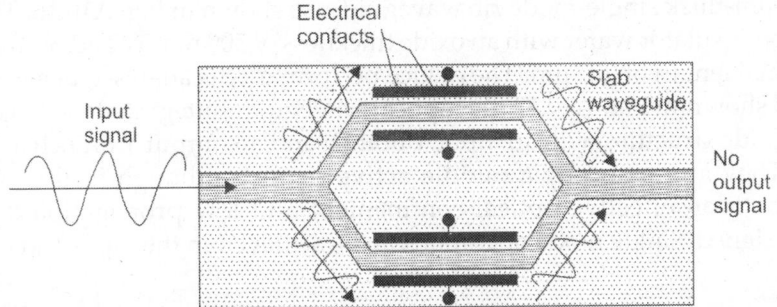

Fig. A10.14: An electro-optic switch using a Mach–Zehnder interferometer

Using the same principle as discussed above, one can built an *electro-optic switch* using two branching waveguides arranged like a 3 dB coupler to switch one input between two outputs. You can replace the one input with two parallel outputs coupled to the pair of switching waveguides by a combining coupler, as shown in Fig. A10.15. An electric field applied to one arm of the waveguide causes a 180° shift in the phase of the signal

Table A10.1. Input and output signals connections	
Voltage	*Connections*
V_1	Port 1 to Port 2 and Port 4 to Port 3
V_2	Port 1 to Port 3 and Port 4 to Port 2

component. The electrical voltage is raised or lowered to shift the delay between waveguides by 180°. This directs the output from one waveguide on the right side to the other output. Because signal interference depends on phase shift, it is possible to further increase the voltage to switch the signal back to the other output. Table A10.1 presents the possible outcomes achieved by applying different voltages across the waveguide arms.

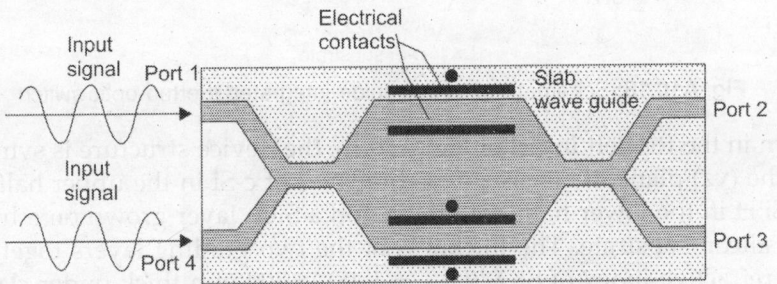

Fig. A10.15: A 2 × 2 electro-optic switch

A10.4 THERMO-OPTIC SWITCHES

A novel rib waveguide-integrated thermo-optic switch has appeared recently. The device is based on the TIR phenomenon and the thermo-optic effect (TOE) in hydrogenated amorphous silicon (a-Si:H) and crystalline silicon (c-Si). It takes advantage of a bandgap-engineered a-Si:H layer to explore the propertis of an optical interface between materials showing similar refractive indexes but different thermo-optic coefficients. In particular, the modern plasma-enhanced chemical vapour deposition techniques, the refractive index of the amorphous film can be properly tailored to match that of c-Si at a given temperature. TIR may be achieved at the interface by acting on the temperature, because the two materials have different dermo-optic coefficients. The switch is integrated in a 4-pm-wide and 3-μm-thick single-mode rib waveguide, as shown in Fig. A10.16. The substrate is a silicon-on-insulator wafer with an oxide thickness of 500 nm. The active middle region has an optimal length of 282 μm. The device performance is analysed at a wavelength of 1.55 μm. As shown in Fig. A10.12, the optical waveguide-integrated switch consists of a 2 × 2 waveguide structure with an input Y branch and an output Y branch and an output Y branch. They are joined by a middle active region, although in this work, which guarantee both an effective optical confinement and low propagation losses. When properly designed, single mode operation can be achieved in the input and output of the Y branches.

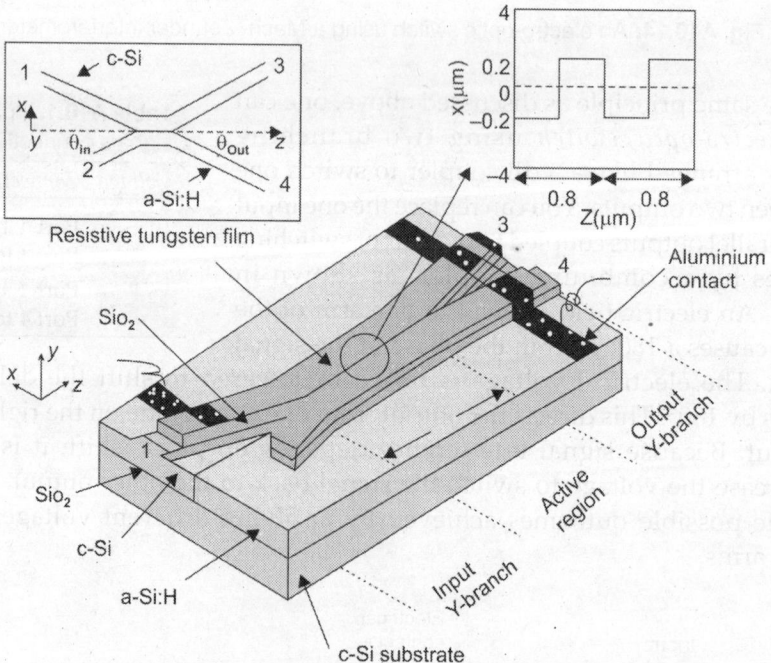

Fig. A10.16: Schematic of a waveguide-integrated thermo-optic switch

As shown in the top-left insert of Fig. A10.16, the device structure is symmetric with respect to the (yz) plane. It consists of a core layer of c-Si in the upper half, and a core layer of a-Si:H in the lower half, both laying on a SiO₂ layer grown on a highly doped crystalline silicon substrate. The thickness of the two guiding layers together is 3 μm. Due to the refractive index of SiO₂ (n_{SiO_2} = 1.48), a 500 mm thick under cladding layer ensures the optical confinement for both waveguides, as suggested by electromagnetic field propagation simulations. In the top-right inset of Fig. A10.16, a detail of the interface between the a-Si:H waveguide and the crystalline Si waveguide in the active region is also shown. The irregular profile at the TIR interface takes into account surface roughness that may result from the fabrication process.

We can exploit the TOE in a SI:H and c-Si by changing the refractive index of the core layers and thereby, switching the light beam at the output of the structure. A 300 nm thick tungsten heating film is introduced on top of the stacked structures. It is separated from the active region by a 100-nm-thick SiO_2 film. This reduces the optical absorption by the electrodes due to the evanescent field of the optical mode. Finally, the heating structure is completed by aluminium bonding pads.

The operating principle of the device is the TIR, which can be activated or dropped by exploiting the different thermo-optic coefficients in a-Si:H and c-Si. In particular, by choosing a proper gas phase composition during the deposition process of a-Si:H, the two materials develop the same refractive index at a given temperature. By changing the device operating temperature, a refractive index discontinuity is created at the (yz) interface, producing the desired optical switching. At room temperature, an incident channel-guided light beam coming from port 1 will encounter a refractive index discontinuity between C-Si and a-Si:H, and the reflection (straight state) exists. Under these conditions TIR will occur and the incident light beam at port 1 will be reflected to port 3.

Another type of thermo-optical switch uses the Mach–Zehnder interferometer for the switching process. This type of thermo-optical switch is used in communication systems. Figure A10.17 illustrates the logic of an 8 × 8 thermo-optical switch. The 8 × 8 optical matrix switch employe Mach–Zehnder interferometer with a thermo-optic phase shifter

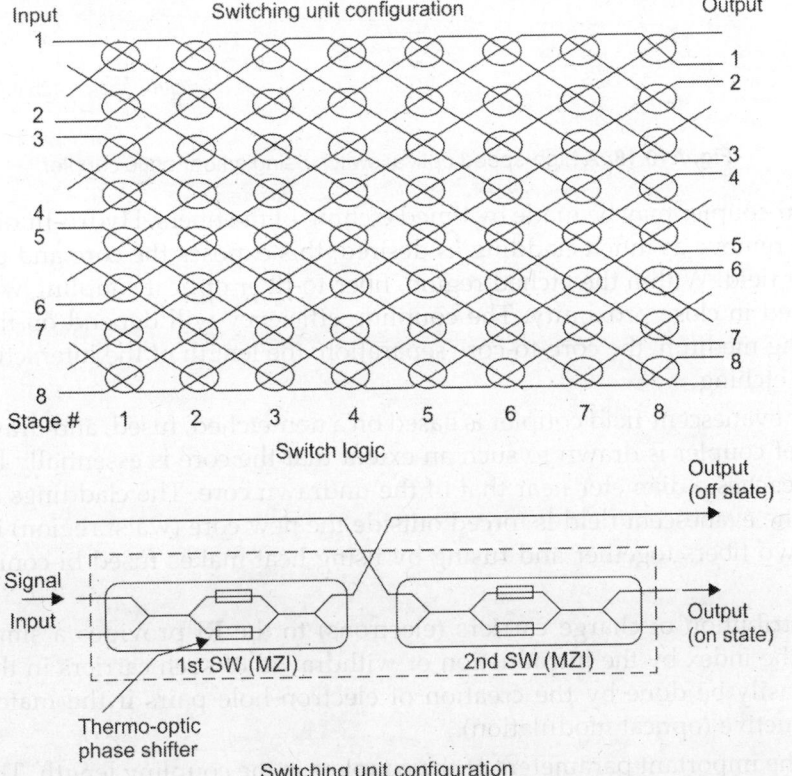

Fig. A10.17: An 8 × 8 thermo-optical switch using Mach-Zehnder interferometer

as the switching mechanism. The small switch offers low loss, low crosswalk, low return loss, excellent stability, high reliability, and low power consumption. Applications of such switches include: space division switching systems (with analog and/or digital signals), wavelength routing (such as cross-connect and add-drop), protective switching, video switching, and inter-module connection.

A10.4.1 Switch Logic

Switching Unit Configuration

A high-speed all-optical switch using a fiber optic coupler and a light-sensitive variable-index material is illustrated in Fig. A10.18. *Refractive index variation with light is the principle of the switch operation.* Evanescent-wave coupling between two mono-mode fibres is extremely sensitive to the RI of the material surrounding the coupling region. Two ground and polished fibers, producing an evanescent field, can be brought in close proximity so that light in one fiber will couple into the other fiber in any desired ratio. Such polished couplers have been constructed to produce very low losses.

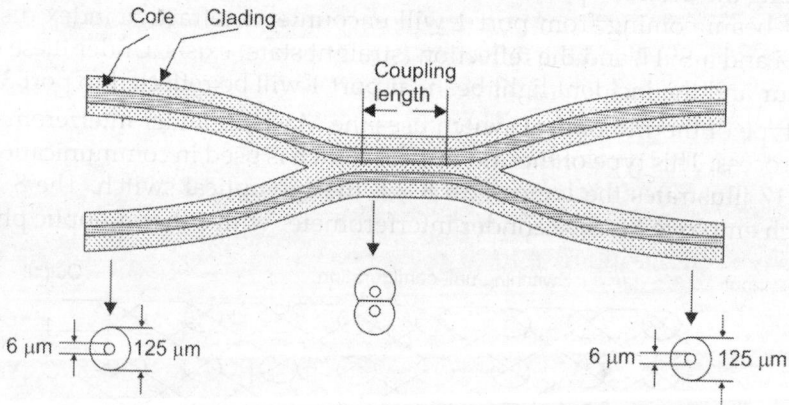

Fig. A10.18: A high-speed optical switch using a fiber optic coupler

A similar coupler may be made by timed etching of the fibers. Hydro-fluoric acid may be used to remove as much cladding as desired; this exposes the core and produces an evanescent field. Within the etched region, fiber-to-fiber optical coupling will occur for fibers placed in close proximity. The coupling efficiency will depend on the RI of the surrounding medium, the core-to-core separation, the length of the interaction, and the amount of etching.

Another evanescent-field coupler is based on a non-etched, fused, and drawn coupler. This type of coupler is drawn to such an extent that the core is essentially lost and the cladding reaches a diameter near that of the undrawn core. The claddings become the core, and the evanescent field is forced outside the new core (waist region) into the air. Twisting two fibers together and fusing by using heat makes fused bi-conical tapered couplers.

The contribution of charge carriers (electrons) to the RI provides a simple way to modulate the index by the introduction or withdrawal of such carriers in the material. This can easily be done by the creation of electron-hole pairs if the material is also photoconductive (optical modulation).

One of the important parameters of the couplers is the coupling length. The coupling length is wavelength dependent. Thus the shifting of power between the two parallel waveguides will take place at different places along the coupler for different wavelengths. Fig. A10.19 shows two wavelengths entering at port 1 and port 2. When coupler length is made exactly to match the wavelength of the signal, the coupler works to combine wavelengths. Combined signals exit from port 2.

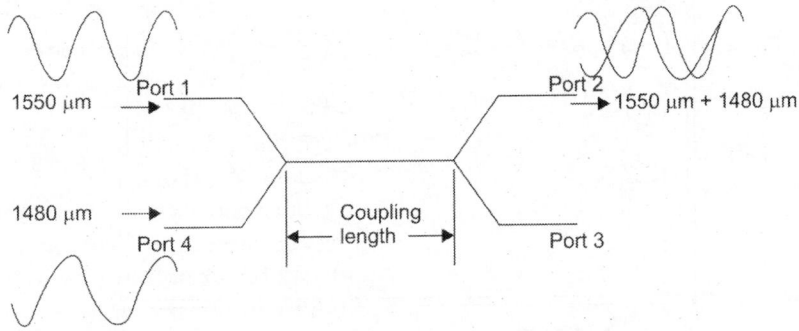

Fig. A10.19: Two wavelengths entering at port 1 and port 2

Figure A10.20 shows the reverse process where two different wavelengths arrive on the same input fiber at port 1. At a particular location along the coupler, the wavelengths will be in different waveguides. Then the wavelengths separate exactly and each wavelength exits from a different port. In this case, one wavelength exits from port 2 and the other from port 3. The processes described in Figs A10.19 and A10.20 are performed in the same coupler. This process is *bi-directional*. The coupler in Fig. A10.19 works as a *splitter*; the same coupler in Fig. A10.20 also works as a *combiner*.

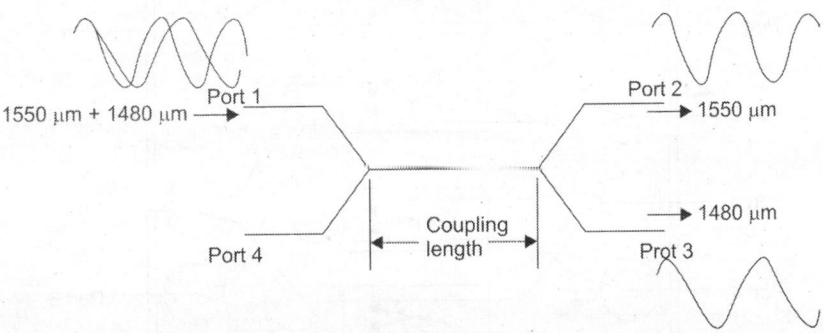

Fig. A10.20: Two wavelengths entering at port 1

There are other types of switches that use the same elements of either the micro-opto-mechanical switch or micro-electro-optical switch. They employ couplers for switching between the inputs and outputs. These types of optical switches are used in communication systems. Figure A10.21 shows the configuration of a 4 × 4 optical space-division switch. The switch is designed to connect any input port to any output port as desired by the user. Any input may be switched to any output; however, two inputs may not go to the same output at the same time. The device is bidirectional such that once a connection has been established between an input port and an output port, that particular connection may be used in either one or both directions. The switches have no moving parts, are very stable, and reliable while exhibiting very low loss; thereby reducing the need for expensive amplifiers.

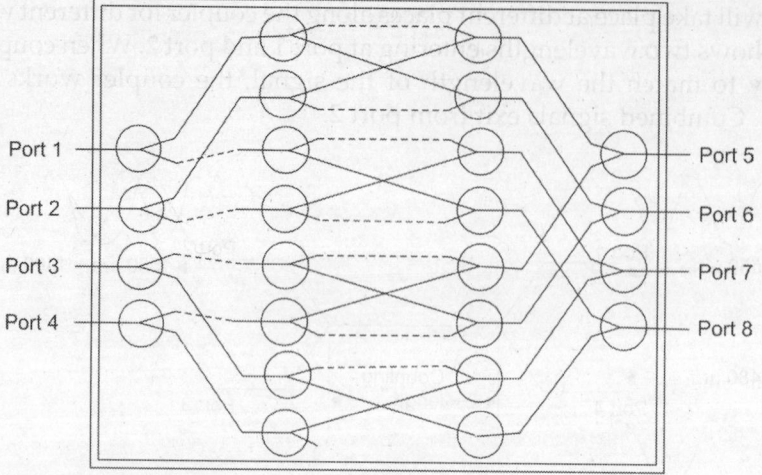

Fig. A10.21: A 4 × 4 optical space-division switch

Figure A10.22 shows the cross connect switch, which selects outputs by optical cross connecting. This results in a significant reduction of overall complexity and number of required elements. These switches are used in protection/backup switching, optical cross-connecting, network testing and monitoring, optical routing, and optical burst switching. A 4 × 4 switch configuration can be cascaded to built 16 × 16–256 × 256 switch configurations.

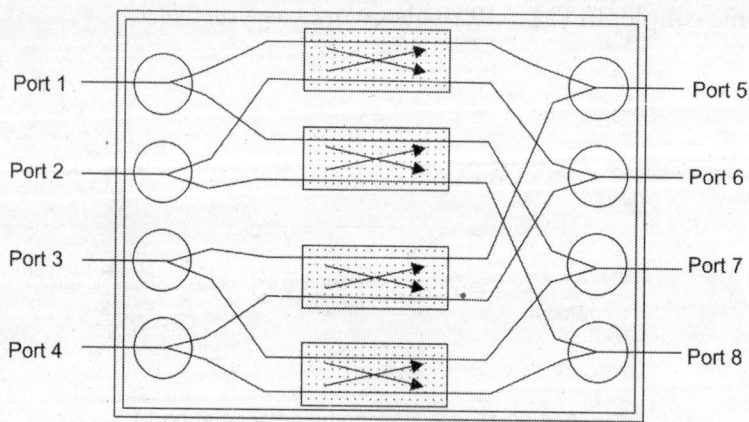

Fig. A10.22: A cross connect switch

A10.5 ACOUSTO-OPTIC SWITCHES

Sound waves are generated when a material is in mechanical vibration mode. They can also be generated by acoustic transducers. Like any light wave, a sound wave is a moving wave, which has a frequency. Light waves travel at the speed of light; sound waves travel at the speed of sound, which is slower than light waves. Sound waves are used to control light transmission in acousto-optic switches and modulators. The refractive index of some optical material is altered by the presence of sound waves. The sound wave causes regular zones of compression and tension within the optical material. This creates a regular pattern of changes in index of refraction n of the optical material; this is called

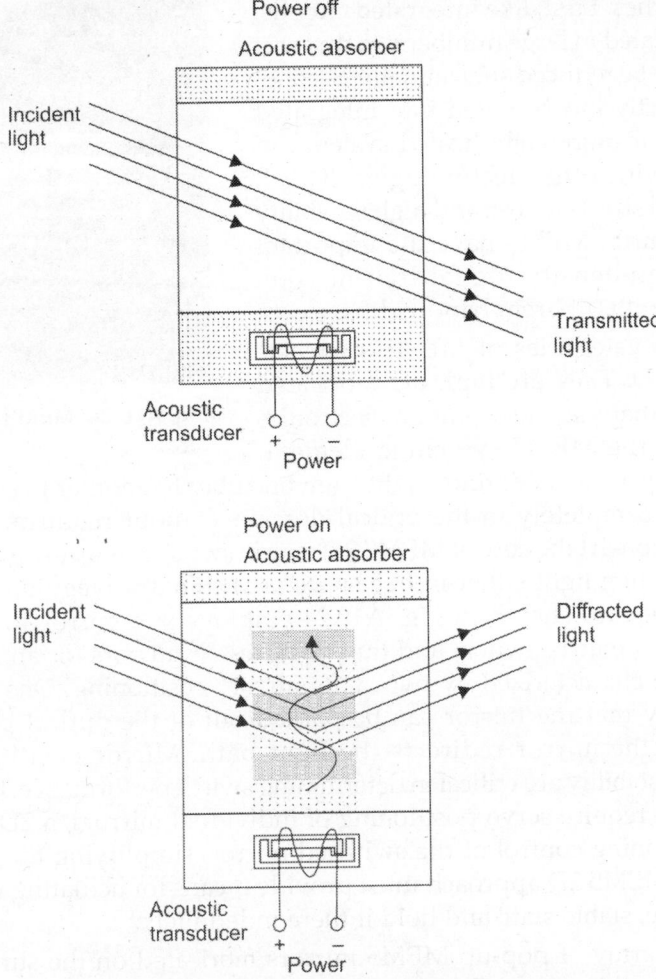

Fig. A10.23: Schematic design of an acoustic-optic switch

a *Bragg diffraction grating*. Within the optical material, there is interference between sound and light waves. The power of the deflected light is controlled by the intensity of the sound wave. The angle of deflection is controlled by the frequency of the sound wave. Figure A10.23 illustrates a design of an acoustic-optic switch, it also shows that an incident light can be controlled by the frequency of the sound wave. The incident light exits the switch from one or more selected output ports depending on the sound wave intensity.

A10.6 MICRO ELECTROMECHANICAL SYSTEM (MEMs)

MEMs is a rapidly growing technology for the fabrication of miniature devices using processes similar to those used in the integrated circuit (IC) industry. MEMSs are widely used in optical switching in telecom networks. The appeal of MEMS goes beyond just switching applications in defense, aerospace, and medical industries. MEMS technology provides a way to integrate electrical, electronic, mechanical, optical, material, chemical, and fluids engineering on very small devices ranging in size from a few microns to one millimeter. MEMS devices have many important advantages over conventional opto-mechanical switches. First, like integrated circuits, they can be fabricated in large numbers, so that cost of production can be reduced substantially. Second, they can be directly incorporated into integrated circuits, so that far more complicated system can be made than with other technologies. Third, MEMS have small size, low cost, and high reliability and stability. Fourth, MEMS have the important capability of high-density digital transmission communication with different bandwidths.

There are two categories of MEMS switches: MEMS 2D and 3D. They are typically fabricated onto a substrate that may also contain electronics needed to drive the MEMS switching element.

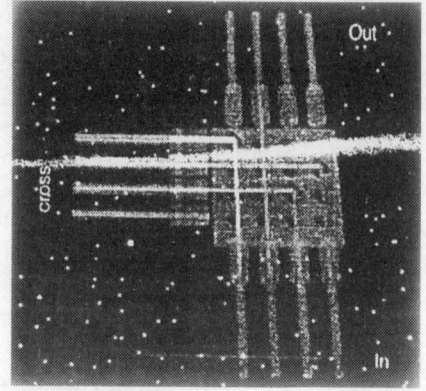

Fig. A10.24: MEMS 2D switch architecture

MEMS-based optical switches route light from one fiber to another to enable equipment to switch traffic completely in the optical domain without requiring any optical-to-electrical conversion. At the core of MEMS 2D matrix switches is an array of micro mirrors capable of redirecting light either in free space or within a waveguide framework. The 2D switch architecture shown in Fig. A10.24 employs one mirror for every possible switched node in a matrix switch, and thus requires N^2 mirrors for an $N \times N$ array. 2D mirror arrays are characterized by two-state mirror positioning. One state is inactive and requires only that the mirror can be parked out of the optical path. During the switching state, the mirror redirects the light path. Mirror positioning accuracy, repeatibility, and stability are critical in determining switch performance. Unlike 3D switch architectures that require servo positioning of individual mirrors, a 2D switch can rely on passive positioning control of the switched mirror, simplifying the control scheme. But a successful MEMS 2D approach must provide means for actuating the mirror into a highly predictable, stable state and hold it there indefinitely.

MEMS use an array of pop-up MEMS mirrors fabricated on the surface of a silicon wafer. The mirror is hinged to allow its rotation off the plane of the substrate to an angle of 90° where it redirects a light channel from the through to cross state, as shown in Fig. A10.25. An addressing scheme is required to select individual mirrors for actuation into the popped-up state and also for positioning them with sufficient accuracy for efficient coupling into the switched channel. The 2D MEMS array described here, called MagOXC, which stands for *"magnetically optical actuated cross-connect"*, uses a combination of magnetic and electrostatic actuation to rotate the mirrors and to select and deselect individual mirrors for clamping into the up or down state.

To rotate unclamped mirrors into the up state, magnetic actuation is implemented globally by applying an external field generated with a small electromagnet. The magnetic signal only needs to be applied momentarily. Using a global field avoids the need to fabricate indiviual magnetic

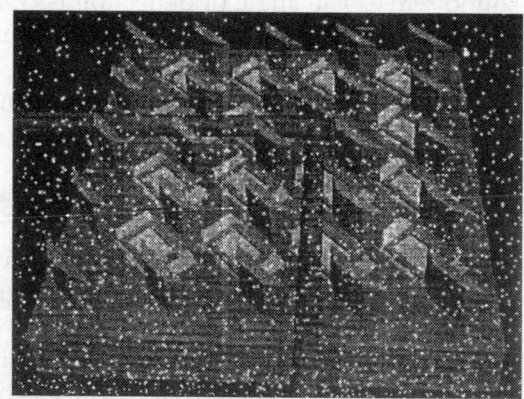

Fig. A10.25: Pop-up mirror array passive mirror alignment

actuators for each chip. Mirrors are fabricated with a layer of attached nickel to produce torque on the mirror hinge in response to the applied field. The nickel plate aligns with the magnetic field lines and generates a magnetostatic torque on the mirror. This lifts the mirror off the substrate and orients it near the desired vertical position, where electrostatic force can take over in setting and holding the final desired mirror position. An electrostatic field is applied mirror by mirror, either to hold the mirror down against the torque produced by the magnet or to hold the mirror in the up position against the restoring force of the elastic hinge. Since the magnetic field is applied globally, all mirrors will attempt to rotate when the field is turned on. Only the mirrors to be rotated into the up position are unclamped; all others are held down electrostatically. Similarly, mirrors clamped in the up state remain so until the electrostatic signal is removed; the magnet is no longer needed to hold the mirror up. The combination of magnetic and electrostatic actuation provides an effective means for configuring a mirror array without resorting to complex individual actuators for each mirror. Since electrostatic clamping of the mirrors requires virtually no current flow, the switch array consumes very little steady state power. Power is consumed only during transitions when the magnet is activated. The components of the switch are packed in a packaging base and lid.

A10.7 3D MEMS BASED OPTICAL SWITCHES

3D MEMS based optical switch route light from any of 80 input fibers to any of 80 output fibers. Designed for fiber-based test and measurement, 10 Gbit/s *Ethernet, high-definition video,* and *telecom* applications, this all-optical micro-photonic subsystem fits in the palm of a hand. The switch design is based on 3D MEMS mirror arrays, which is called *Reflexion*. It can switch signals within 10 ms, which is well within the telecommunications requirement for communications applications. 3D designs have switching elements accommodating hundreds, even thousands of ports, Fig. A10.26 shows a 3D MEMS optical switch. The design ofthe 3D MEMS is simple, solves mechanical and optical issues, is easy to fabricate, and achieves manufacturing tolerances that are accepted by the telecommun ications industry.

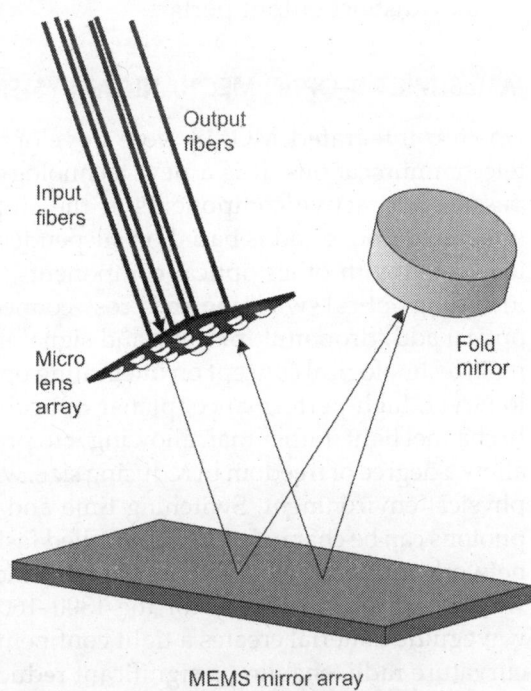

Fig. A10.26: A 3D MEMS optical switch architecture

A 3D MEMS design is shown in Fig. A10.27. A micro-morror array rests atop a single piece of silicon on a ceramic substrate. No bonding pads or other integrated electronics exist on the chip. All routing to the rest of the actuation electronics is done on the back end of the ceramic substrate. Additional electronics is located on a photodetector card, along with constant-delay two-pole *Bessel filters,* and an *analog-to-digital converter* with a conversion-phasing time. Parallel-plate electrostatic actuation of the mirrors, with potentials of about 200 V, is provided by high voltage linear amplifiers.

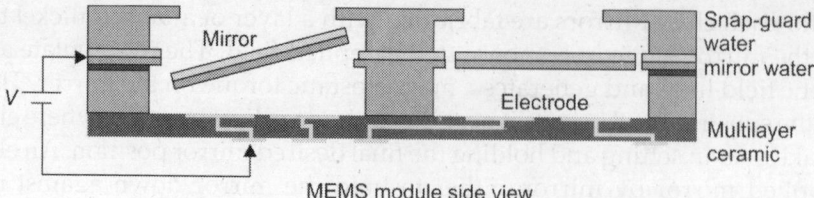

MEMS module side view

Fig. A10.27: A 3D MEMS optical switch design

Figure A10.28 shows a *torsional micro mirror*, which is driven by a vertical bi-directional comb driver (micro electrostatic actuator). Underneath the mirror plate is the substrate electrode. During operation, a voltage is applied to the electrode in order to generate an electrostatic attractive force on the mirror plate. The mirror plate rotates around the supporting axis in two dimensions. Such tilting mirror position can direct light from many distinct input ports to any of many distinct output ports.

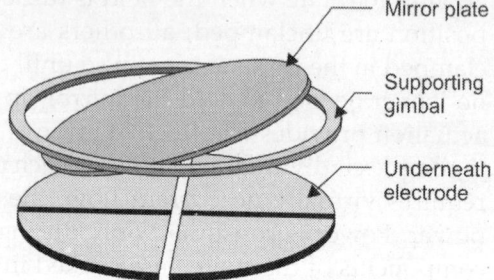

Fig. A10.28: A torsional micro mirror

A10.8 MICRO-OPTIC MECHANICAL SYSTEM (MOMS)

On-chip integrated MOMS were developed for a variety of applications for optical telecommunications. It is a new technology that allows for the integration of multiple passive and active components at the chip level. The technology is an extension of integrated optics and is based on suspended waveguides fabricated on chips, which are integrated with other optical components. It is used for a variety of optical solutions, including optical switching and cross-connect, signal dispersion correction, configurable optical add/drop multiplexers, and signal intensity equalizers. The technology bases its main technological concept on integrating optics at the chip level. The technology explores low-cost, high-performance, planar optical waveguide switches. Waveguides are used to channel light, rather than allowing it to propagate in free-space. The use of waveguides allow a degree of freedom in reducing size, while at the same time operating in a controlled physical environment. Switching time and losses are very low. By using waveguides, photons can be channeled in a controlled fashion, making it possible to lay out a photonic network within the chip with low losses. Since silicon is used as the propagating material, wavelength trans-parency for the 1300–1600 nm is utilized. The use of silicon for the waveguide material creates a tight confinement of light that allows the use of very small curvature radii, enabling a significant reduction of footprint chip size.

11

Advanced Optical Communication Systems and Optical Networks—Wavelength Division Multiplexing (WDM) Technology

11.1 INTRODUCTION

Until the late 1980s, optical fiber communications was mainly confined to transmitting a single optical channel. Due to fiber attenuation, this channel required periodic regeneration which included *detection, electronic processing* and *optical retransmission*. Such regeneration causes a high-speed optoelectronic bottleneck, is bit-rate specific, and can only handle a single wavelength. The need for these single-channel regenerators (i.e. *repeaters*) was replaced when the *erbium-doper fiber amplifier* (EDFA) were developed, enabling high-speed repeaterless single channel transmission. One can think of this single ~Gbits/s channel as a single high speed *lane* in a highway in which the cars represent packets of optical data and highway represents the optical fiber. Single fiber has its low-loss window near 1.55 µm is approximately 25,000 GHz wide. The high-bandwidth characteristic of the optical fiber implies that a single optical carrier at 1.55 µm can be baseband modulated at ~25,000 Gbit/s, occupying this 25,000 GHz bandwidth. Obviously, this bit rate is impossible for present-day optical devices to achieve, given that heroic lasers, external-modulators, switches, or detectors have bandwidths < 100 GHz; we may note that practical data links today would be significantly slower, perhaps no more than 40 Gbit/s per channel. As such, a single high-speed channel takes advantage of an extremely small portion of the available fiber bandwidth. It seems natural to dramatically increase the system capacity by transmitting several different independent wavelengths simul-taneously down a fiber in order to fully utilize this enormous fiber bandwidth. Therefore, the intent was to develop a *multiple-lane highway*, with each lane representing data travelling on a different wavelength. This *highway cartoon* scenario is illustrated in Fig. 11.1.

In addition to high-capacity transmissions, *WDM technology* also enables wavelength routing and switching of data paths in an optical network. By utilizing wavelength-selective component technologies, each data channel's wavelength can be used to determine the routing through the network. Therefore, data can be thought of as travelling not on optical fiber but on wavelength-specific "light paths" from source to destination that can be arranged by a network controller to optimize throughput.

Basic Operation

The practicality of EDFA which can provide gain to many channels simultaneously over a ~THz wavelength range opened the door to multiplexing signals at many wavelengths onto the same optical fiber. This technique, known as WDM, wonderfully enhances an optical system's capacity. Along with the EDFA, WDM is another technology that is the

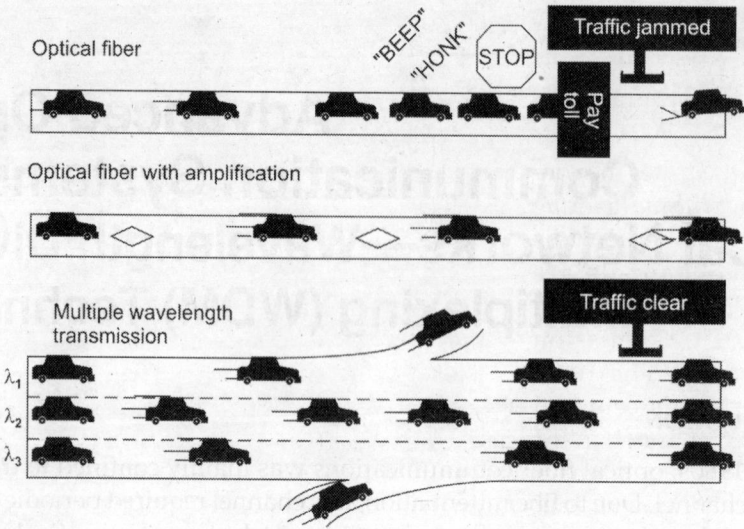

Fig. 11.1: Multiwavelength optical transmission as represented by a multiple-lane highway

key to terabit-per-second optical systems. Conceptually, WDM is the same as the frequency-division multiplexing (FDM) used to place many radio channels on carrier waves of different frequencies. The carrier wave of each optical WDM channel, however, is a million times higher in frequency (terahertz verses megahertz).

In the most basic WDM arrangement as shown in Fig. 11.2, the desired number of lasers, each emitting a different wavelength, are multiplexed together by a wavelength multiplexer (or a combiner) into the same high-bandwidth fiber. After being transmitted through a high-band-width optical fiber, the combined optical signals must be multiplexed by a WDM (or a splitter) at the receiving end by distributing the total optical power to each output port and then requiring that each receiver selectively recover only one wavelength. At the receiver, a narrow-band optical filter is used to select just one of the incoming wavelength, so that only one signal is allowed to pass and establish a connection between source and destination.

It is important to space channel wavelengths an adequate distance apart. The goal is to minimize transmission of unwanted channels through the filter and to accommodate the drift in the wavelength characteristics of optoelectronic components over time—a

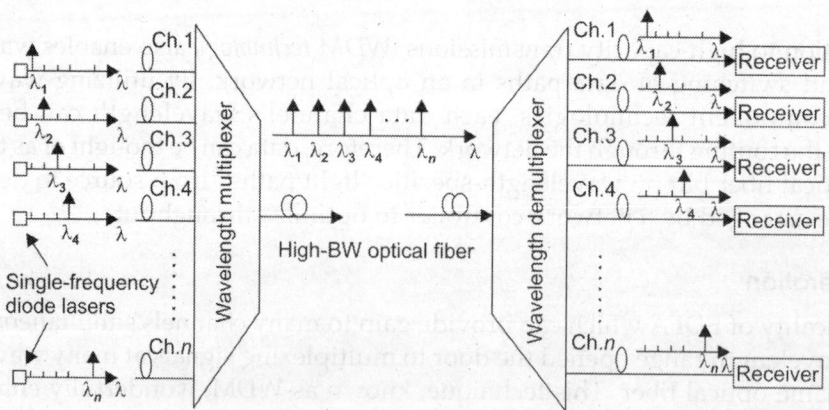

Fig. 11.2: Schematic diagram of a simple WDM system

change in temperature is just one possible cause. Typical channel spacings range from 0.4 nm to 4 nm (50–500 GHz).

Figure 11.3 illustrates the concept of *wavelength demultiplexing* using an optical fiber. In this example, four channels are input to an optical filter which has a nonideal transmission filtering function. The filter transmission peak is centered

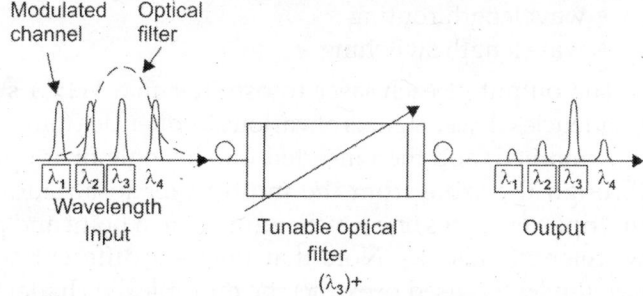

Fig. 11.3: Optical WDM being demultiplexed by an optical filter

over the desired channel, in this case λ_3, thereby transmitting that channel and blocking all other channels. Due to the nonideal filter transmission function, some optical energy of the neighboring channels leaks through the filter causing inter-channel inter-wavelength crosstalk. This crosstalk has the effect of reducing the selected signal's contrast ratio and can be minimized by increasing the spectral separation between channels. Although there is no set definition, a nonstandardized convention exists for defining optical WDM, dense-WDM, and FDM as encompassing a system for which the channel spacing is approximately 10, 1 and 0.1 nm, respectively. However, we will not make any distinction among these system labels.

Obviously, WDM is an optical technology that permits several wavelengths to be coupled into the same fiber cable, effectively increasing the aggregaiton bandwidth per fiber cable. Figure 11.4(a) illustrates the components of a basic communication system. The *de-multiplexer* (de-mux) decouples what the multiplexer has coupled. The de-mux separates several wavelength in a single fiber cable, and directs them individually onto many fiber cables, which are connected to the receiver channels.

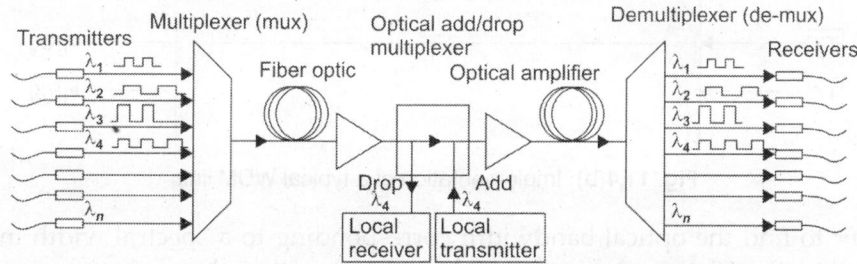

Fig. 11.4(a): A schematic diagram of basic communication system

WDM systems are based on the ability of a fiber cable to carry many different wavelengths without mutual interference. Each wavelength represents an optical channel within the fiber cable. Several optical methods are available to combine individual channels within a fiber cable, and to extract them at appropriate points along a network. WDM technology has evolved to the point that channel wavelength separations can be as small as a few nanometers, giving rise to dense wavelength division multiplexing (DWDM) systems.

Key features:
- capacity upgrade
- transparency (each optical channel can carry any transmission format)

- wavelength routing
- wavelength switching

The output of each laser transmitter in a WDM system is set to one of the channel frequencies. These signals of various frequencies must be then multiplexed (superimposed or combined) and then inserted into a single fiber optic cable. These signals then travel through the cable from the multiplexer to an add-drop multiplexer. The add-drop multiplexer routes one wavelength, λ_4, to a point and picks up another signal at the same wavelength, also λ_4. Note that this is a different signal, as shown in Fig. 11.4(a). A *demultiplexer* is used to extract the multiplexed channels at the receiver end. Multiplexing and demultiplexing devices employ narrowband filters. Multiplexer and demultiplexer devices can be cascaded and combined to achieve the desired results. Several devices exist to perform such filtering, including thin-film fiber *Bragg gratings*, *optic gratings*, *tapered fibers*, *liquid crystal filters*, and *integrated optical* devices. These multiplexing technologies are also used for other optical fiber applications. These applications include telephone and data communications, SONET/SDH networks, inter-exchange networks, and in links for trunk exchange and local exchange hubs.

Implementation of a typical WDM system employing N channels is shown in Fig. 11.4(b). In the shown system *three* wavelengths are multiplexed in one fiber to increase transmission capacity. The light of laser diodes with wavelengths recommended by the ITU is launched into the inputs of a wavelength multiplexer (MUX), where all wavelengths are combined and coupled into a single-mode fiber. When needed, propagating light can be amplified by an optical fiber amplifier and eventually imputed at the wavelength demultiplexer (DMUX), which separates all optical channels and sends them to different outputs.

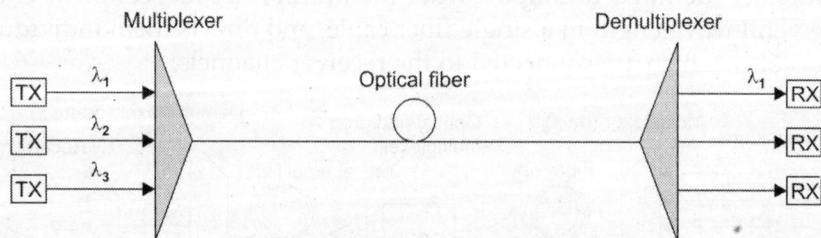

Fig. 11.4(b): Implementation of a typical WDM link

In order to find the optical bandwidth corresponding to a spectral width in optical region, we use the relation $c = \lambda \cdot v$, where λ is wave-length and v carrier frequency and c velocity of light. Differentiating:

$$dv = c \frac{d}{d\lambda} \frac{1}{\lambda} \cdot d\lambda = -\frac{c}{\lambda^2} d\lambda \tag{11.1}$$

or

$$|\Delta v| = \frac{c}{\lambda^2} |\Delta \lambda| \tag{11.2}$$

Equation (11.2) describes the frequency change Δv which corresponds to the wavelength change $\Delta \lambda$ around λ. Using the above formula, we can estimate the usable wavelength range for a standard single-mode fiber. Assuming that telecommunication wavelength range extends from $\lambda_1 = 1280$ nm to $\lambda_2 = 1625$ nm, the ultimate bandwidth of optical fiber is 40 THz. Assuming 50 or 25 GHz channel spacing, there is the possibility to transmit 800–1600 wavelength channels.

11.2 TIME DIVISION MULTIPLEXING

Time division multiplexing (TDM) is a technique for transmitting digitized data, voice, and video signals simultaneously over one fiber cable. This is accomplished by interleaving pulses representing bits from different channels or time slots. The public-switched telephony network (PSTN) is based on the TDM technologies and is often called a *TDM access network*.

The time division multiplexer is a device that uses TDM techniques to combine several slower speed data streams into a single high speed data stream, as shown in Fig. 11.5. Data from multiple sources is broken into portions (bits or bit groups); these portions are transmitted in a defined sequence. The transmission order must be maintained so that the input streams can be reassembled at the destination. Typically, using the same TDM techniques, the same device can also perform the reverse process; decompose the high-speed data streams into multiple low speed data streams, a process called demultiplexing. Therefore, a time division multiplexer and demultiplexer are very often packaged in the same box.

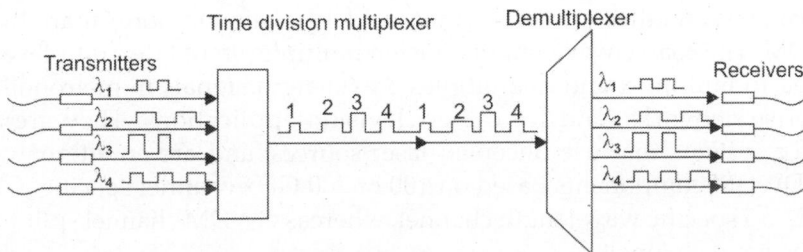

Fig. 11.5: A schematic diagram of time division multiplexing

11.3 FREQUENCY DIVISION MULTIPLEXING (FDM)

Frequency division multiplexing (FDM) is a scheme in which numerous analogue signals are combined for transmission on a single communications line or channel. Each signal is assigned a different frequency (sub-channel) within the main channel. This technology is used in broadcast radio, television, and cable division. Home local area network (LAN) use this technology to ensure compatibility between the different services sharing the same telephone wire, specifically voice, and the home network. To eliminate interference, each service has a frequency spectrum that is different from the others. Traditionally, frequency-division multiplexing is used for analogue signals, but it also can be used for digital signals.

When FDM is used in a communication network, each input signal is sent and received at maximum speed at all times. However, if many signals must be sent along a single long-distance line, the necessary bandwidth is large, and careful design is required to ensure that the system will perform properly. In some systems, time-division multiplexing is used instead.

11.4 DENSE WAVELENGTH DIVISION MULTIPLEXING (DWDM)

DWDM is an acronym for dense wavelength division multiplexing, an optical technology used to increase bandwidth over existing fiber optic backbones. DWDM is a fiber-optic transmission technique that employs light wavelengths to transmit data as parallel bits or a serial string of characters. Using DWDM, up to 80 (and theoretically more) separate wavelength or channels of data can be multiplexed into a single light stream, and then transmitted on a single fiber optic cable. Each channel carries a time division multiplexed (TDM) signal. In a system with each channel carrying data, billions of bits per second, can be delivered by the fiber optic cable. DWDM is also sometimes called wave division multiplexing (WDM). Since each channel is demultiplexed at the end of the transmission back into the original source, different data formats can be transmitted together, at different rates. Specifically, internet data, synchronous optical network (SONET) data, and asynchronous transfer mode (ATM) data can all be transmitted at the same time within the same optical fiber. Utilizing DWDM technology is a suitable solution for high-speed data transmission, without the addition of more fiber cables.

11.5 COARSE WAVELENGTH DIVISION MULTIPLEXING (CWDM)

CWDM is an acronym for coarse wavelength division multiplexing, which is a technology that combines upto 16 wavelengths onto a single fiber. When there are just a few channels (upto 16 channels) and they are spaced more widely (10 nm or more) apart, the system is called CWDM. The coarse wavelength division multiplexer and demultiplexer (CWDM) are designed to multiplex and demultiplex wavelength signals in metropolitan, access and enterprise networks, and for cable television applications. They are a low-cost approach for systems that use uncooled laser sources, and are an alternative to more expensive DWDM components based on 100 or 200 GHz channel spacing. CWDMs are used to isolate a specific wavelength channel, whereas CWDM channel splitters are used to isolate the band channels.

11.6 PASSIVE COMPONENTS

For implementing WDM (or DWDM) various passive and active components are required to combine, distribute, isolate and amplify optical power at different wavelength. The components do not need any external control for their operation.

Passive components are mainly used to split or combine optical signals. These components operates in optical domains. Passive components don't need external control for their operation. Passive components are fabricated by using optical fibers or by planar optical waveguides. Commonly required passive components are: 1. N × N couplers, 2. *Power splitters*, 3. *Power taps*, 4. *Star couplers*.

Most passive components are derived from basic *star couplers*.

Star coupler can perform combining and splitting of optical power. Therefore, star coupler is a multiple input and multiple output port device.

11.6.1 Couplers

Couplers are the simplest passive fiber optic devices. Couplers direct the multiple input light waves to multiple outputs. Normally, couplers split signals into two or more outputs, or combine two or more inputs into one output. Couplers can have more than two inputs or outputs. Couplers work as power splitters, power taps, and wavelength selectors.

(i) 2 × 2 Couplers

A simple 2 × 2 fiber coupler consists of two inputs and two output port as shown in Fig. 11.6.

The arrows indicate the power flow through the coupler. 2×2 coupler can be made by fusing two optical fibers together in the middle and then stretching them so that a coupling region is created. Such devices can be made wavelength independent over a wide spectral range.

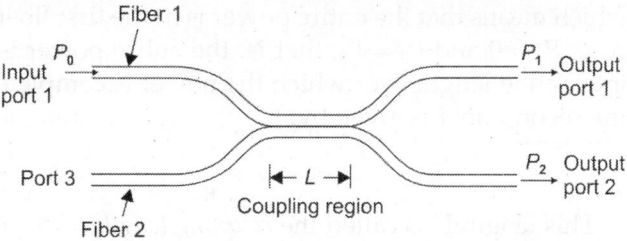

Fig. 11.6: A simple 2×2 fiber-optic coupler

When an optical signal launched at input port 1, it may split into two signals that can be collected at the output ports 1 and 2, based on a set splitting ratio. Ideally, no power will reach port 3, called the isolated port. By convention, the power P_1 emerging from output port 1 is equal to or greater than the power P_2 from output port 2, depending on the designed *splitting ratio* or *coupling ratio* of the coupler. The splitting ratio or coupling ratio is denoted by $P_1:P_2$ or else percentage of power e.g. 1:1 same as 50/50% splits power in half. By careful design, it is possible to achieve coupling ratio from 1:99 to 50:50. A device with a 50:50 coupling ratio is termed as a *3 dB coupler*, as 50% of the input power is coupled to each output port. One can use it as a *splitter*. We may note that a coupler with a coupling ratio of 1:99 can be used as an optical tap.

One can analyse the coupling mechanism using electromagnetic theory for dielectric waveguides. One can easily understand this mechanism in a simple manner also as follows. The V parameter of an optical fiber is given by:

$$V = \frac{2\pi a}{\lambda} n_1 \sqrt{2\Delta} \tag{11.3}$$

where $2a$ is the core diameter, n_1 is the core index, λ is the wavelength of light propagating through the fiber, and Δ is the relative refractive index difference. In the process of manufacturing a coupler, the fibers are heated, fused together, and stretched. Stretching reduces the core diameter and so also the V-parameter. Thus, the optical power propagating through the core of a single-mode fiber (say) will be less confined. If two identical single-mode fibers are used to make a 2×2 coupler, the power in the single mode propagating through the core of the first fiber will couple to that in the core of the second adjacent fiber in the coupling region (fused portion). By controlling the distance between the fibers, it is possible to obtain a desired coupling ratio. Such couplers are called *directional couplers*, because the fibers allow the launched light to pass through them in one direction. It is also possible to make the coupling ratio wavelength selective. Such couplers are used to combine or separate two signals of different wavelengths.

Let us assume that the abovementioned 2×2 coupler is *loss-less* and the *two-single-mode fibers* are identical, the power P_2 coupled from the first fiber into the second fiber over an axial length z is given by:

$$P_2 = P_0 \sin^2 (\kappa z) \tag{11.4}$$

where P_0 is the power launched at input port 1 (Fig. 11.6) and κ is the coupling coefficient describing the interaction between the propagating fields in the two fibers.

Assuming that the power is conserved, one can write the following expression for power P_1 delivered to output port 1:

$$P_1 = P_0 - P_2 = P_0 [1 - \sin^2 (kz)] = P_0 \cos^2 (\kappa z) \tag{11.5}$$

From Eqs (11.4) and (11.5), one can easily infer that there is a periodic exchange of power between the two fibers. Thus, at $z = m\pi / \kappa$, where $m = 0, 1, 2, ..., P_1 = P_0$ and $P_2 = 0$, which means that the entire power is in the first fiber; and at $z = (m + 1/2)(\pi/\kappa)$, $m = 0, 1$, 2, ..., $P_1 = 0$ and $P_2 = P_0$; that is, the entire power is in the second fiber. The minimum interaction length over which the power is completely transferred from the first fiber to the second fiber is given by:

$$z = L_c = \frac{\pi}{\kappa} \tag{11.6}$$

This length L_c is called the *coupling length*.

The main parameters of couplers are optical power losses, i.e. the performance of a directional coupler may be specified in terms of coupling or splitting ratio, defined as follows:

(i) Coupling ratio (%) $= \left(\dfrac{P_2}{P_1 + P_2}\right) \times 100$ \hfill (11.7)

(ii) Coupling ratio (dB) $= -10 \log\left(\dfrac{P_2}{P_1 + P_2}\right)$ \hfill (11.7a)

So far, we have assumed that the coupler is loss-less. However, in a practical device of this type, some power is always lost when the signal passes through it. There are two basic *parameters related to the loss*: (i) *excess loss*, defined as the ratio of the total output power to the input power, and (ii) *insertion loss* (for a specific port-to-port path), defined as the ratio of power at output port j to power at input port i. Thus, in decibels (dB):

$$\text{Excess loss (dB)} = -10 \log\left(\frac{P_1 + P_2}{P_0}\right) \tag{11.8}$$

(Power loss within the coupler)

and $\quad$ Insertion loss (dB) $= -10 \log\left(\dfrac{P_j}{P_i}\right)$ \hfill (11.9)

For a 2×2 coupler, for a path from input port 1 to output port 2, using Eqs (11.7(b)) and (11.8), one can write:

$$\text{Insertion loss} = -10 \log_{10}\left(\frac{P_2}{P_0}\right)$$

$$= -10 \log\left(\frac{P_2}{P_1 + P_2}\right) \times \left(\frac{P_1 + P_2}{P_0}\right)$$

$$= -10 \log\left(\frac{P_2}{P_1 + P_2}\right) - 10 \log_{10}\left(\frac{P_1 + P_2}{P_0}\right)$$

$$= \text{coupling ratio} + \text{excess loss} \tag{11.10}$$

Table 11.1 lists splitting ratio values, throughput loss, and tap loss for several common couplers.

Table 11.1: Characteristics of several common couplers

Coupler description (dB)	Splitting ratio	L_{THP} (dB)	L_{TAP} (dB)
3	1:1	3	3
6	3:1	1.25	6
10	9:1	0.46	10
12	15:1	0.28	12

Here, L_{THP} (dB) is *throughput loss* specifies the transmission loss between the input power P_0 at input port 1 and transmission power P_1 at output port 1, and L_{TAP} (dB) is *tap loss* specifies the transmission loss between the input power P_0 at input port 1 and the tap power P_2 at output port 2.

(ii) 3 dB Couplers

A simple four-port coupler is often called a 3 dB coupler, if the input light splits into two equal portions at the output ports. The signal is split in half (3 dB = half). The 3 dB comes from the

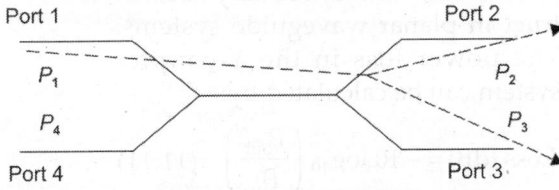

Fig. 11.7: 3 dB coupler

power loss formula: $[-10 \times \log_{10}(P_2/P_1) = -10 \log_{10}(0.5/1.0) = -10 \times (-0.3) = 3 \text{ dB}]$. Half of the light entering at Port 1 will exit at Port 2 and half at Port 3, as shown in Fig. 11.7.

It is often useful to cascade many 3 dB couplers, as shown in Fig. 11.8. The configuration shown is called a *splitter*. This splitter divides a single input into four equal outputs and is denoted as a 1×4 coupler. As might be expected, if the device is perfect, each output port will contain one fourth of the input power.

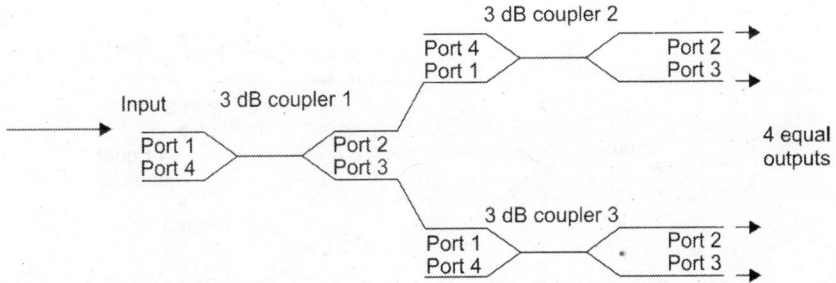

Fig. 11.8: Cascaded 3 dB couplers to produce a 1×4 coupler

Figure 11.9 shows how a 1×8 coupler can be constructed by cascading several 3 dB couplers in a tree configuration. The signal input power will divide into eight equal outputs. Each output port will contain one eighth of the input power.

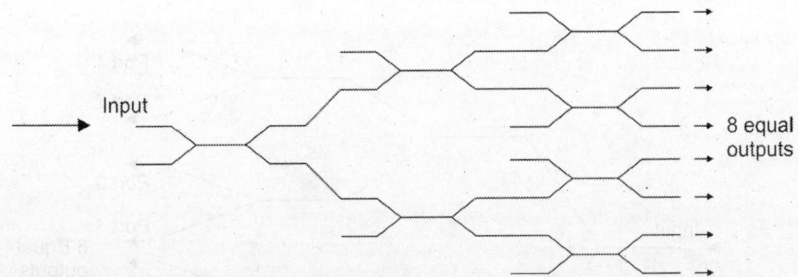

Fig. 11.9: Cascaded 3 dB couplers to produce a 1×8 coupler

(iii) Y-Couplers

Y-couplers or splitters, sometimes called 3 dB couplers, split the light equally. Y-couplers are 3 dB couplers in which Port 4 is not used. In the Y-coupler (splitter), as shown in Fig. 11.10, the light entering Port 1 will be split equally between Ports 2 and 3 with almost no loss. They are extremely efficient at splitting light with little loss. Y-couplers are difficult to construct in fiber optics, but they are easy to construct in planar waveguide systems. The power loss in the Y-coupler system can be calculated by:

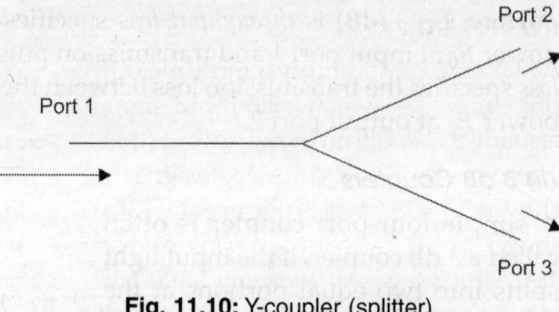

Fig. 11.10: Y-coupler (splitter)

$$Loss\ (dB) = -10 \log_{10} \left(\frac{P_{out}}{P_{in}} \right) \quad (11.11)$$

Y-couplers are very seldom built as separate planar devices; instead they are manufactured on the same substrate as other devices. Connecting Y-couplers to a fiber optic cable is expensive; and significant loss is experienced in the connections. However, Y-couplers of this kind are used extensively in *complex planar devices*.

If is often useful to cascade Y-couplers, as shown in Fig. 11.11. The splitter configuration shown divides a single input into four equal outputs. If the device is perfect, each output port will contain one fourth of the input power. Figure 11.11 shows how a 1 × 4 Y-coupler can be constructed by cascading three 1 × 2 Y-couplers in a tree arrangement.

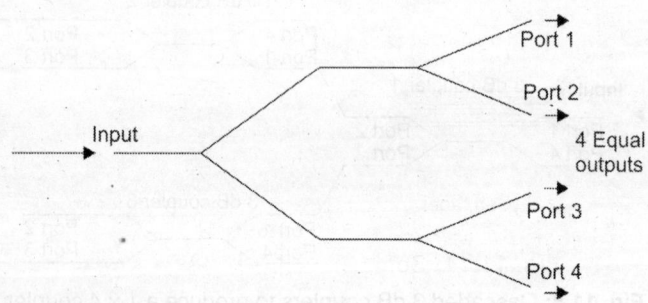

Fig. 11.11: Cascaded 1 × 2 Y-couplers to produce a 1 × 4 coupler

Figure 11.12 shows how a 1 × 8 Y-coupler can be constructed by cascading seven Y-couplers in a tree configuration. The power of the input signal will divide into eight equal outputs. Each output port will contain one eighth of the input power.

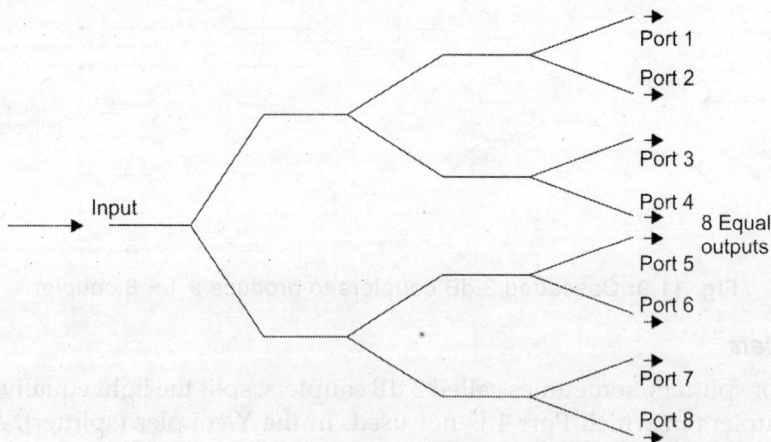

Fig. 11.12: Cascaded Y-couplers to produce a 1 × 8 Y-coupler

(iv) Star Couplers

A star coupler is simply a multiple output coupler in which each input signal is made available on every output fiber. There are two star coupler designs, as shown in Fig. 11.13. Figure 11.13(a) shows an 8 × 8 coupler. *This coupler distributes the power from any input port to all the output ports, splitting equally among the output ports.* This type of coupler is called a *transmission star coupler.* Fig. 11.13(b) shows a reflection star coupler; any input is split equally and is reflected back among all fibers. Star couplers are typically used in *local area networks* (LAN) and *metropolitan area networks* (MAN).

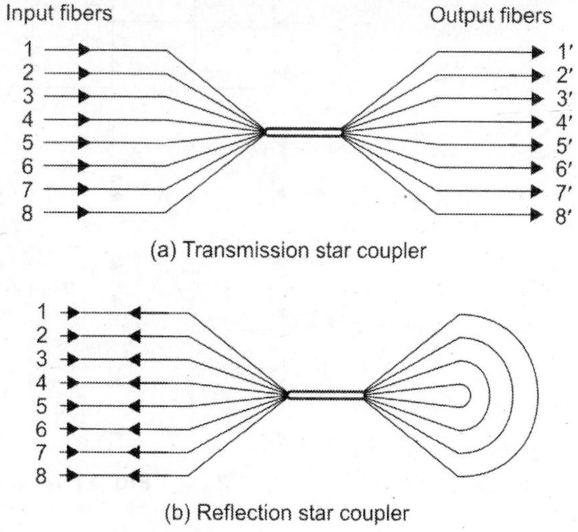

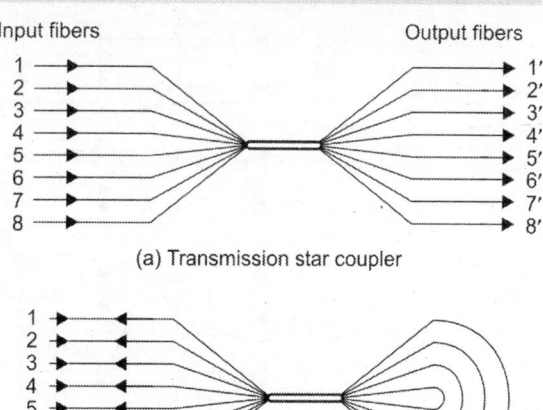

(a) Transmission star coupler

(b) Reflection star coupler

Fig. 11.13: Star couplers

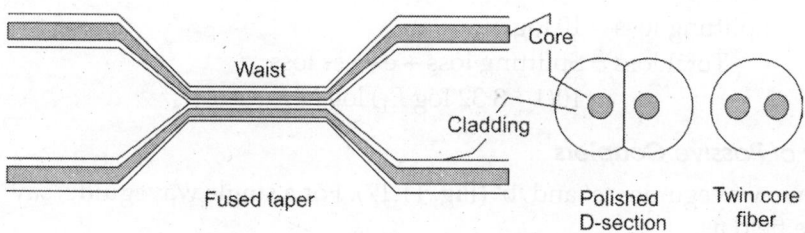

Fig. 11.14: Some coupler configurations

Salient features of a star coupler

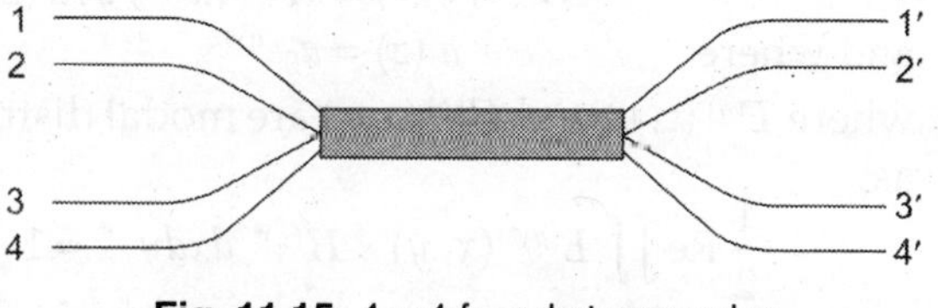

(i) A star coupler is mainly used for combining optical powers from *N*-inputs and divide them equally at *M*-output ports.

Fig. 11.15: 4 × 4 fused star coupler

(ii) For producing *N* × *N* star couplers, the fiber fusion technique is popularly used. Figure 11.15 shows a 4 × 4 fused star coupler.

(iii) The optical power put into any port on one side of coupler is equally divided among the output ports. Ports on same side of coupler are isolated from each other.

(iv) Total loss in star coupler is constituted by splitting loss and excess loss.

$$\text{Splitting loss} = 10 \log\left(\frac{1}{N}\right) = 10 \log N$$

$$\text{Excess loss} = 10 \log\left(\frac{P_{\text{in}}}{\sum\limits_{i=1}^{N} P_{\text{out},i}}\right)$$

(v) An 8 × 8 star coupler can be formed by interconnecting 2 × 2 couplers. It requires twelve 2 × 2 couplers (Fig. 11.16).

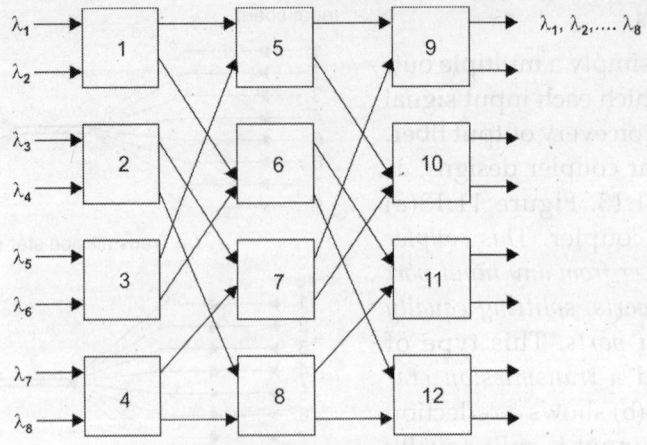

Fig. 11.16: 8×8 coupler

(vi) Excess loss in dB is given as:

$$\text{Excess loss} = 10 \log \left(F_T^{\log_2 N} \right)$$

where, F_T is fraction of power traversing each coupler element.

$$\text{Splitting loss} = 10 \log N$$
$$\text{Total loss} = \text{Splitting loss} + \text{excess loss}$$
$$= 10(1 - 3.32 \log F_T) \log N$$

(v) Theory of Passive Couplers

Consider two waveguides 'a' and 'b' (Fig. 11.17). For a single waveguide, say 'a', one can express the field as:

$$E(x, y, z) = E^{(a)}(x^{(a)}, y) a(z)$$
$$H(x, y, z) = H^{(a)}(x^{(a)}, y) a(z)$$

and where $\quad a(z) = a_0 e^{i\beta az}$

where $E^{(a)}(z, y)$ and $H^{(a)}(x, y)$ are modal distributions in (x, y) plane. They are normalized as:

$$\frac{1}{2} \text{Re} \iint E^{(a)*}(x, y) \times H^{(a)*} \, dxdy \cdot \hat{z} = 1$$

Also $\qquad \dfrac{da(z)}{dz} = i\beta_a a(z)$

Total guided power

$$P = \frac{1}{2} \text{Re} \iint E^{(a)*}(x, y, z) \times H^{(a)*}(x, y, z) \, \hat{z} dxdy = |a(z)|^2$$

For two parallel waveguides, fields in each one are written as:

$$E(x, y, z) = a(z) E^{(a)}(x, y) + b(z) E^{(b)}(x, y) \qquad (11.12)$$
$$H(x, y, z) = a(z) H^{(a)}(x, y) + b(z) H^{(b)}(x, y) \qquad (11.12a)$$

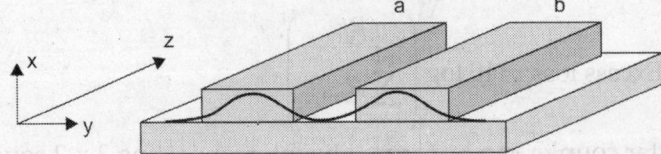

Fig. 11.17: Two coupled optical waveguides (distribution of electric fields is also shown in the figure)

Amplitudes $a(z)$ and $b(z)$ satisfy the following (coupled-mode) equations:

$$\frac{da(z)}{dz} = i\beta_a a(z) + i\kappa_{ab} b(z) \qquad (11.13)$$

$$\frac{da(z)}{dz} = i\kappa_{ba} a(z) + i\beta_b b(z) \qquad (11.14)$$

where κ_{ab} and κ_{ba} are coupling coefficients. Guided power is:

$$P = s_a |a(z)|^2 + s_b |b(z)|^2 + Re\{a(z)b^*(z) C_{ba} + b(z)a^*(z)C_{ab}\} \qquad (11.15)$$

where

$$C_{pq} = \frac{1}{2} \int\limits_{-\infty}^{+\infty} \int E^{(q)}(x,y) \times H^{(p)*}(x,y) \cdot \hat{z} dx dy \qquad (11.16)$$

In the above, s_a, $s_b = +1$ is for propagation in the $+z$ direction and s_a, $s_b = -1$ is for propagation in the $-z$ direction.

Coupled mode equations can be written in a matrix form as:

$$\frac{d}{dz}\begin{bmatrix} a(z) \\ b(z) \end{bmatrix} = i\overline{M}\begin{bmatrix} a(z) \\ b(z) \end{bmatrix} \qquad (11.17)$$

where

$$\overline{M} = \begin{bmatrix} \beta_a & \kappa_{ab} \\ \kappa_{ba} & \beta_b \end{bmatrix} \qquad (11.18)$$

The solution is assumed to be:

$$\begin{bmatrix} a(z) \\ b(z) \end{bmatrix} = \begin{bmatrix} A \\ B \end{bmatrix} e^{i\beta z} \qquad (11.19)$$

After substituting into Eq. (11.17), one finds:

$$\left[\overline{M} - \beta\, \overline{1}\right]\begin{bmatrix} A \\ B \end{bmatrix} = 0 \qquad (11.20)$$

where $\overline{1}$ is an identity matrix. In the full form:

$$\begin{bmatrix} \beta_a - \beta & \kappa_{ab} \\ \kappa_{ba} & \beta_b - \beta \end{bmatrix}\begin{bmatrix} A \\ B \end{bmatrix} = 0 \qquad (11.21)$$

For non-trivial solutions, a determinant must vanish:

$$\det = (\beta_a - \beta)(\beta_b - \beta) - \kappa_{ab}\cdot\kappa_{ba} = 0 \qquad (11.22)$$

From the above, two eigenvalues are found as:

$$\beta = \frac{1}{2}(\beta_a + \beta_b) \pm \gamma \equiv \begin{cases} \beta_+ \\ \beta_- \end{cases} \qquad (11.23)$$

where

$$\lambda = \sqrt{\Delta^2 + \kappa_{ab}\cdot\kappa_{ba}}, \ \Delta = \frac{1}{2}(\beta_b - \beta_a) \qquad (11.24)$$

Eigenvectors are:

$$V_1 = \begin{bmatrix} \kappa_{ab} \\ \Delta - \gamma \end{bmatrix} \text{ or } \begin{bmatrix} \Delta - \gamma \\ \kappa_{ba} \end{bmatrix} \text{ for } \beta_+ \qquad (11.25)$$

and

$$V_2 = \begin{bmatrix} \kappa_{ab} \\ \Delta - \gamma \end{bmatrix} \text{ or } \begin{bmatrix} \Delta - \gamma \\ \kappa_{ba} \end{bmatrix} \text{ for } \beta_- \qquad (11.26)$$

The general solution is therefore:

$$\begin{bmatrix} a(z) \\ b(z) \end{bmatrix} = \vec{V} \begin{bmatrix} e^{i\beta_+ z} & 0 \\ 0 & e^{i\beta_- z} \end{bmatrix} \vec{V}^{-1} \begin{bmatrix} a(0) \\ b(0) \end{bmatrix} \tag{11.27}$$

where matrix V is formed from eigen vectors as:

$$V = [V_1; V_2] \tag{11.28}$$

After some algebra, one finds the final solution as:

$$\begin{bmatrix} a(z) \\ b(z) \end{bmatrix} = S(z) \begin{bmatrix} a(0) \\ b(0) \end{bmatrix} \tag{11.29}$$

with

$$\vec{S}(z) = \begin{bmatrix} \cos \gamma z - i \dfrac{\Delta}{\gamma} \sin \gamma z & i \dfrac{\kappa_{ba}}{\gamma} \sin \gamma z \\ i \dfrac{\kappa_{ba}}{\gamma} \sin \gamma z & \cos \gamma z = i \dfrac{\Delta}{\gamma} \sin \gamma z \end{bmatrix} \cdot e^{\frac{i}{2}(\beta_a + \beta_b)z} \tag{11.30}$$

As a special case, consider a situation when at $z = 0$, the optical power is incident only in waveguide 1, $a(0) = 1$, $b(0) = 0$. One finds in this case:

$$|b(z)|^2 = \left| \frac{\kappa_{ba}}{\gamma} \right|^2 \sin^2 \gamma z$$

At $\gamma z = \dfrac{\pi}{2}, 3\dfrac{\pi}{2}, ..., (2n+1)\dfrac{\pi}{2}$, the power transfer from guide 'a' to guide 'b' is maximum. Since

$$\left| \frac{\kappa_{ba}}{\gamma} \right|^2 = \frac{|\kappa_{ba}|^2}{\left[\dfrac{1}{2}(\beta_b - \beta_a) \right]^2 + |\kappa_{ba}|^2} < 1$$

for $\beta_a \ne \beta_b$ the power transfer between waveguides is never complete.

11.7 MULTIPLEXERS AND DEMULTIPLEXERS

To implement a WDM-based system, a multiplexer is required at the transmitting end to combine optical signals from the several sources into a single fiber, and a demultiplexer is needed at the receiving end to separate the signals into appropriate channels. We may note that optical sources, e.g. an LED or ILD, do not emit significant optical power outside their designated channel width, interchannel cross talk is relatively unimportant at the transmitting end. As regards the design problem, the multiplexing should have low insertion loss. On the other hand, there exists a different requirement for demultiplexers, because photodetectors are generally sensitive over a broad range of wavelengths, which may include all the WDM channels. Obviously, a demultiplexer design must be such that it provides a good channel, isolation of the different wavelengths being used.

On the basis of the above study, we see that these devices are based on the reversible structure. Clearly, any wavelength-division demultiplexer (at least in principle) can also be used as multiplexer by simple exchanging the input and output directions. Therefore, we will restrict to the discussion of wavelength division demultiplexers.

One can classify the commonly used wavelength-division multiplexers (and multiplexers) into two categories: (i) *interference filter based devices*, and (ii) *angular dispersion based devices*.

Figure 11.18 shows the basic configuration of a two-wavelength (or two-channel) interference filter demultiplexer.

An interference filter consists of a thin film obtained by depositing several dielectric layers of alternately low and high refractive index. When light propagates through such a structure, it undergoes multiple reflections, giving rise to either constructive or destructive interference depending on the wavelength. Therefore, a filter can be designed to produce *high transmittance in a given wavelength range and high reflectance outside this range*. In Fig. 11.18(a), appropriate conventional microlenses are used for collimating and focusing light. The incident beam consists of two wavelength, λ_1 and λ_2. The filter transmits the wavelength λ_1 and reflects the wavelength λ_2, thus demultiplexing the two channels. A compact low-loss two-channel demultiplexer (or multiplexer) may be implemented by employing two 0.25 pitch graded refractive index (GRIN) rod lenses as shown in Fig. 11.18(b). These lenses are used for collimating and focusing. The filter is deposited at the interface between these lenses (say, on either of the lens faces). Off-axis entry at the first lens makes it possible to easily separate the reflected beam.

Interference filters can (in principle) be used in series to separate N wavelength channels. However, the complexity involved in cascading the filters and the increase in signal loss that occurs with the addition of each filter generally limit the operation to four or five filters (i.e., four or five channels).

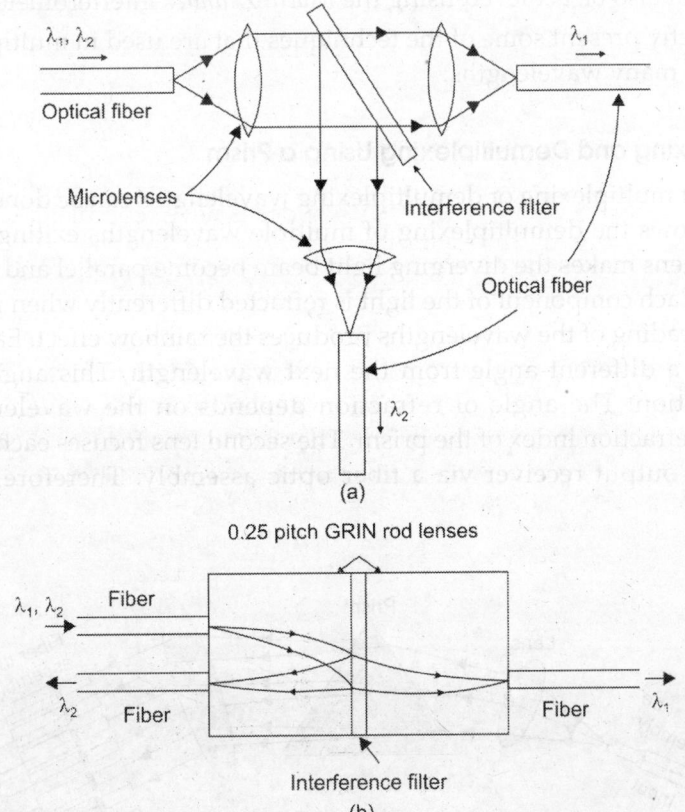

Fig. 11.18: The basic configuration of a two-wavelength (or two-channel) interference filter demultiplexer employing (a) conventional microlenses (b) GRIN rod lenses

The second type of demultiplexers (or multiplexers) are mainly based on angular dispersion. Herein, the input beam (containing several wavelengths) is collimated onto a dispersive element which may be a prism or a grating. The latter angularly separates different wavelengths, the separation depending on the angular dispersion ($d\theta/d\lambda$) of the dispersion element. The separated output beams at different wavelengths are then focused using appropriate optics and collected by separate optical fibers. This type of demultiplexer is more suited to narrow line width sources, such as ILDs.

Three configurations of angular dispersion type demultiplexers are shown in Fig. 11.38 (Example 7). The first one (Fig. 11.38(a)) is a prism-type device. A Littrow prism (a half-prism, with its near surface serving as a reflector) has been used here for compact configuration. A multiwave-length signal from the input fiber is collimated onto the prism and the dispersed wavelengths are focused onto the output fibers by the same lens. Angular separation depends on the refractive index n of the material of the prism, which in turn depends on the wavelength. Suitable materials, giving a high value of $d\theta/dn$, for practical applications in the range 1.3–1.5 μm are not available. Therefore, blazed reflection gratings are normally employed for WDM applications. With a plane grating, the *Littrow mount* is often preferred because it allows the use of only one lens for collimating as well as focusing purposes, thus, reducing the device size. The basic structures of a Littrow grating demultiplexer employing a conventional lens and a 0.25 pitch GRIN rod lens are shown in Figs 11.38(b) and (c), respectively. Wavelength division multiplexing can also be achieved using the *Mach–Zehnder* interferometer.

Now, we briefly present some of the techniques that are used in multiplexing and de-multiplexing of many wavelengths:

11.7.1 Multiplexing and Demultiplexing Using a Prism

A simple way of multiplexing or demultiplexing wavelengths can be done using a prism. Figure 11.19 shows the demultiplexing of multiple wavelengths exiting from the fiber cable. The first lens makes the diverging light beam become parallel and incident on the prism surface. Each component of the light is refracted differently when it exits from the prism. This spreading of the wavelengths produces the rainbow effect. Each wavelength is refracted by a different angle from the next wavelength. This angle is called the angle of refraction. The angle of refraction depends on the wavelength, the apex angle, and the refraction index of the prism. The second lens focuses each wavelength to the designated output receiver via a fiber optic assembly. Therefore, this device is *bidirectional*.

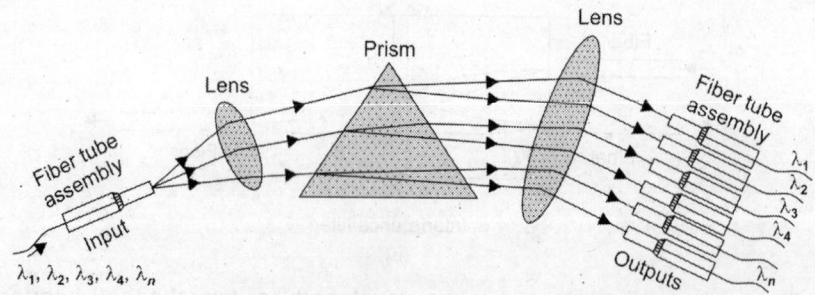

Fig. 11.19: Multiplexing and demultiplexing of wavelengths using a prism

11.7.2 Multiplexing and Demultiplexing Using a Diffraction Grating

Another technology based on the principles of diffraction uses a diffraction grating. When a light source is incident on a diffraction grating, each wavelength is diffracted at a different angle, and therefore, to a different point in space. It is necessary to use a lens to focus the wavelengths onto individual fibers, as shown in Fig. 11.20. Separate wavelengths can be combined onto the same output port, or a single mixed input may be split into multiple outputs, one per wavelength. This device is bidirectional.

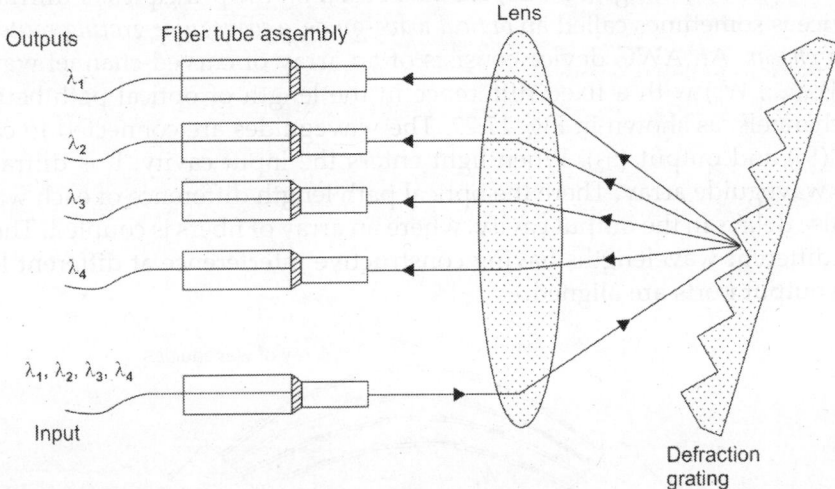

Fig. 11.20: Multiplexing and demultiplexing of wavelengths using a diffraction grating

11.7.3 Optical Add/Drop Multiplexers/Demultiplexers

Figure 11.21 illustrates a schematic representation of a design for an optical add/drop multiplexer/demultiplexer (OADM), which is widely used in communication systems. Between multiplexing and demultiplexing points in a DWDM system, there is a span where multiple wavelengths exist. An OADM removes or inserts one or more wavelengths, the OADM can remove some, while passing others on. OADMs are a key part of moving toward the goal of all-optical networks. The design shown in Fig. 11.21 includes both *pre-* and *post-amplification components* that may or may not be present in an OADM design.

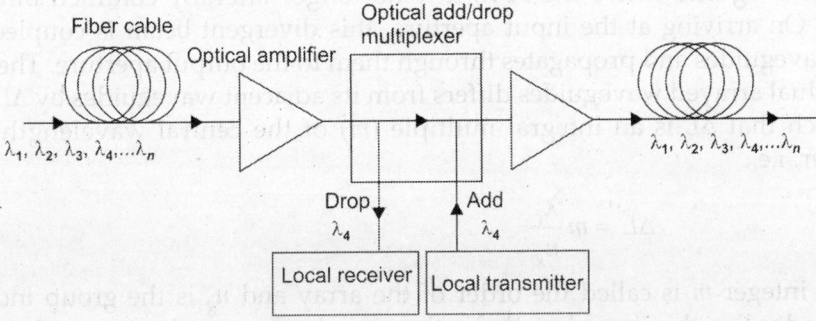

Fig. 11.21: An optical add/drop multiplexer

There are two general types of OADMs. The first generation is a fixed device, physically configured to drop specific present wavelengths while adding others. The second generation is reconfigurable and capable of dynamically selecting which wavelengths are added and dropped. *Thin-film filters* are used for OADMs in metropolitan DWDM systems, because of their low loss, low cost, and high stability. The new third generation of OADMs involves other technologies, such as tunable fiber gratings, fiber Bragg gratings, and circulators.

11.7.4 Arrayed Waveguide Gratings (AWGs)

Arrayed waveguide gratings (AWGs) are also based on the principles of diffraction. An AWG device is sometimes called an *optical wave-guide*, a *waveguide grating router*, a *phase array*, or a *phasar*. An AWG device consists of an array of curved-channel waveguides (W_1, W_2, W_3, ..., W_n) with a fixed difference in the length of optical path between the adjacent channels, as shown in Fig. 11.22. The waveguides are connected to cavities at the input (S_1) and output (S_2). When light enters the input cavity, it is diffracted and enters the waveguide array. There the optical path length difference of each waveguide creates pulse delays in the output cavity, where an array of fibers is coupled. The process results in different wavelengths having constructive interference at different locations, where the output ports are aligned.

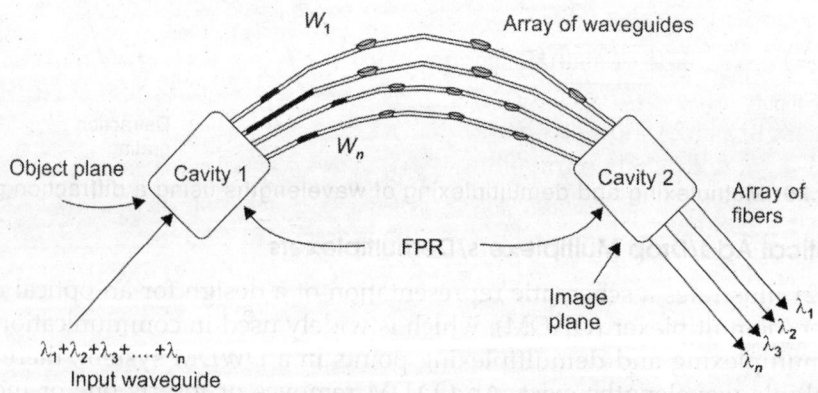

Fig. 11.22: Schematic of an arrayed waveguide grating device

One may understand its operation as follows:

When the optical beam (consisting of wavelengths λ_1, λ_2, ..., λ_N) propagating through the input waveguide enters the FPR, it is no longer laterally confined but becomes divergent. On arriving at the input aperture, this divergent beam is coupled into the array of waveguides and propagates through them to the output aperture. The length of the individual arrayed waveguides differs from its adjacent waveguides by ΔL, which is chosen such that ΔL is an integral multiple (m) of the central wavelength λ_c of the multiplexer, i.e.:

$$\Delta L = m \frac{\lambda_c}{n_g} \tag{11.31}$$

where the integer m is called the order of the array and n_g is the group index of the guided mode. For this wavelength λ_c, the signals propagating through individual waveguides will arrive at the output aperture with equal phase (apart from an integral multiple of 2π), so that the image of the input field in the object plane will be formed at the centre of the image plane. The dispersion is caused by the length increment ΔL of the adjacent array waveguide to vary linearly with signal frequency. Here β is the phase propagation constant of the waveguide mode. As a result, the focal point for different frequencies shifts along the image plane. The spatial shift per unit frequency change (ds/dx) is called the *spatial dispersion D* of the device.

$$D = \frac{1}{v_c} \frac{\Delta L}{\Delta \alpha} \tag{11.32}$$

where v_c is the central frequency of the PHASAR and $\Delta \alpha$ is the divergence angle between adjacent array waveguides nearthe input and output apertures. Substituting ΔL from Eq. (11.31) in Eq. (11.32), one obtains:

$$D = \frac{1}{v_c} \frac{m}{\Delta \alpha} \frac{\lambda_c}{n_g} = \frac{c}{n_g v_c^2} \frac{m}{\Delta a} \tag{11.33}$$

where c is the speed of light in free space. It is clear from Eq. (11.33) that the dispersion is fully determined by the order m and the divergence angle $\Delta \alpha$ between adjacent array waveguides. Thus, by placing the output waveguides at appropriate positions along the image plane, the spatial separation of different wavelengths ($\lambda_a, \lambda_2, ..., \lambda_N$) can be obtained.

11.7.5 Fiber Bragg Grating (FBG)

A Bragg grating is made of a small section of fiber cable, which is modified by exposure to ultraviolet radiation to create periodic changes in the refractive index of the core of the fiber cable. Figure 11.23 shows a fiber Bragg grating fiber cable. The Bragg grating reflects some of the light waves when travelling through it. The reflected waves usually occur at

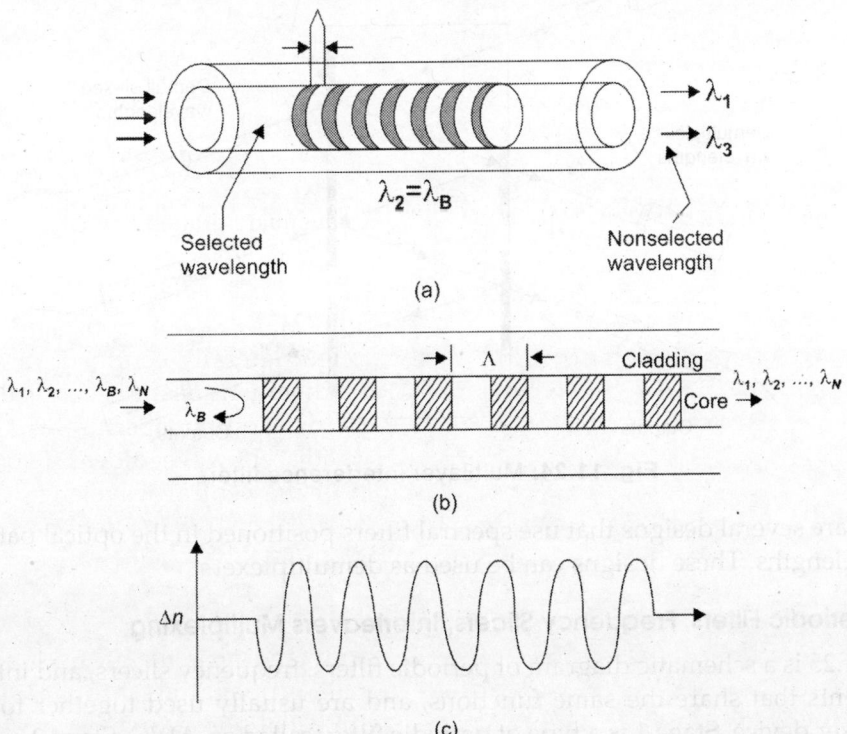

Fig. 11.23: (a) A fiber Bragg grating (b) fiber Bragg grating showing cladding and core (c) periodic variation of the refractive index of the core

one particular wavelength. The reflected wavelength, known as the Bragg resonance wavelength, depends on the change in refractive index that is applied to the Bragg grating fiber. This also depends on the basic parameters of the grating (the grating period, the grating length, and the modulation depth). In such a grating, large coupling may occur between the forward and backward propagating modes if the following Bragg condition is satisfied:

$$\lambda_B = 2\Lambda n_{eff} \tag{11.34}$$

where λ_B is called the Bragg wavelength, Λ is the grating period, and n_{eff} is the effective index of the mode. Thus, proper design can ensure that most of the power is effectively reflected, whereas signals with other wavelengths are transmitted. The advantage of such gratings is that they are fiber-compatible so that the losses generated by connecting them to other fibers are very low.

11.7.6 Thin Film Filters or Multilayer Interference Filters

Figure 11.24 shows one multiplexing technique that uses interference filters in devices called thin film filters, or multilayer interference filters. By positioning the thin filters in the optical path, wavelengths can be distributed. The property of each filter is such that it transmits one wavelength while reflecting others. By arranging the thin filters in a device, a demultiplexer is created, and many wavelengths can be demultiplexed.

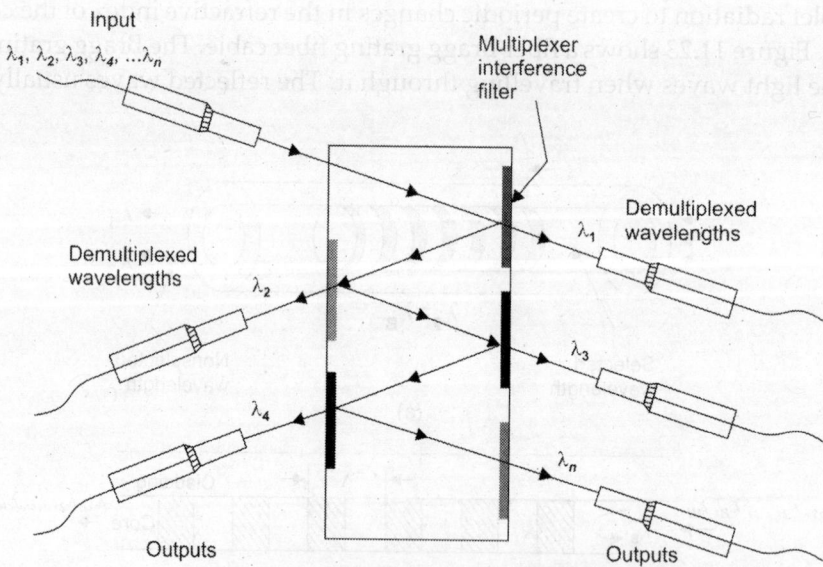

Fig. 11.24: Multilayer interference filters

There are several designs that use spectral filters positioned in the optical path to sort out wavelengths. These designs can be used as demultiplexers.

11.7.7 Periodic Filters, Frequency Slicers, Interleavers Multiplexing

Figure 11.25 is a schematic diagram of periodic filters, frequency slicers, and interleaver components that share the same functions, and are usually used together to make a multiplexer device. Stage 1 is a type of periodic filter, called an AWG. Stage 2 represents a frequency slicer. In this instance, stage 2 is another AWG; an interleaver function on the output is provided by six Bragg gratings. Six wavelengths are received at the input to

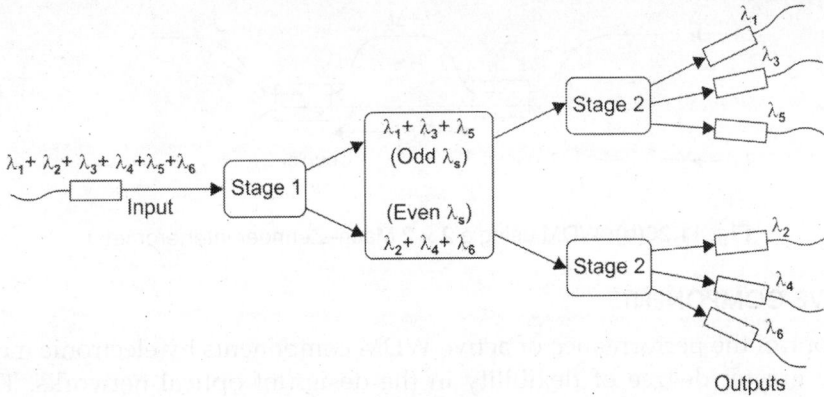

Fig. 11.25: Periodic filters, frequency slicers, and interleaver multiplexing

the AWG at stage 1, which then breaks the wavelengths down into odd and even wavelengths. The odd and even wavelengths go to their respective stage 2 frequency slicer, and then are delivered by the interleaver in the form of six discrete, interference-free optical channels.

11.7.8 Mach–Zehnder Interferometer

Interferometers are based on the interferometric properties of light and the principles of Mach–Zehnder interferometer. Mach–Zehnder inter-ferometers can be used to direct a specific wavelength to a specific output port, as shown in Fig. 11.26(a). The interferometer consists of parallel titanium-diffused waveguides on a lithium niobate substrate. The incoming signal is split evenly along the arms of the Mach–Zehnder interferometer, and then recombined at the output. Electrodes are fixed on the arms of the Mach–Zehnder interferometer, and two couplers are connected to the interferometer. While voltage is applied to the electrodes, a specific wavelength can be directed to either port 2 or 3.

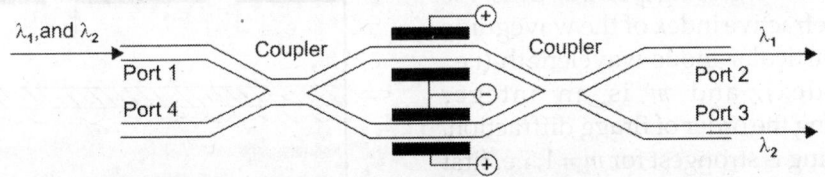

Fig. 11.26(a): Mach–Zehnder interferometer.

This device consists of three parts: (a) 3 dB directional coupler which splits the input signal equally and directs it along two paths having different lengths; (b) a central region consisting of two arms, one arm being longer by ΔL (say) than the other arm, which introduces a phase shift between two wavelengths; and (c) another 3 dB direction coupler which recombines the signals at the output. With this configuration, it is possible to introduce a phase shift in one of the paths so that the recombined signals will interfere constructively at one output port and destructively at the other. The combined (multiplexed) signals will emerge from the port at which constructive interference has occurred. It is possible to make any size $N \times N$ multiplexer (demultiplexer) using basic 2×2 Mach–Zehnder interferometers (Fig. 11.26b).

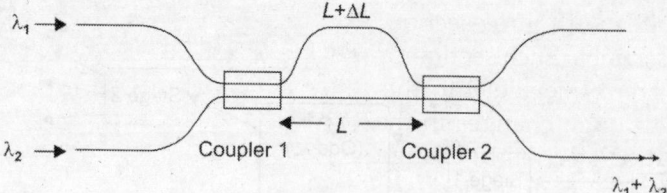

Fig. 11.26(b): WDM using a 2 × 2 Mach–Zehnder interferometer

11.8 ACTIVE COMPONENTS

One can control the performance of active WDM components by electronic means. This provides a greater degree of flexibility in the design of optical networks. The prime components in this category are: (i) tunable sources, (ii) tunable filters, and (iii) optical amplifiers. We will discuss here only tunable sources and tunable filters.

(i) Tunable Sources

In implementing a WDM, it is required to generate several wavelengths (λ_1 to λ_N). One simple way is to use a series of discrete distributed feedback (DFB) or distributed Bragg reflector (DBR) lasers operating at different wavelengths and multiplex their outputs into one fiber using a power combiner or a wavelength multiplexer. But this solution requires a large number of lasers, each of which has to be controlled individually. Further, using a power combiner introduces a loss of at least $10 \log_{10} N$ (dB), where N is the number of wavelength channels. If a multiplexer is used, loss can be reduced, but at the cost of more stringent requirements on the control of emitted wavelengths. Therefore, *wavelength-tunable lasers* are used in modern WDM systems. These devices are based on DFB or DBR structures.

A controlled variation of emission wavelength is possible by changing the effective refractive index of the cavity or a part of it in accordance with the relation:

$$\Lambda = m\lambda_B/2n_e \qquad (11.34a)$$

where Λ is the grating period, n_e is the effective refractive index of the waveguide for that particular mode wavelength (i.e., mode index), and m is an integer representing the order of Bragg diffraction. The coupling is strongest for $m = 1$, i.e. first order diffraction.

At least two independent control currents are needed: (i) in the *active region* and (ii) in the *tuning region*, for the variation of the effective refractive index. Two configurations of lasers using this scheme are shown in Fig. 11.27. The first structure [Fig. 11.27(a)] has a cavity that is subdivided into two to three sections for independent current injection. By controlling the current properly, it is possible to vary the lasing wavelength without altering the output power. A tuning range

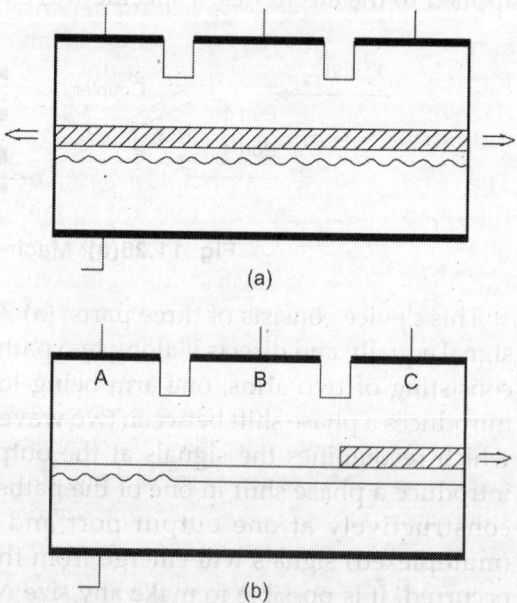

Fig. 11.27: Tunable lasers: (a) multisection DFB laser (b) multisection DBR laser

of 2–3 nm is possible with three-section DFB lasers. The second structure [Fig. 11.27(b)] consists of three sections. Each section can be biased independently by different injection currents. The current injected into the Bragg section (Section A) changes the Bragg wavelength (λ_B) through changes in the refractive index. The current injected into the phase control section (section B) changes the phase of the feedback from the DBR, and current injection in the gain section (section C) controls the output power. Continuous tuning in the range of 10–15 nm with an output power of the order of 100 mW is possible with such lasers. With superstructure grating DBR lasers, a tuning range of up to 100 nm is possible.

(ii) Tunable Optical Filters

Tunable optical filters are versatile devices that are used in many photonic applications. They are essential in wavelength-flexible WDM systems, and they can also play a key role in wavelength-tunable lasers for WDMs.

There is an extensive range of optical tunable filter types. The following filters are available in the market:

- Micron optic fiber Fabry-Perot (FFP) tunable filters.
- Digitally tunable optical filters based on dense wavelength division multiplexer (DWDM) thin film filters and semiconductor optical amplifiers.
- Narrowband tunable optical filters using fiber Bragg gratings.
- High-speed tunable optical filters using a semiconductor double-ring resonator.
- Micromachined in-plane tunable filters using the thermo-optic effect of crystalline silicon.
- Acousto-optic tunable filters (AOTFs).
- Liquid crystal tunable filters (LCTFs).
- Others not listed here.

We will explain some common types of tunable filters.

Optical tunable filter selection depends on various factors, such as fast tuning speed, simple control mechanism, being scalable without additional insertion loss, and long-term operation temperature stability.

(a) Fiber Fabry-Perot tunable filters

The FFP tunable filter principle is based on Fabry–Perot etalon technology. An FFP tunable filter passes wavelengths that are equal to integer fractions of the cavity (etalon) length; all other wavelengths are attenuated or reflected back. The key to the design of the FFP tunable filter is its lensless fiber construction. There are no collimating optics or lenses; thus, the FFP tunable filter achieves high precision, maintains low loss, and good transmission profile. Fig. 11.28 shows a cross-section of an FFP tunable filter design. The design has two pieces of fiber, the ends of which are polished and silvered, so that each end acts like a mirror. The ends are placed precisely opposite one another with a specific gap between them. The fiber assemblies are mounted on two piezo-electric crystals and packaged in a box. By applying a voltage across the crystals, the distance between the fiber ends changes, thus changing the resonant cavity length, and therefore, a change in the wavelength selection.

The design of tunable filter eliminates the *pitfalls* of other Fabry–Perot component technologies, including misalignment and environmental sensitivity. Fiber Fabry–Perot tunable filters have low loss, high isolation, long-term alignment stability, high reliability,

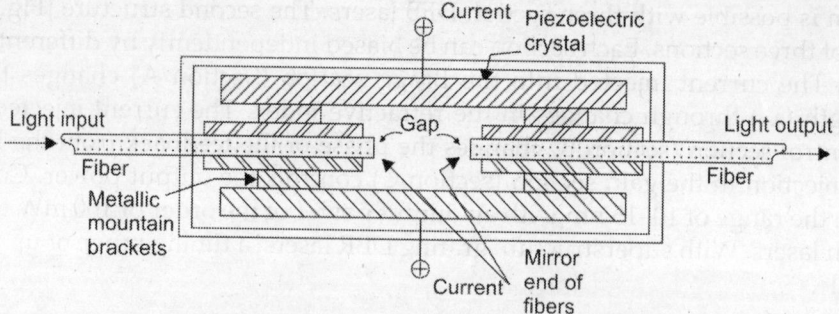

Fig. 11.28: Fiber Fabry–Perot (FFP) tunable filter

and accurate power or wavelength measurements. Fiber Fabry–Perot tunable filters are used in optical performance monitoring, tunable optical noise filtering, dropping of a tunable channel for ultra dense WDM, etc.

The design of FFP tunable filter can be modified by putting a liquid crystal material into the gap between the ends of the two fibers. The index of refraction of the liquid crystal can be changed very quickly, by passing current through the liquid crystal. By changing the index of refraction of the crystal, a change in the wavelengths passing through the crystal can be achieved, thus eliminating unwanted wavelengths.

(b) Mach–Zehnder interferometer tunable filters

The Mach–Zehnder interferometer tunable filter has a ladderlike structure, in which each section resembles a Mach–Zehnder interferometer, as shown in Fig. 11.29. The output waveguide (across the top) and the input waveguide (across the bottom) are joined by regularly spaced linking waveguides, each longer than the previous one by ΔS, as illustrated in Fig. 11.29. For constructive interference to occur at each coupler in the output waveguide, ΔS must be equal to an integral number of wavelengths of the input light. However, similar to a Mach-Zehnder that can be tuned by adjusting the refractive index of one or both arms, this filter can be tuned by adjusting the refractive index of the arms with an injected current.

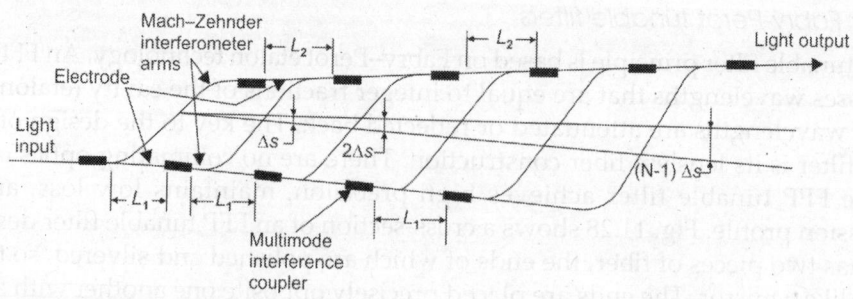

Fig. 11.29: Mach–Zehnder interferometer tunable filter

(c) Fiber grating tunable filters

Fiber grating tunable filters are used in a wide variety of applications within optics and fiber communication systems. They are an important element in wavelength division multiplexer systems for combining and separating individual wavelengths. Fiber–Bragg grating (FBG) transmits one wavelength and reflects all others. Basically, a grating is a periodic structure within an optical material. This variation in the structure of the optical material reflects or transmits light in a certain direction depending on the light wavelength. Therefore, gratings can be categorized as either transmitting or reflecting.

Figure 11.30 shows a design of an in-fiber Bragg grating tunable filter. The filter contains two Bragg gratings and a four-port circulator. The gratings have high reflectance in wavelength bands at specified wavelengths. The Bragg grating fiber is glued to the piezoelectric crystal contacts. Current can be applied on one or two Bragg gratings. The current deforms the crystal, stretching the gratings to match the wavelength of the signals. The wavelength filtered depends on the current level. This type of filter is used in aircraft or spaceborne differential absorption systems that measure water vapour in Earth's atmosphere. It is also used for a unique optical receiver that couples a laser radar signal from a telescope to the in-fiber Bragg grating filter.

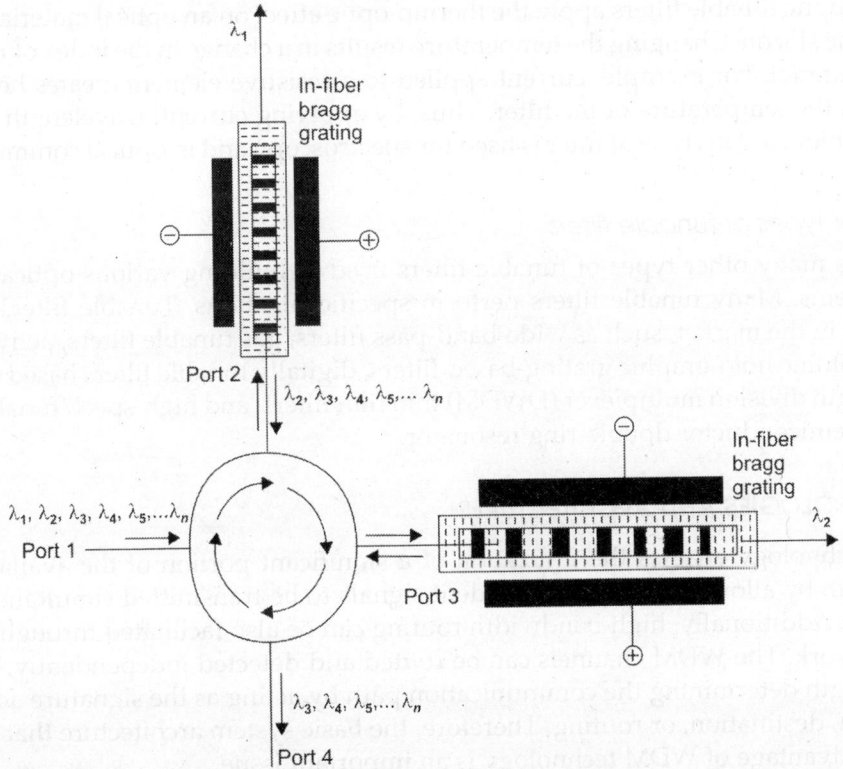

Fig. 11.30: Fiber grating tunable filter

(d) Liquid grating tunable filters

Liquid crystal tunable filters (LCTFs) use electrically controlled liquid crystal elements, which select a specific visible wavelength of light for transmission through the filter. A typical wavelength-selective LCTFs is constructed from a stack of fixed filters that consist of interwoven birefringent crystal/liquid-crystal combinations and linear polarizers. The spectral region transmitted through an LCTF depends upon the choice of polarizers, optical coatings, and the liquid crystal characteristics (nematic, cholesteric, smectic etc.). In general, visible-wavelength devices of this type usually perform in the range of 400–700 nm. This type of filter is ideal for use with electronic imaging devices, such as CCDs, because it offers excellent imaging quality with a simple optical pathway.

(e) Acousto-optic tunable filters

Acousto-optic tunable filters (AOTFs) apply the same technology used in acousto-mechanical switches. An incident beam of light impacts a dioxide crystal of an AOTF. The dioxide crystal is sandwiched between an acoustic transducer and absorber that can be regulated by the acoustic power and acoustic frequency sliders. Upon encouraging the standing wave in the dioxide crystal, a portion of the incident light beam is diffracted into the output port, while the remainder of the beam passes through the crystal and is absorbed by a beam stop. As the slider moves, the amplitudes of the waves passing through the AOTF are increased or decreased. Wavelength selection is controlled by the acoustic frequency slide. Acousto-optic tunable filters are employed to modulate the wavelength and amplitude of incident laser light.

(f) Thermo-optic tunable filters

Thermo-optic tunable filters apply the thermo-optic effect on an optical material, such as crystalline silicon. Changing the temperature results in a change in the index of refraction of the material. For example, current applied to a resistive element creates heat which increases the temperature of the filter. Thus, by applying current, wavelength selection can be achieved. This type of filter is used for spectroscopy and in optical communication systems.

(g) Other types of tunable filters

There are many other types of tunable filters used in building various optical devices and systems. Many tunable filters perform specific functions. Tunable filters are also available in the market, such as wide-band-pass filters, gas tunable filters, active optical filters, volume holo-graphic grating-based filters, digitally tunable filters based on dense wavelength division multiplexer (DWDM) thin film filters, and high-speed tunable filters using a semiconductor double-ring resonator.

11.9 TOPOLOGIES AND ARCHITECTURES

WDM technology enables the utilization of a significant portion of the available fiber bandwidth by allowing many independent signals to be transmitted simultaneously in one fiber. Additionally, high-bandwidth routing can be also facilitated through a multi-user network. The WDM channels can be routed and detected independently, with the wave-length determining the communication path by acting as the signature address of the origin, destination, or routing. Therefore, the basic system architecture that can take the full advantage of WDM technology is an important issue.

11.9.1 Point-to-Point WDM Links

As shown in Fig. 11.31, in a simple point-to-point WDM system, several channels are multiplexed at one node, the combined signals are then transmitted across some distance of fiber, and the channels are demultiplexed at a destination node. This point-to-point WDM link facilitates the high bandwidth fiber transmission without routing or switching in the optical data path.

11.9.2 Wavelength-Routed Networks

Figure 11.32 shows a more complex multiuser WDM network structure, where the wavelength is used as the signature address for either the transmitters or the receivers, and determines the routing path through an optical network. In order for each node to

Point-to-point systems

Optoelectronic routing node

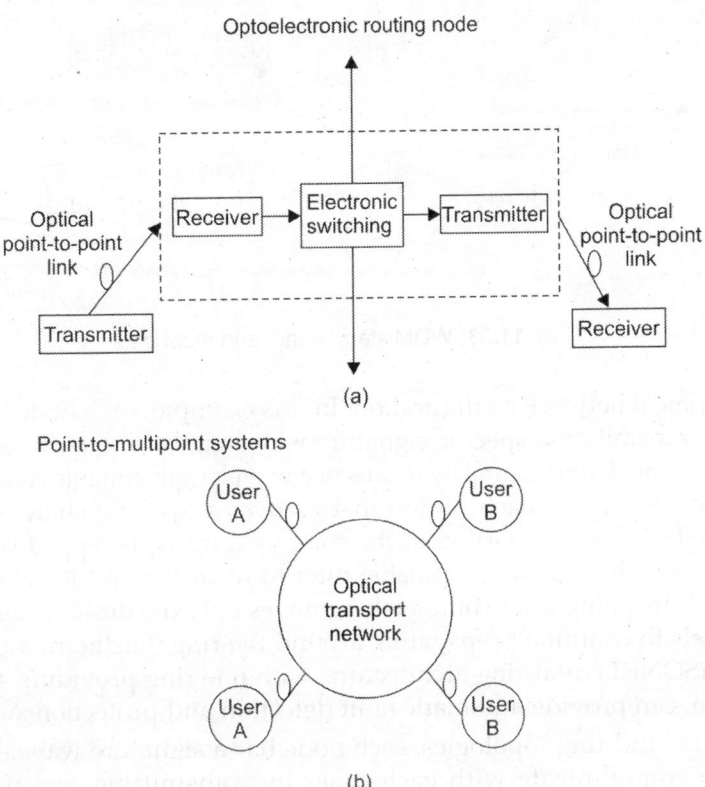

(a)

Point-to-multipoint systems

(b)

Fig. 11.31: Point-to-point and point-to-multipoint optical systems

be able to communicate with any other node and facilitate proper link setup, either the transmitters or the receivers must be wave-length tunable; we have arbitrarily chosen the transmitters to be tunable in this network example. We may note that the wavelength are routed passively in wave-length-routed-networks.

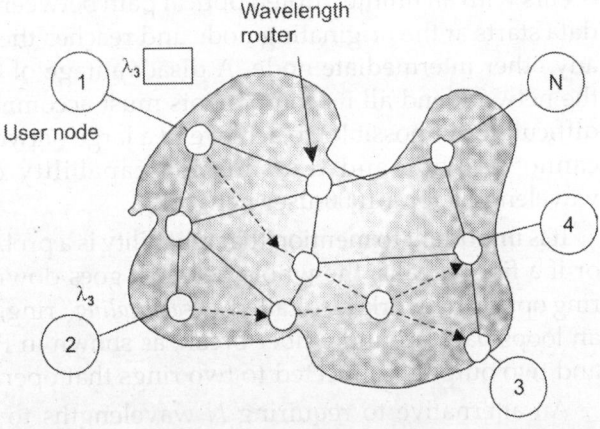

Wavelength-determined routing

Fig. 11.32: A generic multiuser network in which the communication links and routing paths are determined by the wavelengths used within the optical switching fiber

11.9.3 WDM Star, Ring, and Meshes

Three common WDM network topologies are *star*, *ring*, and *mesh* networks. In the star topology, each node has a transmitter and receiver, with the transmitter connected to one of the passive central star's inputs and the receiver connected to one of the star's outputs, as is shown in Fig. 11.33(a). Rings, as shown in Fig. 11.33(b), are also popular because (1) many electrical networks use this topology, and (2) rings are easy to implement

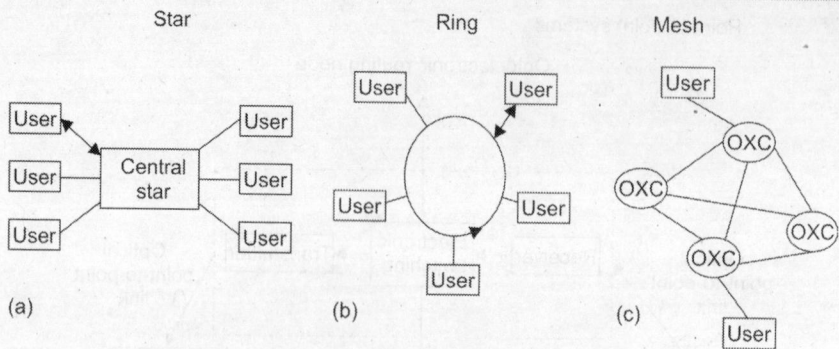

Fig. 11.33: WDM stars, rings, and meshes

for any geographical network configuration. In this example, each node in the unidirectional ring can transmit on a specific signature wavelength, and each node can recover any other node's wavelength signal by means of a wavelength-tunable receiver. Although not depicted in the figure, each node must recover a specific channel. This can be performed (1) where a small portion of the combined traffic is tapped off by a passive optical coupler, thereby allowing a tunable filter to recover a specific channel; or (2) in which a channel-dropping filter completely removes only the desired signal and allows all other channels to continue propagating around the ring. Furthermore, a *synchronous optical network* (SONET) dual-ring architecture, with one ring providing service and the other protection, can provide automatic fault detection and protection switching.

In both the star and ring topologies, each node has a signature wavelength, and any two nodes can communicate with each other by transmitting and recovering that wavelength. This implies that N wavelengths are required to connect N nodes. The obvious advantage of this configuration, known as a single-hop network, is that data transfer occurs with an uninterrupted optical path between the origin and destination; the optical data starts at the originating node and reaches the destination node without stopping at any other intermediate node. A disadvantage of this single-hop WDM network is that the network and all its components must accommodate N wavelengths, which may be difficult (or impossible) to achieve in a large network, i.e. present fabrication technology cannot provide and transmission capability cannot accommodate 1000 distinct wavelengths for a 1000-user network!

It is important to mention that reliability is a problem in fiber ring. If a station is disabled or if a fiber breaks, the whole network goes down. To address this problem, a double-ring optical network, also called a "*self healing*" ring, is used to bypass the defective stations an loops back around a fiber break, as shown in Fig. 11.34. Each station has two inputs and two outputs connected to two rings that operate in opposite directions.

An alternative to requiring N wavelengths to accommodate N modes is to have a multi-hop network (mesh network) in which two nodes can communicate with each other by sending data through a third node, with many such intermediate hops possible, shown in Fig. 11.33(c). In the mesh network, the nodes are connected by reconfigurable optical crossconnects (OXCs). The wavelength can be dynamically switched and routed by controlling the OXCs. Therefore, the required number of wavelengths and the wavelength tunable range of the components can be reduced in this topology. Moreover, the mesh topology can also provide multiple-paths between two nodes to make network protection and restoration easier to realize. If a failure occurs in one of the paths, the

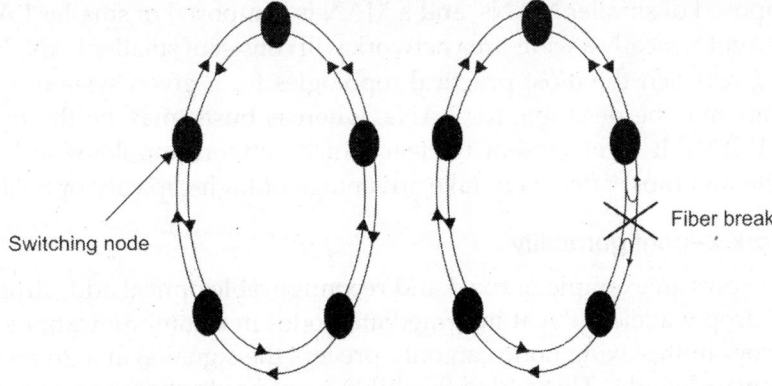

Fig. 11.34: A self-healing ring network

system can automatically find another path and restore communi-cations between any two nodes. However, OXCs with large numbers of ports are extremely difficult to obtain, which limits the scalability of the mesh network.

In addition, there exist several other network topologies, such as a tree network, which is a favourite of broadcast, or distribution, systems. At the "base" of the tree is the source transmitter from which emanates the signal to be broadcast throughout the network. From this base, the tree splits many times into different "branches", with each branch either having nodes connected to it or further dividing into sub-branches. This continues until all the nodes in the network can access the base transmitter. Whereas the other topologies are intended to support bidirectional communication among the nodes, this topology is useful for distributing information unidirectionally from a central point to a multitude of users. This is a very straightforward topology and is in use in many electrical systems, most notably cable television (CATV).

By introducing Fig. 11.35 in which a large network is composed of smaller ones, we have also introduced the subject of the architecture of the network which depends on the network's geographical extent. The three main architectural types are the local-, metropolitan-, and wide-area networks, denoted by LAN, MAN, and WAN, respectively. Although no rule exists, the generally accepted understanding is that a LAN interconnects a small number of users covering a few km (i.e. intra- and inter-building). a MAN interconnects users inside a city and its outlying regions, and a WAN interconnects significant portions of a country (100s of km). Based on Fig. 11.35, the smaller network represents LANs, the larger ones MANs, and the entire figure would represent a WAN. In other words, a

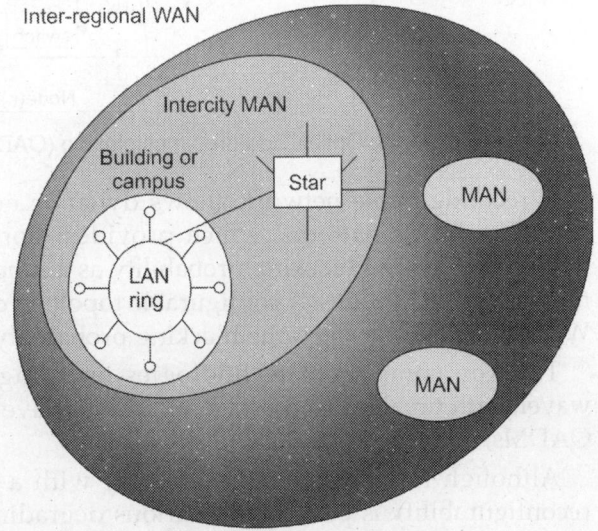

Fig. 11.35: Hybrid network topologies and architectures woven together to form a large network

WAN is composed of smaller MANs, and a MAN is composed of smaller LANs. Hybrid systems exist, and typically a wide-area network will consist of smaller LANs, with mixing and matching between the most practical topologies for a given system. For example, stars and rings may be desirable for LANs, whereas buses may be the only practical solution for WANs. It is, at present unclear which network topology and architecture will ultimately and most effectively take advantage of high-capacity optical systems.

11.9.4 Network Reconfigurability

Figure 11.36 shows an example of fixed and reconfigurable optical add/drop nodes that can add and drop wavelengths at intermediate nodes in a communications network. A fixed add/drop multiplexing node can only process the signal(s) at a given wavelength or a group of wavelengths. This added flexibility would save operating and maintenance costs and would improve network efficiency. In general, a network is reconfigurable if it can provide the following functionality for multi-channel operations: (1) channel add/drop, and (2) path reconfiguration for bandwidth allocation or restoration. It appears that a reconfigurable network is highly desirable to meet the requirements of high bandwidth and bursty traffic in future networks.

Fixed add-drop multiplexing node

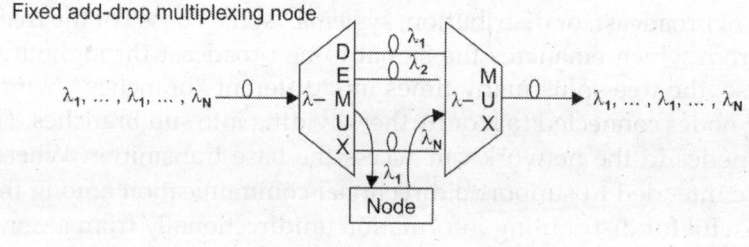

Reconfigurable add-drop multiplexing node

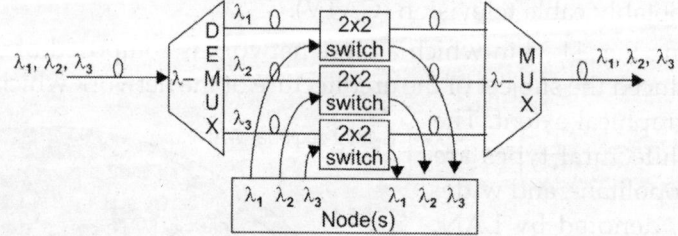

Fig. 11.36: Optical add-drop multiplexing (OADM) systms; fixed vs reconfigurable

A reconfigurable network allows dynamic network optimization to accommodate changing traffic patterns, which provides more efficient use of network resources. Figure 11.37 shows blocking probability as a function of call arrival rate in a WDM ring network with 20 nodes. A configurable topology can support 6 times the traffic of a fixed WDM topology for the same blocking probability.

The key component technologies enabling network reconfigurability include wavelength tunable lasers and laser arrays, wavelength routers, optical switches, OXCs, OADMs, and tunable optical filters, etc.

Although huge benefits are possible with a reconfigurable topology, the path to reconfigurability is paved with various degrading effects. Figure 11.32 shows that the signal may pass through different lengths of fiber links due to the dynamic routing, causing some degrading effects in reconfigurable networks to be more critical than in static networks, such as nonstatic dispersion and nonlinearity accumulation due to reconfigurable paths, EDFA gain transients, channel power nonuniformity.

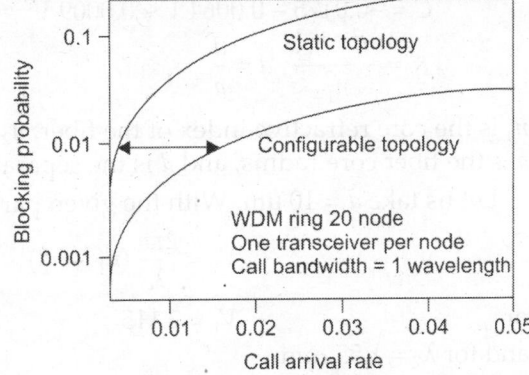

Example 1

For a 2 × 2 fiber coupler, input power is 200 µW, throughput power is 90 µW, coupled power is 85 µW and cross talk power is 6.3 µW. Compute the performance parameter of the fiber coupler.

[B Tech]

Fig. 11.37: Blocking probability as a function of call arrival rate in a WDM ring

Solution

Here P_0 = 200 µW, P_1 = 90 µW, P_2 = 85 µW, and P_3 = 6.3 µW:

(i) Coupling ratio = $\dfrac{P_2}{(P_1 + P_2)} \times 100\% = \dfrac{85}{(90 + 85)} \times 100\% = 48.57\%$

(ii) Excess ratio = $10 \log \left(\dfrac{P_0}{P_1 + P_2} \right)$ dB

$= 10 \log \left(\dfrac{200}{90 + 85} \right)$ dB $= 0.5799$ dB

(iii) Insertion loss (for port 0 to port 1) = $10 \log \left(\dfrac{P_0}{P_1} \right)$ dB

$= 10 \log \left(\dfrac{200}{90} \right) = 3.46$ dB

Insertion loss (for port 0 to port 2) = $10 \log \left(\dfrac{200}{85} \right) = 3.71$ dB

(iv) Cross talk = $10 \log \left(\dfrac{P_3}{P_0} \right) = 10 \log \left(\dfrac{6.3 \times 10^{-3}}{200} \right) = -45$ dB

Example 2

Design a broadband WDM 3 dB coupler which splits at λ = 1310 nm and 1550 nm. The two step-index fibers used to make the coupler are identical and single-moded with a core diameter of 8.2 µm, core index n_1 = 1.45, and cladding index n_2 = 1.446. Calculate the position of the output ports with respect to the input port for the two wavelengths.

[B Tech]

Solution

We know that the interaction length L required to make a 3 dB coupler is $\pi/(4\kappa)$, where κ is the coupling coefficient. Using simple empirical relationship given below may be used to calculate the value of λ:

$$\kappa = \frac{\pi}{2} \frac{\sqrt{\delta}}{a} \exp\left[-(A + Bd + Cd^2)\right]$$

where $A = 5.2789 - 3.663\ V + 0.3841\ V^2$

$B = -0.7769 + 1.2252\ V - 0.0152\ V^2$

$$C = -0.0175 - 0.0064\ V - 0.0009\ V^2$$

$$\delta = \frac{n_1^2 - n_2^2}{n_1^2}, d = \frac{d}{a}$$

n_1 is the core refractive index of the fiber, n_2 is the cladding refractive index of the fiber, a is the fiber core radius, and d is the separation between the fiber axis.

Let us take $d = 10$ μm. With the given parameters, we obtain for $\lambda_1 = 1.31$ μm:

$$V_1 = \frac{2\pi a}{\lambda}(n_1^2 - n_2^2)^{1/2} = \frac{\pi \times (8.2\ \mu m)}{(0.31\ \mu m)}[(1.45)^2 - (1.446)^2]^{1/2}$$

or
$$V_1 = 2.115$$

and for $\lambda_2 = 1.55$ mm:

$$V_2 = 1.787$$
$$d = 5.5096 \times 10^{-3} \text{ and } d = 2.439$$

For coupling coefficient for λ_1 will be:
$$\kappa_1 = 1.0483 \text{ mm}^{-1}$$

And that for λ_2 will be:
$$\kappa_2 = 1.2938 \text{ mm}^{-1}$$

Therefore, the interaction length L_1 and L_2 for $\lambda_1 = 1.31$ μm and $\lambda_2 = 1.55$ μm, respectively, are obtained as:

$$L_1 = \frac{\pi}{4\kappa_1} = \frac{\pi}{4 \times 1.0483} = 0.7488 \text{ mm}$$

and
$$L_2 = \frac{\pi}{4\kappa_2} = \frac{\pi}{4 \times 1.2839} = 0.6114 \text{ mm}$$

Obviously, the output port positioned at 0.6114 mm with respect to the input port will gather signals at $\lambda_1 = 1310$ nm and that positioned at 0.7488 mm will gather signals at $\lambda_2 = 1550$ nm. Therefore, the coupler can be used as a WDM device.

Example 3

A 32 × 32 star coupler is formed by interconnecting 2 × 2 couplers. If 5% of power is lost in each coupler element, calculate total loss in the coupler. **[MSc (Ele)]**

Solution

Here
$$N = 32$$

$$\therefore \qquad F_T = \frac{100 - 5}{100} = 0.95 \ (\because 5\% \text{ power is lost})$$

$$\text{Total loss} = 10\ (1 - 3.322 \log F_T) \log N$$
$$= 10(1 - 3.32 \log 0.95) \log 32 = 16.16 \text{ dB}$$

Example 4

A directional coupler uses two identical single-mode fibers. Determine the interaction length so that the input power P_0 is divided equally at the two output ports. **[B Tech]**

Solution

We have
$$P_1 = P_2 = \frac{P_0}{2}$$

or
$$\sin^2(\kappa L) = \cos^2(\kappa L) = 1/2$$

or
$$kL = \pi/4$$

This gives the interaction length L to be equal to $\pi/2\kappa$. We may note that such a coupler can act as a power divider.

Example 5

Make a PHASAR-based demultiplexer for 16 channels with a channel spacing of 100 GHz. The channels are centred around 1.55 µm. Calculate the required order of the arrayed waveguides. **[B Tech]**

Solution

We know that the dispersion of the PHASAR is due to the difference ΔL in the optical path length of adjacent arrayed waveguides, which causes a phase difference $\Delta\phi = \beta\Delta L$ [where b = $2\pi n_g/\lambda_c = (2\pi n_g/c)\,(v_c)$]. Thus, $\Delta\phi$ increases with frequency. If the change in frequency is such that $\Delta\phi$ increases by 2π, the transfer will be the same as before. Hence, the response of the PHASAR is periodical. This period Δv in the frequency domain is called the *free spectral range* (FSR), and it can be calculated as follows:

$$\Delta\beta\Delta L = 2\pi$$

or

$$\left[\frac{2\pi n_g}{c}(\Delta v_c)_{\text{FSR}}\right] = \Delta L = 2\pi$$

or

$$(Dn_c)_{\text{FSR}} = \frac{c}{n_g \Delta L} = \frac{v_c}{m} \tag{i}$$

Now, a demultiplexer for 16 channels with a channel spacing of 100 GHz should have an FSR of at least 1600 GHz. Since the centre wavelength is 1.55 µm, the corresponding frequency is obtained as:

$$v_c = \frac{c}{\lambda_c} = \frac{3\times10^8}{1.55\times10^{-6}} = 1.935\times10^{14} \text{ Hz}$$

Using Eq. (i), we obtain:

$$m = \frac{v_c}{\Delta v_{\text{FSR}}} = \frac{1.935\times10^{14}}{1600\times10^9} \approx 121$$

This reveals that the PHASAR-based demultiplexer would require an array with an order of at least 121.

Example 6

The LED used in 100 Mb·s^{-1} silica fiber link has a rise time of 8 ns. The wavelength emitted by the LED is 830 nm with a spectral width of 40 nm. The *p-i-n* photodiode has a rise time of 10 ns. The value of $\lambda^2 \dfrac{d^2 n}{d\lambda^2} = 0.024$ for silica fiber.

Calculate the system rise time provided the length of link is 2.5 km. The inter modal dispersion of the fiber is 3.5 nm/km. Estimate the maximum bit rate that may be achieved in the link using RZ and NRZ for solution. **[B Tech]**

Solution

We have:

$$\Delta t_{\text{mat}} = \left(\frac{-L}{c}\right)\left(\frac{\Delta\lambda}{\lambda}\right)\left(\lambda^2 \frac{d^2 n}{d\lambda^2}\right)$$

$$= -\frac{2.5\times10^3}{3\times10^8}\times\frac{40}{830}\times(0.024)$$

$$= -9.64\times10^{-9} \text{ s} = -9.64 \text{ ns}$$

For a 2.5 km link, we have $\Delta t_{modal} = 2.5 \times 3.5 = 8.8$ ns

We have
$$\Delta t_{sys} = 1.1 \sqrt{(\Delta t_s)^2 + (\Delta t_r)^2 + (\Delta t_{max})^2 + (\Delta t_{modal})^2}$$
$$= 1.1 \sqrt{(8)^2 + (10)^2 + (9.6)^2 + (8.8)^2} \text{ ns}$$
$$= 19.8 \times 10^{-9} \text{ s} = 19.8 \text{ ns}$$

(i) $B_T \text{(max)} \dfrac{0.7}{\Delta t_{sys}} = \dfrac{0.7}{19.8 \times 10^{-9}} = 34 \times 10^6$

With RZ format, $B_T \text{(max)} = 34 \times 10^6$

(ii) With NRZ format is used: $B_T \text{(max)} = \dfrac{0.35}{19.8 \times 10^{-9}} = 17 \times 10^6$

Example 7

A multiplexer that uses a plane blazed reflection grating (Fig. 11.38) has to be made. It is required to achieve a channel spacing of 10 nm in the wavelength range of 1500–1600 nm

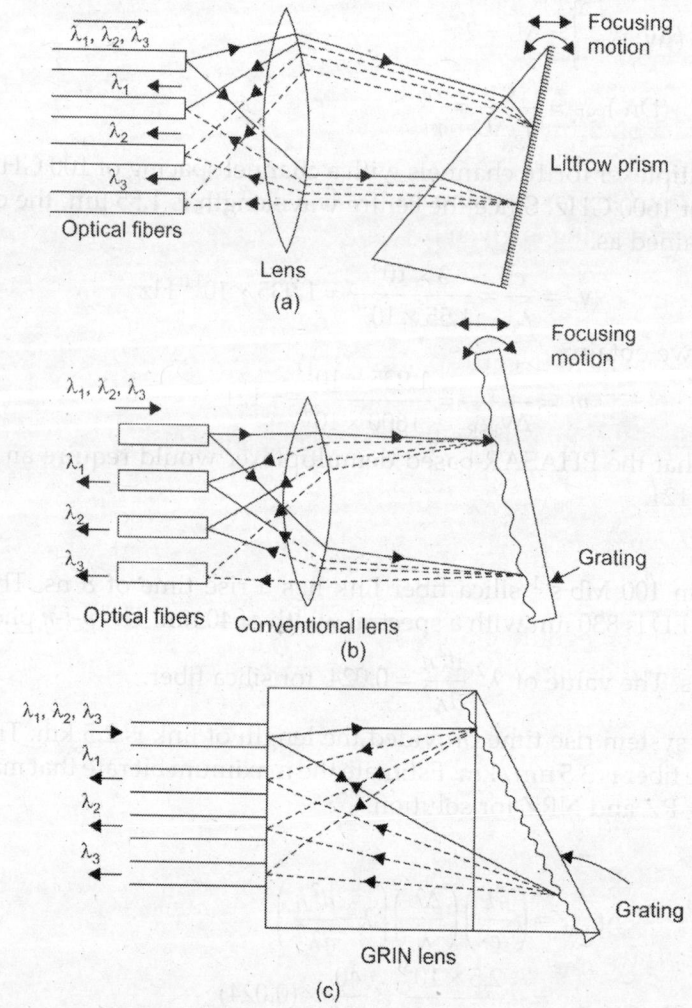

Fig. 11.38: Angular dispersion demultiplexers: (a) Littrow prism type (b) reflection grating type (with a conventional lens) (c) reflection grating type (with a GRIN rod lens)

with a center wavelength of 1550 nm. (a) What should be the grating element if the angle of blaze of the grating is 10°? (b) What should be the focal length of the lens? Assume that the output fibers have a spacing of 150 μm. **[B Tech]**

Solution

A reflection grating has on its surface an array of parallel grooves which are identical in depth and shape, equally spaced, and are provided with a highly reflecting coating (Fig. 11.39). These grooves are inclined at a specific angle (called the angle of blaze, β) with respect to the grating surface. The grating is highly efficient in diffracting wavelengths close to those for which specular reflection occurs. The wavelength for

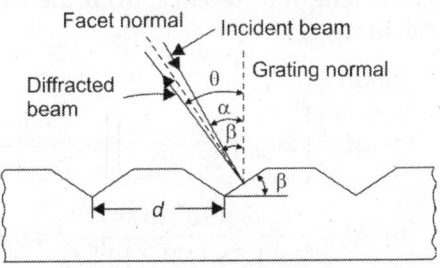

Fig. 11.39: Blazed reflection grating in the Littrow mode

which maximum efficiency is observed is called the blazed wavelength λ_B. When such a grating is used in the Littrow mode, the angle of incidence (α) and angle of diffraction (θ) are nearly equal to the angle of blaze as shown in Fig. 11.39; that is, $\alpha \approx \theta \approx \beta$. The fundamental grating equation, therefore, modifies to, taking the blazed wavelength $\lambda = \lambda_B$.

$$m\lambda_B = d\left[\sin \alpha + \sin \theta\right] \approx 2d \sin \beta \tag{i}$$

where m is the order of diffraction and d is the grating element (i.e. the distance between two grooves).

With such a demultiplexer using a reflection grating in the Littrow mode, the wavelength channel spacing is given by:

$$\Delta\lambda = \frac{x}{f}\left(\frac{d\lambda}{d\theta}\right) = \frac{x}{f}\sqrt{d^2 - \left(\frac{\lambda_2}{2}\right)^2} \tag{ii}$$

where λ_c is central wavelength corresponding to λ_B, x is the spacing of core centres of the output fibers, and f is the local length of the lens.

Here, the required $\lambda_c = 1.55$ μm, so that $\lambda_B = 1.55$ μm, $\beta = 10°$, and $m = 1$ (for first-order diffraction). Using Eq. (i), we get $d = 4.463$ μm. The focal length f of the lens may be obtained by putting $x = 150$ λm, $\Delta\lambda = 10$ nm, and $\lambda_c = \lambda_B = 1.55$ μm in Eq. (ii). This gives $f = 65.92$ mm.

Example 8

Consider an $N \times N$ waveguide grating multiplexer having $L_f = 10$ mm, $x = d = 5$ μm, $n_c = 1.45$, and a central design wavelength $\lambda_c = 1550$ nm. Calculate the waveguide length difference for $m = 1$. **[B Tech]**

Solution

We have: $\Delta L = m\dfrac{\lambda_c}{n_c}$

$\therefore \qquad \Delta L = 1 \times \dfrac{1550}{1.45} = 1069$ μm

Here, $m = 1$, $l_c = 1550$ nm, $n_c = 1.45$.

If $n_s = 1.45$ and $n_g = 1.47$, then:

$$\Delta\lambda = \frac{x}{L_f}\frac{n_s d}{m}\frac{n_c}{n_g} = \frac{5}{10^4} \times \frac{1.45 \times 5}{1} \times \frac{1.45}{1.47}\ \mu m = 3.58\ nm$$

Example 9

(a) Assume that the input wavelengths of a 2 × 2 silicon MZI are separated by 10 GHz (i.e. $\Delta\lambda = 0.08$ nm at 1550 nm). With $n_{eff} = 1.5$ in a silicon waveguide, calculate the waveguide length difference. (b) If the frequency difference is 130 GHz (i.e. $\Delta\lambda = 1$ nm), then calculate ΔL.

Solution

(a) $\Delta L = \left[2n_{eff} \left(\dfrac{1}{\lambda_1} - \dfrac{1}{\lambda_2} \right) \right] = \dfrac{c}{2n_{eff}\, \Delta\nu} = \dfrac{3 \times 10^8 \text{ m/s}}{2 \times 1.5 \times 10^{10}/\text{s}} = 10^{-2}$ m

(b) $\Delta L = \dfrac{3 \times 10^8 \text{ m/s}}{2 \times 1.5 \times (13) \times 10^{10}/\text{s}} = 0.77$ mm

Example 10

The maximum index change of a particular DBR laser operating at 1550 nm is 0.65%. Calculate the tuning rate.

If the source spectral width $\Delta\lambda_{signal} = 0.02$ for a 2.5 Gb/s signal, then find the number of channels that can operate in this tuning range.

Solution

We have
$$DL_{tune} = \lambda\, \dfrac{\Delta n_{eff}}{n_{eff}} = (1550 \text{ nm})(0.0065) = 10 \text{ nm}$$

$$N = \dfrac{\Delta\lambda_{tune}}{\Delta\lambda_{channel}} = \dfrac{10 \text{ nm}}{10 \times 0.02 \text{ nm}} = 50$$

Example 11

An optical power of 100 µW is launched into the input port of a fused biconical tapered fiber coupler. Taking $P_1 = 40$ µW, $P_2 = 35$ µW and $P_3 = 7.5$ nW, estimate the values of coupling ratio, excess loss, insertion loss, and cross-section of the coupler.   **[DTU]**

Solution

We have

(i) Coupling ratio (%) $= \dfrac{P_2}{P_1 + P_2} \times 100$

$= \dfrac{35}{40 + 35} \times 100 = 46.66\%$

We can estimate the excess loss as

(ii) Excess loss (dB) $= 10 \log_{10} \left(\dfrac{P_0}{P_1 + P_2} \right)$

$= 10 \log_{10} \left(\dfrac{100}{40 + 35} \right) = 1.25$ dB

(iii) Insertion loss (input port to output port 1) $= 10 \log_{10} \left(\dfrac{P_0}{P_1} \right)$

$= 10 \log_{10} \left(\dfrac{100}{40} \right) = 3.98$ dB

(iv) Insertion loss (input port to output port 2) $= 10 \log_{10} \left(\dfrac{P_0}{P_2} \right)$

$$= 10 \log_{10} \left(\frac{100}{35} \right) = 4.56 \text{ dB}$$

(v) Cross talk $= 10 \log_{10} \left(\dfrac{P_3}{P_0} \right)$

$$= 10 \log_{10} \left(\frac{7.5 \times 10^{-3}}{100} \right) = -41.25 \text{ dB}$$

Example 12

A 16 × 16 ladder type star coupler is designed by cascading four por (2 × 2) 3 – dB coupler. Find the number of stages and total number of the (2 × 2) couplers required to realize the star coupler. Now, if 90% of the power is transmitted through each element, calculate the excess loss and total loss in dB.   **[MHTU, KTU]**

Solution

The number of stages required for realizing the cascaded (16 × 16) star coupler using four-port (2 × 2) coupler is obtained as

$$M = \log_2(16) = 4$$

Total number of four-port (2 × 2) couplers needed

$$N_c = \frac{16}{2} \times 4 = 32$$

$$\text{Excess loss (dB)} = -10 \log_{10}(F_T^M)$$

$$= -10 \log_{10}[(0.9)^4] = 1.83 \text{ dB}$$

$$\text{Splitting loss (dB)} = 10 \log_{10}(16) = 12.04 \text{ dB}$$

$$\text{Total loss} = 1.83 + 12.04 = 13.87 \text{ dB}$$

We can also compute the total loss using the following relation

$$\text{Total loss (dB)} = 10 \left[1 - \frac{\log_{10}(F_t)}{\log_{10} 2} \right] \log_{10} N$$

Example 13

The tuning current in a DFB laser operating at 1550 nm can cause a maximum change in the effective refractive index of 0.5%. Find the tuning range and compute the number of channels that ca be safely accommodated within this range of WDM applications. You may assume the spectral width of the source as 0.01 nm.   **[MHTU, KTU]**

Solution

The tuning range of the DFB laser operating at 1550 nm is obtained as

$$\Delta\lambda_{\text{tune}} = \lambda \frac{\Delta n_{\text{eff}}}{n_{\text{eff}}} = 1550 \times 0.05 \approx 8 \text{ nm}$$

The channel spacing is obtained as

$$\Delta\lambda_{\text{channel}} = 10 \times 0.01 = 0.1 \text{ nm}$$

The number of channels that can be accommodated within the tuning range

$$N \approx \frac{\Delta\lambda_{\text{tune}}}{\Delta\lambda_{\text{channel}}} = \frac{8 \text{ nm}}{0.1 \text{ nm}} = 80$$

SUMMARY

- Optical signals of different wavelength (1300–1600 nm) can propagate without interfering with each other. The scheme of combining a number of wavelengths over a single fiber is called *wavelength division multiplexing* (WDM), i.e., the oncept of WDM involves simultaneous transmission of several wavelengths (say, λ_1, λ_2, λ_3, ..., λ_N) over the same single optical fiber, effectively increasing the aggregation bandwidth per fiber cable.

- WDM technology has evolved to the point that channel wavelength separations can be as small as a few nms, giving rise to *dense wavelength division multiplexing* (DWDM) *systems.*

- The implementations of WDM or DWDM requires a number of passive and active components. The performance of passive components is fixed whereas that of active components can be controlled electronically.

- To prevent spurious signals to enter into receiving channel, the *demultiplexer* must have narrow spectral operation with sharp wavelength cutoff. The acceptable limit of crosstalk is ~ 30 dB.

- *Passive components* are mainly used to split or combine optical signals. These components operates in optical domains. Passive components don't need external control for their operation. Passive components are fabricated by using optical fibers or by planar optical waveguides. Commonly used passive components are: (i) NXN couplers (ii) Power splitters (iii) Power taps (iv) Star couplers. Most passive components are derived from basic star couplers.

- Star coupler can perform combining and splitting of optical power. Therefore, star coupler is a multiple input and multiple output port device.

- A device with two inputs and two outputs is called as 2×2 coupler.

- Star coupler is mainly used for combining optical powers from N-inputs and divide them equally at M-output ports.

- *Directional couplers* are used to split or combine two signals at different wavelengths. In a directional coupler made up of two identical signal-mode fibers, there is a periodic exchange of power between the two optical fibers. The minimum interaction length over which the power is completely transferred from the first fiber to the second fiber is termed as the *coupling length.*

- The optical power put into any port on one side of coupler is equally divided among the output ports. However, ports on same side of coupler are isolated from each other.

- The performance of a coupler is expressed in terms of the following parameters:

  i. Coupling ratio (%) = $\dfrac{P_2}{P_1 + P_2} \times 100$

  ii. Splitting loss = $-10 \log\left(\dfrac{1}{N}\right) = 10 \log N$

iii. Excess loss (dB) $= +10 \log_{10} \left(\dfrac{P_0}{P_1 + P_2} \right) - 10_{10} \left(\dfrac{P_1 + P_2}{P_0} \right)$

$$= -10_{10} \left(\dfrac{P_{in}}{\sum\limits_{i=1}^{N} P_{out,i}} \right)$$

iv. Insertion loss (dB) $= -10 \log_{10} \left(\dfrac{P_j}{P_i} \right)$

- To implement WDM, a multiplexer is required to combine several wavelengths at the transmitting end, and a demultiplexer is required to isolate the different wavelengths at the receiver end. There are several mechanisms of multiplexing (demultiplexing) studies. Some of these are:

  i. Interference filter devices

  ii. Angular dispersion using a *Littrow* prism or Littrow grating

  iii. Match-Zehnder interferrometer

  iv. Arranged wavelength grating

  v. Fiber Bragg grating

- Many different lasers designs have been proposed to generate the spectrum of wavelength needed of DWDM networks. The use of discrete single-wavelength DFB or DBR lasers is the simplest method. A tuning wavelength range of 10–15 nm is possible with DFB and DBR lasers. For wider ranges, an array of tunable lasers has to be used.

- *Tunable optical filters* are key components for dense WDM optical networks. Two key technologies to make a tunable filters are *MEMS*-based and *Bragg grating* based devices. Tunable filters can be used as add/drop multiplexers in optical networks or demultiplexes in the receiver module.

- *Time division multiplexing* (TDM) is a technique for transmitting multiple digital data, voice, and video signals simultaneously over one fiber cable. This is accomplished by interleaving pulses representing bits from different channels or time slots. The public-switched telephony network (PSTN) is based on the TDM technologies and is often called a TDM access network.

- *Frequency-division multiplexing* (FDM) is a scheme in which numerous analogue signals are combined for transmission on a single communications line or channel. Each signal is assigned a different frequency (sub-channel) within the main channel. This technology is used in broadcast, radio, television, and cable television.

- *Dense wavelength division multiplexing* (DWDM) is an optical technology used to increase bandwidth over existing fiber optic backbones. DWDM is a fiber-optic transmission technique that employs light wavelength to transmit data as parallel bits or a serial string of characters.

- *Coarse wavelength division multiplexing* (CWDM) is a technology that combines upto 16 wavelengths onto a single fiber. When there are just a few channels (upto 16 channels) and they are spaced more widely (10 nm or more) apart, the system is called CWDM.

REVIEW QUESTIONS

1. Draw a neat sketch of WDM scheme and explain it.
2. What is the significance of passive components in WDM?
3. Distinguish between WDM and DWDM. Explain the base frequency and channel spacing specified by ITU for DWDM.
4. Explain the construction and working of 2 × 2 directional fiber coupler and an N × N star coupler.
5. Explain various performance parameters of optical coupler.
6. How one can change the coupling ratio of a 2 × 2 coupler?
7. How many major types of devices are there for multiplexing/demultiplexing? Explain them and compare with merits and demerits.
8. Why tunable sources needed? Explain the principle of at least two types of tunable sources.
9. What are tunable filters? Where they are used?
10. Explain the principle of operation of an AOTF.
11. Mention and explain the possible applications of fiber optic gratings.
12. Write the definitions of following parameters: (a) Insertion loss (B) Channel width (c) Crosstalk of a WDM system.
13. Explain the operation with diagram of a unidirectional WDM. Also explain bidirectional WDM system.
14. Write short notes on:
   (a) Time-division multiplexing (TDM)
   (b) Frequency-division multiplexing (FDM)
   (c) Dense wavelength division multiplexing (DWDM)
   (d) Coarse wavelength division multiplexing (CWDM).
15. Briefly explain the techniques for multiplexing and demultiplexing.

PROBLEMS

1. A 2 × 2 loss-fiber coupler is using identical single mode fibers. Show that the interaction length required to achieve a splitting ratio of 10:90 is $L \approx 1.25/k$.

   [B Tech]

2. How many fibers are required for full duplex communications between two nodes?

   [B Tech]

   [**Hint.** Generally, two fibers are rquired for traffic transmission in each direction. However, it is possible to reduce this to one fiber by using DWDM, WDM or bi-directional coupler technology.]

3. A PHASAR-based demultiplexer with 32 channels spaced at 50 GHz and a central wavelength of 1.55 μm is to be designed. Calculate the FSR and the order of array.

   [B Tech]
   [Ans. 1600 GHz, 121]

4. How one can increase bandwidth (BW, i.e. traffic capacity) economically?

   [B Tech]

[**Hint.** There are number of different ways through which one can economically double fiber capacity. One may use bidirectional couplers that allow traffic transmission in both directions on one fiber. However, installing of bidirectional couplers does not require end mode equipment to be modified.

To enhance the capacity further, one may be able to install passive *cross band WDMS*, DWDMs or CWDMs.]

5. Can you interchange multimode and single mode equipment?

   [**Solution.** Generally no, since multimode and single mode equipment are not interchangeable and also not compatible.]

6. A fiber system uses multimode optical fiber. Can one enhance the capacity of multimode fiber by using WDM or DWDM technology?

   [**Solution.** One can enhance the multimode fiber technology as WDM and DWDM technology is not available for multimode fiber.

7. Using DWDMs, find the maximum number of wavelengths that can be placed onto a fiber. **[NET-SET]**

   [**Solution.** This basically depends on the use of the technology of equipment by manufacturer. With the presently available technology, the maximum number of wavelengths that can be placed onto a fiber using DWDMs lies anywhere from 4 to 80.]

8. A 2 × 2 biconical fiber coupler has an input optical power level of $P_0 = 200\ \mu W$. The output powers at the other three ports are $P_1 = 90\ \mu W$, $P_2 = 85\ \mu W$, and $P_3 = 6.3\ \mu W$. Calculate coupling ratio, excess loss, insertion loss: port 0 to 1 port, port 0 to port 2, return loss. **[B Tech]**

   [**Hint.** We have splitting ratio $= \dfrac{P_2}{P_1 + P_2} \times 100\%$

   (i) Coupling ratio $= \left(\dfrac{85}{90 + 85}\right) \times 100\% = 48.6\%$

   (ii) Excess loss $= 10 \log \dfrac{P_0}{P_1 + P_2} = 10 \log \left(\dfrac{200}{90 + 85}\right) = 0.58$ dB

   (iii) Insertion loss $= 10 \log \left(\dfrac{P_i}{P_j}\right)$

   (a) Port 0 to Port 1 $= 10 \log \left(\dfrac{200}{90}\right) = 3.47$ dB

   (b) Port 0 to Port 2 $= 10 \log \left(\dfrac{200}{85}\right) = 3.72$ dB

   (iv) Return loss $= 10 \log \left(\dfrac{P_3}{P_0}\right)$

   $= 10 \log \left(\dfrac{6.3 \times 10^{-3}}{200}\right) = -45$ dB

9. A symmetric waveguide coupler has a coupling coefficient $\kappa = 0.6\ mm^{-1}$. Find the coupling length for $m = 1$. **[B Tech]**

[**Hint.** We have $L = \dfrac{\pi}{2\kappa}(m+1)$ with $m = 0, 1, 2, ...$

Here $\kappa = 0.6$ mm^{-1}, $m = 1$

$\therefore \qquad L = 5.24$ mm.

10. A 32 × 32 single-mode coupler is made from a cascade of 3 dB fused fiber 2 × 2 couplers, where 5% of the power is lost in each element. Calculate the total loss.

[B Tech]

[**Hint.**

(i) Excess loss $= -10 \log (F_T \log_2 N)$

$\qquad\qquad = -10 \log (0.95 \log 32/\log 2) = 1.1$ dB

(ii) Splitting loss $= -10 \log \dfrac{1}{N} = -10 \log 32 = 15$ dB

$\therefore$ Total loss $= 16.1$ dB.

11. Ten uniformly spaced stations are connected to an optical bus having the following parameters:

C_T	L_T (dB)	L_{thru} (dB)	L_i (dB)	L_c (dB)	α (b/km)
5%	7.5 db	1.0	0.6	1.0	0.5

Considering the separation between the adjacent stations 500 m, prepare a power budget for the optical bus. **[UPTU, PTU]**

[**Hint.** For 10 stations uniformly spaced with a separation of 500 m, we have the power budget

$$10 \log_{10} \left(\frac{P_0}{P_{1,N}} \right) = N \left(\alpha L + 2L_c + L_{thru} + L_i - \alpha L - 2L_{thru} - 2L_T \right)$$

$$= 10 \times \left(0.5 \times \frac{1}{2} + 2 \times 1 + 1 + 0.6 \right) - 0.5 \times \frac{1}{2} - 2 \times 1 + 2 \times 7.4$$

$$= 10 \times 3.85 - 2.25 + 15 = 51.25 \text{ dB}]$$

12. One is interested to design a 3 dB coupler using fused biconical tapered fiber coupler. Show that the coupling length (L) for interaction is $\pi/4k$, where k is the coupling coefficient. **[PTU]**

[**Hint.** For a 3 dB coupler, it is necessary that the available power at each of the output ports 1 and 2 of the coupler should be one-half of the input power. Thus,

$$P_1 = P_0 \cos^2(kz) = \frac{1}{2}P_0$$

Also $$P_2 = P_0 \sin^2(kz) = \frac{1}{2}P_0$$

This situation will arise when the value of z is such that

$$\cos^2(kz) = \sin^2(kz) = \frac{1}{2}$$

or $$kz = \pi/4$$

$\therefore$ The required length of interaction or coupling length, $L = \pi/4k$.]

SHORT ANSWER QUESTIONS

1. What is WDM?

   Ans. Wavelength division multiplexing (WDM) is an optical technology that permits several wavelengths to be coupled into the same fiber cable, effectively increasing the aggregation band-width per fiber fable.

2. What is time-division multiplexing (TDM)?

   Ans. TDM is a technique for transmitting multiple digitized data, voice, and video signals simultaneously over one fiber cable. This is accomplished by interleaving pulses representing bits from channels or time slots.

3. What is frequency-division multiplexing (FDM)?

   Ans. FDM is a scheme in which numerous signals are combined for transmission on a single communication line or channel. Each signal is assigned a different frequency (sub-channel) within main channel. This technology is used in broadcast, radio, television and cable television.

4. What is dense wavelength division multiplexing (DWDM)?

   Ans. DWDM is an optical technology used to increase bandwidth (BW) over existing fiber-optic backbones.

   DWDM works by combining and transmitting multiple signals simultaneously at different wavelengths on the same fibers.

5. What is coarse wavelength division multiplexing (CWDM)?

   Ans. CWDM is a technology that combine upto 16 wavelengths onto a single fiber. When there are just a few channels (upto 16 channels) and they are spaced more widely (10 nm or more) apart, the system is called CWDM.

6. What method allows large number of independent, selectable channels to exist on a single fiber?

   Ans. Frequency division multiplexing (FDM).

7. Explain the concept of dense wavelength multiplexing (DWDM).

   Ans. Typically, the single-channel symbol rates range from 10 G sym/s to 40 G sym/s. A symbol rate beyond 40 G sym/s is hard to achieve in practice because of the speed of electronic components in transmitter of the fiber (1530–1620 nm), it has a bandwidth greater than 10 THz. To utilize the full bandwidth of the fiber, several channels can be multiplexed and they can share the same fiber channel. An EDTA operating in C-band (1530–1565 nm) has a bandwidth of about 4.3 THz and, therefore, several channels can be amplified simultaneousl by a single amplifier. The multiplexing techniques can be of three types: (i) polarization division multiplexing (PDM), (ii) frequency or wavelength division multiplexing (WDM), (iii) time-division multiplexing (TDM).

   In WDM system, multiple optical carriers of different wavelengths are modulated by independent electrical data. These operating wavelengths are so spaced by incorporating gaurd bands that they do not interfere with adjacent channels. The availability of laser sources with extremely small linewidth has made the implementation of WDM possible.

8. What are passive optical couplers?

   Ans. Passive devices operate completely in the optical domain to split and combine light streams. They include $N \times N$ couplers (with $N \geq 2$), power splitters, power taps, and star couplers. These components can be fabricated either from optical fibers or by means of planar optical waveguides using material such as lithium niobate

(LiNbO$_3$), InP, silica, silicon oxynitride, or various polymers.

9. What is splitting ratio or coupling ratio?

Ans. In order to specify the performance of an optical coupler, one usually indicates the percentage division of optical power between the output ports by means of

splitting ratio or coupling ratio, splitting ratio or coupling ratio $= \left(\dfrac{P_2}{P_1 + P_2} \right) \times 100\%$

where P_1 and P_2 are output powers and P_0 being the input power.

10. What is excess loss?

Ans. The excess loss is defined as the ratio of the input power to the total output power. In decibels, the excess loss for a 2 × 2 coupler is:

$$\text{Excess loss} = 10 \log \left(\frac{P_0}{P_1 + P_2} \right)$$

11. What is insertion loss?

Ans. The insertion loss refers to the loss for a particular port-to-port path, e.g. for the path from port i to port j, we have in decibels:

$$\text{Insertion loss } \Delta L = \frac{c\, n_{\text{eff}}}{\Delta \lambda}$$

12. What is cross talk or return loss?

Ans. Return loss measures the degree of isolation between the input at one port and the optical power scattered or reflected back into the other input port, i.e., it is a measure of the optical power level P_3. Thus:

$$\text{Return loss} = 10 \log \left(\frac{P_3}{P_0} \right)$$

13. What are star couplers?

Ans. A star coupler is simply a multiple output coupler in which each input signal is made available on every output fiber. The principal role of all star couplers is to combine the powers from N-inputs and divide them equally (usually) among M output ports. Usual techniques for creating star couplers include fused fibers, gratings, micro-optic technologies, and integrated-optics schemes.

14. What are optical isolators?

Ans. These are devices that allow light to pass through them in only one direction. This is important in a number of instances to prevent scattered or reflected light from travelling in the reverse direction. One common application of an optical isolator is to keep such backward-travelling light from entering a laser diode and possibly causing instabilities in the optical output.

15. What are optical circulators?

Ans. An optical circulator is a non-reciprocal multiport passive device that directs light sequentially from port to port in one direction only. This device is used in optical amplifiers, add/drop multiplexers, and dispersion compensation modules.

16. What are the three common network topologies?

Ans. Star, ring and mesh networks. In the star topology, each node has a transmitter and receiver, with the transmitter connected to one of the passive central star's inputs and receiver connected to one of the star's outputs.

Many electrical networks use ring topology because rings are easy to implement for any geographical network configuration.

In both star and ring topologies, each node has a signature wavelength, and any two nodes can communicate with each other by transmitting and recovering that wavelength.

In the mesh network, the nodes are connected by reconfigurable optical crossconnects (OXCs). The wavelength can be dynamically switched and routed by controlling the OXCs. Therefore, the required number of wavelengths and wavelength tunable range of the components can be reduced in this topology.

17. Mention some generic laudable goals which a WDM-device technologist aims to achieve:

    Ans. i. Large wavelength tuning range
        ii. Multi-user capability
        iii. Wavelength stability and repeatability
        iv. Low crosstalk
        v. High extinction ratio
        vi. Minimum excess losses
        vii. Fast wavelength tunability (especially for packet switching)
        viii. High speed modulation bandwidth
        ix. Low residual chirp
        x. High finesse
        xi. Low noise
        xii. Robustness
        xiii. High yield
        xiv. Potential low cost

18. Write advantages of WDM.

    Ans. Important advantages of WDM are as follows:
    i. *Capacity upgrade*: Since each wavelength supports independent data rate in Gbps.
    ii *Transparency*: WDM can carry fast asynchronous, slow synchronous, synchronous analog and digital data.
    iii. *Wavelength routing*: Link capacity and flexibility can be inserted by using multiple wavelength.
    iv. *Wavelength switching*: WDM can add or drop multiplexers, cross connects and wavelength converters.

19. What are optical couplers?

    Ans. Optical couplers are passive devices which either split optical signal into multiple paths, or combine several signals into one pair. A prime characteristics of couplers is the number of input and output ports, which is typically expressed as an $N \times M$ configuration, where N represents the number of inputs and M represents the number of outputs.

20. The performance of an optical receiver in an intensity modulation (IM)/direct detection (DD) system is greatly constrained by the associated electrical noise. How we can improve the performance of optical fiber communication system?

    Ans. By replacing the conventional IM/DD system by the so called coherent optical fiber communication system. The high sensitivity of the coherent receiver makes coherent optical communication more attractive by enhancing the repeaterless distance between the transmitter and the receiver.

21. Explain the basic concept of polarization division multiplexing (PDM).

Ans. PDM is an effective technique to double the capacity. A single-mode fiber supports two polarizaation modes, one with the electric field aligned with the x-axis and the other with the y-axis. Therefore, it is possible to transmit information using each of these polarization modes. Figure shows the schematic of the PDM.

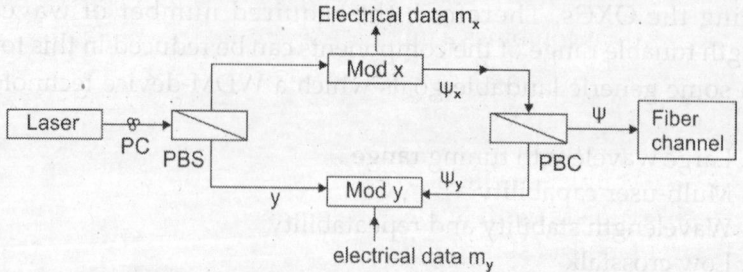

Fig. 11.40: Schematic of polarization-division multiplexing (PDM). PC = polarization controller, PBS = polarization beam splitter, PBC = polarization beam combiner, Mod = optical modulator

22. Explain the concept of diffraction based multi/demultiplexers.

Ans. Diffraction-based multi/demultiplexers make use of Bragg diffraction to isolate/combine the wavelength components. The WDM signal consisting of multiple wavelength components is incident on the grating. Different wavelength components diffract at different angles and they are collected by output fibers. One of the problems with bulk grating-based demultiplexers is that the output fiber core must be larger than the input fiber core in order to obtain the required flat pass band. Instead, an array of optical waveguides acting as grating could be used. Such gratings are known as *arranged-waveguide gratings* or *phased-array demultiplexers*.

23. What is orthogonal frequency-division multiplexing (OFDM) technique?

Ans. WDM is a FDM technique in which the carriers are typically not orthogonal. A special class of FDM in which the carriers (or subcarriers) are orthogonal is known as orthogonal frequency-division multiplexing (OFDM). In a WDM system, if the channel spacing is smaller than the bandwidth of the channels, this leads to cross-talk and performance degradation. However, in an OFDM, if the separation between carriers is smaller than the bandwidth of the data in each carrier, there is significant spectral overlap between the neighbouring channels and yet there would be no cross-task performance degradation because of carrier orthogonality conditions.

OFDM is widely used in wired and wireless communication systems because it is resilient to ISI due to dispersive channels. It has been used for digital audio broadcasting, HDTV terrestrial broadcasting, and wireless LANS.

24. What do you understand by time-division multiplexing?

Ans. In the case of frequency-division multiplexing (FDM), parallel streams of data are modulated by carriers with different frequencies so that the data spectra do not overlap. Instead, the parallel streams of the data can be converted to serial data in such a way that the individual streams do not overlap in time. This type of multiplexing is known as time-division multiplexing.

TDM can be performed in either an electrical or an optical domain. However, as the bit rate increased beyond 40 Fb/s, it becomes hard to do electrical TDM because of the limitations impassed by high-speed electronics. Instead, channels can be multiplexed in the optical domain and such a scheme is known as optical TDM (OTDM). Because of the wide bandwidth of optical devices, OTDM can be used to obtain a total bit rate of several terabits per second.

MULTIPLE CHOICE QUESTIONS

1. The technology that combines a number of wavelengths into the same fiber cable is known as:
   (a) WDM   (b) DWDM
   (c) optical amplifier   (d) optical detector

2. Passive optical couplers include:
   (a) only NXN couplers (with $N \geq 2$)   (b) only power splitters
   (c) only power taps and star couplers   (d) all of the above

3. In general, an NXM couplers has:
   (a) N inputs only   (b) M outputs only
   (c) N inputs and M outputs   (d) none of the above

4. Couplers are devices that are used to:
   (a) combine and split optical signals
   (b) block communication message
   (c) transfer information   (d) none of the above

5. The principal role of all star couplers is to combine the powers from N inputs and divide them usually:
   (a) unequally among M output ports   (b) equally among M output ports
   (c) sometimes equally sometimes unequally among M output ports
   (d) none of the above

6. Which of the following schemes is most suitable for DWDM?
   (a) Arrayed waveguide grating multiplexer
   (b) Mach–Zehnder interferometer
   (c) Fiber Bragg gratings   (d) Blazed reflection gratings

7. Which of the following tunable filters is most suitable for DWDM?
   (a) Mach–Zehnder interferometer   (b) Fabry–Perot filters
   (c) Acousto-optic tunable filters   (d) Fiber Bragg gratings

8. A 2 × 2 durectuibak ciyoker gas an input power level of 100 μW. The power available at output ports 1 and 2 are, respectively, 45 μW and 45 μW. What is the coupling ratio?
   (a) 45%   (b) 50%
   (c) 90%   (d) 100%

9. For the coupler of Question 8, what is the excess loss?
   (a) 3 dB   (b) 1 dB
   (c) 0.5 dB   (d) 0.46 dB

10. For the coupler of Question 8, what is the insertion loss for the path from input port 1 to output port 2?
    (a) 3.46 dB   (b) 5.23 dB
    (c) 6.92 dB   (d) 10 dB

11. A 1×10 coupler has an input signal 0 dB·m. What is the power level at each output port?
    (a) 0 dB·m
    (b) –1 dB·m
    (c) –3 dB·m
    (d) –10 dB·m

12. The function of wavelength-division multiplexer is to:
    (a) separate signals at different wavelengths and couple of them to different detectors
    (b) combine signals at different wavelengths to pass through a single fiber
    (c) tap off part of the energy of the incoming signal
    (d) change the transmission speed of the input signal

13. The scheme of WDM is similar to:
    (a) FDM for *rf* transmission
    (b) TDM
    (c) SDM
    (d) OTDM

14. What is the channel spacing (in nm) specified by the ITU-T recommendation G:692 for DWDM?
    (a) 1.6 nm
    (b) 0.8 nm
    (c) 0.4 nm
    (d) 0.2 nm

15. What is the channel spacing (in GHz) corresponding to the wavelength of Question 14?
    (a) 200 GHz
    (b) 100 GHz
    (c) 50 GHz
    (d) 25 GHz

16. An optical circulator is a nonreciprocal ....
    (a) single-port passive device
    (b) two-port passive device
    (c) 2×2 port passive device
    (d) multiport passive device

17. The conversion from wavelength spectral band to frequency band can be obtained by noting that
    (a) $\Delta v / v = \Delta \lambda / \lambda$
    (b) $\Delta v / v^2 = \Delta \lambda$
    (c) $\Delta v = \Delta \lambda / \lambda$
    (d) $c = v / \lambda$

18. A 2×2 coupler has
    (a) four inputs and two outputs
    (b) two inputs and four outputs
    (c) two inputs and two outputs
    (d) none of the above

19. An NXN coupler has
    (a) N inputs and N^2 outputs
    (b) N^2 inputs and N outputs
    (c) N inputs and N outputs
    (d) N^2 inputs and N^2 outputs

20. For a littrow grating, the blaze angle (θ_B) can be expressed in terms of wavelength (λ) of the incident light, m the diffracted order and the line spacing d on the grating as
    (a) $\theta_B = \sin^{-1}\left(\dfrac{m\lambda}{d}\right)$
    (b) $\theta_B = \sin^{-1}\left(\dfrac{2m\lambda}{d}\right)$
    (c) $\theta_B = \sin^{-1}\left(\dfrac{4m\lambda}{d}\right)$
    (d) $\theta_B = \sin^{-1}\left(\dfrac{m\lambda}{2d}\right)$

21. If n_{eff} is the effective refractive index in the waveguide and Δv is the frequency separation of the two wavelengths λ_1 and λ_2, then the length difference between the arms of Mach–Zehnder (MZ) interferometer can be expressed as

(a) $\Delta L = \dfrac{c}{8n_{eff}\Delta\lambda}$

(b) $\Delta L = \dfrac{c}{n_{eff}^2\Delta\lambda}$

(c) $\Delta L = \dfrac{c}{2n_{eff}\Delta v}$

(d) $\Delta L = \dfrac{cn_{eff}}{\Delta\lambda}$

22. The tuning current DFB laser operating at 1550 nm cause a maximum change in the effective refractive index of 0.5%. The tuning range of the DFB laser is approximately

(a) 8 nm

(b) 16 nm

(c) 4 nm

(d) 2 nm

[**Hint.** $\Delta\lambda_{tune} = \lambda\dfrac{\Delta n_{eff}}{n_{eff}} = 1550 \times 0.005 \approx 8$ nm]

23. In No. 22, if the spectral width is 0.01 nm, then the number of channels that can be safely accommodated within this range for WDM is

(a) 20

(b) 40

(c) 60

(d) 80

[**Hint.** $\Delta\lambda_{channel} = 10 \times 0.01$ nm $\therefore N = \Delta\lambda_{tune}/\Delta\lambda_{channel} = 8nm/0.1$ nm $= 80$]

24. In the bus network topology, each station of the optical network is connected to the main optical fiber cable called

(a) closed loop configuration

(b) bus

(c) central node

(d) point to point link

ANSWERS

1. (a)   2. (d)   3. (c)   4. (a)   5. (b)   6. (a)   7. (a)   8. (b)   9. (d)   10. (a)
11. (d)   12. (b)   13. (a)   14. (b)   15. (b)   16. (d)   17. (a)   18. (c)   19. (c)   20. (d)
21. (c)   22. (a)   23. (d)   24. (b)

12

Fiber Optic Communications

12.1 INTRODUCTION

Optical communications is very old form of data transfer. Line-of-sight primitive digital systems have included lighting bonefire on mountain tops to send a simple one-bit message, smoke signals to send a multiple-bit message, and ship-to-ship road incoherent beam transmission of Morse-code messages. The inventions of *low-loss optical fiber* and the *high-speed semiconductor* laser have caused an explosion in the transmission capacity of optical systems. The availability of information depends on the transmission speed of data, voice, and multimedia across telecommunication networks. Despite new technologies that enable legacy copper telephone lines to carry information more efficiently, optical networks remain the most ideal medium for *high-bandwidth* communications. There are two distinct modes of communications:

(i) *fiber optics* (*fiber optic cable*), and

(ii) *optical wireless* based on free-space optic technology. For long-distance network deployments, nothing is better than fiber. When coupled with the *wavelength division multiplexing* technologies, fiber optic cables are capable of carrying information more densely across the globe.

One of the most basic and undisputed applications of *optical* rather than *electrical communication* is data transmission on long-distance links. Optics is an obvious choice because of the ultra-wide bandwidth (> 25 THz) of low-loss (< 0.2 dB/km) transmission properties of an optical fiber, while the impedance of the electrical cable increases substantially at GHz speeds to > 100 dB/mile. In addition to *ultrawide* bandwidth transmissions, a *wavelength division multiplexing* (WDM) optical network also enables straightforward routing and switching of optical data paths, in which the data travels on wavelength-specific *light-paths* from source to destination that can be arranged by *network controller* to optimize throughput.

The progress in optical communications over the past three decades has been asounding. The advances of optical fiber systems have progressed in five *generation* of technology in the past three decades:

i. The *first generation* of optical fiber system used 0.8 μm GaAs semiconductor lasers and multimode fibers. Other specification of this generation are as under:
Bit rate: 50–100 Mbit/s
Repeater spacing: 10 km in length

ii. *Second generation* employed single mode fibers and 1.3 μm InGaAs and 1.55 μm InGaAsP lasers. Other specifications are:
Bit rate: 100 Mbit/s to 1.7 Gb/s

Repeater spacing: 50 km

Operating wavelength: 1.3 μm

iii. *Third generation* also employed single mode fibers and 1.3 μm InGaAs and 1.55 μm InGaAsP lasers. Other specifications are:

Bit rate: 10 Gb/s

Repeater spacing: 100 km

Operating wavelength: 1.55 μm

iv. *Fourth generation*: The fourth generation systems employed *optical amplifiers* and WDM technologies:

Bit rate: 10 Tbs^{-1}

Repeater spacing: > 10,000 km

Operating wavelength: 1.45 to 1.62 μm

v. *Fifth generation*: Fifth generation uses Roman amplification technique and optical solitons.

Bit rate: 40–160 Gbs^{-1}

Repeater spacing: 24000 km–35000 km

Operating wavelength: 1.53 to 1.57 μm

Today, the high-capacity amplified WDM systems have hundreds of channels at 10 Gbs^{-1} with channel spacing as low as 50 GHz and distances to a few thousand kilometers. Systems operate at 40 Gbs^{-1} channel^{-1} rate already in operation.

The *next generation* systems will be beyond fiber transmission links to optical networks. There are major efforts to promote the concept of Fiber-to-the X (FTTX:X = Curb, Home, Desktop, etc.) to support the demand for voice, data, and internet application across metropolitan areas.

Thus, optical communications is a fairly large and still rapidly-advancing scientific field. The use of wavelength-division multiplexing (WDM) have boosted in transmission capacity. *The basic principle of WDM is to use multiple sources at slightly different wavelengths* to send several independent packets of information data over the same fiber cable. For example, one of many of the world's WDM optical networks the SEA-ME-WE3-cable system. This undersea network runs from Germany to Singapore, connecting many countries in between; hence, the name SEA-ME-WE, which refers to Southeast Asia (SEA), the Middle East (ME), and the West Europe (WE). The network has two pairs of undersea fibers with a capacity of eight STM-16 wavelengths per fiber (equivalent to eight OC-48 which is 8 × 2.5 Gb/s).

Another submarine cable system, the undersea network connects many countries between Portugal (Sesimbra) to Malaysia (Penang). The route distance between these two countries is 23,455 km.

12.2 ESSENTIAL COMPONENTS OF FIBER COMMUNICATION SYSTEM

The basic components of optical fiber communication system are shown in Fig. 12.1(a). The three major components are:

(i) Transmitter,

(ii) Medium (optical fiber cable) or information channel, and

(iii) Receiver.

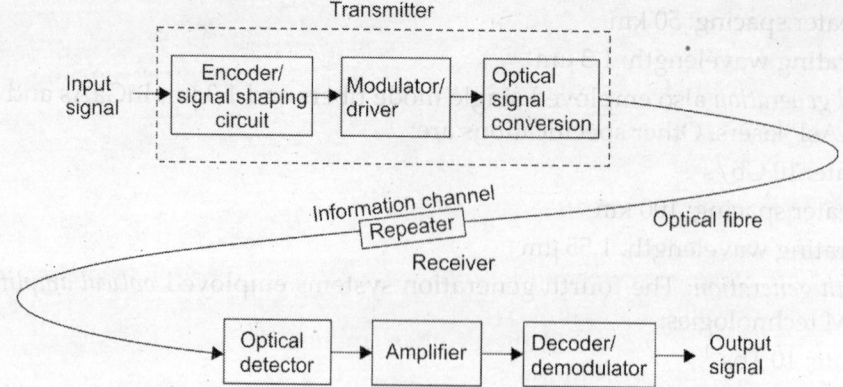

Fig. 12.1(a): Schematic diagram of optical fiber communication

The transmission system consists of encoder, modulator/driver and optical signal converter, the medium or informal channel is optical fiber and receiving system consists of optical detector, amplifier decoder/demodulator circuit.

System design considerations for point to point links: The problems (most) associated with the design of fiber optic communication systems are due to the unique properties of the optical fiber serving as a transmission medium.

Information can be classified in two general forms, *analog* and *digital*. *Analog* signals (Fig. 12.1(b)) represent quantities which can take on any value within an infinite continuum of amplitude and time. This kind of signal is typical of many measured quantities, such as temperature, volume, frequency, dimensions, etc. Analog signals, in theory ultimately accurate. However, to achieve a high-degree of accuracy in signal recovery, the noise must be kept extremely low compared to the signal power (~ –50d). Alternatively, *digital signals* can represent many quantities which may only require measuring of a limiting number of discrete levels at specific bit-time interval. It is only necessary to transmit and detect the difference between discrete levels (i.e. between "O" and "I" levels). Consequently the noise in relation to the signal that can be tolerated for error-free transmission is much higher than in analog transmission and is typically ~ –20 dB.

We may note that in common with other communication systems, the major design criteria for a specific application using either digital or analog techniques

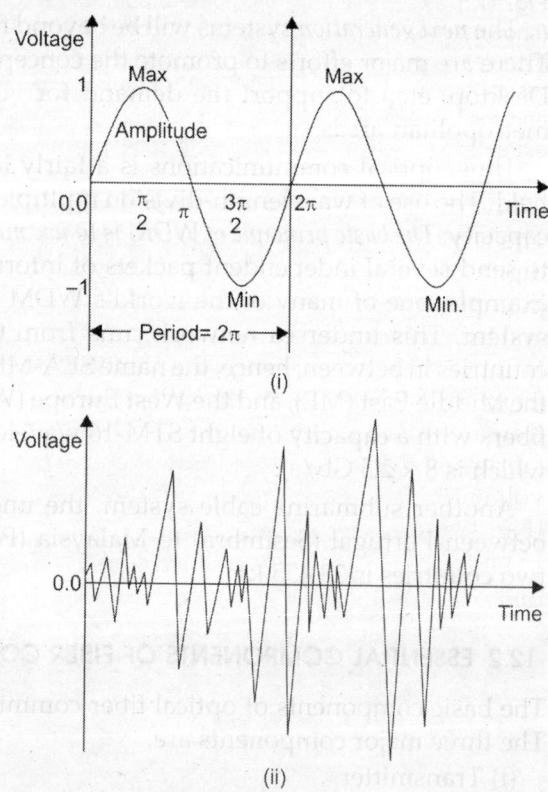

Fig. 12.1(b): Analog signals (i) sine wave (y = sinθ) (ii) analog voice wave

of transmission are the required transmission distance and also the speed of information transfer. These criteria are directly related to two important parameters of optical fibers: (i) *Fiber attenuation*, and (ii) *Fiber dispersion*. Keeping these facts in mind, we will discuss system design consideration for *digital systems* and for *analog systems*.

(a) Digital Systems

The simplest kind of *fiber-optic link* is the simplex (one-directional) point-to-point link having an optical transmitter at one end and an optical receiver at the other (Fig. 12.1(c)). The key system parameters needed to analyse this link are (i) the desired (or possible) transmission distance (without any repeaters), (ii) the data rate, and (iii) a specified bit-error rate (BER). In order to fulfil these requirements, the system designer has many choices. The major ones are as follows:

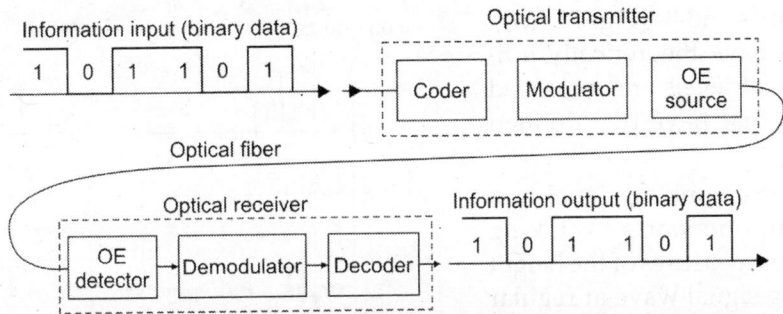

Fig. 12.1(c): A typical simple point-to-point digital fiber-optic link. The information input is binary data (shown as a series of 1's and 0's). A coder in the optical transmitter organizes the 1's and 0's and the modulator acts on this data by producing a current that turns the OE source (LED or ILD) on and off. The resulting pulses of light containing the information are transmitted through the optical fiber. At the receiver end, the OE detector converts the pulses of light into pulses of current. A demodulator-decoder combination extracts the information from the electrical pulses

Converting analog signal to digital signal: The term digital is used frequently because digital circuits are becoming so widely used in computation, robotics, medical science and technology, communications, transportation, etc. Digital electronics developed from the principle that the circuitry of a transistor could be designed and easily fabricated to have an output of one or two voltage levels, based on its input voltage [Fig. 12.1(d)].

Figure (12.1(e)) shows an *analog-to-digital converter* (ADC) used to convert an analog

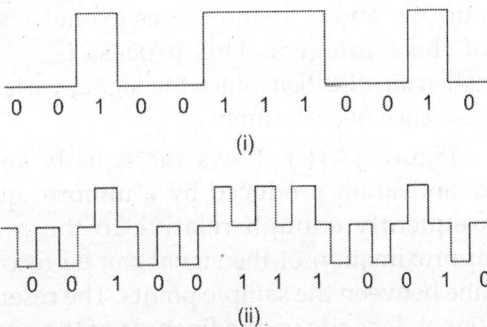

Fig. 12.1(d): Common digital signal configuration (i) digital pulse stream (ii) dipolar return-to-zero pulse

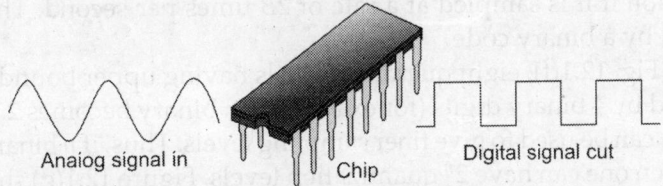

Fig. 12.1(e): A chip used to convert an analog to digital signal

signal into a digital signal. The ADC can be a single chip, or can be one circuit within a chip. The two voltage levels are usually 5 V (high) and 0 V (low); the levels can be represented by 1 and 0.

The binary numbering system (base-2 numbering system) is the main numbering system used in digital electronics. A digital value is represented by a combination of on and off voltage levels, and expressed as a string of 1s and 0s [Fig. 12.1(d)]. Signals that have theoretically infinite number of levels are converted into signals that have two defined levels.

To convert an analog signal to a digital form, one starts by taking instantaneous measures of the height of the analog signal wave at regular interval, this is called sampling the signal. One way to convert these analog samples to a digital format is to simply divide the amplitude of the analog signal into N equally spaced levels, which are designated by integers, and to assign values to one of these integers. This process is

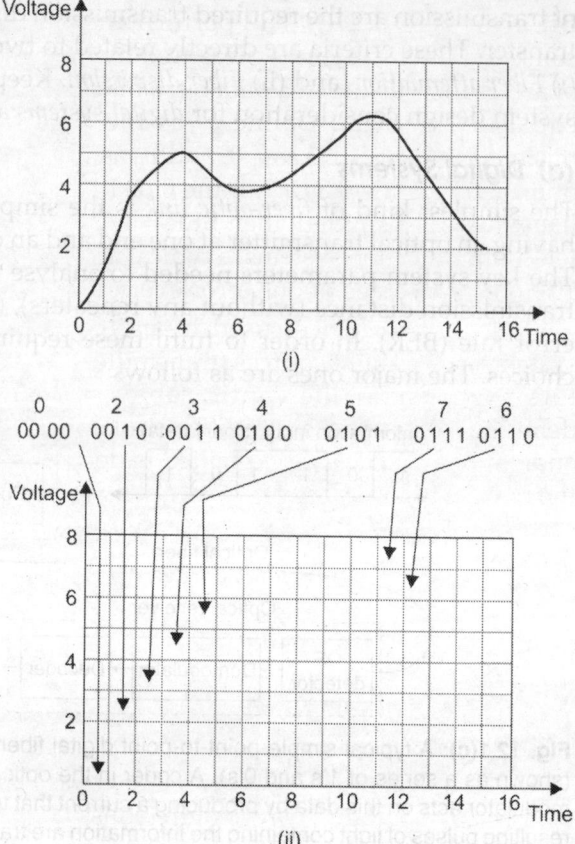

Fig. 12.1(f): Digitization of analog waveforms (i) analog signal varying between 0 to V volts (ii) quantized and sampled digital signal

called *quantization*. Since the signal varies continuously in time, this process generates a sequence of real numbers.

Figure 12.1(f) shows the equally spaced levels that are the simplest method of quantization produced by a uniform quantizer. If the digitization samples are taken frequently enough relative to the rate at which the signal varies, then a good approximation of the signal can be recovered from the samples by drawing a straight line between the sample points. The resemblance of the reproduced signal to the original signal depends on the fineness of the quantizing process, and on the effect of noise and distortion added into the transmission system. If the sampling rate is at least two times the highest frequency, then the receiving device can easily reconstruct the analog signal. Thus, if a signal is limited to bandwidth of B Hz, then the signal can be reproduced without distortion if it is sampled at a rate of $2B$ times per second. These data samples are represented by a binary code.

As shown in Fig. 12.1(f), eight quantized levels having upper bounds, $V_1, V_2, V_3, ... V$, can be described by 4 binary digits (for example 8 in binary becomes $2^3 = 2^3\, 2^2\, 2^1\, 2^0 = 1\,0\,0\,0$). More digits can be used to give finer sampling levels. Thus, if n binary digits represent each sample, then one can have 2^n quantization levels. Figure 12.1(g) shows a conversion process of an analog signal to digital form, and then to bar code.

Bit error rate (BER): The performance of a digital communication system is measured by the probability of an error occurring in a data bit; a bit error rate (BER) equal to 0 is ideal. Define p_1 as the probability of misinterpreting a 1 bit as a 0, and p_0 as the probability of misinterpreting 0 as a 1. If the 0 or 1 bits are equally likely to be transmitted, then BER = $1/2\, p_1 + 1/2\, p_0$. In telecommunication systems, a typical acceptable BER is 10^{-9} (i.e. an average of one error every 10^9 bit).

Optical fiber devices used in any communication system, such as light sources (transmitters) photodetectors (receivers), fiber optic cables, multiplexers, demultiplexers, optiocal amplifiers, isolators, circulators, and optical switches are explained in detail throughout the book.

(i) *Optical fiber*:
   (a) Multimode or single mode,
   (b) Core size
   (c) Refractive index profile
   (d) Attenuation
   (e) Dispersion

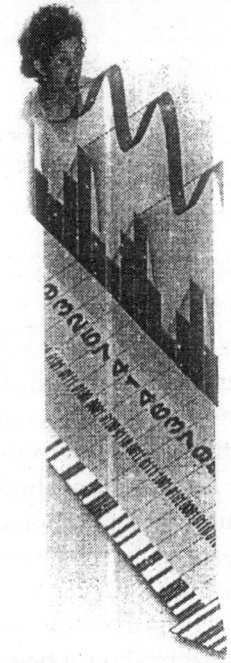

Fig. 12.1(g): Conversion process of an analog signal to digital and to bar code.

(ii) *Optical transmitter*:
   (a) LED or ILD source
   (b) Operating wavelength (emission wavelength of LED or ILD)
   (c) Output power and emission pattern
   (d) Transmitter configuration
   (d) Modulation and coding

(iiii) *Optical receiver*:
   (a) *p-i-n* or avalanche photodiode
   (b) Responsivity at the operating wavelength
   (c) Pre amplifier design (low impedance, or transimpedance front end)
   (d) Demodulation and decoding

We may note that decision regarding the above requirements are interdependent. However, one should kept in mind that the choices are made to optimise the system performance for a particular application.

To ensure that the desired system performance can be met, normally, two types of system analysis are carried out: (i) link power budget analysis, and (ii) rise time budget analysis. The first analysis determines the power margin between the optical transmitter output and the minimum required receiver sensitivity, so that this margin may be allocated to connector, splice, and fiber losses, or to any future degradation of components. The second analysis ensures that the desired overall system performance has been met. We now examine in detail these two types of system analysis.

(i) Link Power Budget Analysis

For optimizing link power budget an optical power loss model is to be studied as shown in Fig. 12.2.

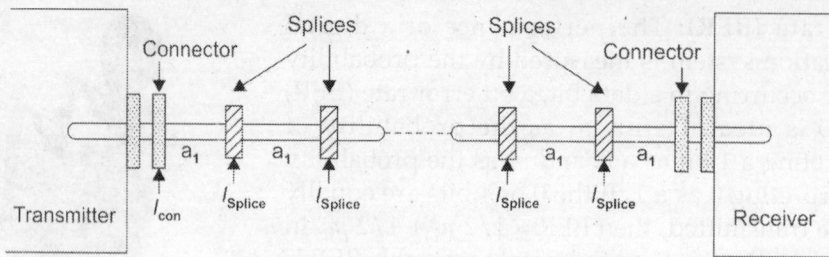

Fig. 12.2: Optical power loss model

The optical power received at the photodetector depends on the amount of optical power coupled into the fiber by the transmitter and on the losses occurring in the optical fiber as well as at the connectors and splices. This means that the power budget is derived from the sequential contributions at all the loss elements in the link. However, in addition to the link loss contributors, a safety margin of 6–8 dB is normally provided to allow for any future degradation of components and/or future addition of splices, etc. Thus, one can assume that the average power supplied by the transmitter is P_{tx}, the sensitivity of the receiver is P_{rx}, the total link loss of channel loss (including the fiber splice and connector losses is P_T, and the system's safety margin is M_s, then one finds that the following relationship should be satisfied:

$$P_{tx} = P_{rx} + C_L + M_s \tag{12.1}$$

The channel loss C_L may be expressed as:

$$C_L = \alpha_f L + \alpha_{con} + \alpha_{splice} \tag{12.2}$$

where α_f is the fiber loss (in dB/km), L is the link length, i.e. the transmission distance, α_{con} is the sum of losses due to all connectors in the link, and α_{splice} is the sum of losses at all the splices in the link. In Eqs (12.1) and (12.2), P_{tx} and P_{rx} are expressed in dB·m, and C_L, M_s, α_{cone} and α_{splice} are expressed in dB. One can use Eqs (12.1) and (12.2) to estimate the maximum transmission distance for a given choice of components.

(ii) Rise-Time Budget Analysis

Rise time gives important information for initial system design. Rise-time budget analysis determines the dispersion limitation of an optical fiber link. Rise time budget analysis is particularly important in the case of digital systems, where it is to be ensured that the system will be able to operate satisfactorily at the desired bit rate. One can define the rise time t_r of a linear system as the time during which the system's response increases from 10% to 90% of the maximum output value when its input changes abruptly (a step function).

We consider a simple RC circuit (Fig. 12.3) as an example of linear system. When the input voltage (V_{in}) across this circuit changes abruptly (i.e. in a step) from 0 to V_0, the output voltage (V_{out}) changes with time in accordance with the relation:

$$V_{out}(t) = V_0 [1 - \exp(-t/RC)] \tag{12.3}$$

where R is the resistance and C the capacitance of the circuit shown in Fig. 12.3. The rise time t_r is expressed as:

$$t_r = 2.2 \, RC \tag{12.4}$$

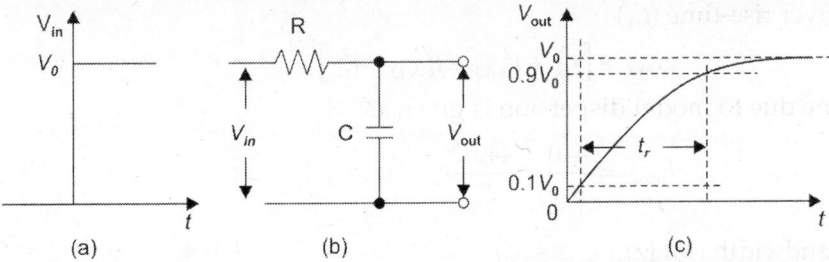

Fig. 12.3: The response of a low-pass RC filter circuit to a voltage step input V_0

Taking *Fourier transform* of Eq. (12.4), one obtains the transfer function $H(f)$ as:

$$H(f) = \frac{1}{(1 + 2\pi jf \, RC)} \tag{12.5}$$

The 3 dB electrical bandwidth Δf for the circuit corresponds to the frequency at which $|H(f)|^2 = 1/2$ and is given by the following relation:

$$\Delta f = \frac{1}{2\pi RC} \tag{12.6}$$

Therefore, using Eqs (12.4) to (12.6a), one can relate t_r to Δf by the relation:

$$t_r = \frac{2.2}{2\pi \Delta f} = \frac{0.35}{\Delta f} \tag{12.6a}$$

In Fig. 12.1(b), we have seen that in a fiber-optic communication system, there are three building blocks, and each block has its own rise time associated with it. Therefore, the total rise time of the system, t_{sys}, is obtained by taking the root-sum-square of rise time of each contributor, i.e. block. If we assume that the rise times associated with the transmitter, fiber, and receiver are respectively t_{tx}, t_f and t_{rx}, then, we can write:

$$t_{sys} = \left[t_{tx}^2 + t_f^2 + t_{rx}^2 \right]^{1/2} \tag{12.7}$$

We must note:

(i) The link components must be switched fast enough and the fiber dispersion must be low enough to meet the bandwidth requirements of the application. Adequate bandwidth for a system can be assured by developing a rise time budget.

(ii) As the light sources and detectors has a finite response time to inputs. The device does not turn-on or turn-off instantaneously. Rise time and fall time determines the overall response time and hence, the resulting bandwidth.

(iii) Connectors, couplers and splices do not affect system speed, they need not be accounted in rise time budget but they appear in the link power budget.

Further, the rise time of the optical fiber include the contribution of *intermodal dispersion* ($t_{intermodal}$) and *intramodal dispersion* ($t_{intramodal}$) through the relation:

$$t_f = \left(t_{intermodal}^2 + t_{intramodal}^2 \right)^{1/2} \tag{12.8}$$

In the absence of mode coupling, $t_{intermodal}$ and $t_{intramodal}$ are normally approximated by the time delays (ΔT) caused by intermodal and intramodal dispersion, respectively.

There are four basic elements that contributes to the rise time are:

- Transmitter rise-time (T_{tx})
- Group-velocity dispersion (GVD) rise time (t_{GVD})
- Modal dispersion rise time of fiber (t_{mod} or t_f)

- Receiver rise-time (t_{tx})

$$t_{sys} = \left[t_{tx}^2 + t_{mod}^2 + t_{GVD}^2 + t_{rx}^2 \right]^{1/2} \tag{12.9}$$

Rise time due to modal dispersion is given as:

$$t_{mod} = \frac{440}{B_M} = \frac{440 L^q}{B_0} \tag{12.10}$$

where,

B_M is bandwidth (MHz),

L is length of fiber (km),

q is a parameter ranging between 0.5 and 1, and

B_0 is bandwidth of 1 km length fiber.

Rise time due to group velocity dispersion is:

$$t_{GVD} = D^2 \sigma_\lambda^2 L^2 \tag{12.11}$$

where,

D is dispersion [ns/(nm·km)],

σ_λ is half-power spectral width of source, and

L is length of fiber

Receiver front end rise-time in nanoseconds is:

$$t_{rx} = \frac{350}{B_{rx}} \tag{12.12}$$

where, B_{rx} is 3 dB-BW of receiver (MHz).

Equation (12.9) can be written as:

$$t_{sys} = \left[t_{tx}^2 + t_{mod}^2 + t_{GVD}^2 + t_{rx}^2 \right]^{1/2}$$

$$t_{sys} = \left[t_{tx}^2 + \left(\frac{440 \, Lq}{B_0} \right)^2 + D^2 \sigma_\lambda^2 L^2 + \left(\frac{350}{B_{rx}} \right)^2 \right]^{1/2} \tag{12.13}$$

We may note that times are in nanoseconds (ns).

The system bandwidth is given by:

$$BW = \frac{0.35}{t_{sys}} \tag{12.14}$$

$$ct_{sys} = \sqrt{(1.75^2 + 3.5^2 + 3.89^2 + 1.00^2 + 1.94^2)}$$

$$t_{sys} = 5.93 \text{ ns}$$

System BW is given by:

$$BW = \frac{0.35}{t_{sys}} = \frac{0.35}{5.93 \text{ ns}} = 59 \text{ MHz} \tag{12.15}$$

We may note that that the optical power generated by the optical transmitter is generally proportional to its *inpout current*, and the *optical power received by the receiver* is proportional to the *power launched into and propagated* by the optical fiber. Finally, the output of the receiver is also proportional to its input. This means that a fiber-optic communication system can be considered to be a *band-limited linear system*, and hence Eq. (12.6) is valid for this system too. Therefore, for a fiber-optic communication system, the *total rise time* t_{sys} may be expressed as:

$$t_{sys} = 0.35 / \Delta f \tag{12.16}$$

Now, the relationship between the electrical bandwidth Δf and the bit rate B depends on the digital pulse format. For the return-to-zero (RZ) format, $\Delta f = B$ and for the non-return-to-zero (NRZ) format $\Delta f = B/2$. Therefore, for digital system, t_{sys} should be below its maximum value given by:

$$t_{sys} \leq \begin{cases} \dfrac{0.35}{B} \text{ for the RZ format} \\[2mm] \dfrac{0.70}{B} \text{ for the NRZ format} \end{cases} \tag{12.17}$$

We may note that the RZ and NRZ formats, to be discussed in the next subsection, are used for signal encoding.

Line coding: There is an important criterion in the design of optical fiber link, i.e. the decision circuit in the receiver should be able to extract precise timing information from the incoming optical signal. The precise timings are desired to (i) allow the signal to be sampled by the receiver at a time when the signal-to-noise ratio is maximum, (ii) maintain proper pulse spacing, and (iii) indicate the start and end of each timing interval. We may remember that channel noise and the distortion mechanism may cause errors in the signal detection process. Obviously, one will desire for the transmitted optical signal to have an inherent error-detecting capability. There is possibility to incorporate these features into the data stream by restructuring or encoding the signal. The main function of time coding is to introduce redundancy into the data stream for the sake of minimizing errors, especially those resulting from channel interference effects.

Let us try to understand line codes. For this purpose, we want to get ourself familiarize with some commonly used terms:

(i) *Digital signal*: This comprises a series of discrete voltage pulses. An individual pulse in the total signal is termed a *signal element*. We may note that *binary* data are transmitted by encoding each data bit into signal elements. The element may be a positive or negative voltage pulse. However, when a signal consists of both positive and negative voltage pulses, it is termed as *bipolar*. When only one polarity of voltage pulse is present, the signal is called *unipolar*.

(ii) *Data rate (R)*: R is the transmission rate of data in bits per second.

(iii) *Bit duration* $(T_b = 1/R)$: T_b is the time taken by the transmitter to transmit one bit. One can use a variety of wave shapes (signal elements) to represent binary data.

(iv) *Encoding*: The mapping of binary data bits to signal elements is termed as encoding. There are three popular encoding schemes as shown in Fig. 12.4.

   (a) *NRZ*: The simplest NRZ code is the NRZ level (or NRZ-L) as shown in Fig. 12.4(a), in which 1's or 0's of a serial data stream are represented by high voltage level and a 0 represented by low voltage level. Obviously, for a 1, there will be a light pulse filling the entire bit period, and for a 0, no light pulse will be transmitted. We may note that these codes are easier to generate and decode but do not possess an *inherent error-monitoring* capability. However, they make efficient use of bandwidth.

   (b) *RZ*: This code differs from NRZ codes in that only half the bit period is used for data, while the voltage is zero in the secondhalf of the bit period. Obviously, in a unipolar RZ data format (Fig. 12.4(b)), a 1 is represented by a half-period optical pulse that occurs in the first half of the bit period and a 0 is represented by no signal during the bit period. We may note that the disadvantages of the unipolar RZ format are that it requires double the

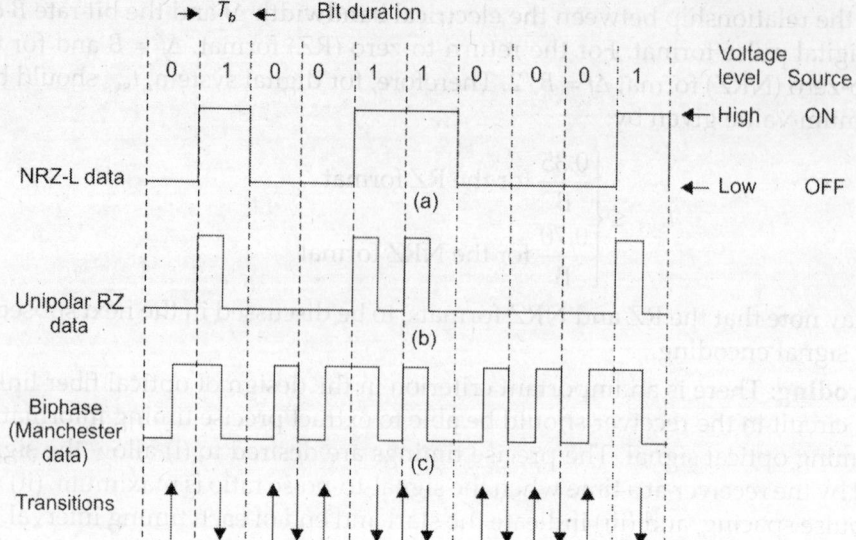

Fig. 12.4: Three popular encoding schemes: (a) NRZ, (b) RZ, and (c) biphase

bandwidth of NRZ-*L* format, and a long string of 0's can cause loss of timing information.

(c) *Biphase-L*: This is a data format which possesses the virtues of easy time synchronization, no *dc* component, and some inherent facility for error detection. Biphase-*L* is also called as the *optical Manchester code* shown in Fig. 12.4(c). In biphase-*L* code, there is a transition in the middle of the bit interval, the voltage level is high for a 1 and low for a 0. In this scheme, obviously, a transition from high to low in the middle of the bit interval represents a 1 and a transition from low to high represents a 0. We may note that these codes are widely used in fiber-optic systems.

(b) Analog Systems

For long-haul communication links, digital systems with single-mode fibers are normally considered superior, even with their expensive terminal equipment for coding, multiplexing, timing, etc. The main reason for this is that an analog fiber-optic system required 20–30 dB higher signal-to-noise ratio as compared with that required for a similar digital fiber-optic system. However, for *short-haul* and *medium-haul links*, analog fiber-optic systems can be very attractive, especially for the transmission of video signals, because of their simplicity and cost effectiveness. There are several other application of analog systems. It is reported that for most applications, analog transmitters use *laser diodes*. In the design implementation of an analog system, the main parameters that need to be considered are carrier-to-noise ratio, bandwidth, and the signal distortion resulting from non-linearities in the transmission system. In such system, carrier-to-noise ratio analysis is used instead of signal-to-noise ratio, because the information signal is normally superposed on an *rf* carrier.

Figure 12.5 shows the basic elements of two types of analog fiber-optic links. In the first system [Fig. 12.5(a)], the optical transmitter contains either an LED or ILD as the optical source. The output intensity of the source is directly changed or modulated by the information-carrying analog signal. It is necessary to first set a bias point on the

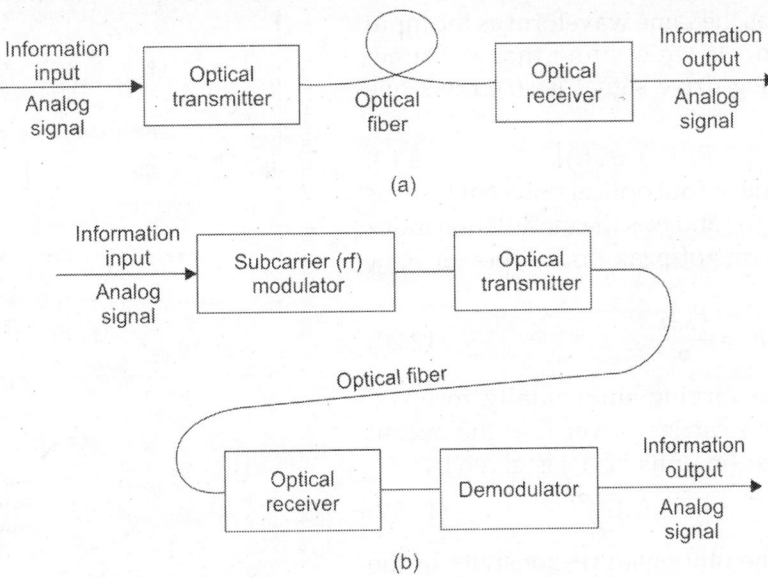

Fig. 12.5: An analog fiber-optic communication system: (a) type I—optical intensity is directly modulated by the analog signal (b) type II—A subcarrier is modulated by the analog signal

source approximately in the middle of the linear output region. The analog signal can then be transmitted using one of the several modulation techniques, the simplest one being direct intensity modulation. In this scheme, the optical output from the source is modulated by varying the current around the bias point in proportion to the level of the information signal. Thus, the signal is directly transmitted in the baseband. The modulated signal travels down the optical fiber and is demodulated at the receiver.

There also exists a more efficient way of modulation in which the base-band signal is first translated into an electrical (subcarrier prior to intensity modulation as shown in Fig. 12.5(b). This is accomplished using standard techniques of amplitude modulation (AM), frequency modulation (FM), or phase modulation (PM). These modulation techniques are employed when there is a need to send multiple analog signals over the same fiber as in the case of broadband common antenna television (CATV) supetrunks.

The performance of analog systems is normally analysed by calculating the carrier-to-noise ratio (CNR) of the system. It is defined as the ratio of the rms carrier power to the rms noise power (resulting from the source, detector, amplifier, and intermodulation) at the output of the receiver, thus:

$$CNR = \frac{\text{rms carrier power}}{\text{rms noise power}} \tag{12.18}$$

For single-channel transmission the noise contributions of the source, detector, and amplifier are considered, whereas for the transmission of multiple information channels through the same fiber, the inter-modulation factor is also considered. Here, we are examining a simple single-channel amplitude-modulated signal sent at baseband frequencies.

In order to determine carrier power, let us consider a laser transmitter. The optical signal variation by the source is caused by the drive current (through the source), which is a sum of the fixed bias and an analog input signal (a time-varying sinusoid), as shown in Fig. 12.6. An ILD acts as a *square-law device*, so that the envelope of the output optical power $P(t)$ has the same waveform as the input drive current. If we assume that the time-varying analog drive signal is $s(t)$, then, one may write:

$$P(t) = P_B [1 + ms(t)] \qquad (12.19)$$

where P_B is the output optical power at the bias current level (I_B) and m is the modulation index defined in terms of peak optical power P_{peak} as follows:

$$m = \frac{P_{peak}}{P_B} \qquad (12.20)$$

For a time-varying sinusoidally received signal, the rms carrier power C at the output of the receiver (in units of A^2) is given by:

$$C = \frac{1}{2}(mRM\overline{P})^2 \qquad (12.21)$$

where R is the unity gain responsivity of the photodetector, M is the gain of the APD ($M = 1$ for p-n and p-i-n photodiodes), and $\overline{P}$ is the average received optical power.

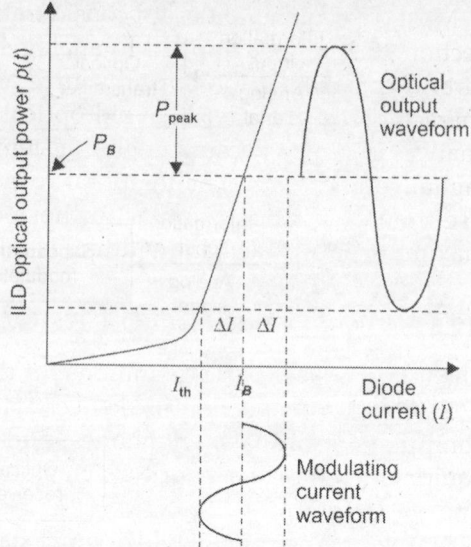

Fig. 12.6: Schematic representation of the biasing conditions of an ILD and its response to analog signal modulation

The rms noise power in Eq. (12.18) is the sum of the noise powers arising due to the source, photodetector, and preamplifier. The source noise, in the present case, will be given by:

$$\langle i_{source}^2 \rangle = RIN(R\overline{P})^2 \Delta f \qquad (12.22)$$

where RIN is the laser relative intensity noise measured in dB/Hz and is defined by:

$$RIN = \frac{\langle (\Delta P_L)^2 \rangle}{\overline{P_L}^2} \qquad (12.23)$$

where $\overline{P}_L$ is the average laser light intensity and $\langle (\Delta P_L)^2 \rangle$ is the mean square intensity fluctuation of the laser output. Δf is the effective noise bandwidth. This type of noise decreases as the injection current level increases.

The photodiode noise arises mainly due to shot noise and bulk dark current noise. Thus, combining the two, one obtains an expression for photodiode noise as follows:

$$\langle i_N^2 \rangle = 2e(I_p + I_d)M^2 F(M)(\Delta f) \qquad (12.24)$$

Here, $I_p = R\overline{P}$ is the primary photocurrent, I_d is the bulk dark current of the detector, M is the detector's gain with the associated noise figure $F(M)$, and Δf is the effective noise bandwidth of the receiver. The thermal noise of the photodetector and the noise of the pre-amplifier may be combined in the expression:

$$\langle i_T^2 \rangle = \frac{4kT}{R_{eq}}(\Delta f)F_t \qquad (12.25)$$

where R_{eq} is the equivalent resistance of the photodiode and the preamplifier, and F_t is the noise factor of the pre-amplifier.

Substituting the values of the rms carrier power from Eq. (12.21) and the rms noise power [which is a sum of expressions (12.22), (12.24), and (12.25)] into Eq. (12.18), one obtains the CNR for a single-channel AM fiber optic system as:

$$CNR = \frac{(1/2)(mRm\overline{P})^2}{RIN(R\overline{P})\Delta f + 2e(I_p + I_d)M^2 F(M)\Delta f + 4kT(\Delta f)F_t/R_{eq}} \qquad (12.26)$$

Most of the general design considerations for digital fiber-optic systems described in Section 12.2 may be applied to analog systems as well. However, one must take extra care to ensure that the optical source and the photodetector have linear input-output characteristics, in order to avoid optical signal distortion. A careful link power budget analysis is a must because analog system require a higher SNR at the receiver than their digital counterparts. The temporal response of analog systems may be determined by rise-time calculations similar to those done for digital systems. In this case too, the maximum attainable bandwidth Δf is related to t_{sys} by Eq. (12.16).

12.3 BASIC COMMUNICATION SYSTEM

The following are basic definitions for the networks used in communication systems:

Station is a collection of devices with which users wish to communicate. such as computers, terminals, telephones, and videos. Stations are also called data terminal equipment (DTE) in network systems, and they can be connected directly to a transmission line.

Network is a group of two or more stations linked or interconnected by a transmission medium, such as a fiber optic cable or coaxial cable.

Topology is the logical manner or structure in which nodes/devices are linked together in information-transmission channels to form a network.

Switching is the transfer of information from source to destination through a series of intermediate nodes. A switch is a device that filters and forwards packets between *network segments*. Switches operate at the data link layer (layer 2) and sometimes at the network layer (layer 3) of the open system interconnection (OSI) reference model. A description of the layers is presented later in this chapter. Switches support any pocket protocol.

Routing is the process of moving a packet of data from the source to the destination by the selection of a suitable path through a network. Routing is usually performed by a dedicated device called a router.

Protocol is an agreed-upon format for transmitting data between two devices. The protocol determines the following items:

- Type of error checking to be used;
- Data compression method, if any; and
- Hand shaking, how the device indicates when finished sending a message.

A popular protocol used in optical LANs is the fiber distributed data interface (FDDI) protocol; SONET/SDH protocols are used in optical networks in metro or wider areas. Logical topologies are bound to the network protocols that direct how the data moves across a network. The Ethernet protocol is a common logical bus topology protocol.

12.4 TYPES OF TOPOLOGIES

Topology refers to the shape of a network, or the network's layout. There are different nodes in a network which communicate by the network's topology. Topologies are either physical or logical. Connections between the nodes are via optical couplers. The five most common network topologies are (i) bus topology, (ii) ring topology, (iii) star topology, (iv) mesh topology, and (v) tree topology.

(i) Bus Topology

In a bus topology, all stations are connected to a central cable which is called the bus or backbone, as shown in Fig. 12.7.

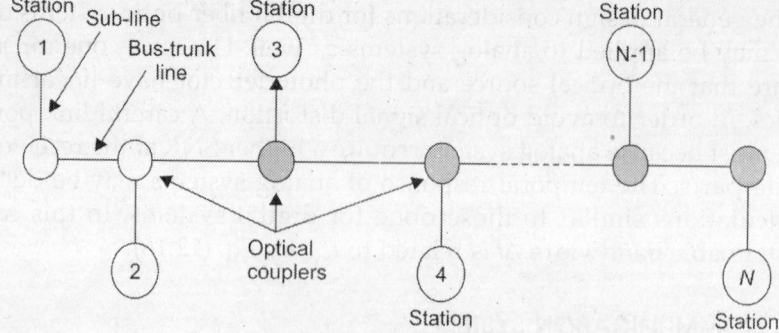

Fig. 12.7: Bus topology

(ii) Ring Topology

In a ring topology, all stations are connected to one another in the shape of a closed loop, so that each station is connected directly to two other stations on either side, as shown in Fig. 12.8.

(iii) Star Topology

In a star topology, all stations are connected to a central hub, which is an optical star coupler. Stations communicate across the network by passing data through the hub, as shown in Fig. 12.9.

(iv) Mesh Topology

In a a mesh topology, all stations are connected via many redundant interconnections, as shown in Fig. 12.10. In a true mesh topology, every station has a connection to every other station in the network.

(v) Tree Topology

In a tree (hybrid) topology, all stations are connected by various topologies, as shown in Fig. 12.11. Groups of star-configured networks are connected to a linear bus backbone.

12.5 TYPES OF NETWORKS

Networks are divided into five types based on the size of the area that the network covers: (i) home-area net-

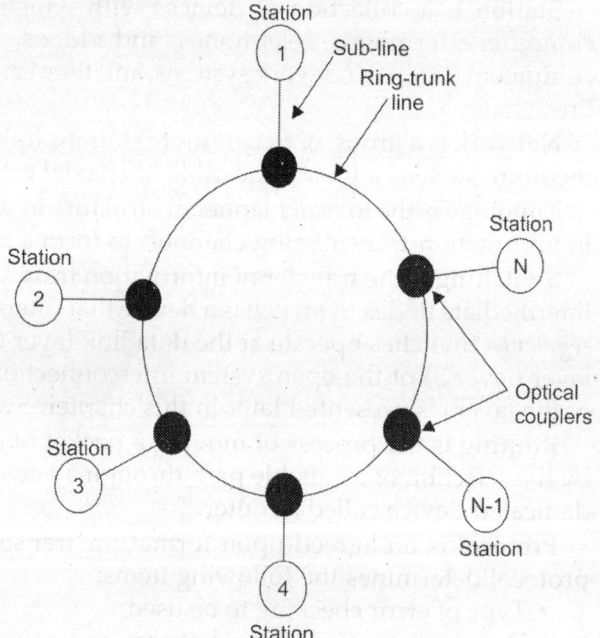

Fig. 12.8: Ring topology

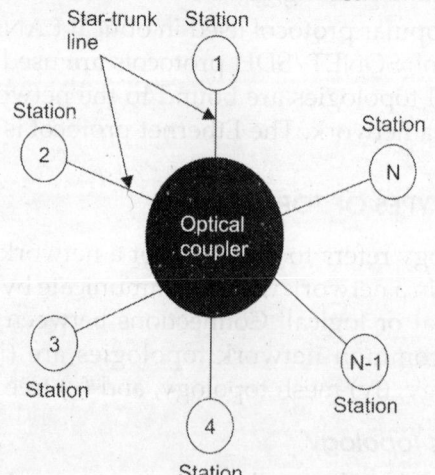

Fig. 12.9: Star topology

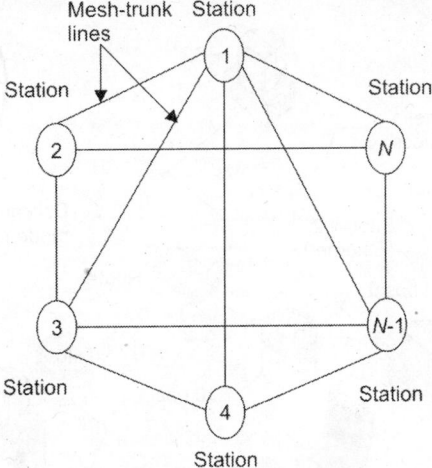

Fig. 12.10: Mesh topology

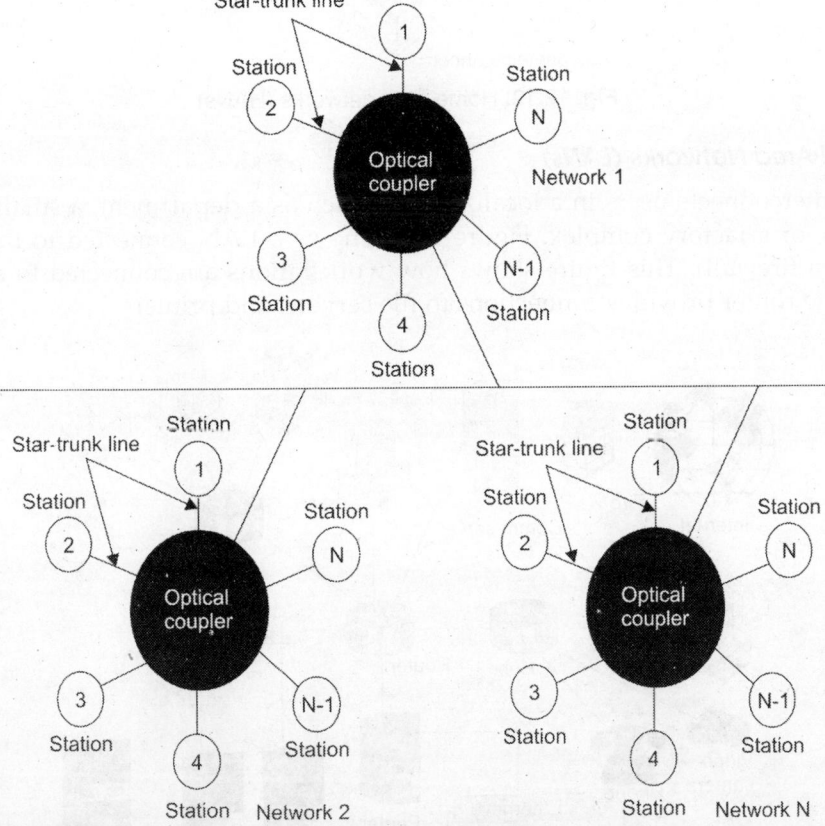

Fig. 12.11: Tree topology

works (HANs), (ii) local-area network, (iii) campus-area networks (CANs), (iv) metropolitan area networks (MANs) and (v) Wide area networks (WANs).

(i) Home Area Networks (HANs)

As shown in Fig. 12.12, a HAN is a network that connects the digital devices to computers, which are contained within an individual user's home.

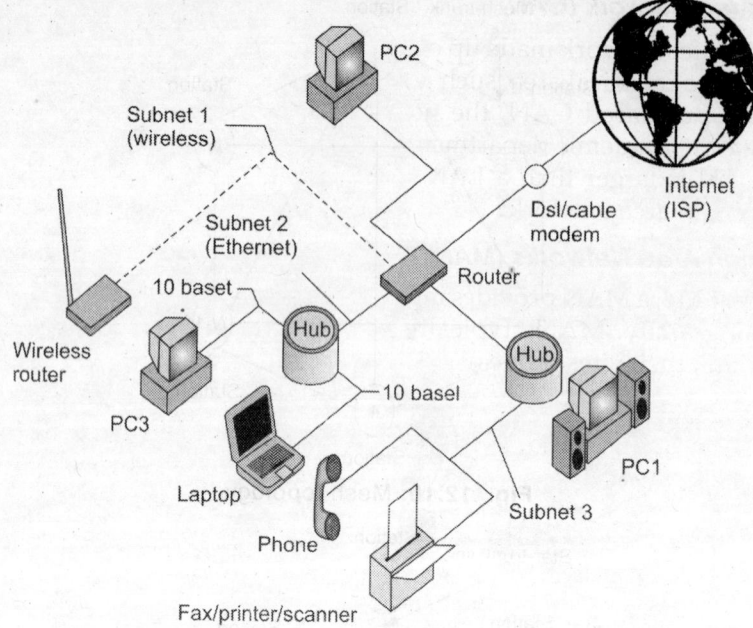

Fig. 12.12: Home-area networks (HANs)

(ii) Local Area Networks (LANs)

A LAN interconnects users in a localized area such as a department, a small group of buildings, or a factory complex. Figure 12.13 shows a LAN connected to the internet (through a firewall). This figure shows how workstations are connected to a hub and router. The router provides connections to file servers, and printers.

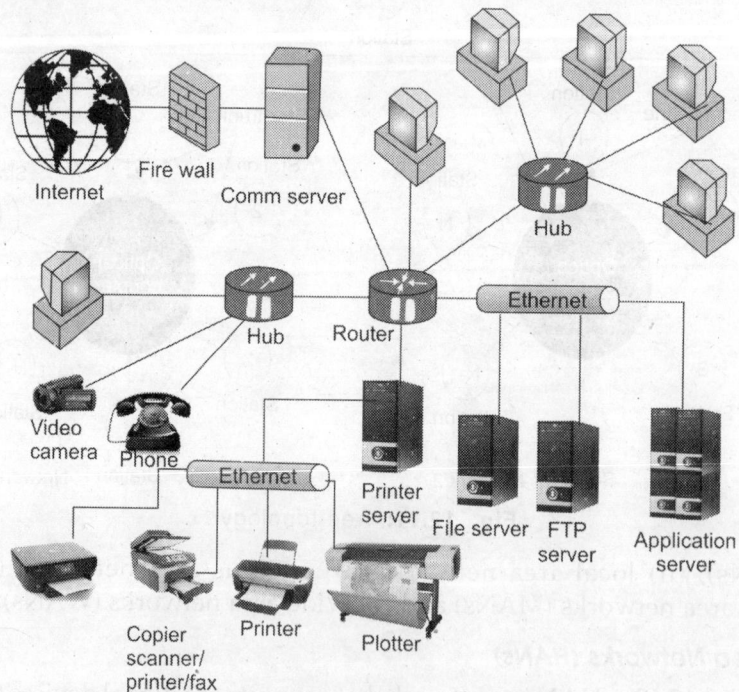

Fig. 12.13: Local-area network (LAN)

(iii) Campus Area Network (CAN)

A CAN is a computer network made up of an interconnection of LANs which are located within a limited geographical area, such as a university or college campus. In the case of a university campus-based CAN, the network is likely to link a variety of campus buildings, including academic departments, the university library, and student halls of residence. A CAN is larger than a LAN, but smaller than a MAN. In addition, CAN stands for corporate-area network.

(iv) Metropolitan Area Networks (MANs)

As shown in Fig. 12.14, a MAN provides interconnections within a city or in a metropolitan area surrounding a city. MANs typically use wireless infrastructure or optical fiber connections to link their sites (nodes).

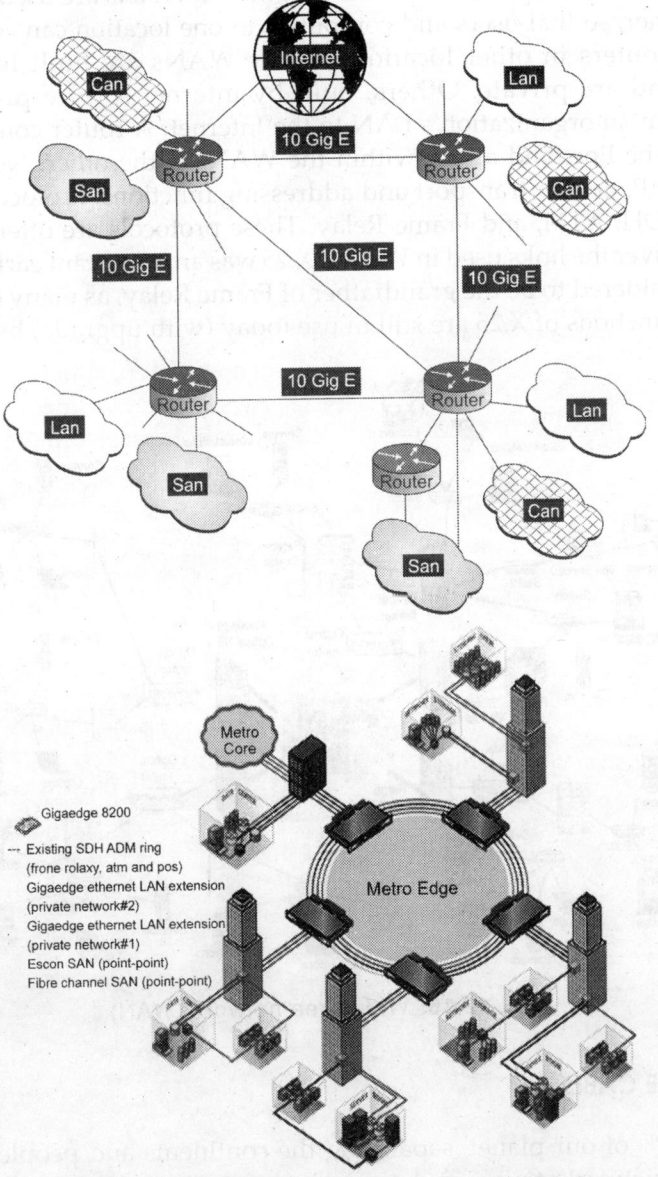

Fig. 12.14: Metropolitan area network (MAN)

For instance, a university or college may have a MAN that joins together many of their LANs, which are situated in a site whose area is less than a square kilometer. Beyond that, the MAN could have several WAN links to other universities or the internet.

Some of the technologies used for this purpose are asynchronous transfer mode (ATM) and fiber distributed data interface (FDDI). These older technologies are in the process of being displaced by ethernet-based MANs (e.g. metro ethernet) in most areas. MAN links between LANs have been built without cables, by using microwave, radio, or infra-red free-space optical communication links.

(v) Wide Area Networks (WANs)

A WAN covers a large geographical area connecting cities, countries and continents (Fig. 12.15). The best example of a WAN is the *internet*. WANs are used to connect LANs or MANs together, so that users and computers in one location can communicate with users and computers in other locations. Many WANs are built for one particular organization and are private. Others, built by internet service providers, provide connections from an organization's LAN to the Internet. A router connects to the LAN on one side of the line, and a hub within the WAN on the other. Network protocols, including TCP/IP, deliver transport and addressing functions. Protocols include Packet over SONET/SDH, ATM, and Frame Relay. These protocols are often used by service providers to deliver the links used in WANs. X.25 was an important early WAN protocol, and is often considered to be the grandfather of Frame Relay, as many of the underlying protocols and functions of X.25 are still in use today (with upgrade) by Frame Relay.

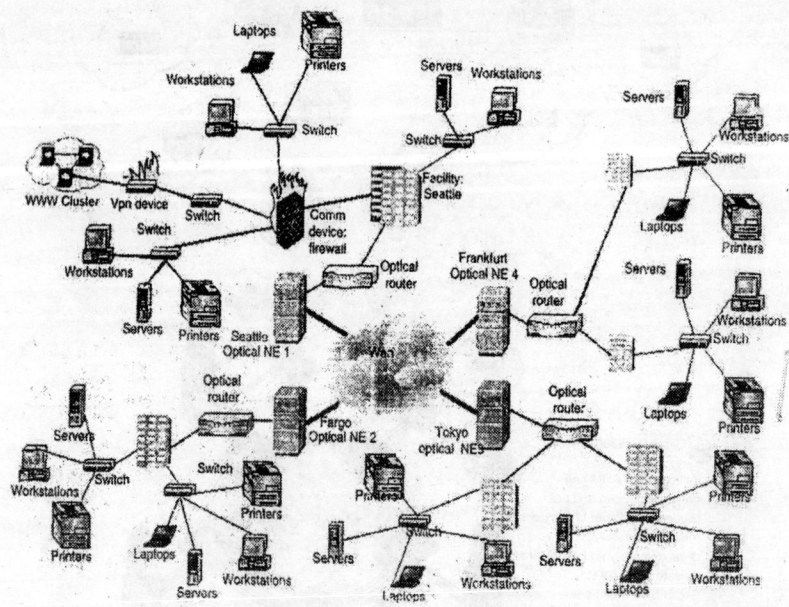

Fig. 12.15: Wide-area network (WAN)

12.6 SUBMARINE CABLES

Oceans cover 70% of our planet, separating the continents and people. People rely on submarine cable networks for voice, data and internet communication. Extreme demands between continents for network reliability and high capacity is achieved by using submarine networks that are reliable and well designed. Submarine cables are sometimes known as *underwater cables*. The world-leading supplier of submarine networks connected every continent from Europe to Japan, the length of the Americas, and across the Pacific. For high capacity, dense wavelength division multiplexer (DWDM) technology is used in tele-communication systems.

12.7 OPEN SYSTEM INTERCONNECTION (OSI)

An OSI is a model that defines a networking framework used for implementing protocols in seven layers of communications. Control is passed from one layer to the next, starting at the application layer in one station, and proceeding through to the optical bottom layer. Control passes over the channel (in optical pulses) to the next station and back up the hierarchy. Figure 12.16(a) shows the layers of OSI and data process, while Fig. 12.16(b) shows the host and media layers located in the OSI model.

(i) Physical (Layer 1)

This layer conveys the bit stream (electrical impulse, light, or radio signal) through the network at the electrical and mechanical level. This is transmission of raw data over a communication medium. It provides the hardware means of sending and receiving data on a carrier which includes defining cables, cards, and physical aspects. SONET/SDH, Fast Ethernet, RS232, and ATM are protocols with physical layer components.

(ii) Data Link (Layer 2)

Layer 2 includes transfer of data frames/packets, addressing, and error connection. At this layer, data packets are encoded and decoded into bits. Layer 2 furnishes transmission protocol knowledge and manage-ment, and handles errors in the physical layer, flow control, and frame synchronization. The society of electrical and electronic engineers formed the 802 committee which was responsible for dividing the data link layer into two sublayers: the media access control (MAC) layer and the 802.2 logical link control (LLC) layer. The MAC sublayer controls how a computer on the network gains access to the data and permission to transmit it. The LLC layer controls frame synchronization, flow control, and error checking.

(iii) Network (Layer 3)

This layer provides switching and routing functions, creating logical paths, known as virtual circuits (e.g. X.25 connection), for transmitting data from node to node. Other functions of this layer are routing and forwarding, as well as addressing, internetworking, error handling, congestion control, and packet sequencing. Routing of data packets across networks provides software interface between the physical and data link layers.

(iv) Transport (Layer 4)

This layer provides transparent transfer of data between end systems, or hosts, and is responsible for end-to-end error recovery and flow control. It ensures complete data transfer.

(v) Session (Layer 5)

This layer establishes, manages, and terminates internode connections between applications and uses standards to move data between the applications. The session layer

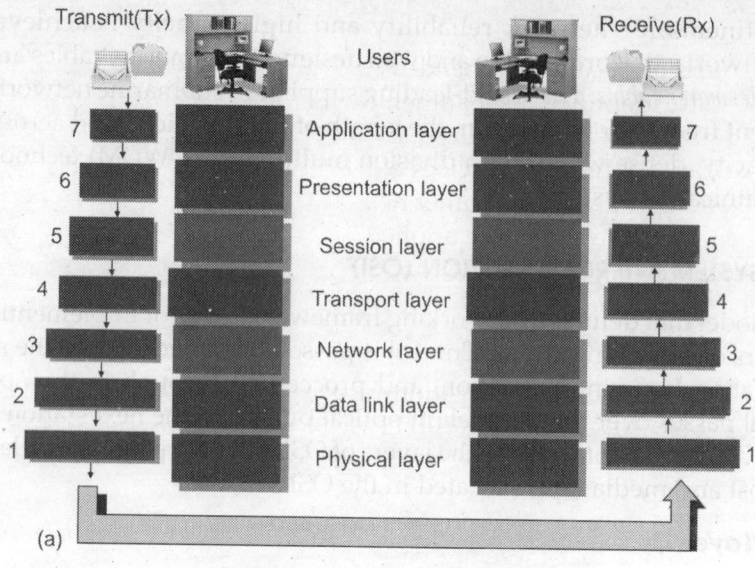

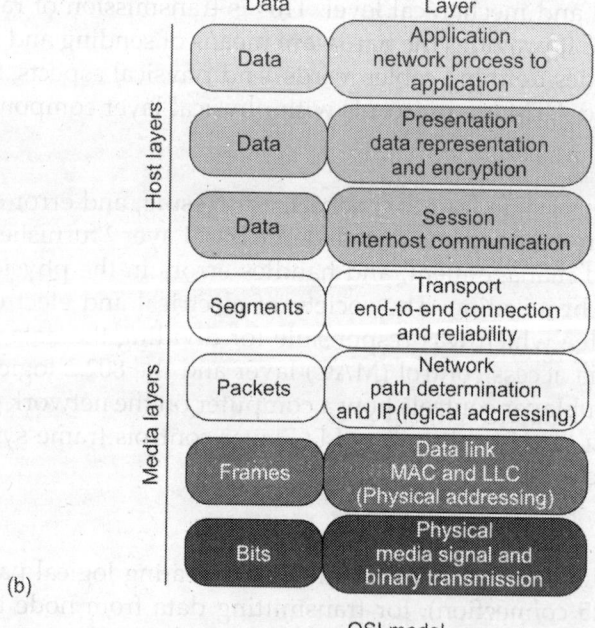

Fig. 12.16: Open system interconnection (OSI) (a) OSI and data process (b) OSI model

sets up, coordinates, and terminates conversations, exchanges, and dialogues between the application at each end. It deals with session and connection coordination.

(vi) Presentation (Layer 6)

This layer involves data formatting, character conversion, security, and coding. It provides independence from differences in data representation (e.g. encryption) by translating from application to network format, and vice versa. The presentation layer transforms data into the form that the application layer can accept. This layer formats and encrypts data to be sent across a network, providing freedom from compatibility problems. It is sometimes called the *syntax layer*.

(vii) Application (Layer 7)

This layer supports application and end-user processes. Communication partners and quality of service are identified, user authentication and privacy are considered, and any constraints on data syntax are recognized. Everything at this layer is application specific. This layer provides application services for file transfers, e-mail, network operating systems, application programs, and other network software services. Telnet and FTP are applications that exist entirely in the application level. Tiered application architectures are part of this layer.

12.8 SYSTEM ARCHITECTURES

One can classify fiber-optic communication systems into three broad categories: (i) *Point-to-point links*, (ii) *Distribution networks* (iii) *Local area networks* (LANs).

12.8.1 Point-to-point Links

We have mentioned in our previous discussion of digital and analog fiber optic communication systems that these are based on essentially point to point links. Their role is to transport information from one point to another as accurately as possible. For short-haul applications (say, less than 10 km), the attenuation, dispersion, and bandwidth of optical fibers are not of major concern. In such cases, optical fibers are used primarily because of their immunity to electromagnetic interference and radio frequency interference. However, for long-haul applications, e.g. transoceanic light wave systems, the low loss, low dispersion, and large bandwidth of optical fibers are important factors. Therefore, whenever the link length exceeds a certain value, it becomes essential to compensate for the fiber loss and/or dispersion. Such a compensation is normally carried out by *optical amplifiers*, dispersion-compensating fibers, or other means.

12.8.2 Distributed Networks

Distributed networks are preferred when data is to be transmitted to a group of subscribers. The transmission distance is relatively short (< 50 km). Examples of distributed networks are – broadcast of video channels over cable TV, telephone and FAX, commonly used topologies for distributed networks are: (i) Hub topology, (ii) Bus topology.

(i) Hub Topology

In hub topology channel distribution takes at hubs or central locations. Hub facilitates the cross-connect switched channels in electrical domain. Fig. 12.17 shows hub topology.

(ii) Linear Bus Topology

Linear bus configuration is similar to *ethernet topology* using co-axial cable. Fig. 12.18 shows linear bus configuration.

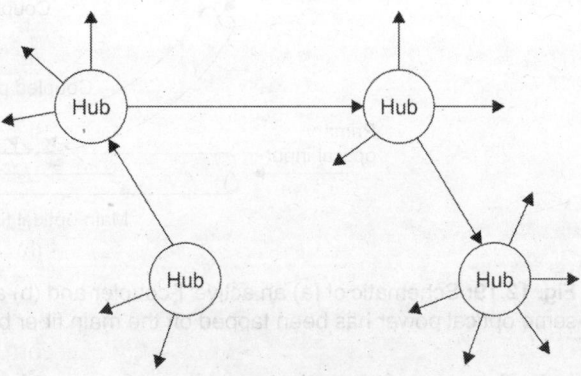

Fig. 12.17: Hub topology

A single fiber cable carries the multichannel optical signal throughout the area of service. Distribution is done by using optical taps which divert a small fraction of optical power to each station.

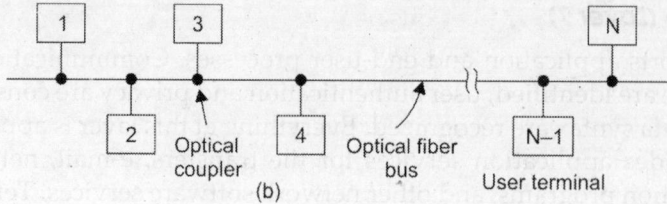

Fig. 12.18: Linear bus topology

A problem with bus topology is that the signal loss increases exponentially with number of taps for stations. This limits the number of stations or subscribers that can be served by a single optical fiber bus.

Use of optical amplifiers can boost the optical power of bus and therefore, large number of stations can be connected to linear bus as long as the effect of fiber dispersion is negligible.

As compared with the coaxial cable bus, an optical fiber based bus network is more difficult to implement. The main problem is the ready availability of bidirectional optical taps which can efficiently couple optical signals into and out of the main optical fiber trunk. Access to an optical data bus is normally achieved by means of either an *active* or a *passive coupler*, as shown in Fig. 12.19.

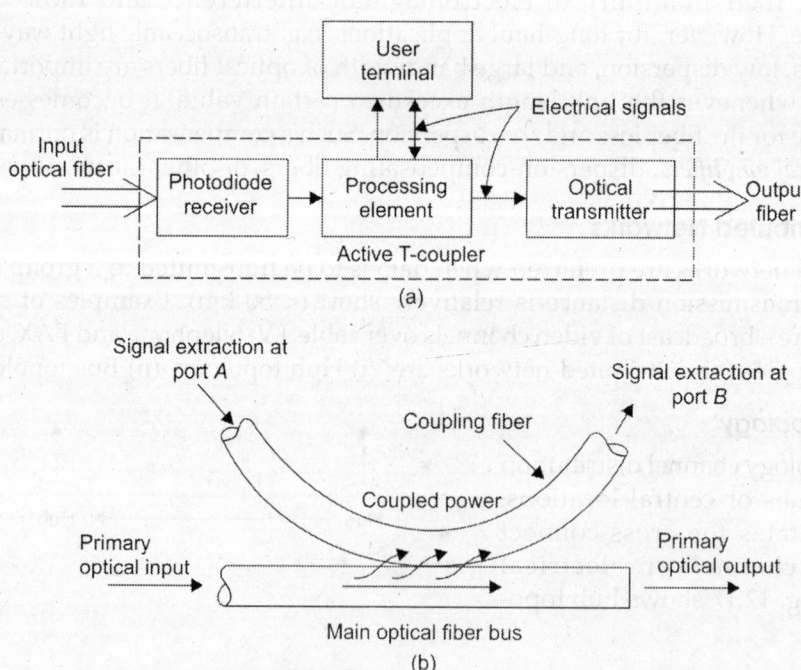

Fig. 12.19: Schematic of (a) an active T-coupler and (b) a passive T-coupler. The tilted arrows show that some optical power has been tapped off the main fiber bus into the receiver at port B

In the case of an active coupler, a front-end photodiode receiver converts the optical signal from the bus into an electrical signal. The processing element removes or copies a part of this signal for transmission to the user terminal and sends the remainder to optical trans-mitter. The latter, in turn, converts the electrical signal back into the optical bit stream, while gets coupled into the output fiber that is connected to the next terminal.

The advantage of such a linear fiber bus network is that every accessing terminal acts as a repeater. Therefore, at least in principle, an active bus can accommodate an unlimited number of terminals. However, the reliability of each repeater is critical to the operation of a *single-fiber bus network*. The failure of any one repeater will stop all the traffic. This problem may be overcome by using some bypass scheme, so that if one repeater fails, the bypass ensures optical continuity from the preceding transmitter to the next terminal.

However, in the case of a *passive coupler* no repeaters are used. At each terminal node a passive coupler is used to remove a fraction of the optical signal from the main fiber bus trunk line or to inject additional optical signals into the trunk. A major problem with this type of coupler is that the *optical signal is not regenerated at each terminal node*. Therefore, optical losses at each tap coupled with the fiber losses between the taps limit the size of the network to a small number of terminals.

(iii) Local Area Networks (LAN)

Many applications of fiber optic communication technology require networks in which a large number of users within local campus are interconnected in such a way that any user can access the network randomly to transmit data to any other user. Such networks are called **local area networks (LANs).**

Fiber optic cables are used in implementation of networks. Since the transmission distance is relatively short (less than 10 km), fiber losses are not at much concern for LAN applications. Use of fiber optic offers large bandwidth.

The commonly used topologies for LANs are: (a) ring topology (b) star topology.

(a) Ring topology

In a ring topology consecutive nodes are connected by point to point links to form a closed ring. Fig. 12.20 shows ring topology.

Each node can transmit and receive the data by using a transmitter receiver pair. A token (predefined bit sequence) is passed around the ring. Each node monitors the bit stream to listen for its own address and to receive the data.

The use of ring topology for fiber optic LANs is known as fiber distributed data interface (FDDI). FDDI operates at 100 Mb/s by using 1.3 µm multimode fibers and LED based transmitters. It can provide backbone services, e.g. interconnection of lower speed LAN.

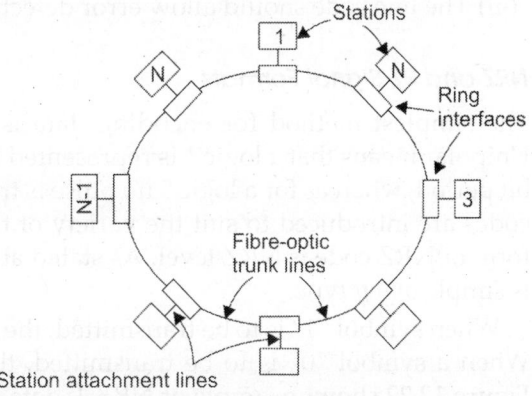

Fig. 12.20: Ring topology

(b) Star topology

In a star topology, all nodes are connected through point-to-point link to central node called a central nod or hub. Figure 12.21 shows star topology.

The central node may be an active or a passive device. In an active central node, all incoming optical

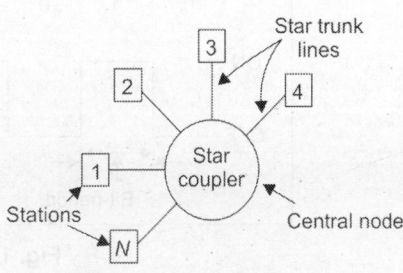

Fig. 12.21: Schematic of star LAN topology

signals are converted into electrical signals through photodiode receivers. The electrical signal is then distributed to drive different node transmitters. One can also perform the switching operation at this node. In a star configuration with a passive central node the distribution takes place in the optical domain, through devices such as directional couplers. In this case, the input from one node is distributed to many output nodes, and hence the power transmitted to each node depends on the number of users.

The network topologies discussed above are also used by metropolitan area network (MANs), which connect users within a city or in a metropolitan area around the city, and wide area networks (WANs), which provide user interconnection over a large geographical area. We have already discussed MANs and WANs in Section 5.

12.9 LINE CODING IN OPTICAL LINKS

Line coding or channel coding is a process of arranging the signal symbols in a specific pattern. Line coding introduces redundancy into the data stream for minimizing errors. There are three types of line codes used in optical fiber communication. These are:

(i) Non-return-to-zero (NRZ)

(ii) Return-to-zero (RZ)

(iii) Phase-Encoded (PE)

The following properties of line codes are desirable:

(i) The line code should contain timing information.

(ii) The line code should be immune to channel noise and interference.

(iii) The line code should allow error detection and correction.

NRZ and RZ Signal Formats

The simplest method for encoding data is the unipolar *nonzero*-to-zero (NRZ) code. Unipolar means that a logic 1 is represented by a voltage or light pulse that fills an entire bit period, whereas for a logic 0 no pulse is transmitted. Although different types of NRZ codes are introduced to suit the variety of transmission requirements, but the simplest form of NRZ code is NRZ level. As stated above, it is a unipolar code, i.e. the waveform is simple *on-off* type.

When symbol "1" is to be transmitted, the signal occupies high level for full bit period. When a symbol "0" is to be transmitted, the signal has zero volts for full bit period. Figure 12.22 shows example of NRZ-L data pattern.

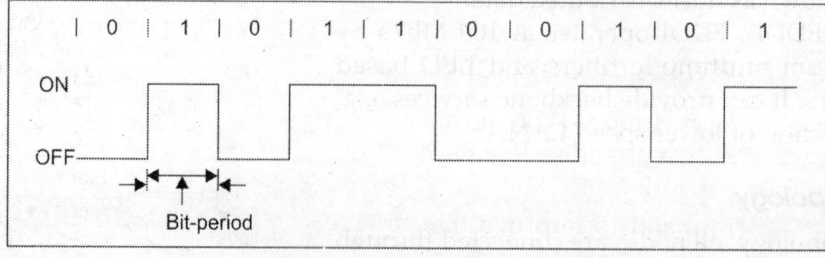

Fig. 12.22: NRZ-level data pattern

Since this process turns the light signal on and off, it is also known as *amplitude shift keying* (ASK) or *on-off keying* (OOK). If 1 and 0 pulses occur with equal probability, and if the amplitude pulse is A, then the average transmitted power for this code is $A^2/2$. In optical system one typically describes a pulse in terms of its optical power level. Thus, in this case the average power for an equal number of 1 and 0 pulses is $P/2$, where P is the peak power in a 1 pulse.

Salient features of NRZ codes

(i) Simple to generate and decode.

(ii) No timing (self-clocking) information.

(iii) No error-monitoring or correcting capabilities.

(iv) NRZ coding needs minimum BW (band width)

We may note that the lack of timing capabilities in an NRZ code can lead to mis-interpretation of the bit stream at the receiver.

If an adequate bandwidth margin exists, the timing problem associated with NRZ encoding can be alleviated with a *return-to-zero* (RZ) code.

In unipolar RZ data pattern a 1-bit is represented by a *half-period* in either *first* or *second half of the bit-period*. A 0-bit is represented by zero volts during the bit period. Fig. 12.23 shows RZ data pattern.

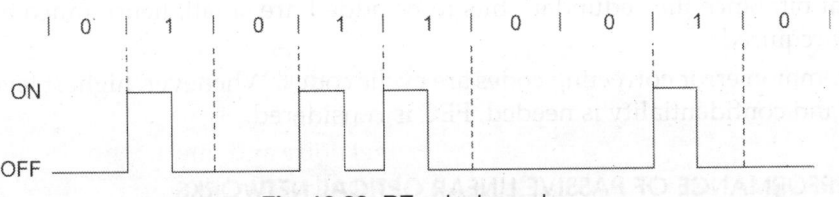

Fig. 12.23: RZ unipolar codes

Salient features of RZ codes

(i) The signal transition during high-bit period provides the timing information.

(ii) Long strings of 0 bits can cause loss of timing synchronization.

(iii) The RZ code has an amplitude transition at the beginning of each bit interval when a binary 1 is transmitted and no transition for a binary 0. Obviously, for a RZ pulse a bit occupies only part of the bit interval and returns to zero in the remainder of the bit interval. No pulse is used for a 0 bit.

(iv) Although the RZ pulse nominally occupies exactly half a bit period in electronic digital transmission systems, in an electronic communication link the RZ pulse might occupy only a fraction of a bit period. A variety of RZ formats are used for links that send data at the rates of 10 Gb/s and higher.

12.10 ERROR CONTROL OR CORRECTION

In any digital transmission system, errors are likely to occur when there is a sufficient signal-to-noise ratio to provide a low bit rate. The acceptance of a certain level of errors depends on the network user.

To control errors and to improve the reliability of communication line, first, it is necessary to be able to detect the errors and then either to correct them or restransmit the information. Error detection methods encode the information stream to have a specific pattern. If the segments in the received data stream violate this pattern, then errors have occurred.

The two basic schemes for error correction are *automatic repeat request* (ARQ) and *forward error correction* (FEC).

In *ARQ scheme*, the information word is coded with adequate redundant bits so as to enable detection of errors at the receiving end. If an error is detected, the receiver asks the sender to retransmit the particular information word.

Each retransmission adds one round trip time to latency. Therefore, ARQ techniques are not used where low latency is desirable. Figure 12.24 shows the scheme of *ARQ error correction scheme*.

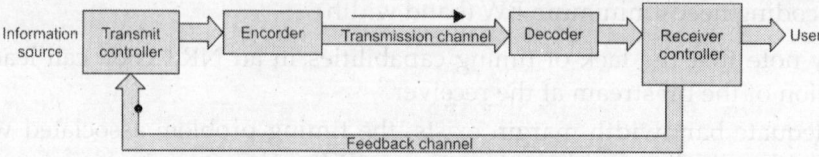

Fig. 12.24: ARQ error correction scheme

Forward Error Correction (FEC) system adds redundant information with the original information to be transmitted. The error or lost data is used reconstructed by using redundant bit. Since the redundant bits to be added are small, hence much additional BW is not required.

Most common error correcting codes are cyclic codes. Whenever, highest level of data integrity and confidentiality is needed, FEC is considered.

12.11 PERFORMANCE OF PASSIVE LINEAR OPTICAL NETWORKS

To evaluate the performance of passive linear networks, consider the fraction of optical power (F_C) lost at a particular interface or component along the transmission path, as shown in Fig. 12.25. The power ratio (A_0) over an optical fiber of length (x) will be:

$$A_0 = \frac{P_{(x)}}{P_{(0)}} = 10^{-\alpha x/10} \qquad (12.27)$$

where $P_{(x)}$ is the power received, $P_{(0)}$ is power transmitted, and a is the fiber attenuation (dB/km).

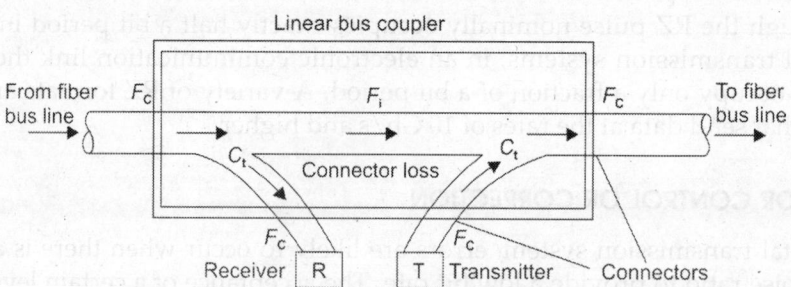

Fig. 12.25: Losses in a passive linear-bus coupler consisting of two cascaded directional couplers

If F_C is lost at each port of the coupler, then the connecting loss (L_C) will be:

$$L_C = 10 \log (1 - F_C) \qquad (12.28)$$

For example, if $F_C = 20\%$, then $L_C = -0.9691$ dB. The optical power gets reduced by the L_C of 1 dB at any connection junction.

The power extracted from the bus is called tap loss (L_{tap}), and is given by:

$$L_{tap} = 10 \log C_T \qquad (12.29)$$

where C_T is the fraction power removed from the bus and delivered to the detected port.

Then, the throughput coupling loss (L_{thru}) is given by:

$$L_{thru} = 10 \log (1 - C_T)^2 = 20 \log (1 - C_T) \qquad (12.30)$$

In addition to the losses L_C and L_{tap}, there is an intrnisic loss (L_i) associated with each bus coupler. If the fraction of power lost in the coupler is F_i, then:

$$L_i = 10 \log (1 - F_i)$$

All losses are measures in decibels (dB).

A linear bus configuration, as shown in Fig. 12.26, consisted of a number of stations (N) separated by a various lengths. For simplicity, assume a constant distance L.

The fiber attenuation between two adjacent stations is given by:

$$L_{fiber} = 10 \log A_0 = \alpha L \qquad (12.31)$$

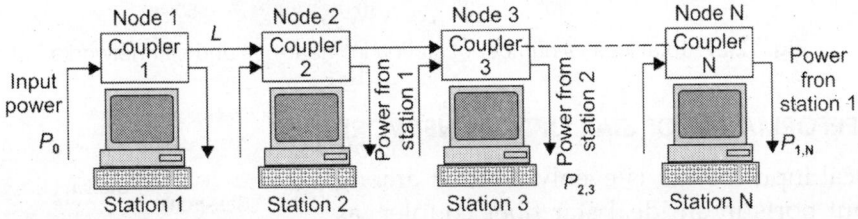

Fig. 12.26: Topology of a simplex linear bus consisting of N uniformly speed stations

12.11.1 Power Budget Calculation

To calculate the power budget of a fiber link consisting of N stations, as shown in Fig. 12.26, the fractional power losses F_c should be examined first.

12.11.2 Nearest-Distance Power Budget

If P_0 is the optical power launched from the optical source at station 1, then the optical power detected $P_{1,2}$ at the station 2 is given by:

$$P_{1,2} = A_0 C_T^2 (1 - F_C)^4 (1 - F_i)^2 P_0 \qquad (12.32)$$

Then the power budget (considering all losses) between stations 1 and 2 is:

$$10 \log \left(\frac{P_0}{P_{1,2}} \right) = \alpha L + 2L_{tap} + 2L_c + 2L_i \qquad (12.33)$$

12.11.3 Largest-Distance Power Budget

If P_0 is the optical power launched from the optical source at station 1, then the optical power detected $P_{1,N}$ at the station N is given by:

$$P_{1,N} = A_0^{N-1} (1 - C_T)^{2(N-2)} C_T^2 (1 - F_c)^{2N} (1 - F_i)^N P_0 \qquad (12.34)$$

Then the power budget (considering all losses) between stations 1 and N is:

$$10 \log \left(\frac{P_0}{P_{1,N}} \right) = N(\alpha L + 2L_c + L_{thru} + L_i) - \alpha L - 2L_{thru} + 2L_{tap} \qquad (12.35)$$
$$= [\text{fibre} + \text{connector} + \text{coupler throughput}$$
$$+ \text{ingress/egress} + \text{coupler intrinsic}] \text{losses}$$

As shown in Fig. 12.27, the losses (in dB) of a linear bus configuration in Fig. 12.26 increase linearly with the number of stations N.

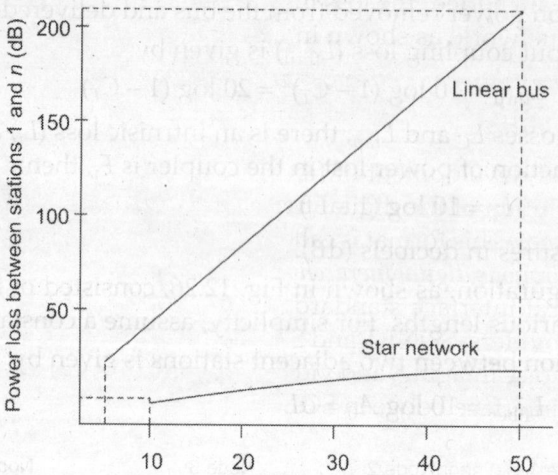

Fig. 12.27: Total loss vs number of station in linear-bus and star networks

12.12 PERFORMANCE OF STAR OPTICAL NETWORKS

The optical input power is evenly divided among the output ports in an ideal star fiber coupler, as shown in Fig. 12.28.

The total optical power loss of the coupler consists of its splitting loss and the excess loss in each path through the star configuration. The splitting loss (L_{split}) among the N stations is given by:

$$L_{split} = 10 \log\left(\frac{1}{N}\right) = 10 \log N \qquad (12.36)$$

The star fibre coupler excess loss (L_{excess}) is defined as the ratio of the single input power (P_{in}) to the total output power ($P_{out,\,i}$) of the N stations ($i = 1....N$).

$$L_{excess} = 10 \log\left(\frac{P_{in}}{\sum\limits_{i=1}^{N} P_{out,\,i}}\right) \qquad (12.37)$$

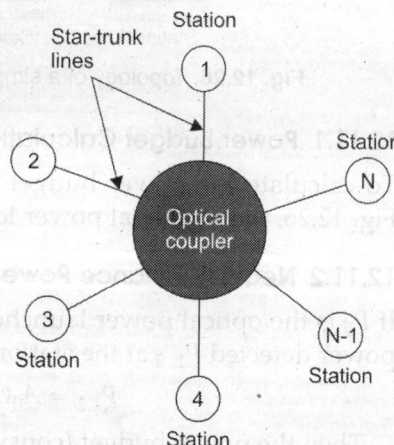

Fig. 12.28: A star coupler

The total loss within the fiber star coupler is given by:

$$\text{Total loss} = L_{split} + L_{excess} \qquad (12.38)$$

The optical power balance equation between any two stations in a star network, include all losses, and is defined as:

$$P_S - P_R = L_{excess} + \alpha(2L) + 2L_c + L_{split}$$

$$= L_{excess} + \alpha(2L) + 2L_c + 10 \log N \qquad (12.39)$$

where P_S is the fiber coupled output power from source in dBm; P_R is the minimum optical power required at the receiver; L_{excess} is the star fiber coupler excess loss; L_{split} is the splitting loss; L_C is the connector loss; L is the distance from the star coupler, assuming all stations at the same distance; and α is the fiber attenuation.

As more stations are added, the loss in a star network increases much slower than the loss in a linear bus network, as shown in Fig. 12.27.

12.13 SONET AND SDH

With the advent and development of fiber optic cables and optical fiber amplifiers, the next important evolution of the digital time-division multiplexing (TDM) scheme was a standard signal format. This format is called *synchronous optical network* (SONET) in North America, and *synchronous digital hierarchy* (SDH) in other parts of the world. SONET and SDH are both optical interface standards that allow inter-networking of services from multiple service providers. SONET and SDH are almost identical standards dedicated to transporting data, voice imaging, and video over optical networks. Figure 12.29 illustrates a standard optical interface between SONET and SDH network.

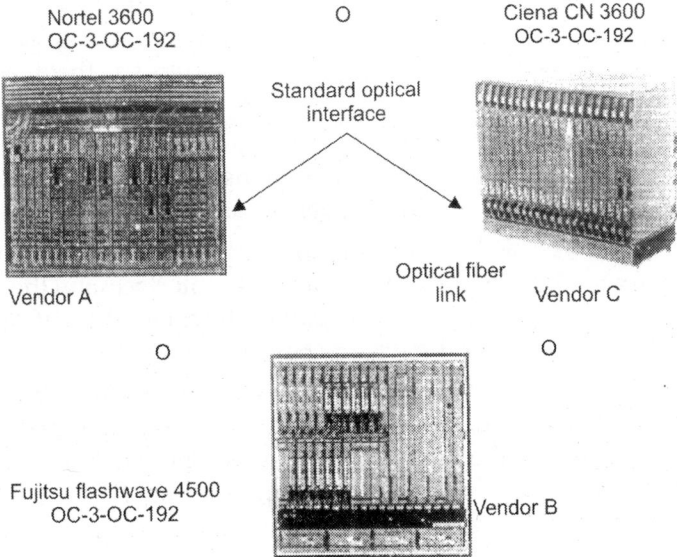

Fig. 12.29: SONET/SDH

SONET was specified primarily by Bellcore (now Telcordia) in the late 1980s. It was submitted to the international standards bodies as a proposed international standard. After some negotiation, SDH emerged as the international standard, of which SONET can be considered a complete subset. The standards define a hierarchy of high-speed transmission rates, which currently range from 51.84 Mb/s (SDH at 155 Mb/s) up to 40 Gb/s.

The standard specifies the physical interfaces, such as the optical wavelengths, pulse shapes, and link budgets. For some of the lower rates in the hierarchy, electrical interfaces are specified as well, including line coding and electrical pulse shapes. The organization of the digital information crossing the interface is defined by specifications for frame structures, payload mappings, and overhead assignments. In addition, special signals are specified which allow communication between the two optical network elements for the purpose of operations, administration, maintenance, and provisioning (OAM&P). The OAM&P of SONET/SDH networks rely on the telecommunication management Network architecture (TMN) as defined by the ITU. SONET/SDH network elements are managed by using translation language 1 (TL1) protocol.

Purposes and Features of SONET/SDH

There are several purposes for implementing SONET or SDH. Some of the purposes and features are as follows:

(i) *Multi-vendor networks*: The primary motivation for developing the SONET standard was to allow the deployment of multi-vendor optical networks. Prior to SONET, fiber optic transport systems could only be deployed in point-to-point configurations, resulting in a lot of unnecessary equipment to terminate the proprietary interfaces. With SONET, a completely optical transport network is envisaged whereby high capacity fibers interconnect network elements that provide access to the transport network and manage the fiber bandwidth (BW).

(ii) *Cost reduction*: It was also assumed that the resulting network would be cheaper due to the consolidation of network functions, elimination of unnecessary functions, and increased competition between vendors. Network providers feel that they no longer have to lock themselves into a single vendor's proprietary (non-standard) solution.

(iii) *Survivability and availability*: With the increasing concern over network reliability and robustness, SONET also provides the ability to build survivable networks; networks that can restore traffic within 50 ms, in the event of fiber cuts and equipment failure.

(iv) *New high-speed services*: The demand for higher bandwidth pipes continues to increase. SONET provided the opportunity to define an interface, and therefore, a network that was capable of carrying a variety of payload types with differing bandwidth requirements, including broadband payloads beyond 50 Mb/s.

(v) *Bandwidth (BW) management*: SONET manages bandwidth by introducing the concept of the payload envelope, into which all pay-loads are mapped as they enter the SONET network. This allows the infrastructure to be concerned only with transporting the envelops, regardless of their contents. A limited number of envelops are defined, with payload capacities ranging from 1.5 Mb/s to 10 GB/s. In addition, different envelops may be combined on the same fiber.

(vi) *Network management/Single-ended operations*: Each rate in the SONET/SDH hierarchy is an integer multiple of a basic rate. For SONET, this basic rate is 51.84 Mb/s; for SDH, it is 155.52 Mb/s. The signal format at each level is created by synchronously multiplexing the basic format. This format is called the synchronous transport signal-level 1 (STS-1) in SONET and the synchronous transport module-level (STM-1) in SDH. Synchronous multiplexing simplifies bandwidth management, allowing access to individual tributaries within the fiber signal without having to completely de-multiplex the fiber signal. The creation of an all-optical network enables management of the network bandwidth using automated techniques. Spare bandwidth on one route may be reallocated to another route, and new connections between end offices can be created quickly when required. SONET includes overhead allocations for a variety of OAM&P functionality. Examples include a data communications channel to allow network elements to be monitored from a central operations system, and integrity checks to allow single-ended performance monitoring of fiber systems and end-to-end networks.

12.14 MULTIPLEXING TERMINOLOGY AND SIGNALING HIERARCHY

12.14.1 Existing Multiplexing Terminology and Digital Signalling Hierarchy

In order to understand the role that the SONET standard plays, it is first necessary to understand what interface standards existed pre-viously. In North America, the standard pre-SONET digital hierarchy consisted mainly of digital signals of several levels. The digital signal-level 1 (DS1), is capable of transmitting and receiving data at a bit rate of 1.544 MB/s (150 MB/s) and the DS3 has the capability of 44.736 Mb/s, as shown in Fig. 12.30. The DS2 really only exists as an inter-mediate step in the DS1–DS3 multiplex. The DS1 is the main interface to digital voice switches and channel banks, whereas the DS3 is the main interface to fiber optic transmission systems. The M13 multiplexer links the two together, and is named for its ability to multiplex DS1 into a DS3. This hierarchy is based on time division multiplexing (TDM).

A similar hierarchy, called electrical signal E, exists in most of the rest of the world. The 2.048 MB/s interface is the key digital switch interface, whereas most pre-standard fiber optic transmission systems carry the 139 MB/s signal. 2.048 MB/s is called E1, and the hierarchy is based on multiples of 4 EIs:

E2 = 4 × E1 = 8 Mb/s
E3 = 4 × E2 = 34 Mb/s
E4 = 4 × E3 = 140 Mb/s
E5 = 4 × E4 = 565 Mb/s

The E3 tributaries are faster than the E2 tributaries, while the E2 tributaries are faster than the E1 tributaries, and so forth. To synchronize with other tributaries, extra bits, called justification bits, are added. These tell the multiplexers which bits are data and which are spare. Multiplexers on the same level of the hierarchy remove the spare bits, and are synchronized with each other at that level only. Multiplexers on one level operate on a different timing from multiplexers on another level. For instance, the timing between primary rate muxes (which combine 30 × 64 Kb/s channels into 2.048 Mb/s E1) will be different from the timing between 8 Mbit muxes (which combine up to 4 × 2 Mb/s into 8 Mb/s.

DSI is sometimes called *transport level-1* (T1). T1 is the optimal rate for accessing low-level devices. It is a type of telephone service capable of transporting the equivalent of 24 conventional telephone lines, using only two pairs of wires. T1 uses two pairs of copper wires (four indi-vidual wires) to carry up to 24 simultaneous conversations (channels) that would normally need one pair of wires each. Each 64 Kbit/s channel can be configured to carry voice or data traffic. Most telephone companies allow customers to buy just some of these individual channels, a service called fractional T1. Typically, fractional T1 lines are sold in increments of 56 Kbps (the extra 8 Kbps per channel are used for administration purposes). One of the most common uses of a T1 line is an Internet T1. This connection is used to provide Internet access to businesses of all sizes, assisting of data at speed of 256 Kbit/s, 512 Kbit/s, 1.544 Mbit/s, and sometimes 3 Mbit/s.

12.14.2 SONET Multiplexing Terminology and Optical Signaling Hierarchy

Table 12.1 presents the optically transmitted SONET signal which is referred to as an optical carrier-level N (OC-N). The OC-N is essentially the optical equivalent of the STS-N; however, the STS-N terminology is used when referring to the SONET format. As shown in Fig. 12.31, the STS-N consists of a synchronous multiplex of N STS-1s. The

Table 12.1: SONET terminology	
Optical carrier-level N (OC-N)	Optical SONET signal at N times the basic rate of 51.84 Mb/s
Synchronous transport signal-level N (STS-N)	The electrical SONET signal, or SONET format, at N times the basic rate of 51.84 Mb/s, consists of a multiplex of N STS-1s
Synchronous transport signal-level 1 (STS-1)	Electrical SONET signal at 51.84 Mb/s, also used to refer to the SONET format
Synchronous payload envelope (SPE)	In SONET, all payloads are mapped into several types: the VT SPEs carry 1.5-Mb/s payloads, the STS-1 SPE carries 50 Mb/s pay-loads, and the STS-Nc SPE carries 150 Mb/s and higher payloads
Virtual tributary group (VTG)	A logical grouping of VTs prior to multiplex-ing into the STS-1 SPE
Virtual tributary (VT)	The unit into the STS-1 SPE can be subdivided to carry payloads that require much less than 51.84 Mb/s

STS-1 has a bit rate of 51.84 MB/s, therefore, the STS-N and OC-N have a bit rate of N times 51.84 Mb/s.

In SONET, all payloads are mapped into synchronous payload envelopes (SPE) at the edge of the SONET network, as shown in Fig. 12.30. The core of the SONET network transports the envelopes. Carried within the STS-1 is the STS-1 SPE, which has a payload capacity of approximately 51.85 Mb/s. N STS-1s may be concatenated to carry an STS-Nc SPE, which has a payload capacity of N × 51.84 Mb/s, as shown in Table 12.1.

12.14.3 SDH Multiplexing Terminology and Optical Signalling Hierarchy

As discussed previously, a European standard, SDH, was developed parallel to the SONET standard. SDH uses a different terminology, as shown in Table 12.2 and Fig. 12.32. Aside from the terminology, most other features of SONET can be extended to SDH.

Table 12.2: SDH terminology	
Synchronous transport module-level N (STM-N)	A synchronous multiplex of N STM-1s
Synchronous transport module-level 1 (STM-1)	The basic rate (155.52 Mb/s) and format of the SDH hierarchy; also refers to the optical signal
Administrative unit group (AUG)	A logical grouping of like AUs
Administrative unit (AU)	Similar to the TU; consists of a higher order VC and a payload pointer
Tributary unit group (TUG)	A logical grouping of like TUs
Tributary unit (TU)	A logical element consisting of a lower order VC and a payload pointer
Virtual container (VC)	The SDH structure into which all payloads are mapped

12.15 SONET AND SDH TRANSMISSION RATES

Although the SONET multiplexing scheme would in theory allow any multiple of STS-1s, only certain rates are defined as standard trans-mission rates. Physical (photonic) interfaces are specified for these rates. Table 12.3 lists the most commonly supported SONET rates with their SDH equivalents.

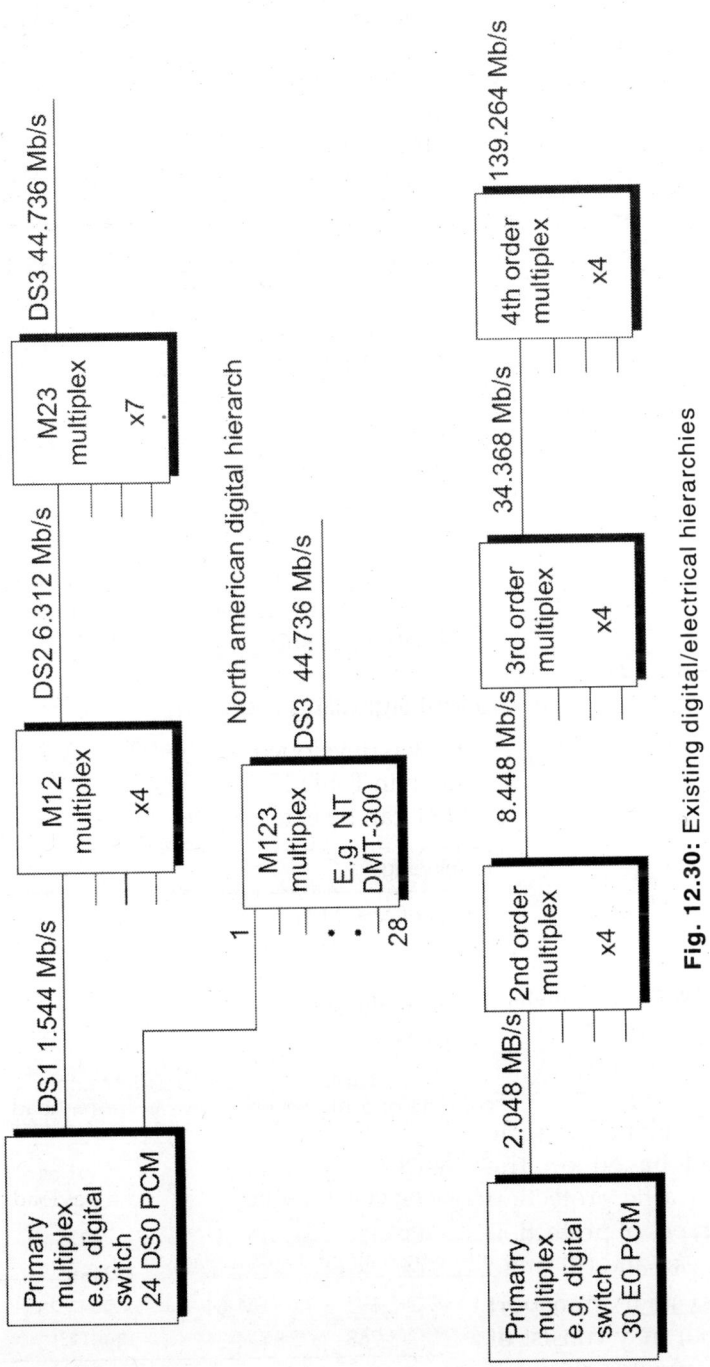

Fig. 12.30: Existing digital/electrical hierarchies

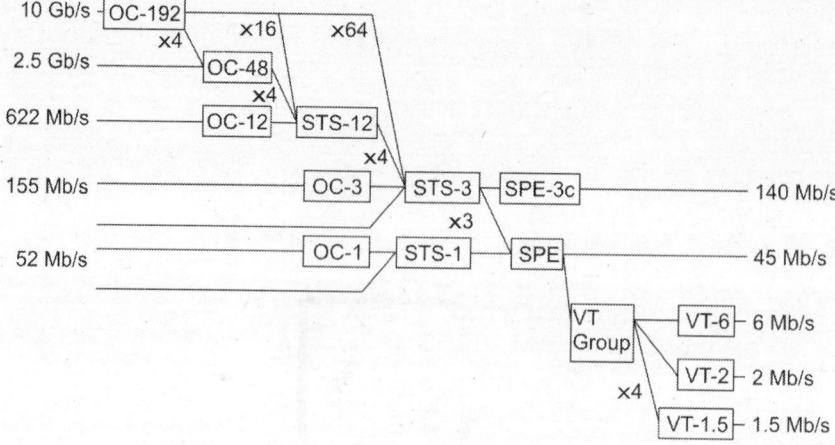

Fig. 12.31: SONET multiplexing hierarchies

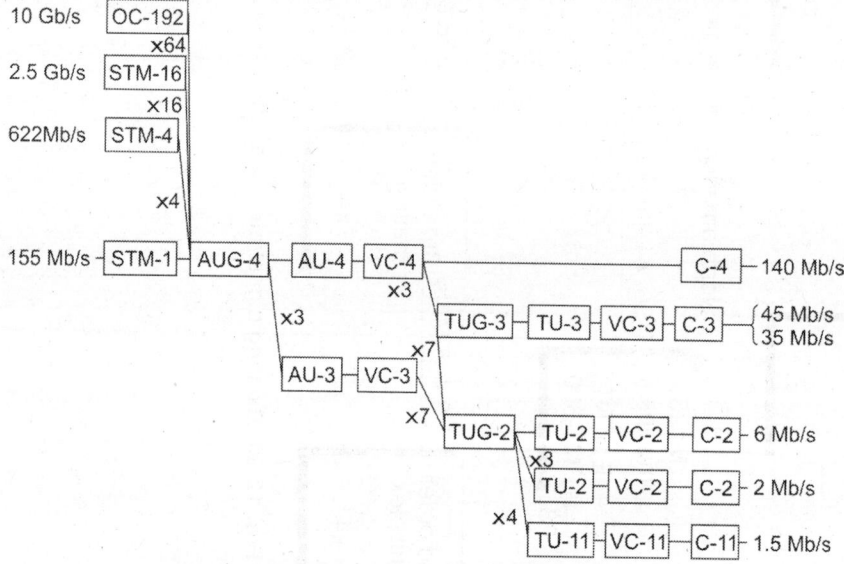

Fig. 12.32: SDH multiplexing hierarchies

12.16 SONET SYSTEMS

SONET network elements are combined to create systems that are classified based on the mechanism used to provide traffic protection and survivability. Two main types of protection provides in SONET are: (i) linear, and (ii) ring.

(i) *Linear systems*: Linear systems transport traffic along a single route that may consist of one or more working fibers. A one plus one (1 + 1) system has one protection fiber and one working fiber, as shown in Fig. 12.33. The traffic is permanently bridged onto both fibers, so that the receiving end can autonomously choose the fiber that is operating better.

Table 12.3: SONET/SDH rates

SONET	SDH	Rate (Mb/s)
OC-1	STM-0	51.84
OC-3	STM-1	155.52
OC-12	STM-4	622.08
OC-48	STM-16	2488.32
OC-192	STM-64	9953.28
OC-768	STM-256	39813.12

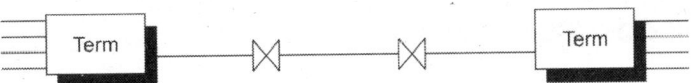

Fig. 12.33: Linear SONET system

(ii) *Ring system*: Ring systems transport traffic around a ring, allowing traffic to be added and dropped anywhere along the ring, as shown in Fig. 12.34. Spare capacity is allocated around the ring so that when a failure occurs at any one point, the affected traffic can be restored using the spare capacity. In a unidirectional path switched ring (UPSR), traffic added to the ring is bridged onto both directions, such that the drop node can autonomously select the better path. In a bidirectional line switched ring (BLSR), the traffic affected by a failure at any point on the ring is rerouted the other way around the ring. A protocol operating around the ring coordinates this action.

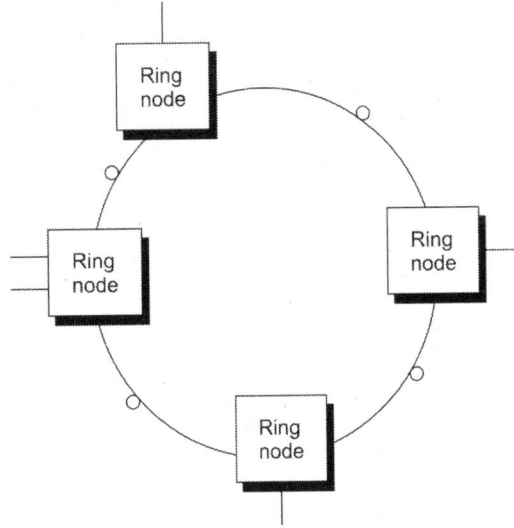

Fig. 12.34: SONET ring system

12.17 METRO AND LONG-HAUL OPTICAL NETWORKS

Metro optical networks can be thought of as consisting of *core networks* and *access* networks, as shown in Fig. 12.35. SONET/SDH metro and long-haul core networks are typically configured as point to point or ring connections that are spaced in tens or thousands of kilometers apart. The metro optical network consists of optical links between the end users and central office (CO). The ring configuration shown in Fig. 12.35 contains three or four modes.

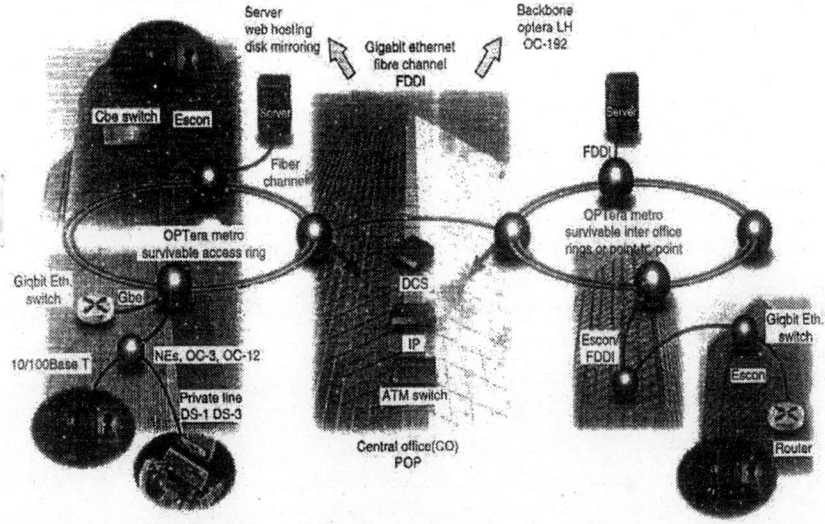

Fig. 12.35: Metro and long-haul optical networks

12.18 NETWORK CONFIGURATION

12.18.1 Automatic Protection Switching (APS)

Ring automatic protection switching (APS) provides an increased level of survivability for SONET/SDH networks by allowing as much traffic as possible to be restored, even in the event of a cable cut or node failure.

12.18.2 SONET/SDH Ring Configurations

SONET/SDH networks has two main types of ring configurations: (i) a UPSR, and (ii) a bidirectional line switched ring (BLSR).

A UPSR consists of two fibers on each span transmitting in opposite directions between adjacent nodes.

There are two types of *bidirectional line switched ring* (BLSR): (a) *two-fiber BLSR*, and (b) *four fiber BLSR*. In the two-fiber BLSR, there are two fibers transmitting in opposite directions between adjacent nodes. In the four-fiber BLSR, there are four fibers between adjacent nodes, with two fibers transmitting in one direction and other two fibers in the opposite direction. The four-fiber BLSR supports more traffic.

For a UPSR network, the selection of data path is made on a per path basic using the path layer integrity information. Thus, the ring is called path switched. In the case of a BLSR network, the decision to switch to the other path is made by the nodes adjacent to the failure using line layer integrity information. Thus, the ring is called *line switched*.

(a) Two-Fiber UPSR Configuration

Figure 12.36 shows a two-fiber UPSR network. By convention, in a unidirectional ring, the normal working traffic travels clockwise around the ring on the primary (working) path, e.g. the connection from the node 1 to node 3 uses links 1 and 2, whereas the traffic from the node 3 to node 1 traverses links 3 and 4. In a UPSR ring, the counterclockwise path is used as an alternate route for protection against link or node failures. This protection path (links 5–8) is indicated by dashed lines. The signal from a transmitting node is dual-fed into both the primary and protection fibers. This establishes a designated

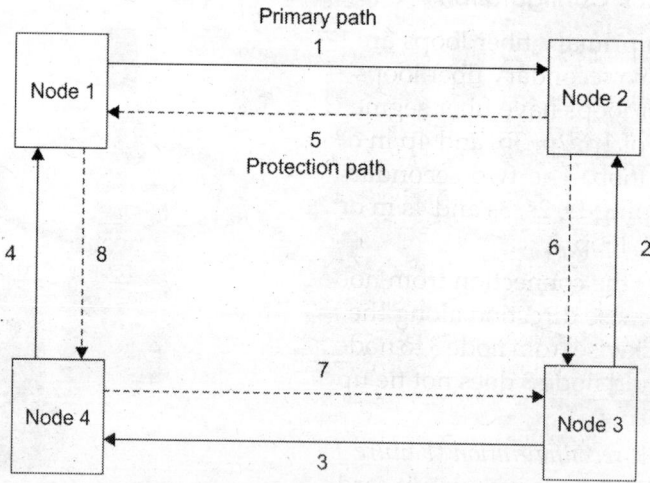

Fig. 12.36: A 2-fiber unidirectional ring with a counter-rotating protection path

protection path on which traffic flow counterclockwise, namely, from node 1 to node 3 via protection links 8 and 7.

Two-fiber UPSR configuration (Traffic flow): In Fig. 12.37, two signals from node 1 arrive at their destination at node 3 from opposite directions. The receiver at node 3 selects the signal from the primary (working) path. However, if the quality of received signal on the primary path is poor, then it selects the signal from the protection path. In case of any failure in the node 2 equipment or on the primary path 2, node 3 will switch to the protection path via node 4 to receive the signal from node 1.

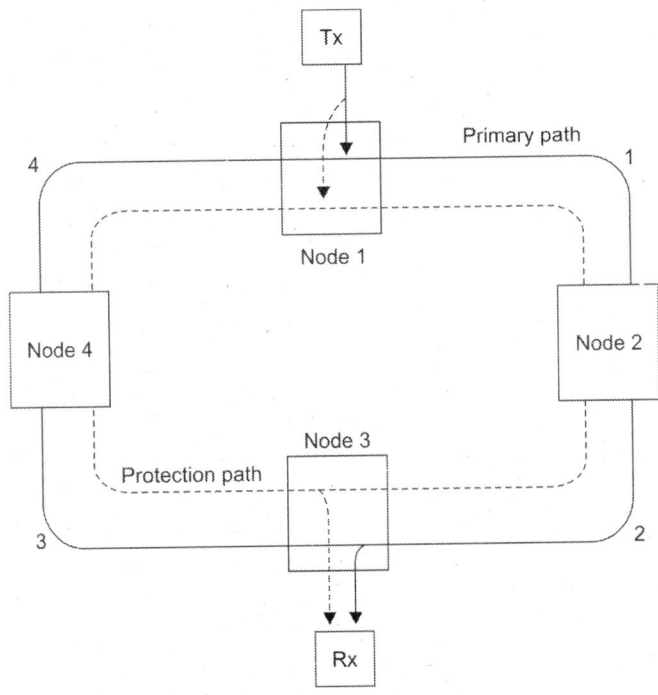

Fig. 12.37: Flow of primary and protection traffic from node 1 to node 3

(b) Four-Fiber BLSR Configuration

In Fig. 12.38, two primary fiber loops are used for normal bidirectional communication while the other two secondary fiber loops are standby links for protection purposes. The two primary fiber loops have fiber segments labeled 1p through 8p, which provides for an arrange-ment of 1p, 2p, 3p, and 4p in one primary loop, and 8p, 7p, 6p, and 5p in the second primary loop. The two secondary fiber loops have fiber segments labeled 1s through 8s, grouping 1s, 2s, 3s and 4s in one secondary loop, and 8s, 7s, 6s, and 5s in the second secondary loop.

Let us consider the connection from node 3 to node 1. The traffic from node 1 to node 3 flows in a clockwise direction along the links 1p and 2p. The traffic in the return path flows counterclockwise from node 3 to node 1, along links 6p and 5p. Thus, the information between node 1 and node 3 does not tie up any of the primary channel bandwidth in the other half of the ring.

Four-fiber BLSR reconfiguration (Failure 1): Consider the scenario shown in Fig. 12.39, where a transmitter or receiver circuit card used on the primary ring gails (in either node 3 or 4, in this case). In this case the affected nodes detect a lose-of signal (LOS) condition

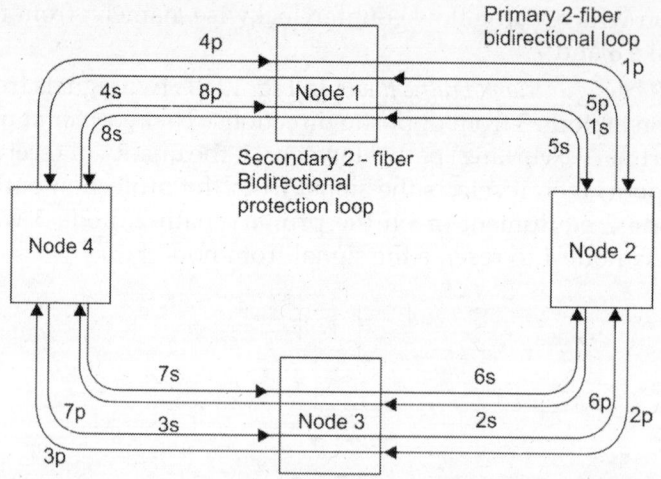

Fig. 12.38: Four-fiber bidirectional line switched ring network

and switch both primary fibers, connecting them to the secondary protection pair. The protection between these nodes (3 or 4, in this case) now becomes part of the primary bidirectional loop.

Four-fiber BLSR reconfiguration (Failure 2): The exact same reconfiguration scenario as in failure 1 will occur when the primary fiber connecting two nodes (in this case, nodes 3 and 4 breaks, as in Fig. 12.39. Note that in any case, the other links remain unaffected.

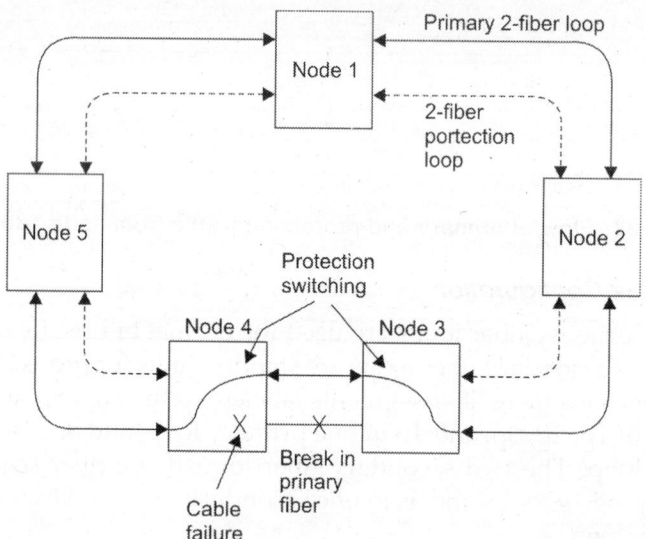

Fig. 12.39: Reconfiguration under transceiver card or line failure

Four-fiber BLSR reconfiguration (Failure 3): In Fig. 12.40, consider the scenario where an entire node fails (in this case node 3), or both the primary and the protection fibers in a given span are severed, which could happen if they are in the same cable between 2 nodes (in this case nodes 3 and 4). In this scenario, the nodes on either side of the failed internal span will internally switch the primary path connection from their receivers and transmitters to the protection fibers, in order to loop traffic back to the previous node.

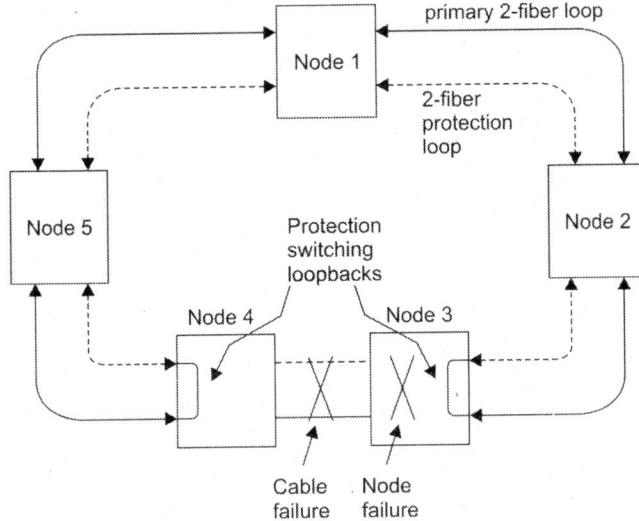

Fig. 12.40: Reconfiguration under node or fiber cable failure

(c) Generic SONET Network

SONET/SDH architecture allows the interconnections and interoper-ability of a variety of network configuration, as shown in Fig. 12.41. One can build point-to-point links, linear chains, UPSR, bidirectional link switched rings (BLSR), and interconnected rings. Each of the individual configuration has their own failure-recovery and protection mechanism, and SONET/SDH network management procedures.

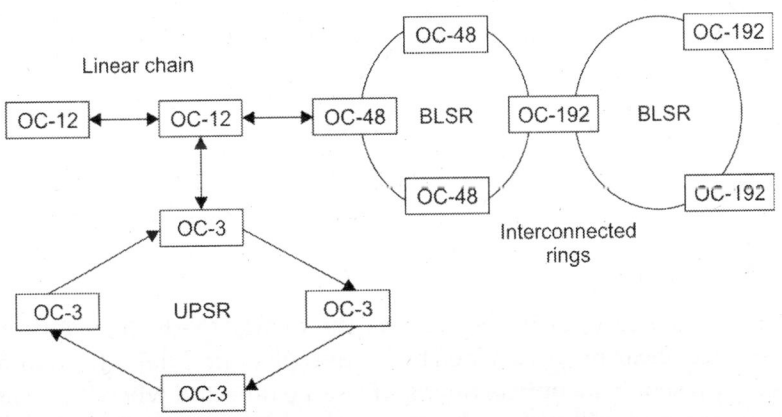

Fig. 12.41: Generic configuration of large SONET network consisting of various types of interconnected systems

(d) SONET ADM

One of the important features in SONET/SDH architecture is the add/drop multiplexer (ADM), as shown in Fig. 12.42. Various pieces of equipment are fully synchronized, and a byte-oriented multiplexer is used to add and drop sub-channels within an OC-N stream. Here, various OC-12s and OC-3s are multiplexed into OC-48 stream. Upon entering an ADM, these multiplexed sub-channels can be individually dropped by the ADM, and others can be added.

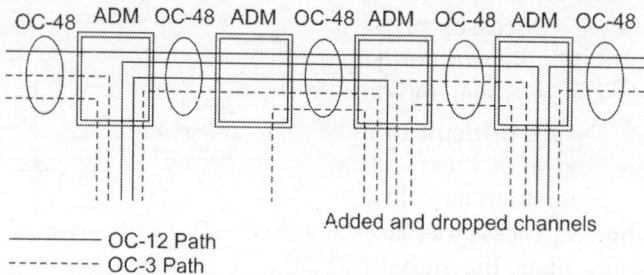

OC-12 Path
OC-3 Path

Fig. 12.42: Functional concept of an add/drop multiplexer (ADM) for SONET applications

(e) Dense WDM Deployment

SONET/SDH architecture can also be implemented with wavelengths. Figure 13.43 shows an example of dense wavelength division multiplexer (DWDM) deployment on an OC-192 trunk ring for n wavelengths (e.g. one could have $n = 16$). The different wavelength outputs from each OC-192 transmitter are first passed through the variable attenuator (VA) to equalize the out powers. These are then fed into a wavelength multiplexer, possibly amplified by a post optical amplifier, and sent out over the transmission fiber. Additional optical amplifiers might be located at intermediate points or at the receiver end.

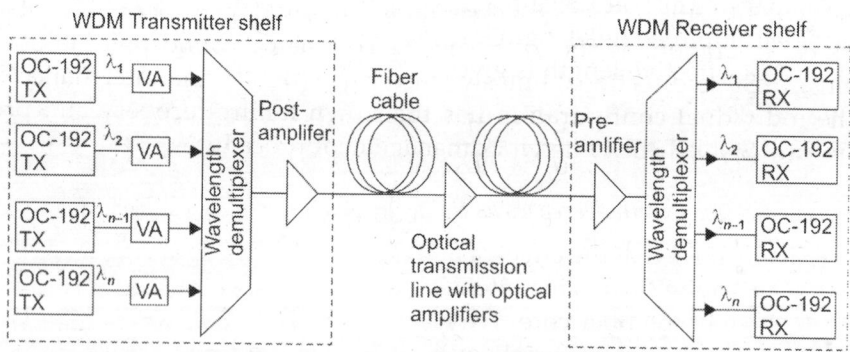

Fig. 12.43: DWD deployment of n wavelengths in an OC-192 trunk ring

12.19 NONLINEAR EFFECTS

Nonlinear phenomena in optical fiber affects the overall performance of optical fiber networks. These nonlinearities arise when high-strength optical fields from different signal wavelengths are present in an optical fiber at the same time and when these fields interact with acoustic waves and molecular vibrations.

The nonlinearities arise above a certain optical power threshold, and hence, the effect becomes negligible, once the signal has become sufficiently attenuated after travelling a distance along the fiber. Some important nonlinear effects are as follows:

(i) Group velocity dispersion (GVD)
(ii) Non-uniform gain for different wavelength
(iii) Polarization mode dispersion (PMD)
(iv) Reflection from splices and connectors
(v) Non-linear inelastic scattering processes
(vi) Variation in reflactive index in optical fiber.

The major nonlinear processes physically affect system performance. These non-linearities are stimulated *Raman scattering*, stimulated *Brillouin scattering*, *self-phase modulation, cross-phase modulation,* and *four wave mixing* (FWM).

Non-linear processes are difficult to model because they depend on various factors, such as the *transmission length, cross sectional area of the fiber, transmitted power level,* etc. The problem can be understood as follows. If the signal power is assumed to be constant, the effect of a non-linear process increases with distance. However, we know that due to attenuation within the fiber, the signal power does not remain constant but decreases with distance. As a consequence, the non-linear process diminishes in magnitude. In practice, therefore, it is fairly reasonable to assume that the power is constant over a certain effective fiber length, which is less than the actual length of the fiber, and also take into account the exponential decay in power due to absorption. The effective length L_{eff} is given by:

$$L_{eff} = \frac{1}{P_0} \int_0^L P(z)\,dz = \frac{1}{P_0} \int_0^L P_0 e^{-\alpha z}\,dz = \frac{1 - e^{-\alpha L}}{\alpha} \tag{12.40}$$

where L is the actual length of the fiber, α is the attenuation coefficient, P_0 is the power at the input end of the fiber, and $P(z)$ is the power at a distance z. For large values of L, $L_{eff} \to 1/\alpha$. Thus, if we take α to be typically around 0.22 dB km^{-1} (which is equivalent to a coefficient of 0.0507 km^{-1}) at 1.55 µm, $L_{eff} \approx 20$ km. If the link incorporates optical amplifiers and the total amplified link length is L_A and the total span length of the fiber between amplifiers is L, the effective length is given approximately by the following relation:

$$L_{eff} = \frac{1 - e^{-\alpha L}}{\alpha} = \frac{L}{L_A} \tag{12.41}$$

Thus, the *total effective length decreases as the amplifier span increases.*

It has been said above that the effect of non-linear processes increases in light intensity transmitted through the fiber. This intensity, however, is inversely proportional to the cross-sectional area of the fiber core. We have seen earlier that for a single-mode fiber, this power is not distributed uniformly over the entire cross-sectional area of the core. In practice, therefore, it is convenient to use an effective cross-sectional area A_{eff}. If the mode field radius is w, $A_{eff} \approx \pi w^2$. Typical effective areas for a conventional single-mode fiber (CSF), dispersion-shifted fiber (DSF), and dispersion-compensating fiber (DCF) are 80 µm^2, 50 µm^2, and 20 µm^2, respectively.

12.19.1 Stimulated Raman Scattering

Stimulated Raman scattering (SRS) is the result of the inelastic scattering of a light wave (propagating through a silica-based optical fiber) by silica molecules. When a photon energy $E_1 = h\nu_1$ (where the symbols have their usual meaning) interacts with a silica moleule, some of its energy, depending on the vibrational frequency of the molecule, is absorbed by the latter and the photon is scattered. As the original photon has lost some energy, the energy of the scattered photon becomes less, say, $E_2 = h\nu_2$. This change in the frequency of the interacting photon ν_1 and ν_2 ($\nu_1 > \nu_2$) is called *Stoke's shift*. Since the light wave propagating through the fiber is a source of interacting photons, it is normally called a *pump wave*. This process generates scattered light at a wavelength longer than the pump wave ($\lambda_2 > \lambda_1$ as $\nu_2 < \nu_1$). If two or more signals at different wavelengths are simultaneously injected into the fiber, SRS can cause power to be transferred from the

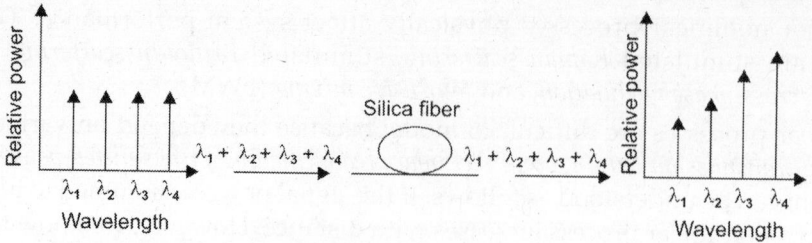

Fig. 12.44: The effect of stimulated Raman scattering (SRS)

lower wavelength signals to the higher wavelength signals. This effect is shown in Fig. 12.44. As a consequence, SRS can severely affect the performance of a multi-channel fiber-optic communication system by transferring energy from shorter wavelength channels to other longer wavelength channels. This effect occurs in both the directions.

The effect of SRS can be estimated following Buck (1995) as follows. Consider a WDM system with N equally spaced channels, 0, 1, 2, ... $(N-1)$, with a channel spacing of $\Delta\lambda_2$. With the assumptions that the same power is transmitted in all the channels, the Raman gain increases linearly, and that there is no interaction between other channels, the fraction of power coupled from channel 0 to channel i is given approximately by:

$$F(i) = g_R \frac{i\Delta\lambda_s}{\Delta\lambda_c} \frac{P_0 L_{\text{eff}}}{2 A_{\text{eff}}}$$

where g_R is the *peak Raman gain coefficient*, $\Delta\lambda_c$ is the *total channel spacing*, and the other symbols have their usual meaning. Therefore, the fraction of power coupled from channel 0 to all the other channels is given by:

$$F = \sum_{i=1}^{N-1} F(i) = \frac{g_R \Delta\lambda_s}{\Delta\lambda_c} \frac{P_0 L_{\text{eff}}}{2 A_{\text{eff}}} \frac{N(N-1)}{2} \qquad (12.42)$$

The power penalty for channel 0 is then $-10 \log_{10}(1-F)$. Thus, in order to keep this penalty below 0.5 dB, the fraction F should be less than 0.1.

SRS is not a serious problem in systems with small number of channels. However, it can create severe problems in WDM systems with large numbers of wavelength channels. In order to alleviate the effect of SRS, (i) the channels should be spaced as closely as possible, and (ii) the transmitted power level in each channel should be kept below the threshold (in other words, the distance between the optical amplifiers in the link should be reduced).

12.19.2 Stimulated Brillioun Scattering (SBS)

Stimulated Brillioun scattering (SBS) may be viewed as the scattering of a pump wave by an acoustic wave (generated by the oscillating electric field of the pump wave). This process creates a *Stokes' wave* of lower frequency, which travels in the backward direction. The Stokes' wave experiences gain at the expense of the depletion of the signal power of the forward propagating signal (i.e. the pump wave). The frequency shift due to SBS is called the Brillioun shift and is given by:

$$\nu_B = 2n V_A/\lambda_p \qquad (12.43)$$

where n is the mode index of the fiber, V_A is the velocity of the acoustic wave, and λ_p is the wavelength of the pump wave. If we take typical values of $n = 1.46$ for the silica fiber, $V_A = 5960$ m·s^{-1}, and $\lambda_p = 1.55$ μm, then $\nu_B = 11.22$ GHz. This interaction occurs over a very narrow line width of $\Delta v_B = 20$ MHz at $\lambda_p = 1.55$ µm. There are two important features of SBS: (i) it does not cause any interaction between different wave-lengths, as long as the wavelength spacing is much greater than 20 MHz, and (ii) its effect can create significant distortion within a single channel, especially when the amplitude of the scattered wave is comparable with the signal power.

A simple criterion for determining the impact of SBS is to consider the SBS threshold P_{th}, which is defined as the signal power at which the backscattered power equals the fiber input power. It is given by the following approximate expression:

$$P_{th} = \frac{21bA_{eff}}{g_B L_{eff}} \left[1 + \frac{\Delta v_{source}}{\Delta v_B} \right] \tag{12.44}$$

where Δv_{source} is the line width of the source, g_B is the *Brillioun gain*, and the value of b lies between 1 and 2, depending on the relative polarizations of the pump and Stokes' waves. Thus P_{th} increases with increase in the source line width.

12.19.3 Four-Wave Mixing

In a WDM system, if three waves with angular frequencies ω_i, ω_j, and ω_k co-propagate inside a *silica fiber* simultaneously, then the non-linear susceptibility of the silica fiber generates new waves at angular frequencies $\omega_i \pm \omega_j \pm \omega_k$. This phenomenon is known as *four-wave mixing* because three waves at frequencies, ω_i, ω_j, ω_k combine to produce a fourth wave at a frequency $\omega_i \pm \omega_j \pm \omega_k$. In principle, several frequencies corresponding to the combinations of plus and minus signs are possible. However, most of them do not build up due to the lack of a *phase-matching condition*. The frequency combinations of the $\omega_i + \omega_j + \omega_k$ (with $i, j \neq k$) are often troublesome for WDM systems, as they can become phase matched when the wavelength channels are closely spaced or are spaced near the dispersion zero of the fiber. Such frequency combinations can be defined as:

$$\omega_{ijk} = \omega_i + \omega_j + \omega_k \ (i, j \neq k) \tag{12.45}$$

For N wavelength channels co-propagating through the fiber, the number of generated frequencies is given by

$$M - \frac{N^2}{2}(N-1) \tag{12.46}$$

If the wavelength channels are equally spaced, the new waves overlap the original injected frequencies. This causes severe crosstalk and the depletion of the original signal waves, thus degrading the system performance.

In general, the penalty due to four-wave mixing can be reduced by (i) making the channel spacing unequal, (ii) increasing the channel spacing, and (iii) using a non-zero dispersion-shifted fiber instead of a dispersion-shifted fiber.

12.19.4 Self- and Cross-Phase Modulation

Self-phase modulation (SPM) arises because the refractive index n of the fiber depends on the intensity I (which is equivalent to the power per unit effective area of the fiber). The relation is as follows:

$$n = n_0 + n_2 I = n_0 + n_2 \left(\frac{P}{A_{eff}} \right) \tag{12.47}$$

where n_0 is the ordinary refractive index of the fiber core and n_2 is the non-linear index coefficient, P is the optical power and A_{eff} is the effective area of the fiber. Depending on the dopant, the value of n_2 for a silica fiber varies from 2.2 to 3.4×10^{-8} µm^2/W.

To understand the effect of SPM, let us consider a *Gaussian pulse propagating* through a fiber with a non-linear index of refraction given by Eq. (12.47). The pulse shape is shown in Fig. 12.45. The time axis is normalized to the time parameter t_0, the pulse half-width measured at $1/e$ intensity point. As is evident from the figure, the intensity of the pulse first rises from zero to a maximum and then falls to zero again. Because the refractive index of the fiber is dependent on intensity, it will also vary with time. This variation of n with t will give rise to a temporally varying phase change in exactly the same fashion. Thus, different parts of the pulse undergo different phase shifts, which gives rise to what is known as *frequency chirping*; that is, the rising edge of the pulse shifts towards higher frequencies (red shift) and the

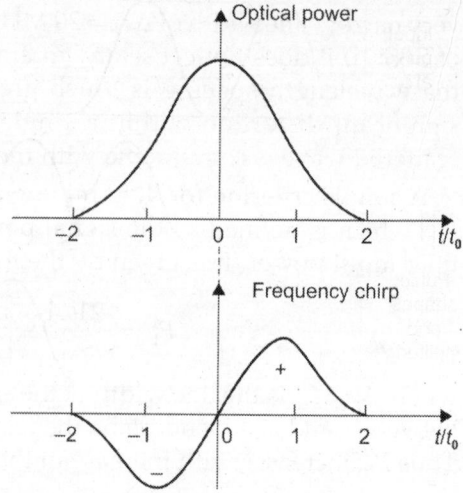

Fig. 12.45: SPM-induced frequency chirp for a Gaussian pulse

trailing edge shifts towards lower frequencies (blue shift). This pulse chirping, in turn, enhances the group velocity dispersion (GVD) induced pulse broadening. Moreover, this effect is proportional to the transmitted signal power, and hence, SPM effects are more pronounced in long-haul systems where the transmitted powers are high.

In WDM systems, the intensity-dependent refractive index of the fiber gives rise to another kind of non-linear effect, called cross-phase modulation (CPM). In this process, the power fluctuation in one channel produces phase fluctuations in other co-propagating channels. The effect can be significant if the system is using dispersion-shifted fibers and is operating above 10 Gb/s. The effect may be reduced by employing non-zero dispersion single-mode fibers.

12.20 DISPERSION

The pulse gets distorted as it travels along the fiber lengths. Pulse spreading in fiber is referred as *dispersion*. Dispersion is caused by difference in the propagation times of light rays that takes different paths during the propagation. The light pulses travelling down the fiber encounter dispersion effect because of this the pulse spreads out in time domain. Dispersion limits the information bandwidth. The distortion effects can be analyzed by studying the group velocity in guided mode.

12.20.1 Information Capacity Determination

Dispersion and attenuation of pulse travelling along the fiber is shown in Fig. 12.46(a).

Figure 12.46(a) also shows, after travelling some distance, pulse starts broadening and overlap with the neighbouring pulses. At certain distance, the pulses are not even distinguishable and error will occur at receiver. Therefore, the information capacity is specified by bandwidth-distance product (MHz·km). For step index bandwidth distance produce is 20 MHz·km and for graded index, it is 2.5 GHz·km.

12.20.2 Group Delay

Consider a fiber cable carrying optical signal equally with various modes and each mode contains all the spectral components in the wavelength band. All the spectral components

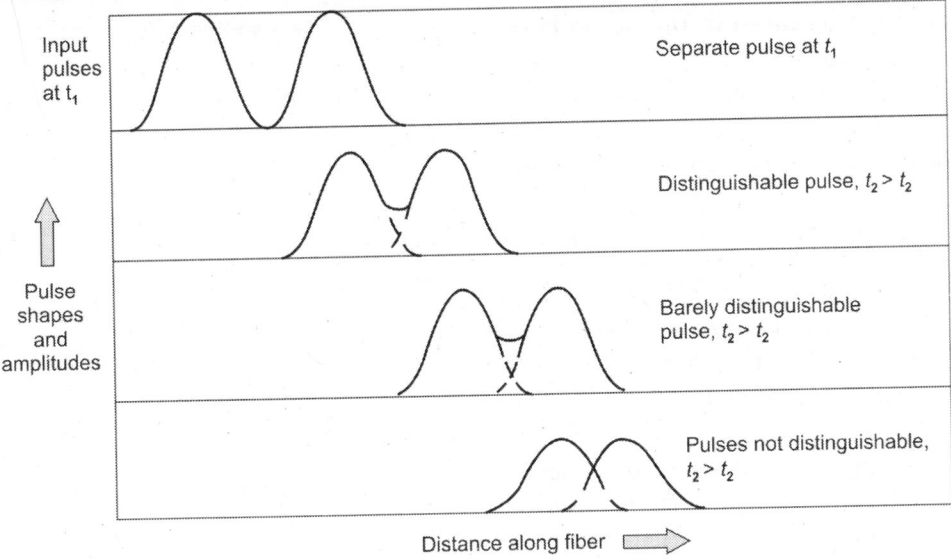

Fig. 12.46(a): Dispersion and attenuation in fiber

travel independently and they observe different **time delay** and **group delay** in the direction of propagation. The velocity at which the energy in a pulse travels along the fiber is known as a **group velocity**. Group velocity is given by:

$$V_g = \frac{\partial \omega}{\partial \beta} \tag{12.48}$$

Thus different frequency components in a signal will travel at different group velocities and so will arrive at their destination at different times, for digital modulation of carrier, this results in dispersion of pulse, which affects the maximum rate of modulation. Let the difference in propagation times for two side bands is $\delta\tau$.

$$\delta\tau = \frac{d\tau}{d\lambda} \times \delta\lambda \tag{12.48a}$$

where $\delta\lambda$ = Wavelength difference between upper and lower sideband (spectral width)

$\dfrac{\delta\tau}{d\lambda}$ = Dispersion coefficient (D)

Then,
$$D = \frac{1}{L} \cdot \frac{d\tau}{d\lambda} \quad \text{where, } L \text{ is length of fiber}$$

$$D = \frac{d}{d\lambda}\left(\frac{1}{V_g}\right) \quad \text{As } \tau = \frac{1}{V_g} \text{ and considering unit length } L = 1$$

$$\frac{1}{V_g} = \frac{d\beta}{d\omega}$$

$$\frac{1}{V_g} = \frac{d\lambda}{d\omega} \times \frac{d\beta}{d\lambda}$$

$$\frac{1}{V_g} = \frac{-\lambda^2}{2\pi c} \times \frac{d\beta}{d\lambda}$$

$$\therefore \qquad D = \frac{d}{d\lambda}\left(\frac{-\lambda^2}{2\pi c} \cdot \frac{d\beta}{d\lambda}\right) \tag{12.48b}$$

Dispersion is measured in picoseconds per nanometer per kilometer.

Material dispersion (MD) occurs because the index of refraction (n) varies as a function of the optical wavelength (λ). As a consequence, since the group velocity (V_g) of a mode is a function of n, the various spectral component of a given mode will travel at different speeds, depending on λ. Obviously, *material dispersion* is, therefore, an *intermodal* dispersion effect, and is of particular importance for single-mode waveguides for LED system (since an LED has a broader output spectrum than a laser diode).

Material dispersion is also called as **chromatic dispersion**. Material dispersion exists due to change in index of refraction for different wavelengths. A light ray contains components of various wavelengths centered at wavelength λ_0. The time delay is different for different wavelength components. This results in time dispersion of pulse at the receiving end of fiber. Figure 12.46(b) shows index of refraction as a function of optical wavelength.

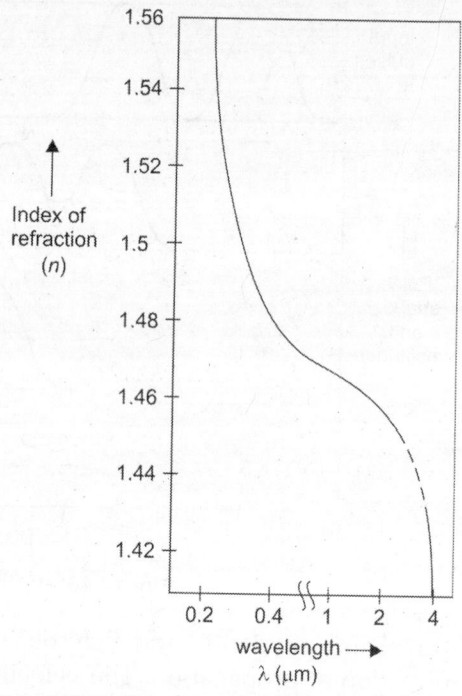

Fig. 12.46(b): Index of refraction (n) as a function of wavelength (λ)

The material dispersion for unit length ($L = 1$) is given by:

$$D_{mat} = \frac{-\lambda}{c} \times \frac{d^2 n}{d\lambda^2} \qquad (12.48c)$$

where c = Light velocity
λ = Centre wavelength

$\dfrac{d^2 n}{d\lambda^2}$ = Second derivative of index of refraction with respect to wavelength

Negative sign shows that the upperside band signal (lowest wavelength) arrives before the power side band (highest wavelength).

A plot of material dispersion and wavelength is shown in Fig. 12.46(c).

The unit of dispersion is: ps/nm·km.

For single mode fibers, *waveguide dispersion* (WD) is of importance and can be of the same order of magnitude as material dispersion. The pulse spread σ_{wg} occurring over a distribution of wavelengths σ_λ is obtained from the derivative of the group delay (τ_{wg}) with respect to λ:

$$\sigma_{wg} \approx \left| \frac{d\tau_{wg}}{d\lambda} \right| \sigma_\lambda = L \, | D_{wg}(\lambda) | \, \sigma_\lambda \qquad (12.48d)$$

where $D_{wg}(\lambda)$ is the *waveguide dispersion*.

(i) Waveguide dispersion is caused by the difference in the index of refraction between the core and cladding, resulting in a 'drag' effect between the core and cladding portions of the power.

(ii) Waveguide dispersion is significant only in fibers carrying fewer than 5–10 modes.

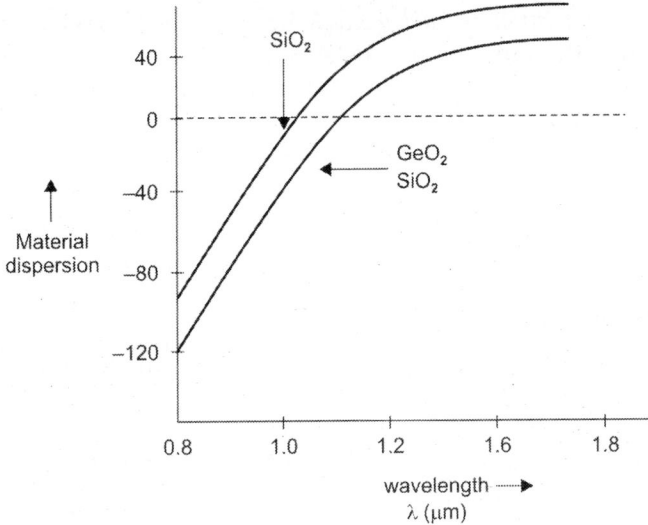

Fig. 12.46(c): Material dispersion as a function of λ

Since multimode optical fibers carry hundreds of modes, they will not have observable waveguide dispersion.

(iii) The group delay (τ_{wg}) arising due to waveguide dispersion.

$$\tau_{wg} = \frac{L}{c}\left[n_2 + n_2\,\Delta\,\frac{d\,(kb)}{dk} \right] \tag{12.48e}$$

where, b = Normalized propagation constant

$k = 2\pi/\lambda$ (group velocity)

Normalized frequency υ:

$$\nu = k\,a\left(n_1^2 - n_2^2\right)^2 = k\,a\,n_2\,\sqrt{2\Delta}\ \text{ (For small }\Delta\text{)}$$

$\therefore$
$$\tau_{wg} = \frac{L}{c}\left[n_2 + n_2\,\Delta\,\frac{d(V_b)}{dV} \right] \tag{12.48f}$$

The second term $\dfrac{d(V_b)}{dV}$ is waveguide dispersion and is mode dependent term.

Polarization-mode dispersion (PMD): The effects of fiber birefringence on the polarization states of an optical signal are another source of pulse broadening. This is particularly critical for high-rate long haul trans-mission links (e.g. 10 and 40 Gb/s over tens of kilometers), i.e.:

(i) Different frequency component of a pulse acquires different polariation states (such as linear polarization and circular polari-zation). This results in pulse broadening is known as *polarization-mode dispersion* (PMD).

(ii) PMD is the limiting factor for optical communication system at high data rates. The effects of PMD must be compensated.

A varying birefringence along its length will cause each polarization mode to travel at a slightly different velocity. The resulting difference in propagation times $\Delta\tau_{\text{PMD}}$ between the two orthogonal polarization modes will result in pulse spreading. This is *polarization-mode* dispersion (PMD). If the group velocities of two orthogonal polarization modes are

V_{gx} and V_{gy}, then the *differential time delay* $\Delta\tau_{PMD}$ between the two polarization components during propagation of the pulse over a distance L is:

$$\Delta\tau_{PMD} = \left| \frac{L}{V_{gx}} - \frac{L}{V_{gy}} \right| \tag{12.49}$$

We may note that, in contrast to chromatic dispersion, which is relatively stable phenomenon along a fiber, PMD varies randomly along a fiber. Typical values of D_{PMD} range from 0.05 to 1.0 ps/$\sqrt{km}$.

12.20.3 Modal Dispersion

As only a certain number of modes can propagate down the fiber, each of these modes carries the modulation signal and, each one is incident on the boundary at a different angle, they will each have their own individual propagation times. The net effect is spreading of pulse, this form of dispersion is called *modal dispersion*.

Modal dispersion takes place in multimode fibers. It is moderately present in graded index fibers and almost eliminated in single mode step index fiber.

Modal dispersion is given by:

$$\Delta t_{modal} = \frac{n_1 Z}{c} \left(\frac{\Delta}{1-\Delta} \right) \tag{12.49a}$$

where Δt_{modal} = Dispersion,

n_1 = Core refractive index,

Z = Total fiber length,

c = Velocity of light in air, and

Δ = Fractional refractive index.

Putting $\Delta = \dfrac{NA^2}{2n_1^2}$ in above equation:

$$Dt_{modal} = \frac{(NA)^2 Z}{2n_1 c} \tag{12.49b}$$

The modal dispersion Δt_{modal} describes the optical pulse spreading due to modal effects. Optical pulse width can be converted to electrical rise time through the relationship.

$$t_{r\,mod} = 0.44\,(\Delta t_{modal}) \tag{12.49c}$$

12.20.4 Signal Distortion in Single Mode Fibers

The pulse spreading σ_{wg} over range of wavelengths can be obtained from derivative of group delay with respect to λ:

$$\sigma_{wg} = \left| \frac{d\tau_{wg}}{d\lambda} \right| \sigma_\lambda = L \,| D_{wg}\,(\lambda)|\sigma_\lambda = \frac{V}{\lambda} \left| \frac{d\tau_{wg}}{d\lambda} \right| \sigma_\lambda$$

$$= \frac{n_2 L\Delta\sigma_\lambda}{c\lambda} \left[V \frac{d^2\,(Vb)}{dv^2} \right] \tag{12.49d}$$

where $$D_{wg}\,(\lambda) = \frac{-n_2\Delta}{c\lambda} V \left[\frac{d^2\,(Vb)}{dV^2} \right] \tag{12.49e}$$

This is the equation for waveguide dispersion for unit length.

12.20.5 Higher Order Dispersion

Higher order dispersive effective effects are governed by dispersion slope S.

$$S = \frac{dD}{d\lambda}$$

where, D is total dispersion.

Also,

$$S = \left(\frac{2\pi c}{\lambda^2}\right)^2 \beta_3 + \left(\frac{4\pi c}{\lambda^3}\right)\beta_2$$

where, β_2 and β_3 is second and third order dispersion parameter.

Dispersion slope S plays an important role in designing WDM system.

12.20.6 Dispersion Induced Limitations

The extent of pulse broadening depends on the width and the shape of input pulses. The pulse broadening is studied with the help of wave equation.

12.20.7 Basic Propagation Equation

The basic propagation equation which governs pulse evolution in a single mode fiber is given by:

$$\frac{\partial A}{\partial z} + \beta_1 \frac{\partial A}{\partial t} + \frac{i\beta_2}{2} \cdot \frac{\partial^2 A}{\partial t^2} - \frac{\beta_3}{6} \frac{\partial^3 A}{\partial t^3} = 0$$

where, β_1, β_2 and β_3 are different dispersion parameters.

12.20.8 Chirped Gaussian Pulses

A pulse is said to be **chirped** if its carrier frequency changes with time.

For a Gaussian spectrum having spectral width σ_ω, the pulse broadening factor is given by:

$$\frac{\sigma^2}{\sigma_0^2} = \left(1 + \frac{C\beta_2 L}{2\sigma_0^2}\right)^2 + (1 + V_\omega^2)\left(\frac{\beta_2 L}{2\sigma_0^2}\right)^2 + (1 + C + V_\omega^2)^2 \left(\frac{\beta_3 L}{4\sqrt{2}\,\sigma_0^3}\right)^2$$

where, $V_\omega = 2\sigma_\omega \sigma_0$

12.20.9 Limitations of Bit Rate

The limiting bit rate is given by:

$$4B\sigma \leq 1$$

The condition related to bit-rate distance product (BL) and dispersion (D) is given by

$$BL\,|D|\,\sigma_\lambda \leq \frac{1}{4}$$

$$BL\,|S|\,\sigma_\lambda^2 \leq \frac{1}{\sqrt{8}}$$

where, S is dispersion slope.

Limiting bit rate for a single-mode fibers as a function of fiber length for $\sigma_\lambda = 0, 1$ and 5 nm is shown in Fig. 12.46(d).

12.20.10 Dispersion Management

Erbium-doped fiber amplifiers have opened a new era of optical transmission technology, allowing one to use WDM or DWDM with compact as well as economical approaches.

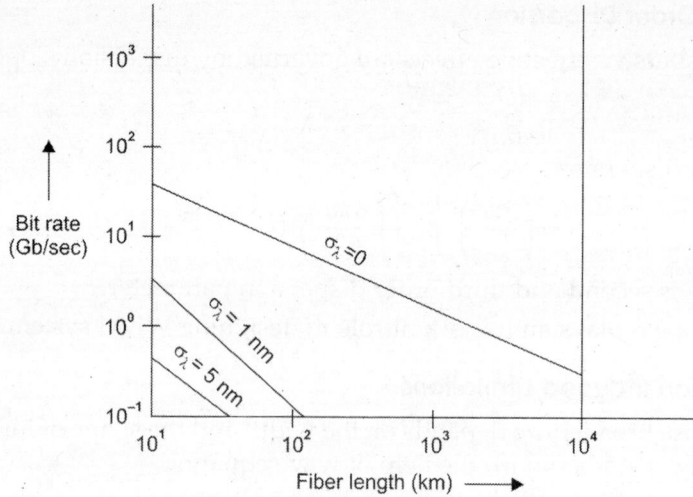

Fig. 12.46(d): Dependence of bit rate on fiber length

However, the price that has to be paid for this success is the *combat* with the accumulated impact of the dispersive or non-linear effects of the transmission fiber, which grows with the transmission distance. Dispersion management techniques have been developed to solve this problem. The basic idea is to use two types of fibers with opposite signs of dispersion to produce a sawtooth pattern of the dispersion map as shown in Fig. 12.47. The relation for perfect dispersion compensation is:

$$D_1 L_1 + D_2 L_2 = 0 \qquad (12.50)$$

where D_1 and D_2 are the dispersion of the two types of fibers and L_1 and L_2 are their respective lengths. A special type of fiber called the *dispersion-compensating fiber* (DCF) has been developed for this purpose. Typically, a small length of the DCF may be placed just before the optical amplifier. If the transmission fiber has a low positive dispersion, the DCF should have a large negative dispersion. With this approach, the total cumulative dispersion is made zero (or small) so that the dispersion-induced penalties are negligible, but the dispersion is non-zero everywhere along the link so that the penalties due to non-linear effects are also reduced.

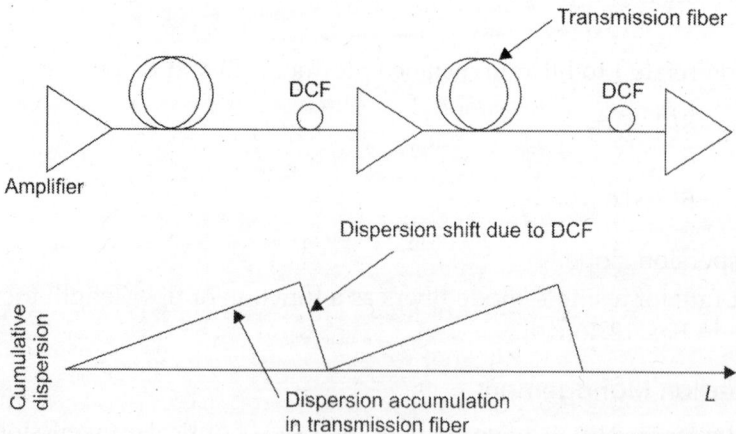

Fig. 12.47: Dispersion management using dispersion compensating fiber (DCF)

12.21 SOLITONS

12.21.1 Nonlinear Effects, i.e. Nonlinear Optical Susceptibility

Soliton refers to special kinds of waves that propagate undistorted over long distances and remain unaffected after collision with each other. Solitons exist due to *nonlinearity* and *dispersion*. Optical responses including nonlinear effects are described as:

$$P(t) = \epsilon_0 \left\{ \chi^{(1)} E(t) + \chi^{(2)} E^{(2)}(t) + \chi^{(3)} E^3(t) + \ldots \right\} \tag{12.50a}$$

$$\equiv P^{(1)}(t) + P^{(2)}(t) + P^{(3)}(t) + \ldots$$

where, we have expressed polarization $P(t)$ as a power series in the field strength $E(t)$. The quantities $\chi^{(1)}$, $\chi^{(2)}$, $\chi^{(3)}$ are known as suscepti-bilities; $\chi^{(1)}$ is a linear susceptibility and $\chi^{(2)}$ and $\chi^{(3)}$ are known as the second order- and third-order nonlinear susceptibilities respectively.

For a typical solid-state system $\chi^{(1)}$ is of the order of unity whereas $\chi^{(2)}$ is the order of $1/E_{at}$ and $\chi^{(3)}$ of the order of $1/E_{at}^2$, where $E_{at} = e/(4\pi \epsilon_0 a_0^2)$ is the characteristic atomic electric field strength and $a_0 = 4\pi\epsilon_0 h^2/me^2$ is the Bohr radius of the hydrogen atom. Explicitly.

$$\chi^{(2)} \simeq 1.94 \times 10^{-12} \text{ m/V}$$

$$\chi^{(3)} \simeq 3.78 \times 10^{-24} \text{ m}^2/V^2$$

Formal expression for the third-order susceptibility is:

$$P_1(\omega_0 + \omega_n + \omega_m) = \epsilon_0 \, D \sum_{jkl} \chi_{ijkl}^{(3)} (\omega_0 + \omega_n + \omega_m, \omega_0, \omega_n, \omega_m) \times E_j(\omega_0) \, E_k(\omega_n) \, E_1(\omega_n)$$

where i, j, k, l refer to the Cartesian components of the fields and the degeneracy factor D represents the number of distinct permutations of the frequencies ω_0, ω_m, ω_m.

$\chi^{(j)}$ ($j = 1, 2, \ldots$) is the j-th order susceptibility. The linear susceptibility $\chi^{(1)}$ contributes to the linear refractive index n_0 (real and imaginary parts; the imaginary part being responsible for attenuation). The second-order susceptibility $\chi^{(2)}$ is responsible for the second harmonic generation. For SiO_2, the second-order nonlinear effect is negligible since SiO_2 has the inversion symmetry. Therefore, optical fibers normally do not show the second-order nonlinear effects.

The third-order susceptibility $\chi^{(3)}$ is responsible for the *lowest order nonlinear effects in optical fibers*. Generally, it manifests itself as the change in the refractive index with optical power or as a scattering pheno-menon. It is linked with the *optical Kerr effect*, four-wave mixing, third-harmonic generation, stimulated Raman scattering etc.

Assuming linear polarization of propagating light and neglecting tensorial character of $\chi_{ijkl}^{(3)}$, one finds the following relation for the nonlinear polarization:

$$P^{NL}(\omega) = 3 \epsilon_0 \, \chi^{(3)} (\omega = \omega - \omega - \omega) | E(\omega) |^2 \, E(\omega)$$

Total polarization, which consists of linear and nonlinear parts, is written as:

$$P(\omega) = \epsilon_0 \, \chi^{(1)} E(\omega) + 3 \epsilon_0 \, \chi^3 | E(\omega) |^2 \, E(\omega) = \epsilon_0 \, \chi_{\text{eff}} E(\omega)$$

The effective susceptibility is field dependent as:

$$\chi_{\text{eff}} = \chi^{(1)} + 3\chi^{(3)} | E(\omega) |^2$$

and it is linked to refractive index as:

$$n = 1 + \chi^{(3)} \equiv n_0 + n_2 I \tag{12.50b}$$

Here I denotes the time-averaged intensity of the optical field. The main features of nonlinear effects are as follows:

12.21.2 Main Nonlinear Effects

Kerr effect: Kerr in 1875 found that a transparent liquid becomes *doubly* refracting (birefringent) when placed in a strong electric field. Generally, Kerr effect described situations where refractive index depends on electric field as:

$$n\,(\omega, |\, E^2\, |) = n_0\,(\omega) + n_2\,(\omega)\, E\,|^2$$

Here n_2 is known as Kerr coefficient and it is related to susceptibility as:

$$n_2(\omega) = \frac{3}{4\pi}\chi^{(3)}_{xxx} \tag{12.50c}$$

for a linearly polarized wave in the x direction. For silica, its value is approximately $1.3 \times 10^{-22}\ \mathrm{m^2/V^2}$. Kerr effect originates from the *non-harmonic motion of electrons bound in molecules*. Consequently, it is fast effect, the response time of the order of 10^{-15} s.

12.21.3 Stimulated Raman Scattering

Scattering phenomena are responsible for Raman and Brillouin effects. During those scatterings, the energy of the optical field is transferred to local phonons: in Raman sacttering optical phonons are generated whereas in the Brillouin scattering the acoustic phonons.

12.21.4 Derivation of the Nonlinear Schödinger Equation

Solitons in optical fibers are described by the so-called nonlinear Schrödinger (NSE) equation. In the derivation, we use the concept of the Fourier spectrum of the propagating pulse (Fig. 12.48).

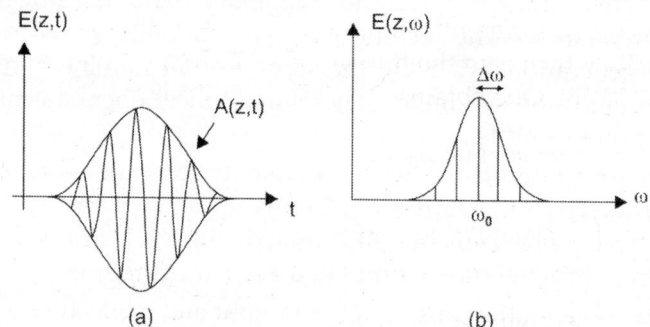

Fig. 12.48: (a) Illustration of the propagating modulated pulse (b) and its spectrum

A medium where solitons propagate exhibits Kerr nonlinearity. In such a medium, refractive index depends on intensity of electric field $I(t)$ given by Eq. (12.50), again reproduced here:

$$n(t) = n_0 + n_2 \cdot I(t) \tag{12.51}$$

where $$I(t) = 2n_0\varepsilon_0 c\,|\,A(z, t)\,|^2 \tag{12.52}$$

Here $A(z, t)$ is the slowly varying envelope connected to the optical pulse described by the optical pulse $E(z, t)$ as shown in Fig. 12.47.

$$E(z, t) = A(z, t) e^{i(\omega_0 t - \beta_0 z)} \tag{12.53}$$

Fourier transform of the optical field is:

$$E(z, t) = \int_{-\infty}^{+\infty} d\omega \, \tilde{E}(z, \omega) e^{i(\omega t - \beta z)} \tag{12.54}$$

where $\tilde{E}(z, \omega)$ is the Fourier spectrum of the pulse, β propagation constant and ω_0 the frequency at which the pulse spectrum is centered (also known as carrier frequency) (Fig. 12.47).

For quasi-monochromatic pulses with $\Delta\omega \equiv \omega - \omega_0$, it is useful to expand propagation constant $\beta(\omega)$ in a Taylor series:

$$\beta(\omega) = \beta_0 + \beta_1 \cdot (\omega - \omega_0) + \frac{1}{2} \beta_2 \cdot (\omega - \omega_0)^2 + \Delta\beta_{NL} \tag{12.55}$$

where we have neglected higher order derivatives. Here $\Delta\beta_{NL} = n_2 k_0 I$ is the nonlinear contribution to the propagation constant.

Substituting expansion of Eq. (12.54) into Eq. (12.55), one obtains

$$E(z, t) = e^{-i\beta_0 z} \int_{-\infty}^{+\infty} d(\Delta\omega) \, \tilde{E}(z, \omega) \exp\left(i\omega t - i\beta_1 z \Delta\omega - \frac{1}{2} i\beta_2 z \Delta\omega^2 - i \cdot z \cdot \Delta\beta_{NL} \right)$$

$$= e^{-i(\omega_0 t - \beta_0 z)} \int_{-\infty}^{+\infty} d(\Delta\omega) \, \tilde{E}(z, \omega_0 + \Delta\omega) \times \exp\left(it \Delta\omega - i\beta_1 z \Delta\omega - \frac{1}{2} i\beta_2 z \Delta\omega^2 - i \cdot z \cdot \Delta\beta_{NL} \right)$$

$$\equiv e^{i(\omega_0 t - \beta_0 z)} A(z, t)$$

where we have introduced

$$A(z, t) = \int_{-\infty}^{+\infty} d(\Delta\omega) \, \tilde{E}(z, \omega_0 + \Delta\omega)$$

$$\times \exp\left(it \Delta\omega - i\beta_1 z \Delta\omega - \frac{1}{2} i\beta_2 z \Delta\omega^2 - i \cdot z \cdot \Delta\beta_{NL} \right)$$

$$A(z, t) \equiv \int_{-\infty}^{+\infty} d(\Delta\omega) \, \tilde{E}(z, \omega_0 + \Delta\omega) e^{ig(z, t)} \tag{12.56}$$

Now, we will obtain a differential equation describing evolution of the amplitude $A(z, t)$ from Eq. (12.56) which is in the integral form. To do this, one needs to take partial derivatives of Eq. (12.56). One obtains:

$$\frac{\partial A(z, t)}{\partial t} = \int_{-\infty}^{+\infty} d(\Delta\omega) \, \tilde{E}(z, \omega_0 + \Delta\omega) \, i\Delta\omega \, e^{ig(z, t)}$$

$$\frac{\partial A(z, t)}{\partial t^2} = \int_{-\infty}^{+\infty} d(\Delta\omega) \, \tilde{E}(z, \omega_0 + \Delta\omega) \, (i\Delta\omega)^2 \, e^{ig(z, t)}$$

$$\frac{\partial A(z, t)}{\partial z} = \int_{-\infty}^{+\infty} d(\Delta\omega) \, \tilde{E}(z, \omega_0 + \Delta\omega) \left(-i\beta_1 \Delta\omega - \frac{1}{2} i\beta_2 \Delta\omega^2 - i\Delta\beta_{NL} \right) e^{ig(z, t)}$$

While evaluating time derivatives, we have assumed in the above that $I(t)$ does not depend on time. Addition of the above combination of derivatives produces:

$$\frac{\partial A(z, t)}{\partial z} + \beta_1 \frac{\partial A(z, t)}{\partial z} - i\frac{1}{2}\beta_2 \frac{\partial A(z, t)}{\partial z^2} = \int_{-\infty}^{+\infty} d(\Delta\omega) \, \tilde{E}(z, \omega_0 + \Delta\omega) \times \left[\left(-i\beta_1 \Delta\omega - \frac{1}{2} i\beta_2 \Delta\omega^2 \right. \right.$$

$$\left. \left. - i \cdot \Delta\beta_{NL} \right) + \beta_1 i\Delta\omega - i\frac{1}{2}\beta_2 (i\Delta\omega)^2 \right]$$

The term in the bracket is, $[...] = -i \cdot \Delta \beta_{NL} = in_2 k_0 I$. Thus, Eq. (15.9) gives:

$$\frac{\partial A(z,t)}{\partial z} + \beta_1 \frac{\partial A(z,t)}{\partial t} - i\frac{1}{2}\beta_2 \frac{\partial^2 A(z,t)}{\partial t^2} = \int_{-\infty}^{+\infty} d(\Delta\omega)\, \tilde{E}(z, \omega_0 + \Delta\omega)\, (-in_2 k_0 I)\, e^{ig(z,t)}$$

$$= -ink_0 I \int_{-\infty}^{+\infty} d(\Delta\omega)\, \tilde{E}(z, \omega)\, e^{ig(z,t)}$$

$$= in_2 k_0 I A\,(z,t) \qquad (12.57)$$

The final equation describing solitons is therefore:

$$\frac{\partial A(z,t)}{\partial z} + \beta_1 \frac{\partial A(z,t)}{\partial t} + i\frac{1}{2}\beta_2 \frac{\partial^2 A(z,t)}{\partial z^2} = i\gamma\,|A(z,t)|^2\,A(z,t) - \frac{\alpha}{2} A(z,t) \qquad (12.58)$$

where we have defined nonlinear coefficient γ as:

$$\lambda = \frac{2\pi n_2}{\lambda A_{\text{eff}}} \qquad (12.59)$$

Here A_{eff} is the effective core area.

Our interest lie here in the pulse evolution during propagation and not in the time of pulse arrival. We can, therefore, simplify the above equation by transforming it to a coordinate system which moves with group v_g. In this moving frame, new time T and new coordinate Z are:

$$Z = z \qquad (12.60)$$
$$T = t - b_1 z$$

To obtain the transformed equation, we must evaluate derivatives with respect to new variables as follows:

$$\frac{\partial A}{dt} = \frac{\partial A}{dT}\frac{\partial T}{dt} + \frac{\partial A}{\partial/Z}\frac{\partial Z}{\partial t} = \frac{\partial A}{\partial T}$$

since $\dfrac{\partial A}{\partial t} = 1$ and $\dfrac{\partial Z}{\partial t} = 0$. From the above one finds:

$$\frac{\partial^2 A}{\partial t^2} = \frac{\partial^2 A}{\partial T^2}$$

Using the above results, one has:

$$\frac{\partial A}{\partial z} = \frac{\partial A}{dT}\frac{\partial T}{\partial z} + \frac{\partial A}{\partial/Z}\frac{\partial Z}{\partial Z} = -\beta_1 \frac{\partial A}{dT} + \frac{\partial A}{\partial/Z}$$

The last result is used in Eq. (12.58) to replace $\dfrac{\partial A}{\partial t}$. The transformed equation is:

$$\frac{\partial A}{\partial z} + i\frac{1}{2}\beta_2 \frac{\partial^2 A}{dT^2} - i\gamma\,|A|^2\,A + \frac{1}{2}\alpha A = 0 \qquad (12.61)$$

where in the final step, we replaced Z by z. It is known as a *nonlinear Schrödinger equation* (NSE).

To further analyse NSE, we will introduce two characteristic lengths describing dispersion (L_D) and nonlinearity (L_{NL}). Those are defined as:

$$L_D = \frac{T_0^2}{|\beta_2|} = \frac{T_0^2\, 2\pi c}{|D|\lambda^2} \qquad (12.62)$$

and

$$L_{NL} = \frac{1}{\gamma P_0} \qquad (12.63)$$

where P_0 is the peak power of the slowly varying envelope $A(z, T)$ and T_0 is a temporal characteristic value of the initial pulse, which is often defined as full width half maximum (the pulse 3 dB width). Those two lengths characterize how far a pulse must propagate to show the respective effect. Physically, L_D is the propagation length at which a Gaussian pulse broadens by a factor of $\sqrt{(2)}$ due to *group velocity dispersion* (GVD).

GVD dominates pulse propagation in fibres whose length L is $L \ll L_{NL}$ and $L \geq L_D$. In such situation, the nonlinearity in NLSE can be ignored and the equation can be solved analytically. Nonlinear effects dominate in fiber where $L \ll L_D$ and $L \geq L_{NL}$. In this limit, the dispersion term can be ignored.

Typical values of parameters for solitons are summarized in Table 12.4. The numerical analysis normalize variables:

$$U = \frac{1}{\sqrt{P_0}} A \quad \text{and} \quad \tau = \frac{T}{T_0} \tag{12.64}$$

Table 12.4: Typical parameters for solitons

Parameter	Symbol	Value	Unit
Wavelength	λ	1.55	μm
Nonlinear coeff.	γ	1.3	1/km·W
GVD	β_2	15×10^{-24}	s²/km
Width parameter	T_0	100	ps
Peak power	P_0	0.15	mW
Losses	α	0.01	dB/km^{-1}
Chirp parameter	c	1.2	dimensionless
Soliton period	z_0	1047.2	km

The width parameter T_0 is related to the full-width at half-maximum (FWHM) intensity of the input pulse. Specifically:

$$T_s = 2T_0 \ln(1 + \sqrt{(2)}) \approx 1.763 T_0 \tag{12.65}$$

After simplification, Eq. (12.61) takes the form:

$$\frac{\partial U}{\partial z} - i \frac{\sin(\beta_2)}{2L_D} \frac{\partial^2 U}{\partial \tau^2} + i \frac{1}{L_{NL}} |U|^2 U + \frac{1}{2} \alpha U = 0 \tag{12.66}$$

Another normalized form of the Schrödinger equation exists in the literature. We obtain it in the lossless case, i.e. $\alpha = 0$. To derive it, normalize the z coordinate as follows:

$$\xi = \frac{z}{L_D} \tag{12.67}$$

After a few algebraic steps, one obtains:

$$\frac{\partial U}{\partial \xi} - i \frac{\sin(\beta_2)}{2} \frac{\partial^2 U}{\partial \tau^2} + iN^2 |U|^2 U = 0 \tag{12.68}$$

where N is known as soliton order and is defined as:

$$N^2 = \frac{L_D}{L_{NL}} = \frac{\gamma P_0 T_0^2}{|\beta_2|} \tag{12.69}$$

The last form of the NLSE is found by introducing u as:

$$u = NU = \left(\frac{\gamma P_0 T_0^2}{|\beta_2|} \right)^{1/2} A \tag{12.70}$$

Equation (12.68) then takes the form:

$$\frac{\partial u}{\partial \xi} - i\frac{\sin(\beta_2)}{2}\frac{\partial^2 u}{\partial \tau^2} - i|u|^2 u = 0 \qquad (12.71)$$

We will now discuss the numerical solution of the nonlinear Schrödinger equation (NSE) which describes propagation of optical solitons using the so-called *split-step Fourier method* (SSFM).

The SSFM is a numerical technique used to solve nonlinear partial differential equations like the NSE. The method relies on computing the solution in small steps and on taking into account the linear and nonlinear steps separately. The linear step (dispersion) can be made in either frequency or time domain, while the nonlinear step is made in the time domain. The method is widely used for studying nonlinear pulse propagation in optical fibers.

A nonlinear Schrödinger equation, Eq. (12.61) contains dispersive and nonlinear terms. To introduce SSFTM, write the NLSE equation in the following form:

$$\frac{\partial A(z,T)}{\partial z} = (\hat{L} + \hat{N})A(z,t) \qquad (12.72)$$

where

$$\hat{L}A = -\frac{\alpha}{2} - \frac{i}{2}\beta_2\frac{\partial^2 A}{\partial T^2} \qquad (12.73)$$

contains losses and dispersion in the linear medium and nonlinear term:

$$\hat{N}A = i\gamma|A|^2 A \qquad (12.74)$$

accounts for the nonlinear effects in the medium.

The basis of the SSFM is to split a propagation form z to $z + h$ (h is a small step) into two operations (assuming that they act independently): during first step nonlinear effects are included and in the second step one accounts for linear effects (Fig. 12.49).

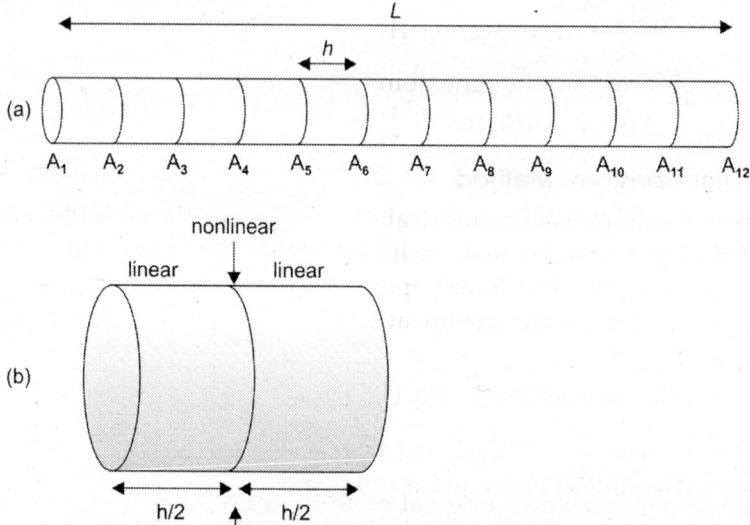

Fig. 12.49: Illustration of a split-step Fourier method (a) division of optical fiber into N regions (here N = 11) of equal lengths (b) illustration of operation of linear and nonlinear operations at arbitrary segments

Formal solution of Eq. (12.72) over a small step h is thus:

$$A(z + h, t) = e^{h(\hat{L} + \hat{N})} A(z, t) \qquad (12.75)$$

In the first-order approximation, the above formula can be written as:

$$A(z + h, t) = e^{h\hat{L}} e^{h\hat{N}} A(z, t) + O(h^2) \qquad (12.76)$$

The basis of this approximation is established by Baker–Hausdorf lemma, which is:

$$e^{\hat{A}} e^{\hat{B}} = e^{\hat{A} + \hat{B}} e^{1/2[\hat{A}, \hat{B}]} \qquad (12.77)$$

given that operation $\hat{A}$ and $\hat{B}$ commute with $[\hat{A}$ and $\hat{B}]$.

The basis of the method is suggested by Eq. (12.76). It tells us that $A(z + h, t)$ can be determined by applying the two operators independently. The propagation from z to $z + h$ is split into two operations: first the nonlinear step and then the linear step assuming that they act independently. If h is sufficiently small, Eq. (12.76) gives good results.

The value of step h can be determined by assuming that the maximum phase shift ϕ_{max} = $g|A_p|^2 h$, where A_p is the peak value of $A(z, t)$ due to the nonlinear operator is smaller than the predefined value. Iannone showed that $\phi_{max} \leq 0.05$ rad.

For a practical implementation of the SSFM, we need to establish practical expressions for dispersive and nonlinear terms. In the following, we will, therefore, analyse the effect of both terms independently neglecting losses.

Let us analyse the effect of the dispersive term alone. For that, we temporarily switch off the nonlinear term. After Fourier transform, the 'linear equation' becomes:

$$\frac{\partial \tilde{A}(z, \omega)}{\partial z} = -\frac{i}{2} \omega^2 \beta_2 \tilde{A}(z, \omega)$$

which has the solution:

$$\tilde{A}(z, \omega) = \tilde{A}(0, \omega) e^{-i\omega^2 \beta_2 z/2}$$

The action of the nonlinear term alone is described by the equation:

$$\frac{\partial A(z, t)}{\partial z} = i\gamma |A(z, t)|^2 A(z, t)$$

The 'natural' solution is in the time domain. It produces:

$$A(z, t) = A(0, t) e^{i\gamma|A|^2 A}$$

Split-Step Fourier Transform Method

The propagation medium (say, cylindrical optical fiber) is divided into small segments, each of length h (Fig. 12.49). Further, each individual segment of length h is subdivided into two of equal lengths. The linear operator operates over each subsegment in the frequency domain, whereas the nonlinear operator operates only locally at the central point.

Operation of the linear operator $\hat{L}$, Eq. (12.73) over first subsegment is done as follows:

$$e^{h\hat{L}/2} A(z, t) = F^{-1} \left\{ e^{h\hat{L}/2} F\{A(z, t)\} \right\} \qquad (12.78)$$

i.e. one must Fourier transform original amplitude from time domain into frequency domain, apply linear operator $\hat{L}$ and then, apply inverse Fourier transform to get the amplitude back to time domain.

The operation of nonlinear operator defined by Eq. (12.74) is as follows:

$$A_{i+1/2, L}(z, t) = A_{i+1/2, R}(z, t) e^{h\hat{N}} \qquad (12.79)$$

where $A_{i+1/2, L}$ is the value of field amplitude at an infinitesimal point left from $i + 1/2$. Finally the operation of linear operator over second subsegment of length $h/2$ is done exactly the same way as over the first segment.

To summarize, the method over each segment of length h consists of three steps:

Step 1 $\begin{cases} \tilde{A}_i(z, \omega) = F\{A_i(z, t)\} \\ \tilde{A}_{i-}(z, \omega) = \tilde{A}_i(z, \omega) \cdot \exp\left(-i\dfrac{1}{2}\omega^2\beta_2 h\right) \\ A_{i-}(z, t) = F^{-1}\{\tilde{A}_{i-}(z, \omega)\} \end{cases}$

Step 2 $A_{i+}(z, t) = A_{i-}(z, t) \cdot \exp\left(-i\gamma |A|^2 Ah\right)$

Step 3 $\begin{cases} \tilde{A}_{i+1}(z, \omega) = F\{A_{i+1}(z, t)\} \\ \tilde{A}_{i+1}(z, \omega) = \tilde{A}_{i+1}(z, \omega) \cdot \exp\left(-i\dfrac{1}{2}\omega^2\beta_2 h\right) \\ A_{i-}(z, t) = F^{-1}\{\tilde{A}_{i+}(z, \omega)\} \end{cases}$

where F indicates Fourier transform (FT) and F^{-1} inverse FT.

Symmetrized Split-Step Fourier Transform Method (SSSFM)

The simulation time of Eq. (12.76) essentially depends on the size to step h. To reduce simulation time, a new method was invented which allows us to use larger steps, h.

Mathematically, one uses the following second-order approximation:

$$A(z, +h, t) = e^{1/2h\hat{L}} \exp\left\{\int_z^{z+h} N(z')dz'\right\} e^{1/2h\hat{L}} A(z, t) + O(h^3) \qquad (12.80)$$

In this approach, one assumes that the nonlinearities are distributed over h, which is more realistic. For small h, one can approximately evaluate:

$$\int_z^{z+h} \hat{N}(z')dz' \approx \frac{h}{2}\left[\hat{N}(z) + \hat{N}(z+h)\right]$$

In the SSSFM algorithm Eq. (12.79) is replaced by:

$$A_{i+1/2, L}(z, t) = A_{i+1/2, R}(z, t) e^{h[\hat{N}(z) + \hat{N}(z+h)]} \qquad (12.81)$$

The above scheme requires iteration to find A_{i+1} since it is not known at $z + \dfrac{1}{2}h$. Initially $\hat{N}(z + H)$ will be assumed to be the same as $\hat{N}(z)$.

Single Solitons

In analysis, we used fiber and pulse parameters summarized in Table 12.2. The input soliton was considered to be in the form:

$$A_{in}(\xi = 0, T) = \sqrt{A_0}\, \text{sec}h\left(\frac{T}{T_0}\right) \qquad (12.82)$$

where N is the soliton order given by Eq. (12.69). In Fig. 12.49, we illustrated the propagation of $N = 1$ soliton without damping and in Fig. 12.50, the evolution of the same soliton with damping ($\alpha = 0.01$ dB km^{-1}).

A higher-order soliton with $N = 3$ is defined as:

$$A_{in}(\xi = 0, T) = N^3 \sqrt{A_0}\, \text{sec}\, h\left(\frac{T}{T_0}\right) \qquad (12.83)$$

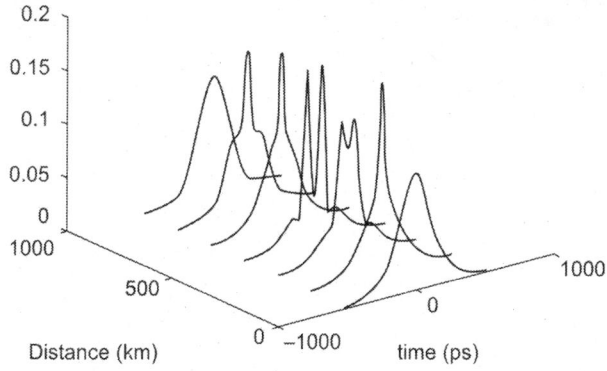

Fig. 12.50: Evolution in time over one soliton period for N = 1 soliton

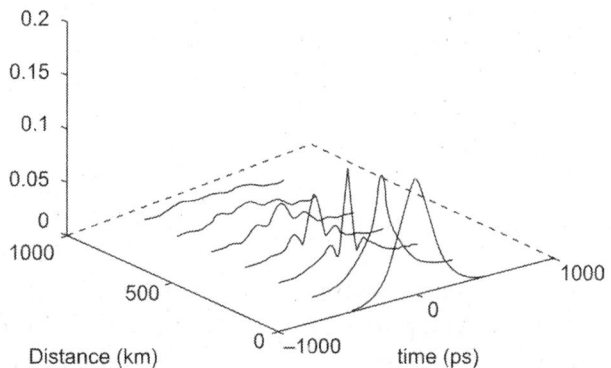

Fig. 12.51: Evolution in time over one soliton period for N = 1 soliton with damping

Propagation of higher-order soliton with $N = 3$ is shown in Fig. 12.52 (no damping) and in Fig. 12.53 (with damping). One can observe periodic evolution of the undamped soliton.

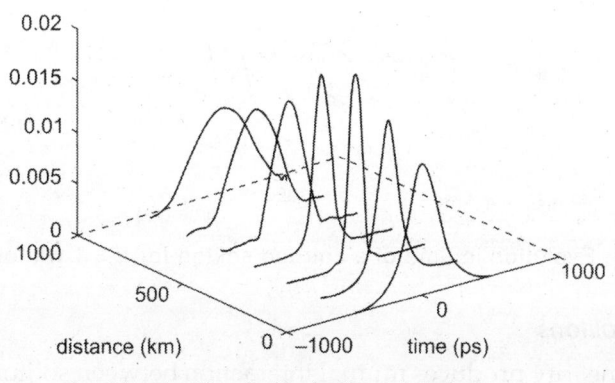

of a chirped soliton for N = I without damping

Fig. 12.52: Evolution in time over one soliton period for N = 3 soliton. Note soliton splitting near $z_0 = 0.5$ and its recovery beyond that point

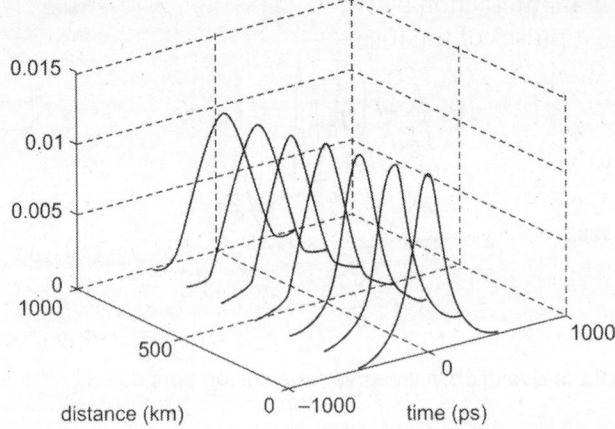

Fig. 12.53: Evolution in time over one soliton period for $N = 3$ soliton with damping

Chirped Solitons

Here, we analyse how chirp affects single soliton propagation. We assume the following input:

$$A_{in} (\xi = 0, T) = \sqrt{A_0} \sec h\left(\frac{T}{T_0}\right) \exp\left[-iC/2\left(\frac{T}{T_0}\right)^2\right] \qquad (12.84)$$

where C is the chirped parameter. Evolution of such soliton in the case of $N = 1$ and $C = 1.6$ is shown in Fig. 12.54. The pulse is initially compressed and then broadens.

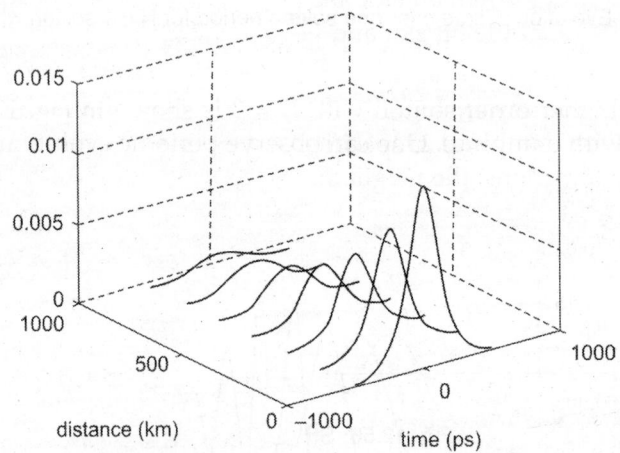

Fig. 12.54: Evolution in time of a chirped soliton for $N = 1$ without damping

Two Interacting Solitons

The effect of nonlinearity produces mutual interaction between soliton pulses, if they are launched close together. This interaction is important from a practical point of view and also from a fundamental perspective related to soliton propagation. For example, it was shown that nonlinear interaction between solitons can result in a bandwidth reduction by a factor of 10.

First, we consider an interaction between two solitons of the same strength and $N = 1$. We assume the initial pulses of the form:

$$A_{in} (\xi = 0, T) = \sqrt{A_0} \ \sec h \left(\frac{T}{T_0} - 1 \right) + \sqrt{A_0} \ \sec h \left(\frac{T}{T_0} + 1 \right) \tag{12.85}$$

The result of two interacting solitons is shown in Fig. 12.55.

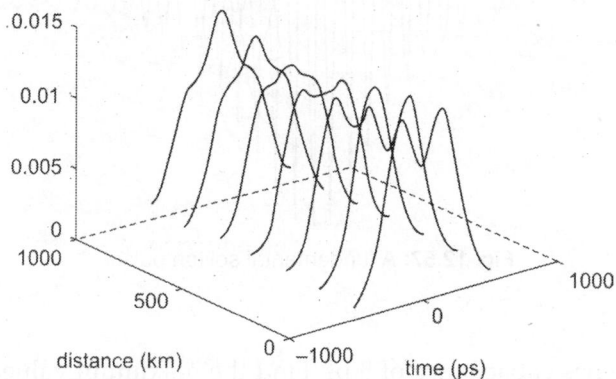

Fig. 12.55: Evolution in time of two interacting solitons without damping

An important application of solitons is in the transmission of information in optical fiber systems. Soliton pulses are stable when they propagate over long distances. Losses in fibers are an important limiting factor, so it becomes necessary to compensate periodically for fiber loss. This can be done by using EDFA.

In the transmission of information, solitons are considered like linear pulses. In a bit stream each soliton has its own bit slot and it represents logical one or zero (Fig. 12.56). Here T_B is the duration of the bit slot and it is related to bit rate B as:

$$T_B = \frac{1}{B} = 2aT_0 \tag{12.86}$$

where T_0 is the soliton width and $2a$ specifies the distance between neighbouring solitons. To prevent their interactions, the neighbouring solitons should be well separated.

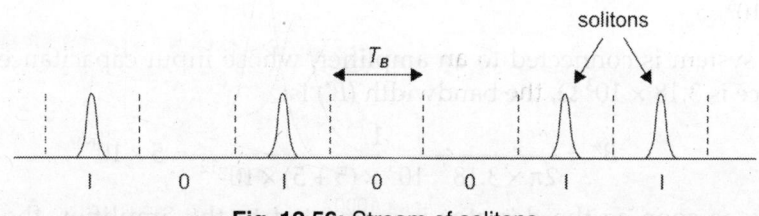

Fig. 12.56: Stream of solitons

The shape of fundamental solitons that are being experimented upon along with optical amplifiers for communication is shown in Fig. 12.57. In fact the solitons overcome the detrimental effect of chromatic dispersion, and optical amplifiers negate the attenuation. Hence, using the two together offers the promise of very high bit rate transmission with large repeaterless distances.

Solitons are very well suited for *long-haul communication* because of their high information carrying capacity and the possibility of periodic amplification. However, soliton systems are still waiting for the full field deployment.

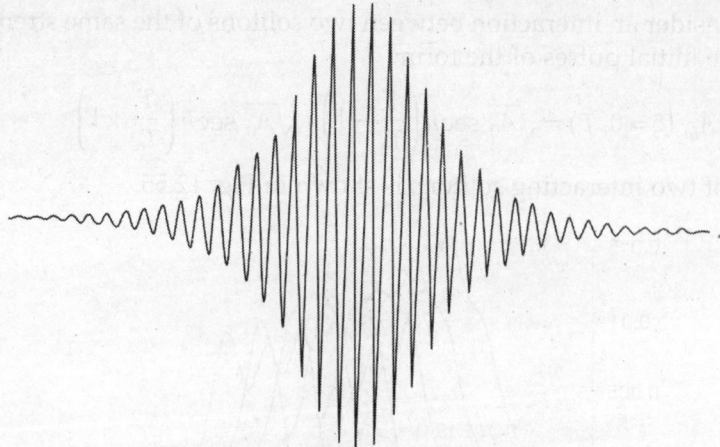

Fig. 12.57: A fundamental soliton pulse

Example 1

A *p-i-n* photodiode has capacitance of 5 pf. Find the maximum value of load resistance R_L which will make the post detection bandwidth (B) of 10 MHz and also calculate the decrease in bandwidth with the same load resistance when the amplifier has a input capacitance of 5 pf.

Solution

The maximum bandwidth is given by:

$$C = \frac{1}{2\pi R_L C_d}$$

or

$$R_L = \frac{1}{2\pi B C_d} = \frac{1}{2\pi \times 10 \times 10^6 \times 5 \times 10^{-12}} = 3.18 \times 10^3 \ \Omega$$

Here

$C_d = 5 \text{ pf} = 5 \times 10^{-12} \text{ f}$

$B = 10 \times 10^6$

When the system is connected to an amplifier, whose input capacitance is 5 pf and load resistance is $3.18 \times 10^3 \ \Omega$, the bandwidth ($B'$) is:

$$B' = \frac{1}{2\pi \times 3.18 \times 10^3 \times (5+5) \times 10^{-12}} = 5 \times 10^6$$

Obviously, as soon as the detector is connected to the amplifier, the bandwidth decreases to 5 MHz.

Example 2

A digital fiber link operating at 850 nm requires a BER of 10^{-9}. Show that the quantum limit in terms of quantum efficiency is 20.7 hv/η.

Solution

Probability of error:

$$P_r(0) = e^{-N} = 10^{-9}$$

Here, $\lambda = 850 \text{ nm} = 850 \times 10^{-9} \text{ m}$

$\quad\quad$ BER $= 10^{-9}$

$\therefore \quad\quad \overline{N} = 9 \log 10 = 20.7$

where $\overline{N}$ represents electron-hole pair generated. Quantum efficiency (η), photon energy (hv) and energy received (E) are related by:

$$N = \frac{\eta E}{h\upsilon}$$

or $\quad\quad E = N \frac{h\upsilon}{\eta} = 20.7 \times \frac{h\upsilon}{\eta} = 20.7 \frac{h\upsilon}{\eta}$

Example 3

A high input impedance amplifier is used in an optical fiber receiver. The effective input resistance of the amplifier is 5 mΩ matched with the bias resistance of the detector of the same value. Calculate: (i) The maximum bandwidth that may be obtained without equalization if the total capacitance (C_T) = 5 pf. (ii) The mean square thermal noise current per unit bandwidth generated by this high input impedance configuration when operating at 27°C. (iii) Compare the values obtained in (i) and (ii) with those values obtained when the high input amplifier is replaced by a trans-impedance amplifier having feedback resistor R_F = 100 kΩ and open loop gain of 400. You may assume $R_F \ll R_{TL}$ and total capacitance (C_T) = 5 pf.

Solution

(i) We have:

$$R_{TL} = \frac{R_b R_a}{R_b + R_a}$$

$\quad\quad$ where $\quad R_b$ is detector's load resistance

$\quad\quad\quad\quad\quad\quad R_a$ is input resistance of the amplifier

Now, $\quad\quad\quad R_{TL} = \frac{5 \times 10^6 \times 5 \times 10^6}{5 \times 10^6 + 5 \times 10^6} = 2.5 \text{ m}\Omega$

Here, $R_b = 5 \times 10^6$ W, $R_a = 5 \times 10^6$ W

$\therefore$ Maximum bandwidth

$$B = \frac{1}{2\pi R_{TL} C_T} = \frac{1}{2\pi \times 2.5 \times 10^6 \times 5 \times 10^{-12}} = 1.27 \times 10^4 \text{ Hz}$$

Obviously, the maximum bandwidth that may be obtained without equalization is 1.27×10^4 Hz.

(ii) The mean thermal energy noise current per unit bandwidth for the high impedance configuration:

$$\langle i_{amp}^2 \rangle = \frac{4 k_B T}{R_{TL}} = \frac{4 \times 1.38 \times 10^{-23} \times 300}{2.5 \times 10^6} = 6.62 \times 10^{-27} \text{ A}^2 \text{ Hz}^{-1}$$

Here $B = 1$ Hz, $T = 273 + 27 = 300$ K

(iii) The maximum bandwidth without equalization for the trans-impedance configuration:

$$B = \frac{A}{2\pi R_F C_F} = \frac{400}{2\pi \times 10^5 \times 5 \times 10^{-12}} = 1.24 \times 10^8 \text{ Hz}$$

Obviously, the bandwidth with transimpedance is 124 MHz.

Now, assuming $R_F \ll R_{TL}$, the mean square thermal noise current per unit bandwidth for the transimpedance configuration can be obtained as:

$$\langle i_{th}^2 \rangle = \frac{4k_B T}{R_F} = \frac{4 \times 1.38 \times 10^{-23} \times 300}{10^5} = 16.56 \times 10^{-25} \text{ A}^2 \text{ Hz}$$

Example 4

Consider the design of a typical digital fiber-optic link which has to transmit at a data rate of 20 Mb/s with a BER of 10^{-9} using the NRZ code. The transmitter uses a GaAlAs LED emitting at 850 nm, which can couple on an average 100 μW (–10 dBm) of optical power into a fiber of core size 50 μm. The fiber cable consists of a graded-index fiber with the manufacture's specification as follows: $a_f = 2.5$ dB/km, $(\Delta T)_{mat} = 3$ ns/km, $(\Delta T)_{modal} = 1$ ns/km. A silicon p-i-n photodiode has been chosen, for detecting 850-nm optical signals, for the front end of the receiver. The detector has a sensitivity of –42 dBm in order to give the desired BER. The source along with its drive circuit has a rise time of 12 ns and the receiver has a rise time of 11 ns. The cable requires splicing every 1 km, with a loss of 0.5 dB/splice. Two connectors, one at the transmitter end and the other at the receiver end, are also required. The loss at each connector is 1 dB. It is predicted that a safety margin of 6 dB will be required. Calculate the maximum possible link length without repeaters and the total rise time of the system for accessing the feasibility of the desired system. **[B Tech]**

Solution

We have $C_L = \alpha_f L + \alpha_{con} + \alpha_{spice}$. The total channel loss C_L may be calculated as follows:

$C_L = \alpha_f L +$ (splice loss per km) $\times L +$ (loss per connector) $\times$ no. of connectors

$= (2.5$ dB/km$) \times L$ (km) $+ (0.5$ dB/splice$) \times (1$ splice/km$) \times L$ (km) $+ (1$ dB$)$

$= (3L + 2)$ dB

Here, $P_{tx} = -10$ dBm, $P_{rx} = -42$ dBm, and $M_s = 6$ dB. Substititing the values of P, P_{rx}, C_L, and M_S in Eq. $P_{tx} = P_{rx} + C_L + M_S$, we get:

$$-10 = -42 + (3L + 2) + 6$$

or
$$L = 8 \text{ km}$$

Obviously, a maximum transmission path of 8 km is possible without repeaters.

Let us now calculate the total rise time t_{sys} using following Eqs:

$$t_{sys} = \left[t_{tx}^2 + t_f^2 + f_{rx}^2 \right]^{1/2} \tag{i}$$

and
$$t_f = \left[t_{intermodal}^2 + t_{intramodal}^2 \right]^{1/2} \tag{ii}$$

It is given that $t_{tx} = 12$ ns, $t_{rx} = 11$ ns. In the case of multimode fibers, intramodal dispersion, primarily due to material dispersion, and hence $t_{intramodal} \approx t_{mat}$:

$$t_{mat} = (3 \text{ ns/km}) \times L = (3 \text{ ns/km}) \times (8 \text{ km}) = 24 \text{ ns}$$

$$t_{intermodal} = (1 \text{ ns/km}) \times L = (1 \text{ ns/km}) \times 8 \text{ (km)} = 8 \text{ ns}$$

$\therefore$
$$t_{sys} = [(12)^2 + (24)^2 + (8)^2 + (11)^2]^{1/2} = 30 \text{ ns}$$

The maximum allowable rise time t_{sys} for our 20-Mb/s NRZ data stream from Eq. (i):

$$t_{sys} \leq \frac{0.35}{B} \text{ for the RZ format}$$

$$\frac{0.70}{B} \text{ for the NRZ format}$$

$$\therefore \qquad t_{sys} \leq \frac{0.70}{B} = \frac{0.70}{20 \times 10^6} \text{ s} = 35 \text{ ns}$$

Since t_{sys} (= 30 ns) for the proposed link is less than the maximum allowable limit, the choice of components is adequate to meet the system design criteria.

Example 5

A transmitter has an output power of 0.1 mW. It is used with a fiber having following specifications:

$$\text{NA} = 0.25, \text{ attenuation of 6 dB/km, and length} = 0.5 \text{ km}$$

The link contains two connectors of 2 dB average loss. The sensitivity (minimum acceptable power) of the receiver is –35 dB m. The designer kept a 4 dB margin. Find link power budget.

Solution

$$\text{Coupling loss} = -10 \log (\text{NA}^2) = -10 \log (0.25)^2 = 12 \text{ dB}$$

Here, Source power, $P_S = 0.1$ mW

$$P_S = 10 \text{ dBm}$$
$$\text{NA} = 0.25$$

$$\text{Fiber loss} = \alpha_f L$$
$$\therefore \qquad l_f = (6 \text{ dB/km}) (0.5 \text{ km}) = 3 \text{ dB}$$
$$\text{Connector loss} = 2 (2 \text{ dB})$$
$$l_c = 4 \text{ dB}$$
$$\text{Design margin } P_m = 4 \text{ dB}$$
$$\therefore \quad \text{Actual power output } P_{out} = \text{Source power} - (\Sigma \text{ losses})$$
or
$$P_{out} = 10 \text{ dBm} - [12 \text{ dBm} + 3 + 4 + 4]$$
$$= -13 \text{ dBm}$$

Since receiver sensitivity is given = – 35 dB m, i.e. P_{min} = –35 dB·m.

We note that $P_{out} > P_{min}$, i.e. the system will perform adequately over the system operating life.

Example 6

Calculate the total power that should be transmitted over 32 channels of a WDM system that are spaced 0.8 nm apart at 1.55 μm for a repeater-less distance of 80 km. Take $L_{eff} = 20$ km, $\Delta\lambda_c = 125$ nm, $g_R = 6 \times 10^{-14}$ m/W, and $A_{eff} = 55$ μm^2. **[B Tech]**

Solution

Let us assume that the power penalty is to be kept below 0.5 dB, obviously, we must have $F \leq 0.1$. Therefore, from Eq.

$$F = \frac{g_R \, \Delta\lambda_s}{\Delta\lambda_c} \frac{P_0 L_{eff}}{2 \, A_{eff}} \frac{N \, (N-1)}{2}$$

where $\Delta\lambda_c$ is total channel spacing, $\Delta\lambda_s$ is channel spacing, g_R is peak Raman gain coefficient, N are equally spaced channels, 0, 1, 2, ..., $(N-1)$ in a WDM system, P_0 is power at the input end of the fiber, L_{eff} is effective length and A_{eff} is effective cross-sectional area.

We can calculate the total transmitted power P_{tot} as follows:

$$P_{tot} = NP_0 = \frac{4F\,\Delta\lambda_c\,A_{eff}}{g_R\Delta\lambda L_{eff}\,(N-1)}$$

or

$$P_{tot} = \frac{0.1\,(125\text{ nm}) \times 4 \times (55 \times 10^{-12}\text{ m}^2) \times (10^{-3}\text{ km/m})}{(6 \times 10^{-14}\text{ m/W}) \times (0.8\text{ km}) \times (20\text{ nm}) \times (32-1)}$$

$$= 0.0924\text{ W} = 92.4\text{ mW}$$

The transmitted power per channel, P_0, therefore, should be less than 2.887 mW. In this calculation, it has been assumed that there is no dispersion in the system.

Example 7

In a fiber link, the laser diode output power is 5 dBm, source-fiber coupling loss = 3 dB, connector loss = 2 dB and has 50 splices of 0.1 dB loss. If fiber attenuation loss for 100 km is 25 dB, compute the loss margin for (i) APB receiver having sensitivity –40 dBm, (ii) Hybrid PINFET high impedance receiver with sensitivity –32 dBm.   **[M Tech]**

Solution

Calculations for power budget:

Source output	5 dBm
Source fiber coupling loss	3 dB
Connector loss	2 dB
Splicing loss (50 × 0.1)	5 dB
Fiber attenuation	25 dB
Total loss	35 dB

Now, available power to receiver: (5–35) dBm = –30 dBm:

   (i) APD sensitivity = – 40 dBm

      Loss margin = [–40 – (–30)] dBm = 10 dBm

  (ii) Hybrid (H) - PINFET high-impedance receiver = –3 dBm

      Loss margin = [–32 – (–30)] = 2 dBm.

Example 8

A college campus CATV system uses an optical bus to distribute video signals to the subscribers. The transmitter couples 0 dB·m (1 mW) of optical power into the bus. Each receiver has a sensitivity of –40 dB·m. Each optical tap couples 5% of optical power to the subscriber and has a 0.5 dB insertion loss. How many subscribers can be added to the optical bus before the signal needs in-line amplification?   **[B Tech]**

Solution

With reference to Fig. 12.58, if we neglect the optical loss within the bus (the optical fiber itself), the power available at the Nth tap is given by:

$$P_N = P_T C\,[(1-\delta)\,(1-C)^{N-1}$$

where P_T is the transmitted power, C is the fraction of optical power coupled out at each tap, and δ is the fractional insertion loss (assumed to be the same) at each tap, and N is the number of subscribers.

Here, $P_T = 1$ mW, $P_N = -40$ dB·m $= 10^{-4}$ mW, and $C = 0.05$. δ may be calculated as follows: the insertion loss (in dB):

$$L = -10 \log_{10} (1 - \delta)$$

Here $L = 0.5$ dB, therefore $d = 0.11$. Thus, one obtains:

$$10^{-4} = 1 \times 0.05 [(1 - 0.11) (1 - 0.05)]^{N-1}$$

This gives $N = 38$. That is, at the most 38 subscribers may be added to the bus without any in-line amplification of the signal.

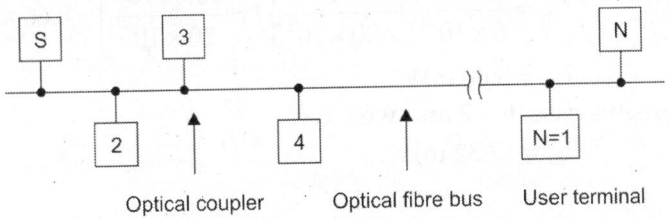

Fig. 12.58: Configuration of distribution network: Bus topology

Example 9

For a multimode fiber, calculate system rise time by using following values of various parameters:

(i) Rise time of LED with drive circuit = 15 ns
(ii) LED spectral width = 40 nm
(iii) Material dispersion related rise time degradation = 21 ns over 6 km link
(iv) Receiver bandwidth = 25 MHz
(v) Model dispersion rise time = 3.9 ns   **[B Tech]**

Solution

We have:

$$t_{rx} = \frac{350}{B_{rx}}$$

∴
$$t_{rx} = \frac{350}{25} = 14 \text{ ns}$$

Here, $t_{tx} = 15$ ns, $t_{mat} = 21$ ns, $t_{mod} = 3.9$ ns

Now:

$$t_{sys} = \left(\sum_{i=1}^{N} t_{ri}^2 \right)^{1/2}$$

∴
$$t_{sys} = [15^2 + 21^2 + 3.9^2 + 14^2]^{1/2} = 29.6 \text{ ns}$$

Example 10

Calculate the SBS threshold power for the worst and best possible cases if the line width of the source is 100 MHz, $g_B = 4 \times 10^{-11}$ m/W, $A_{eff} = 55 \times 10^{-12}$ m^2, $L_{eff} = 20$ km, and $\lambda_p = 1.55$ μm.   **[B Tech]**

Solution

We have at $\lambda_p = 1.55 \mu m$, $\Delta v_B = 20$ MHz. For the worst case, $b = 1$. Therefore, using SBS threshold power, we get:

$$P_{th} = \frac{21 \, b \, A_{eff}}{g_B \, L_{eff}} \left[1 + \frac{\Delta v_{source}}{\Delta v_B} \right]$$

where Δv_{source} is line width of the source, g_B is the Brillion gain, Δv_B very narrow line width, A_{eff} is effective cross-sectional area and the value of b lies between 1 and 2.

$$P_{th} = \frac{21 \times 1 \times 55 \times 10^{-12}}{6 \times 10^{-11} \times 20 \times 10^3} \left[1 + \frac{100 \times 10^6}{20 \times 10^6} \right] = 8.66 \times 10^{-3} \text{ W}$$

or

$$P_{th} = 8.66 \text{ mW}$$

For the best possible case, $b = 2$ and we have:

$$P_{th} = 17.32 \text{ mW}$$

Example 11

Using the following data related to fiber link, compute the system rise time and bandwidth:

Component	BW (MHz)	Rise time (t_r in ns)
Transmitter	200	1.75
LED (850 nm)	100	3.50
Fiber cable	90	3.89
Pin detector	350	1.00
Receiver	180	1.94

[B Tech]

Solution

We have,

$$\text{System rise time} \quad t_{sys} = \left(\sum_{i=1}^{N} t_{ri}^2 \right)^{1/2}$$

or

$$t_{sys} = \sqrt{1.75^2 + 3.5^2 + 3.89^2 + 1.00^2 + 1.94^2} = 593 \text{ ns}$$

Now, system BW is given by:

$$\text{BW} = \frac{0.35}{t_{sys}} = \frac{0.35}{5.93 \text{ ns}} = 59 \text{ MHz}$$

Example 12

For a single mode fiber, $n_2 = 1.48$ and $\Delta = 0.2\%$ operating at $A = 1320$ nm, compute the waveguide dispersion if $V \cdot \dfrac{d^2(Vb)}{dv^2} = 0.26$.

Solution

Here $n_2 = 1.48$,

$$\Delta = 0.2, \text{ and}$$
$$\lambda = 1320 \text{ nm}.$$

Waveguide dispersion is given by:

$$D_{wg}(\lambda) = \frac{-n_2\Delta}{c\lambda}\left[V\frac{d^2\,(Vb)}{dV^2}\right] = \frac{-1.48\times0.2}{3\times10^5\times1320}[0.20]$$

$$= -1.943 \text{ picosec/nm}\cdot\text{km}$$

Example 13

A digital baseband binary optical communication link working at 100 Mbps offers a signal-to-noise ratio of 20. Estimate the bit-error rate (BER) for the system assuming all associated noise components for the system are Gaussian in nature.   **[KTU]**

Solution

Under the given condition, we have

$$\text{BER} = \frac{1}{2}\left[1 - erf\left(\frac{V}{2\sqrt{2}\sigma}\right)\right]$$

$$= \frac{1}{2}\left[1 - erf\,\frac{(S/N)^{1/2}}{2\sqrt{2}}\right]$$

Signal-to-noise ratio is generally measured in terms of power rather than current or voltage ratio unless stated otherwise. Thus, we have

$$\text{BER} = \frac{1}{2}\left[1 - erf\,\frac{\sqrt{20}}{2\sqrt{2}}\right] = \frac{1}{2}[1 - erf\,(1.6)]$$

$$= \frac{1}{2}[1 - 0.9763] = 11.83\times10^{-3}$$

Example 14

An optical fiber link of 5 km length is established by end-to-end splicing of ten pieces of fibers of length 500 m each. If the splice loss at each joint is 0.2 dB and the average loss of the optical fiber at the operating wavelength is 2 dB km^{-1}, calculate the total loss over the link. Assume that the connector losses at the transmitter and receiver end are 2 dB each.
                                             [PTU, DTU]

Solution

We have the number of splices between the ten pieces of fiber is
$$n = 10 - 1 = 9$$
The total splice loss over the link is obtained as
$$S_l = 0.2\times9 = 1.8 \text{ dB}$$
The connector losses are
$$C_i = C_r = 2 \text{ dB}$$
The overall loss of the link is obtained as
$$\mathcal{I} = 2\times5 + 1.8 + 2 + 2$$
$$= 15.8 \text{ dB}$$

Example 15

An average optical power of −6 dBm is launched by the transmitter of an optical fiber data link operating at 100 Mbps. The receiver uses an avalanche photodiode with a sensitivity of 50 dBm. If the average loss introduced by the fiber is 0.5 dBkm^{-1} and the splice loss is 0.2 dB per splice, calculate the repeaterless link length by assuming that the link contains 20 splices and the connection loss at the transmitter and the receiver ends are 2.5 dB and the system requires a safety margin of 8 dB.   **[MHTU, PTU]**

Solution

The total fiber loss over the link is obtained as

$$L_f = 0.5 \times L \text{ dB}$$

The total splice loss is obtained as

$$S_i = 0.2 \times 20 = 4 \text{ dB}$$

Therefore, we have

$$-6 - (-50) = 0.5 \times L + 4 + 2.5 + 2.5 + 8$$

or

$$L = \frac{44 - 17}{0.5} = \frac{27}{0.5} = 54 \text{ km}$$

Example 16

A 30 km long digital optical fiber data link operating at 1330 nm uses an injection laser diode with a spectral width of 0.2 nm. The transmitter offers a rise time of 20 ps. The APD based receiver operates at 2 GBps. The multimode graded-index fiber used in the link offers a chromatic dispersion and modal dispersion of 5 ps and 7 ps respectively over the entire length of the link. Estimate the system rise-time.   **[RTU, DTU]**

Solution

We have the receiver rise-time (assuming NRN format)

$$T_R = \frac{350}{2000} = 0.175 \text{ ns}$$

$$T_{sys} = [(0.02 \text{ ns})^2 + (0.007 \text{ ns})^2 + (0.005 \text{ ns})^2 + (0.175 \text{ ns})^2]^{1/2}$$
$$= 0.175 \text{ ns}$$

This reveals that the overall system rise-time in this case is decided by the rise-time of the receiver circuit.

GLIMPSES

- *Fiber optic communication* has the advantage of high available band-widths and hence, high data rates. Optical communication was enhanced by the invention of lasers and fibers. High cost and special advanced mechanisms to couple and direct light are some of the limitations of fiber-optic communication.
- The important components of a fiber optic communication system are: transmitter, information channel, and receiver.
- System design considerations for point-to-point links are related to two important transmission parameters of optical fibers: (i) fiber attenuation, and (ii) fiber dispersion.
- To ensure that the designed system performance has been met, two types of system analysis are performed: (i) link power budget analysis, and (ii) rise time budget analysis.

Following relation can be used to estimate maximum repeaterless transmission-distance:

$$P_{tx} = P_{rx} + C_L + M_S$$

where P_{tx} is average power supplied by the transmitter, P_{rx} is the sensitivity of the receiver, C_L is total link loss or channel loss (including the fiber splice and connector losses) and M_S is system safety margin.

For the desired bit rate, the *total rise time* (t_{sys}), the digital system should be below its maximum value given by:

$$t_{sys} \leq \begin{cases} \dfrac{0.35}{B} \text{ for RZ format} \\ \dfrac{0.70}{B} \text{ for NRZ format} \end{cases}$$

where RZ stands for return-to-zero (RZ) format, $\Delta f = B$ and NRZ stands for the non-return-to-zero (NRZ) format $\Delta f = B/2$.

The performance of analog systems is normally analyzed by calculating the carrier-to-noise ratio (CNR) of the system.

- *Optical sources*: *Optical transmitter* converts electrical input signal into corresponding optical signal. The optical signal is then launched into the fiber-optical source is the major component in an optical transmitter.

  LED and semiconductor laser diodes (LD) are popularly used optical transmitters.

- *Attenuation*: Attenuation is a measure of decay of signal strength or loss of light power that occurs as light power propagate as light pulses through the length of the fiber.

  In optical fibers the attenuation is mainly caused by two physical factors: absorption and scattering losses. Absorption is because of fiber material and scattering due to structural imperfections within the fiber.

- *Optical receiver*: An optical system converts optical energy into electrical signal, amplify the signal and process it. The important blocks of optical receiver are: Photodetector/Front end, Amplifier/Linear channels, Signal processing circuitry/Data recovery.

- Fiber optic communication systems may be classified into three broad categories: (i) the point-to-point link, (ii) distribution networks, and (iii) local area networks.

- *Point-to-point links*: A point to point link comprises of one transmitter and a receiver system. This is the simplest form of optical communication link and it sets the basis for examining complex optical communication links. For analyzing the performance of any link, important aspects are: (i) distance of transmission, (ii) channel data rate, and (iii) bit error rate.

- *Distributed networks* are preferred when data is to be transmitted to a group of subscribers. The transmission distance is relatively short (< 50 km). Examples of distributed networks are – broadcast of video channels over cable TV, telephone and FAX, commonly used topologies for distributed network are: Hub topology, Bus topology.

- *Local area networks (LAN)*: Several applications of fiber optic communication technology require networks in which a large number of users within local campus are interconnected in such a way that any user can access the network randomly to transmit data to any other user. The commonly used topologies for LANs are: (i) Star topology, (ii) Ring topology.

- In *ring topology*, consecutive nodes are connected by point-to-point links to form a closed link.

- In *star topology*, all nodes are connected through point-to-point link to central node called a hub.

- *WDM*: Optical signals of different wavelength (1300–1600 nm) can propagate without interfering with each other. The scheme of combining a number of wavelengths over a single fiber is called *wavelength division multiplexing* (WDM).

- *Star coupler* is mainly used for combining optical powers from N-inputs and divide them equally at M-output ports.

- *Optical amplifier*: An optical amplifier is nothing but a laser without feedback. Optical gain is achieved when the amplifier is pumped optically or electrically to achieve population inversion. Optical amplification depends on: (i) frequency (or wavelength) of incident signal, and (ii) local beam intensity.

  Optical amplifiers are mainly classified into two types: (i) Semi-conductor optical amplifiers (SOA), and (ii) doped fiber amplifier (DFA).

- There are two types of optical nonlinear effects that place limitations on system performance particularly at high transmitted power levels or at high bit rates exceeding 10 Gb/s: (i) non-linear inelastic process, e.g. SRS and SBS, and (ii) non-linear effects arising from the intensity-independent variation in the refractive index of fiber core, e.g. SPM, CPM, and FWM.

- *Material dispersion* occurs because of refraction varies as a function of the optical wavelength. Dispersion defines pulse spread as a function of wavelength and is measured in picoseconds per kilo-meter per nanometer [ps/(nm·km)]. Dispersion in long haul systems can be compensated using two types of fibers with opposite signs of dispersion.

- *'Soliton'* refers to special kinds of waves that can propagate undistorted over long distances and remain unaffected after collisions with each other. In an optical communication system, solitons are very narrow, high frequency optical pulses that retain their shape through the balancing pulse dispersion with the nonlinear properties of an optical fiber.

Solitons are very narrow optical pulses with high peak powers that retain their shapes as they propagate along the fiber. Owing to GVD, the pulse propagating through the fiber gets broadened. In the anomalous regime (where chromatic dispersion is positive, say, above 1.32 μm in silica-based optical fibers), SPM causes the pulse to narrow, thereby partly compensating the chromatic dispersion. If the relative effects of SPM and GVD for an appropriate pulse shape are controlled properly, the compression of the pulse resulting from SPM can exactly balance the broadening of the pulse due to GVD. Therefore, the pulse shape either does not change or changes periodically as the pulse propagates down the fiber. The family of pulses that do not undergo any change in shape are called *fundamental solitons* and the pulses that undergo periodic changes are known as higher order solitons.

Fundamental solitons along with optical amplifiers offer the promise of very high bit rate transmission over large repeaterless distance.

REVIEW QUESTIONS

1. Draw a relevent diagram showing signal path through optical data link via transmitter, fiber and receiver and describe the nature of the signal wave forms.

2. Give the block diagram of a receiver showing different types of noise generated and derive the expression for each type of noise.

3. Using steady-state amplifier equations and appropriate approximations, derive an analytical expression for an optimum length of fiber which gives maximum amplification.

4. Explain link power budget and rise-time budget analyses? Perform these analyses for a fiber-optic link that uses a conventional single-mode fiber that has been upgraded by DCF loops and optical amplifiers.

5. Mention different types of a system architectures and discuss them. Suggest the application of each of these topologies.

6. Explain non-linear effects observed in optical fibers. Also explain, why do these effects become pronounced at high power levels?

7. Write and define the networks used in communication systems.

8. How many types of topologies are there? Explain each topology.

9. How many types of networks are there based on the size of the area that the network covers? Explain briefly each of them.

10. Explain, how passive linear optical networks perform?

11. Explain the performance of star optical networks.

12. What are transmission links in an optical communication system. Explain each of them.

13. Define and explain SONET and SDH. What do you understand by SONET and SDH transmission rates?

14. What is four-fiber BLSR configuration? Explain briefly.

15. What is FWM? Mention negative effects of FWM in WDM systems. Can it be used in a beneficial way? If yes, how?

16. Define SPM and CPM and explain how SPM can be used to produce fundamental solitons? Write unique properties of solitons.

PROBLEMS

1. Calculate the minimum power required to maintain a bit error of 10^{-6} achieved with a photodiode detector with a responsivity 0.4 A/W. Assuming that the signal-to-noise ratio is limited by thermal noise with 50 W load, 400 K noise temperature and a 10 MHz noise bandwidth. **[Ans. $P_{min} = 1.587\,\mu W$]**

   [**Hint.** we have:

$$20 \log \frac{\langle i_s \rangle}{\langle i_n \rangle} = 19.6 \text{ dB}$$

$$\therefore \quad \frac{\langle i_s \rangle}{\langle i_N \rangle} = 9.55$$

Since $\langle i_N \rangle = \sqrt{\langle i_N \rangle^2}$

Now, $\langle i_s \rangle = 9.55 \langle i_N \rangle^2 = 9.55 \sqrt{\dfrac{4kTB}{R}}$

$$= 9.55 \sqrt{\dfrac{4 \times 1.38 \times 10^{-23} \times 400 \times 10^7}{50}}$$

$$= 6.35 \times 10^{-7} = 635 \text{ NA}$$

Now, $P_{\min} = \dfrac{\langle i_s \rangle}{R} = \dfrac{635 \times 10^{-9}}{0.4} = 1.587 \times 10^{-6} \text{ W} = 1.587 \text{ μW}]$

2. Design an optical fiber link for transmitting 15 Mb/s of data for a distance of 4 km with BER of 10^{-9}.

   [**Hint.** Bandwidth × length = 15 Mb/s × 4 km = (60 Mb/s) km

   (i) *Optical source*: LED at 820 nm is suitable for short distances. LED generates 120 dB·m optical power.

   (ii) *Optical detector*: PIN-FET optical detector is reliable and has 50 dB·m sensitivity.

   (iii) *Optical fiber*: Step index multimode fiber can be selected. This fiber has bandwidth length product of 100 (Mb/s) km.

   Link power budget: We assume:

   Splicing loss = 0.5 dB/slice

   Connector loss = 1.5 dB

   System link power margin, $P_m = 8$ dB

   Fiber attenuation, $\alpha_f = 6$ dB/km

   Actual total loss $= (2 \times l_c) + \alpha_f L + P_m$

   or $P_T = (2 \times 1.5) + (6 \times 4) + 8 = 35$ dB

   Maximum permissible system loss

   $P_{\max}$ = Optical source output power – Optical receiver sensitivity

   $\quad = -10 \text{ dB·m} - (-50 \text{ dB·m}) = 40 \text{ dB·m}$

   We see that actual losses in the system are less than the allowable loss, hence the system is functional.

3. A type-I intensity-modulated fiber-optic link employs a laser trans-mitter which couples a mean optical power of 0 dB·m into a multi-mode optical fiber cable. The cable exhibits an attenuation of 3.0 dB/km with splice losses estimated at 0.5 dB/km. A connector at the receiver end shows a loss of another 1.5 dB. The *p-i-n* photodiode receiver has a sensitivity of –25 dB·m for a CNR of –50 dB with a modulation index of 0.5. A safety margin of 7 dB is required. The rise times of ILD and *p-i-n* diode are 1 ns and 5 ns, respectively, and the intermodal and intramodal rise times of the fiber cable are 9 ns/km and 2 ns/km, respectively. (i) What is the maximum possible link length without repeaters? (ii) What is the maximum permitted 3-dB bandwidth of the system? **[B Tech]**

   [**Hint:**

   (i) *Link power budget*: The mean optical power coupled into the fiber cable by the laser transmitter $(P_{tx}) = 0$ dB·m, the mean optical power required at the *p-i-n* receiver $(P_{rx}) = -25$ dB·m, and the total system margin $(P_{tx} - P_{rx}) = 25$ dB.

   Let us assume that the repeaterless link length is L. Then, using following Eq.

   $$C_L = \alpha_f L + \alpha_{con} + \alpha_{splice}$$

where α_f is the fiber loss in (dB/km), L is link length, α_{con} is the sum of the losses at all the connectors in the link, and α_{splice} is the sum of the losses at all the splices in the link. C_L, α_{con} and α_{splice} are expressed in dB, the total channel loss C_L may be calculated as follows:

C_L = (attenuation/km) $\times$ L + (splice loss/km) $\times$ L + connector loss

$\quad$ = (3 dB/km) $\times$ L + (0.5 dB/km) $\times$ L + 1.5 dB

$\quad$ = (3.5 L + 1.5) dB

Therefore, from Eq. $P_{tx} = P_{rx} + C_L + M_S$

or $\quad P_{tx} - P_{rx} = C_L + M_S$, we obtain

$\qquad$ 25 dB = [(3.5 L + 1.5) + 7] dB

or $\qquad L = \dfrac{16.5}{3.5} = 4.7$ km

(ii) *Rise-time budget*:

$$t_f^2 = [(9 \text{ ns/km} \times 4.7 \text{ km})^2 + (2 \text{ ns/km} \times 4.7 \text{ km})^2]$$
$$= 1877.65 \text{ ns}^2$$

$$t_{sys} = (t_{tx}^2 + t_f^2 + t_{rx}^2)^{1/2} = \{(1 \text{ ns})^2 + 1.877.65 \text{ ns}^2 + (5 \text{ ns})^2\}^{1/2}$$
$$= 43.63$$

The system bandwidth:

$$\Delta f = \frac{0.35}{t_{sys}} = \frac{0.35}{43.6 \times 10^{-9}} \text{ Hz} = 8 \times 10^6 \text{ Hz} = 8 \text{ MHz}$$

Thus, the proposed link length without repeaters is 4.7 km with a 3 dB bandwidth of 8 MHz.]

SHORT ANSWER QUESTIONS

1. Write the names of important parts of an optical transmitter?
   Ans. (i) Interface circuit, (ii) Source driver circuit, (iii) An optical source.
2. What is an optical fiber receiver?
   Ans. An optical fiber receiver is an electro-optic device that accepts optical signals from an optical fiber and converts them into electrical signals.
3. What is an optical detector?
   Ans. An optical detector is a device that converts optical signal into electrical signal. The electrical signal is proportional to the intensity of the optical radiation.
4. What are the basic applications of optical amplifiers (OAs)?
   Ans. OAs can be used to boost signal power after multiplexing, or before demultiplexing, or at any point in modern optical net-works. OAs are ideal for metro and long-haul dense wavelength multiplexing (DWDM) as well as single wavelength applications.
5. What is wavelength division multiplexing (WDM)?
   Ans. WDM is an optical technology that permits several wavelengths to be coupled into the same fiber cable, effectively increasing the aggregation bandwidth per fiber cable.
6. What is an optical receiver?
   Ans. Optical receivers are an essential part of a communication system. An optical receiver converts an optical signal, transmitted through an optical fiber cable into an electrical signal suitable for a receiving device installed at the other end of the communication system. The conversion process in the receiver is performed by two

essential parts: (i) a detector (ii) an electronic signal processor. The detector converts the optical signal into an electrical signal. The electronic signal processor converts the raw detector signal into a form decipherable by the receiving device, such as a telephone, camera, or scanner.

7. What are the important parameters which define the performance of an optical receiver?

   Ans. (i) Receiver sensitivity (ii) Bandwidth and (iii) Dynamic range.

8. How the signal is carried in fiber optic cable?

   Ans. Through photons. Photon is a quanta of energy ($E = h\upsilon$). Photon energy depend only on the frequency υ.

9. Why the optical fiber cables are not used for point to point transmiossion?

   Ans. We know that transmission through metal wires requires simple circuitry. Point to point transmission from one device to another using metal wire is much simple than using optical fibers as they don't require the use of transmitter and receiver. However, optical fibers are preferred when data rates becomes too high.

10. What is the speed of laboratory optical fiber local area networks (LANs)?

    Ans. Hundreds of megabits per second. Optical fibers and LANs are the hottest communication technologies now. The main problem in optical fibers is the implementation of couplers and extra cost of optical fiber equipment. We know that metal wires and coaxial cables can operate from 1 Mb/s to 10 Mb/s. Optical fiber connec-ted Lans which were tested, were operating at 100 Mb/s and up and so far not exceeded far from this value.

11. What is dispersion?

    Ans. Dispersion is caused by the expansion of light pulses as they travel through optical components. This occurs because the speed of light through the optical medium is dependent on the wavelength, the propagation mode, and the optical properties of the material along the light path. Dispersion is given by:

    $$D = \frac{1}{L}\frac{d\tau_g}{d\lambda} = \frac{d}{d\lambda}\left(\frac{1}{V_g}\right) = \frac{2\pi c}{\lambda^2}\beta_2$$

    The factor $\beta_2 = d^2b/d\omega^2$ is the GVD parameter, which determines how much a light pulse broadens as it travels along an optical fiber. Dispersion defines the pulse spread as a function of wavelength and is measured in picoseconds per kilometer per nano-meter [ps/(nm·km)].

12. What is the speed of laboratory fiber optic local area networks?

    Ans. Hundreds of megabits per second. Presently, fiber optics and LANs are the hottest communication technologies. The main problem in the optical fibers is the implementation of couplers and the extra cost of fiber optic equipment. Metal wires and coaxial cables can operate from 1 Mb/s to 10 Mb/s. Optical fibers connected LANs which were tested operating at 100 Mb/s and up but so far not exceeded this figure.

13. What are solitons?

    Ans. Solitons are very narrow optical pulses with high peak powers that retain their shapes as they propagate along the fiber.

    Group velocity dispersion (GVD) causes most pulses to broaden in time as they propagate through an optical fiber. However, a soliton takes advantage of nonlinear effects in silica, particularly, *self phase modulation* (SPM), resulting from Kerr nonlinearity, to overcome the pulse-broadening effects of GVD.

The term *soliton* refers to special kind of waves that can propagate undistorted over long distances and remain unaffected after collisions with each other. In an optical communication system, solitons are very narrow, high-intensity optical pulses that retain their shape through the interaction of balancing pulse dispersion with the nonlinear properties of an optical fiber.

14. What stands FTTB?

Ans. FTTB means *"Fiber to the building"* and refers to installing optical fiber from the telephone company central office to a specific building such as a business or apartment house.

15. What stands FITH?

Ans. FITH means *"fiber to the home"* is network technology that deploys fiber optic cable directly to the home or business to deliver voice, video or data services.

16. What stands FTTC?

Ans. FTTC stands for *"fiber to the curb"* and refers to the installation and use of optical fiber cable directly to the curbs near homes or any business environment as replacement for plain old telephone service (POTS).

17. What is SONET?

Ans. SONET is synchronous optical networking. General SONET equipment uses one wavelength to carry an OC level, which can be divided into time slots for individual circuits. In Europe and Asia, SONET is known as SDH (synchronous digital hierarchy).

18. What is HFC?

Ans. Hybrid fiber coax (HFC) is a way of delivering video, voice telephony, data and other interactive services over coaxial and fiber optic cables.

An HFC network consists of a headend office, distribution center, fiber nodes, and network interface units.

19. What is dense wavelength division multiplexing (DWDM)?

Ans. DWDM is an optical technology used to increase bandwidth over existing fiber-optic backbones.

DWDM works by combining and transmitting multiple signals simultaneously at differen wavelengths on the same fibers.

20. Write the names of different components of an optical fiber communication system.

Ans. (i) Optical transmitter, (ii) Fiber channel, (iii) Optical amplifier, (iv) Optical detector.

21. What makes optical fibers immune to EMI?

Ans. Optical fibers transmit signals in a light rather than electric current. This is the main reason that optical fibers are immune to EMI, which is a type of noise that originates with one of the properties of electromagnetism. We know that EMI is induced when magnetic field lines are cut across a conductor.

22. What is topological reconfiguration?

Ans. Topological reconfiguration relies on the capability of the transmission subsystem to establish an alternate data path in case of failure by changing its basic topology. This reconfigured topology should allow the live stations to operate normally despite the fault condition. We may note that this is very effective for protection against fiber breaks and applies specifically to an active structure.

23. Which method permits large number of independent, selectable channels to exist on a single fiber.

Ans. Frequency division multiplexing (FDM). Using FDM, multiple frequencies of light, i.e. multiple channels can coexist on a single optical fiber.

MULTIPLE CHOICE QUESTIONS

1. One aspect of SONET that has allowed it to survive during a time of tremendous changes in network capacity needs is its:
   (a) functionality
   (b) capability
   (c) versatility
   (d) scalability

2. The key requirement/requirements needed in analyzing a link is/are
   (a) data rate
   (b) distance of transmission
   (c) bit-error rate
   (d) All of the above

3. The bit duration of a 2.5-Gbits/s signal is:
   (a) 2.5 ns
   (b) 1 ns
   (c) 0.4 ns
   (d) 0.1 ns

4. For a passive star network, the total optical power supplied by the central node is 1 mW and that received at the terminal nodes is 0.1 μW. If the fractional insertion loss at each coupler is 0.05, what is the number of subscribers (nodes)?
   (a) 50
   (b) 100
   (c) 250
   (d) 500

5. Which of the following is a non-linear inelastic process?
   (a) SRS
   (b) SPM
   (c) CPM
   (d) FWM

6. Which of the following non-linear effects arise from the intensity-dependent variation of the refractive index of a fiber?
   (a) SPM
   (b) CPM
   (c) FWM
   (d) All of these

7. Assuming the fiber link span to be large, what will be its effective length if the attenuation per unit length is taken to be 0.20 dB/km?
   (a) 95.6 km
   (b) 50.2 km
   (c) 22.2 km
   (d) 10 km

8. A typical standard dispersion-shifted fiber has a dispersion parameter of 16 ps·nm^{-1}·km^{-1}. The repeaterless fiber length is 50 km. What should be the dispersion parameter of a DCF of length 2 km in order to compensate for the accumulated dispersion of the DSF for a repeaterless distance?
   (a) 180 ps·nm^{-1}·km^{-1}
   (b) −80 ps·nm^{-1}·km^{-1}
   (c) −200 ps·nm^{-1}·km^{-1}
   (d) −400 ps·nm^{-1}·km^{-1}

9. A fiber-optic link of length 50 km has two splices each exhibiting a loss of 1 dB. The fiber itself has a rated 0.2 dB/km loss. If the minimum power required to run a photodetector is 20 nW, what power must be supplied by the optical source?
   (a) 20 nW
   (b) 0.317 μW
   (c) 0.317 mW
   (d) 0.90 mW

10. A fiber used in a typical link has $(\Delta T)_{mat} = 3$ ns/km and $(\Delta T)_{modal} = 1$ ns/km. The link length is 8 km. The rise times of the transmitter and receiver are 12 ns and 11 ns, respectively. The total rise time of the system is:
    (a) 30 ns
    (b) 35 ns
    (c) 23 ns
    (d) 57 ns

11. The channel loss C_L may be expressed by the following equation (symbols have usual meanings):
    (a) $C_L = \alpha_f L + \alpha_{con} + \alpha_{splice}$
    (b) $C_L = \alpha_f - \alpha_{con} + \alpha_{splice}$
    (c) $C_L = \alpha_f L - \alpha_{con} - \alpha_{splice}$
    (d) $C_L = \alpha_f L + \alpha_{con} - \alpha_{splice}$

12. For a fiber-optic communication system, the total rise time t_{sys} in terms of electrical bandwidth Δf may be written as:
    (a) $t_{sys} = \dfrac{0.65}{\Delta f}$
    (b) $t_{sys} = \dfrac{0.35}{\Delta f}$
    (c) $t_{sys} = \dfrac{1}{\Delta f}$
    (d) $t_{sys} = \dfrac{0.1}{\Delta f}$

13. Which of the following relation for t_{sys} for digital system is correct?
    (a) $t_{sys} \leq \begin{cases} \dfrac{0.65}{B} & \text{for RZ format} \\ \dfrac{0.75}{B} & \text{for NRZ format} \end{cases}$
    (b) $t_{sys} \leq \begin{cases} \dfrac{0.35}{B} & \text{for RZ format} \\ \dfrac{0.70}{B} & \text{for NRZ format} \end{cases}$
    (c) $t_{sys} \leq \begin{cases} \dfrac{0.70}{B} & \text{for RZ format} \\ \dfrac{0.35}{B} & \text{for NRZ format} \end{cases}$
    (d) $t_{sys} \leq \begin{cases} \dfrac{0.15}{B} & \text{for RZ format} \\ \dfrac{0.65}{B} & \text{for NRZ format} \end{cases}$

14. If the number of wavelength channels in a WDM system is 10, what will be number of frequencies created by four-wave mixing?
    (a) 300
    (b) 1000
    (c) 450
    (d) 900

15. Which of the following process is used to compensate for the GVD-induced dispersion in a soliton?
    (a) FWM
    (b) SPM
    (c) CPM
    (d) All of the above

16. The carrier-to-noise ratio (CNR) for the performance of analog system is defined as:
    (a) $CNR = \dfrac{\text{rms carrier power}}{\text{rms noise power}}$
    (b) $CNR = \dfrac{\text{carrier frequency}}{\text{noise frequency}}$
    (c) $CNR = \dfrac{\text{carrier power}}{\text{noise power}}$
    (d) None of the above

17. For N wavelength channels copropagating through the optical fiber, the number of generated frequencies is:
    (a) $M = \dfrac{N^2}{2}$
    (b) $M = \dfrac{N}{2}(N-1)$
    (c) $M = \dfrac{N^2}{2}(N-1)$
    (d) $M = N(N-1)^2$

18. If D_1 and D_2 are the dispersion parameters of the two types of fibers and L_1 and L_2 are their respective lengths, then the condition for perfect dispersion compensation is:
(a) $D_1L_1 + D_2L_2 = 1$ (b) $D_1L_1 + D_2L_2 = 100$
(c) $D_1L_1 + D_2L_2 = 0$ (d) $D_1L_1 + D_2L_2 = 1000$

19. Scattering related non-linear effects in single channel and multichannel optical fibers respectively are:
(a) stimulated Brillouin scattering, stimulated Raman scattering
(b) stimulated Raman scattering, stimulated Brillouin scattering
(c) self phase modulation, cross-phase modulation: four wave mixing
(d) none of the above

20. If n_0 is the ordinary refractive index of the optical material, then the dependence of refractive index of many optical materials exhibiting weak dependence on optical intensity (equal to the optical power (P) per effective area A_{eff}) having n_2 as nonlinear index coefficience is governed by the relation:
(a) $n = n_2 I = n_2 \dfrac{P}{A_{eff}}$ (b) $n = n_0 + n_2 I = n_0 + n_2 \dfrac{P}{A_{eff}}$
(c) $n = n_0 \dfrac{P}{A_{eff}}$ (d) $n = \dfrac{n_0}{n_2} I = \dfrac{n_2}{n_0} \dfrac{P}{A_{eff}}$

21. Four-wave mixing (FWM) in silica fibers is:
(a) single-order nonlinearity   (b) second-order nonlinearity
(c) third-order nonlinearity   (d) none of the above

22. A 75 km link of dispersion-shifted fiber carrying two wavelengths at 1540.0 nm and 1540.5 nm. The new frequencies generated due to FWM are:
(a) 1539.5 nm, 1541.0 nm   (b) 1540.5 nm, 1540.0 nm
(c) 1541.0 nm, 1542.0 nm   (d) 1539.0 nm, 1540.0 nm
[**Hint:** $v_{112} = 2v_1 - v_2 = 2\,(1540.0\text{ nm}) - 1540.5\text{ nm} = 1539.5\text{ nm}$,
and $v_{221} = 2v_2 - v_1 = 2\,(1540.5\text{ nm}) - 1540.0\text{ nm} = 1540\text{ nm}]$

ANSWERS

1. (d)   2. (d)   3. (c)   4. (d)   5. (a)   6. (d)   7. (c)   8. (d)   9. (b)   10. (a)
11. (a)   12. (b)   13. (b)   14. (d)   15. (c)   16. (a)   17. (c)   18. (c)   19. (a)   20. (b)
21. (c)   22. (a)

13

Fiber Optic Measurement and Testing

13.1 INTRODUCTION

In this chapter, we are primarily concerned with the successful implementation of optical fiber communication system which need careful design, measurement, and testing of various optoelectronic devices and components. We have read that the major components of a typical optical fiber communication system/network include:
- Optical fibers/cables
- Optical sources
- Optical detectors
- Optical amplifiers
- Optical splitters/couplers/connectors.

We have also read that in optical fiber communication systems, both single mode and multimode fibers are used. The selection of the optical fiber to be used generally depends on the nature of the application.

13.2 MEASUREMENT STANDARDS

There are large number of manufacturers of optical fibers and devices with slightly different characteristics. All these components and devices need to maintain certain standards for their deployment in optical fiber system networks.

Several international organizations and bodies, e.g. National Institute of Standards and Technology in USA, National Physical Laboratory, UK, etc. are involved for standardization. Various national level standardizations are available in different countries for testing and characterization of fundamental parameters of optical fibers, e.g. attenuation, dispersion, bandwidth, mode-field diameter, etc.

There are several international bodies and organizations, e.g. Telecommunication Industries Association (TIA) in association with Electronic Industries Alliance (EIA) in the form of TIA/EIA; American National Standard Institute (ANSI); International Electrotechnical Association (IEC); Institute of Electrical and Electronic Engineers (IEEE), etc. are involved in setting up standards for testing optical fiber components and optical devices and also formulate procedures for calibration of optical measuring and testing equipment. Table 13.1 provides a list of a few reference number published in TIA publication, 2000 (TIA, 2000) for standard measurement and testing procedures.

ANSI, ITU-T, and IEEE have prescribed the system standards for optical links and networks. Table 13.2 provides some of recent recommendations for optical links and networks prescribed by the said agencies.

Table 13.1: TIA/EIA standards (TIA, 2000)	
Reference Number	*Specification items*
ANSI/EIA/TIA-455-A-1994	Standard test procedures for optical fibers, cables, transducers, sensors, connectors and other components and terminal devices.
ANSI/TIA/EIA-526-7-1998	Optical power loss measurements of installed single mode fiber cable
ANSI/TIA/EIA-526-14-A-1998	Optical power loss measurements of installed multimode fiber cable
ANSI/TIA/EIA-598-A-1995	Optical fiber cable color coding
ANSI/TIA/EIA-604-3-1997	Fiber optic connector intermateability standard

Table 13.2: Some prescribed recommendations for ITU-T standard terms of reference for optical links and networks

Recommendation reference	*Year*	*Relevant Network Aspect*
ITU-T G.652	2003	Characteristics of single-mode optical fiber
ITU-T G.982	1996	Optical access networks to support services up to the ISDN primary rate
ITU-T G.983.3	2001	Broadband optical access system with increased service capability by wavelength allocation
ITU-T G.984.2	2003	Gigabit-capable passive optical networks (GPON): Physical media dependent (PMD) layer specification
ITU-T G.984.3	2008	Gigabit-capable passive optical networks (GPON): Transmission convergence layer specification
ITU-T G.691	2006	Optical interfaces for single channel STM-64 and other SDH systems with optical amplifiers
ITU-T G.694.1	2002	Spectral grids for WDM applications: DWDM frequency grid
ITU-T G.709/Y.1331	2012	Interfaces for the optical transport network
ITU-T G.783	2006	Characteristics of synchronous digital hierarchy (SDH) equipment functional blocks
ITU-T G.872	2001	Architecture of optical transport networks
ITU-T G.873.1	2006	Optical transport network (OTN): Linear protection
ITU-T G.874	2008	Management aspects of optical transport network elements
ITU-T G.957	2006	Optical interfaces for equipments and systems relating to the synchronous digital hierarchy
ITU-T G.959.1	2009	Optical transport network physical layer interfaces

13.3 TESTING PHOTONIC COMPONENTS

The testing of optical fiber devices is based on two different measurements aspects of light output: *power* and *frequency*. Power measurements refer to light intensity, as measured by photosensitive devices, usually called photodetectors (e.g. photodiodes and photosensors). The photodetectors generate an electrical signal proportional to the intensity (or power) of the incident light, thus allowing measurement of the light power. Photosensitive devices will not, however, react differently to different light frequencies. They will be more sensitive to certain frequencies while not being able to detect others. Because of this frequency dependence, power meters are calibrated for predetermined frequencies only. To ensure accurate readings, it is very important to verify the calibration of the power meter, before making any power measurements.

Photodetectors also depend on the polarization of the incident light. Different polarizations will generate different current intensities in the photosensitive devices, thus affecting the power readings during measurement. Polarization effects can be seen when measuring light power for a fibre optic device while moving the fibres or optical components. Movements will change the polarization of the light passing into the device, causing the power readings to fluctuate slightly. For this reason, fibers and/or optical components should not be moved during test measurements.

Polarization measurements require more complex calculations than power measurement alone. Many methods have been developed over the years to calculate the polarization dependent loss (PDL) of optical fiber devices. For each state of polarization, a device will absorb varying amounts of light. Thus, in order to determine the PDL of a device, the device needs to be illuminated with all possible polarization states while measuring the loss for each. Then the maximum difference in loss for all the polarization states can be calculated. This process is tedious and time-consuming. However, another calculation method, known as the Mueller matrix, allows the calculation of the PDL with enough accuracy using only four basic polarization states (linear 0, 90, 45° and circular polarizations). Using this matrix calculation method significantly reduces the time required to measure the PDL of any device. This algorithm is used in most PDL meters today to perform measurements.

The frequency of light refers to the colour of the light. Colours cannot be determined simply with the use of a photosensitive cell alone. Instead, comparison methods are used to determine the colour of light. A reference beam of light (a laser with a known and fixed single wavelength, such as a HeNe laser or another gas laser) is combined with the beam of light to be tested. From the interference of the two beams, the frequency of the incident beam can be determined. This method requires a more complex test circuit and more components (e.g. reference laser) than power measurements. This is why wavelength meters are more expensive and bigger than power meters. Furthermore, the alignment between the test beam and the reference beam is a critical factor in analysing the interference of the two beams. Thus, it is crucial to exercise caution when handling wavelength meters, to avoid misalignment of the internal optical components of the wavelength meter.

Calibration is always an issue in measurement practices for optical devices. The calibration of a power meter involves knowledge of the electrical properties of photodetectors. From this knowledge, calculations can establish the relationship between the current generated by the photodetector and the intensity of the test beam measured at a specific light wavelength. Lasers with adjustable light intensity are used to calibrate power meters with respect to a master power meter. The power measured by the power meter has to be equal to the power detected by the master power meter. Any deviation is recorded, and the values (constants) are adjusted in the calculation algorithms of the power meter. Power meters need to be calibrated on a regular basis, because the properties of the photodetectors are known to change over time. Power meters can be calibrated in a very short time using software.

Wavelength meters also need to be calibrated for power measurements. They too use photodetectors, which measure the power of the interfering beam of light in order to determine the light colour. Improper power calibration could result in incorrect readings.

Frequency measurements do not, however, only require power calibration in terms of seconds; they also require proper optical alignment. Thus, full calibration of this equipment requires opening the device box and realigning the internal optical components. Further calibration of a wavelength meter requires the skills of a qualified technician for aligning the optical parts.

As explained earlier, the optical fibre measurements can be divided into two types:

(i) Optical power measurements (intensity I in watts)
(ii) Optical frequency measurements (wavelength λ in metres)

13.4 OPTICAL POWER MEASUREMENTS (INTENSITY)

13.4.1 Optical Power Measurement Units

Three common units are used in optical power measurements:

- *Linear* (mW): The milliwatt is the standard unit of measurement. For example, typical communications lasers used are in the range of 1–10 mW.
- *Logarithmic* (*absolute*) (dBm): In the absolute scale, 0 dBm = 1 mW.

$$P_{dBm} = 10 \times \log_{10}(P_{mW}) \tag{13.1}$$

- *Logarithmic* (*relative*) (dB): Indicates a change in power level independent of the absolute power at the input,

$$L_{dB} = P_{in}(dBm) - P_{out}(dBm) \tag{13.2}$$

13.4.2 Optical Power Loss Measurements

Insertion Loss (IL)

Insertion loss (IL) occurs in all optical fiber devices, such as fibre optic cables, optical passband filters, and optical switches, which are discussed in more detail throughout the text.

Consider an optical switch as an example. An optical switch redirects the optical signal in one or another direction or path, with low attenuation (loss) of the light. Thus, a very important parameter to test for a switch is the IL. Internal components of a switch (such as lenses, mirrors, or prisms) will always attenuate the light intensity, because of either absorption, diffraction, diffuse reflection, or scattering. Thus, the power transmitted out of the switch is less than the power incident on the switch. Thus, IL is never zero. For best switch performance, the IL should be as low as possible for all the paths of the switch.

A common procedure is used in testing optical fibre devices for IL. Using a single-wavelength laser source, the IL can be measured with a power meter calibrated for that wavelength. All optical testing procedures described below are based on this IL test. The procedure remains more or less the same; only the test parameters will change.

The intensity of light at one of the output ports, specified in dB, is attenuated, relative to the input signal power. The general light-loss formula is used to calculate the insertion loss, as given in the following equation:

$$IL(dB) = -10 \log_{10} \frac{P_{out}}{P_{in}} \tag{13.3}$$

A perfect optical device would have no internal losses and would transmit 100% of the incident light ($P_{in} = P_{out}$). In other words, IL = 0 dB in ideal device.

Figure 13.1 shows the basic test set up for using the insertion loss technique to measure attenuation of cables that have attached connectors, where the launch and detector couplings are made through connectors. The wavelength-tunable light source is coupled to a short length of fiber that has the same basic characteristics as the fiber to be tested. For multimode fibers, a mode scrambler is used to ensure that the fiber core contains an equilibrium-mode distribution. In single-mode fibers, a cladding-mode stripper is employed so that only the fundamental mode is allowed to propagate along the fiber. A wavelength-selective device, such as an optical filter, is generally included to find the attenuation as a function of wavelength.

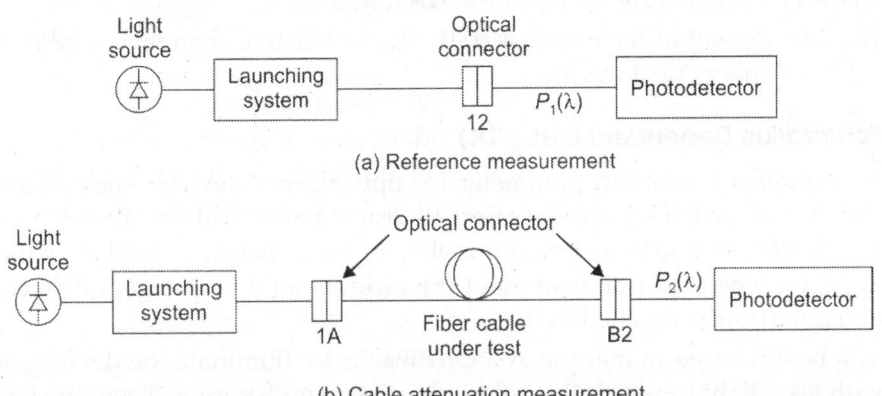

(a) Reference measurement

(b) Cable attenuation measurement

Fig. 13.1: Test setup for using the insertion-loss technique to measure attenuation of cables that have attached connectors

To carry out the attenuation tests, the connector of the short-length launching fiber is attached to the connector of the receiving system and the launch-power level $P_1(\lambda)$ is recorded. Next, the cable assembly to be tested is connected between the launching and receiving systems, and the received-power level $P_2(\lambda)$ is recorded. The attenuation of the cable in decibels is then

$$A = 10 \log \frac{P_1(\lambda)}{P_2(\lambda)} \tag{13.4}$$

This attenuation is the sum of the loss of the cabled fiber and the connector between the launch connector and the cable.

13.4.3 Crosstalk

The purpose of an optical switch, as mentioned above, is to redirect the light in one, and only one, direction (channel). Ideally, when activating a switch, all the incoming light will go through one specific output port (active port), and no light at all will go through any other output port (inactive port). Therefore, in addition to measuring the IL for the active path, the loss for all the inactive paths must be measured, in order to discover if light leaks to other channels. In theory, all light is transmitted through the active channel, and absolutely no light goes through the inactive channels. In practice, however, this is not always the case. Diffuse reflection, diffraction or backreflection of the incident light on an internal component of a switch will redirect the light elsewhere inside the switch. This light can escape from the package by any other input or output port of the switch, depending on where the light is headed. This leakage of light into another channel can be measured in a manner similar to that used for the IL; the IL for the inactive channel (through which no light should be traveling) can be measured. The same procedure as used for the IL test is employed here, except that the optical path chosen is not the active path. The leak towards a wrong or inactive output port is calculated with the same formula used to calculate the IL of the active port, but P_{out} is measured at an inactive output port.

Crosstalk (XT) is the leakage from the active channel into the inactive channel. Crosstalk between channels (ports) occurs in optical devices, such as filters, wavelength separators, and switches. Crosstalk is critically detrimental in wavelength division multiplexer systems. When signals from one channel arrive in another undesired channel, they become noise in the other channel. This can have serious effects on the signal-to-noise ratio, and, hence, on the error rate of the communication system.

A perfect device would have no crosstalk (P_{out} of inactive channel = 0 mW). In other words, XT = $-\infty$ in a perfect device.

13.4.4 Polarization Dependent Loss (PDL)

The PDL is another important parameter for optical fiber devices, such as an optical switch. An optical switch should not affect or distort the optical signal, only re-route it. Therefore, the PDL should be as low as possible for the active path. The loss in the switch should not vary when the polarization of the incident light is changed. Any change in loss due to polarization is called PDL.

PDL can be measured in many ways. One way is to illuminate the device under test (DUT) with laser light in which the polarization state is changing. Then, the loss for all possible states of polarization can be measured. However, as mentioned earlier, this method consumes too much time and too many resources to be cost-effective for companies to use routinely.

In order to measure the PDL property of a device, one of the most popular techniques used in manufacturing is the Mueller method. Mueller discovered that, by using the four basic light polarization states of the light (linear 0, 45, 90°, and circular polarization), the PDL can be calculated with great accuracy in a few seconds. Quite complex, the calculations take the form of the *Mueller matrix*. Most PDL meters use this matrix to calculate the PDL of a device.

PDL meters have a built-in laser source of known polarization, combined with a power detector, and also include polarizing filters, which can be moved in and out of the laser path to vary the polarization.

Because the components included in the PDL meter are expensive and their alignment needs to be precise, the cost of a PDL meter is much higher than that of a power meter. Also, because the PDL meter has to adjust the polarization of the light to take four measurements and then perform a calculation, it takes approximately 1s before the PDL value is refreshed on the display. Further-more, any change in the light path can modify the PDL value, so it is very important that the components and fibres do not move during the measurement. If the fibre optic cables of the device are moving during testing, the PDL values will change on the display unit and will not be as accurate.

There are three other polarization effects: *polarization dependent gain* (PDG) in optical amplifiers; *polarization mode dispersion* (PMD) in optical fibers; and *polarization dependent modulation* (PDM) in electro-optic modulators. These polarization effects occur in almost all other optical fibre devices transmitting polarized light. Such devices are *polarizing beam-splitter devices* and *erbium doped fiber amplifiers*.

We may note that in contrast to chromatic dispersion which is relatively a stable phenomenon along a fiber, PMD varies randomly along a fiber, because of the randomness of the underlying geometric and stress irregularities. Thus statistical predictions are needed to account for its effects. A useful means of characterizing PMD is in terms of the mean or the expected value of the differential group delay average over time:

$$\langle \Delta \tau_{pol} \rangle_\lambda = \frac{kN_e \, \lambda_{start} \, \lambda_{stop}}{2\,(\lambda_{start} - \lambda_{stop})\,c} \tag{13.5}$$

where λ_{start} and λ_{stop} are in beginning and end, respectively, of the wavelength measurement sweep, N_e represents the number of extrema occuring in the scan, and c is the speed of light. The dimensionless mode-coupling factor k statistically the polarization states. The value of k is 0.84 for randomly mode-coupled fibers and 1.0 for non-mode coupled fibers and devices.

13.4.5 Return Loss (RL) or Backreflection

The return loss (RL) of the DUT should be as high as possible, depending on the definition of loss. This is because having a large amount of incident light reflecting back into the system is not desired. Light reflected back towards the light source can damage the source, especially when laser light is employed.

A small portion of incident light will always be reflected due to a change in the refractive index between two adjacent surfaces. This reflection can be reduced when an antireflective coating is applied to one of the surfaces, or by using angled surfaces along the path of light. It is difficult, however, to eliminate any undesired reflection completely. Furthermore, a microbend in a fiber optic cable, glue joint, or anywhere else along the path of light, will create backreflection.

In order to measure the backreflection, the path of light must be terminated. A situation must be created in which all the transmitted light in the device will dissipate or diffract in the fiber and escape the device. To achieve this situation, the fiber needs to be coiled into fiber loops of a very small diameter (usually around 1–2 cm). This is the only situation in which it is acceptable to coil the fiber in very small loops. Careful coiling of the fibers is important so as not to coil part of the fiber onto another fiber loop. This coiling could crush the fiber underneath and create damage.

13.4.6 Temperature Dependent Loss

In most cases, an optical device, such as an optical switch, is used inside a module containing many other devices. These can include optical devices (e.g., couplers and filters) and electrical devices (e.g. switch controller, power supply, and fan). Because of the electronic components creating heat inside the module, the temperature can rise and/ or fluctuate, so that the switch will almost never operate at ambient temperature. Therefore, the temperature properties of the DUT need to be measured.

The temperature dependent losses (TDL) are measured through the use of a test called the thermal gradient stability test, which consists of cycling the temperature of the DUT and measuring the optical losses of the DUT over the temperature range.

Usually, the operating temperature range of an optical module is small, varying from –10 to –40°C, to less than + 100°C. Under these small temperature changes he properties of the materials composing the switch will only change slightly (on the order of microns), and the effect on the optical properties will be small. Such a small loss, usually less than 1 dB, is significant for the IL and PDL, but are not significant for XT or RL. This is wh usually only the IL and sometimes PDL are measured over the temperature range for a switch.

However, only the steady state losses are measured to calculate the TDL; the transient losses are not considered. Thus, the measurements are performed when the temperature has been achieved and the losses stabilized. Then a simple subtraction (maximum loss value achieved over the temperature range minus the minimum loss value achieved over the temperature range) is calculated.

The parameters most affected by temperature are the IL and PDL, as mentioned above. The variation of IL over temperature is called TDL. However, the PDL difference over the temperature range is not measured; instead, the maximum PDL value achieved over the temperature range is given, and it is called Max PDL over temperature.

13.4.7 Wavelength Dependent Loss

Because of the properties of the antireflection (AR) coating on the lens and other optical components of an optical fiber device, the IL can vary depending on the wavelength of the incident light. The variation of IL over a wavelength range is called the wavelength dependent loss (WDL). It is also sometimes called the wavelength flatness or transmission curve. The WDL is a direct consequence of any coating or physical properties of the materials composing the optical fiber device.

In an optical switch, the AR coating must be able to transmit all the wavelengths with the same efficiency and have a WDL as low as possible. Thus, the difference between the IL measured at 1310, 1480 or 1550 nm should be near zero.

13.4.8 Chromatic Dispersion

All forms of dispersion degrade a light wave signal, reducing the data-carrying capacity through pulse broadening. Chromatic dispersion results from a wavelength-dependent variation in propagation delay and is affected by materials and dimensions of the waveguide of an optical fiber device or the fiber. Chromatic dispersion measurements characterize the way in which the velocity of propagation changes with wavelength, while traveling down the length of the fiber or through the waveguide of optical components.

The concept of optical phase should be considered in a discussion of chromatic dispersion. A mathematical relationship exists between optical phase and chromatic dispersion or group delay. It is important to mention optical phase before any explanations of chromatic dispersion or *group delay*. Group delay is defined as the first derivative of optical phase with respect to optical frequency. Chromatic dispersion is the second derivative of optical phase with respect to optical frequency. These quantities are represented as follows:

$$\text{Group Delay} = \frac{\partial \varphi}{\partial f} \tag{13.6}$$

$$\text{Chromatic Dispersion} = \frac{\partial^2 \varphi}{\partial f^2} \tag{13.7}$$

where Optical phase φ is the measured modulation in degrees. Optical frequency f is measured in Hz or THz. For example, a typical communications wavelength is 1550 nm = 193.4 THz.

Both of these phenomena occur because all optical signals have a finite spectral width, and different spectral components propagate at different speeds along the length of the fiber. One cause of this velocity difference is that the index of refraction of the fiber core is slightly different for different wavelengths. This condition is called *material dispersion*; it is the dominant source of chromatic dispersion in single-mode fibers.

Another cause of dispersion is the wavelength dependence of the cross-sectional distribution of light within the fiber. Shorter wavelengths are more completely confined to the fiber core, while a larger portion of the optical power at longer wavelengths propagates in the cladding. Since the index of the core is greater than the index of the cladding, the wavelengths in the core travel slightly more slowly. Thus, this difference in spatial distribution causes a change in propagation velocity among the wavelengths. This phenomenon is known as *waveguide dispersion*, which is relatively small compared to material dispersion.

Chromatic dispersion can also cause bit errors in digital communications, distortion, and a higher noise in analogue communications. These outcomes can pose a serious problems in high-bit-rate systems, if its dispersion is not measured accurately, and if some form of dispersion compensation is not employed.

Figure 13.2 shows a set up for measuring chromatic dispersion by the modulation phase-shift method. An electric signal generator intensity modulates the output of a narrowband, tunable optical source by means of an external modulator. After detecting the transmitted signal with a photodiode receiver, a vector voltmeter is used to measure the phase of the modulation of the received signal relative to the electrical modulation source. The phase measurement is repeated at wavelength intervals $\Delta\lambda$ across the spectral band of interest. Using the measurements at any two adjacent wavelength, the change in group delay (in ps) over the wavelength interval between them is

$$\Delta\tau_\lambda = \frac{\phi_{\lambda+\Delta\lambda/2} - \phi_{\lambda-\Delta\lambda/2}}{360 f_m} \times 10^6 \tag{13.8}$$

where λ is the wavelength at the center of the interval, f_m is the modulation frequency in MHz, and ϕ is the phase of the measured modulation in degrees.

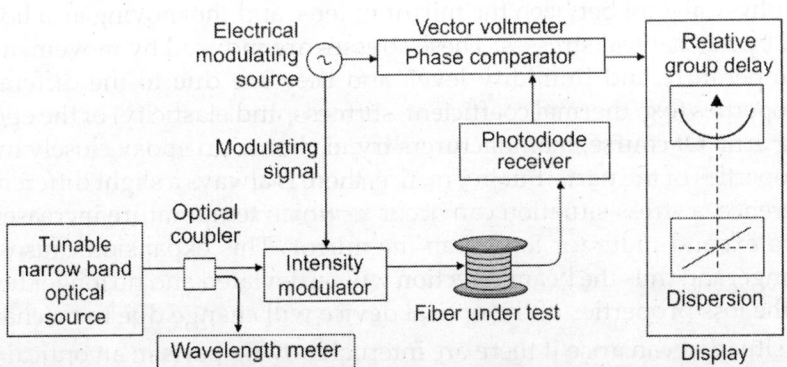

Fig. 13.2: Schematic illustration of test setup and display output for measuring chromatic dispersion by the phase shift method

These data points are then plotted to a yield the typical curve shown in Fig. 13.2. The dispersion can be calculated by applying the curve-fitting equations to the pulse-delay data.

13.4.9 Optical Frequency Measurements

The relation between light wavelength λ and frequency f is given by the following equation:

$$\lambda = \frac{c}{nf} \tag{13.9}$$

where λ is the light wavelength in nm, c is the seed of light in a vacuum in m/s, f is the light frequency in Hz or THz, and n is the index of refraction of an optical material.

Optical measurements are typically calibrated to the light wavelength in a vacuum ($n - 1$). Therefore, when $n = 1$, Eq. (13.9) can be rewritten as:

$$\lambda = \frac{c}{f} \tag{13.10}$$

13.5 TESTING OPTICAL FIBER SWITCHES

The following are the most common tests on optical fiber switches required by industry standards and consumers. These tests stimulate the conditions that may be present during the switch's lifetime operation in the field.

There are a few reasons why testing of the optical performance is not the only important factor in testing an optical device. Mechanical, electrical, and environmental tests of devices are as important as optical testing, before delivering the devices to the market.

13.5.1 Mechanical Tests

Mechanical tests are carried out to test the durability of the moving mechanical parts inside optical devices, such as switches. Inside an optical switch, there usually is a moving part (either a moving mirror, moving prism, or moving lens) that is moved in and out of the optical path; this changes the direction of the optical path (e.g. if the mirror is out of the optical path, the light will pass straight through the device, unaffected, to one output port; if the mirror is placed in the optical path, the light will be reflected by the mirror into a different output port).

Like all other devices, optical components wear out with time. For example in an optical switch, the physical joint between the mirror or lens, and the moving arm holding them, are affected by mechanical stresses. These stresses are induced by movement, change in ambient temperature and humidity level, and they are due to the different intrinsic physical properties (e.g. thermal coefficient, stiffness, and elasticity) of the epoxy, mirror, and moving arm. Of course, manufacturers try to choose an epoxy closely matching the physical properties of the parts, but in practice, there is always a slight difference. Because of this difference, a stress situation can occur in which temperature increases will cause the epoxy to expand more (or less) than the mirror. This expansion causes the mirror angle to change, and thus the beam direction will be deviated and no longer be optimized. Therefore, the loss properties of the optical device will change due to mechanical stress.

Another situation can arise if there are internal moving parts in an optical device. The physical joint between moving parts, for example, between a mirror and the arm to which it is attached, can become weak after many movement cycles. This weakness causes the mirror to move a little with each cycle and induces instability in the beam deviation, and this weakness will of course affect the optical properties of the device.

Still another factor that needs to be taken into consideration concerns the device's electrical properties. Although it is not obvious, when dealing with the mechanical properties of a device, electrical signals are often linked to the observed mechanical defects. As an example, take an actuator with a coil creating a magnetic field used to move an arm up and down, depending on the orientation of the electric signal. A mirror is glued to the tip of the moving arm. The mirror can be moved either in or out of the optical path of a beam of light, forming an electro-optical switch. If the amplitude of the electrical current changes, the magnetic field will change accordingly, and thus will make the arm move more quickly or more slowly. This will affect the speed at which the mirror moves in and out of the optical path. Such factors can seem insignificant, but in some applications where the speed of the transmission of a signal is important (and customers always want faster components), this variation in time can become a real problem.

13.5.2 Environmental Tests

Industries standards require that a representative number of samples of a product be subjected to a programme of environmental challenges including high and low temperature storage, temperature cycling, and humidity. An environmental testing procedure might consist of three to six stages of temperature and humidity tests on selected devices. The characteristics of a DUT must be measured before and after each test stage. In some cases, continuous or interval testing is conducted during each test stage.

Environmental test systems are usually integrated in an automated test system, which is intended for long-term reliability testing of optical components under environmental stress conditions. Such stress conditions are listed in Telcordia specifications GR-326-CORE, GR1209-CORE, and GR-1221-CORE. The Telcordia GR-xxx-CORE standards are quality standards used in the fiber optic industry, and they are more complete and restrictive than the ISO quality standards.

Devices under test are subjected to a range of environmental stress conditions in a test chamber, usually over a period of many weeks. Chamber conditions are recorded at specified time intervals during the environmental tests, and the required parameters for each DUT are measured. User selected parameters are calculated from these responses and recorded along with the time and environmental data.

Switches combined with the appropriate source and monitoring hardware along with software can create fully automated measurement systems. An optional polarization controller is installed when PDL measurements are required. A computer is used to set up the tests, control the measurements, and monitor the test conditions and results.

For measuring IL and PDL, the optical component environmental test system (OCETS) uses a combination of up to three internal Fabry–Perot lasers, and a broadband source (BBS) with a filter or an external source. The light from any of these sources can be routed to either end of each DUT. The power meter measures either the insertion loss through the DUT, in either direction, or the back-reflection from either end. A polarization controller enables PDL to be measured. Second and subsequent tests can be added for additional sets of DUTs, up to the switch capacity limit, while the first test is running. In this way, an environmental chamber running a long-term test (on a first prototype, for example) could evaluate the performance of product improvements, by installing later devices in the chamber and configuring a second test to run with the same conditions and measurements.

13.5.3 Repeatability Test

If there are moving parts in the optical path, the optical signal may change slightly each time the parts move from one position to another. This change in optical signal, or loss variation at each cycle, is a measure of repeatability. The difference in performance between test cycles is due to the physical properties of the components in the optical device. Minimal difference between the cycles indicates good repeatability. For example, the repeatability test for an optical switch measures the maximum IL variation, for a given optical path, over number of cycles, at a given constant temperature. The results of repeatability tests are often displayed as a graph. This graph enables a quick view of the readings stability, and it allows determination of the occurrence of spikes or non-regular variations.

The repeatability test is usually very sensitive to external vibrations (such as someone walking near the test station or banging on the table) because such vibrations induce additional movement to the internal parts of the DUT. This test can also be affected by the orientation of the DUT (due to gravitational forces on the DUT's internal moving parts). It is also important to keep the temperature constant during this test, because the physical properties of the materials composing the DUT change the temperature. This induces additional measurement variations, which are not due to the moving parts themselves.

13.5.4 Speed Test

Moving parts do not move instantly; they need an amount of time to react to the signal that controls them in order to move. The time elapsed between the application of the control pulse and the moment when the optical signal achieves its steady state is called the *switching time* for optical switches (also often called speed time for switches).

For an optical switch, the switching time is usually defined as the time between the application of the activation pulse and the time when the optical signal reaches 90% of its steady state, at a given constant temperature. In order to measure the switching time, a very fast optical power meter (OPM) is required. The sampling speed of the OPM should be at least ten times faster than the switching speed to be measured. For example, if a switching time in the order of milliseconds is to be measured, the sampling speed of the OPM should be at least 0.1 ms faster.

The results of this test are often displayed as a graph to see if the steady state of the optical signal is flat and high enough, and if the dynamic range between light-on signal and light-off signal is good.

This test is very sensitive to fluctuations of the laser light source. For example, a variation in optical signal could be perceived as unwanted movement inside of a switch. Also, when the OPM is set in the fast-reading mode, it is very sensitive to the power level of the laser because the response time of the OPM detector varies with the power of light: the lower the power, the slower the response time. Poor OPM performance results in additional noise in the measurements. However, if the laser power is too high, the detector will saturate and give inaccurate readings. Thus, it is important to find the acceptable power range for optimum response time of the OPM detector for this test.

Temperature is also an important factor for this test, because the properties of the materials will change with temperature (electrical current moves faster at higher temperatures, for example). So the temperature should be kept constant during the speed test.

The orientation of the DUT is also a factor to be considered. If the moving parts of the DUT are heavy, then gravitational forces will not be negligible and will have an effect on the speed. Thus, it is important to perform some tests to determine if the orientation of the DUT will have an effect on the speed test measurements.

13.6 LIGHT WAVELENGTH MEASUREMENTS

Wavelength measurements provide various information about most optical fiber devices. In these measurements, optical properties, such as IL, are measured over a wide range of wavelengths. For example, WDL is the variation in insertion loss over a specified wavelength range shown in a spectral plot.

From the spectral plot (IL versus λ), many device parameters can be measured:

1. Flatness (WDL)
2. Passband width (bandwidth, BW)
3. Full width half maximum (FWHM) (–3 dB BW)
4. Cross-channel isolation to reduce crosstalk
5. Maximum/minimum loss in passband
6. Free spectral range (FSR)

Light wavelength measurements can be achieved using either a tunable laser source with fixed detector or a broadband light source with an OSA. In addition, advanced wavelength measurement systems conduct different measurements, including different types of losses.

13.7 DEVICE POWER HANDLING TESTS

There are two categories of power-handling failures that occur during the power-handling test of an optical fiber device:

1. Increasing the input optical power until a device failure occurs: this happens in an epoxy joint, when the epoxy ruptures and the surface coating burns: in this case, a graph of loss versus power shows the results for each DUT.
2. Applying a higher than normal input optical power over a prolonged period of time, until a device failure occurs: in this case, a graph of losses versus time for different input powers shows the results for each DUT.

13.8 TROUBLESHOOTING

The main sources of problems that can arise during any of the preceding tests are:

1. Unwanted reflections occur when the refractive index along the light path changes, for example, at a glass-air interface, dirty and/or damaged connectors, and terminated reflections from unused fiber ends. Reflection between two parallel optical surfaces can be prevented, by using non-perpendicular surface angles.
2. Unstable laser source occurs if laser temperature is fluctuating, light is reflected back into the laser source (which can be solved by installing an isolator device after the laser source). It also occurs because of dirty and/or damaged connectors, damaged jumpers, or a sharply bent or too tightly coiled cable. It can also occur if the power meter is in fast-sampling mode.
3. Inaccurate power measurements occur when the power meter needs calibration, or are caused by stray light (low power measurement can be affected by room light; therefore, connections must be properly shielded). It also occurs due to dirty and/or damaged connectors or detectors or poor switch repeatability. It can also occur because of the connection to the detector differs between the reference and measurement.

When a problem arises during testing and troubleshooting is required, one must first ensure that these abovementioned problems are not present at the test station before calling the DUT a failure. Even if none of these situations occurs during testing, there are other sources of errors, intrinsic to any test system, that must be taken into account.

13.9 SOURCES OF ERROR DURING FIBER OPTIC MEASUREMENTS

The following are the main categories for sources of error in a test system:

13.9.1 Resolution

Resolution is defined as the size of the smallest increment or unit in which the instrument can read. The resolution of the system should be ≤ 1/10 of the total tolerance width. The resolution of equipment is an intrinsic property of the equipment's internal components, which the person performing the test has no control over (unless, of course, that person decides to buy another piece of equipment with a better resolution). Consider a *ruler*: the smallest divisions are millimeters. The human eye can differentiate, without the use of a magnifier, details as small as one tenth of a millimeter. However, when measuring the length of a line, it would be difficult to say whether the measurement is 11.2 or 11.3 mm. Therefore, the resolution of the human-eye-and-ruler system is ± 0.5 mm. Another example is a *digital meter*: the resolution of the digital meter is ± the last digit; if the meter gives a reading of 0.67 dB, then the resolution of the measurement is ± 0.01 dB.

13.9.2 Accuracy

Accuracy is defined as the difference between the observed average for a series of measurements and the true value being measured. The true value is measured using a reference measurement system, a master power meter. A master power meter has been referenced and calibrated with the world's master power meter located at the National Institute of Standards and Technology, and used to calibrate all the master power meters in the world (not that many). This reference ensures that any power meter in any facility worldwide, when calibrated with a master meter, will give the same measurement result for a given device. The accuracy of a power meter therefore usually depends on how long ago the meter was calibrated. Likewise, when measuring wavelength, the reference is a master wavelength meter.

13.9.3 Stability (Drift)

Stability is defined as the change in measurements over time. Measurement readings will vary over time, because the equipment wears out with time, dust can accumulate, and temperature and humidity, along with other factors, can affect the readings. If a device remains connected to a power meter for a long time and measurements are repeatedly performed at predetermined time intervals, the reading will vary over time. Most of the time, the readings variation follows a cycle, such as a sinusoid curve or a series of abrupt changes (steps). This pattern can be caused by instability in, for example, electrical components and heating components. In fact, the instability is closely related to inaccuracy. Stability can be considered a measure of the variation in accuracy over time. The more time that passes, the greater the likelihood that a drift will occur in the readings. This is why periodic calibration has to be performed on any measurement equipment.

13.9.4 Linearity

Linearity is defined as the difference in accuracy values over the expected operating range. Some electrical and optical components will not have linear response depending on the intensity of electric current or incident light. Linearity is the linear correlation of an input power or signal to the corresponding optical power output. A mathematical formula is used to calculate the linearity value of a device. The correlation between electric current and light power, for an optical diode, is not perfectly linear; the correlation graph will usually be a curve. The more the curve bends, the worse the linearity is. This means that for a power value near the middle of the measurement range of the apparatus, the readings will be closer to the real value than when the power value is close to one end of the curve. The linearity and the correlation coefficients are adjusted during calibration of the meter of equipment.

13.9.5 Repeatability Error

Repeatability error is defined as the consistency of a given system, making repeated measurements of the same part, using the same measurement instrument. It is a measure of the inherent variation in the system. Basically, to determine the repeatability error of a measurement system (a complex automated system or a simple power meter and an operator), a number of devices (between five and thirty, but usually around ten to fifteen) have to be selected and tested. The selected devices should have measured values covering the entire range of probable results. These devices should include those that have both passed and failed testing. All of the devices are tested, and the test results are recorded as the first set of results. The order of the device testing is changed. Then, a new test is performed, and the results are recorded. This procedure can be repeated a number of times (between two times and five times, usually three to five times), and each time the testing order of the devices is changed. After each test, the results are correlated to identify all of the devices throughout the tests. Once all the series of tests are performed, the results can be recorded in a table, wherein each row corresponds to a device and the columns contain the test results for each measurement performed for each device. From the difference in test results for each device, analysis can be performed to determine the repeatability error of the test system.

13.9.6 Reproducibility

Reproducibility is defined as consistency of different operators measuring the same part using the same measurement instrument. To determine the reproducibility error of a measurement system, a number of devices (between five and thirty, usually around ten to fifteen) have to be selected and tested. The same devices used for the repeatability-error test can be used for this. Selected devices should have measured values covering the entire range of probable results, and the devices should include those that passed and failed testing. A number of people are then selected (between two and five) to perform the tests. The devices are identified with a code, and one person is asked to test all of the devices and record the test results. This is the first set of results. Then the ID codes of the devices are changed, and another person tests the devices again and records the results. The same procedure continues until all the selected persons have tested the devices. The results can be recorded in a table, wherein each row corresponds to a device, and the columns correspond to the test results obtained for each person. From the difference between person-to-person results for each device, analysis can be performed to determine the reproducibility error of the test system.

The following points should be considered, when examining the sources of measurement errors.

1. The errors stem mostly from the measurement system and not only from the persons performing the test. If the test system were perfect, it would always give exactly the same results regardless of test operator or the number of tests. But systems are never perfect, and there will always be variations in the test results or errors. It is possible to minimize error occurrence by using experienced persons. System error itself can be reduced with more frequent calibration and a more-stable or better-designed system.

2. The repeatability and reproducibility errors will almost always be the major source of error in any test system. It is important to characterize these two sources of error, in order to determine if the results obtained from the test system are reliable or not. The measurement tool is sometimes called gauge. The most common way to determine the repeatability and reproducibility error factors of a system is to perform a *gauge capability study* (GCS) of the system, also known as *gauge repeatability* and *reproducibility study* (Gauge R&R Study). This GCS study includes simultaneously performing repeatability and reproducibility studies.

3. If the gauge R&R results show a systematic error in the measurements (results are always lower/higher than the real value), then this can be reduced by a proper calibration and increasing the frequency of calibrations.

4. If the gauge R&R results show random errors in the measurement results, then it is better to add a guardband to the test results. For example, if the test specification for the IL value is less than 1.0 dB, and the system gives a random error of ± 0.05 dB, then the test must fail any device that has an IL higher than 0.95 dB.

5. The resolution, accuracy, stability and linearity sources of error are quoted in technical equipment specifications. These values can be improved with the calibration of the equipment.

13.10 OPTICAL SYSTEM TEST EQUIPMENT/INSTRUMENTS

Table 13.3 summarizes some widely used basic optical-system test instruments and their functions.

13.10.1 Optical Power Meter

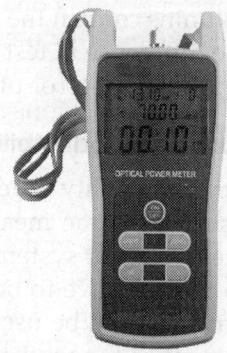

Optical power meter (Fig. 13.3) is the basic instrument for all types of optical fiber communication applications and it is a must just like multimeters for electronic circuits. It measures the optical power level available at the tip of the fiber or pigtail end of an optical source. The power is coupled to the input port of power meter through a connector or adaptor. Further, both single mode and multimode fibers can be connected to the input port by using different connectors. Figure 13.4 shows the schematic block diagram of internal units of an optical power meter.

Fig. 13.3: Optical power meter

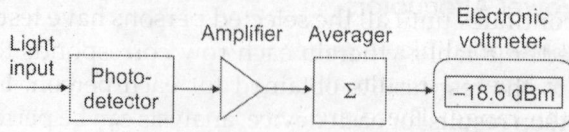

Fig. 13.4: Block diagram of the internal units of an optical powermeter

Table 13.3: Some widely used basic optic-system test instruments and their functions

Test instrument	Function
Test-support laser (multiple-wavelength or broadband)	Assist in tests that measure the wavelength-dependent response of an optical component or link
Optical spectrum analyzer	Measures optical power as a function of wavelength
Multifunction optical test system	Factory or field instruments with exchangeable modules for performing a variety of measurements
Optical power attenuator	Reduces power level to prevent instrument damage or to avoid overload distortion in the measurements
Conformance analyzer	Measures optical receiver performance in accordance with standards-based specifications
Visual fault indicator	Uses visible light to give a quick indication of a break in an optical fiber
Optical power meter	Measures optical power over a selected wavelength band
BER test equipment	Uses standard eye-pattern masks to evaluate the data-handling ability of an optical link
OTDR (field instrument)	Measures attenuation, length, connector/splice losses, and reflectance levels; helps locate fiber breaks
Optical return loss tester	Measures total reverse power in relation to total forward power at a particular point

The optical power meters are available either in the table-top form or as a hand-held instrument. However, the field applications hand-held power meters are more convenient. The optical power meter can display the optical power directly in mW or µW depending on the capability and selected range of the meter. The power meter uses a photodetector at the input port to convert the optical signal into electrical signal which is subsequently amplified as processed to measure the corresponding electrical energy. The power meters can be operated either by the normal electric supply by using an adaptor or using the built in battery. Generally, the power meters are calibrated over different wavelength ranges depending on the type of photodetector used. A Ge photodetector can be used at the input port for measuring optical power in the range of 780–1600 nm and InGaAs photodetector at the input port for the range of 840–1650 nm.

There are various models of optical power meters available in the market from different manfacturers. The major features of power meter from UNIWAY (Fig. 13.1) include easy operation (hand-held and battery operated), large measurement range (−50 to +26 dBm), LCD display, absolute power measurement, wavelength selectivity (980, 1310, 1490, and 1350 nm), relative optical power measurement, quite high accuracy (+0.15 dB). FPM-600 optical power meter from Anstel is more advanced power meter. This power meter is an ideal tool for link and system testing and certification. This meter has a memory capacity of 1000 data items alongwith converter software to facilitate data management and data transfer to a PC via USB connection. There are several advanced tools in the form of hand-held optical testers, e.g. FOT-930 optical teaser from ANSTEL, etc.

13.10.2 Fiber Optical Power Attenuators

These are used in the fiber optic links to reduce the optical power to a desired level, i.e., to bring down the power level (if it is far above the measuring range of a normal power meter) to match with the range. There are various types of optical fiber attenuators, including LC, SC, ST and FC are available. Commonly used optical attenuators come as female male type called a plug fiber attenuator. These optical fiber attenuators come with ceramic ferrules and there are also various types to fit different kinds of fiber connectors. Attenuators can be a fixed type or variable type. We may note that fixed value fiber optic attenuators can reduce the optical light power by a fixed factor, e.g. a 3 dB attenuator reduces the power by a factor of 2. Fiber optic attenuators are available for large value, e.g. 60 dB which corresponds to the reduction of power by a factor of 10^6. There are also variable attenuator which allows one to adjust the attenuation in a continuous manner. The fiber attenuators are basically required to meet TIA/EIA standards.

13.10.3 Test-Support Lasers: Tunable Laser Sources

Tunable laser sources are important instruments for measurements of the wavelength-dependent response of an optical instrument or link. The characteristics of two such instruments used for test support are listed in Table 13.4. Generally, a tunable laser source consists of a single-mode laser source with an external cavity. To tune the laser source, a tunable filter in the form of a movable diffraction grating is used. Depending on the source and grating combination, an instrument may be tunable over (for example) the 1280-to-1330-nm, the 1370-to-1945-nm, or the 1460-nm band. Wavelength scans, with an output power that is flat across the scanned spectral band, can be done automatically. The minimum output power of such an instrument usually is −10 dBm and the absolute wavelength accuracy is typically ± 0.01 nm (± 10 pm).

Table 13.4: Characteristics of laser-source instruments used for test support

Parameter	Tunable source	Broadband source
Spectral output range	Selectable, e.g. 1370–1945 nm or 1460–1640 nm	Peak wavelength ± 25 nm
Total optical output power	Up to 8 dBm	> 3.5 mW (5.5 dBm) over a 60 nm range
Power stability	< ± 0.02 dB	< ± 0.05 dB
Wavelength accuracy	< ± 10 pm	(Not applicable)

A broadband incoherent light source with a high output power coupled into a single-mode fiber is desirable to evaluate passive DWDM components. Such an instrument can be realized by using the amplified spontaneous emission (ASE) of an erbium-doped fiber amplifier. The power spectral density of the output is up to one hundred times (20 dB) greater than that of edge-emitting LEDs and up to 100,000 times (50 dB) greater than white-light tungsten lamp sources. The instrument can be specified to have a total output power of greater than 3.5 mW (5.5 dBm) over a 50-nm range with a spectral density of − 13 dBm/nm (50 µW/nm). The relatively high-power spectral density allows test personnel to characterize devices with medium or high insertion loss. Peak wavelengths might be 1200, 1310, 1430, 1550, or 1650 nm.

13.10.4 Optical Spectrum Analyzer (OSA)

To study the amplitude spectra (amplitude of various frequency components) of a signal a general purpose optical spectrum analyzer (OSA) is used. OSA measures optical power as a function of wavelength. The most common implementation uses a diffraction-grating based optical filter, which yields wavelength resolutions to less than 0.1 nm. One can achieve the higher wavelength accuracy (± 0.001 nm) with wavelength meters based on *Michelson interferometry*.

The operation of a grating based optical spectrum analyzer is illustrated in Fig. 13.5. Light emerging from a fiber is collimated by a lens and is directed onto a diffraction grating that can be rotated. The exit slit selects or filters the spectrum of the light from the grating. Thus, it determines the *spectral resolution* of the OSA. The term *resolution bandwidth* describes the width of this optical filter. Typical OSAs have selectable filters ranging from 10 nm down to 0.1 nm. The optical filter characteristics determine the

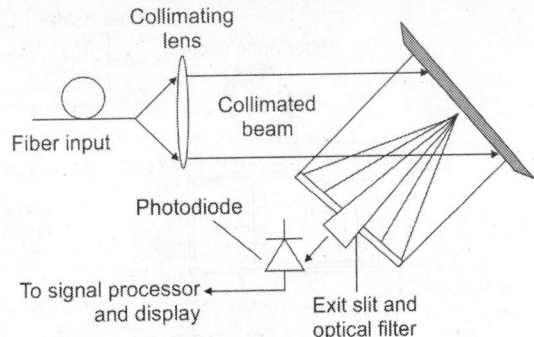

Fig. 13.5: Schematic illustration of the operation of a grating-based optical spectrum analyzer

dynamic range, which is the ability of the OSA to simultaneously view large and small signals in the same sweep. The bandwidth of the amplifier is a major factor affecting the sensitivity and sweep time of the OSA. In the O-band through L-band the photodiode is usually an InGaAs device.

The OSA normally sweeps across a spectral band making measurements at discretely spaced wavelength points. This spacing depends on the bandwidth-resolution capability of the instrument, and is known as the *trace-point spacing*.

The basic principle of operation of OSA is shown with the help of basic building blocks constituting the analyzer (Fig. 13.6). We can see that the input test signal passes through a monochromator. The optical bandpass filter restricts the light within a narrow wavelength slot. A photodetector defects the output light to convert the signal into the electrical signal (O/E conversion). The electrical signal is subsequently amplified and converted to a digital signal with the help of a D/A converter as shown in the Fig. 13.6. The electronic signal is then fed to the y-axis control of an oscilloscope. The x-axis control of the oscilloscope is swept across in synchronism with the wavelength setting of the FP filter.

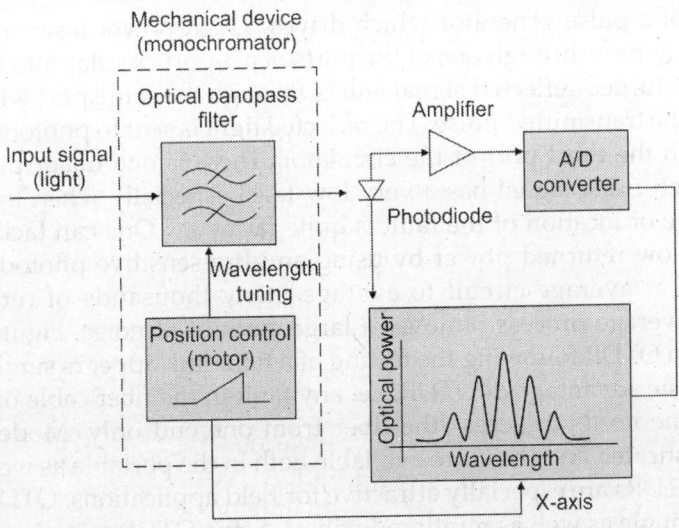

Fig. 13.6: Schematic illustration of internal functional building block of a optical spectrum analyzer (OSA)

Experimental setup to test a optical fiber cable using an OSA is shown in Fig. 13.7.

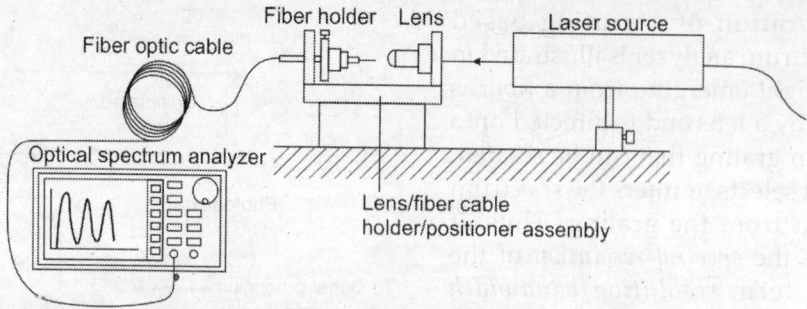

Fig. 13.7: Fiber optic cable testing using an OSA

13.10.5 Optical Time Domain Reflectometer (OTDR)

OTDR can be used to examine, test and measure numerous parameters related to an optical fiber link, e.g. the length of the fiber, attenuation of the whole fiber link in dB, connector and splice losses, location of connector joints, and fault in the optical fiber.

Figure 13.8 shows the functional block diagram of a typical OTDR.

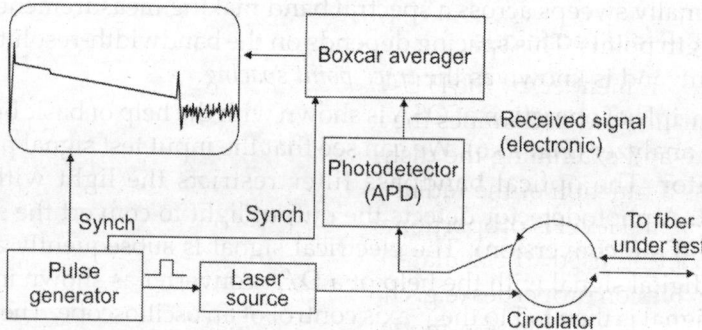

Fig. 13.8: Functional block diagram of a typical OTDR

OTDR consists of a pulse generator which drives a high power laser source. The light pulse is allowed to pass through one of the ports of a 3-port circular into the optical fiber under test. The returned reflected signal enters through the same port which also acts as the exit port for the transmitted pulse. The reflected light is sent to photodetector (usually an APD) through the third port of the circulator. There is one major problem with an OTDR, i.e. the returning signal has a very low level especially when the length of the fiber is very large or location of the fault is quite far away. One can tackle the problem associated with low returned power by using an ultra-sensitive photodetector, e.g. an APD and a boxcar average circuit to average many thousands of returning pulses. Obviously, the average process removes a large amount of noise. Figure 13.9 shows a typical trace of an OTDR following the testing of a fiber link appears similar to it. We see that there is a basic advantage of OTDR, i.e. any fault in the fiber cable or measurement of attenuation one needs to access the fiber from one end only. Modern OTDRs are extremely sophisticated and these are available both in the portable as well as bench-top form. Portable OTDRs are especially attractive for field applications. OTDRs can be used for testing both single as well as multimode fibers. Some OTDRs are also equipped with additional laser source and optical power meter. The model T-BERD 6000 of OTDR is a compact and lightweight portable test instrument for installation and maintenance of optical fiber communication networks.

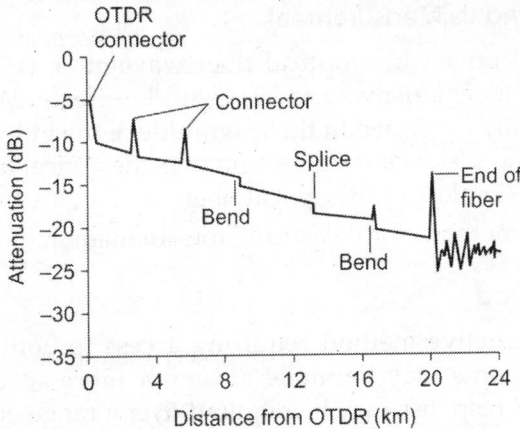

Fig. 13.9: Typical OTDR test result in the form of a trace exhibiting the presence of various discontinuities due to connector, splices, bend, etc. in the optical fiber

13.11 CHARACTERIZATION TECHNIQUES OF OPTICAL FIBER

• Refracted Near-Field Technique

This method is recommended by the ITU-T and TIA for determining the refractive-index profile (RIP). This method determines the index profile by moving a focused laser across the fiber end face and examining the distribution of the light that is refracted sideways out of the core as a function of the radial position of the laser spot. The variation in the detected optical signal level is proportional to the index change at the fiber end face. The RIP parameter can be used to calculate the geometrical parameters of a fiber and to estimate all transmission properties (e.g. chromatic dispersion and the cut-off wavelength) except attenuation and polarization-mode dispersion.

Transmitted Near-Field Technique

This method is recommended by the ITU-T and TIA for measuring mode-field characteristics. Knowledge of the mode-field diameter (MFD) is important since it describes the radial optical field distribution across the fiber core. Detailed information of the MFD enables one to calculate characteristics such as source-to-fiber coupling efficiency, splice and joint losses, microbending loss, and dispersion. A transmitted near-field scan directly provides the intensity distribution $E^2(r)$ at the fiber exit. From this distribution one then can calculate the MFD. MFD can be expressed in terms of the near-field intensity distribution as

$$\text{MFD} = 2\sqrt{2} \left[\frac{\int_0^\infty E^2(r)\, r\, dr}{\frac{1}{4} \int_0^\infty \frac{1}{E^2(r)} \left(\frac{d(E^2)}{dr} \right)^2 r\, dr} \right]^{1/2} \tag{13.11}$$

One can easily program this equation, the measurement equipment software can then calculate the MFP directly from the near field data.

13.11.1 Attenuation and Its Measurement

Attenuation of optical power in a optical fiber waveguide is a result of absorption processes, scattering mechanisms, and waveguide effects. We may note that the manufacturer is generally interested in the magnitude of the individual contributions to attenuation, whereas the system engineers who uses the optical fiber is more concerned with the total transmission loss of the optical fiber.

There are two basic methods for measuring the attenuation of an optical fiber:

(i) The Cut-back Method

This method is a destructive method requiring access to both ends of optical fiber (Fig. 13.10). Measurements may be made at one or more specific wavelengths, or, alternatively, a spectral response may be required over a range of wavelengths. To find the transmission loss, the optical power is first measured at the output (or far end) of the fiber. Then, without disturbing the input condition, the fiber is cut off a few meters from the source, and the output power at this near end is measured. If P_F and P_N represent the output powers of the far and near ends of the fiber, respectively, the average loss α in decibels per kilometer is given by

$$\alpha = \frac{10}{L} \log \frac{P_N}{P_F} \tag{13.12}$$

where L (in kilometers) is the separation of the two measurement points. The reason for following these steps is that it is extremely difficult to calculate the exact amount of optical power launched into a fiber. By using the cutback method, the optical power emerging from the short fiber length is the input power to the fiber of length L.

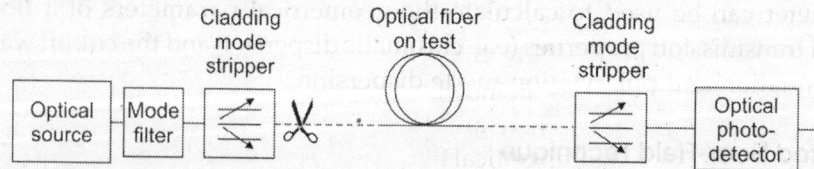

Fig. 13.10: Schematic experimental set-up for attenuation measurement by cut-back method

In carrying out this measurement technique, special attention have to be paid to how optical power is launched into the fiber. This is because, in a multimode fiber, different launch conditions can yield different loss value. The effects of modal distributions in the multimode fiber that result from different numerical apertures (NA) and spot sizes on the launch end of the fiber are shown in Fig. 13.11. If the spot size is small and its NA is less than that of the fiber core, the optical power is concentrated in the center of the core [Fig. 13.11(a)]. In this case, the attenuation contribution arising from higher-order-mode power loss is negligible. In Fig. 13.11 the spot size is larger than the fiber core and the spot NA is larger than that of the fiber. For this overfilled condition, those parts of the incident light beam that fall outside of the fiber core and outside of the fiber NA are lost. In addition, there is a large contribution to the attenuation arising from higher-mode power loss.

Steady-state equilibrium-mode distributions are typically achieved by the *mandrel-wrap* method. In this method, excess higher-order cladding modes that are launched by initially overexciting the fiber are filtered out by wrapping several turns of fiber around

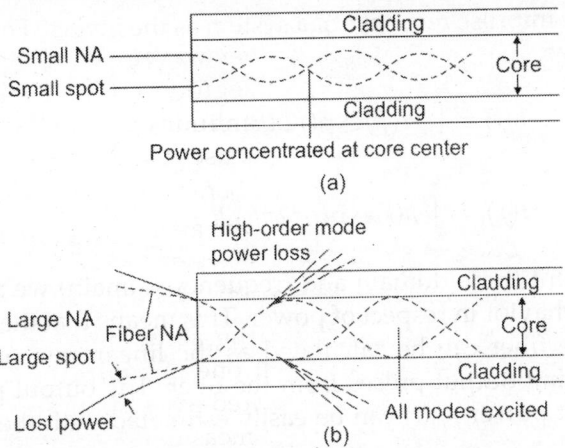

Fig. 13.11: The effects of launch numerical aperture (NA) and spot size on the modal distribution (a) underfilling the fiber excites only lower-order modes (b) an overfilled fiber has excess attenuation from higher-order mode loss

a mandrel, which is about 1.0–1.5 cm in diameter. In single-mode fibers, this type of mode filter is used to eliminate cladding modes from the optical fiber.

One can also use this method to study the dependence of attenuation with the wavelength of light by making use of tunable laser as source.

(ii) Insertion-Loss Method

See Section 13.4.2.

13.11.2 Dispersion Measurement

Measurements of dispersion give an indication of the distortion to optical signals as they propagate down optical fibers. There are three basic forms of dispersion produce pulse broadening of lightwave signals in optical fibers, thereby limiting the information-carrying capacity. In multimode fibers, intermodal dispersion arises from the fact that each mode in an optical pulse travels a slightly different distance and thus arrives at the fiber end at slightly offset times. Chromatic dispersion stems from the variation in the propagation speed of the individual wavelength components of an optical signal. Polarization-mode dispersion arises from the splitting of a polarized signal into orthogonal polarization modes, each of which has a different propagation speed.

There are many ways to measure the various dispersion effects. Here, we will study at some common methods.

Intermodal Dispersion

For practical purposes in evaluating intermodal dispersion, the fiber can be considered as a filter characterized by an impulse response $h(t)$ or by a power transfer function $H(f)$, which is the Fourier transform of the impulse response. Either of these can be measured to determine the pulse dispersion. The impulse-response measurements are made in the time domain, whereas the power transfer function is measured in the frequency domain.

Both the time-domain and frequency-domain dispersion measurements assume that the optical fiber behaves quasi-linearly in power; that is, the individual overlapping output pulses from an optical waveguide can be treated as adding linearly.

We may write the impulse response of a system as the inverse Fourier transform of the transform function as

$$h(t) = \int_{-\infty}^{\infty} H(f)\exp(j2\pi ft)df \tag{13.12}$$

or conversely,

$$H(f) = \int_{-\infty}^{\infty} h(t)\exp(-j2\pi ft)dt \tag{13.12a}$$

In the measurement (time-domain and frequency domain) we assume that the fiber has a quasi-linear behavior in respect of power. This means that the total power received at the output of the fiber can be calculated as the linear sum of the contribution of individual overlapping output pulses from the fiber. The output power of the fiber in response to an input power $p_{in}(t)$ can be easily estimated with the help of convolution integral given by

$$p_{out}(t) = h(t) * p_{in}(t) = \int_{-T/2}^{T/2} p_{in}(t)h(t-\tau)d\tau \tag{13.13}$$

where, T is the period between the input pulses.

Now, taking Fourier transform on both sides of Eq. (13.13), one may write,

$$P_{out}(f) = H(f)\, P_{in}(f) \tag{13.14}$$

where $P_{in}(f)$ and $P_{out}(f)$ are the Fourier transforms of the input and output pulse responses of the fiber considered as a filter. Therefore, we have

$$P_{out}(f) = \int_{-\infty}^{\infty} P_{out}(t)\exp(j2\pi ft)dt \tag{13.15}$$

$$P_{in}(f) = \int_{-\infty}^{\infty} P_{in}(t)\exp(j2\pi ft)dt \tag{13.16}$$

The above transfer function of a optical fiber cable gives important information about the bandwidth of the system.

Time-domain Intermodal Dispersion

Figure 13.12 shows an experimental set up for measuring the pulse dispersion in time domain. One can estimate the pulse broadening caused by an optical fiber in a simplest way by launching a narrow optical pulse at one end of the fiber and detect the broaden pulse at the other end with the help of the above set up. Here, output pulses from a laser source are coupled through a mode scrambler into a test fiber. The output of the fiber is measured with a sampling oscilloscope that has a built-in optical receiver, or the signal

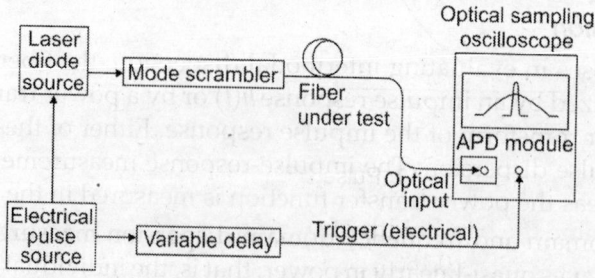

Fig. 13.12: Schematic of measurement setup for making pulse-dispersion measurements in the time domain

can be detected with an external photodetector and then measured with a regular sampling oscilloscope. Further, the shape of the input pulse is measured the same way by replacing the test fiber with a short reference fiber that has a length less than 1% of the test fiber length. This reference fiber can be a short length cut from the test fiber or it can be a fiber segment that has similar properties. The variable delay in the trigger line is used to offset the difference in delay between the test fiber and the shorter reference fiber.

From the output pulse shape, an rms pulse width, σ, as defined in Fig. 13.13 can be calculated with the help of following relation:

$$\sigma = \left[\frac{\int_{-\infty}^{\infty} (t - \bar{t})^2 \, p_{out}(t) \, dt}{\int_{-\infty}^{\infty} p_{out}(t) \, dt} \right]^{1/2} \tag{13.17}$$

where the center time $\bar{t}$ of the pulse is given by

$$\bar{t} = \frac{\int_{-\infty}^{\infty} t \, p_{out}(t) \, dt}{\int_{-\infty}^{\infty} p_{out}(t) \, dt} \tag{13.18}$$

The evaluation of Eq. (13.18) requires a numerical integration. An easier method is to assume that the output response of a fiber can be approximated by a *Gaussian function* given by

$$p_{out}(t) = \frac{1}{\sigma\sqrt{2\pi}} \exp\left(-\frac{t^2}{2\sigma^2}\right) \tag{13.19}$$

where the parameter σ (rms width) determines the pulse width, as shown in Fig. 13.13. This figure also shows the parameter t_{FWHM}, which is the full width of the pulse at its half-maximum value. This is equal to $2\sigma(2 \ln 2)^{1/2} = 2.355\sigma$.

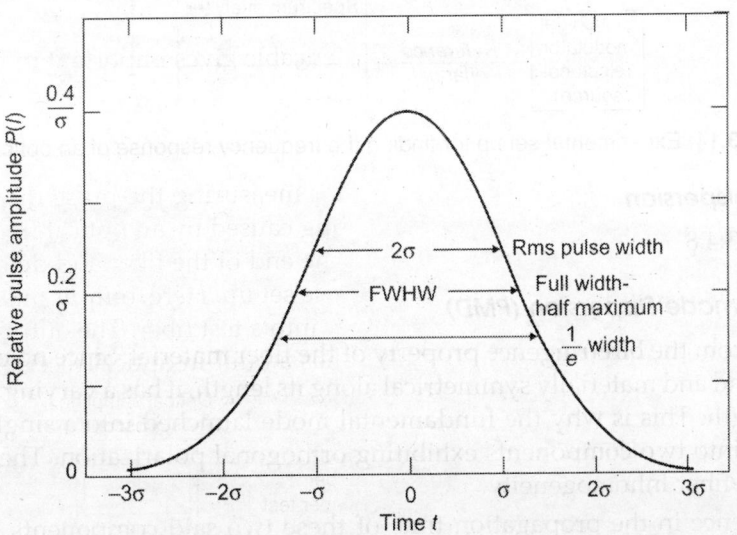

Fig. 13.13: Pulse shape for estimation of σ

One can determine the bandwidth of the fiber using the following relation

$$B = \frac{0.186}{\sigma} \text{ Hz} \tag{13.20}$$

Frequency-domain Intermodal Dispersion Measurement

One can also estimate the bandwidth of the test fiber by making the measurement in the frequency domain. We may note that the frequency domain intermodal dispersion directly yields the amplitude versus frequency as well as phase versus frequency of the optical fiber. Figure 13.14 shows a experimental test set up arrangement for measurement of frequency domain intermodal dispersion of the optical fiber. The light from a linewidth CW laser source is sinusoidally modulated about a fixed level and the signal is launched into the fiber one obtains. The frequency response of the fiber from the ratio of the amplitudes of the sinusoidally modulated wave at the input end and the output end of the fiber. At the exit end of the optical fiber a photodetector is used to convert the intensity modulated optical signal to corresponding electric power $P_{out}(f)$ as a function of frequency. The input signal power $P_{in}(f)$ is subsequently measured by replacing the test fiber by a short-length reference fiber. The transfer function of the fiber under test can be obtained from the measurement with the help of relation for baseband frequency response

$$H(f) = \frac{P_{out}(f)}{P_{in}(f)}$$

(13.21)

As the modulation frequency is increased, the optical power level at the fiber output will eventually start to decrease. The fiber bandwidth is defined as the lowest frequency at which the baseband frequency response, $H(f)$ has been reduced to 0.5.

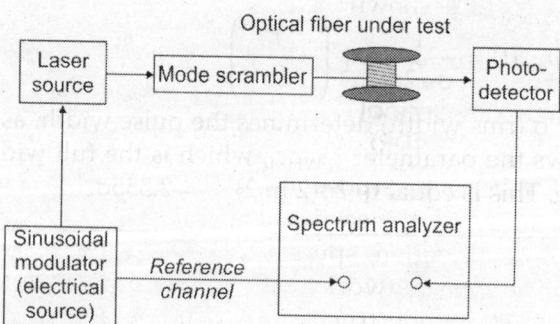

Fig. 13.14: Experimental set up for finding the frequency response of an optical fiber

Chromatic Dispersion

See Section 13.4.8

Polarization-mode Dispersion (PMD)

PMD arises from the birefringence property of the fiber material. Since no optical fiber is perfectly round and materially symmetrical along its length, it has a varying birefringence along its length. This is why the fundamental mode launched into a single mode fiber decomposes into two components exhibiting orthogonal polarization. The main reason for this is the fiber inhomogeneity.

The difference in the propagation time of these two said components lead to pulse spreading and is termed *polarization mode dispersion* (PMD). PMD limits the ultimate bandwidth of a single mode fiber. There are different methods of measuring polarization mode dispersion of a fiber. Here we will discuss the *fixed analyzer method*. The measurement set up for polarization mode dispersion of a single mode fiber is shown in Fig. 13.15. It consists of a broadband polarized source and polarized (variable) optical spectrum analyzer. The mean period of the intensity modulation is measured from the power fluctuations spectrum. This is done by measuring the rate at which the state of polarization changes as wavelength changes. This corresponds to the

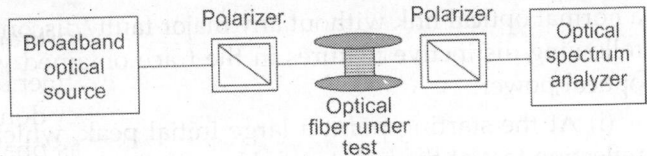

Fig. 13.15: Schematic experimental set up for measurement of polarization mode dispersion (PMD)

number of maxima and minima. Using this value the *mean differential group delay* is estimated as following:

$$\langle \Delta \tau_{pol} \rangle = \frac{k N_e \lambda_{start} \lambda_{stop}}{2(\lambda_{start} - \lambda_{stop})c} \tag{13.22}$$

where, λ_{start} and λ_{stop} are the wavelengths corresponding to the starting and ending of the wavelength sweep used in the measurement, N_e is the number of extrema (maxima and minima) within the scanning range and c is the velocity of light and k is the mode coupling factor. The value of k is 0.84 for randomly mode-coupled fibers and 1.0 for non-mode coupled fibers and devices.

A typical spectrum analyzer trace exhibiting the transmitted power level as a function of the wavelength is shown in Fig. 13.16.

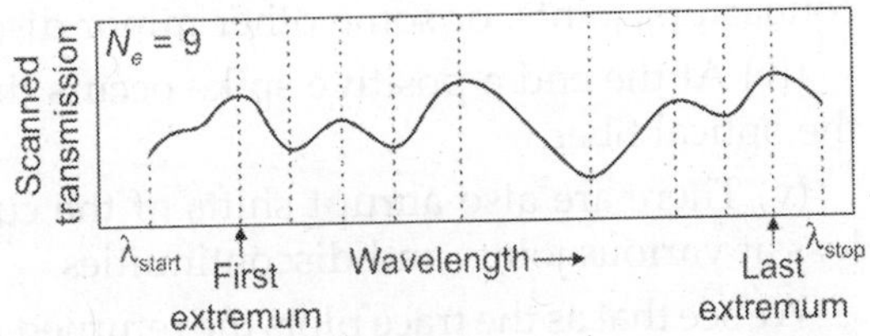

13.11.3 Measurements with Optical Time Domain Reflectometer (OTDR)

One can use the OTDR, a multipurpose

Fig. 13.16: Typical OSA trace for PMD exhibiting transmitted power level as a function of wavelength

instruments to make single-ended measurement of optical power link. One can measure the parameters such as attenuation, splice loss, connector loss, return loss, chromatic dispersion, etc. of an optical network for installed optical fiber link. Further, the measurement is completely non-destructive. One of the major applications of OTDR is to detect the location of any fault in the link arising out of optical fiber damage or rupture.

Figure 13.17 shows a typical trace on the screen of an OTDR for an installed optical fiber link. We can see that OTDR acts like an optical RADAR which sends intense optical pulse of narrow linewidth through the optical fiber. The ordinate of the display screen represent the back-reflected optical power in dB whereas the abscissa corresponds to the distance between the instrument and the measurement point in the optical fiber link. For

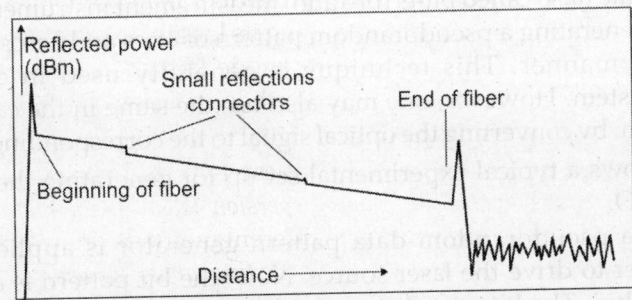

Fig. 13.17: Typical display on an OTDR screen exhibiting back scattered optical power

a normal optical link without any major fault/discontinuity one finds that it exhibit the following distinctive features in the trace obtained with the help of the back-reflected optical power:

(i) At the starting point a large initial peak, which can be attributed to the Fresnel reflection loss at the input end. Now, if the light enters from air to the optical fiber, we have the Fresnel reflection coefficient

$$R = \left(\frac{n_1 - 1}{n_1 + 1} \right)^2 \tag{13.22a}$$

where n_1 is the refractive index of the optical fiber core at the operating wavelength.

One can estimate the back reflected power as

$$P_{ref} = P_o R \tag{13.23}$$

(ii) There is a long decaying task till the end of the trace. This is mainly due to the Rayleigh scattering of the back reflected wave in the reverse direction as the wave advances through the optical fiber.

(iii) There appears small peaks in between. These peaks are attributed to strong reflections of the light resulting in large power of the back-reflected light arising from connectors, joints, or some other minor discontinuities in the optical fiber link.

(iv) At the end a positive spike occurs due to Fresnel reflection from the back end of the optical fiber.

(v) There are also abrupt shifts of the curve, which are caused by additional optical loss at various joints and discontinuities.

We see that as the trace plots the returned power against distance, the OTDR instrument helps one to pin point the position of joints, connectors, splices, any discontinuity in the fiber, etc.

In addition to the measurement of various parameters, e.g., attenuation, dispersion, splice loss, component loss, etc. one can also use ODTR to detect the location of any fault in the optical fiber link arising out of any damage/break in the optical fiber. Any major break or damage of optical fiber will appear as an additional spike in the trace and one can read the distance directly.

13.12 EYE DIAGRAM TESTS

One can best adjudge the data handling capability of an optical fiber with the help of eye diagram for digital transmission system. The use of an *eye diagram* is a traditional technique for quickly and intuitively assessing the quality of a received signal. We may note that modern bit-error-rate (also called bit-error-ratio) measurement instruments construct such eye diagrams by generating a pseudorandom pattern of ones and zeros at a uniform rate but in a random manner. This technique is generally used in digital electrical communication system. However, one may also use the same in the case digital optical transmission system by converting the optical signal to the corresponding electrical signal.

Figure 13.18 shows a typical experimental set up for generating the eye diagram on the screen of a CRO.

The output of a pseudorandom data pattern generator is applied to the optical transmitter in order to drive the laser source. Now, the bit pattern is allowed to travel through the test fiber. The bits get distorted while traveling through the optical fiber.

The optical fiber distorted optical pulses are converted to electrical bit pattern which is subsequently applied to the vertical input of the oscilloscope. The data rate of the pseudorandom bit generator is used to trigger the time base circuit of the oscilloscope. This results in the formation of the eye pattern or eye diagram. A typical eye diagram is shown in Fig. 13.19. The eye diagram provides the following important information on the system performance:

Pseudorandom bit pattern generator
Data Bit
Cathode ray oscilioscope (CRO) vertical trigger
Optical Tx
Optical Rx

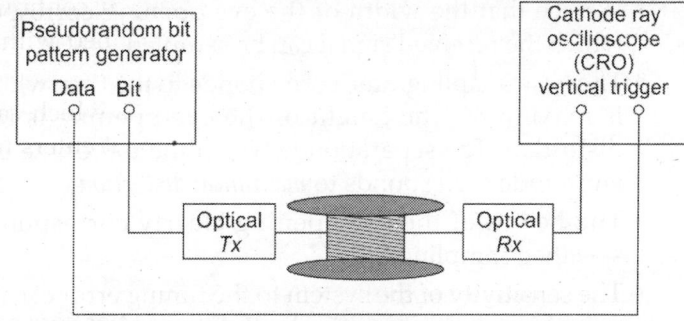

Fig. 13.18: A typical experimental set up for generating eye diagram

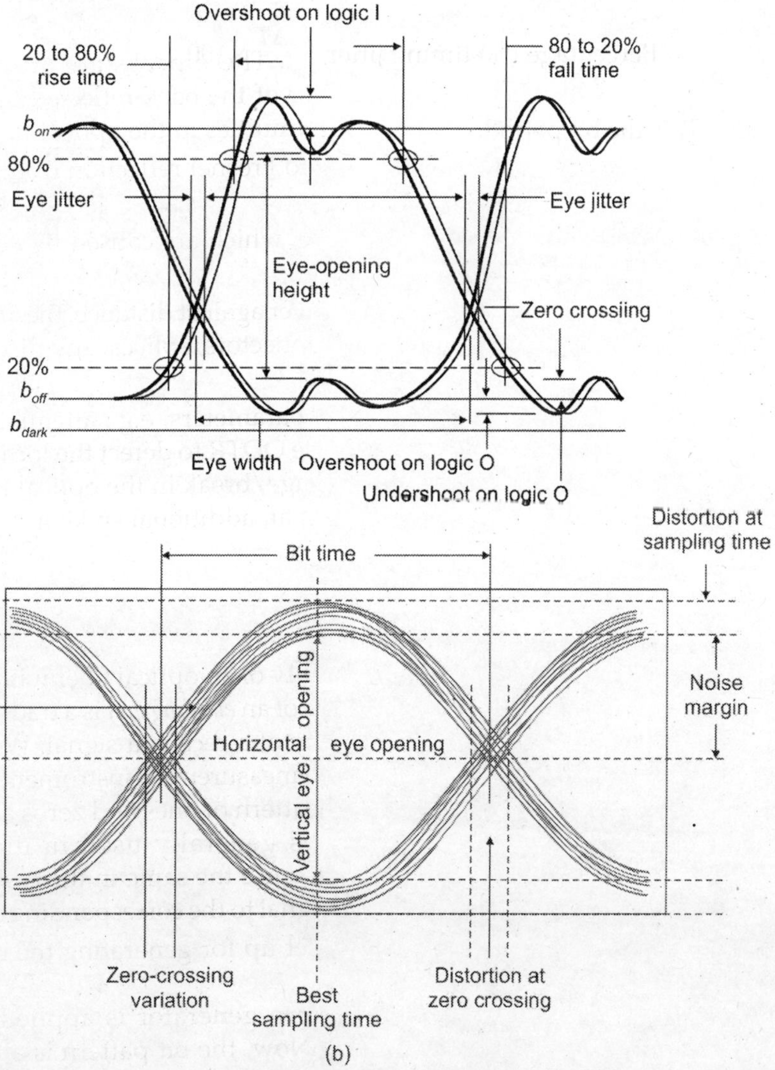

Overshoot on logic I
20 to 80% rise time
80 to 20% fall time
b_{on}
80%
Eye jitter
Eye jitter
Eye-opening height
Zero crossiing
20%
b_{off}
b_{dark}
Eye width
Overshoot on logic O
Undershoot on logic O
Distortion at sampling time
Bit time
Slope = sensitivity of timing
Noise margin
Horizontal eye opening
Vertical eye opening
Threshold level
Zero-crossing variation
Best sampling time
Distortion at zero crossing
(b)

Fig. 13.19: Eye diagrams exhibiting the key performance pattern and definitions of fundamental measurement parameters

- We see that the width of the eye opening corresponds to the time interval over which the received signal can be sampled.
- The best sampling time corresponds to the time when the height of the eye opening is maximum. The height of the eye opening is reduced because of amplitude distortion. The separation between the top of the eye opening and the maximum amplitude corresponds to *maximum distortion.*
- The height of the eye opening clearly corresponds to the noise margin at the specified sampling time.
- The sensitivity of the system to the timing error can be easily determined by the rate at which the eye closes, i.e. by the slope of the eye pattern side.
- Time jitter arising out of the noise introduced by the optical receiver and pulse distortion introduced by the fiber. Now, if the signal is sampled at the middle of the bit period then the amount of distortion at the threshold level clearly indicates the amount of jitter, we have

$$\text{Percentage (\%) timing jitter} = \frac{\Delta T}{T_b} \times 100 \tag{13.24}$$

where, T_b is the bit period.

Suggested Reading

- S.L. Kakani and Shubhra Kakani, *Photonics*, CBS Publishers and Distributors, New Delhi-2 (2017).
- G.P. Agrawal, *Nonlinear Fiber Optics*, 2nd Ed., Academic Press, New York (1995).
- J. Grower, *Optical Communication Systems*, Prentice Hall, Englewood Cliffs, New Jersey (1984).
- G. Keiser, *Optical Fiber Communications*, McGraw Hill International Edition, Singapore (2000).
- J.M. Senior, *Optical Fiber Communications: Principles and Practice*, 3rd Ed. Pearson Education Limited (2009).
- F.C. Allard, *Fiber Optic Handbook for Engineers and Scientists*, McGraw Hill Education, New York (1989).
- S.L. Kakani and Priyanka Pungalia, *Communication Systems*, New Age International Publishers, New Delhi-2 (2017).
- S.L. Kakani and C. Hemrajani, *Electromagnetics*, CBS Publishers, New Delhi-2 (2016).
- M.N.O. Sadiku, *Elements of Electromagnetics*, Oxford University Press, New York, 2nd Ed. (1995).
- E.G. Cullwick, *The Fundamentals of Electromagnetism*, 3rd Ed., Cambridge University Press (1966).
- S.R. de Groot, *The Maxwell's Equations*, North Holland, Amsterdam (1969).
- H. Kogelnik, 'Theory of Optical Waveguides' In Tamir T, Ed. Springer Series in Electronics and Photonics. Guided Wave Optoelectronics, Vol. 26, pp. 7–88, Springer (1988).
- T.E. Midwinter, *Optical Fibers for Transmission*, Wiley (1979).
- K. Okamoto, *Fundamentals of Optical Waveguides* (2nd Ed.), Academic Press (2006).
- C.W. Yeh, *Optical Waveguide Theory*, IEEE Trans. Circuit Syst. CAS-26 (3.12), pp. 1011–1019 (1979).
- A Marcuse, *Theory of Dielectric Optical Waveguides*, Academic Press (1974).
- G.P. Agrawal, *Nonlinear Fiber Optics*, 2nd Ed., Academic Press, New York (1995).
- F.C. Allard, *Fiber Optics Handbook for Engineers and Scientists*, McGraw Hill Education, New York (1989).
- A.W. Synder and J.D. Love, *Optical Waveguide Theory*, Chapman and Hall, London (1983).
- G. Keiser, *Optical Fiber Communications*, Tata McGraw Hill, 4th Ed. (2008).

- P.E. Green, *Fiber Optic Networks*, Prentice Hall, Englewood Cliffs, New Jersey (1993).
- S. Kumar and M. Jamal Deen, *Fiber Optic Communications: Fundamentals and Applications*. John Wiley (2014).
- Le Nguyen Binh, *Optical Fiber Communications Systems*, CRC Press, Taylor and Francis Group (2010).
- A. Al-Azzawi, *Fiber Optics: Principles and Practices*, CRC Press (2014).
- Palais, Joseph C., *Fiber Optic Communications*, 4th Ed., Prentice Hall Inc., Englewood, Cliffs, NJ (1998).
- S.L. Kakani and C. Hemrajani, *Mathematical Physics*, CBS Publishers, New Delhi-2, 3rd Ed. (2018).
- S.L. Kakani and Amit Kakani, *Material Science*, New Age International Publishers, New Delhi-2, 3rd Ed. (2016).
- V. Degiorgio, and I. Cristiani, *Photonics*, Springer (2014).
- S.L. Kakani and K.C. Bhandari, *Optics*, 2nd Ed., Sultan Chand, New Delhi-2 (2002).
- S.L. Kakani and Shubra Kakani, *Advances in Optics*, New Age International Publishers (2018).
- D. Marcuse, *Theory of Dielectric Waveguide*, Academic New York, 2nd Ed. (1991).
- R.M. Gagliardi and S. Karp, *Optical Communication*, John Wiley (1976).
- E.G. Neumann, *Single Mode Fibers: Fundamentals*, Springer (1988).
- N.K. Dutta and G.P. Agrawal, *Semiconductor Lasers*, Van Nostrad Reinhold, 2nd Ed. (1993).
- P. Bhattacharya, *Semiconductor Optoelectronic Devices*, 2nd Ed. Pearson Prentice Hall, New Delhi (2007).
- B.G. Streetman and S. Banerjee, *Solid State Electronic Devices*, 6th Ed. Pearson Education, New Delhi (2008).
- S.M. Sze, *Physics of Semiconductor Devices*, John Wiley, 2nd Ed., New York (2003).
- A Yariv, *Quantum Electronics*, John Wiley, 3rd Ed. (1989).
- S.L. Kakani and C. Hemrajani, *Solid State Physics*, Sultan Chand, New Delhi-2, 4th Ed. (2005).
- S.L. Kakani and Shubhra Kakani, *Modern Physics*, Viva Book, New Delhi-2, 2nd Ed. (2013).
- S.L. Kakani and K.C. Bhandari, *Electronic Devices and Circuits*, Viva Books, New Delhi-2, 2nd Ed. (2018).
- S.L. Kakani and Shubra Kakani, *Classical and Quantum Electrodynamics*, CBS Publishers, New Delhi-2 (In Press).

Appendices

APPENDIX A: LIST OF ABBREVIATIONS

Abbreviation	Meaning
A/D	Analog to digital
AGC	Automatic gain control
AM	Amplitude modulation
APD	Avalanche photodiode
ASK	Amplitude shift keying
ATM	Asynchronous transmission mode
BER	Bit error rate
CATV	Common antenna television
CCITT	International Telephone and Telegraph Consultative Committee
CCTV	Closed circuit television
CNR	Carrier-to-noise ratio
CWDM	Coarse wavelength division multiplexing
D/A	Digital to analog
DBR	Distributed Bragg reflector
dBm	Decibel with reference to 1 mW power
D-IM	Direct intensity modulation
DC	Depressed cladding
DC	Direct current
DF	Dispersion flattened
DFB	Distributed feedback
DH	Double heterostructure
DPSK	Differential phase shift keying
DS	Dispersion shifted
DSB	Double sideband
DWDM	Dense wavelength division multiplexing
EDFA	Erbium doped fiber amplifier
ELED	Edge-emitter light emitting diode
EMI	Electromagnetic interference
FA	Fiber amplifier
FBT	Fiber biconical taper
FDM	Frequency division multiplexing
FM	Frequency modulation
FOTP	Fiber optic test procedure
FPA	Fabry–Perot amplifier
FSK	Frequency-shift keying
FWHP	Full width half power
FWHM	Full-width half maximum
GI	Graded index (fiber)
GRIN	Graded-index (rod lens)
HB	High birefringence
HBT	Heterojunction bipolar transistor
HEMT	High electron mobility transistor
He-Ne	Helium-Neon (laser)
ILD	Injection laser diode
IM-DD	Intensity modulation direct detection
IO	Integrated optics
I/O	Input-output
ISDN	Integrated services digital network
ISI	Intersymbol interference
LAN	Local area network
LB	Low birefringence

LED	Light-emitting diode	RAPD	Reach-through avalanche photodiode
LP	Linearly polarized	SAM	Separate absorption and multiplication (APD)
LPE	Liquid phase epitaxy		
MAN	Metropolitan area network	SAW	Surface acoustic wave
MBE	Molecular beam epitaxy	SBS	Stimulated Brillouin scattering
MC	Matched cladding		
MCVD	Modified chemical vapor deposition	SC	Subcarrier connector
MESFET	Metal semiconductor field effect transistor	SCM	Subcarrier multiplexing
		SDH	Synchronous digital hierarchy
MFD	Mode field diameter		
MISFET	Metal insulator field effect transistor	SDM	Space division multiplexing
		SHF	Super high frequency
MMF	Multimode fiber	SLA	Semiconductor laser amplifier
MOSFET	Metal-oxide field effect transistor		
		SLD	Semiconductor laser diode
MOVPE	Metal organic vapor phase epitaxy	SLED	Surface emitting LED
		SMF	Single mode fiber
MQW	Multiquantum well	SNR	Signal-to-noise ratio
MSM	Metal-semiconductor-metal	SONET	Synchronous optical network
NRZ	Non-return-to-zero		
OEIC	Optoelectronic integrated circuit	SOP	State of polarization
		SQW	Single quantum well
OFDM	Optical frequency division multiplexing	SRS	Stimulated Raman scattering
OOK	On-off keying	TDM	Time-division multiplexing
OTDR	Optical time domain reflectometer	TDMA	Time-division multiple access
OVPO	Outside vapor phase oxidation	TE	Transverse electric
		TEM	Transverse electromagnetic
PCM	Pulse code modulation	TM	Transverse magnetic
PCS	Plastic clad silica (fiber)	TWA	Traveling wave amplifier
PCVD	Plasma-activated chemical vapour deposition	UHF	Ultra high frequency
		VAD	Vapour axial deposition
PDF	Probability distribution function	VCO	Voltage controlled oscillator
		VHF	Very high frequency
PIN-FET	PIN photodetector followed by FET	VPE	Vapour phase epitaxy
		VSB	Vestigial sideband
PLL	Phase locked loop	WDM	Wavelength-division multiplexing
PM	Phase modulation		
PMF	Polarization maintaining fiber	WKB	Wenzel–Kramer–Brillouin (method)
PoLSK	Polarization shift keying		
PON	Passive optical network	ZMD	Zero material dispersion
PSK	Phase-shift keying	ZTD	Zero total dispersion

APPENDIX B: PHYSICAL CONSTANTS

Quantity	Symbol	Value
Electronic charge	q	$1.60217733 \times 10^{-19}$ C
Rest mass of electron	m_0	$9.10938975 \times 10^{-31}$ kg
Rest mass of proton	m_P	$1.67262311 \times 10^{-27}$ kg
Speed of light in vacuum	c	2.99792458×10^8 m/s
Avogadro's number	L	$6.02213673 \times 10^{23}$/mole
Permeability of vacuum	μ_0	$4\pi \times 10^{-7}$ H/m
Permittivity of vacuum	ϵ_0	$8.854187817 \times 10^{-12}$ F/m
Planck constant	h	$6.62607554 \times 10^{-34}$ J.s
Reduced Planck constant ($h/2\pi$)	$\hbar$	1.05458×10^{-34} J.s
Boltzmann constant	k or k_B	$1.38065812 \times 10^{-23}$ J/K
Electronic volt	eV	$1.60217733 \times 10^{-19}$ J
Thermal voltage (300K)	V_T	0.02585 eV
Gas constant	R	1.98719 cal/mol-K

APPENDIX C: STANDARD INTERNATIONAL (SI) UNITS

Quantity	Unit	Symbol	Dimension
Mass	kilogram	kg	
Length	meter	m	
Time	second	s	
Temperature	Kelvin	K	
Current	Ampere	A	C.s
Electric Charge	Coulomb	C	A.s
Frequency	Hertz	Hz	s^{-1}
Force	Newton	N	$kg.m/s^2$
Pressure	Pascal	Pa	N/m^2
Energy	Joules	J	N.m
Potential	Volt	V	J/C
Resistance	Ohm	Ω	V/A
Capacitance	Farad	F	C/V
Inductance	Henry	H	Wb/A
Conductance	Siemens	S	A/V
Magnetic flux	Weber	Wb	V.s
Magnetic induction	Tesla	T	Wb/m^2

APPENDIX D: BESSEL FUNCTIONS

Bessel Function of the First Kind

The Bessel function of the first kind of order n and argument x, denoted by $J_n(x)$ is defined as follows:

$$J_n(x) = \frac{1}{2\pi} \int_{-n}^{n} \exp(jx \sin\theta - jn\theta)\, d\theta \tag{D1}$$

$$= \frac{1}{\pi} \int_0^n \cos(x \sin\theta - n\theta)\, d\theta \tag{D2}$$

Bessel function defined by (D1) and (D2) can be expanded in power series as follows:

$$J_n(x) = \sum_{m=0}^{\infty} \frac{(-1)^m \left(\frac{1}{2}x\right)^{n+2m}}{m!(n+m)!} \tag{D3}$$

The various orders of Bessel function of the first kind can be written using Eq. (D3) as follows:

$$J_0(x) = 1 - \frac{x^2}{2^2} + \frac{x^4}{2^2 \cdot 4^2} - \frac{x^6}{2^2 \cdot 4^2 \cdot 6^2} + \ldots \tag{D4}$$

$$J_1(x) = \frac{x}{2} - \frac{x^3}{2^2 \cdot 4} + \frac{x^5}{2^2 \cdot 4^2 \cdot 6} \tag{D5}$$

and

$$J_2(x) = \frac{x^2}{2.4} - \frac{x^4}{2^2 \cdot 4 \cdot 6} + \frac{x^6}{2^2 \cdot 4^2 \cdot 6 \cdot 8} - \ldots \tag{D6}$$

Properties of Bessel function:

(i) $\qquad\qquad J_n(x) = (-1)^n J_{-n}(x) \tag{D7}$

(ii) $\qquad\qquad J_n(x) = (-1)^n J_n(-x) \tag{D8}$

(iii) $\quad J_{n-1}(x) - J_{n+1}(x) = \dfrac{2n}{x} J_n(x) \tag{D9}$

(iv) $\quad J_{n-1}(x) - J_{n+1}(x) = 2J_n'(x) \tag{D10}$

(v) $\qquad\qquad J_n'(x) = J_{n-1}(x) - \dfrac{n}{x} J_n(x) \tag{D11}$

(vi) $\qquad\qquad J_n'(x) = -J_{n-1}(x) + \dfrac{n}{x} J_n(x) \tag{D12}$

(vii) For small values of x, we have

$$J_n(x) = \frac{x_n}{2^n n!} \tag{D13}$$

$$J_0(x) \approx 1 \tag{D14}$$

$$J_1(x) \approx x/2 \tag{D14a}$$

$$J_n(x) \approx 0 \quad \text{for} \quad n > 1 \tag{D14b}$$

(viii) For large values of x, we have

$$J_n(x) = \sqrt{\frac{2}{\pi x}} \cos\left(x - \frac{\pi}{4} - \frac{n\pi}{2}\right) \tag{D15}$$

(ix)
$$\sum_{n=-\infty}^{\infty} J_n^2(x) = 1 \text{ for all } x \tag{D16}$$

where $J_n'(x)$ is the first derivative of $J_n(x)$ with respect to x.

Bessel Function of the Second Kind

The Bessel function of the second kind can be expressed in the integral form as follows:

$$K_0(x) = \frac{1}{\pi} \int_0^\pi \exp\left(\pm x \cos\theta\right) \left[\gamma + \ln\left(2x \sin^2\theta\right)\right] d\theta \tag{D17}$$

where $\gamma = 0.57722$ is the Euler's constant, we have

$$K_n(x) = \frac{\pi^{\frac{1}{2}} \left(\dfrac{x}{2}\right)^m}{\Gamma\left(n + \dfrac{1}{2}\right)} \int_0^\infty \cos^{-x \cos ht} \sin h^{2n} t\, dt \tag{D18}$$

where $\Gamma(z)$ is the Gamma function given by,

$$\Gamma(z) = \int_0^\infty t^{z-1} \exp(-t)\, dt$$

For integer n, we have
$$\Gamma(n + 1) = n!$$

For fractional values, we have

$$\Gamma\left(\frac{1}{2}\right) = \pi^{\frac{1}{2}} = \left(-\frac{1}{2}\right)! \approx 1.77245$$

$$K_0(x) = \int_0^\infty \cos\left(x \sin ht\right) dt = \int_0^\infty \frac{\cos(xt)}{\sqrt{t^2 + 1}}\, dt \ (x > 0) \tag{D19}$$

$$K_n(x) = \sec\left(\frac{n\pi}{2}\right) \int_0^\infty \cos\left(x \sin ht\right) \cos h(nt)\, dt \ (x > 0) \tag{D20}$$

Recurrence Relation

Let
$$L_n = \exp\left(j\pi n\right) K_n$$

$$L_{n-1}(x) - L_{n+1}(x) = \frac{2n}{x} L_n(x) \tag{D21}$$

$$L_n'(x) = L_{n-1}(x) - \frac{n}{x} L_n(x) \tag{D22}$$

$$L_{n-1}(x) + L_{n+1}(x) = 2L_n'(x) \tag{D23}$$

$$L_n'(x) = L_{n+1}(x) + \frac{n}{x} L_n(x) \tag{D24}$$

Values of Bessel Function of the First Kind, $J_n(x)$

$\downarrow x$ $\overrightarrow{n}$	0	1	2	3	4	5	6	7	8	9	10	11
0.00	1.00											
0.10	0.997	0.050	0.001									
0.20	0.990	0.099	0.005									
0.30	0.978	0.148	0.011	0.001								
0.40	0.960	0.196	0.020	0.000								
0.50	0.938	0.242	0.031	0.002								
0.60	0.912	0.287	0.044	0.004								
0.70	0.881	0.329	0.059	0.007								
0.80	0.846	0.369	0.076	0.010	0.001							
0.90	0.807	0.406	0.095	0.014	0.002							
1.0	0.765	0.440	0.115	0.019	0.002							
1.25	0.646	0.511	0.171	0.037	0.006	0.001						
1.50	0.512	0.558	0.232	0.061	0.012	0.002						
1.75	0.370	0.580	0.294	0.092	0.021	0.004						
2.00	0.224	0.577	0.353	0.129	0.034	0.007	0.001					
2.50	−0.048	0.497	0.446	0.217	0.074	0.019	0.004	0.001				
3.00	−0.260	0.339	0.486	0.309	0.132	0.043	0.011	0.003				
3.50	−0.380	0.137	0.459	0.387	0.204	0.080	0.025	0.007	0.002			
4.00	−0.397	−0.006	0.364	0.430	0.281	0.132	0.049	0.015	0.004	0.001		
4.50	−0.321	−0.231	0.218	0.425	0.348	0.195	0.084	0.030	0.009	0.002		
5.00	−0.178	−0.328	0.047	0.365	0.391	0.261	0.131	0.053	0.018	0.005	0.001	
5.50	−0.007	−0.341	−0.117	0.256	0.397	0.362	0.187	0.087	0.034	0.011	0.003	0.001
6.00	0.151	−0.277	0.243	0.115	0.358	0.374	0.246	0.130	0.056	0.021	0.007	0.002
6.50	0.260	−0.154	−0.307	−0.035	0.275	0.348	0.300	0.180	0.090	0.037	0.013	0.004
7.00	0.300	−0.005	−0.301	−0.168	0.158	0.283	0.339	0.234	0.128	0.059	0.024	0.008
7.50	0.266	0.135	−0.230	−0.258	0.024	0.186	0.354	0.283	0.174	0.089	0.039	0.015
8.00	0.171	0.234	−0.113	−0.291	−0.105	0.067	0.338	0.321	0.223	0.126	0.061	0.026
8.50	0.042	0.273	0.022	−0.263	−0.208	0.055	0.287	0.338	0.269	0.169	0.089	0.041
9.00	−0.091	0.245	0.145	−0.181	−0.65	−0.055	0.204	0.327	0.305	0.215	0.125	0.062
9.50	−0.194	0.161	0.227	−0.06	−0.269	−0.161	0.009	0.287	0.323	0.258	0.165	0.090
10.0	−0.245	0.044	0.255	−0.058	−0.220	−0.234	−0.014	0.217	0.318	0.0290	0.207	0.213

APPENDIX E: SOME USEFUL MATHEMATICAL RELATIONS

(i) Trigonometric Identities

$$e^{\pm j\theta} = \cos\theta \pm j\sin\theta$$
$$\sin^2\theta + \cos^2\theta = 1$$
$$\cos^2\theta - \sin^2\theta = \cos 2\theta$$
$$4\sin^3\theta = 3\sin\theta - \sin 3\theta$$
$$4\cos^3\theta = 3\cos\theta + \cos 3\theta$$
$$8\sin^4\theta = 3 - 4\cos 2\theta + \cos 4\theta$$
$$8\cos^4\theta = 3 + 4\cos 2\theta + \cos 4\theta$$
$$\sin(\alpha \pm \beta) = \sin\alpha\cos\beta \pm \cos\alpha\sin\beta$$
$$\cos(\alpha \pm \beta) = \cos\alpha\cos\beta \mp \sin\alpha\sin\beta$$
$$\tan(\alpha \pm \beta) = \frac{\tan\alpha \pm \tan\beta}{1 \mp \tan\alpha\tan\beta}$$

(ii) Vector Analysis

The symbols e_x, e_y, and e_z, or $\hat{i}$, $\hat{j}$, and $\hat{k}$ denote units vectors lying parallel to the x, y, and z axes, respectively, of the rectangular coordinate system. Similarly, e_r, e_ϕ, and e_z, are unit vectors for cylindrical coordinates. The unit vectors e_r and e_ϕ vary in direction as the angle ϕ changes. The conversion from cylindrical to rectangular coordinates is made using the relationships

$$x = r\cos\phi \quad y = r\sin\phi \quad z = z$$

(iii) Rectangular Coordinates

$$\text{Gradient } \nabla f = \frac{\partial f}{\partial x}e_x + \frac{\partial f}{\partial y}e_y + \frac{\partial f}{\partial z}e_z$$

$$\text{Divergence } \nabla.\mathbf{A} = \frac{\partial A_x}{\partial x} + \frac{\partial A_y}{\partial y} + \frac{\partial A_z}{\partial z}$$

$$\text{Curl } \nabla \times \mathbf{A} = \begin{vmatrix} e_x & e_y & e_z \\ \dfrac{\partial}{\partial x} & \dfrac{\partial}{\partial y} & \dfrac{\partial}{\partial z} \\ A_x & A_y & A_z \end{vmatrix}$$

$$\text{Laplacian } \nabla^2 f = \frac{\partial^2 f}{\partial x^2} + \frac{\partial^2 f}{\partial y^2} + \frac{\partial^2 f}{\partial z^2}$$

(iv) Cylindrical Coordinates

$$\text{Gradient } \nabla f = \frac{\partial f}{\partial r}e_r + \frac{1}{r}\frac{\partial f}{\partial \phi}e_\phi + \frac{\partial f}{\partial z}e_z$$

$$\text{Divergence } \nabla.\mathbf{A} = \frac{1}{r}\frac{\partial(rA_r)}{\partial r} + \frac{1}{r}\frac{\partial A_\phi}{\partial \phi} + \frac{\partial A_z}{\partial z}$$

$$\text{Curl } \nabla \times \mathbf{A} = \begin{vmatrix} \dfrac{1}{r}e_r & e_\phi & \dfrac{1}{r}e_z \\ \dfrac{\partial}{\partial r} & \dfrac{\partial}{\partial \phi} & \dfrac{\partial}{\partial z} \\ A_r & rA_\phi & A_z \end{vmatrix}$$

$$\text{Laplacian } \nabla^2 f = \frac{1}{r}\frac{\partial}{\partial r}\left(r\frac{\partial f}{\partial r}\right) + \frac{1}{r^2}\frac{\partial^2 f}{\partial \phi^2} + \frac{\partial^2 f}{\partial z^2}$$

(v) Vector Identities

$$\nabla \times (\nabla \times \mathbf{A}) = \nabla(\nabla \cdot \mathbf{A}) - \nabla^2 \mathbf{A}$$

$$\nabla^2 \mathbf{A} = \nabla^2 A_x e_x + \nabla^2 A_y e_y + \nabla^2 A_z e_z$$

(vi) Useful Integrals

$$\int \sin x\, dx = -\cos x$$

$$\int \cos x\, dx = \sin x$$

$$\int \sqrt{a^2 - x^2}\, dx = \frac{1}{2}\left(x\sqrt{a^2 - x^2} + a^2 \arcsin \frac{x}{a} \right)$$

$$\int x\sqrt{a^2 - x^2}\, dx = -\frac{1}{3}(a^2 - x^2)^{3/2}$$

$$\int x^2 \sin^2 x\, dx = \frac{x^3}{6} - \left(\frac{x^2}{6} - \frac{1}{8} \right) \sin 2x - \frac{x \cos 2x}{4}$$

$$\int \frac{dx}{\cos^n x} = \frac{1}{n-1} \frac{\sin x}{\cos^{n-1} x} + \frac{n-2}{n-1} \int \frac{dx}{\cos^{n-2} x}$$

$$\int u\, dv = uv - \int v\, du$$

$$\int e^{ax} dx = \frac{1}{a} e^{ax}$$

$$\int \sin^2 x\, dx = \frac{x}{2} - \frac{1}{4} \sin 2x$$

$$\int \sin^n x\, dx = -\frac{\sin^{n-1} x \cos x}{n} + \frac{n-1}{n} \int \sin^{n-2} x\, dx$$

$$\int \cos^2 x\, dx = \frac{x}{2} + \frac{1}{4} \sin 2x$$

$$\int \cos^n x\, dx = \frac{1}{n} \cos^{n-1} x \sin x + \frac{n-1}{n} \int \cos^{n-2} x\, dx$$

$$\int_{-\infty}^{\infty} \frac{e^{jpx}}{(\beta + jx)^n}\, dx = \begin{cases} 0 & \text{if } p < 0 \\ \dfrac{2\pi (p)^{n-1} e^{-\beta p}}{\Gamma(n)} & \text{if } p \geq 0 \end{cases} ; \text{ where } \Gamma(n) = (n-1)!$$

$$\int_{-\infty}^{\infty} e^{-p^2 x^2 + qx}\, dx = e^{q^2/4p^2} \frac{\sqrt{\pi}}{p}$$

$$\int_{-\infty}^{\infty} \frac{1}{1 + (x/a)^2}\, dx = \frac{\pi a}{2}$$

$$\frac{2}{\sqrt{x}} \int_0^t e^{-x^2}\, dx = \text{erf}(t)$$

(vii) Series Expansions

$$(1 + x)^n = 1 + nx + \frac{n(n-1)}{2!} x^2 + \frac{n(n-1)(n-2)}{3!} x^3 + \cdots \text{ for } |nx| < 1$$

$$e^x = 1 + x + \frac{x^2}{2!} + \frac{x^3}{3!} + \cdots$$

$$\sin x = x - \frac{x^3}{3!} + \frac{x^5}{3!} - \cdots$$

$$\cos x = 1 - \frac{x^2}{2!} + \frac{x^4}{4!} - \cdots$$

Index

A

Absorption 92
  loss 239
Acceptance angle 71
Acceptors 317
Active glass fibers 134
Acousto-optic switches 609
Adaptor 154
Amplifier
  gain 570
  ripple 554
Amplitude shift keying (ASK) 688
Analog
  systems 674
  to digital converter 667
Antireflection coating 43
Array waveguide gratings 667
Attenuation 93, 237, 238
Avalanche photodiodes 520

B

Band gap 313
Band limited linear system 672
Bandwidth 434
Bessel function 204
Bending loss 246
Bit error rate (BER) 527, 669
Bit rate transparency 491
Bragg
  grating 336
  mirrors 44
Brewster's angle 43
Brillouin scattering 105
Broadband incoherent light source 762
Buffer jacket 144
Bus topology 677

C

Campus area network 681
Catastrophic degradation 427

Chalcogenide glass fibers 135
Chromatic dispersion 256, 710, 752
Chirped solitons 724
Circularly and elliptically polarized waves 39
Cladding 64
  modes 192
Core 64
  cladding loss 249
Conductors 313
Compound semiconductors 325
Coherent light 328
Coarse
  phase modulation 559
  wavelength division multiplexing 620
Couplers 620
Connectors 149
  testing 157
Cosine power distribution 312
Critical angle 66
Crosstalk 749
Cylindrical waveguides 202

D

Decibles 73
Dense wavelength division multiplexing 546
Depletion region 490
Demodulation techniques 9
Digital systems 667
Directionality 340
Direct band gap materials 321
Dispersion 253, 707
  flattened fibres 279
  intermodal 69, 253, 671
  intramodal 253, 268, 671, 767
  material 258
  modal 712
  profile 264
  shifted fiber 94, 278
Doping 318
Double heterostructure laser 346, 360

E

Edge emitting LED 445
Electric boundary conditions 315
Electrical communication system 3
Electromagnetic
    waves 36
    bypass switches 597
Electro-optic switches 602
Electronic signal processor 488
Energy band diagram 313
Environmental tests 755
Erbium-doped fiber optical amplifiers 565
Etalon effect 595
Excess loss 250
Extrinsic absorption 242
Eye diagram tests 772

F

Fiber
    attenuation 667
    Bragg grating (FBG) 633
    connectors 151
    dispersion 667
    glass 131
    graded index 211
    optic connectors 96
    optic communication 664
    optic power attenuators 961
    splicing 158
    waveguide 65
    fluoride 133
Four-fiber BLSR
    configuration 701
    reconfiguration 702
Four wave mixing 707
Fresnel
    coefficients 40
    reflection loss 152
Frequency
    chirping 382
    modulation 675
Fusion splices 159

G

Group velocity 257
    dispersion 213, 258
Guided modes 191

H

HBT based photoreceiver 502
Heterostructures 368
Heterofunction lasers 347
Holey fiber 144
Home area network 679

Homogeneous p-n junction 368
Hub topology 685

I

Index
    matching fluid 68
    profile 76
Indirect band gap materials 322
Injection
    electroluminescence 440
    laser diode 311
Infrared emitting diode 458
Insertion loss 152, 748
Insulators 313
Intermodal dispersion 69, 253, 268, 671, 767
Intrinsic
    absorption 239
    semiconductor 316

J

Jacket 65

K

Kerr nonlinearity 131

L

Laser
    diode 311
    rate equations 351
Leaky modes 192
LED indicator circuits 457
Light
    waveguide 63
    emitting diode (LED) 311, 427, 437
Line coding 673
Linear
    bus topology 685
    optical amplifiers 269
    scattering loss 243
Link power budget analysis 669
Local area network 271, 680
LP modes 202

M

Magnetic boundary conditions 35
Macroscopic bends 246
Macrobending loss 247
Mach–Zehnder interferometer 561, 602, 635
Maxwell's equations 31
Meridional rays 70
Metal
    semiconductor detectors 513
    semiconductor field effect transistor (MESFET) 498

Mesh topology 636
Metropolian area network 681
Metro and long-haul network 699
Mie scattering 244
Microbending loss 246
Microscopic bends 246
Mode coupling 277
Monochromaticity 340
Muller matrix 750
Multicolour LEDs 457
Multisegment LED displays 458
Multifiber connectors 156
Multimode
    graded index fiber 80
    step index fiber 77

N

Network 677
Nonlinear effects 283
Noise equivalent power 435
Nonradiative recombination 350
Nonlinear optical susceptibility 715
Nonlinearly effects 104
Nonzero-to-zero (NRZ) code 688
Normalized frequency parameter 196
NRZ and RZ signal formats 688
n-type semiconductor 316
Numerical aperature 67

O

On-off keying (OOK) 688
Optical
    amplifier 545
    confinement methods 357
    fiber 62, 64
    fiber cables 143
    feedback 33
    gains 369, 561
    power meter 760
    receiver 490
    switches 594
    spectrum analyzer 762
    time domain reflectometer 764
Optoelectronics 183
Optomechanical switches 594
Organic light emitting diode 456
Orthogonality 199

P

Phase
    modulation 675
    velocity 88
Photodetector 505
    noise 521

Photoreceiver 501
Photoconductor 432
Photoconductive
    effect 429
    mode 429
Photoemissive effect 428
Photovoltaic effect 430
Photonics 63
Photonic
    band gap fibers 215
    crystal fibers 213, 214
Photoelectric effect 23
Phototransistors 511
Photovoltaics 512
p-n junction 320
p-n photodiode 515
p-i-n photodiodes 516
p-type semiconductor 317
Planar optical waveguide 188
Plastic
    clad silica fibers 136
    optical fiber 136
Planar waveguide optical amplifiers 577
Polarization 101
    dependent loss 750
    maintaining fibers 282
    mode dispersion 253, 266, 711, 750, 769
    of light 27
    waves 38
Power budget calculation 691
Poynting theorem 44
Population inversion 331, 548
Point-to-point WDM links 640
Protocol 677
Pulse amplification 557

Q

Quantum
    dot LED 456
    dot lasers 362
    efficiency 428, 433, 507
    limit 525
    noise 525
    theory 23
    well lasers 361
    yield 428

R

Radiation mode 246
Raman
    fiber optical amplifiers 565, 573
    scattering 243
Rayleigh scattering 243
Repeatability text 755

Resonant
  electromagnetic cavity 329
  cavity LEDs 454
Responsivity 434, 507
Ring topology 678, 687
Rise-time budget analysis 670
RMS
  width 91
  pulse broadening 271
Routing 677

S

SDM 693
Semiconductor
  lasers 343
  optical amplifier 546
  photodiode 489
Shot noise 573
Silica glass 133
Signal degradation 92
Single mode
  fibers 1
  step index fiber 77
Single
  pass amplifier gain 554
  soliton 722
Skew rays 71
Smart design 237
Snell's law 25
Solar cell 430
Solitons 106
  propagation 284
SONET 693
  ADM 703
  and SDH transmission rates 696
Splices 149
  loss 250
Spring groove 160
Speed test 756
Spontaneous emission 327
Square law device 675
Star
  couplers 625
  topology 678, 687
Stimulated
  absorption 327
  Raman scattering 705, 716
  Brillioun scattering 706
Submarine cables 682
Super luminescence LED 446
Surface emitting LED 442

Switch logic 607
Switching 677

T

TE modes 195
TE polarization 40
Testing photonic components 746
Temporal coherence 340
Thermal noise 523
Thermo-optic switches 606
Thin film filters 632, 634
Time
  harmonic fields 37
  domain intramodal dispersion 768
TM modes 195
TM polarization 41
Topology 677
Total internal reflection 27, 63, 66
Tree topology 678
Troubleshooting 757
Tunable
  laser sources 762
  optical filters 637
  sources 636
Two fiber UPSR configuration 700

V

Valence electrons 313
V-groove 159
V-parameter 75

W

Wave
  equation 35
  –particle duality 24
Waveguide
  loss 249
  dispersion 258, 260, 710, 753
Wavelength
  division multiplexing technology 615, 664
  routing 618
  routed networks 640
Wide area network 682

Y

Y-couplers 623

Z

ZBLAN glass 133